The Advanced Practice Nurse Cardiovascular Clinician

Kelley M. Anderson, PhD, FNP, is an assistant professor of nursing at Georgetown University School of Nursing & Health Studies. She has been a faculty member in the Family Nurse Practitioner (FNP) program and the Doctor of Nursing Practice program since 2007, serving as the assistant director of the FNP program from 2011 to 2013 and as the coordinator of the FNP Georgetown campus cohort since 2011. Dr. Anderson is certified as a family nurse practitioner and has held a clinical position as a nurse practitioner at Medstar, Georgetown University Hospital in the Division of Cardiology since 2002. In 2013 she began collaborating with the Arlington Street People Assistance Network (A-SPAN) to provide primary health care services to the homeless in Arlington, Virginia.

Dr. Anderson received her BSN from the University of Virginia, Charlottesville, her MSN from the University of Texas, Austin, post-MSN FNP certificate from the University of Florida, Gainesville, and a PhD from The Catholic University of America, Washington, DC. She has peer-reviewed publications in *Heart & Lung: The Journal of Acute and Critical Care, Clinical Scholars Review: The Journal of Doctoral Nursing Practice, American Journal of Critical Care, Journal of the American Academy of Nurse Practitioners, Journal of Nursing Education, Journal of the American Association of Nurse Practitioners, Journal of Cardiovascular Nursing,* and *OJIN: The Online Journal of Issues in Nursing.* Dr. Anderson is a reviewer for three scholarly journals and received the 2013 Certificate of Excellence in Reviewing from *Heart and Lung: The Journal of Acute and Critical Care.* She is a member of the American Association of Heart Failure Nurses, serving on the Education Committee; the Northern Virginia Council of Nurse Practitioners, serving on the Nominations and Awards Committee; Sigma Theta Tau, serving as graduate counselor for the Tau Chapter; and member of the American Academy of Nurse Practitioners, the American Heart Association, and the National Organization of Nurse Practitioner Faculties.

The Advanced Practice Nurse Cardiovascular Clinician

Kelley M. Anderson, PhD, FNP

EDITOR

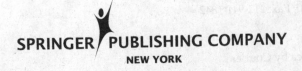

SPRINGER PUBLISHING COMPANY

NEW YORK

Springer Publishing Company, LLC
11 West 42nd Street
New York, NY 10036
www.springerpub.com

Acquisitions Editor: Margaret Zuccarini
Composition: Westchester Publishing Services

ISBN: 978-0-8261-3857-6
e-book ISBN: 978-0-8261-3858-3

15 16 17 18 / 5 4 3 2 1

The author and the publisher of this Work have made every effort to use sources believed to be reliable to provide information that is accurate and compatible with the standards generally accepted at the time of publication. Because medical science is continually advancing, our knowledge base continues to expand. Therefore, as new information becomes available, changes in procedures and drug administration protocols become necessary. We recommend that the reader always consult current research, current drug references, and specific institutional policies before performing any clinical procedure or administering any drug by any route. The author and publisher shall not be liable for any special, consequential, or exemplary damages resulting, in whole or in part, from the readers' use of, or reliance on, the information contained in this book. The publisher has no responsibility for the persistence or accuracy of URLs for external or third-party Internet websites referred to in this publication and does not guarantee that any content on such websites is, or will remain, accurate or appropriate.

Library of Congress Cataloging-in-Publication Data

The advanced practice nurse cardiovascular clinician / Kelley M. Anderson, editor.
    p. ; cm.
Includes bibliographical references.
ISBN 978-0-8261-3857-6 (hardcopy : alk. paper) — ISBN 978-0-8261-3858-3 (ebook)
I. Anderson, Kelley M., editor.
[DNLM: 1. Cardiovascular Nursing–methods.   2. Advanced Practice Nursing.
3. Cardiovascular Diseases—nursing.   WY 152.5]
RC674
616.1'0231—dc23

2015020700

Printed in the United States of America by Courier.

Contents

Contributors

Kelley M. Anderson, PhD, FNP, Georgetown University School of Nursing & Health Studies and Medstar, Georgetown University Hospital, Washington, DC

Rachel Barish, MSN, RN, ANP-BC, Medstar, Georgetown University Hospital, Washington, DC

Linda Briggs, DNP, ANP-BC, ACNP-BC, George Washington University, School of Nursing, Washington, DC

Helen F. Brown, MS, ACNP-BC, FNP-BC, Georgetown University School of Nursing & Health Studies, Washington, DC; Doctors Emergency Services, PA, Emergency Department, Anne Arundel Medical Center, Annapolis, Maryland

Samantha J. Bullock, BS, CVT, Medstar, Georgetown University Hospital, Washington, DC

Brian C. Case, MD, Medstar, Georgetown University Hospital, Washington, DC

Dev Chatterji, PharmD, BCPS, Medstar, Georgetown University Hospital, Washington, DC

Erin K. Coughlin, MS, RN, FNP-C, Pediatric Primary Care, Kailua, Hawaii

Ladan Eshkevari, PhD, CRNA, Georgetown University School of Nursing & Health Studies, Washington, DC

Dana E. Haggett, MS, RN, FNP-BC, OCN, Brookline, Massachusetts

Bernard J. Horak, PhD, FACHE, CPHQ, Georgetown University School of Nursing & Health Studies, Washington, DC

Catherine Horvath, MSN, CRNA, Georgetown University School of Nursing & Health Studies, Washington, DC

Donna M. Jasinski, PhD, CRNA, Georgetown University School of Nursing & Health Studies, Washington, DC

Patricia Matticola, MS, RN, ACNP, Medstar, Georgetown University Hospital, Washington, DC

Robert L. McSwain, MD, Virginia Heart, Fairfax, Virginia

John N. Meriwether, MD, Medstar, Georgetown University Hospital, Washington, DC

Brittany C. Moore, MS, BSN, FNP, Medstar, Georgetown University Hospital, Washington, DC

Dorothy L. Murphy, MS, FNP-BC, Liberty University, Lynchburg, Virginia

Jonathan Richard E. Puhl, PharmD, Medstar, Georgetown University Hospital, Washington, DC

Venkatesh K. Raman, MD, FACC, Georgetown University School of Medicine and Medstar, Georgetown University Hospital, Washington, DC

Constance Ryjewski, MSN, ACNS-BC, Advocate Lutheran General Health, Park Ridge, Illinois

Monvadi B. Srichai, MD, MS, Georgetown University School of Medicine and Medstar, Georgetown University Hospital, Washington, DC

Denise H. Tola, MSN, CRNA, Georgetown University School of Nursing & Health Studies, Washington, DC

Lauren Wenhold, MS, BSN, FNP, Medstar, Georgetown University Hospital, Washington, DC

Lois A. Wessel, RN, FNP-BC, Georgetown University School of Nursing & Health Studies, Washington, DC

Connie H. Yoon, PharmD, BCPS, University of Maryland School of Pharmacy, Baltimore, Maryland

Preface

Almost every clinician requires a basic knowledge of cardiovascular care. Given the complexities of cardiovascular care practices, opportunities for growth and learning are both ever-present and essential. Although this book is grounded in scientific knowledge and practice guidelines, a vital element of cardiovascular care is the clinical judgment that is born from experience and based on our daily interactions with patients, their families, and students. It is through our work for and with these individuals that we learn to deliver care that is effective, individualized, and innovative, which has informed our writing of this book.

I have come to appreciate that learning is enhanced through clear organization and clarification of difficult topics through images, lists, tables, and algorithms. This book endeavors to deliver clinically relevant, applicable content in an interesting and accessible manner. Ultimately, regardless of the discipline, understanding of these cardiology care topics helps health care professionals achieve our overarching goal to improve outcomes for patients and their families. The philosophical underpinning of this book is that it is our collective efforts that ensure our successful attainment of this goal.

The impact of cardiovascular illness in our society is tremendous and will continue to be so for the foreseeable future. All of the authors of this text have aspired to provide the most current and relevant information on daily cardiovascular topics. However, we practice in a field that is always changing and evolving with discoveries that will improve the health and the quality of life for our patients. Yet despite all of the advances, we remain humbly aware that there is no substitute for forming partnerships with patients and families and providing essential care through a thoughtful health history and comprehensive examination. These activities are the cornerstones of care practices. We are also knowledgeable that the fundamental aspects of a healthy lifestyle are the basis of prevention and treatment to improve overall heart health.

The book is organized with an overview of cardiovascular care topics progressing to cardiovascular conditions, both chronic and acute. These topics are followed by common cardiovascular diagnostics, then cardiovascular therapeutic management options and interventions. The book concludes with a table of cardiovascular guidelines as a reference.

Essentially, I wanted to create a work that would be helpful to all of us: for the more experienced clinician as a daily resource and especially for those who are beginning in the field of cardiovascular care, as you are our future. I hope our lessons learned will serve to inform your practice.

Kelley M. Anderson

Acknowledgments

I would like to thank Edilma Yearwood, Carol Taylor, Jane Fall-Dickson, and Peggy Compton for their continuous support and encouragement. Much gratitude for the kind efforts and contributions of Anna Cardall, Raffaele Girlanda, Alice Karr, Allen Taylor, and John V. White. A special thank you to Roseanne Geisel for her advisement and endless efforts. My sincere appreciation to the Georgetown Campus Family Nurse Practitioner Students from 2007 to 2015 for all they have taught me.

And to my family—Michael, Ellyse, Pam McKeta, Mia French, Robert, and Hideko Mcketa—with my love and gratitude.

Overview of Cardiovascular Care

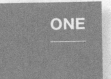

ONE

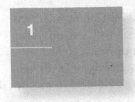

The Interprofessional Team: Focus on Quality

LOIS A. WESSEL, BERNARD J. HORAK, KELLEY M. ANDERSON, AND SAMANTHA J. BULLOCK

Optimal health care results when a multidisciplinary team enhances and values each member's expertise to deliver patient-centered care. The effectiveness and efficiency of these teams are increased by interprofessional collaboration, in which two or more professional disciplines combine their perspectives and strengths to deliver enhanced high-quality health care. Gone are the days when a single provider could manage all the requirements for patients in both the inpatient and outpatient settings, and act as the leader with sole decision-making authority. Our understanding of the complexities of patient care, including an appreciation of the essential components of social determinants of health, health literacy, and patient empowerment, have increased the responsibilities of the health care team, patients, and families. A multifaceted comprehension of health and disease, along with technical advances including electronic health records, has fostered a restructuring of a formerly hierarchical system into a team-based approach, which builds on the strengths of all members. Although the concept is not new as evidenced by the 1972 report from the Institute of Medicine (IOM) on "education for the health team," there is a renewal in the interest of multidisciplinary teams amid the need to transform health care delivery in the United States.

Ideally, patients and providers are better served when all caregivers collaborate to encourage communication, coordination, and optimal patient care. While numerous studies on interdisciplinary care exist and primary care remains the cornerstone of care coordination, the focus of this book is cardiovascular care and the integration of these specialty services within the context of the care continuum. Interprofessional collaboration has demonstrated effectiveness in improving patient and provider satisfaction and quality of care in numerous venues of specialty cardiovascular care practices, while promoting care across health care services.

HEALTH CARE DELIVERY SYSTEM REDESIGN

Currently, the health care delivery system in the United States is undergoing redesign, and consistently the concepts of multidisciplinary teams and interdisciplinary care are components of this change. The need for and effectiveness of teamwork, particularly to address system failures and patient safety, has been reported in a number of studies by the IOM (1999, 2001, 2012). The Institute for Healthcare Improvement (IHI, 2014), a Cambridge, Massachusetts–based independent, nonprofit organization, fosters research, innovation and collaboration to improve outcomes, care delivery, cost-effectiveness, and wellness for individuals and populations worldwide. This organization has developed an approach to improving health system performance. The IHI reasons that new designs must be developed to simultaneously pursue three dimensions, which are referred to as the "Triple Aim":

- Improving the patient experience of care, both quality and satisfaction
- Improving the health of populations
- Reducing the cost of health care per person

The IHI asserts that the Triple Aim approach will strengthen medical homes and accountable care organizations (ACOs), which are encouraged under the Patient Protection and Affordable Care Act (PPACA) to improve quality and reduce health care costs. These reforms focus on appropriate use of technology, organizations of care, and interprofessional team-based care.

The concept of ACOs is defined as a set of health care providers—specialists, primary care providers, mental health clinicians, and hospitals—that work together to collectively account for the costs and the quality of care delivered to patients. The Patient-Centered Medical Home (PCMH) model, originally proposed by the American Academy of Pediatrics, the American College of Physicians, and the American Osteopathic Association in 2007, is an enhanced primary care delivery model that focuses on improved access, partnerships between the patient and the medical team, and coordination and communication with specialists. The ACO is analogous to the medical neighborhood, whereas the PCMH is the home. While the PCMH model is primary care focused, ACOs include specialists and hospitals, and both of these are important facets of health care reform, which require and support interprofessional collaboration.

The concept of team-based care is an integral part of the PCMH model where roles and responsibilities of the clinical staff members are modified to increase provider efficiency and improve patient satisfaction and care. For example, medical assistants are empowered to provide screening and document findings into the electronic health record; nurses may lead chronic-disease group visits; and community health workers provide home visits linking patients to appropriate community resources. Each member of the team provides care to the full scope in which they are trained and licensed to deliver, and through collaboration and communication, care is optimized.

While interprofessional collaboration can result in improved outcomes with lower costs, it also provides a level of support for clinicians that can reduce provider fatigue and burnout. In one study, nurses participated in patient rounds at the bedside with the medical team, resulting in improvements in workflow, communication, and job satisfaction (Sharma & Klocke, 2014). The PCMH model that requires interprofessional collaboration can be a protective factor from the high levels of burnout reported by a significant proportion of the primary care workforce. In a study of more than 4,000 clinicians from 588 Veterans Administration (VA) hospitals, lower levels of self-reported burnout were associated with medical homes with increased collaboration among team members (Helfrich et al., 2014). Similarly, another study of clinicians and staff members at public health and university-based primary care clinics in San Francisco demonstrated that working in a tight team structure was associated with less exhaustion among staff

(Willard-Grace et al., 2014). Providing comprehensive team-based care when working in an outpatient or inpatient setting with patients who have been diagnosed with cardiac disease can be an essential part of improving health care delivery and improving clinical work satisfaction.

Still, barriers exist to the implementation of team-based care. The health care community is facing new rules and regulations from the PPACA concerning electronic medical records and the expanded role of advanced practice nurses, community health workers, and others on the team. New models of care are challenging to establish because both patients and the health care team are required to reframe the view of the care-delivery structure. However, with the increasing prevalence of chronic disease and the aging of the population, the current health care delivery system requires redesign to control costs and improve outcomes.

INTERPROFESSIONAL COLLABORATION

The benefits of multidisciplinary teams that strengthen interprofessional collaboration have gained support nationally and internationally. In 2012, a private–public partnership created the National Center for Interprofessional Practice and Education (NCIPE) at the University of Minnesota to coordinate and evaluate team-based health care education and patient delivery models. This partnership is comprised of three private foundations—the Robert Wood Johnson Foundation, the Josiah Macy Jr. Foundation, and the Gordon and Betty Moore Foundation—with a federal agency, the Health Resources and Services Administration (HRSA) of the U.S. Department of Health and Human Services. Five core domains are identified for the NCIPE: leadership; collaborative practice and health system transformation; education and training; research, evaluation, and scholarship; and innovative and novel models. Part of the vision for the center encourages "strengthening the alignment of health professions education and health care practice . . . by advancing the field of interprofessional practice and education . . . (to) produce a positive impact on Triple Aim outcomes."

The nine goals specified by HRSA in the original funding announcement, and adopted by the NCIPE, are to:

1. Provide unbiased, expert guidance to the health care community on issues related to interprofessional education and collaborative practice (IPECP)
2. Provide supporting evidence to build the case for IPECP as an effective care delivery model to engage patients, families, and communities in their own health care
3. Identify exemplary IPECP environments to serve as exemplar training sites where IPECP competencies can be modeled, learned, and practiced
4. Prepare academic and practice faculty and preceptors to teach interprofessional competence through curriculum development and ongoing quality improvement activities
5. Collect, analyze, and disseminate data metrics to assess the effectiveness of IPECP models
6. Coordinate IPECP scholarly, evaluation, and dissemination efforts to share innovative, evidence-based, best practice IPECP models

7. Evaluate the impact of team-based care on patient, family, and community health and health care outcomes
8. Develop new, and support and/or enhance existing, team-based IPECP programs across the United States
9. Convene and engage IPECP thought leaders, educators, practitioners, and policy makers to build consensus and bring national attention to IPECP agenda (HRSA, 2012; NCIPE, 2013)

The University of Minnesota Academic Health Center Information Exchange also contains the National Center Data Repository focused on IPECP outcomes with de-identified data.

In 2010, the WHO published the "Framework for Action on Interprofessional Education and Collaborative Practice." The report highlights the status of interprofessional collaboration around the world and outlines a series of action items local health systems can implement to move from the fragmentation of care to coordination with the goal to provide better services and improved health outcomes (WHO, 2010). Collaborative practice requires three interdependent mechanisms of institutional support, work culture, and the environment to optimize health services; these components are described in Table 1.1.

TABLE 1.1 Mechanisms for Collaborative Practice

Institutional support	Governance models
	Structured protocols
	Shared operating resources
	Personnel policies
	Supportive management practices
Working culture	Communication strategies
	Conflict resolution policies
	Shared decision-making processes
Environment	Built environment
	Facilities
	Space design

Source: WHO (2010).

Interprofessional Education

Interprofessional collaboration in both the hospital and outpatient setting is an essential part of the changing health care environment nationally and internationally; in addition, professional training and education for health care providers is integral to changing practice patterns. Ideally, interprofessional training should occur as a fundamental component of basic professional training within each discipline; however, turf and scheduling issues often become barriers in the academic setting. Students in training can benefit from exposure to interprofessional collaboration in community and hospital settings and may observe and participate in team meetings as part of their clinical hours. Training sessions may include nursing, medical assistants, pharmacists, social workers, nutritionists, physical therapists, health-administration staff, and many other disciplines functioning together to discuss professional roles and review patient case studies to enhance the concept of team-based care. Training is occurring across the country in educational settings and in hospitals, clinics, and private practices.

The IOM landmark report titled *The Future of Nursing: Leading Change, Advancing Health* placed emphasis on the importance of early, continual interprofessional education (IOM, 2010). In addition, the WHO (2010) endorsed the concept in its report, which discusses the world shortage of health care workers and the innovative strategies policy makers are evaluating to increase the collaborative practice-ready global health workforce through the interaction between health and education systems with interprofessional education (Figure 1.1). Table 1.2 suggests mechanisms to enhance interprofessional education, and the key learning domains include teamwork; roles and responsibilities; communication; learning and critical reflection; relationship with the patient; and ethical practice (WHO, 2010).

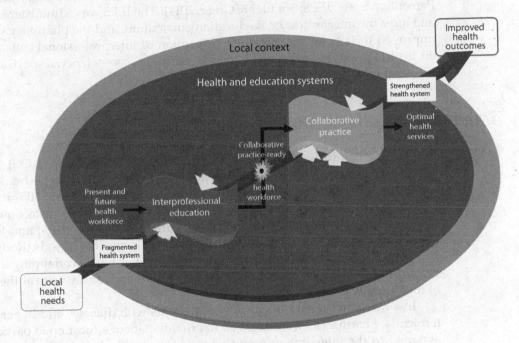

FIGURE 1.1 Health and education systems.
Source: WHO (2010).

TABLE 1.2 Mechanisms for Interprofessional Education

Educator	Curricular
Staff training	Logistics and scheduling
Champions	Program content
Institutional support	Compulsory attendance
Managerial commitment	Shared objectives
Learning outcomes	Adult learning principles
	Learning methods
	Contextual learning
	Assessment

Source: WHO (2010).

As part of training, the next generation of primary care providers, nurse practitioners, and medical residents round together at San Francisco's VA Medical Center (UCSF, 2014). The morning "huddle" of students, attending physicians, and nurses has the aim of fostering better communication and coordination among the team of professionals responsible for care, as well as the innovative training of primary care providers in the model of team-based care.

The South Carolina College of Pharmacy has incorporated interprofessional activities into their doctor of pharmacy (PharmD) program. In one study, the 71 third-year pharmacy students participating in multiple interprofessional educational activities with medical, nursing, and physician-assistant students completed a validated survey to measure the perceptions on this collaboration. The authors reported that incorporating such activities into the training significantly changed pharmacy students' perception of interprofessional collaboration as demonstrated by improvement in knowledge on the Interdisciplinary Education Perception Scale (IEPS; Shrader & Grigg, 2014). The IEPS was administered before and after the interprofessional education curriculum, and the pharmacy students improved their knowledge on their perception of interprofessional collaboration on 16 of 18 questions, focusing on the contributions, competency, respect, and professional regard among different disciplines.

Collaborative Interprofessional Practices in Cardiology

In a survey conducted by the American College of Cardiology (ACC), 63% of health care professionals working in team-based settings reported increased efficiency in care delivery, 53% reported improved quality of care, 50% reported increased patient satisfaction, and 36% reported increased staff satisfaction. These teams were also more likely to implement patient education (69%) and internal communications (63%) as part of standard of care protocols (Brinds, Rodgers, & Hanberg, 2011). Each team member has specific duties with overlapping interests toward the shared goal of ensuring that the patient and family were at the center of high-quality care.

In a randomized controlled study of patients with diabetes and hypercholesterolemia, pharmacists were engaged to provide patient education to participants assigned to the intervention group who had received pharmacologic treatment from a prescriber. The patients in the intervention group were more likely to achieve low-density lipoprotein cholesterol target values than those in the control group (Pape et al., 2011).

At Yale New Haven Hospital, daily multidisciplinary rounds instituted for care of the heart transplant patient demonstrated enhanced communication, an 85% decrease in time to complete a transplant evaluation, a 37% decrease in median post-transplantation stay, and a 33% reduction in the 30-day readmission rate (Roussel, Gorham, Wilson, & Mangi, 2013). In another study, 79 pediatric cardiac surgery patients were followed to determine if the implementation of a handover protocol based on a team approach could reduce the number of errors occurring in transitions from the operating room to the intensive care unit. This study reported that a structured handover process reduced medical errors and improved teamwork and collaboration (Joy et al., 2011).

Walsh et al. (2006) performed a systematic review of 44 studies to evaluate strategies for hypertension management that included provider and patient education and reminders, relaying of clinical information, self-management, audit and feedback, team change, and financial incentives. Strategies were not evaluated equally and were dependent on the data of the original studies; however, team change, which incorporated the assignment of specific responsibilities to health care professionals in addition to the patient's physician, was associated with the most beneficial blood pressure outcomes (Walsh et al., 2006).

The Specialist Nurse-Led Clinics to Improve Control of Hypertension and Hyperlipidemia in Diabetes trial (SPLINT) was a randomized controlled trial, enrolling 1,407 participants (BP $n = 406$, BP control $n = 429$, lipid $n = 317$, lipid control $n = 310$), in an inner city with participants of low socioeconomic status (Mason, Freemantle, Gibson, & New, 2005). Participants with elevated blood pressure, elevated total cholesterol, or both, were randomly assigned to usual care or usual care plus an invitation to attend clinics led by registered nurses (Mason et al., 2005). Nurse-led clinics included discussions of lifestyle factors, evaluations for change readiness, and development of individualized plans of care, including medication titration, according to protocols. This study incorporated cost-effectiveness Markov modeling based on a quality-adjusted life year; the authors reported the nurse-led clinics were beneficial in improving lipid levels and blood pressure control in the diabetic patient population in a cost-effective manner (Mason et al., 2005).

Collaborative Practice Opportunities for Patients With Hypertension

In May 2012, the Community Preventive Services Task Force, a component of the Centers for Disease Control and Prevention (CDC), recommended team-based care for improving blood pressure control, based on 77 studies that indicated systolic and diastolic blood pressure control improved when care was provided by a team of health professionals rather than by a single physician. A team was comprised of a primary care provider supported and complemented by the activities of a pharmacist, nurse, dietitian, social worker, or community health worker. The most significant improvements in blood pressure control occurred with team members who could independently change medications, or with the approval of the primary care provider.

Team-based care interventions in this population typically included activities to:

- Improve medication management
- Facilitate communication and coordination of care
- Enhance use of evidence-based guidelines
- Establish structured follow-up mechanisms
- Actively engage patients in self care by providing them with education about hypertension medications, adherence support, blood pressure monitoring, reducing sodium in the diet, and increasing physical activity (CDC, 2012)

Collaborative Practice Opportunities for Patients With Heart Failure

Heart failure is a growing medical concern, and its prevalence will increase as our population ages. It is the leading cause of hospitalization among adults older than 65 in the United States, and readmission rates following a heart-failure hospitalization remain high. In evaluating practices to reduce costs and improve care, readmission rates have been targeted in numerous quality-improvement projects. Since 2009, reducing hospital readmissions for heart failure has been a national priority of the Centers for Medicare & Medicaid Services (CMS) and part of the National Quality Strategy of the Department of Health and Human Services. Reporting of readmissions fulfills a federal mandate to improve hospital outcomes and efficiency measures. The PPACA, commonly called the ACA, established financial penalties for hospitals with high readmission rates during the first 30 days after discharge.

The complex management of this common, disabling, and costly disease can be addressed through interprofessional collaboration, improving the quality of patient care, reducing medical costs, and increasing the care team's satisfaction. A heart-failure patient's quality of life may be diminished by problems with physical and social functioning. Care may involve lifestyle changes, medication, implantable defibrillators, pacemakers, left ventricular assist devices, and other treatment options. Most patients have co-morbidities that increase the risk of complications and polypharmacy. Among elderly patients, problems with vision, hearing, housing, and resources contribute to the complexity of managing heart failure. Integration of lifestyle changes through multidisciplinary teams is important in improving adherence and quality of life (Jaarsma, 2005). Cardiologists, family-practice providers, nurse practitioners, physician assistants, internists, geriatricians, nutritionists, social workers, nurses, physical therapists, pharmacists, and other professionals may provide treatment to heart failure patients.

Hospitals that have improved readmissions rates have implemented an interdisciplinary approach to care that identifies patients at highest risk for readmission and assigns members of the care teams to address specific needs. Low-income patients are linked by social workers to programs that provide free or reduced-cost medication or to community health clinics. Patients with limited English proficiency (LEP) utilize interpreter services to communicate with the care team. Pharmacists and nurses provide individualized education to patients and families that address health literacy. Discharge nurses use telemonitoring devices to assess critical information, informing relevant providers as necessary. In a study by the Commonwealth Fund, four top-performing hospitals with low 30-day readmission rates in different regions of the country were examined to highlight the best practices that led to improved care. For all of the hospitals in the study, workforce redesign that supported nurses and pharmacists working with care coordinators and hospitalists to manage patient needs led to improved outcomes (Silow-Carroll, Edward, & Lashbrook, 2011). Specifically, the WHO has identified that implementing multidisciplinary strategies for the management of patients with heart failure results in benefits to the health system and a reduction in costs (McAlister, Stewart, Ferrua, & McMurray, 2004; WHO, 2010).

CARDIOVASCULAR TEAM MEMBERS

The multidisciplinary cardiovascular team is comprised of a diverse and extensive group of individuals with various roles, responsibilities, and contributions. Each member provides different and complementary health care services to the patient and his or her family, working together to improve outcomes and overall health care goals. In Table 1.3, general members of the cardiovascular team are described, including degrees or certifications and general roles. The descriptions are general, and many individuals obtain additional certifications and specializations to reflect advanced knowledge and expertise from certifying organizations, for example, the American Association of Heart Failure Nurses' Certified Heart Failure Nurse designation.

There are a variety of cardiovascular tests performed to provide diagnostic, prognostic, and management information for patients with cardiovascular disease. These evaluations may include electrocardiograms, Holter monitors, event monitors, tilt table testing, exercise stress tests, pharmacologic stress tests, transthoracic and transesophageal echocardiograms, nuclear myocardial perfusion

TABLE 1.3 General Cardiovascular Team Members

Advanced practice registered nurses Four roles—certified registered nurse anesthetist, certified nurse midwife, clinical nurse specialist, and certified nurse practitioner. usually certified nurse practitioner in cardiology practice	Board certified advanced practice registered nurse Graduate-level education; required master of science in nursing or master of science (MSN or MS), or doctor of nursing practice (DNP) BLS and ACLS required Must maintain continuing education credits for certification Licensure and prescription privileges vary by state; licensed independent providers	Nurse specializing in providing cardiac care in a variety of cardiac settings. Clinical interest in diagnosing cardiac disease, treatment and management with medication, and diet and exercise. Depending on experience and educational preparation, may practice in specialized areas. Provides health promotion and disease prevention to patients with cardiovascular disease.
Health system administrators	Master of health systems administration (MHSA) or master of business administration in health care (MBA)	Administrator providing support to the clinical team including budgets for equipment, scheduling systems, and information technology. Conducts strategic planning, marketing, and workflow/process improvements. Ensures regulatory and accrediting standards are met.
Licensed practical nurse (LPN)	Must be a registered LPN Completion of state-approved LPN training program Knowledgeable of basic nursing skills, medical terminology, pharmacology, and cardiovascular care; on-the-job experience working in a cardiovascular unit or related allied health care field; must maintain continuing education credits; licensure privileges vary by state	Licensed practicing nurse specializing in providing cardiac care in a variety of cardiac settings under the direction of a physician. Responsibilities include recording patient vital signs, reporting medical history, recording patient symptoms, performing a variety of tests as ordered by cardiologist, and collects samples as ordered.

(continued)

TABLE 1.3 General Cardiovascular Team Members (*continued*)

Medical assistant	High school diploma or GED (required)	Assistant who provides initial patient assessments involving vital signs, performs physical exam, obtains patient's medical history, and collects lab samples. Responsible for recording information into the patient's record.
	Completion of an accredited certified medical assistant (CMA) program (preferred)	
	Knowledgeable of medical terminology, procedural protocols, cardiovascular and secondary co-morbidity care; on-the-job training in the area of cardiovascular care, diagnosis, intervention, and/or rehabilitation	
		Performs any tests requested by a provider, follows protocols.
	Must maintain continuing education credits	
	Licensure privileges vary by state	
Physician cardiologist	Board certified cardiologist	Physician who diagnoses, manages, and prevents the progression of heart disease. Specializes in hypertension, lipid disorders, acute coronary syndrome, coronary heart disease, cardiac conduction disturbances, and heart failure.
	Completion of cardiology fellowship (3 years), completion of Internal medicine training (3 years residency)	
	Graduate of 4-year medical school	
	Must maintain continuing education credits for certification	
		Provides lifestyle modification information to patients with cardiovascular disease.
	BLS and ACLS required	
Registered nurse	Board certified registered nurse (required)	Registered nurse specializing in providing cardiac care in a variety of cardiac settings. Responsibilities include obtaining health history, conducting physical examination, evaluating symptoms, and performing a variety of tests. Clinical interest is in helping to diagnose, recover, and rehabilitate patients with cardiovascular disease.
	Bachelor of science in nursing (BSN) or associate degree in nursing (ADN)	
	Master of science in nursing (MSN) or MS in nursing (optional)	
	On-the-job training in the area of cardiovascular and secondary co-morbidity care, diagnosis, intervention, and/or rehabilitation	
		Provides lifestyle modification information to patients with cardiovascular disease.
	Must maintain continuing education credits	
	BLS and ACLS required	
	Licensure privileges vary by state	

ACLS, advanced cardiac life support; BLS, basic life support.

imaging studies, multiple gated acquisition scans, CT studies, MRI, PET, and other tests. In order to complete the diagnostic studies, team members (Table 1.4) are required to have specialized skills and training.

In certain situations, the invasive use of diagnostic and interventional cardiovascular and peripheral vascular evaluations plays a role to further diagnose, treat, and manage patients with atherosclerotic cardiovascular disease. These procedures may include diagnostic cardiac catheterization, coronary angiogram, peripheral angiograms, percutaneous coronary interventions (PCI), ventriculograms, peripheral interventions, electrophysiology studies, pericardiocentesis, arrhythmia ablations, and various other studies. Invasive cardiovascular and vascular team members for these specialized procedures are described in Table 1.5, including degrees or certifications and general roles.

Cardiac rehabilitation programs are indicated after percutaneous interventions, coronary artery bypass surgery, and myocardial infarction, as well as in heart failure with reduced ejection fraction. Cardiac rehabilitation is a professionally supervised three-phase process, with Phase I promptly beginning in the hospital setting. The cardiac rehabilitation team is comprised of a variety of health care specialists including physicians, nurses, and therapists. Phase II is a 36-session outpatient program

TABLE 1.4 Noninvasive Cardiac Testing Team Members

Profession	Degree or Certification	Role
Exercise physiologist (EP)	Master's degree in kinesiology or applied health physiology (optional) Bachelor's degree in exercise science (required) BLS and ACLS required On-the-job training in the area of cardiovascular and secondary co-morbidity care, diagnosis, intervention, and/or rehabilitation Must maintain continuing education credits Licensure will vary depending on states	Physiologist who oversees the analysis, improvement, and maintenance of health and fitness; rehabilitation of heart disease and various other chronic diseases/illnesses and disabilities. Develops exercise regimens to improve athletic performance, overcome injury, or improve daily lifestyles. Knowledgeable in the field of coronary disease and secondary co-morbidities.
Noninvasive cardiovascular technician (CVT)	Graduate from accredited program with bachelor's degree in exercise science or kinesiology Associates degree On-the-job training in the area of cardiovascular and secondary co-morbidity care, diagnosis, intervention, and/or rehabilitation BLS and ACLS required Must maintain continuing education credits	Technician who performs diagnostic exams and therapeutic interventions of the heart or vascular system at the request or direction of a provider. Able to perform diagnostic tasks using noninvasive procedural testing and knowledgeable in educating patients on cardiovascular health, exercise, and dietary intake.
Nuclear medicine physician	Board certified in the field of nuclear medicine by the American Board of Radiology Completion of (3 years) residency in nuclear medicine; training in allied health sciences such as nuclear physics, radiopharmaceutical chemistry, radiation biology, instrumentation, and/or computer sciences Must complete 1–2 years of preparatory training and 2–3 years of nuclear medicine residency Graduate of a 4-year medical school Must maintain continuing education credits	Physician who uses radiopharmaceuticals (tracers) for the diagnosis and therapy of diseases. Studies the physiologic and metabolic processes of the body.
Nuclear medicine technologist (NMT)	Bachelor's degree in nuclear medicine technology (required) Professional certification from an accredited nuclear medicine program recognized by the NMTCB and/or ARRT(N) Must have completed 1000+ hr in nuclear medicine training BLS required. ACLS is optional, but preferred Must maintain continuing education credits Licensure will vary depending on states *In January 2016, only graduates who have graduated from an accredited program will be able to sit for the NMTCB exam	Technologist who prepares and administers radiopharmaceuticals to patients for the purpose of diagnostic testing. Trained in using special technology to obtain images. Monitors the characteristics and functions of tissue and organs in which the radiopharmaceutical localizes. With additional training and certifications, technologist may also operate CT, MRI, and PET.
Registered cardiac sonographer (RCS)	Bachelor's degree in cardiovascular technology or equivalent & diagnostic medical sonography (preferred) Associates degree (optional) BLS required, ACLS optional, but preferred Must maintain continuing education credits Licensure will vary depending on states	Sonographer performs echocardiograms to evaluate and assist in diagnosing heart disease in collaboration with physicians for the purpose of identifying heart disease and vascular conditions. Understands and evaluates different aspects of the heart and its function, as well as identifies abnormalities.

(continued)

TABLE 1.4 Noninvasive Cardiac Testing Team Members (*continued*)

Profession	Degree or Certification	Role
Registered diagnostic cardiac sonographer (RDCS)	Bachelor's degree in cardiovascular technology and diagnostic medical sonography (preferred) Associates degree (optional) Licensure will vary depending on states BLS required, ACLS optional, but preferred Must maintain continuing education credits Licensure will vary depending on states	Sonographer performs echocardiograms to evaluate and assist in diagnosing heart disease in collaboration with physicians for the purpose of identifying heart disease and vascular conditions. Understands and evaluates different aspects of the heart and its function, as well as identifies abnormalities.

ACLS, advanced cardiac life support; ARRT, American Registry of Radiologic Technologists; BLS, basic life support; NMTCB, Nuclear Medicine Technology Certification Board.

TABLE 1.5 Invasive Cardiac Procedures Team Members

Profession	Degree or Certification	Role
Cardiac electrophysiologist physician (EP)	Board certified clinical cardiac electrophysiology Board certified cardiologist Completion of clinical electrophysiology fellowship (2–3 additional years) Completion of cardiology fellowship (3 years) Completion of 3 years internal medicine training (residency) Graduate of 4-year medical school BLS and ACLS required Must maintain continuing education credits	Cardiologist who diagnoses and manages complex cardiac conduction disorders with medications, cardiac ablation, cardiac-implanted electronic devices, 3D mapping of arrhythmias, temporary pacemaker wires, pacemaker and defibrillator implantations and explanations. Knowledgeable in sterile technique, radiation safety, ECG, and EGM interpretation and stimulation.
Cardiovascular interventionalist physician	Board certified cardiologist Board certified interventional cardiology Completion of cardiology fellowship (3 years) Completion of fellowship training in interventional cardiology (additional 1 year) Completion of 3 years internal medicine training (residency) Graduate of 4-year medical school BLS and ACLS required Must maintain continuing education credits	Cardiologist who performs catheter-based treatment in the diagnosis and treatment of coronary heart disease, congenital heart defects, heart failure, structural heart disease, and valvular disorders. Knowledgeable in sterile technique and radiation safety, cardiac pathology, cardiac arrhythmias, and advanced cardiac ECG.
Invasive cardiovascular technician (CVT)	Bachelor's degree in exercise science or kinesiology (preferred) Master's degree in kinesiology or applied health physiology (optional) Clinical work experience in the field of cardiology and have prior allied health training, and recent related work experience BLS and ACLS required Must maintain continuing education credits Licensure will vary depending on states	Technician who assists a physician in invasive procedures to diagnose cardiac disease and/or circulatory disease. Performs IV placement, hemodynamic, and ECG monitoring, and has knowledge of cardiac medications. Assists physician with interventional procedures such as angioplasty and/or stent, and intra-aortic balloon pumps.

(*continued*)

TABLE 1.5 Invasive Cardiac Procedures Team Members (*continued*)

Profession	Degree or Certification	Role
Registered nurse (RN)	Board certified registered nurse (required) Bachelor of science in nursing (BSN) or associate degree in nursing (ADN) Master of science in nursing (MSN) or MS in nursing (optional) Knowledge and experience with conscious sedation procedures and protocol Clinical work experience in the field of cardiology and recent work-related experience BLS and ACLS required Must maintain continuing education credits Licensure privileges vary by state	Registered nurse specializing in providing cardiac care in a diagnostic and invasive cardiac setting. Responsibilities include recording patient vital signs, evaluating medical history and symptoms, performing a variety of tests, and being knowledgeable of the conscious sedation protocol. Knowledgeable in sterile technique, radiation safety, cardiac pathology, cardiac arrhythmias, and ECG interpretation. Clinical interest in helping to prepare and enabling patients to recover with cardiovascular diagnostic or interventional procedures.
Registered cardiac electrophysiologist specialist (RCES)	National licensure for RCES Bachelor's degree in exercise science Master's degree in kinesiology or applied health physiology (optional) Must complete 600+ in-hospital based case studies or complete educational training program Must have prior allied health training and recent work-related experience Licensure will vary depending on state BLS and ACLS required Must maintain continuing education credits	Specialist who assists the electrophysiology physician in procedures such as cardiac ablations, 3D mapping of arrhythmias, temporary pacemaker wires, pacemaker and defibrillator implantations, and explanations. Knowledgeable in sterile technique, radiation safety, cardiac pathology, cardiac arrhythmias, and ECG and EGM interpretation and stimulation. Performs hemodynamic and ECG monitoring and has knowledge of cardiac arrhythmia medications.
Registered cardiac invasive specialist (RCIS)	National licensure for RCIS Bachelor's degree in exercise science (required) Master's degree in kinesiology or applied health physiology (optional) Must complete 600+ in-hospital case studies and/or completion of an educational training program Must have prior allied health training and recent work-related experience Licensure will vary depending on states BLS and ACLS required Must maintain continuing education credits	Specialist who assists the cardiologist and/or vascular surgeon with catheter-based procedures. Knowledgeable in sterile technique and radiation safety, cardiac pathology, cardiac arrhythmias, and advanced cardiac ECG recognition and intervention. Performs hemodynamic and ECG monitoring and has knowledge of cardiac medications. Assists physicians with interventional procedures such as angioplasty and/or stent, and intra-aortic balloon pumps.
Radiologic technologist (RT)	National licensure for RT (required) Must complete at least 2 years of an accredited hospital based training program or 2- to 4-year educational training program Must have prior allied health training and recent work-related experience Must maintain continuing education credits BLS and ACLS required Licensure will vary depending on states	Technologist who specializes in the field of diagnostic imaging using machines such as x-ray, MRI, CT, and arteriogram/angiograms (specific to cardiac testing) and administer radiation therapies. Specialized in cardiovascular-interventional radiology, sterile technique, and radiation safety. Able to use techniques such as fluoroscopy to help guide catheters during cardiac catheterizations. Assist physicians in deploying angioplasty and/or stents.

(*continued*)

TABLE 1.5 Invasive Cardiac Procedures Team Members (*continued*)

Profession	Degree or Certification	Role
Vascular surgeons	Board certified vascular surgeon Board certified general surgeon Completion of vascular surgery training program (fellowship) (2 years) Completion of general surgery (residency) (3 years) Graduate of 4-year medical school Must maintain continuing education credits BLS and ACLS required	Physician who specializes in all elements of clinical evaluation, management, and operative treatment for vascular disease processes. Specialized in noninvasive testing including plethysmography, duplex ultrasonography, magnetic resonance, vascular ultrasonography, diagnostic CT scans, angiography, and various other diagnostic tests used for diagnosing vascular disease. Specializes in operative treatment such as peripheral intervention, peripheral bypass procedures, and extremity amputation, if necessary. Provides drug therapy and risk factor modification information to patients with vascular disease.

ACLS, advanced cardiac life support; BLS, basic life support.

TABLE 1.6 Cardiac Rehabilitation Team Members

Profession	Degree or Certification	Role
Medical director-cardiologist	Board certified cardiologist Completion of cardiology fellowship (3 years) Completion of internal medicine training (3 years) Graduate of 4-year medical school BLS and ACLS required Must maintain continuing education credits	Physician who makes a diagnosis, treats/manages, and prevents progression of heart disease. Specializes in myocardial infarctions, coronary heart disease, heart rhythm disturbances, and heart failure. Provides lifestyle modification information to patients with cardiovascular disease.
RN Cardiac care	Bachelor of nursing (BSN) or associated degree in nursing (ADN) (required) Master of science in nursing (MSN) or MS in nursing (optional) Must have prior allied health training and recent work-related experience BLS and ACLS required Must maintain continuing education credits Licensure will vary by state	Nurse specializing in providing cardiac care in a variety of cardiac settings. Has experience in acute coronary care settings such as post-coronary intervention, coronary bypass surgery, myocardial infarctions, valve replacement/repair surgeries, left ventricle assist device, pacemaker/defibrillator placements, and heart failure. Clinical interest to assist in managing cardiac disease, with lifestyle interventions and educating patients and families. Interprets daily ECG information during patient exercise. Monitors throughout the 36-session program.
Registered exercise specialist/physiologist	Bachelor's degree in allied health, exercise physiology or kinesiology (required) Master's in allied health, exercise physiology, or kinesiology (preferred) Must have prior allied health training and recent work-related experience BLS and ACLS required Must maintain continuing education credits Licensure will vary by state	Physiologist who provides analysis, improvement, and maintenance of health and fitness; rehabilitation of heart disease and various other chronic diseases/illnesses and disabilities. Clinical interest to assist in managing cardiac disease, diet, and exercise in coordination with the physician. Develops exercise regimens for improving athletic performance, overcoming injury, or enhancing daily lifestyles. Knowledgeable in the field of coronary disease and secondary co-morbidities.

ACLS, advanced cardiac life support; BLS, basic life support.

executed by a variety of health care professionals ranging from physicians, nurses, exercise specialists, physiologists, dieticians, and social workers who help in improving the health and well-being of patients with heart problems through a comprehensive approach. Patients are provided education to further reduce risk factors by modifying lifestyles. Cardiac rehabilitation team members are described in Table 1.6, including degrees or certifications and general roles.

In many circumstances, the general team may also include social workers, medical interpreters, clergy, physical or occupational therapists, or others deemed valuable to ensure quality, patient-focused care. Not all potential members of the health care team are listed in Table 1.7. Additional members may include anesthesiologists,

TABLE 1.7 Additional Cardiac Care Team Members

Profession	Degree or Certification	Role
Chaplain	Bachelor's degree in counseling, psychology, theology, or related field Master of divinity (optional, but preferred) Endorsed by a religious institution, demonstrates additional training or certification from a recognized institution or professional organization	Religious professional who assists a diverse population with spiritual concerns, counseling patients, and supporting end-of-life issues. Offers support to patient, family, and friends. Demonstrates strong interpersonal skills, and is compassionate, approachable, and friendly. Provide support to hospital staff and care providers if needed.
Occupational therapist	Graduate of 3 year master's degree in occupational therapy (required) Bachelor's degree in allied health sciences or related field (required) Postgraduate training (1–2 years residency—optional) CPR and basic life support (BLS) required Must maintain continuing education credits Licensure will vary depending on states	Assists with helping patients learn to take care of themselves post acute-coronary or vascular care. Activities include learning how to drive, eating, talking, and problem solving by engaging patients in meaningful activities. Assists patients within their environments to ensure an easier transition to performing daily routines. Primarily focuses on patients with mental or emotional disorders.
Pharmacist	Graduate of 4-year doctor of pharmacy program (PharmD) (required) Post graduate training (1–2 years residency—optional) Maintain licensure requirements according to national association of boards of pharmacy (NABP) Must maintain continuing education credits Licensure will vary depending on states	Licensed health care provider who is dedicated to provide patients with education and information regarding their medications. Assists in monitoring patients' progress with medications and informs prescribers regarding medications.
Physical therapist	Doctorate of physical therapy (DPT) accredited program (required) Master of physical therapy (MPT)—no longer offered as an entry degree Postgraduate training—2 years residency (optional) BLS required Must maintain continuing education credits Licensure will vary depending on states	Therapist who assists with regaining or obtaining strength, physical mobility, balance, and flexibility and manages pain post acute coronary or vascular care. Works with patients through an inpatient and outpatient setting. Prescribes pain-management techniques to patients to further improve daily routines.

(continued)

TABLE 1.7 Additional Cardiac Care Team Members (*continued*)

Profession	Degree or Certification	Role
Physician assistant	Graduate of an accredited physicians' assistant program (required) Bachelor's or master's degree in allied health sciences or related field (required) Clinical work experience in the field of cardiology and recent work-related experience (required) BLS required Must maintain continuing education credits Licensure and prescription privileges vary by state	Assistant who provides care under the supervision and direction of a cardiologist in diagnosing, treating/managing, and preventing progression of heart disease. May also assist in procedures specializing in diagnostic and interventional coronary or vascular procedures. Improves access to timely care to patients and acts as vital communication between hospital staff, family, patients, and physicians. Provides medication therapy and risk factor modification information to patients with cardiovascular and peripheral vascular disease.
Registered dietician (RD) or Registered dietitian nutritionist (RDN)	Bachelor's degree in dietetics approved by Academy of Nutrition and Dietetics Holds national dietetic and nutrition licensure Holds certification in specialized areas such as diabetes, renal, and pediatrics Must maintain continuing education credits Licensure will vary by state	A food and nutrition expert who specializes in the area of post-acute coronary care. Provides information to patients about healthy diets to improve health and prevent disease. Has the ability to facilitate facts from fads and translate national science into useful information. Assists patients in reducing their risks for developing and/or preventing heart disease and various co-morbidities.
Social worker	Bachelor of social work (BSW) (preferred) or psychology, sociology, and/or education degrees (optional) Master of social work (MSW) for therapy services is required Licensure will vary by state	Professional who assists patients to improve their quality of life and subjective well-being after a life-changing event. Worker is able to teach coping mechanisms to patients dealing with disabilities, mental and physical illness, and social disadvantages.
Certified medical interpreter	Degree and certification vary but most hospitals require national certification from a variety of accreditation boards	Health care interpreters facilitate communication between patients and families with limited English proficiency and their physicians, nurses, lab technicians, and other health care providers.

certified registered nurse anesthetists, dentists, chiropractors, complementary health care providers, psychiatrists and psychologists, community health workers, and others.

Each health care setting will have a distinct composition of the health care team. The diverse education, training, and experiential opportunities of the various disciplines contribute to the enhancement of the multidisciplinary team.

TECHNIQUES FOR IMPLEMENTATION OF INTERDISCIPLINARY COLLABORATION WITH THE HEALTH CARE TEAM

A number of approaches or techniques can be implemented to improve the effectiveness of teams. One training approach is that of TeamSTEPPS (Strategies and Tools to Enhance Performance and Patient Safety) from the Agency of Healthcare Research and Quality (AHRQ, 2014). The following are the three phases of this approach and the steps within each phase.

Phase 1: Assess the Need

1. Establish an organizational-level change team consisting of representatives of the multidisciplinary group
2. Conduct an assessment of teamwork deficiencies
3. Identify the recurring problems that affect patient safety and the intervention that would address these issues as a team
4. List the goals for the intervention, identifying whose behavior would change and when the change would occur

Phase 2: Planning, Training, and Implementation

1. Define the TeamSTEPPS intervention in detail
2. Develop a plan for determining the intervention's effectiveness
3. Develop an implementation plan, identifying the level of training, who will conduct the training, and where and when the training will take place
4. Gain leadership commitment to the plan
5. Develop a communications plan to disseminate information about the training
6. Prepare the group by describing how the new knowledge and skills will impact their job
7. Implement the training

Phase 3: Sustaining the Intervention

1. Provide opportunities to practice
2. Ensure leaders emphasize the new skills
3. Provide regular feedback and coaching
4. Celebrate improvements in teamwork
5. Measure success
6. Update the plan

TeamSTEPPS is one of a number of ways to enhance team functioning. Table 1.8 lists and describes 10 common approaches to improve teamwork. In deciding which approach to use, first decide on the purpose of a team intervention. For example, if a team is taking on additional tasks or is confused about "who will do what"—the technique of responsibility charting (#8) would be most appropriate.

TABLE 1.8 Techniques to Improve Teamwork

Technique	Purpose	Method/Steps
1. TeamSTEPPS (Strategies and Tools to Enhance Performance and Patient Safety) Training (AHRQ, 2014)	To improve teamwork, in particular to address quality and patient safety issues	TeamSTEPPS is a systematic and comprehensive team development program that consists of three phases: 1. A pretraining assessment 2. Planning, training, and implementing the TeamSTEPPS program 3. Sustainment (e.g., providing feedback and coaching) Note: Further information can be found at http://teamstepps .ahrq.gov

(continued)

TABLE 1.8 Techniques to Improve Teamwork (*continued*)

Technique	Purpose	Method/Steps
2. Ground rules	To set behavioral expectations for the practice, particularly interactions among team members	The group brainstorms, then comes to consensus on a set of 6–12 ground rules by doing the following: 1. First ask: "Think about an ideal practice and past issues in working together, either here or in other places—what would be good ground rules to follow in our practice?" 2. Then ask: "Given this brainstorm list, what are 6–12 ground rules that should be given top priority and posted in our meeting or conference rooms?" Note: An example is found in Table 1.9.
3. Survey of team effectiveness	To assess and improve on the current level of teamwork across key dimensions of team effectiveness	1. The group rates (on a 1–5 scale) key variables of teamwork (leadership, communication, participation, collaboration, conflict management, trust, and level of mutual support). 2. The group then focuses on the three variables, scoring the lowest, and discusses ways to address issues underlying each variable.
4. Observations and feedback by a third party, usually a consultant	To provide impartial feedback to the team based on observations of team interactions	1. The consultant observes team interactions during daily work and team meetings. 2. The consultant then provides feedback on observations and engages the team to develop strategies/approaches to improve future teamwork.
5. Meeting postmortems	To improve meeting effectiveness and group interactions during staff meetings	After a meeting, the following questions are asked: 1. What was effective? 2. What should we do differently the next time we meet? 3. What lessons did we learn about teamwork today?
6. Experiential exercises (games)	To use an exercise or game that will assess and improve the team's ability to work together	1. Appoint an observer. 2. Play a game or conduct an exercise. For example, have the team build a plane from Lego blocks or have the group complete a sentence by having each member of the team add a word. 3. After the completion of the game/exercise, have each team member identify lessons in teamwork. 4. After each team member responds, have the observer comment on team interactions and summarize the overall lesson learned.
7. Role clarification	To create understanding and appreciation for the roles of other disciplines	1. Each discipline meets separately and identifies their skills and what they can contribute to the team. 2. A spokesperson from each discipline then reports to large group. 3. After the report is read out, the group discusses ways to integrate the skills and contributions from all disciplines.
8. Responsibility charting	To delineate responsibilities (who will do what on the team) in different situations	1. Identify the situation or setting (e.g., outpatient clinic). 2. Create a matrix that consists of the names of team members in the first column and specific tasks or actions that must be taken for a specific situation in the other columns. 3. Assign (through checkmarks or abbreviations) who has primary responsibility (PR) and who will provide support (SU) for the task.

(continued)

TABLE 1.8 Techniques to Improve Teamwork (*continued*)

Technique	Purpose	Method/Steps
9. Team "Dos & Don'ts"	To create a list of acceptable and unacceptable behaviors	The list is created by asking two questions: 1. What behaviors have you seen that were effective in promoting teamwork? 2. What behaviors have you observed that hindered teamwork? Note: See example in Table 1.10.
10. Work style preferences	To identify how each member of the team wishes to be approached or communicated with as part of the team	The facilitator asks the team to: 1. Express their pet peeves or "turn-offs" in how others have approached or worked with them in the past. 2. Describe what approaches work best in communicating or working with them on the team.

TABLE 1.9 Examples of Ground Rules for Working Together

1. Go about your work as though this was your own solo practice.
2. Value, appreciate, and respect differences and each partner's role on the team.
3. Maximize individual strengths for the benefit of the group.
4. Go directly to the person with whom you have an issue.
5. Deal with conflict among partners away from nonpartners and staff.
6. Realize that each person has a role and obligation to resolve an interpersonal conflict.
7. Develop frameworks or systems (for decision making, communication, etc.) on which everyone agrees.
8. Set the example and tone for nonpartners (e.g., explain the rationale for decisions, speak with a common voice on decisions that were made).
9. Communicate face-to-face or voice-to-voice when possible, realizing that this communication strengthens the fabric of the practice and greatly increases trust.
10. Seek clarification and understanding of the viewpoint of others.
11. Strive for increased self-insight and self-awareness in order to be more effective as a member of the group.
12. Ensure openness/input in decisions and, when practical, solve major problems as a group.
13. Maintain confidentiality on issues with others.

Each group or organization should develop specific ground rules based on its particular setting. Table 1.9 provides some examples of commonly agreed-upon ground rules.

Regardless of the setting or situation, there are particular behavioral characteristics that improve or hinder the effectiveness of team functioning. Table 1.10 describes some of these characteristics.

FOCUS ON QUALITY

Collaborative practice improves the health care system, health care services, and, therefore, health outcomes. Research has demonstrated that treatment by collaborative teams results in higher levels of patient satisfaction, improved acceptance of care, and better health outcomes, as shown in Table 1.11 (WHO, 2010). In addition, chronically ill patients who received team-based care in their homes reported improved satisfaction and overall good health with fewer clinic visits and symptoms (WHO, 2010).

TABLE 1.10 Examples of Effective and Ineffective Team Behaviors

Effective Behaviors
- Use the person's name
- Maintain eye contact, smile
- Have positive body language
- Use pleasant tone of voice
- Provide timely information
- Keep an open mind
- Accept input without being threatened
- Ask for clarification
- Know the person personally
- Use SBAR in handing off care (situation, background, assessment, recommendation)

Ineffective Behaviors
- Not communicating
- Withholding information
- Not acknowledging or avoiding the other person
- Not having eye contact
- Having pursed lips, tight body, hands on hips, eye rolling
- Speaking abruptly and defensively
- "Bashing" the other person
- Jumping to conclusions, assuming a malicious intent
- Not supporting others, not backing up one another

TABLE 1.11 Outcomes of Collaborative Practice

Improvement	Decrease
Access to health care services	Total patient complications
Coordination of health care services	Length of hospital stay
Appropriate use of specialists	Tension and conflict among caregivers
Improved outcomes in chronic disease	Staff turnover
	Hospital admissions
	Clinical error rates
	Mortality rates

Source: WHO (2010).

Listed in Table 1.12 are practice and educational organizations that focus on interprofessional concepts and initiatives.

TABLE 1.12 Interprofessional Practice and Educational Organizations and Initiatives

National Center for Interprofessional Practice and Education
Institute for Health care Improvement
Interprofessional Education Collaborative
National Academies of Practice
Institute of Medicine Global Forum on Innovation in Health Professional Education
World Health Organization
Alliance for Continuing Health Professions Education
Institute for Health care Improvement Open School
Health Resources and Services Administration, Bureau of Health Professions
Geriatric Interdisciplinary Team Training Program

For full reference citations to this chapter, please see "Section References" in the back of the book, under the heading "Section I."

2

The Cardiovascular History

ERIN K. COUGHLIN, DANA E. HAGGETT,
AND KELLEY M. ANDERSON

The patient's medical history is the key to clinical evaluation, management, and diagnosis. The purpose of the comprehensive cardiovascular history is to collect general health information from the patient, with a focus on obtaining specific details pertinent to the patient's cardiovascular status. A comprehensive history, driven by careful questioning, requires active listening and effective communication skills. The patient interview is an opportunity to assess the patient's overall health and perception of illness, and create a trusting patient–provider relationship. Often an accurate diagnosis is obtained from the history alone.

Prior to obtaining the health history, first establish whether the patient is experiencing a condition associated with a life-threatening problem, such as acute chest pain, requiring immediate evaluation. In an urgent or emergent situation, obtain only the most pertinent, problem-focused information to determine the relevant treatment plan, referral, and required interventions. In the new patient who presents with non-acute cardiac complaints and appears medically stable, obtain a comprehensive cardiac history. The initial history is often longer in duration than the history of an established patient. If the patient's medical history or previous diagnostic results are available, review the information prior to the patient encounter.

This chapter's methodical framework provides an approach to the patient history by determining patient concerns and identifying important data that requires further exploration. Although not every component of the health history is relevant for each patient, this comprehensive framework provides a starting point to initiate the interview process. Each patient encounter should begin with introductions in an environment that is conducive to the interview—private, comfortable, and free from distractions. Adopt behaviors to create a rapport with the patient by sitting down, displaying relaxed body language, being respectful, and paying attention. In the outpatient setting, consider obtaining the history prior to asking the patient to change into a gown for the physical examination.

Remember the patient's history is subjective, and it is important to precisely document all details of the patient encounter. Additionally, the patient's history serves as a permanent, legal document as well as a reference for other clinicians involved in the patient's care. To be both legally protective and to facilitate continuity of care among the patient's health care team, it is crucial to be well organized, accurate, and concise while documenting the history.

IDENTIFYING INFORMATION

Start the comprehensive cardiac health history by obtaining some simple identifying information. Document the patient's name, date of birth, age, gender, and ethnicity.

Age and Gender

Age and gender are important nonmodifiable factors potentially placing a patient at risk for certain cardiovascular illnesses. For example, according to the American Heart Association (AHA), high blood pressure is more prevalent in older men and women when compared with younger patients (Roger et al., 2012). Until age 45, men are more likely to have higher blood pressure than women. From age 45 through 64, the prevalence of high blood pressure is comparable in men and women; and in patients 65 and older, women are more frequently affected by hypertension than men (Roger et al., 2012).

Ethnicity

Ethnicity is also an important nonmodifiable factor when assessing a patient's risk for cardiovascular disease, as many disorders have differing prevalence and disease progression depending on ethnic groups. Again using hypertension as an example, the AHA states the prevalence of hypertension in African Americans is greater than in Caucasians (Roger et al., 2012). Additionally, when compared with Caucasians, African Americans are more likely to develop hypertension at a younger age and have higher blood pressures, thus increasing their risk for such complications as cerebral vascular accidents and chronic kidney disease (Roger et al., 2012).

The Historian

The historian providing the health information during the visit should be noted. Assess and record the reliability of the historian in a nonjudgmental manner. This can be documented as "the patient appears to be a reliable historian" or "the patient appears to be a poor historian." A family member or caregiver may be present during the patient encounter and speak on behalf of the patient. Both family members and caregivers can provide thoughtful insight into a patient's condition. For example, the patient's partner may verify that the patient experiences episodes of snoring and apnea due to frequent disruptions during the night.

For patients who speak a foreign language, it is best to obtain services with a certified medical interpreter to translate the medical history rather than a family member (Swartz, 2014). If an interpreter is utilized, document the interpreter's name and the language spoken during the patient encounter.

CHIEF CONCERN

Inquire about the reason the patient is seeking medical attention. The chief concern or complaint should be a brief statement of the symptom or problem and the duration of these symptoms, ideally expressed in the patient's own words (Seidel et al., 2011; Woods, Froelicher, Motzer, & Bridges, 2010). Common cardiovascular chief complaints include, but are not limited to, chest pain, shortness of breath, heart palpitations, edema, syncope, and fatigue (Bonow, Mann, Zipes, & Libby, 2012). Remember, the patient may not vocalize the problem using medical terminology. Rather, the patient may use the word "swelling" to indicate edema or state "I felt lightheaded and dizzy, like I was going to pass out" to describe a near-syncopal episode. In these situations, the chief complaint should be documented using quotation marks to capture the patient's exact statement of the problem. Often patients and families may be confused by medical terminology; during the interview, evaluate the patient's health literacy and adapt questions and answers based on the patient's level of understanding.

Determine if the patient has sought recent medical evaluation or treatment. Discern who provided the care and in what type of facility, for example, emergency department, urgent care center, or clinic setting. Decide if it would be helpful to have the patient's recent health records and obtain them as indicated.

HISTORY OF PRESENT ILLNESS

To elicit a thorough history of present illness (HPI), begin with open-ended questions: "What brings you in today? What seems to be the problem? How may I help you?" Alternatively, probe into the documented chief concern. Actively listen and allow the patient to comfortably tell the story. One caveat—some patients ramble when given the opportunity; these patients need to be guided with more direct questioning. Direct questions clarify earlier details provided by the patient. Often times, direct questions seek a yes or no answer or a brief response. Successful interviewing requires a balance between eliciting important information and forgoing less relevant data. There is no single best way to interview all patients; it is a give-and-take between the provider and the patient, with the patient's answers guiding the logic of subsequent questions.

When a patient complains of a specific symptom, it is necessary to investigate all characteristics of that symptom during the HPI. The mnemonic **OLDCARTS** (Table 2.1) is helpful to assess the patient's symptoms.

Inquire about the *onset* of the symptom. If possible, document the exact date and time the problem began. Additionally, determine what the patient was doing when the problem started. Was the patient eating? Exercising? Sleeping? Furthermore, was the onset gradual or sudden?

In the patient complaining of pain, *location* is an important factor. Is the pain generalized or more localized to a specific part of the body? Does the pain stay in one area or does it radiate to another location? If the patient has difficulty describing the pain location, ask the patient to point with one finger to the area of pain. If the patient complains of radiating pain, ask the patient to indicate the path of radiation (Woods et al., 2010).

TABLE 2.1 OLDCARTS Patient Symptoms

Onset
Location
Duration
Character
Aggravating/**A**ssociated factors
Relieving factors
Temporal factors
Severity

Inquire about the *duration* of the symptom. How long has the problem been going on? Has the problem been continuous since it started or more intermittent? How long does an episode of the problem last—minutes, hours, or days? Is it similar to a problem in the past?

Character of the symptom refers to the nature of the problem. If the patient is having chest pain, is it dull or sharp in quality? The patient might have a unique way of describing this pain, and in that case, it is best to document the description using the patient's own words within quotation marks (Woods et al., 2010).

Detail the factors that *aggravate* the problem. Does the patient's discomfort worsen with food or activity? Ask the patient, "What makes it worse?" Find out if a specific position or movement aggravates the symptom. Additionally, does the patient experience any *associated* constitutional symptoms such as nausea, vomiting, fever, or chills with the presenting symptom? If the patient does report associated symptoms, these problems should be further evaluated, again using OLDCARTS.

Is there anything the patient has done that has helped *relieve* the symptom? Does resting make the shortness of breath go away? Does changing position alleviate the chest pain? Has the patient tried any prescribed or over-the-counter (OTC) medications? Has the patient tried any home remedies or complementary therapies?

When assessing *temporal* factors, ask how frequently the patient is experiencing the symptom. For example, does the patient experience shortness of breath every time on climbing two flights of stairs or was it just one time? Furthermore, ask the patient to describe a typical attack (Seidel et al., 2011). Has the symptom improved or gotten worse since the initial episode? Does the symptom occur at a certain time of day, or on specific days? How does this compare with 6 months ago? If changing, better or worse, what is the rate of change? Is there something new or different today?

Severity can be measured with a scale or the impact on the patient's daily activities. Determine how bothersome the problem is to the patient. Severity of pain can be measured on a scale from 0 to 10, 0 indicating no pain and 10 indicating the worst pain the patient has ever experienced. For comparison, ask the patient to describe the 10—a broken limb, urinary stone, or childbirth? Determining how the problem is impacting the daily life of the patient is another measure of severity. For example, is the patient unable to go to work due to the increasing discomfort? How has the problem affected the patient's quality of life or sleep?

In the HPI, it is important to document pertinent positives as well as pertinent negatives (Woods et al., 2010). For example, if the patient is complaining of shortness of breath with activity, note whether the patient denies other respiratory symptoms such as wheezing or a productive cough to help differentiate between cardiovascular and respiratory etiologies.

If the patient presents with an explicit cardiovascular complaint with prior cardiac history, document the patient's cardiac history in the HPI as well as the patient's established cardiology provider (Holler, 2008). Ask if the patient has ever experienced a similar cardiovascular episode, and if so, what was done to resolve the issue. In addition, evaluate relevant cardiac risk indicators such as smoking status, family history of cardiovascular disease, and personal history of cardiovascular risk factors (Holler, 2008). Cardiac-specific laboratory testing, diagnostic imaging results, noninvasive testing, and invasive cardiac interventions should also be noted in the HPI (Woods et al., 2010).

PAST MEDICAL HISTORY

The past medical history (PMH) is a compilation of the patient's previous medical illnesses, diagnoses, and the patient's general health throughout the life span. Inquire about any medical problems and provide some prompts if the patient has difficulty answering the question. Determine if the patient has any chronic conditions and proceed to name a few if needed. What type of medical care has the patient received? Has the care been continuous or episodic?

Inquire about the dates of diagnosis and duration of the illness. The length of an illness provides insight into the trajectory of disorders that are generally progressive in nature. Patients living with chronic illnesses for many years may be severely disabled or limited by the illness. A patient with a chronic illness may differ from that of a patient newly diagnosed with the same condition. Thus, the disorder must be understood within the context of the patient's disease progression. For example, the patient with a 10-year history of heart failure with worsening dyspnea on exertion may be unable to climb stairs at home and determine it is necessary to move to an apartment without stairs. Conversely, the patient newly diagnosed with heart failure might not yet appreciate how limiting a heart failure exacerbation can be when attempting to complete activities of daily living (ADL).

There are defined cardiovascular conditions that are important aspects to determine from the PMI. These conditions include hypertension, lipid metabolism disorders, coronary heart disease (CHD), heart failure, valvular heart disease, cardiac conduction abnormalities, peripheral vascular disease, and cerebrovascular disease. Any bodily system can have implications for cardiovascular health; similarly, cardiovascular health can influence the function of many other systems. An understanding of the complete health history is essential to the understanding of the cardiovascular history. For example, renal disease is related to hypertension and cardiovascular diseases; malignancies can predispose individuals to pericardial effusions and thrombophilia; and thyroid disorders affect cardiac conduction. In addition, the following systemic disorders predispose patients to a variety of cardiovascular conditions: scleroderma, systemic lupus erythematosus, amyloidosis, anemia, hemochromatosis, HIV, Lyme disease, rheumatic fever, and pulmonary hypertension.

Congenital and Childhood History

Determine if the patient has any known congenital heart diseases, generally classified as cyanotic or non-cyanotic. Examples of cyanotic congenital heart diseases include tetralogy of Fallot, transposition of the great vessels, tricuspid atresia, truncus arteriosus, pulmonary atresia, hypoplastic left heart, and Ebstein's anomaly. Non-cyanotic congenital heart diseases include patent ductus arteriosus, atrial and ventricular septal defects, pulmonic stenosis, coarctation of the aorta, atrioventricular canal defect, and aortic stenosis. In the history, determine the interventions or surgeries conducted for the disorders mentioned earlier. Bicuspid aortic valve is a congenital disorder that may or may not result in valvular heart disease later in life. Genetic and chromosomal syndromes associated with a higher incidence of various cardiac diseases include Down, DiGeorge, Marfan, Noonan, and Turner syndromes, and Trisomy 13.

Major childhood illnesses should be evaluated to include measles, mumps, pertussis, varicella, scarlet fever, rheumatic fever, Kawasaki, diphtheria, Lyme disease, and polio (Seidel et al., 2011). According to the World Heart Federation (2012), untreated rheumatic fever can lead to fibrosis of heart valves as well as valvular heart disease, heart failure, and even death. Kawasaki syndrome predisposes patients to mitral regurgitation, arrhythmias, myocarditis, and vasculitis of coronary arteries, which may lead to coronary aneurysm development. Untreated Lyme disease can result in conduction disorders and arrhythmias. Therefore, knowing the patient's history of congenital and childhood illnesses may suggest the need to evaluate the patient's risk for developing future cardiovascular complications.

Adult Illnesses and Hospitalizations

Significant illnesses and conditions are evaluated in the PMH. When obtaining a PMH from the patient with a cardiovascular concern, ask the patient specifically about the following cardiovascular illnesses, events, or devices: CHD, hypertension, lipid metabolism disorders, myocardial infarction, cardiac arrhythmias, valvular heart disease, or placement of pacemakers, recorders, or defibrillators. If the patient reports a history of any of the aforementioned conditions, document the managing providers. If the patient has a history of cardiac conditions requiring invasive interventions, obtain the names of the patient's cardiologist, cardiac surgeon, and electrophysiologist (Holler, 2008). Be sure to also document any hospitalizations with the date, reason for admission, diagnosis, name of the hospital, and any complications experienced (Seidel et al., 2011).

Other systemic disorders associated with cardiovascular diseases include human immunodeficiency virus, diabetes mellitus, cerebrovascular disease, renal artery stenosis, chronic kidney disease, pulmonary hypertension, pulmonary fibrosis, malignancy, thyroid dysfunction, anemia, gout, systemic lupus erythematosus, and connective tissue disorders. When the patient reports a history of malignancy, document the type of malignancy as well as the treatment the patient received because some chemotherapeutics can cause cardiovascular complications. For example, Doxorubicin, an anthracycline-based chemotherapeutic utilized in the treatment of breast cancer and several hematologic malignancies, is potentially cardiotoxic by reducing cardiac function (Lotrionte et al., 2013). Additionally, the patient who has undergone radiation therapy to the mediastinum as part of cancer treatment is at an increased risk of developing a spectrum of cardiovascular complications such as radiation-induced atherosclerosis, pericardial disease, myocardial disease, endocardial disease, valvular disease, and conduction disturbances (Yusuf, Sami, & Daher, 2011).

In patients with chronic kidney disease, evaluate the most recent or baseline serum creatinine and glomerular filtration rate. The intravenous contrast administered during cardiovascular studies, such as coronary angiography and cardiac computed tomography, can worsen impaired renal function (Hung, Lin, Hung, Huang, & Wang, 2012).

Considerations in Women

For the comprehensive cardiovascular history, women require certain considerations based upon the reproductive status and gender specific conditions. Obtain an obstetric and gynecologic history of the female patient including gravity, parity, and the outcome of each pregnancy. Complications of pregnancy, including preeclampsia, gestational diabetes, and pregnancy-induced hypertension and a history of polycystic ovary syndrome portend future CHD in women (Mosca et al., 2011). In patients of childbearing age, inquire if the patient is currently pregnant, breastfeeding, or if she desires pregnancy in the near future. Evaluate cardiovascular medications in regards to reproductive status, as certain pharmaceuticals, such as angiotensin-converting enzyme inhibitors, are contraindicated in pregnancy. Furthermore, if she does not desire pregnancy, inquire and document her pregnancy prevention method. Use caution in prescribing combined oral contraceptive pills in patients older than 35 with uncontrolled hypertension or in those with concomitant tobacco use, as these conditions may increase the patient's risk of developing venothromboembolism, myocardial infarction, or stroke (Bonnema, McNamara, & Spencer, 2010). In women with children, evaluate for a history of postpartum cardiomyopathy.

Determine if the female patient is postmenopausal due to age or after oophorectomy, as these patients have an increased risk for developing CHD when compared with younger women. Evaluate for a current or past usage of estrogen replacement therapy. Additionally, determine if there is a history of systemic autoimmune collagen vascular disease, including systemic lupus erythematosus or rheumatoid arthritis, as these conditions are more common in women and are risk factors for future CHD (Mosca et al., 2011).

Mental Health History

Mental health disorders, such as depression and anxiety, not only influence the cardiology patient's lifestyle choices, but recent studies suggest they also increase the patient's risk for adverse cardiac events (Rozanski, Blumenthal, Davidson, Saab, & Kubzansky, 2005). Ask the patient about a history of a mental health illness and current treatment. Discuss methods of cardiovascular management that support the patient's psychological needs and initiate appropriate referrals to mental health and behavior specialists who can become involved with the patient's care.

PAST PROCEDURAL AND SURGICAL HISTORY

Ask the patient about any previous surgical procedures or interventions completed, even in childhood. Document the specific procedure or surgery, year of completion, surgeon, hospital, and whether the surgery was medically necessary or if it was an elective procedure. Specifically gather data regarding percutaneous coronary interventions with or without drug eluting or bare metal stents; coronary artery bypass grafts, including the number and location; vascular procedures, including the anatomy and interventions; cardiac valvular procedures; electrophysiology studies or procedures; and devices, including bioprosthetic or mechanical valves, pacemakers, implantable cardioverter defibrillators, and implanted monitoring devices. Also note if the patient underwent anesthesia, and if so, whether the patient experienced any adverse effects from anesthesia including hypertension or hyperthermia. Address any complications the patient suffered during or after the procedure or surgery, such as myocardial infarction, cerebral vascular accident, arrhythmia, or excessive bleeding requiring a blood transfusion. If the patient is unsure of the type of procedure or operation, determine the reason why the intervention was performed.

REVIEW OF SYSTEMS

In conducting a comprehensive review of systems (ROS), review each organ system in a systematic manner to ensure all symptoms and disorders are evaluated (Table 2.2). The ROS serves as a screening tool to identify any important conditions that may go unrecognized without prompts to the patient. Target specific questions of the ROS based on the individual patient characteristics, risk factors, and PMH. For example, inquire about prostate disease symptoms in men older than 50 years of age.

Encourage the patient to answer yes or no during the ROS to identify if he or she does or does not experience specific symptoms. Further investigate any positive findings. If the patient reports having experienced weight gain, for example, ask about the quantity of weight gain, if it was intentional, and over what period of time. According to the AHA (2012), sudden weight gain or weight loss can be an indicator that the patient is developing heart failure or that a patient's existing heart failure is worsening. Advise patients with heart failure to weigh themselves at the same time daily (the best time is in the morning before eating breakfast and after urinating; AHA, 2012). Any daily weight gain of 3 pounds or more and weekly weight gain of 5 pounds or more requires a report by the patient to his or her health care provider (AHA, 2012).

Information previously obtained in the HPI does not need to be readdressed, unless further clarification of the symptoms is necessary (Swartz, 2014). For example, in the patient presenting with chest pain, a further review of the patient's respiratory and cardiovascular systems is not necessary if sufficient information about this complaint was already documented in the HPI. In this example, when documenting the respiratory and cardiovascular systems under the ROS, it is acceptable to write "see HPI."

TABLE 2.2 Review of Systems

System	Questions
Constitutional	Fever? Fatigue? Weight change? Loss or gain? Change in appetite? Difficulty sleeping? Malaise? Night sweats? Chills? Pain? Feeling poorly? General state of health? Exercise intolerance?
Head	Masses or growth? Headache? Migraines? Head trauma? Dizziness? Syncope? Loss of consciousness? Pre-syncope?
Eyes	Vision changes? Blurred vision? Double vision? Eye discharge? Cataracts? Glaucoma? Sensitivity to light? Eye pain? Red eye? Contact lenses or glasses? Recent eye exam?
Ears	Change in hearing acuity? Ear pain? Drainage or discharge from ears? Ringing in ears? Vertigo?
Nose	Nasal discharge or post-nasal drip? Change in sense of smell? Frequency of colds or sinus infections? Nosebleeds? Sinus tenderness?
Throat and mouth	Sore throat? Gingival bleeding? Taste disturbance? Painful swallowing? Neck/thyroid masses? Sores or non-healing ulcers in or around mouth? Change in voice? Hoarseness? Tooth pain? Dental problems? Lump in throat? Difficulty swallowing?
Cardiovascular	Chest pain or pressure? Palpitations—rapid or irregular heart beat? Shortness of breath—at rest or with exertion? Orthopnea—shortness of breath lying down? Paroxysmal nocturnal dyspnea (PND)—shortness of breath awakens patient from sleep? Edema or swelling—shoes or jewelry fitting more tightly? Calf or leg pain with walking? Loss of consciousness? Wounds or ulcers on legs or feet?
Respiratory	Cough (productive, nonproductive)? Sputum quality? Hemoptysis? Dyspnea? Shortness of breath—at rest or with exertion? Chest discomfort? Cyanosis? Wheezing? Stridor? Snoring? Stop breathing? Breathing quickly?
Gastrointestinal	Change in appetite? Nausea? Vomiting? Diarrhea? Constipation? Bowel regularity? Trouble swallowing? Pain with swallowing? Regurgitation? Indigestion or heart burn? Abdominal pain? Jaundice? Abdominal swelling or distention? Change in stool consistency or color? Hemorrhoids? Black or tarry stools?
Genitourinary	Urinary frequency? Urgency? Pain with urination? Urinating at night? Incomplete emptying? Blood in urine? Hesitancy? Decreased force of stream? Need to urinate soon after urinating? Flank pain? Dribbling? Incontinence—unintentional loss of urine? Urinary retention?
Musculoskeletal	Loss of strength? Joint pain? Joint swelling? Joint stiffness? Fractures? Dislocations? Muscle pain or muscle ache? Restriction of motion? Pain or swelling—lower back, knees, hands, elbows, hips, shoulder?
Integumentary	Color change? Skin eruptions or rashes? Itching? Excessive sweating? Excessive dryness? Unusual hair growth? Changes in nail contour or growth? Hair loss? Lesions changing in size, shape, or color? New growths?
Neurologic	Headache? Change in memory? Loss of consciousness? Altered sensation or coordination? Weakness? Paralysis? Syncope? Dizziness? Lightheadedness? Seizures? Tremors? Vertigo? Speech changes? Balance problems? Numbness?
Endocrine	Polyuria? Polydipsia? Polyphagia? Goiter? Thyroid enlargement or tenderness? Heat/cold intolerance? Unexplained weight changes? Changes in facial hair? Change in sex characteristics? Inability to conceive? Fatigue?
Hematologic/lymphatic	Pallor? Abnormal bleeding? Abnormal bruising? Swollen lymph nodes? Recurrent infections? Anemia? Prior blood transfusions? Fatigue? Fever? Chills? Unexplained weight loss? Night sweats? New growing mass? Hypercoagulability? Blood clots?
Allergic/immunologic	Wheezing? Urticaria? Angioedema? Pruritus? Rhinorrhea? Recurrent infections?

(continued)

TABLE 2.2 Review of Systems (*continued*)

System	Questions
Reproductive	Male—Testicular pain? Libido? Infertility? Hernia? Penile sores or discharge?
	Female—Menstruation—history, regularity, duration, amount of flow? Irregular bleeding? Postmenopausal bleeding? Vaginal discharge? Breast pain, tenderness, discharge, bumps, galactorrhea?
Peripheral vascular	Pain with walking—frequency and duration? (Calf = superficial femoral artery, thigh = common femoral artery or external iliac artery, buttock = common iliac artery or distal aorta). Edema or swelling? Varicose veins? Loss of hair on legs? Blood clots? Discoloration of extremities? Non-healing wounds? Changes in veins?
Mental health	Depression? Anxiety? Memory problems? Confusion? Change in mood? Difficulty concentrating? Nervousness? Anxiety? Panic attacks? Irritability? Agitation? Stress? Tension? Suicidal or homicidal ideations? Hallucinations? Delusions? Sleep disturbances? Personality changes?

Adapted from Seidel et al. (2011).

The Centers for Medicare & Medicaid Services (CMS, 2010) recognizes the following systems for ROS documentation purposes: constitutional symptoms; eyes; ears, nose, mouth, and throat; cardiovascular; respiratory; gastrointestinal; genitourinary; musculoskeletal; integumentary; neurologic; endocrine; hematologic and lymphatic; and allergic and immunologic. The peripheral vascular system is an additional system to consider reviewing in the patient presenting with a cardiovascular complaint.

CMS has established criteria for three different types of ROS: problem pertinent, extended, and complete (2010). A problem-pertinent ROS is specific to the problem outlined in the HPI and addresses only one system, whereas an extended ROS addresses the specific system identified in the HPI as well as two to nine additional systems (CMS, 2010). The complete ROS reviews the problematic system from the HPI to address the chief concern, as well as 10 additional organ systems (CMS, 2010).

ALLERGIES AND REACTIONS

An essential component of the medical record is a list of the patient's allergic reactions to medications, foods, environmental agents, and latex. These allergies should be reviewed during the initial cardiology visit and at each subsequent visit. Pay close attention to medications and the type of reaction described by the patient. A true allergy occurs when the immune system reacts to an allergen. The manifestations of this reaction include hives, rash, redness, blisters, serum sickness, fever, chills, joint pain, swollen glands, or anaphylaxis, which is a severe systemic, potentially life-threatening reaction. Penicillin is a common cause of drug allergies. Other common medication classes causing allergic reactions include antiepileptics, sulfa, antithryoid, contrast agents, vaccinations, and certain blood pressure medications. Treatment includes avoiding the class of medications that caused the reaction and symptom relief with antihistamines and steroids. In severe cases (anaphylaxis), emergency care is required. Many patients confuse a drug's adverse side effect or intolerance, such as nausea, with an allergy. Electronic medical records typically permit medication reactions to be categorized as allergic (hives) or as adverse side effects (nausea) allowing improved accuracy in prescription management.

Identify any allergies to medications commonly used during emergencies and diagnostic cardiac tests such as morphine and lidocaine (Woods et al., 2010). Specifically determine the patient's reaction to intravenous contrast agents during previous procedures. A shellfish allergy does not increase a patient's risk of a reaction to intravenous contrast (Schabelman & Witting, 2010). When determining adverse effects of radiocontrast administration and premedication protocols, focus on the patient's atopic disposition, such as asthma and multiple true allergies, and on the patient's previous history of contrast reactions (Schabelman & Witting, 2010).

If the patient has a "no known drug allergy" (NKDA) status, verify this information during each patient encounter. Confirmation of the patient's allergy status may also be necessary after a recent illness, hospitalization, or surgery, due to increased medication exposure.

MEDICATION HISTORY

Current Medications

Current medications should be listed with the name, dose, route, frequency, indication, and start date. Obtain the name and contact information of the dispensing pharmacy or pharmacies. Determine how the patient is taking the medications, and determine if the patient is taking them as prescribed, especially with complex medication regimens. If the patient is missing doses or not taking medications as directed, determine the reason—cost, side effects, or misunderstanding. Specifically discuss OTC medications, vitamins, herbal supplements, home remedies, and other "nontraditional" therapies. Check interactions between herbal supplements and prescription medications. Supplements used as complementary therapies may greatly impact the pharmacologic effects of cardiac medications (Tachjian, Maria, & Jahangir, 2010). Examples of those effects include:

- Increased bleeding risks from warfarin when used with alfalfa, fenugreek, garlic, ginger, and ginkgo
- Increased effects of antihypertensives with use of fumitory, Irish moss, kelp, and lily of the valley
- Digoxin levels affected with use of aloe vera and St. John's wort (Tachjian et al., 2010)

Note the patient's reason for taking nonprescription drugs and therapies. Each cardiology visit presents an opportune time for the patient to bring all prescription medications, OTC medications, and supplements to the appointment for proper review and documentation. Provide the patient with an updated medication list at each visit and urge him or her to have the list available at all times. Encourage patients on anticoagulants to wear identification of the medication on a bracelet or necklace to identify themselves as individuals at risk for bleeding.

Cardiac Medication History

A specific cardiac medication history includes the evaluation of current medications such as antihypertensives, antiplatelet therapy, cholesterol-lowering agents, and the use of symptom-relieving medications, such as nitroglycerin sublingual tablets. The frequency of the administration of medications to relieve patient symptoms is an indicator of the patient's stability. Ask the patient to identify the duration of therapies and who originally prescribed his or her medications, and if the provider continues to monitor the patient's cardiovascular status. Some medications are potentially harmful to the cardiovascular system, and it is important to review prior or current administration of these medications in appropriate patients. Potentially harmful medications include phen-fen, anti-retrovirals, nonsteroidal anti-inflammatory drugs, cyclooxygenase inhibitors, estrogens, and certain chemotherapeutic agents.

Relevant Medication History

The relevant medication history should include previous medications and the reason for their discontinuation, such as limited response, intolerance, adverse side effects, or resolution of illness. Also include a history of chemotherapy treatment detailing the medication name, reason, and duration of therapy. Proper documentation of the patient's past medication history minimizes valuable time spent determining the reason for a medication's discontinuation.

HEALTH PROMOTION AND DISEASE PREVENTION

Ask about the patient's general state of health and wellness. Discuss whether or not the patient is satisfied with the current management of symptoms and if the patient is adhering to treatment recommendations. Specify the conditions that the patient finds to be the greatest health asset and the most debilitating. Detail what has improved the patient's health or has caused the most functional impairment.

The typical cardiology patient presents with multiple co-morbidities managed by health care generalists and specialists. Ask the patient to provide a record of immunizations, preventative health screenings, and a list of health care providers managing the patient's medical care. Complementary or alternative therapy used for symptom management should also be listed, as approximately 38% of American adults and 12% of children use complementary and alternative medicine (Barnes, Bloom, & Nahin, 2008). Avoid terms such as "unorthodox therapy" or "unconventional medicine" when addressing this topic (Swartz, 2014).

Immunizations

See the Centers for Disease Control and Prevention (CDC) for appropriate vaccinations based on age, risks, and health conditions. Review and collect dates of the following immunizations for the cardiology patient:

- Influenza
- Pneumococcal
- Tetanus
- Diphtheria
- Pertussis
- Varicella
- Zoster
- Meningococcal
- Hepatitis A and B
- *Haemophilus influenzae* type b (Hib)

Screening

Determine appropriate screening recommendations based on age, gender, and risk factors. The U.S. Preventive Services Task Force provides recommendations for preventative screenings. Review and collect dates of the following preventative health screening exams including date, interval, indication, and screening results:

- Colonoscopy
- Mammography
- Bone density scan
- Cervical cancer screening
- Low-dose chest computerized tomography scan
- Abdominal aortic aneurysm ultrasound
- Fasting blood sugar and HbA1C
- Fasting lipid panel
- Vision and hearing
- Chest x-ray

COLLABORATORS

In order to provide comprehensive and integrated care, evaluate the utilization of other health care providers and specialists. Patients with significant co-morbidities or longstanding chronic diseases may have a team of caregivers, and understanding these elements will ensure intra- and interdisciplinary collaborations and appropriate referrals.

Collaborative Providers

Obtain names and contact information for the following providers in the following health care areas:

- Primary care
- Pulmonology
- Endocrinology or diabetes specialist

■ Gastroenterology
■ Urology
■ Nephrology
■ Gynecology
■ Surgeons
■ Ophthalmologist or optometrist
■ Psychology or other mental health providers
■ Other specialists
■ Physical therapist
■ Nutritionist or dietician

Complementary or Alternative Therapy

As necessary or relevant, consider obtaining information for the following health providers:

■ Chiropractic
■ Homeopathy
■ Naturopathy
■ Guided imagery
■ Meditation therapy

FAMILY HISTORY

The family history serves two main purposes. First, it is an evaluation of the patient's overall family health status. Second, it is an assessment of the patient's health risks by identifying the presence or absence of specific heritable illnesses (Woods et al., 2010). Common heritable conditions in the United States are cardiovascular diseases, diabetes mellitus, lipid metabolism disorders, and certain malignancies. Determine the onset of the disorder in the affected family member, as this may have important prognostic implications for the patient. For example, a myocardial infarction at age 40 is of more concern than when it is at age 80. Also, determine if there are any unusual, rare, or congenital disorders in the family. Start the conversation by asking, "Are you aware of any medical conditions or illnesses that run in your family?" The patient may be able to list specific disorders such as high blood pressure or diabetes. However, the patient may only be able to describe an illness in general terms such as: "My grandfather and brother have bad hearts," or "My older sister and uncle have memory problems." Obtain as specific information as possible.

A three-generation pedigree of first-degree family members and their health status should be listed in the family history. If possible, include parents, grandparents, siblings, and children. Also note if a patient or family member is adopted. Record the following data: living family member's age, medical conditions, and, if deceased, the age and cause of death, if known (Swartz, 2014). As generations of family members are added to the patient's history, pay close attention to trends and consider possible genetic or environmental causes of specific diseases. Electronic medical records typically allow documentation of the family history in a list format. A diagram or family pedigree, however, may prove more useful when assessing for possible inherited disorders. The recognition of illnesses commonly occurring in a family may assist in the assessment and management of the patient's current and future health (Woods et al., 2010).

Specific medical conditions worth identifying in the family history include hypertension, CHD, lipid-metabolism disorders, premature cardiovascular disease, diabetes mellitus, kidney disease, stroke, thrombophilia or coagulopathies, tuberculosis, arthritis, asthma or lung disease, seizure disorders, mental illness, suicide, alcoholism, and substance abuse (Bickley & Szilagyi, 2009; Woods et al., 2010). Also ask about the occurrence of cancer in the family. List the type of cancer or at least specify its location, such as colon, lung, breast, ovarian, prostate, or brain, and the age of onset (Swartz, 2014).

Cardiovascular Family History

Many cardiovascular disorders have familial tendencies. The cardiovascular family history should be obtained in both the acute setting and during cardiovascular screening and assessment. With the patient who is acutely ill, for example, only briefly address any family history of myocardial infarction or heart failure. Alternatively, the child or adolescent who presents for a cardiology screening prior to sports participation requires a more detailed cardiovascular family history. With this patient, inquire about a family history of sudden cardiac death or, in surviving relatives, a family history of hypertrophic cardiomyopathy, long QT syndrome, Marfan syndrome, implanted devices, or arrhythmias (Lyznicki, Nielsen, & Schneider, 2000). For the new cardiology patient, also include a detailed family history of CHD, as it is a significant predictor of subclinical atherosclerosis in asymptomatic patients (Pandey et al., 2013). Review of the cardiovascular family history can identify potential risk factors in not only the unstable or chronic patient but also the young, healthy patient who may benefit from early screening and potentially preventative therapies.

SOCIAL HISTORY

View the social history as an opportunity to learn more about the patient's life, as these aspects may determine the success or failure of medical management and therapeutic interventions. A detailed assessment of psychosocial influences can help explain the patient's presentation of symptoms, reason for seeking care, and adherence to medical treatments (Cole & Bird, 2014). Some topics may come up naturally in conversation, while other more personal topics require questions to be asked in a sensitive and objective manner. Consider during the exam how the patient's cultural beliefs and socioeconomic status may influence the patient's daily habits and understanding of his or her health or illness. Elements of the social history should include the patient's lifestyle, education and occupation, home environment, safety, and support.

Lifestyle

Major elements of the patient's social history relate to the patient's day-to-day activities and habits. Guide the interview to include the following topics: spiritual considerations, nutrition, physical activity, sleep, substance use, and sexual health.

Spiritual Considerations

Spirituality provides many patients with meaning and purpose in life, often framing the patient's perception of health and illness (Puchalski & Romer, 2000). Integrate the patient's spiritual framework into health care decision making and, when necessary, make the appropriate referrals to chaplains, spiritual leaders, and community resources. The FICA Spiritual Assessment Tool© created by Dr. Christina Puchalski in 1996, for example, assists in the evaluation of spirituality during the patient's medical care. The tool provides structured questions and recommendations to help begin the conversation of spiritual considerations, based on F = Faith, belief, and meaning; I = Importance and influence; C = Community; A = Address and action in care.

- What things do you believe in that give meaning to your life?
- How have your beliefs influenced your behavior during this illness?
- Are you part of a spiritual or religious community?
- How would you like me, your health care provider, to address these issues in your health care? (Puchalski & Romer, 2000)

Nutritional Intake

Understanding the patient's nutritional intake is often dependent upon self-reported dietary intake and dietary logs. Evaluate nutritional intake by asking the patient to describe normal dietary patterns including any specialty diets, food restrictions, or food allergies. Patients with known cardiovascular disease may adhere to diets, including the Dietary Approaches to Stop Hypertension (DASH), a Mediterranean diet, a low-sodium diet, a low-cholesterol/-fat diet, or a diet restricting daily fluid intake or carbohydrates. Determine who conducts the food shopping and prepares the meals, and how often meals are prepared at home. Prepared foods and foods consumed outside the home are generally higher in dietary sodium. With elderly patients, identify how meals are obtained and how frequently they are provided. To gain a better understanding of the patient's dietary habits, ask the patient to describe meals consumed within the previous day, a 24-hour recall, or provide a dietary log for the next visit. Another strategy is to ask the patient to identify how many servings are consumed on an average day in the following categories.

- Calcium—milk, yogurt, and cheese
- Protein—poultry, pork, fish, and beef
- Carbohydrates—breads and pasta
- Vegetables and fruits

- Processed/prepared foods and snacks
- Restaurant and fast food
- Soda and juice
- Caffeine
- Fiber
- Water
- Dietary supplements
- Desserts—high-sugar foods

Physical Activity

Evaluate daily physical activity and ask the patient to specify the type, duration, and difficulty of the fitness routine. Highlight the benefits of exercise on overall cardiovascular health, praise positive achievements, and assess the patient's desire to introduce more physical activity into daily life. Determine how illness may affect the patient's ability to exercise. Is the patient concerned physical activity will cause chest pain? Does the patient notice decreased exercise tolerance during activities? Evaluate for opportunities to provide suggestions to modify physical activities and for the suitability of additional services such as physical therapy or cardiac rehabilitation.

Sleep Patterns

The patient's sleep pattern is an indicator of both physical and psychological health. Evaluate the usual sleep and wake cycles, where the patient sleeps, and how frequently the patient wakes up during the night. The patient's partner may be able to provide an account of the patient's sleep habits by identifying periods of snoring, apnea, sleepwalking, and daily naps. Screen the patient for prescription and OTC sleep aids, alcohol, stimulant intake, caffeine, and nicotine. If the sleep pattern is causing concern, also evaluate food intake, exercise, exposure to natural light, sleep environment, and bedtime routines related to the patient's sleep hygiene.

Alterations in the sleep pattern may prompt further investigation of the patient's cardiovascular, pulmonary, mental health, and other related conditions. The patient with heart failure or pulmonary disease may demonstrate disrupted sleep with orthopnea, a condition causing shortness of breath in a reclined position due to pulmonary congestion. This patient typically sleeps in an elevated position with multiple pillows or sits in a chair to improve breathing. Determine the patient's sleep habits with orthopnea such as number of pillows and where the patient sleeps to reduce breathlessness. The heart failure patient may also experience paroxysmal nocturnal dyspnea, a sudden awakening from sleep usually 1 to 2 hours after falling asleep. This patient may notice that obtaining an upright position provides relief. The patient with heart failure, diabetes, or urinary conditions may also experience disrupted sleep due to nocturia. For example, in heart failure, nocturia occurs due to the redistribution of fluid volume in the recumbent position. Mental health conditions may also result in a variety of sleep disorders from hypersomnolence to insomnia.

Substance Use

The use of a variety of substances—tobacco, alcohol, and illicit drugs—needs to be assessed at each visit to determine increased or decreased use and its impact on the patient's cardiovascular status. Tobacco use is detrimental to cardiac, vascular, and pulmonary function and is a risk factor for a multitude of cardiovascular conditions. The history for tobacco use includes the type of tobacco and the duration of use. One pack contains 20 cigarettes; therefore, the patient who smokes one pack per day smokes 7,300 cigarettes per year. The data for cigarette use is generally recorded in number of pack-years and is calculated by multiplying number of packs per day by the number of years of use (Swartz, 2014). For example, the patient who smoked two packs of cigarettes per day for 15 years has a 30 pack-year smoking history. If the patient has discontinued smoking, reinforce the positive behavior and note the prior pack-year smoking history and the date of last tobacco exposure. Approximations have been derived for other forms of tobacco to include cigars, pipes, loose tobacco, and cigarillos, which are small, thin cigars (Table 2.3), (Wood, Mould, Ong, & Baker, 2005). The implications of electronic cigarette use are currently unknown.

TABLE 2.3 Approximations of Tobacco Products

Tobacco Type	Quantity	Equivalent Number of Cigarettes
Cigarillo	1	2
Pipe	1	2.5
Cigar	1	4
Loose tobacco	25 grams, 1 ounce	50

Source: Wood et al. (2005).

Determine the patient's alcohol consumption by asking about alcohol type, quantity, duration, and frequency of use. Moderate alcohol consumption is defined as one drink per day for women and one to two drinks per day for men (AHA, 2014). Educate the patient on the amount of alcohol which constitutes one drink, as restaurant and bar serving sizes may be significantly larger (Table 2.4). Medical literature continues to debate the benefits of alcohol, especially red wine, on cardiovascular health. The AHA highlights that although some research suggests potentially small increases in high-density lipoprotein (HDL) cholesterol with alcohol and red wine consumption, there is no recommendation for initiating alcohol consumption for cardioprotective measures (2014). Rather, encourage the patient to

TABLE 2.4 Definition of One Alcoholic Drink

Type of Alcohol	Amount of Alcohol (oz)
Beer	12
Wine	4
80-proof spirits	1.5
100-proof spirits	1

Source: American Heart Association (2014).

focus on lifestyle factors such as physical activity, a well-balanced diet, lowering blood pressure and cholesterol, and maintaining a healthy weight to reduce cardio-vascular risks (AHA, 2014).

To elicit an accurate account and minimize defensive behavior when obtaining the patient's alcohol consumption history, a skilled interview technique is required. The well-established CAGE questionnaire is an example of one such screening tool to help identify the patient who struggles from alcoholism by addressing the social and behavioral impacts of the patient's alcohol use (Ewing, 1984). Two or more positive responses to the four areas of inquiry suggest a history of alcoholism. The four questions include feelings that the patient should cut down on drinking; feeling annoyed by others who criticize the amount of drinking; feeling bad or guilty about the drinking; and consuming a drink first thing in the morning (eye-opener) to steady nerves or relieve a hangover (Ewing, 1984).

Illicit drug screening includes the identification of both recreational drug use and abuse of prescription medications. Any drug use, past or present, should be determined. Preface the need to identify the patient's drug use due to the potential of these substances having serious health complications, especially in relation to cardiovascular disease, medication combinations, and surgery. For example, cocaine use has been associated with acute coronary syndrome (ACS), and the incidence of cocaine-induced ACS has increased with the increased use of this illicit substance (Gurudevan et al., 2013). Endocarditis of the tricuspid valve is highly linked to intravenous drug use due to the direct introduction of pathogens into the vascular space. On occasion, the patient may prefer to not answer these questions; respect the patient's wishes and address the topic of substance abuse at a later time.

Sexual Health

Obtain a comprehensive sexual history when appropriate. This includes asking the patient about relationships and intimate physical contact with a partner, sexual preferences, use of contraception and condoms, sexual problems or issues with performance, and history of a sexually transmitted infection. Women with cardio-vascular disease may require counseling for issues related to pregnancy and contraceptive alternatives (Levine et al., 2012). The patient with cardiovascular disease may have specific concerns regarding sexual activity after a myocardial infarction or will report sexual dysfunction. The AHA developed a scientific statement regarding sexual health and cardiovascular disease with specific recommendations for individuals with CHD, heart failure, valvular heart disease, arrhythmias, pacemakers, implanted cardioverter defibrillators, congenital heart disease, and hypertrophic cardiomyopathy (Levine et al., 2012). General recommendations in the guidelines include the appropriateness of the health history and physical examination for the evaluation to initiate or resume sexual activity in patients with cardio-vascular disease. Patients who can undergo three to five metabolic equivalents of energy expenditure during exercise without ischemia have a very low risk of ischemia during sexual activity (Levine et al., 2012). Additionally, patients with unstable or decompensated symptoms should defer sexual activity until further evaluation and stabilization.

Certain medications, including beta-adrenergic blocking agents and diuretics, have anecdotal evidence of causing reduced sexual function. However, there are no clear studies to document these relationships. It is recommended to continue cardiovascular medications in situations that improved survival and symptoms, despite potential changes in sexual function, including erectile dysfunction (Levine et al., 2012). Prescribing of phosphodiesterase-5 inhibitors for erectile dysfunction is recommended with caution in certain cardiovascular conditions, including severe aortic stenosis, and should not be used with concomitant nitrate administration.

Education and Occupation

Assessment of the patient's educational level provides information regarding health literacy, reading level, and occupation. Past and current occupations offer clues to the patient's exposure to health hazards and stress level. Diseases caused by occupational and environmental conditions do not typically appear immediately after exposure, thus increasing the probability of being misdiagnosed (Swartz, 2014). Occupational hazards in relation to the risk of cardiovascular disease are not well known (National Institute for Occupational Safety and Health [NIOSH], 2013). The CDC identifies exposure to chemicals such as carbon disulfide, carbon monoxide, nitroglycerin chemical compound, and environmental tobacco smoke, along with occupations causing excessive stress or requiring shift work, as possible risk factors in the development of CHD (2010). Occupations that may expose the patient to the aforementioned chemicals and stressors include: truck drivers, tunnel and bridge officers or construction workers, munitions workers, bartenders, nurses, and business executives. Patients who undertake international travel may be exposed to various infectious diseases. Additionally, patients with military service may have experiences of physical trauma, mental health issues, and unusual exposures to toxins and infections.

Home Environment

Evaluating the home environment offers insight into the patient's social support system and family dynamics. Determine who resides with the patient at home—grandparents, parents, children, grandchildren, or other individuals. *Family structure* includes marital status and number of children, along with family roles, relationships, and dynamics. Eliciting information about the patient's family structure aids in categorizing the family as a system. *Environmental factors* surrounding the home environment can suggest health hazards and safety concerns. Consider assessing the patient's home environment in depth in patients with conditions that cause concern, for example, repeat hospitalizations for heart failure or failure to adhere to pharmacologic management. The following are some questions to ask to begin the conversation about the home environment.

- Who lives with you?
- Is there anyone at home to help you with your health care?
- Describe where you live. How many steps?

- What is your source of heat and air conditioning?
- Do you have access to a scale to weigh yourself?
- Do you have difficulty entering and leaving your home?
- What is your neighborhood like? Do you feel safe?
- Who has access to your home?

Safety

For safety screening, inquire about the patient's use of a seatbelt, helmet, sunscreen, and home smoke detectors. Address the safety concerns appropriately by providing education on why these safety measures are important. *Fall risk* should be a safety concern for all patients who are elderly, chronically ill, or receiving anticoagulation therapy. Ask if the patient has a history of falls or has fallen recently. A positive response suggests the need for further investigation of the patient's gait, balance, sensation, and cognitive status. *Intimate partner and elder-abuse screening* is necessary for all patient encounters, due to the potential for the abuse to go unrecognized and impact chronic illnesses. It is estimated that only one in five elderly-adult abuse cases in the United States are actually reported (U.S. Preventive Services Task Force, 2013). The initiation of this topic may vary with each patient and can be addressed when evaluating the patient's home environment, support systems, or with general screening. It is preferable to pose these questions when alone with the patient. Approach physical, sexual, emotional, and financial abuse screening with open-ended questions, highlighting the fact that every patient is screened. Start the conversation by stating: "I talk with all my patients about their safety. Have you ever felt unsafe at home or in the workplace? Tell me more about this experience." Possible screening tools to be used in practice include:

- Hurt, Insult, Threaten, Scream (HITS)
- Ongoing Abuse Screen/Ongoing Violence Assessment Tool (OAS/OVAT)
- Slapped, Threatened, and Throw (STaT)

Psychosocial Support

Various systems of support or lack of support can greatly impact the patient's cardiovascular disease outcomes. The cardiology patient with low social support may live alone, have limited financial resources, and lack family support. Recent research suggests this type of patient is at an increased risk of cardiac death (Rozanski et al., 2005). Chronic life stressors may become apparent as the patient's social history is obtained. Due to the complexity of cardiology patients, evaluate the support systems and resources available to the patient, especially during periods of illness and disability. Support systems to assess include family members, financial resources, access to health care, and community services.

COGNITIVE AND FUNCTIONAL ABILITIES

Cognitive Abilities

Assess the patient's cognitive abilities and impairments. This can include assessing the patient's understanding of the disease process and treatment along with asking about any noticeable decline in hearing, vision, and memory. Changes in memory and cognitive function may be due to normal aging, mild cognitive impairment, delirium, or various types of dementia, such as Alzheimer's disease and vascular dementia (Sloane et al., 2012). Consider the patient's risks for cognitive decline and dementia in relation to vascular and cardiac disease. For example, lowering blood pressure in the middle-aged and young elderly (< 80 years) adult patient may help prevent late-life dementia (Gorelick et al., 2011). Cognitive decline in memory, executive function, psychomotor skills, and attention span is common in the patient with heart failure (Dardiotis et al., 2012). Thus, when assessing end-organ damage due to cardiovascular disease, include an assessment of the patient's cognitive function. This assessment may prove to be extremely beneficial in the identification of early cognitive changes and guide the modification of therapeutic interventions (Gorelick et al., 2011).

Possible cognitive screening tools are listed here. Positive screening results require advanced assessment and diagnostic testing by a specialist.

- Mini-Cog Test
- AD8 Dementia Screening Interview
- Mini-Mental State Examination (MMSE)
- Rey Auditory Verbal Learning Test

Activities of Daily Living

Assessment of the patient's functional capabilities is an evaluation of the patient's ability to live an independent life and manage chronic illness. Struggles with daily activities can greatly impact the patient's physical and mental health, potentially leading to poor cardiovascular outcomes. Issues with basic care abilities can be a source of embarrassment for the patient and may not be initially discussed by the patient during the HPI. With the older or more disabled adult, ask about ADL and then assess higher levels of function with instrumental activities of daily living (IADL). The patient's ADL include bathing, dressing, toileting, transferring, continence, feeding, and managing money. The patient's IADL include using the telephone, shopping, preparing food, housekeeping, laundry, transportation, and taking medication (Bickley & Szilagyi, 2009). The patient who struggles with elements of ADL or IADL will require support services in order to improve quality of life.

PATIENT EXPECTATIONS, GOALS, AND VALUES

In order to provide comprehensive care, an understanding of the patient as a person is essential in guiding care and treatment decisions.

Perceptions and Expectation of Health

Discuss current and future health and lifestyle expectations with the patient. How does the patient perceive, for example, hypertension or heart failure as impacting daily-life activities? What are the patient's expectations for current medication treatments or surgical interventions? Answers to these questions help to evaluate the patient's understanding of a chronic illness and sets the stage to discuss the patient's health care goals.

Patient's Goals

Emphasize the need for shared decision making with the patient. By setting goals, the patient must verbalize lifestyle preferences in relation to illness management. For example, the elderly adult with multiple co-morbidities may want to focus on symptom management rather than survival (Pacala, 2012). The patient's goals and preferences can drastically impact the choices made in medical management of cardiovascular diseases. Ask the patient to list top lifestyle priorities when coping with a chronic illness and what the patient would like to accomplish in 3, 6, or 12 months.

Values for End-of-Life Care

Discuss end-of-life care considerations before the patient becomes too ill. This is a difficult topic to address in any setting for the patient, family, and health care team. Educate the patient on the progression of cardiac conditions, options for short-term interventions, and more invasive procedures such as life support. Highlight options that can maximize comfort, function, and quality of life. With the new cardiology patient, obtain living wills, advance directives, and preferences on palliative and hospice care when necessary (Dahlin, 2013). For additional information on palliative care, see the National Consensus Project (NCP) *Clinical Practice Guidelines for Quality Palliative Care* online at www.nationalconsensusproject.org.

CARDIOVASCULAR RISK STRATIFICATION AND DIAGNOSTIC REASONING

Obtaining a thorough and comprehensive history is essential for evaluating cardiovascular risk, differentiating common cardiovascular complaints, and determining certain cardiovascular diagnoses. Although confirmation of many cardiovascular disorders is based on physical examination findings and diagnostic testing, most are highly dependent upon the clinical evaluation obtained during the health history. For example, during an evaluation of angina symptoms, the pretest probability of coronary artery disease is determined by the evaluation of age, gender, and angina characteristics, with the patient categorized as very low, low, intermediate, or high risk based on these findings (Gibbons et al., 1997). The Framingham criteria for the diagnosis of heart failure is based on a constellation of historical and physical examination findings. In this criteria, important historical features include weight loss, paroxysmal nocturnal dyspnea, nocturnal cough, and dyspnea on exertion. The New York Heart Association (NYHA) functional classification for heart failure is dependent on the information obtained from the patient during the health history, as this classification is based upon the patient's perceived exertion at various levels of activity. The atherosclerosis cardiovascular disease pooled risk equation is utilized to evaluate the appropriateness of cholesterol-lowering medications. This risk equation accounts for several features from the patient history, including age, gender, ethnicity, history of diabetes mellitus, treatment for hypertension, and history of smoking, as well as blood pressure and cholesterol values. The cardiovascular history is an integral component of the evaluation, diagnosis, and management of cardiovascular risks and disorders.

CODING THE VISIT

After the patient's interview and exam, account for the encounter by coding the visit. Coding for inpatient services can be completed using the International Classification of Diseases (ICD). Continue to employ the ICD-9-Clinical Modification diagnosis and procedure codes for inpatient services until the mandated implementation of the International Classification of Diseases, 10th Revision, Clinical Modification/Procedure Coding System (ICD-10-CM/PCS) (CMS, 2010, p. 5).

In the outpatient setting, Current Procedural Terminology (CPT) coding requires the patient encounter to be assigned a level 1 through a level 5 office visit. A level 1 code is considered a problem-focused visit, while a level 5 code is a comprehensive, highly complex visit. The CPT codes differ for new patients and established patients (Table 2.5). To determine the proper coding level, the former Health Care Financing Administration's (now the Centers for Medicare & Medicaid Services) "Documentation Guidelines for Evaluation and Management Services" and the American Medical Association define the medical history, physical exam, and medical decision-making process as the three core elements of documentation necessary to justify billing (Moore, 2010).

TABLE 2.5 CPT Outpatient Codes

CPT Level	New Patient	Established Patient
Level 1	99201	99211
Level 2	99202	99212
Level 3	99203	99213
Level 4	99204	99214
Level 5	99205	99215

CPT, Current Procedural Terminology.

The comprehensive history is considered the highest level of history and requires the completion of three components: HPI; ROS; and past medical, family, and social history (PFSH). Of note, documentation of the chief complaint (CC) is necessary for all levels of CPT coding (CMS, 2010). To satisfy the requirements of the comprehensive cardiology history with an evaluation and management (E/M) code consistent with a level 4 (99204, 99214) or level 5 (99205, 99215) outpatient visit, specific elements of the HPI, ROS, and PFSH must be addressed (Table 2.6).

TABLE 2.6 General Guidelines for Levels of Evaluation and Management Services for Outpatient Patient History Requirements

Type of History	CC	HPI	ROS	Past, Family, and/or Social History
Problem focused	Required	*Brief* ■ One to three HPI elements	Not required	Not required
Expanded problem focused	Required	*Brief* ■ One to three HPI elements	*Pertinent problem* ■ System directly affected by problem in HPI	Not required
Detailed	Required	*Extended* ■ Four or more HPI elements (1995 documentation guidelines) ■ At least four HPI elements for present CC *or* status of at least three chronic or inactive conditions (1997 documentation guidelines)	*Extended* ■ System directly affected by problem in HPI plus two to nine additional systems	*Pertinent* ■ Review of history directly affected by problem in HPI ■ Must include at least one element from any of the three history areas
Comprehensive	Required	*Extended* ■ Four or more HPI elements (1995 documentation guidelines) ■ At least four HPI elements for present CC *or* status of at least three chronic or inactive conditions (1997 documentation guidelines)	*Complete* ■ System directly affected by problem in HPI plus at least 10 organ systems	*Complete* ■ Review of two or all three history areas, depending on E/M category

CC, chief complaint; E/M, evaluation and management; HPI, history of present illness; ROS, review of systems.
Adapted from CMS (2010).

The CMS describe two types of HPIs: a brief HPI and an extended HPI (2010). To qualify as a brief HPI, CMS states that one to three HPI elements must be documented. For example, a brief HPI may detail the onset, location, and duration of a symptom (2010). A brief HPI is consistent with CPT levels 2 and 3 or E/M codes 99212 and 99213 for established patients (Hill, 2011). According to the 1997 documentation guidelines, a comprehensive HPI includes reviewing and recording four or more elements that relate to the acute problem (location, quality, severity, duration, timing, context, modifying factors, and associated signs and symptoms) *or* the status of three or more chronic diseases (CMS, 2010). The extended HPI is consistent with CPT level 4 or E/M code 99214 for an established patient (Hill, 2011).

The ROS for a detailed history requires the documentation of between two and nine systems, while a comprehensive history includes a review of at least 10 systems. The PFSH, although an extremely broad section of a patient's medical history, requires only two elements to be addressed during an established-patient visit and three elements during a new-patient visit (Hill, 2011).

Coding of the patient history for an inpatient hospitalization is dependent on several factors, including whether the visit is an initial, follow-up, or discharge visit, and the complexity of the patient encounter (Table 2.7).

TABLE 2.7 General Guidelines for Levels of Evaluation and Management Services for Hospitalized, Inpatient Patient History Requirements

Encounter Type	Code	History Requirement
Initial inpatient	99221	Detailed or comprehensive
	99222	Comprehensive
	99223	Comprehensive
Subsequent inpatient	99231	Interval-problem focused
	99232	Interval-problem focused
	99233	Interval detailed
Hospital discharge	99238	Management services ≤ 30 minutes
	99239	Management services > 30 minutes
Same-day admission and discharge	99234	Detailed or comprehensive
	99235	Comprehensive
	99236	Comprehensive

PRIVILEGE AND CHALLENGES

The opportunity to work professionally with patients and families is a privilege. In order to ensure comprehensive care and a therapeutic relationship, in-depth and intimate questions are required throughout the patient interview. Proceed in a manner that respects the patient's dignity and privacy while acknowledging certain topics may generate feelings of discomfort. Maintain a sense of professionalism and confidence to not only enhance the patient–provider interview process but also allow the patient to feel a sense of normalcy during an otherwise stressful experience.

For full reference citations to this chapter, please see "Section References" in the back of the book, under the heading "Section I."

The Comprehensive Cardiovascular Physical Examination

KELLEY M. ANDERSON

Cardiovascular examination is a key component of the evaluation, diagnosis, and management of cardiovascular concerns and conditions. The physical examination strategy is informed by the comprehensive history, during which the clinician will assess relevant health history, changes in health status, recent procedures or operations, and family history that may influence the evaluation. Past physical examination findings, especially abnormal findings, will be reassessed to determine if there are conditions that require follow-up or reevaluation during the current encounter. Examination findings are an integral component to assess for a change in status of an individual over time, the progress of therapies, or advancement of disease.

Although the focus is on cardiovascular conditions, the examination is performed in the context of the entire patient. Cardiovascular conditions may have systemic manifestations, and disorders in other organs can result in a variety of cardiac conditions. Therefore, the cardiovascular examination is a comprehensive examination with a focus on the heart and the vasculature.

Examination findings vary in significance. Examinations may reveal normal findings and variations of normal that may have no substantial implications. Abnormalities, including both typical variations and noteworthy changes that require attention, are recorded and inform further evaluation. Patients who present with acute symptoms and significant clinical findings require an expedited evaluation, with a focused examination accompanied by rapid triage and management. Routine examinations entail a detailed and comprehensive approach.

This chapter provides a comprehensive cardiovascular examination. It is incumbent upon the cardiovascular clinician to be knowledgeable of all techniques and the circumstances that require their use. In clinical practice, a parsimonious and considerate examination must be tailored to the patient's specific needs, so the examiner does not perform all examination techniques for each patient. The comprehensive health history informs the physical examination. In general, a nonsignificant history and normal physical findings result in a complete, although less complex physical examination. When the history is notable for particular disorders, or when abnormalities are discovered on examination, further evaluation through additional techniques is necessary. For example, an examination of the extremities is performed in all cardiovascular assessments, although in a patient with bacterial endocarditis, the extremities are specifically assessed for Osler's nodes, Janeway lesions, and splinter hemorrhages in the nail beds.

Physical examination techniques relevant to the cardiovascular system must be paired with enhanced clinical judgment to aid the clinician in the interpretation of findings through advanced diagnostic reasoning. The examination is a significant component of the art of diagnostic decision making, informing the development of differential diagnosis, and appraising the evaluation of patients over the trajectory and natural history of cardiovascular disorders. However, in contemporary clinical cardiovascular practice, diagnostic testing has improved the ability to objectively diagnose and manage cardiovascular conditions. With these advances in technology and imaging, clinicians have become less reliant on physical examination findings for establishing diagnosis and guiding management. Rather, examination findings often direct which diagnostic test to order. Nonetheless, the examination continues to be an essential component of care practices, and one cannot provide care unless there is engagement in these physical processes. In several cardiovascular conditions, the examination findings are an essential component of the diagnosis. For example, the Framingham criteria for heart failure incorporates findings from the cardiac sounds, neck veins, pulmonary sounds, hepatic size, and peripheral edema as components of the diagnostic criteria. Similarly, the Duke criteria for bacterial endocarditis incorporate fever, vascular, and immunologic examination findings as a component of the minor diagnostic criteria. In other conditions, the examination findings are clearly linked to the diagnosis. For example, the diagnoses of obesity and hypertension are based on the body mass index (BMI) and blood pressure (BP) findings, respectively. These findings are necessary components to establish the diagnosis of these particular disorders and to monitor progress over time.

Before beginning the examination, prepare by washing hands and gathering any necessary equipment—warm stethoscope, ophthalmoscope, or ruler. Obtain a quiet setting and ensure proper lighting, as inspection of the movement of skin surfaces is best evaluated with tangential lighting. While performing the examination, ensure that you maintain patient modesty, exposing the minimum amount necessary to provide a thorough evaluation. However, a thorough examination requires direct contact. Examination through clothing or a gown demonstrates poor technique and can compromise the quality of the examination findings. Explain what you are planning to examine, and if appropriate, why you are doing so. The examination should be performed in a systematic manner with inspection, palpation, auscultation, and then percussion. Auscultation is a significant and necessary component of all cardiovascular examinations. Over time, the examiner will become more fluid in the multiple components of the examination and evaluate many complementary systems simultaneously while minimizing disruptions and energy for both the patient and provider.

THE GENERAL SURVEY

The general survey includes an evaluation of the overall patient appearance and the measure of the patient's vital statistics. During the general survey, observe the patient as a whole person—evaluate for anxiety, pain, agitation, discomfort, general mood, and overall affect. Body habitus can be visualized for general weight, overweight, obesity, dress, hygiene, poor nutrition, cachexia, and stature. Cardiac cachexia is a finding in some end-stage cardiovascular conditions, including heart failure. Tall stature with arachnodactyly is observed in individuals with Marfan syndrome.

Overall cognitive and mental status is assessed by evaluating the patient's appropriateness in answering questions, affect, grooming, attire in relationship to the weather, and level of consciousness. Evaluate for indicators of distress including anxiety, pain, dyspnea, and skin-color changes such as pallor or cyanosis. The *Levine sign* is the classic hand movement of myocardial ischemia of a clenched fist over the substernal area, demonstrating constriction.

Vital Signs

Prior to obtaining vital signs, the patient should be seated with feet uncrossed on the floor and allowed to rest for at least 5 minutes. Basic vital signs include the measurement of pulse, BP, respirations, and temperature. Evaluate the actual measurement number, the quality, and associated findings, especially if there is an abnormality. For example, the respiratory rate is measured in breaths per minute and can be characterized as tachypneic, eupneic, or bradypneic. The quality of the respirations should be evaluated—deep, normal, or shallow. Any associated findings such as irregular, agonal, easy, or labored breathing should also be noted. Through the evaluation of basic vital signs, the clinician can rapidly identify acute conditions of febrile illness, hypertensive urgency, arrhythmia, or chronic conditions.

Pulse

A normal pulse is between 60 and 90 beats per minute. However, this range is a generalization, and a true normal rate is dependent on the individual patient, as a low rate may be present in a well-conditioned athlete. The pulse is best palpated with the pads of the second and third fingers placed on arteries close to the surface and over bony structures. Pulses are palpable in the carotid, brachial, radial, femoral, dorsalis pedis, and posterior tibialis arterial locations. In addition to the rate, evaluate the rhythm, symmetry, strength, and waveform. Normally the rhythm is regular, and there is symmetry between the right and left sides of the body. Strength or amplitude is graded on a 0 to 4 scale, with 0 indicating a nonpalpable pulse; 1 indicating a diminished, barely palpable pulse; 2 indicating an expected pulse; 3 indicating a full, increased pulse; and 4 indicating a bounding pulse. The general waveform of the pulse is smooth, round, and dome shaped.

Simultaneously, compare the peripheral pulsation with auscultation, as these findings indirectly inform the examiner about several factors: the ability of the aorta and large arteries to distend, the blood viscosity, the rate of cardiac emptying, the cardiac rhythm, and the peripheral arteriolar resistance. Certain disturbances prevent adequate filling of the ventricles, resulting in smaller stroke volume and low impulse that may not be palpable or may be difficult to palpate. By evaluating the volume of the pulsation, an assessment of the stroke volume is obtained. In hypovolemia a weak, thready pulse is noted. While auscultating the lungs and palpating the pulse concurrently, determine if there is pulse variation with respirations. Variability with deep breathing—tachycardia on inspiration with bradycardia on expiration—may be consistent with a sinus arrhythmia, which is generally a normal finding if the difference in the pulse during the respiratory cycle is less than 9 beats per minute.

Blood Pressure

Arterial BP is the general force of blood flow against the wall of the arteries as the ventricles contract and relax, resulting in the two components of systolic and diastolic blood pressure. Systolic blood pressure (SBP), which reflects cardiac output and blood volume, measures the force of blood flow against arterial walls when the ventricles contract. Diastolic blood pressure (DBP), which measures the filling and relaxed state of the ventricles, is primarily an indication of peripheral vascular resistance. BP can be measured directly with an arterial line or indirectly using a mercury-based manometer, known as a sphygmomanometer. Although in contemporary practice clinicians use aneroid manometers, electronic devices, and digital-mechanical manometers instead of mercury, the measurement remains, by convention, in millimeters of mercury or mmHg.

The normal BP range is between 100/60 and 140/90 mmHg, and the measurements should be equal bilaterally. The normal values for ambulatory BP are less, with a normal daytime level of less than 135/85 mmHg, a nighttime level of less than 120/70 mmHg, and a 24-hour average of 130/80 (Pickering et al., 2005). BP arm differences greater than 20 mmHg between arms may suggest abdominal aortic aneurysm, coarctation of the aorta, subclavian steal syndrome, or other vascular disorders.

To measure BP, ensure that the patient is in a sitting position, arms are at the sides at heart level, and both feet are on the floor with legs uncrossed. Allow the patient to rest for a minimum of 5 minutes. Avoid obtaining BP in a postmastectomy or arteriovenous fistula arm, as possible lymphedema can occur in the former, and restricted blood flow may result in thrombus formation in the latter. There are several circumstances that can interfere with an accurate BP measurement. An arm that is too high will result in an artificially lowered BP, and an arm that is too low artificially elevates BP. Smoking, caffeine ingestion, and medications with sympathomimetic activity will raise BP.

Cardiac arrhythmias, particularly bradyarrhythmias and tachyarrhythmias, as well as irregular impulses and extremes of size, such as obesity, can pose a challenge in obtaining accurate BP and can result in altered measurements. A cuff size that is too large for the circumference of the patient's arm will artificially reduce BP. In contrast, a cuff that is too small will artificially elevate BP. The bladder width and length should be 40% and 80% of the circumference of the limb, respectively (Levine, 2010). Table 3.1 provides general guidelines of arm circumference and corresponding cuff sizes.

In 1905, Nikolai Korotkoff detailed his findings for the measurement of arterial BP in his dissertation titled, "Experiments for Determining the Strength of Arterial Collaterals" (Shevchenko & Tsitlik, 1996). This ausculatory method of obtaining BP

TABLE 3.1 Arm Size and Corresponding Blood Pressure Cuff Size

Arm Size (cm)	Cuff Category	Cuff Size (cm)
22–26	Small adult	12 × 22
27–34	Adult	16 × 30
35–44	Large adult	16 × 36
45–52	Adult thigh	16 × 42

Source: Pickering et al. (2005).

measurement has remained relatively unchanged since the dissemination of his finding, and the sounds generated from obtaining the BP are attributed to his name, Korotkoff sounds.

When auscultating BP, use the bell of the stethoscope, as it is more effective than the diaphragm for hearing the low-pitched sounds of Korotkoff. Korotkoff sounds are classified into five phases:

- Phase I—During this initial stage, the clinician begins to hear clear tapping sounds corresponding to a palpable pulse. These sounds indicate systolic pressure.
- Ausculatory Gap—A pause can occur between Phase I and II that can be delayed for up to 40 mmHg. This gap occurs most often in situations with reduced velocity of arterial flow including venous distention, hypertension, and severe aortic stenosis (AS) (Pickering et al., 2005).
- Phase II—During this time, the sounds become softer and longer and have no clinical significance.
- Phase III—The sounds now become crisper and louder and, again, have no clinical significance.
- Phase IV—In this phase the sounds become muffled and softer.
- Phase V—During this final phase, the sounds disappear completely. This absence of sound corresponds with diastolic pressure. However, the Phase V sound is not always the last audible sound, especially in hyperkinetic states such as hyperthyroidism, exercise, pregnancy, and aortic insufficiency. In these situations, there may be a Phase VI, which is the true diastolic pressure (Levine, 2010; Pickering et al., 2005).

In clinical practice, BP is primarily evaluated for elevations, with circumscribed values corresponding to classifications of hypertension. Prehypertension is defined as an SBP of 120 to 139 mmHg or DBP of 80 to 90 mmHg; Stage 1 hypertension is defined as an SBP of 140 to 159 mmHg or DBP of 90 to 99 mmHg; Stage 2 hypertension is defined as an SBP that is equal to or greater than 160 mmHg or DBP equal to or greater than 100 mmHg. In general, BP increases with age. Individuals older than 50 years may develop increased SBP, while the DBP may decrease (Pickering et al., 2005). These physiologic changes reflect arterial stiffening, and current hypertension guidelines allow more lenient SBP goals, equal to or less than 150 mmHg for those aged 60 years or older and those aged 80 years or older, from the Eighth Joint National Committee and the American Society of Hypertension/International Society of Hypertension, respectively (James et al., 2014; Weber et al., 2013).

During hypotension and shock states, the BP may be low, with values of less than 90/60 mmHg associated with decreased blood flow, oxygen supply, and cerebral and peripheral perfusion. For BP values that are unobtainable in the normal manner, due to reduced peripheral perfusion, an SBP may be obtained with palpation or Doppler. This SBP is reported as the systolic value over *p* for palpation or *d* for Doppler; for example, 80/*p* or 80/*d*. Alternatively, measurements can be obtained from the thigh or forearm, due to inaccessibility of the upper extremities. Although these locations are less desirable due to the lack of standard normal values, they can be useful in monitoring BP trends over time. In the acute care setting, an invasive arterial line provides continuous arterial BP measurements.

Orthostatic or Postural Vital Signs

Orthostatic is defined as related to, or caused by, an upright posture. A normal physiologic response occurs upon rising from a lying to standing position, when 300 to 800 mL of blood is gravitationally redistributed to the lower extremities and splanchnic vasculature, reducing cardiac preload (Freeman et al., 2011). Muscle contraction compresses veins, resulting in an autonomic response of the baroreceptors in the aorta and carotids. These baroreceptors sense BP change and prompt the sympathetic nervous system to stabilize BP by increasing vascular tone, heart rate (HR), and cardiac contractility. Ordinarily, there is a transient reduction of equal to or less than 10 mmHg SBP, equal to or less than 5 mmHg DBP, or an increase of 5 to 20 beats per minute in HR with this position change. Positive orthostatic findings are consistent with a sustained reduction of equal to or greater than 20 mmHg SBP, equal to or greater than 10 mmHg DBP, or an increase equal to or greater than 30 beats per minute in HR within 3 minutes of standing, with or without symptoms (Freeman et al., 2011).

Symptoms of orthostatic hypotension are generally consistent with presyncopal or syncopal findings associated with cerebral hypoperfusion, including lightheadedness, dizziness, weakness, blurring of vision, and loss of consciousness. In general, patients are more symptomatic with more relevant findings of changes in HR or BP parameters. Clinically relevant causes for orthostasis may include hypovolemia, response to medications, autonomic nervous system dysfunction, acute blood loss, and inadequate vasoconstriction mechanism. However, the etiology may be difficult to determine at times. Changes with aging can contribute to the increased incidence of orthostasis due to reductions in vasoconstrictor response, inefficiency of the skeletal muscle pump, loss of cardiac and vascular compliance, blood volume, and changes in baroreflex function (Freeman et al., 2011).

To obtain orthostatic vital signs, measure HR and BP after the patient is supine for 5 to 10 minutes. As an intermediary step, measurements in the sitting position may be performed, serving as a screening and safety evaluation in some patients. If significant orthostasis is noted, it may be unnecessary for the patient to stand. However, the absence of orthostasis in the seated position does not rule out orthostatic hypotension. After the patient stands, the measurements are repeated, and the patient is monitored for symptoms. If after several minutes no orthostasis is noted on the first standing evaluation or if the patient becomes symptomatic, the provider measures HR and BP again in the standing position. If this usual maneuver does not illicit symptoms or vital sign changes, the provider may request that the patient demonstrate the movement that causes symptoms and obtain measurements with these position changes.

Pulse Pressure

Pulse pressure is an indirect measurement of cardiac output and is an indication of stroke volume, vascular resistance, and the velocity of ejected blood. Pulse pressure is measured by subtracting the difference between the systolic and diastolic blood pressures, and is normally between 30 and 40 mmHg. Table 3.2 describes conditions that are associated with narrow and wide pulse pressures.

TABLE 3.2 Conditions Associated With Altered Pulse Pressure

Wide >40 mmHg	Narrow <30 mmHg
Ischemic heart disease	Tachycardia
Aortic regurgitation	Severe aortic stenosis
Patent ductus arteriosus	Mitral stenosis
Aortic coarctation	Mitral regurgitation
Arteriovenous fistula	Peripheral vasoconstriction
Thyrotoxicosis	Constrictive pericarditis
Anemia	Pericardial effusion
Abdominal aortic aneurysm	Reduced ejection velocity
Ventricular hypertrophy	Heart failure
Sinus bradycardia	Shock
Complete heart block	Hypovolemia
Anxiety	
Fever	
Exercise	
Aging	
Hypertension	

Paradoxical BP

As with HR, BP changes with physiologic changes in the thorax associated with respirations. SBP is lower with inspiration, higher with expiration. The reduction of BP with inspiration is due to increased blood flow to the right heart, increased right ventricular output, and pulmonary venous capacity with reduced left ventricular stroke volume. The changes normally amount to less than 10 mmHg between the SBP on inspiration and expiration. A 10 mmHg or greater SBP reduction with respirations between inspiration and expiration is a paradox and can be noted in cardiac tamponade, constrictive pericarditis, pulmonary embolism, cardiogenic shock, chronic obstructive pulmonary disease (COPD), and restrictive cardiomyopathy.

Respirations

Respirations are evaluated in breaths per minute, with a normal rate between 12 and 20 breaths in adults. A respiratory rate greater than 20 breaths per minute is considered tachypneic, and a rate less than 12 breaths per minute is considered bradypneic. The quality of respiration is normally even, regular, and unlabored. The majority of cardiac conditions that contain a respiratory component as a part of the clinical syndrome have respiratory manifestations in rate and quality. There are several respiratory patterns that are primarily associated with metabolic and neurologic conditions. Biot's respirations occur in an irregular pattern with varying depth and periods of apnea. Cheyne-Stokes respirations have a crescendo and decrescendo pattern, with deep breathing followed by apnea intervals in an alternating pattern. Cheyne-Stokes respirations may be noted in severe heart failure. Kussmaul respirations are deep, rapid, and require an increased respiratory effort that is evidenced by the use of accessory muscles, pursed lips, and upright and forward leaning positions. Severe distress with Kussmaul pattern is accompanied by retraction of the intercostal spaces (ICSs).

Temperature

The internal thermometer is maintained by the hypothalamus, set at 98.6°F or 37°C, with a diurnal variation slightly lower in the morning and higher in the afternoon. The normal temperature varies somewhat by device. Core temperatures measured in the urinary bladder, pulmonary artery, rectum, or tympanic membrane are somewhat higher than oral temperatures. An increase in temperature is a normal physiologic reaction to infection and many illnesses and stress states, including myocardial infarction. Fever is defined as a temperature greater than 100.4° to 101.5°F or 38° to 38.5°C. Infectious cardiovascular conditions associated with fever are bacteremia, endocarditis, rheumatic fever, scarlet fever, and myocarditis. In adults, fever with temperature above 103°F or 39.4°C may be dangerous and indicate a serious illness. The older adult may be less likely to manifest with a febrile presentation than the younger individual, and infection may be present without the temperature exceeding the usual values that define fever.

Oxygen Saturation

Oxygen saturation (SaO_2) with a pulse oximeter is a noninvasive measure of red blood cell oxygen-carrying capacity and an indirect measurement of gas exchange. The SaO_2 value, which represents the relative amount of dissolved oxygen, is measured as the percentage of hemoglobin-binding sites bound with oxygen. A normal value is between 95% and 100%. There is a precipitous fall in arterial oxygen content, measured as the partial pressure of oxygen (PaO_2) with lower saturation levels, as the affinity of oxygen for hemoglobin is not linear. Table 3.3 demonstrates this relationship. The normal PaO_2 is between 75% and 100%. Conditions that will falsely decrease SaO_2 are severe anemia, poor perfusion, vasoconstriction, hypotension, reduced blood flow, hypothermia, and Raynaud's syndrome. Disorders that inaccurately elevate SaO_2 are severe dehydration, carbon monoxide poisoning, methemoglobinemia, and tachypnea.

TABLE 3.3 Comparison of PaO_2 and SaO_2

Partial Pressure of Oxygen (PaO_2) (mmHg)	Oxygen Saturation (SaO_2) (%)
100	97.5
60	90
40	75

Height, Weight, BMI, and Waist Circumference

The assessment of body size and weight is important in the diagnosis and management of cardiovascular conditions. Obtain the weight of the patient when in a gown or light clothes, preferably early in the morning after voiding and before eating or drinking. Height is measured without shoes. Weight changes are particularly important for the management of fluid status in individuals with heart failure, especially patients on diuretic therapy. Primary reasons to measure weight, BMI, and waist circumference are the diagnosis of overweight and obesity and the monitoring of lifestyle interventions. Excess weight and body size are the main reasons why these measures are evaluated; however, individuals with end-stage cardiovascular disease may present with weight loss in association with cardiac cachexia. Measuring the weight of these patients is important to evaluate for untoward weight reduction.

BMI is the relative body size to height, and is generally a reliable indicator for the measurement of body fat. Other methods to measure body fat include caliper skinfold thickness measurements, underwater weighing, bioelectrical impedance, dual-energy x-ray absorptiometry, and isotope dilution (Garrow & Webster, 1985; Mei et al., 2002). These methods are expensive and more difficult to obtain. BMI is a calculated equation. The metric system formula is defined by weight (kg)/ [height (m)]^2. Height is commonly measured in centimeters divided by 100 to obtain height in meters. The conventional system formula is calculated as weight (lb)/[height (in.)]^2 ×703, 703 being a conversion factor. A patient with a BMI less than 18.5 is underweight; between 18.5 and 24.9 is healthy; between 25 and 29.9 is overweight; and greater than 30 is obese. Muscle mass in athletic individuals may cause an overestimation of BMI. The loss of muscle mass in individuals such as older adults can cause an underestimation of BMI. At the same BMI, women have more body fat than men, and older individuals have more body fat than younger patients.

Waist circumference is a measure of central abdominal adiposity, a risk factor for diabetes, metabolic syndrome, and cardiovascular disorders. Risk is associated with a waist size greater than 35 inches for women or greater than 40 inches for men. Measure the waist circumference in the standing position with a measuring tape around the waist above the hipbones, and obtain the measurement after exhalation.

CARDIOVASCULAR ASSESSMENT

Carotid Artery

The best sequence to evaluate the carotid arteries is to begin with inspection, carotid auscultation, and then palpation. Carotid upstroke refers to the normal full and prompt inflow of blood into the carotid arteries from the left ventricle. Evaluate the quantity and timing of the carotid upstroke while simultaneously auscultating the apical impulse on the precordium. The pulsations should be strong with no delay. A delayed pulsation is referred to as tardus, and a diminished pulse is called parvus. The medical term *pulsus tardus et parvus* is a sign of reduced cardiac output and describes a pulse that is delayed and weak, with a small amplitude that rises slowly. Reduced vigor of the pulsation may indicate AS, significant left ventricular impairment, or atherosclerosis. Corrigan's or water-hammer pulse is evidenced by a jerky pattern with a large amplitude that rises rapidly, falls abruptly, and is classically associated with aortic regurgitation (AR), severe mitral stenosis (MS), patent ductus arteriosus, hypertrophic cardiomyopathy, essential hypertension, thyrotoxicosis, and anemia (Chizner, 2002). *Pulsus bisferiens* (bifid) is a double systolic peaked pulse, associated with hypertrophic cardiomyopathy or combined AS and regurgitation. Diminished amplitude of the carotid pulsation is often associated with carotid stenosis related to atherosclerosis.

Carotid auscultation provides insight into aortic valve and outflow-tract disorders that may manifest in findings in the carotid arteries. Auscultation of the carotid arteries prior to palpation allows for the evaluation of carotid bruits and signs of obstruction, in which case the clinician may consider forgoing or exercising caution during carotid palpation. To differentiate bruits with radiating aortic murmurs, murmurs will be audible in both carotids and increase in intensity as you listen toward the chest. When auscultating the carotid arteries, the patient should be instructed to hold the breath momentarily so that the clinician may clearly differentiate the vascular sounds, rather than air movement with respirations. In relationship to the cardiac cycle, the timing of the palpation of the carotid impulse should occur simultaneously with S_1.

Palpate carotid arteries, one at a time, at the lower third of the neck to avoid the carotid sinuses and to prevent bradycardia, arrhythmia, or diminished cerebral blood flow. Locate the arteries by placing the second and third fingers alongside the thyroid cartilage, also known as the Adam's apple, and sliding the fingers along the side of the trachea. There is a groove between the trachea and the surrounding soft tissue, and the carotid pulsation is palpable here. Although the pulsation is generally easy to palpate, the clinician may need to increase the firmness of pressure for patients with significant subcutaneous neck fat.

Jugular Venous Distention or Pressure

The internal jugular (IJ) vein communicates linearly with the right atrium and can function as an indirect manometer. Distention of the jugular vein indicates an elevation of central venous pressure, a marker of increased intravascular volume and cardiac function. Jugular venous distention (JVD) is a sign of heart failure, with a role in both heart failure diagnosis and evaluation of management. The assessment of the distention of the IJ vein provides insight into the activities of the right heart that is transmitted back through the jugular veins as a pulse with three peaks (a wave, c wave, v wave) and two descending slopes (x slope, y slope). These peaks and slopes are notable in sinus rhythm, although altered or absent with tricuspid regurgitation (TR), atrial fibrillation, cardiac tamponade, and constrictive pericarditis. In cardiac tamponade, the y descent is diminished or absent due to the reduction of diastolic filling of the ventricles, although the JVD remains elevated (Khandaker et al., 2010). The a, c, and v waves are subtle and more consistent with a flicker rather than a pulsation. The jugular venous pulse contour patterns are as follows (Figure 3.1):

■ a wave = right atrial systole, increased right atrial pressure due to retrograde blood flow into the superior vena cava and jugular veins; upon simultaneous auscultation of the heart, the a wave will occur just before or synchronous with S_1, and follow the P wave on the ECG as a sharp rise followed by rapid descent; this finding is absent in atrial fibrillation; an elevated a wave will occur with increased right ventricular diastolic pressure—pulmonary hypertension, pulmonary emboli, left ventricular failure, tricuspid stenosis

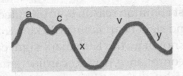

FIGURE 3.1 The jugular venous pressure waveform.
Source: Wikimedia Commons (2011).

- x descent = right atrial diastole, emptying and relaxation; then the fall of the right atrial pressure during early right ventricular systole; the most prominent motion of the normal jugular venous pulsation; begins during systole and ends just before S_2
- c wave = carotid arterial impulse; tricuspid valve closure, during x descent
- v wave = atrial filling, ventricular systole; tricuspid valve closed; increase in right atrial pressure; upon simultaneous auscultation of the heart, this wave will occur immediately after the arterial pulse; an elevated v wave will occur in TR or increased venous volume; second major positive wave; begins in late systole and ends with early diastole
- y descent = tricuspid valve opens and reduced right atrial volume; a slow y descent occurs in tricuspid stenosis, pericardial disease, or cardiac tamponade with impaired atrial emptying; a rapid y descent occurs with TR or increased venous volume; begins and ends during diastole

The IJ vein lies deep in the skin and soft tissue and is lateral to the carotid artery. The transmitted venous impulse in the IJ is weak compared with the adjacent pulsating carotid artery and has a single upstroke synchronized to the radial arterial pulsation. Ordinarily, the IJ is not visible and the clinician cannot feel a pulsation, whereas the adjacent carotid pulsation is palpable. When attempting to palpate the IJ, do not apply excessive pressure to avoid obliterating the upstroke of the IJ. The external jugular (EJ) vein is usually directly visible across the sternocleidomastoid muscle in an oblique manner. A Valsalva maneuver may cause distention of the EJ. However, the EJ is not a reliable indicator of intravascular volume, due to the valves in the EJ that prevent retrograde blood flow and the circuitous route of the EJ from the right atrium to the central venous system.

To evaluate jugular venous pressure (JVP), place the patient in a supine position with the head of the bed elevated to 45 degrees, which is the conventional position for this measurement. A flat, supine position raises the height of the IJ, whereas a sitting position lowers the height. The JVP remains the same despite the patient's position, but the vein's relationship to other structures differs according to the patient's position. Stand to the right side of the patient and use tangential light to identify the highest level of undulation of the IJ vein. Turn the head to the left, evaluate the IJ area, and search for the top of the pressure wave. Position a card or other straight rigid object parallel to the floor (horizontal) and level with the peak of the jugular vein undulation. Place a centimeter ruler perpendicular to the floor (vertical) with the zero edge touching the sternal angle, the Angle of Louis. The Angle of Louis is the junction between the manubrium and the sternum—the manubriosternal junction—usually 4 to 5 cm below the suprasternal notch. Note the number of centimeters at the intersection between the card and the ruler. The estimated JVP is the number of centimeters above the sternal angle *plus* 4 to 5 cm—the distance from the sternal angle to the right atrium. Traditionally, this value is recorded as cm H_2O. Values higher than 9 to 10 cm H_2O are considered elevated and may reflect pericardial disorders, tricuspid valve stenosis, superior vena cava obstruction, or right ventricular stiffness, although the most common reason is an elevated venous pressure associated with volume overload and right heart failure (Bickley & Szilagyi, 2008). An increased JVP with inspiration, known as the Kussmaul sign, can be an indication of decreased right ventricular compliance due to cardiac tamponade, right-sided heart failure, right ventricular infarct, or constrictive pericarditis (Khandaker et al., 2010).

Hepatojugular Reflux/Abdominojugular Reflux

Apply hepatic pressure to the abdomen in the right upper quadrant while simultaneously evaluating the IJ vein. Normally, the venous column will elevate briefly, although it will return to normal due to a compliant right ventricle. The column will remain elevated with continuous abdominal pressure due to a poorly compliant right ventricle or obstruction to right ventricular filling. A positive hepatojugular reflux occurs when a rise of 3 cm or more in the IJ is apparent and sustained with this maneuver. The reflux occurs as pooled blood in the liver fills the IJ in a retrograde manner.

Precordium

Examine the precordium by inspection first, then by palpation, percussion, and auscultation. Inspection is primarily used to evaluate for abnormal physical features or movement in the precordial area. Place the patient in a supine position and use tangential lighting to improve visualization of chest wall movements. Obesity and breast tissue may limit the evaluation. Inspect the chest wall for physical deformities, including pectus excavatum and findings associated with mediastinal radiation. Left ventricular aneurysms may result in paradoxical movements of the precordium.

Inward movements of the chest wall are called retractions and outward movements are called pulsations. The point of maximal impulse (PMI), at the apical area, is normally visualized as a rapid upstroke at the 5th ICS at the midclavicular line or just medial. Displacement of the apical impulse lateral to the midclavicular line or below the 5th ICS by more than one ICS is abnormal and can be indicative of pathology. Abnormalities associated with a displaced PMI include left ventricular enlargement due to mitral insufficiency or left ventricular failure. A PMI located at the 2nd right ICS may be consistent with an aortic aneurysm, and pulsations in the 2nd ICS may be associated with increased filling pressure or pulmonary artery blood flow.

Palpate the precordium systematically in five areas: at the apex, left sternal border, base, right sternal border, and epigastrium or axillae. The fingertips are best to palpate localized pulsations; the base of the fingertips for thrills; and the palm for the PMI, heaves, or lifts. Place the palm of the right hand, using the base of the hand and fingertips, directly under the left breast, placing the index finger against the inferior breast. Evaluate the location and width of the apical impulse. The impulse is typically 1 cm in diameter, or the size of a dime. Palpation is usually completed in the supine position, although it may be completed with the patient sitting or leaning forward. A vigorous or accentuated impulse may be described as a heave or thrust. This accentuated impulse may be the result of left ventricular hypertrophy, exertion, increased sympathetic stimulation, or thyrotoxicosis.

A thrill, or palpable murmur, is a fine, palpable vibratory sensation produced by turbulent blood flow, often due to blood moving rapidly through a narrow space into a larger area (Levinson, Meehan, Schwartz, & Griffith, 1956). Generally thrills are palpated at the base in the right or left ICS and their location depends upon the corresponding structural heart condition. Thrills are not present with an innocent murmur and are generally associated with valvular abnormalities, although they can be associated with septal defects. A thrill at the lower left sternal border may be consistent with tricuspid valve abnormality, at the apex with mitral regurgitation (MR), at the 2nd left ICS with pulmonary valve abnormality, at the 4th left ICS with ventricular septal defect, and at the 2nd left and right ICS with aortic valve abnormality. Upon auscultation, grades IV to VI heart murmurs are associated with thrills, although thrills are generally uncommon findings.

In addition to being visualized, the PMI can be palpated. The PMI represents ventricular systole, when the apex of the left ventricle rotates forward to the chest wall, normally palpated after the first heart sound. A diastolic pulsation is unusual and may indicate impaired ventricular filling. There is generally no pulsation in the right ventricular area or epigastrium, and a pulsation in these areas may indicate right ventricular enlargement. If the PMI is nonpalpable, the patient can be moved to the sitting, forward leaning, or left-lateral decubitus position and reevaluated. Although the location is dependent on the body habitus of the patient, the usual location to palpate the PMI is the 5th ICS, 7 to 9 cm left of the middle of the sternum, which is approximately medial to the midclavicular line. In a slender person, the heart may be more vertical and central, whereas a stocky, larger person, or a pregnant woman, may have a heart that is more horizontal and to the left.

The apical impulse should produce a tapping sensation; and the examiner will note the location, size, and amplitude. Evaluate for findings suggestive of a shift in position of the impulse, an enlarged impulse, or an accentuated impulse. A shift to the left may suggest an enlarged myocardium consistent with cardiomyopathy or heart failure, and PMIs near the axilla indicate significant enlargement. A shift to the right may indicate a left pneumothorax. An enlarged impulse may be suggestive of left ventricular hypertrophy, AS, or outflow tract obstruction. Loss of a palpable apical pulse may indicate fluid or air in the precordium or displacement of the impulse. Obesity or COPD may limit the ability to locate a defined pulsation. Accentuated or prolonged impulses may occur in ventricular hypertrophy or with ventricular hypercontractility due to increased stroke volume, compensated MR, or aortic insufficiency.

When palpating the chest wall, determine if the patient is experiencing any chest discomfort with the assessment. Costochondritis is consistent with reproducible pain with palpation due to inflammation of a costochondral junction of ribs or chondrosternal joints of the anterior chest wall. Costochondritis is a common syndrome and pain is usually present at multiple sites on the chest wall, usually at the 2nd through 5th joints. In addition to palpation, movement of the arm on the affected side will often increase the pain. Bosner et al. (2010) completed a study of 1,212 patients with chest pain and evaluated for predictive variables to diagnose chest wall pain. Four clinical predictors demonstrated reliability to exclude or include the diagnosis of chest wall pain; for patients with two or more criteria, the positive predictive value for the diagnosis of chest wall pain was 77% (Bosner et al., 2010).

Chest wall pain criteria (one point for each of the four criteria)

- Localized muscle tension
- Stinging pain
- Pain reproducible by palpation
- Absence of cough

Interpretation: Likelihood of chest wall pain

- Score 0–1 = 82% negative predictive value
- Score 2–4 = 77% positive predictive value (Bosner et al., 2010)

Tietze's syndrome is an uncommon disorder with a presentation similar to that of costochondritis. This syndrome generally occurs in adults younger than age 40, and presents with focal pain, visible swelling, and tenderness. The swelling and tenderness are usually located at the 2nd or 3rd costochondrial spaces, often affecting a single rib area. Tietze's syndrome is generally a manifestation of an underlying malignancy, rheumatologic process, or infectious disease (Proulx & Zryd, 2009).

Percussion of the precordium for heart size is a somewhat limited examination due to the rib structures and is not commonly conducted in clinical practice, as the heart size estimation by percussion is less accurate than diagnostic tests, including chest radiograph. Percussion of a change from a resonant to a dull note marks the cardiac border. This examination technique may be useful in the diagnosis of dextrocardia, although this is a rare condition.

Cardiac Auscultation

The auscultation of the heart is an essential component of the cardiac examination, providing indispensible information about anatomic, physiologic, and potentially pathologic conditions. Cardiac sounds are generated from mechanical events and are of low frequency, less than 1,000 hertz, with the human ear most sensitive between 1,000 and 5,000 hertz (Levine, 2010). The diaphragm is most suitable to evaluate high-pitched sounds and to filter sounds of lower frequency. The diaphragm should be pressed firmly to the chest wall and is most useful to auscultate S_1, S_2, high-frequency murmurs, and lung sounds. The bell enhances low-pitched sounds and should be held lightly to the chest. The bell is most useful to evaluate diastolic filling sounds and low-frequency murmurs, including mitral or tricuspid stenosis. To hone auscultation skills, consider the general anatomic location of cardiac structures (Table 3.4) and link findings with the physiology of the mechanical events occurring in the heart. In addition, compare auscultation findings with more experienced clinicians and the results from diagnostic imaging studies, including an echocardiogram or cardiac catheterization, to confirm findings.

The patient will breathe normally, unless instructed otherwise, as certain respiratory maneuvers augment specific auscultatory findings. Sounds may differ from person to person, so evaluate the sounds within each individual. Listen for the

TABLE 3.4 General Anatomic Location of Cardiac Structures

Left ventricle	5th ICS MCL, or slightly medial to MCL	Primarily positioned posteriorly, evaluate on anterior chest at the cardiac apex
Right ventricle	4th–5th ICS at LSB	Under the sternum
Right atrium	4th–5th ICS at RSB	Right, lateral of sternal border
Ventricular outflow tracts	3rd left ICS	Erb's point
Pulmonary artery	2nd left ICS	
Ascending aorta	2nd right ICS	

ICS, intercostal space; LSB, left sternal border; MCL, midclavicular line; RSB, right sternal border.

rate, rhythm, normal heart sounds S_1 and S_2, splitting, extra systolic sounds, extra diastolic sounds, clicks, murmurs, pericardial friction rubs, and gallops. Differentiate the various sounds by the sound quality, the timing within the cardiac cycle, and the location of the placement of the stethoscope. Normal findings include a HR of 60 to 90 beats per minute that is regular with clear S_1 and S_2 and no murmurs, rubs, or gallops present.

A systematic approach is recommended with the examiner inching the stethoscope along the chest wall. By convention, a suggested sequence is to begin at the aortic area (Figure 3.2), followed by the pulmonic, tricuspid, and mitral areas (Table 3.5). Add additional areas if abnormalities are found or suspected by following the direction of sounds in small increments along the precordium, noticing the intensity of sounds and radiation. An alternative sequence is to auscultate in the direction of blood flow, beginning laterally in the mitral area at the cardiac apex and focusing on the first heart sound, then moving upward and toward the right.

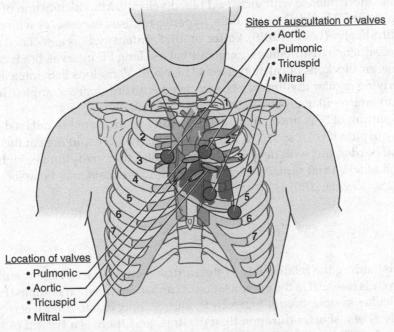

Sites of auscultation of valves
• Aortic
• Pulmonic
• Tricuspid
• Mitral

Location of valves
• Pulmonic
• Aortic
• Tricuspid
• Mitral

FIGURE 3.2 Cardiac auscultation locations. See color insert.

TABLE 3.5 Conventional Auscultation Sequence

Area	Intercostal Space	Location
Aortic	2nd right ICS	Right sternal border
Pulmonic	2nd left ICS	Left sternal border
Second pulmonic	3rd left ICS	Left sternal border, Erb's point
Tricuspid	4th left ICS	Left sternal border
Mitral (Apical)	5th left ICS	Midclavicular line

ICS, intercostal space.

Although examination techniques are reviewed separately, patients can have more than one condition, complicating the interpretation of examination findings and requiring additional skill and mastery of auscultation. In addition, coexisting diseases, including COPD, can increase the difficulty of the auscultation evaluation due to air trapping and lung hyperinflation that rotates the heart away from the chest wall into a posterior–inferior cardiac rotation. Pulmonary diseases also increase the likelihood of additional pulmonary sounds that may interfere with the ability to appreciate cardiac sounds. To improve auscultation in patients with pulmonary disease, position the patient to lean forward, instruct the individual to exhale fully, and then hold the breath while the clinician listens to the heart.

S_1 is the "lub" and indicates the beginning of systole. If S_1 is difficult to distinguish, especially with significant tachycardia, ask the patient to hold the breath on expiration and listen for S_1 while palpating the carotid pulse, which will coincide or immediately follow S_1. The S_1 sound is generated from the movement of blood against the closure of the atrioventricular valves, the mitral and tricuspid valves. S_1 is loudest at the apex, and S_2 is best heard at the base and at Erb's point. At the apex, S_1 is clearer and the duration is longer than S_2; the relative intensity of the sounds compared to one another is helpful to distinguish between them. S_1 may become more intense with increased blood velocity, MS, calcification of the mitral valve, short PR interval, tachycardia, hyperthyroidism, exercise, or with a mechanical mitral valve (Levine, 2010). Softer, or lower-intensity, S_1 is associated with chest wall conduction disturbances, immobile valves, long PR interval, bradycardia, beta adrenergic blockers, or calcium channel blockers. Variations in S_1 intensity with an underlying regular rhythm may be associated with 3rd-degree complete heart block or with an irregular rhythm including atrial fibrillation.

Splitting of S_1 is uncommon, and generally is attributed to delayed closure of the tricuspid valve. A split S_1 is most distinct in the tricuspid area at the lower-left sternal border and with deep inspiration. Ventricular arrhythmias, right bundle-branch block, atrial septal defect, and tricuspid stenosis may be associated with a split S_1 (Levine, 2010).

Cardiac Cycle

Understanding the relationship of the cardiac sounds in association with the cardiac cycle is essential in the interpretation of cardiac auscultation findings (Figure 3.3). Ventricular systole occurs between S_1 and S_2, and diastole between S_2 and S_1. Systole is of a shorter duration than diastole, and there is a typical cadence and pattern. In tachycardia, the duration of systole and diastole equalize. Normally there

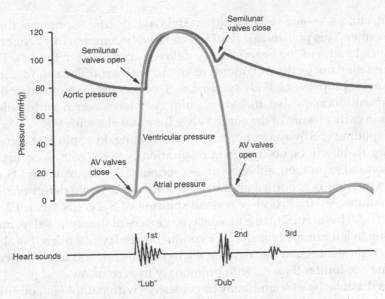

FIGURE 3.3 The association of the cardiac cycle and heart sounds.

Source: Wikimedia Commons (2013).

are no sounds during systole; however, the examiner must listen for extra sounds or murmurs; murmurs that occur during this time period are systolic murmurs. Extra systolic heart sounds that have a high-pitched clicking quality are classified as early ejection sounds, as well as mid- to late-systolic clicks. Early ejection sounds occur shortly after S_1 and are associated with opening of the aortic and pulmonic valves. Aortic ejection sounds have a high pitch and are heard best with the diaphragm at the base. Pathologic processes associated with an early aortic ejection sound are AS or a dilated aorta. Pulmonic ejection sounds are also high pitched and best heard with the diaphragm at the 2nd or 3rd ICS. Pulmonary stenosis, pulmonary hypertension, or dilation of the pulmonary artery can cause a pulmonic ejection sound. A mid- to late-systolic click is a frequent finding with mitral valve prolapse (MVP), and may be followed by a murmur. To elicit the mid- to late-systolic click, listen with the diaphragm with the patient in a seated or supine position.

The S_2 "dub" signifies the end of systole and the beginning of diastole. This sound is associated with closure of the aortic and pulmonic valves and is therefore clearest at the aortic and pulmonic areas at the base. A loud S_2 is associated with hypertension, aortic mechanical valve, or ascending aortic aneurysm. A loud P2 suggests the presence of pulmonary artery hypertension. A softer or lower intensity S_2 is consistent with heart failure, or pulmonary embolism. Diastole begins with S_2, and this period must be evaluated for extra sounds or murmurs, as diastolic murmurs are more suggestive of an underlying pathologic process than systolic murmurs.

A split S_2 is usually due to closure of the aortic valve (A2), which has a louder component, followed by the pulmonic valve (P2), which is softer. A split S_2 is loudest at the pulmonic site, the 2nd left ICS. Splitting of S_2 is best auscultated when the patient inhales deeply in the sitting position. A physiologic split S_2 occurs on inspiration when venous return to the heart is enhanced due to an increase in lung volumes during inspiration, which prolongs the ejection of blood from the right ventricle, and pulmonic valve closure is delayed; during expiration, the sounds occur together. This physiologic finding is relatively common in younger patients with the right side of the heart slightly delayed compared to the left. The splitting sound may not be distinct, more consistent with a muffled sound, rather than two separate components. Wide splitting of S_2 occurs in conditions that delay closure of the pulmonic valve, including pulmonic stenosis or right bundle branch block, or in early closure of the aortic valve, for example, with MR.

The splitting of S_2 may also be an abnormal finding. In a split S_2 associated with pathology, there will be no change in respiration pattern, with S_2 occurring with inspiration and expiration, although more pronounced with expiration. S_2 splitting during expiration is abnormal and may indicate atrial septal defect or right ventricular failure. A paradoxical or reverse splitting of S_2 occurs when P2 is heard first, then A2. This is attributable to a delayed closure of the aortic valve, most commonly due to left bundle branch block conduction delay, although it is also noted with AS, right ventricular pacing, systolic hypertension, and left ventricular failure. P2 may be louder than A2 with pulmonary hypertension.

Extra diastolic heart sounds may be consistent with pathologic conditions and include an S_3, S_4, summation gallop, and mitral valve opening snap. A gallop is a diastolic filling sound, which is an extra heart sound usually identified as an S_3 or S_4. The sounds occur in sequence with the usual S_1, S_2, followed by S_3 and/or S_4 occurring in diastole, with S_3 occurring early in diastole immediately following S_2, and S_4 in late diastole, immediately prior to the subsequent S_1. S_3 has a galloping rhythm consistent with Ken-TUCK-y or lub-dub-*ta*. In children and adults between 20 and 30 years of age, a physiologic S_3 gallop may represent a variation of a normal finding, although these sounds are generally pathologic in an older adult. In pathologic conditions, an S_3 represents passive ventricular filling as ventricular relaxation ends and there is a reduction in wall motion that is related to a deceleration of blood flow, generally due to filling of a noncompliant ventricle. The sound is associated with ventricular failure; pulmonary hypertension with cor pulmonale; mitral or TR; or aortic insufficiency due to blood from the atrium moving into an overfilled ventricle during early diastolic filling. The low-pitched sounds of S_3 and S_4 are both heard best with the bell, and the sounds can be soft. Position the bell of the stethoscope at the apex for the left ventricle and over the lower-left sternal border for the right ventricle. The left-lateral recumbent position brings the apex closer to the chest wall and improves the ability to hear left ventricular S_3.

The galloping rhythm of S_4 is consistent with the sound of TEN-nes-see, *ta*-lub-dub, with S_4 occurring late in diastole. In pathologic conditions, an S_4 represents the active, rapid ventricular filling associated with atrial contraction, and the sound is associated with blood entering a noncompliant, stiff ventricle during atrial contraction, which produces a rapid elevation in ventricular pressure. An S_4 will not be apparent with conduction disorders that disrupt synchronized atrial contraction, including atrial fibrillation. Clinically, S_4 is often a manifestation of significant hypertension and associated left ventricular hypertrophy; other causes can include heart failure, prior myocardial infarction, angina, coronary heart disease, hypertrophic cardiomyopathy, and AS (Levine, 2010). To evaluate S_4, listen with the bell at the apex for the left ventricle and the lower left-lateral sternal border with the patient in a supine or left-lateral recumbent position for the right ventricle. A summation gallop is the presence of S_1 and S_2, then both S_3 and S_4. During slower heart rates, the examiner may hear four distinct sounds—although it is difficult to assess four separate sounds with normal heart rates and tachycardia—and then the S_3 and S_4 combine to form a summation gallop. A summation gallop is generally associated with heart failure due to the combination of volume overload and non-compliant ventricles.

A mitral valve opening snap occurs when the mitral valve is restricted or delayed during opening, with the primary associated pathology of mitral valve stenosis. An opening snap occurs in early diastole and is a high-pitched sound that can radiate or be loud. This sound is heard best by examining medial to apex, at the 2nd left ICS. An opening snap of the mitral valve is a high-frequency sound that is heard better with the diaphragm, while the S_3 is a low-frequency sound.

Pericardial Friction Rub

A pericardial friction rub is an extra heart sound that generally occurs through-out the cardiac cycle, during both systole and diastole. Classically there are three components: (a) atrial systole, (b) ventricular systole, and (c) ventricular diastole, although rubs with only one or two components have also been documented. A friction rub is associated with inflammation or infiltration of the pericardium and associated with pericarditis, pericardial effusion, and cardiac tamponade. The rub can be associated with or without an effusion. Pericardial friction rubs are specific for pericarditis, occurring in 85% of patients (Khandaker et al., 2010). The etiology of the rub may be idiopathic, viral, infectious or related to a myocardial infarction, malignancy, metabolic disorder, autoimmune condition, myocarditis, adjacent struc-tures, medications, radiation, trauma, or after a procedure.

The pericardium is comprised of the fibrous pericardium, which is the outer sac; the parietal pericardium, which is the serous layer that lines the fibrous pericardium; the pericardial cavity between the parietal and visceral pericardium, which nor-mally contains 15 to 50 mL of ultrafiltrated plasma; and the epicardium, which is the visceral pericardium or the serous layer lining the heart. The friction rub is generated by the inflammation of the two pericardial layers with the movement of the heart within the sac. A pericardial friction rub is a continuous high-pitched grat-ing, scraping, scratching sound that is usually widely audible, and clearest near the apex and at the left sternal border. To enhance the sound, listen with the diaphragm when the patient is sitting up and leaning forward during exhalation, which brings the parietal and pericardial layers closer. Variations in the rub occur over time, even between short intervals, and the patient should be reexamined frequently. To differ-entiate a pericardial friction rub from a pleural rub, request that the patients hold their breath; a rub that continues to be audible while the breath is held is pericardial. Generally, a pericardial friction rub is an uncommon finding, although its absence is commonly reported in the typical cardiac physical examination.

Patient Positioning

Most cardiac auscultation is conducted with the patient in the supine position. The supine position allows clear identification of anatomic positions and evalua-tion of S_1 and S_2. This position also enhances a split S_2, S_3, S_4, and most systolic murmurs except hypertrophic obstructive cardiomyopathy (HOCM). Alternative positions can improve the ability to auscultate specific sounds, and the patient may be moved from a supine position if these conditions are suspected from the initial examination. Sitting up and leaning slightly forward can improve the clarity of high-pitched sounds, including the click of an MVP. Low-pitched sounds can be improved with the supine left-lateral recumbent or left-lateral decubitus position in which the patient lies on the left side with his or her left arm under the head and the knees bent. The right-lateral recumbent position is ideal for right-rotated hearts or dextrocardia.

Dynamic Maneuvers

Dynamic patient maneuvers, standing, squatting, Valsava, isometric exercises, and respiratory effects are utilized to alter circulatory dynamics by increasing or decreasing filling pressures to improve the interpretation of heart sounds. To decrease venous filling and venous return, the patient can be requested to stand or the Valsalva maneuver can be performed. Sudden standing reduces venous return and quiets most murmurs, although this maneuver will accentuate the systolic murmur of HOCM and enhance the murmur and click of an MVP.

For the Valsalva maneuver, request that the patient bears down, or place a hand on the abdomen and ask the patient to strain against the hand. Straining changes the intrathoracic pressure, resulting in a reduction of right and then left ventricular filling and a rise in HR. As with the standing maneuver, any decrease in preload and ventricular volume causes all murmurs to be quieter, except those caused by hypertrophic cardiomyopathy and MVP. Decreasing the preload also narrows S_2, and a split S_2 will be less apparent with standing or Valsalva. Once the patient has adjusted to the standing position or the intrathoracic pressure from the Valsalva is released, then venous return increases along with ventricular filling, which widens the A2-P2 interval, increasing the split S_2, and the A2-P2 interval along with the murmur of a hypertrophic cardiomyopathy will increase.

Maneuvers to increase venous return include squatting and isometric exercises, including hand grips. An increase in venous return to the heart results in increased blood volume in the ventricles and systemic vascular resistance, which enhances S_3, S_4, and most murmurs, including AS. The increased blood volume reduces the murmur of HOCM because the additional blood volume moving through the hypertrophied ventricular walls reduces the obstruction of the outflow tract. The murmur of MVP is reduced as the increased volume reduces the prolapse.

Variations in the respiratory cycle change intrathoracic pressures and blood flow through the heart, altering cardiac auscultation findings. Patients can be requested to exacerbate inspiration and expiration to augment heart sounds. Expiration increases left heart venous return and ventricular diastolic filling pressure and stroke volume, which enhance paradoxical split S_2, S_3, S_4, mitral opening snaps, and left heart murmurs. Right heart ausculatory findings are enhanced with inspiration; this increases right heart venous return and right ventricular diastolic filling pressure and stroke volume while reducing pulmonary vascular impedance, resulting in an increased pulmonary vascular capacitance. The Muller maneuver is a prolonged inspiratory effort against the closed glottis and enhances the findings of a physiologic split S_2, right ventricular S_3, S_4, tricuspid opening snaps, and right heart murmurs. Usually three to four cardiac cycles are required for blood volume to move through the pulmonary vasculature (Levine, 2010).

Cardiac Murmurs

Cardiac murmurs occur as a result of normal and abnormal blood flow patterns and may be innocent, physiologic, or represent an underlying pathologic process. Innocent murmurs are common findings in infants and children and are created due to flow-related phenomena. These murmurs are characterized as short, soft, systolic murmurs at the left sternal border with normal S_1 and S_2 (Table 3.6). By changing the patient's position and altering blood flow, the intensity of the murmur will change; the murmur should be evaluated with the patient supine, sitting, standing, squatting, and with a Valsalva maneuver (Biancaniello, 2005). The innocent murmur will change with position changes and quiet with the Valsalva maneuver. Common innocent murmurs are Still's, pulmonary flow, systemic flow, and venous hums. Physiologic murmurs occur due to an increase in blood flow related to metabolic conditions including fever, anemia, hyperthyroidism, exercise, or pregnancy. Pathologic murmurs have varying degrees of clinical importance and are caused by an underlying cardiac structural or cardiovascular disorder, including flow into a dilated vessel, for example, the aortic root; retrograde flow, valve regurgitation or septal defect; flow through a partial obstruction, valve stenosis; flow to an area of resistance, pulmonary or systemic hypertension; or flow across an abnormal valve with or without obstruction, MVP, bicuspid aortic valve, and aortic sclerosis. Murmurs can be attributed to congenital abnormalities or acquired disease, rheumatic fever and infections, or cardiac conditions that distort the valves, including myocardial infarction, heart failure, arrhythmias, hypertension, and age-related changes. Pulmonic murmurs are difficult to hear due to low pressures in the right heart and are rare in adults.

TABLE 3.6 General Characteristics of Benign or Pathologic Murmur Findings

Characteristic	Benign	Pathologic
Grade	I or II	III–VI
Timing	Early or mid-systolic	Diastolic, mid-late systolic, holosystolic
Location	Left sternal border or pulmonic area	Radiation to carotid arteries, neck, or axilla
Associated findings	Absent	Regurgitant murmurs, associated with click, abnormal 2nd heart sound
Cardiopulmonary symptoms	Absent	Present
Significant family history	Absent	Present
Physical examination	Otherwise normal	Cardiopulmonary findings
Exacerbated by valsalva	No	Yes

Murmurs are characterized based on the intensity, pattern, quality, duration, pitch, timing in the cardiac cycle, and associated features, including thrills or radiation. The intensity of a murmur is conventionally graded where it is most audible on a six-point scale, I to VI, and often noted with the auscultated intensity as the numerator and VI the denominator, for example, a grade two murmur is II/VI. As a general relationship, a louder murmur is associated with increased pathology, although there are exceptions. In severe AS or cardiogenic shock, the murmur can become quieter due to the overall reductions in blood flow. Although subject to significant interlistener variability, the following is a guideline for the six grades.

I = barely audible, localized sound
II = quiet although heard immediately
III = moderate
IV = moderately loud, barely palpable thrill
V = loud with palpable thrill
VI = loud with visible and palpable thrill

Murmurs can be enhanced or quieted with dynamic maneuvers (Table 3.7). Understanding the characteristic responses assists in determining the causes of the murmur. Murmurs have a longer duration than heart sounds and may have a pattern described as crescendo, decrescendo, plateau, crescendo–decrescendo or diamond, or a variable, uneven pattern. A murmur that peaks near midsystole with a quiet gap before S_2 is most commonly associated with HOCM or AS. The pitch of a murmur may be high, medium, or low, and the quality may be harsh, rumbling, blowing, squeaking, musical, or mechanical due to a prosthetic valve. Murmurs may be associated with a thrill or radiation that may extend to the neck, carotids, back, or axilla. The murmur of AS may radiate, although aortic sclerosis does not. The duration of the murmur is often combined with the relationship to the cardiac cycle and whether the murmur occurs early, late, or continuously in systole, diastole, or both (Table 3.8).

Dynamic changes in heart sounds over time or the onset of new murmurs may be of concern and require further evaluation, particularly if there are associated clinical findings of bacterial endocarditis, papillary muscle dysfunction, or aortic insufficiency. Papillary muscle dysfunction may occur in the setting of cardiac

TABLE 3.7 Murmurs and Associated Changes With Dynamic Maneuvers

Murmur	Increased Venous Return Increased Preload (Leg Raise or Squat)	Decreased Venous Return Decreased Preload (Valsalva or Standing)	Increased Afterload (Handgrip)
Mitral stenosis	↑	↓	↑
Aortic stenosis	↑	↓	↓
Mitral regurgitation	↑	↓	↑
Aortic regurgitation/insufficiency	↑	↓	↑
Ventricular septal defect	↑	↓	↑
Hypertrophic obstructive cardiomyopathy	↓	↑	↓
Mitral valve prolapse	↓	↑	↓

TABLE 3.8 Timing of Murmurs in the Cardiac Cycle and Associated Disorders

Mid-Systolic Ejection	Mid-Late Systolic	Holosystolic	Early Diastolic	Mid-Diastolic	Continuous
Aortic stenosis	Mitral valve prolapse	Mitral regurgitation	Aortic regurgitation	Mitral stenosis	Patent ductus arteriousus
Aortic sclerosis	Papillary muscle dysfunction	Tricuspid regurgitation	Aortic dissection	Tricuspid stenosis	Aortic septal defect
Hypertrophic cardiomyopathy		Ventricular septal defect	Congenital bicuspid valve	Atrial tumors	Pulmonary coarctation
Aortic coarctation			Pulmonic regurgitation		
Pulmonic stenosis			Ventricular septal defect		
Atrial septal defect					
Ventricular septal defect					
Pulmonary artery dilation					

ischemia or with acute coronary syndromes. These muscles contract to ensure closure of the atrioventricular valves, and in the setting of ischemia, the muscles may not function properly and the closure of the valves can be compromised, permitting the retrograde flow of blood through the valve, often the mitral valve of the left ventricle. Generally the murmur with papillary muscle rupture is soft, with a high pitch of a crescendo–decrescendo pattern, occurring in early to midsystole or holosystolic, associated with angina or heart failure. Infarction of these muscles may lead to papillary muscle rupture and clinically significant compromise. New onset murmur associated with aortic insufficiency should be further evaluated for acute aortic dissection or dehiscence of the valve after coronary artery bypass surgery or aortic valve replacement. This murmur of aortic insufficiency occurs in early diastole at the 2nd or 3rd left ICS with radiation toward the apex.

Systolic Murmurs

Systolic murmurs may be related to a benign condition or an abnormality. The murmur may occur early, midsystole, late systole, or throughout systole—holosystolic or pansystolic. Systolic murmurs are attributed to turbulence from an increased flow across a normal semilunar valve, increased flow into a dilated great vessel, flow across an abnormal semilunar valve, flow across a narrowed ventricular outflow tract, flow across an incompetent atrioventricular valve, or flow across the interventricular septum. In adults, abnormal systolic murmurs are commonly due to semilunar valve stenosis, atrioventricular valve regurgitation, or ventricular septal defects. In the older adult, systolic murmurs are frequently related to aortic sclerosis from thickening of the leaflets of the aortic valve, which represents mild calcification without any significant pathology and the valve is functionally normal. Hypertrophic cardiomyopathy may result in a systolic murmur without radiation and is associated with double-peaked, bifid, carotid upstrokes. Holosystolic murmurs are pathologic, beginning immediately with S_1 until S_2. Holosystolic murmurs are associated with blood moving from a high- to a low-pressure chamber through a structure that should be a closed, ventricular septal defect, or MR or TR.

Aortic Stenosis

AS is an ejection murmur in which blood flow is obstructed due to the irregular valve that does not open fully. Typically this is a harsh, midsystolic murmur with a crescendo–decrescendo pattern, with greater stenosis associated with a longer crescendo phase, later peak, and shorter decrescendo. The murmur of AS is loudest in the aortic area at the base in the 2nd right ICS and will become softer in the lower and lateral areas toward the axilla. This murmur may radiate to the bilateral carotid arteries. The intensity of the murmur varies with cardiac output, and A2 decreases as the stenosis worsens. Palpation of the PMI may demonstrate lateral and posterior displacement in the presence of severe AS and left ventricular failure. Concurrent palpation of the PMI and the carotid artery may demonstrate a delay in carotid pulsation in severe AS. Auscultation may also reveal a single or paradoxically split S_2. A thrill is highly specific for severe AS and is often palpable in the right- and/or left-second ICS.

The *Gallavardin effect* is a phenomenon that can be noted with AS in which the murmur sounds harsh in the aortic region and musical at the apical area, due to transmission through solid tissue rather than the flow of blood. The murmur has a similar shape in the sound, and transmission to the apical area may be confused with MR (Giles, Martinez, & Burch, 1974). The Gallavardin effect is also noted with papillary muscle dysfunction (Giles et al., 1974).

A subaortic stenosis is a growth of septal tissue in the region of the aortic outflow tract. A similar crescendo–decrescendo murmur will be heard with a subaortic stenosis as in AS, although the murmur tends to be louder along the left sternal border and toward the apex, without radiation to the carotids. The dynamic obstruction varies depending on ventricular filling, whereas AS obstruction is fixed at the time of auscultation and is less likely to vary. The murmur of subaortic stenosis is louder with Valsalva or handgrip, which decreases venous return and increases the murmur; this is unlike AS, in which these maneuvers decrease the murmur. The subaortic stenosis murmur will become softer with increased ventricular filling as more blood moves the abnormal septum away from the opposite wall, decreasing the obstruction.

Mitral Regurgitation

Cardiac examination of an individual with chronic MR often reveals a holosystolic, soft-blowing murmur, which is loudest at the apex. The murmur does not have a harsh quality and is typically described as a "shshshshsh" sound that may radiate to the base, axilla, or back. The location of the radiation is dependent on the regurgitant jet—a flail of the posterior leaflet will result in an anterosuperior jet with radiation to the base, and a flail of the anterior leaflet will result in a posterior jet with radiation to the axilla and back. Chronic MR may reveal a soft S_1 or be associated with a systolic thrill. Hemodynamically significant MR may produce an S_3. Continue to listen to the murmur as the patient is moved into the left-lateral decubitus position. The lateral position enhances the ability to hear MR as the left atrium, which is receiving the volume from the regurgitation, is brought closer to the stethoscope; as a result, the murmur is appreciated and accentuated. Maneuvers that decrease the left ventricular volume, such as sudden standing, will decrease the regurgitation and murmur. Maneuvers that increase the left ventricular volume, such as squatting and handgrip, will increase the regurgitation and murmur.

Rupture or dysfunction of papillary muscles is a significant complication of myocardial infarction; this event can lead to the systolic murmurs of TR or MR. TR due to myocardial infarction is rare. In acute myocardial infarction, MR can result in heart failure, significantly increasing mortality.

Mitral Valve Prolapse

The physical findings of MVP may be normal if the prolapse is mild and MR is absent. General physical examination findings that should elicit suspicion for MVP include thoracic malformations, including pectus excavatum in which up to 25% of patients have associated MVP (Jaroszewski, Notrica, McMahon, Steidley, & Deschamps, 2010). The classic cardiac examination finding of MVP is a midsystolic click that is best auscultated with the diaphragm of the stethoscope at the apex or the left lower sternal border. The midsystolic click results from the movement of the mitral valve apparatus as the leaflet prolapses into the left atrium during systole and may be followed by a late systolic medium- to high-pitched murmur. Maneuvers that decrease the left ventricular volume produce an early-systolic click or murmur; alternatively, maneuvers that increase the pressure produce a late-systolic click or murmur.

Tricuspid Regurgitation

TR can be related to an isolated right heart condition or a result of left side or pulmonic pressure changes that are transmitted to the right side. Often there are no physical examination findings suggestive of TR, even severe TR. However, TR may produce a short, medium-pitch, blowing systolic murmur, audible at the right and left lower sternal borders. In individuals with severe TR that coincides with pulmonary hypertension, physical examination often reveals JVD, murmur, and hyperdynamic right ventricular impulse upon palpitation of the chest wall. The intensity of TR can be accentuated by increasing venous return and preload, including inspiration with auscultation.

Diastolic Murmurs

In general, diastolic murmurs are softer and less obvious, because diastole is a passive phase of the cardiac cycle without the movement or pressure generated by ventricular contraction. Diastolic murmurs are almost always pathologic. In adults, common diastolic murmurs are due to regurgitation or insufficiency of semilunar valves and stenosis of atrioventricular valves.

Aortic Regurgitation or Aortic Insufficiency

In patients with AR, palpation of the PMI may be prominent and laterally displaced if there is associated left ventricular volume overload, hypertrophy, or dilation. Auscultation of an early diastolic, low-pitched, rumbling murmur at the 2nd ICS is highly predictive of AR. The direction of the regurgitation is indicative of the underlying pathology, with a murmur at the left sternal border associated with primary valvular disorder and at the right sternal edge with aortic root disorders. The pattern of AR is generally a decrescendo murmur, which quiets toward the end of diastole. The sound of AR can be enhanced in the sitting position and in the forward leaning position. Individuals with chronic, severe AR may demonstrate increased carotid upstroke as a result of the increased preload due to the regurgitant volume. The manifestation of the increased upstroke is a bisferiens or a double-peaked carotid pulsation and *Corrigan's pulse* with a rapid rise and fall of the carotid impulse. Additional findings associated with severe AR are *Hill's sign* with a lower extremity SBP greater than 20 mmHg higher than arm SBP and *de Musset sign*, head bobbing with ventricular systole.

The Austin Flint murmur is a middiastolic to presystolic murmur audible with chronic, severe AR. The murmur is of a low frequency, with little radiation and loudest at the apex. This murmur mimics rheumatic MS, and may result in a functional MS, as the mitral valve is influenced by the regurgitant jet from the aortic valve and the movement of blood from the left atrium to the left ventricle. One distinguishing feature with the Austin Flint murmur is the absence of a mitral opening snap.

Mitral Stenosis

In MS, cardiac auscultation may reveal an accentuated S_1 with an opening snap that is a soft, low-pitched sound from the opening or snapping of the thickened, calcified mitral valve. The murmur of MS is a middiastolic murmur that occurs during rapid ventricular filling or just presystolic during atrial contraction. The presystolic sound will not be heard with concurrent atrial fibrillation. The murmur is a low-pitched diastolic rumble best heard over the apex or axilla with the bell of the stethoscope. The sound does not usually radiate. Mild MS may be loudest when auscultated in the left-lateral decubitus position.

Pulmonary Regurgitation

Pulmonary murmurs are generally difficult to hear. A Graham Steell murmur is an early diastolic murmur that is notable with pulmonary hypertension due to the high velocity of regurgitant flow across the pulmonary valve. Pulmonary hypertension is often associated in patients with cor pulmonale due to COPD. The Graham Steell murmur is loudest at the 2nd left ICS at the sternal border on deep inspiration.

Continuous Murmurs

Patent ductus arteriosus is generally diagnosed in early childhood, and presents as a harsh, machinelike quality murmur due to blood flowing from the aorta into the pulmonary artery. This is a continuous murmur, although there is greater flow during systole than diastole.

Mammary soufflé is a systolic and diastolic murmur related to arterial flow during the late third trimester of pregnancy and postpartum lactation due to increased blood volume to gravid breasts. The murmur is of a high-pitched blowing quality and unaffected by the Valsalva maneuver.

Cervical venous hum is more notable in children, although it is evident in adults and is usually heard best just above the clavicle, lateral to the clavicular head of the sternocleidomastoid muscle on the right side of the neck. The venous hum is related to the flow of blood into the IJ vein from the cerebrovascular circulation that causes a vibration or humming sound. The importance of this finding is to distinguish this sound from AR, carotid artery stenosis, patent ductus arteriosus, and arteriovenous aneurysms (Rivin, 1966). The venous hum is audible throughout the cardiac cycle and will decrease with compression of the IJ vein.

Additional Sounds

Hamman's sign is substernal crepitance, usually synchronous with the heartbeat. This sound results in a crunching, cracking sound, which can be caused by mediastinal emphysema; pneumopericardium; air in the mediastinum; or pneumothorax (Baumann & Sahn, 1992).

CARDIOVASCULAR-RELATED FINDINGS IN OTHER BODY AREAS AND SYSTEMS

Eyes

There are specific and nonspecific findings of the eyes in relationship to cardiovascular conditions. The appearance of corneal arcus senilis, a thin gray circle around the iris, is a normal finding in an older adult, although in younger persons it may be an indication of elevated lipids. Arcus senilis is more prevalent in African Americans. Another finding of lipid metabolism disorders is the occurrence of xanthelasmas, which are yellow, slightly raised, well-circumscribed plaques that often are found on the nasal side of eyelids, unilaterally or bilaterally.

The fundoscopic examination allows direct visualization of the blood vessels by evaluating a small portion of the retina with the ophthalmoscope. Evaluate the general size, shape, color, and distribution of the vessels and look for any lesions on the retina. Follow the blood vessels to the disc, and the vessels will enlarge closer to the disc. Assess the round optic disc for clarity. The nasal aspect of the optic disc may normally be blurred. The disc should be yellow in color, or occasionally pink to orange, and have a physiologic cup, a light depression centrally located in the optic disc. The presence of optic disc edema is related to increased intracranial pressure or significant hypertension.

Changes in the vasculature occur with hypertension, dyslipidemia, and diabetes mellitus, and these changes can be visualized through a fundoscopic examination. The retinal arteries are actually arterioles, because they do not have a muscular lining. These arterioles are approximately two-thirds smaller than the veins and are normally light red with a bright light reflex. Retinal veins are larger, darker in color, and duller. Retinal changes in chronic hypertension include arteriolosclerosis with generalized narrowing of vessels; copper or silver wiring; arteriovenous nicking; retinal hemorrhages; vascular tortuosity; and microaneurysms. With chronic hypertension, the arterioles thicken and there is an increase in the reflection of the light, resulting in a shiny appearance due to luminal narrowing from intimal and subintimal fibrosis. Initially the light reflection has a red-brown colored sheen, referred to as copper wiring; with progressive hypertension, the reflection over time becomes more white, silver wiring. The Scheie classification defines retinal and light reflex changes noted with hypertension (Table 3.9). In hypertension, the extent of focal arterial narrowing is related to the control of BP. Improved control of hypertension has been correlated with a reduction in microvascular abnormalities in a study by Wang et al. (2012) of 2,058 participants who were evaluated for progression or regression of changes over 5 years. Evaluate the areas where the arteries and veins cross, that is, the arteriovenous crossing points. In chronic hypertension, the arteries stiffen and displace the more pliable veins—resulting in an hourglass appearance, termed arteriovenous (AV) nicking or the Gunn sign. As the arteriole continues to harden, the course of the vein will change; Salus' sign.

Microinfarcts of the small retinal arterioles are yellow-white spots, termed cotton wool spots because they may have a fluffy appearance. Cotton wool spots occur from hypertension, diabetes, hypercoagulable states, connective tissue disorders, severe anemia, and many other causes. Cotton wool spots are most commonly located in the posterior area and may fade after 36 weeks. A Roth's spot is a cotton wool spot with a white center due to an ischemic condition and surrounded by a hemorrhage from ischemic changes that ruptures the arteriole. Roth's spots can occur due to many conditions, although they are often attributed to bacterial endocarditis. Other causes of these spots are hard exudates of lipid residue from damaged capillaries associated with diabetes, and malignant hypertension associated with optic disc edema.

TABLE 3.9 Scheie Classification of Arteriolosclerotic Changes With Hypertension

Stage	Retinal Changes	Light Reflex Changes
0	No visible abnormalities	Normal
1	Diffuse arteriolar narrowing No focal constriction	Broadening of light reflex Minimal arteriovenous compression
2	More pronounced arteriolar narrowing with focal constriction	Light reflex changes and crossing changes more prominent
3	Focal and diffuse narrowing, with retinal hemorrhage	Copper-wire appearance with more prominent arteriolovenous compression
4	Retinal edema, hard exudates, and optic disc edema	Silver-wire appearance, severe changes at arteriolovenous crossing

Source: Scheie (1953).

Neck

Palpate the thyroid for goiter or masses. Hypothyroidism and hyperthyroidism have implications for cardiovascular risk and disease. Additionally, evaluate the thickness of the neck for findings that may be consistent with the Pickwickian syndrome or an enlarged neck consistent with obstructive sleep apnea.

Pulmonary

The evaluation of the pulmonary system includes inspection, palpation, percussion, and auscultation comparing the anterior, lateral, and posterior areas from top to bottom and side to side. In general, the posterior chest is evaluated sitting upright followed by the anterior assessment with the patient lying down or sitting. Posteriorly, the examiner is able to assess the upper and lower lobes; in order to assess the right middle lobe, the right lateral and anterior chest must be assessed. Evaluate the chest and back for abnormalities, including pectus excavatum, kyphosis, or kyphoscoliosis, and abnormal spinal curvatures that may inhibit normal lung expansion. The normal transverse diameter of the chest is twice the size of the anteroposterior (AP) diameter. With a barrel chest, the transverse and AP diameter are about equal, resulting in decreased lung resiliency with increased stiffness and loss of muscle strength in the diaphragm. Evaluate the thorax for symmetry in chest wall movement, including costal or diaphragmatic breathing, the use of accessory muscles, and retractions. Also assess chest excursion as unequal expansion may be indicators of pneumothorax, extrapleural air, fluid, or a mass. Use of accessory muscles, such as the scalene and sternocleidomastoid muscles, indicates more significant respiratory distress. Paradoxical movement of the abdominal muscles, outward with expiration, is a sign of respiratory fatigue. These distressing signs can be due to exacerbations of cardiac or pulmonary diseases, or other causes of respiratory failure.

To evaluate breath sounds, request that the patient breathes through the mouth with deep and slow breaths, and listen from side to side for a full breath in each location. Use the diaphragm of the stethoscope, pressing firmly to evaluate airflow, obstruction, and adventitious sounds. Normal breath sounds are clear with high-pitched, loud bronchial sounds over the trachea; bronchovesicular sounds over the major mainstem bronchi; and vesicular, soft, low-pitched, low-intensity, blowing sounds in smaller airways. The bronchial and bronchovesicular sounds are louder and of high to moderate pitch, and it is abnormal to hear these sounds in other locations. Absent breath sounds are always a clinically important finding and may be consistent with poor airway exchange with asthma or pneumothorax, or severe respiratory distress. Adventitious sounds are superimposed over normal breath sounds and must be evaluated in terms of several elements: timing in the respiratory phase, location, duration, pitch, loudness, and continuous or intermittent pattern. Stridor is a high-pitched sound during inspiration, consistent with an obstruction. Crackles, or inspiratory rales, are discrete, discontinuous, fine sounds, typically located in the bases due to the gravitational effect on fluid, although they may be audible in the higher lung areas when associated with fluid in the alveoli. Common conditions associated with crackles are heart failure, atelectasis, postoperative recovery, and other periods of difficulty taking deep breaths.

Prominent pulmonary findings in acute heart failure and resultant pulmonary edema are inspiratory crackles, dyspnea, orthopnea, and paroxysmal nocturnal dyspnea. Usually crackles are first noted in the bases of one or both lungs, with more severe pulmonary edema manifested by extensive crackles, tachypnea, and respiratory distress. Pink frothy sputum is sometimes associated with severe pulmonary edema. Rhonchi are rumbling sounds due to airway secretions and narrowing. These sounds are more pronounced on expiration, prolonged, continuous, and less discreet than crackles. A wheeze is a musical, high-pitched, continuous sound with a whistling character that occurs during inspiration and expiration, but is commonly isolated to expiration. A wheeze is a result of air movement through constricted airways due to intermittent obstructive lung disease, asthma, pulmonary edema, or an underlying pulmonary disease exacerbated with beta adrenergic blocking agents. A continuous wheeze is associated with a fixed characteristic, including a mass or tumor in the endobronchial airway. A pleural friction rub is a coarse, grating, dry, low-pitched sound that occurs outside the respiratory tree. The friction rub is due to pleuritis, which is an inflammation of the pleura, and occurs during inspiration and expiration. To differentiate from a pericardial friction rub, the patient will hold the breath, and the pleural friction rub will no longer be audible. The Hamman sound, a mediastinal crunch, is a loud crackle, clicking, or gurgling sound associated with mediastinal emphysema.

Vocal resonance is the transmission of voice sounds that are ordinarily muffled and indistinct into sounds that are louder or clearer than normal due to the consolidation of lung tissues. Vocal resonance can be assessed through auscultation of the lung fields with the following maneuvers: bronchophony, when spoken words are louder and clearer on auscultation of the lungs; whispered pectoriloquy, when a whisper can be heard distinctly; and egophony, when the voice intensity increases and has a nasal quality.

Assess for any associated cough, including its quality, pitch, frequency, onset, sputum production, postural influences, and loudness. A dry cough may be consistent with angiotensin-converting enzyme (ACE) inhibitor use; and in heart failure, a cardiac cough may accompany sputum production with pink, frothy sputum as an indication of pulmonary edema.

Pulmonary toxicity occurs in 2% to 5% of individuals on amiodarone therapy (Wolkove & Baltzan, 2009). Evaluation for this side effect is important, because if pulmonary toxicity occurs, the medication should be discontinued and the patient may begin therapy to reverse the disorder. Common manifestations of amiodarone pulmonary toxicity are progressive shortness of breath, nonproductive cough, pleuritic chest pain, and systemic symptoms of malaise and fever.

The pulmonary system is palpated for tenderness, crepitus, and vocal or tactile fremitus. Fremitus is a palpable vibration during speech due to the transmission of the sounds and vibrations through the bronchopulmonary system. Use the palm or ulnar surface of the hand on the posterior chest while the patient is repeating words—words such as "ninety-nine" are typically used—and normal chest wall vibrations should be symmetrical. An area of decreased fremitus is associated with air or fluid in the pleural space or by an obstructive bronchus, due to certain disease states, including emphysema. Tactile fremitus is increased with conditions that cause lung consolidation, including pneumonia. The level of the diaphragm can be determined by evaluating for fremitus, and is generally between the 10th and 12th ribs with deep inspiration. An elevated diaphragm occurs with pleural effusion or atelectasis. The thorax should expand evenly, assessed by placing the thumbs parallel to the 10th ribs on both sides of the spine during deep inhalation, evaluating the movement and displacement of the thumbs. The displacement should be even and symmetrical.

Percussion causes vibrations and is usually evaluated posteriorly because of anterior breast tissue and anterior dullness due to the cardiac chambers and the liver. Evaluate percussion sounds to determine if the underlying area is primarily air, fluid, or solid. Percuss by pressing the middle finger of one hand over an area and striking the distal interphalangeal joint with the middle finger of the other hand. Evaluate from side to side and at intervals a few centimeters apart to determine diaphragmatic excursion, normally a 3 to 6 cm difference between inspiration and expiration. Normal percussion findings are resonant sounds with air-filled lungs; dullness occurs with fluid, solid tissue, or lung consolidation. Hyperresonant sounds are due to emphysema and air trapping. Table 3.10 contrasts clinical findings to differentiate effusion from consolidation by the physical examination.

TABLE 3.10 Clinical Findings to Differentiate Pulmonary Effusion From Consolidation

	Effusion	Consolidation
Auscultation	Decreased or absent breath sounds	Bronchial breath sounds
Percussion	Dull	Dull
Tactile fremitus	Decreased	Increased
Egophony	Absent	Present

Abdominal

The abdominal exam should be performed with inspection and auscultation before percussion or palpation to prevent changes in bowel sounds from increasing or diminishing. Inspect the abdomen for symmetry, visible peristalsis, ascites, and the general contour—flat, round, concave, or distention. Auscultate the abdomen with the diaphragm over all four quadrants; audible sounds may be heard without a stethoscope, known as *borborygmi*. Listen for the bowel sounds, which are usually clicks or gurgles that may occur in a variable pattern of 5 to 30 sounds in a minute. To determine that there are no sounds or reduced sounds, listen for several minutes. Hyperperistalsis is noted with diarrhea and early intestinal obstruction; decreased or absent sounds are noted with peritonitis or paralytic ileus. Evaluate for bruits in the abdomen, abdominal aorta, and renal artery areas, while considering the evaluation for femoral bruits at the same time.

Palpate the abdomen while the patient exhales, by placing the right hand under the right costal margin and palpate upward. The liver edge will be palpable with inhalation and should be a smooth, firm edge that is nontender. Palpate the abdomen for liver and spleen size and for urinary distention. The liver may be enlarged with heart failure due to hepatic congestion. If there is pain in the abdomen, evaluate the quadrants without pain first. Percussion is useful to evaluate for tympany and liver size; the usual range is 6 to 12 cm below the costal angle. At the right midclavicular line, evaluate for the area of resonance, which is consistent with the lungs; then move downward to find the dullness of the liver. Pleural effusion or lung consolidation will result in dull pulmonic sounds. To find the lower edge of the liver, locate the tympanic sounds consistent with the intestines, and move upward to an area of dullness. The area of dullness provides an approximation of the liver size. Bladder distention will be located from umbilicus down and result in suprapubic dullness. Ascites is the accumulation of fluid in the peritoneal area, usually due to portal hypertension, although it is also associated with heart failure. The patient can be examined in the supine position or on the lateral side, with the dependent area of ascites associated with dullness rather than tympany.

The abdominal examination may be benign in many cardiovascular conditions. However, patients with cardiogenic shock may have hypoactive to absent bowel sounds due to impaired mesenteric circulation. Patients with longstanding heart failure may have hepatomegaly or liver engorgement, with discomfort on palpation. In addition, nonalcoholic fatty liver disease and medications that result in hepatic impairment may result in liver discomfort and enlargement. Hepatojugular reflux occurs earlier in heart failure and is assessed by applying gentle pressure with the examiner's right hand over the right upper abdominal quadrant from 10 to 60 seconds, noting the difference in the level of jugular venous pulsations before and during the application of the pressure. An increase of more than 3 cm is considered positive for heart failure.

Integument

The integument can provide important evidence of cardiovascular conditions and associated co-morbidities for cardiovascular illness. The nails may reveal clubbing, which occurs in pathologic conditions of congenital heart disease, bacterial endocarditis, severe pulmonary conditions including lung cancer, and disease states that result in chronic hypoxia. Evaluate for clubbing by inspecting the side of the fingernails for changes in the hyponychial angle, which is the angle between the base of the nail and the distal phalangeal tissue. Determine the angle by evaluating the distal digital crease to the cuticle in comparison with the cuticle to the hyponychium. The usual angle is 192 degrees; an angle greater than 195 degrees is consistent with nail clubbing (Sarkar, Mahesh, & Madabhavi, 2012). In addition, the depth of the interphalangeal tissue is normally shorter than the depth of the distal phalangeal, but in clubbing, the distal phalangeal depth is larger; the nail may also be unstable, and upon palpation of the nail base, the tip of the nail may move, referred to as a floating nail. In the nail beds, brown, linear streaks, which are splinter hemorrhages, may appear with infectious endocarditis.

Cyanosis, a blue discoloration of the skin or mucous membranes, can be an indicator of decreased SaO_2 of the blood supplying an affected area. However, cyanosis is an unreliable indicator of hypoxemia due to influencing factors, such as anemia. In order for cyanosis to be detected, at least 5 g/dL of deoxygenated hemoglobin must be in the capillary bed. If the quantity of circulating hemoglobin is decreased, as in anemia, a much lower level of arterial SaO_2 to partial PaO_2 is required for cyanosis to be evident. Peripheral arterial vasoconstriction due to reduced peripheral blood flow in fingers and toes can also cause cyanosis, which can be due to anxiety, a cold environment, or pathologic states, including peripheral occlusive disease or cardiogenic shock. Peripheral cyanosis can be evaluated in the nose, lips, and earlobes. Central cyanosis can be appreciated in the buccal mucosa and associated with significant right to left shunts, as well as COPD and fibrosis.

The autonomic nervous system controls moisture and temperature, and changes may be evident in acute conditions when a normal, warm, and dry integument becomes cool, moist, cold, or clammy. Among patients with suspected acute coronary syndrome, pallor and diaphoresis are suspicious for decreased circulation. Pallor could also be the result of anemia that is provoking a cardiac ischemic event due to decreased oxygen delivery to the myocardium.

The skin can provide evidence of past surgical procedures and metabolic conditions. *Acanthosis nigricans* is the darkened, velvety discoloration in skin folds and a marker for glucose metabolism disorders; jaundice is an indication of hepatic disorders and may be elevated with hepatic engorgement in heart failure; and xanthelasmas are markers of lipid metabolism disorders. Petechiae may be a result of an underlying coagulation disorder or a complication of antiplatelet and antithrombotic medications. In infectious bacterial endocarditis, integumentary manifestations may result in Janeway lesions and Osler's nodes. Janeway lesions are nontender hemorrhagic lesions of the palms and soles, and Osler's nodes are purple, tender nodules that occur in the fingerpads.

Peripheral Pulsations and Circulation

Arterial pulsations are evaluated centrally with a femoral or carotid pulse or peripherally with the radial, ulnar, brachial, popliteal, posterior tibial, or dorsalis pedis pulse. The popliteal pulse may be difficult to palpate, requiring more pressure due to the quantity of the surrounding tissue. The popliteal pulsation may be absent, although this is not generally clinically important if distal pulses are identified. The palpation of pulses is graded on a subjective 0 to 4 scale: 0 = nonpalpable; 1 = diminished, barely palpable; 2 = expected, normal; 3 = full, increased; and 4 = bounding. When palpating pulses, evaluate the skin surrounding the area and assess for bruits as indicated. A bruit is evaluated with auscultation, and the sound is a low-pitched murmur sound due to turbulent blood flow or stenosis in arteries. Typically the carotid artery is evaluated for bruits while the patient is holding his or her breath. Other areas to auscultate for bruits are the temporal, subclavian, renal, iliac, femoral, and abdominal aorta regions. For individuals with atrioventricular fistulas, evaluate the fistula site and ensure there is a bruit and thrill, which is a normal finding, and palpate the pulses in the surrounding area and distal to the fistula.

According to the Advanced Trauma Life Support guidelines, in hypotension, palpable pulses are an approximate indicator of BP (Table 3.11). Deakin and Low (2000) performed a study evaluating 20 patients with hypovolemia for pulse and BP obtained with arterial lines. From their findings, these authors report that the guidelines may overestimate BP.

The characteristic of peripheral pulses can be a sign of cardiovascular disorders. *Pulsus alternans* is an alternating strong and weak pulse that is an indication of heart failure and left ventricular systolic dysfunction. *Pulsus paradoxus* is a diminished pulse and reduction of greater than 10 mmHg in BP with respiratory inspiration. Pulsus paradox may be a finding with cardiac tamponade, constrictive pericarditis, severe heart failure, severe chronic obstructive or restrictive pulmonary disease, pericardial effusion, MS with right heart failure, hypovolemia, cardiac amyloidosis, and pulmonary embolism (Khandaker et al., 2010).

TABLE 3.11 Palpable Pulse and Relationship to Systolic Blood Pressure

Palpable Pulse	Minimum Systolic Blood Pressure (mmHg)
Carotid	60–70
Carotid and femoral	70–80
Radial	>80

The Allen test is an evaluation of the collateral circulation of the wrist and hand that is performed prior to puncture of the radial artery to avoid the risk of hand ischemia. Indications for radial artery puncture are arterial blood sampling; arterial cannulation with an indwelling arterial line; or procedures that require arterial access, such as cardiac angiogram. Approximately 3% of patients have inadequate collateral blood flow to the hand, which may be an anatomic variant or due to overuse syndromes, such as the hypothenar hammer syndrome.

To perform the Allen test:

- Request that the patient create a fist while elevating the hand for 20 to 30 seconds.
- Maintain the fist and position the hand in a neutral position.
- Firmly apply pressure to compress both the radial and ulnar arteries.
- Instruct the patient to open the hand; the hand should be blanched.
- Release the compression of the ulnar artery.
- The hand should flush within 5 seconds for a normal result. The hand that remains blanched until the radial compression is released is evidence of an abnormal result.

Alternatively, an assessment of the radial artery may be performed with a Doppler ultrasound or the Barbeau test (Barbeau, Arsenault, Dugas, Simard, & Lariviere, 2004). To perform the Barbeau test:

- Place a pulse oximetry on the patient's index finger or thumb.
- Occlude the radial artery while the ulnar artery oximetry tracing and saturation numbers are noted.
- If there is no dampening of the tracings or dampening followed by recovery within 2 minutes, this confirms dual circulation of the hand.
- A waveform that is lost and continues to be absent after 2 minutes is considered to be an abnormal test and requires a repeat test on the radial artery. If the abnormality is confirmed, consider not accessing the radial artery.

Peripheral Vasculature

The peripheral vasculature is assessed for alterations in arterial and venous blood flow by inspection, palpation, and comparing for symmetry. Evaluation must be completed with bare legs and feet without shoes or socks to evaluate the dorsal and plantar surfaces of the foot and between the toes. Peripheral arterial disease (PAD) will manifest with alterations in pulses that will be weak or absent. In addition, bruits may be present and the extremity cool or cold with pigment color changes and pallor, cyanosis, or mottling. Inspect the integument for hair distribution, ulcerations, thickened nails, smooth shiny skin, dependent rubor, scars, or atrophy. Sensation may be decreased with PAD and associated with paresthesia, tenderness, or pain. In arterial disease, pain is often relieved with the extremity in the dependent position that improves blood flow; in contrast, venous disease pain is often improved with elevation. Peripheral neuropathy from diabetes mellitus and other disease states will result in abnormal pain sensations to the lower extremities. Evaluate arterial insufficiency by visualizing blood return in the leg by placing the patient in a supine position, raising the leg, and noticing the amount of blanching. Then place the extremity in a dependent position, evaluating the duration of time for the color to normalize. The color should return as soon as the leg is dependent. Arteriosclerosis obliterans of the extremities occurs in the older adult and is an occlusive atherosclerotic process due to fibrosis of the tunica intima and calcification of the tunica media that affects the small- and medium-sized arteries of the lower extremities and the abdominal aorta. In this condition, the lower-extremity pulses, popliteal, posterior tibial, and dorsalis pedis may be absent. In acute presentations, evaluate for the four Ps of pulselessness, pallor, pain, and paralysis, which require immediate referral and consultation. Gangrenous tissue is nonviable and the skin becomes black in color.

For chronic venous insufficiency, evaluate the venous pattern for superficial veins, venous distention, and tortuous dilation of the veins. Inspect the skin for temperature, color changes, swelling, edema, engorgement, inflammation, and ulcerations, commonly occurring near the lateral or medial malleolus. Color changes of venous insufficiency can be dark blue or purple, and the changes are enhanced in a dependent position. Longstanding venous stasis is evident by a dark, speckled appearance due to the deposit of hemosiderin over time. Erythema is most consistent with cellulitis. Evaluate for pain and tenderness, which may be evidence of a deep vein thrombosis (DVT). Few clinical examination findings have high sensitivity or specificity for thrombus, including the Homans' sign, which is positive for pain with dorsiflexion of the foot, although a negative finding does not exclude DVT. The Pratt's sign is an indication of deep venous obstruction and is positive if dilated veins do not collapse with the elevation of the leg. Thighs and calves should be symmetrical and a difference greater than 2 cm is suggestive of vein thrombosis. The Trendelenburg test examines the varicose veins to evaluate the competency of the superficial and deep vein valves by evaluating venous insufficiency.

- In the supine position, raise the leg to 90 degrees, flexing the leg at the hip to empty the great saphenous vein.
- Apply a tourniquet around the upper thigh to compress the superficial veins, without occluding the deeper veins or the arterial pressure; alternatively, place the tourniquet above the knee to assess the mid-thigh perforators or below the knee to assess the competence of the short saphenous vein to the popliteal vein.
- Lower the leg and the patient will stand.
- There is valvular incompetence in the deep veins if the superficial veins fill rapidly; this is a positive test indicating incompetence in the communicating veins; normally, the superficial saphenous vein will fill slowly over 30 seconds.

■ After 20 to 30 seconds, if there was no rapid filling, release the tourniquet; sudden filling is evidence that the communicating veins are competent, although the superficial veins are incompetent, and again is an abnormal finding.

Capillary Refill

The capillary bed joins the venous and arterial systems to allow exchange between the vascular and interstitial spaces; capillary refill time is the duration required for the capillary bed to fill after occluded by pressure and provides an indication of the health of the capillary system. The test generally is performed on the nail beds. Apply pressure to blanch the nail, release the pressure, and note the time to return to full color. Normal is instantaneous, less than 2 seconds; longer duration indicates reduced peripheral circulation, hypovolemia, or heart failure with low cardiac output.

Edema

Edema is the abnormal interstitial accumulation of lymphatic fluid. The movement of lymphatic fluid occurs in a closed circuit with the cardiovascular systems and is dependent on the cardiovascular system for movement. The lymphatic fluid and proteins move from the bloodstream to the interstitial spaces and merge into the venous system through ducts at the subclavian vein; if there is an obstruction, low flow, or low protein levels, the fluid movement decreases. Obstruction may be due to local venous insufficiency, lymphatic obstruction, or obesity. Although edema may be evident in the face, abdomen, and upper extremities, the dependent location of the lower extremities is a typical area for assessment. Edema is often evaluated in clinical practice; however, changes in fluid distribution by the monitoring of weight may be a better estimation of fluid overload. In the lower extremities, assess for edema by pressing the index finger over the bony prominence of the medial malleolus or tibia for several seconds. Edema may be pitting, and is assessed by pressing the thumb over the bony surface—dorsal surface of feet, shins, medial malleolus, or sacrum. The degree of pitting is subjectively graded by severity: 0 = none, 1+ for slight pitting with rapid disappearance to 4+ for deep pitting that remains for 2 or more minutes. Anasarca indicates generalized edema and is related to a systemic disorder, including heart failure, whereas a unilateral edema is consistent with a localized disorder.

Auxiliary Manometer

Fluid status may also be evaluated with the hand as an auxiliary manometer. Place the patient in a sitting or supine position with head elevated 45 degrees and the hand at the heart level. Palpate the veins of the hands to ensure they are compressible, and then slowly raise the arm and hand until the veins appear collapsed. Measure the distance between the hand and the midaxillary line at the level of the nipple; the vertical distance is an approximate mean JVD.

FUNCTIONAL CAPACITY

The evaluation of functional capacity is essential in the comprehensive management of patients with cardiovascular disorders, especially chronic disorders that adversely affect the overall quality of life. Understanding the overall functional capacity allows for the monitoring of progress over time, for preoperative risk assessment, and to determine the need for multidisciplinary consultation in patients that require assistance. Functional capacity can be assessed by objective measurements including, but not limited to, evaluations of activities of daily living, the New York Heart Association functional classification, a 6-minute walking test, metabolic equivalents (METs), and the Duke Activity Status Index (Table 3.12). Functional capacity can be characterized as excellent, good, moderate, and poor at greater than 10, 7 to 10, 4 to 6, or less than 4 METs, respectively (Fleisher et al., 2014). The Duke Activity Status Index is a self-administered 12-question tool to evaluate functional status and quality of life by providing an estimate of oxygen uptake (Hlatky et al., 1989).

TABLE 3.12 Duke Activity Status Index

Can you take care of yourself, that is, can you eat, dress, bath, or use the toilet?	2.75
Can you walk indoors, such as around your house?	1.75
Can you walk a block or two on level ground?	2.75
Can you climb a flight of stairs or walk up a hill?	5.50
Can you run a short distance?	8.00
Can you do light work around the house such as dusting or washing dishes?	2.70
Can you do moderate work around the house such as vacuuming, sweeping floors, or carrying in groceries?	3.50
Can you do heavy work around the house such as scrubbing floors or lifting or moving heavy furniture?	8.00
Can you do yardwork such as raking leaves, weeding, or pushing a power mower?	4.50
Can you have sexual relations?	5.25
Can you participate in moderate recreational activities like golf, bowling, dancing, doubles tennis, or throwing a baseball or football?	6.00
Can you participate in strenuous sports like swimming, singles tennis, football, basketball, or skiing?	7.50

Duke Activity Status Index (DASI) = sum _____

VO_2 peak = $(0.43 \times DASI) + 9.6$

VO_2 peak = _____ mL/kg/min divided by 3.5 mL/kg/min = _____ METs

Reprinted from Hlatky et al. (1989), with permission from Elsevier.

POPULATION CONSIDERATIONS

Pregnant women will have an increase of 40% to 50% in total blood volume from 12 to 34 weeks with an increase of 30% to 40% in cardiac output. The blood volume returns to prepregnancy levels in approximately 4 weeks after delivery. The enlarged uterus and developing fetus move the diaphragm and the heart position upward, horizontally with a slight axis rotation. Cardiac auscultation may reveal more audible splitting and murmurs. In pregnancy, hormonal changes result in vasodilation of the blood vessels, and in normal pregnancy, the BP drops in the early stage and rises during the third trimester. There is venous pooling and increase in venous pressure, which may result in lower extremity edema and varicosities.

There are normal age-related variations in the older adult. In general, HR slows and stroke volume and cardiac output decrease as the exercise capacity diminishes with a delayed response to stress and a less efficient response to increased oxygen demand. The myocardium becomes less elastic, and the endocardium thickens with fibrosis and sclerosis of the sinoatrial node and heart valves. The heart becomes more transverse. Tachycardia is less tolerated, and the return to a resting HR is prolonged. There is also an increase in vagal tone, while the arterial walls lose elasticity and vasomotor tone, which causes a diminished ability of the arteries to adjust to changes in pressure and volume. The baroreceptors lose sensitivity. There is an increase in cardiac conduction with changes including blocks, ST-T wave abnormalities, and atrial fibrillation. In the frail elderly, adaptive examination strategies may be required, including examining the patient in the chair or supine position.

BILLLING AND CODING

The completeness of the physical examination has implications for appropriate coding of patient visits, billing practices, and reimbursement issues. The physical examination involves a number of components, which must be evaluated in order to justify the level of examination, which is combined with the history and medical decision making to determine the overall level of the visit (Hill, 2011). The Centers for Medicare & Medicaid Services (CMS) guidelines for documentation titled "Evaluation and Management Services Guide" (2010), which details Medicare's description of the requirements for coding and billing purposes. The document reviews the level of examination performed and required documentation to justify a specific visit level (Table 3.13). To document a normal finding, a brief statement or notation of "negative" or "normal" is adequate. A finding described as "abnormal" requires an explanation and description.

TABLE 3.13 General Guidelines for Levels of Evaluation and Management Services From the Centers for Medicare & Medicaid Services

Type of Examination	Description of Examination	Systems	Identified Elements
Problem focused	Limited examination of the affected body area or organ system	≥1	1–5 elements
Expanded problem focused	Limited examination of the affected body area or organ system and other symptomatic or related organ system(s)	≥1	≥6 elements
Detailed	Extended examination of the affected body area(s) and other symptomatic or related organ system(s)	≥2 OR ≥6	≥12 elements OR ≥2 elements
Comprehensive	Multi-system examination or complete examination of a single-organ system and other related systems	≥9	All elements and document ≥2 elements for each system

The following body systems are recognized: head, including face; neck; chest, including breasts and axillae; abdomen; genitalia, groin, buttocks; back, including spine; and each extremity. The organ systems in Table 3.14 are recognized by CMS for general multisystem physical examination.

TABLE 3.14 General Multi-System Physical Examination

Constitutional	General appearance of the patient Measurement of any three of the following seven items—sitting or standing blood pressure, supine blood pressure, pulse rate and regularity, respiration, temperature, height, weight
Eyes	Inspection of conjunctivae and lids Examination of pupils and irises Ophthalmic examination of optic discs
Ears, nose, mouth, and throat	External inspection of ears and nose Otoscopic examination of external canals and tympanic membranes Assessment of hearing Inspection of nasal mucosa, septum, and turbinates Inspection of lips, teeth, and gums Examination of oropharynx
Neck	Examination of neck Examination of thyroid
Cardiovascular	Palpation of heart Auscultation of heart Examination of carotid arteries Examination of abdominal aorta Examination of femoral arteries Examination of pedal pulses Examination of extremities for edema or varicosities
Respiratory	Respiratory effort Percussion of chest Palpation of chest Auscultation of lungs
Chest	Inspection of breasts Palpation of breasts and axillae
Gastrointestinal	Inspection and palpation of abdomen Examination of liver and spleen Evaluation for hernia Examination of anorectal area Stool sample for occult blood
Genitourinary—male	Examination of scrotum Examination of penis Digital rectal examination of prostate gland
Genitourinary—female	Examination of external genitalia Examination of urethra Examination of bladder Examination of cervix Examination of uterus Examination of adnexa/parametria

(continued)

TABLE 3.14 General Multi-System Physical Examination (*continued*)

Musculoskeletal	Examination of gait and station
	Inspection or palpation of digits and nails
	Inspection, palpation, range of motion, stability, strength, and tone of:
	Head and neck
	Spine, ribs, and pelvis
	Right upper extremity
	Left upper extremity
	Right lower extremity
	Left lower extremity
Skin	Inspection of skin and subcutaneous tissue
	Palpation of skin and subcutaneous tissue
Neurologic	Cranial nerve test
	Deep tendon reflexes
	Examination of sensation
Psychiatric	Patient judgment and insight
	Orientation to time, place, and person
	Recent and remote memory
	Mood and affect
Lymphatic	Palpation of lymph nodes in:
	Neck
	Axillae
	Groin
	Other

Single-organ system examinations are cardiovascular; ears, nose, mouth, and throat; eyes; genitourinary; hematologic, lymphatic, immunologic; musculoskeletal; neurologic; psychiatric; respiratory; and skin. The single-organ system for the cardiovascular examination as described by CMS includes the elements described in Table 3.15. For the cardiovascular examination, the level of examination performed and documentation should include:

- Problem Focused = one to five elements identified
- Expanded Problem Focused = at least six elements identified
- Detailed = at least 12 elements identified by a bullet
- Comprehensive = every element for the systems constitutional, respiratory, cardiovascular, gastrointestinal, and neurologic/psychiatric; and at least one element for eyes, ears/nose/mouth/throat, neck, musculoskeletal, extremities, skin

TABLE 3.15 Cardiovascular Examination: Single-Organ System

Constitutional	Measurement of any three of the following seven vital signs: (1) sitting or standing blood pressure, (2) supine blood pressure, (3) pulse rate and regularity, (4) respiration, (5) temperature, (6) height, (7) weight
	General appearance of patient—development, nutrition, body habitus, deformities, attention to grooming
Eyes	Inspection of conjunctivae and lids (xanthelasma)
Ears, nose, mouth, and throat	Inspection of teeth, gums, and palate
	Inspection of oral mucosa with notation of presence of pallor or cyanosis

(*continued*)

TABLE 3.15 Cardiovascular Examination: Single-Organ System (*continued*)

Neck	Examination of jugular veins—distention; a, v, or cannon a waves Examination of thyroid—enlargement, tenderness, mass
Respiratory	Assessment of respiratory effort—intercostal retractions, use of accessory muscles, diaphragmatic movement Auscultation of lungs—breath sounds, adventitious sounds, rubs

Cardiovascular	Palpation of heart—location, size, and forcefulness of the point of maximal impact; thrills; lifts; palpable S_3 or S_4
	Auscultation of heart including sounds, abnormal sounds, and murmurs
	Measurement of blood pressure in two or more extremities when indicated aortic dissection, coarctation
	Examination of:
	   Carotid arteries—waveform, pulse amplitude, bruits, apical-carotid delay
	   Abdominal aorta—size, bruits
	   Femoral arteries—pulse amplitude, bruits
	   Pedal pulses—pulse amplitude
	   Extremities for peripheral edema and/or varicosities

Musculoskeletal	Examination of the back with notation of kyphosis or scoliosis Examination of gait with notation of ability to undergo exercise testing and/or participation in exercise programs Assessment of muscle strength and tone—flaccid, cog wheel, spastic—with notation of any atrophy and abnormal movements
Extremities	Inspection and palpation of digits and nails—clubbing, cyanosis, inflammation, petechiae, ischemia, infections, Osler's nodes
Skin	Inspection and/or palpation of skin and subcutaneous tissue—stasis dermatitis, ulcers, scars, xanthomas
Neurologic/Psychiatric	Brief assessment of mental status including Orientation to time, place, and person Mood and affect—depression, anxiety, agitation

For full reference citations to this chapter, please see "Section References" in the back of the book, under the heading "Section I."

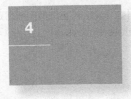

Preoperative Cardiovascular Risk Assessment and Evaluation for Noncardiac Surgery

LADAN ESHKEVARI, CATHERINE HORVATH,
DENISE H. TOLA, AND DONNA M. JASINSKI

Cardiovascular clinicians frequently care for patients who require evaluation and screening prior to noncardiac surgical procedures. Preoperative risk assessment promotes the ability of the health care team to provide the safest care, while ensuring the most favorable perioperative and postprocedure outcomes for patients. Annually, more than 1 million out of the 200 million people who have noncardiac surgery die within 30 days of their procedure, often due to cardiac complications (Devereaux et al., 2012). Indeed, an estimated 10 million are believed to suffer significant myocardial injury after noncardiac surgery, with myocardial ischemia a frequent cause of perioperative cardiac complications (Devereaux et al., 2011). Therefore, it is of utmost importance for clinicians who evaluate patients preoperatively to understand the risk factors associated with intraoperative cardiac morbidity, and to optimize patients for surgical procedures, whenever possible. Toward that end, this chapter describes the comprehensive cardiovascular preoperative assessment for noncardiac surgery. The aim is to assist the clinician in determining preoperative risk by evaluating the patient's condition in the context of the anticipated surgical procedure and by determining the stability and severity of any underlying condition. For patients who require urgent or emergent surgical procedures, the ability to conduct a comprehensive evaluation is limited and dictated by the surgical requirements of the patient.

Cardiac complications with surgery and anesthesia can range from minimal alterations in vital signs to life-threatening situations. Given that anesthetic agents and surgery can cause physiologic stress responses, fluid shifts, pain, temperature changes, immobility, and alterations in perfusion and oxygenation, assessment is aimed at ascertaining the capability of the patient to adjust to these physical and metabolic challenges. Thus, preoperative cardiac risk assessment is paramount to enhancing patient outcomes.

One significant risk factor associated with perioperative cardiac events is patient age, with patients older than the age of 65 demonstrating the greatest risk (Botto et al., 2014). In the United States, as in most Western nations, the population is aging, with an estimated 13.7% of the current population older than 65 years of age. The percentage of U.S. citizens older than the age of 65 is forecasted to reach 20% by 2030 (United States Bureau of the Census, 2008). The longer people live, the more likely they are to have surgery, with an estimated 30% to 40% of all surgeries in the United States performed on patients in this age group. Although age is a risk factor, emerging data suggest that it is not necessarily the greatest risk factor, as patient history and co-morbidities play an important role in cardiac-related mortality after noncardiac surgical procedures (Botto et al., 2014).

PREOPERATIVE INTERVIEW

Preoperative patient evaluation is a key component in identifying potential risk factors that are associated with increased risk in patients undergoing anesthesia for surgery. The preoperative evaluation should include a medical record review, patient interview, a physical examination of the patient, and considerations for diagnostic testing (Marley, Calabrese, & Thompson, 2014). A general history should begin with an evaluation of the patient's past medical history, surgical history, and prior exposure to anesthetics. If the patient has had no prior anesthetic complications, it is likely that he or she will have an uneventful anesthesia experience unless there has been a significant change in his or her history.

Complications with anesthesia experienced by blood relatives should be included in the history, because several critical anesthetic complications can be caused by inherited traits. These complications include malignant hyperthermia, acute intermittent porphyria, and plasma-cholinesterase deficiency. Prolonged periods of mechanical ventilation postoperatively lead to complications; it is prudent to investigate the reason for the extended period of mechanical ventilation (Marley et al., 2014). All of the aforementioned inherited patient conditions have the potential to require prolonged mechanical ventilation postoperatively, and each requires specific anesthesia techniques or combinations of medications to avoid complications (Marley et al., 2014).

Allergies

Evaluation of all allergies to medications, foods, or substances such as latex is another important aspect of the patient history. Patients who are chronically exposed to latex products or who report an intolerance to latex products such as balloons, dental dams, rubber gloves, or condoms are at higher risk for latex allergy. Allergies to certain foods such as avocado, banana, kiwi, mango, passion fruit, and chestnuts are associated with a higher risk of latex allergy (Marley et al., 2014). A skin-prick test can be performed to confirm the diagnosis of latex allergy, but diagnosis is usually made through confirmation by the health history (Marley et al., 2014). Accommodations to the operating room environment, timing of the scheduled procedure, and the use of latex-free equipment are indicated for patients with known latex allergy or those at high risk (Marley et al., 2014).

Medications

Current prescription and nonprescription medications are important to evaluate for the appropriate care of the presurgical patient. Most antihypertensive medications and antiarrhythmic agents are continued throughout the perioperative period. Angiotensin-converting enzyme inhibitors (ACEI) and diuretics may be held the

TABLE 4.1 General Cardiac Medication Recommendations With Anesthesia

Medication	Intraoperative Concerns	Recommendations
Angiotensin-converting enzyme inhibitors	Hypotension	Discontinue on day of surgery if used solely for treatment of hypertension
Beta adrenergic blocking agents	Hypotension Bradycardia	Continue, including day of surgery
Calcium channel blockers	Hypotension Mild bradycardia	None
Diuretics	Hypokalemia Hypovolemia (hypotension)	Consider discontinuation the day of surgery
Antiarrhythmics	Cardiac depression Hypotension	Continue, including day of surgery
Aspirin	Increased bleeding Altered platelet function	Cardiology consultation, highly recommended
Coumadin	Increased bleeding	Cardiology consultation, highly recommended
Novel anticoagulants—fondaparinux, apixaban, rivoraxaban	Increased bleeding	Cardiology consultation, highly recommended

morning of surgery if their only indication is hypertension, as these agents can cause labile blood pressures intraoperatively (Marley et al., 2014). Solid clinical judgment, based on current recommendations in the literature and consideration for the patient's condition, is paramount. Table 4.1 enumerates some of the current recommendations regarding discontinuation of cardiac-related medications prior to anesthesia and surgery (Marley et al., 2014).

Herbal Supplements

Herbal supplements vary in their effects on bodily systems. Some of these supplements may interact with medications during the administration of anesthesia or can potentiate hemorrhage during surgery. For example, kava can potentiate the sedative effects of anesthetics and should be stopped at least 24 hours prior to surgery. Herbal supplements, including garlic supplements, should be stopped at least 7 days prior to surgery due to their inhibition of platelet aggregation and other effects. Ginseng lowers blood glucose and should also be discontinued at least 7 days prior to surgery. Ginkgo inhibits platelet-activating factor and should be stopped a minimum of 36 hours prior to surgery. Ephedra or ma-huang has direct and indirect sympathomimetic effects and should be discontinued a minimum of 24 hours prior to scheduled surgery (Marley et al., 2014). Herbal supplements that have no pharmacokinetic information available should be discontinued 2 weeks prior to surgery. However, in the same-day surgery environment where the patient is often not evaluated until the day of surgery, it is incumbent upon the anesthesia practitioner to understand potential risks of herbal supplements and prepare the necessary adjustments to care (Fisher, Bader, & Sweitzer, 2010).

Tobacco, Alcohol, and Other Substances

A social history inquiring about tobacco, alcohol, or other recreational substances is included in the preoperative history. Nicotine increases heart rate, blood pressure, myocardial oxygen consumption, and peripheral-vascular resistance causing a suboptimal myocardial oxygen supply and demand ratio (Marley et al., 2014). In addition, carbon monoxide has a 250 to 300 times greater affinity than oxygen for hemoglobin, and patients who smoke tobacco have a sixfold increase in incidence of pulmonary complications postoperatively. Smoking cessation of short durations can improve the patient's surgical condition with cessation 12 hours prior to surgery resulting in reduced heart rate, blood pressure, and carboxyhemoglobin levels in the blood. Smoking cessation of 8 weeks or more improves ciliary function, decreases mucous production, and reduces risk of pulmonary complications (Marley et al., 2014).

Obtain an accurate history about the amount, frequency, and type of alcohol a patient normally consumes. Patients who drink alcohol chronically or excessively are at risk for withdrawal syndromes, arrhythmias, and infections during the perioperative period (Marley et al., 2014). The chronic alcohol user that has a tolerance to alcohol may have a higher anesthetic requirement due to a cross-tolerance with hypnotics and opioids. Alcohol-induced hepatic disease may result in enzymatic dysfunction and reduced albumin levels. Consequently, the metabolism of certain anesthetic medications is altered or a greater amount of circulating drug is available, which results in prolonged drug effects. Postoperative morbidity and mortality are higher in alcoholic patients as a result of poor wound healing, bleeding, infection, and overall multisystem organ deterioration (Marley et al., 2014). The major concerns for anesthesia practitioners are acute intoxication and withdrawal syndrome; in either situation, it is recommended that surgery be delayed (Marley et al., 2014).

Patients using illegal recreational substances may not reveal this information; nonetheless, the practitioner should inquire and evaluate for clues that may be indicative of illegal substance use. For instance, thrombotic vessels, skin abscesses, scarring from frequent self-injection, and malnourishment are a few physical traits that should raise suspicion. Cocaine and amphetamines inhibit the uptake of sympathomimetic neurotransmitters, causing tachycardia and elevation in blood pressure, which in turn result in erratically unstable hemodynamics intraoperatively. Opioid and heroin users will have a tolerance to opioid analgesia medications. Marijuana smokers incur the same risks as tobacco smokers, and additionally may experience tachycardia, dysrhythmias, and EKG abnormalities of ST segment and T wave changes (Fisher et al., 2010). Patients on methadone maintenance should continue their medication regimen throughout the perioperative period, and addiction counselors and acute pain-management services should be consulted for the management of postoperative pain and avoidance of relapse if significant pain is expected (Fisher et al., 2010).

Functional Capacity

For the patient without significant cardiac history or symptoms, the focus should be the patient's risk factors such as advanced age, functional capacity, and comorbid conditions that are associated with cardiac disease. The patient's functional capacity can be ascertained through questions about physical activity. For instance, if the patient is not able to go up one flight of steps, bicycle, or rake leaves, that is, cannot perform activities that equate to four to five metabolic equivalents (METs) of functional capacity or average activity level, then he or she is at increased risk for perioperative complications (Fisher et al., 2010).

Co-morbid Conditions

Although advanced age beyond 70 is associated with greater risk, it may not be as significant in determining perioperative risk as comorbid conditions including diabetes mellitus, peripheral-vascular disease, hypertension, and renal insufficiency, which are frequently accompanied by cardiovascular disease (Fisher et al., 2010). For example, diabetes increases the risk for coronary heart disease and contributes to a greater risk for developing ischemia, myocardial infarction, or heart failure postoperatively (Fisher et al., 2010; Hata & Hata, 2013). Sequelae of diabetes, renal compromise, and autonomic neuropathy have been identified as risk factors for perioperative cardiac morbidity (Hata & Hata, 2013). Autonomic dysfunction usually affects multiple systems and may or may not be manifested clinically. Abnormalities such as resting tachycardia, orthostatic hypotension, gastroparesis, neurogenic bladder, and erectile dysfunction may suggest autonomic dysfunction (Vinik, Maser, Mitchell, & Freeman, 2003). Cardiovascular autonomic neuropathy is particularly important, as the risk of silent myocardial infarction with this condition doubles (Vinik et al., 2003), and these patients should be evaluated for prior infarct before undergoing elective surgery (Hata & Hata, 2013).

Hypertension is also associated with coronary heart disease and with increased incidence of silent myocardial ischemia (Hata & Hata, 2013). For every 20 mmHg increase in systolic blood pressure over 115 mmHg and every 10 mmHg increase in diastolic pressure over 75 mmHg, the risk for the development of cardiovascular disease is doubled in patients 40 to 70 years old. The focus of preoperative evaluation for hypertensive patients is to establish the disease duration, the presence of end-stage organ damage, and the effectiveness of current treatment (Fisher et al., 2010). Left ventricular hypertrophy with a strain pattern on the ECG is suggestive of a chronic ischemic state and may warrant further preoperative cardiac testing (Hata & Hata, 2013). Patients should continue their antihypertensive medication regimen throughout the perioperative period, with the exception of diuretics, and perhaps ACEI (Table 4.1). However, diuretic therapy should continue throughout the perioperative period if the medication is indicated for renal insufficiency or heart failure (Marley et al., 2014). Contradictory data exist in the literature regarding ACEI, as these medications may intensify the cardiovascular effect of general anesthesia. In general, ACEI are withheld the morning of surgery if the primary indication is hypertension, although they can be restarted in the immediate postoperative period to prevent rebound hypertension (Whinney, 2009).

Renal insufficiency is linked to higher risk for cardiac incident following major noncardiac surgery and it may be prudent to consider further preoperative cardiac studies for these patients (Fleisher et al., 2014). Preoperative evaluation should evaluate the homeostatic condition of the patient by evaluating the cardiovascular system and fluid and electrolyte balance. For patients with end-stage renal disease with dialysis, evaluate the dialysis type and schedule. Surgery is often scheduled within 24 hours of dialysis, as surgery immediately after hemodialysis has been associated with electrolyte imbalances and volume depletion that can complicate the intraoperative course (Fisher et al., 2010).

Peripheral vascular disease is commonly associated with coronary heart disease risk factors of tobacco use and hyperlipidemia, as well as other diseases including diabetes mellitus and hypertension. Coronary heart disease occurs with a prevalence of 75% in patients with known peripheral vascular disease (Fisher et al., 2010). In addition, the presence of peripheral claudication with this disease often limits physical activity, and consequently masks symptoms of ischemic conditions (Fisher et al., 2010). Therefore, it is important to inquire about claudication and the tolerated level of activity, as a sedentary status limits the ability to assess functional capacity or activity, and further cardiac testing may be warranted.

Pulmonary complications occur with an incidence of 5% to 10% of patients having major noncardiac surgical procedures (Hata & Hata, 2013). Complications include aspiration, atelectasis, exacerbation of existing disease, and respiratory failure necessitating mechanical ventilator support. Routine chest radiograph and pulmonary function testing are not recommended, because they have a limited ability to predict pulmonary complications and rarely alter anesthetic management (Hata & Hata, 2013). However, for the patient with existing pulmonary disease, preoperative evaluation is directed at understanding the type and severity of the pulmonary disease, any circumstances that precipitate an exacerbation of respiratory symptoms, and the effectiveness of current treatment. Baseline oxygen saturation by pulse oximetry may be useful in determining if further testing is indicated. Corticosteroid and bronchodilator therapy should continue throughout the perioperative period, including the day of surgery (Fisher et al., 2010; Hata & Hata, 2013).

Obstructive sleep apnea (OSA) is often suspected in the obese patient population, those with a neck circumference greater than 16 inches, severely hypertrophic tonsils, or airway abnormalities. The patient and family should be questioned about the patient snoring, frequent arousals from sleep with a choking sensation, and daytime somnolence. Left untreated, OSA can lead to pulmonary hypertension and right heart failure. If possible, formal sleep studies should be completed prior to surgery to initiate treatment with continuous positive airway pressure (CPAP) as necessary. For outpatient surgical procedures, prolonged care is mandated in the postanesthesia care unit (PACU) for patients with OSA, and the patient must maintain oxygen saturation on room air without stimulation or prompting prior to discharge (Hata & Hata, 2013). Patients prescribed CPAP therapy should bring their machine and devices to the preoperative area for use during the postoperative period.

Cardiac History

The targeted cardiac history aims to identify those at risk for ischemic heart disease, since the disease is often undiagnosed in about half of men and more than half of women, until an acute coronary event occurs. Traditional risk factors of age, smoking, and family history are important when determining if chest pain or ECG changes are significant, although less important in determining the perioperative risk of cardiac events (Fisher et al., 2010). History of prior ischemic heart disease, heart failure, cerebrovascular disease, diabetes mellitus, and renal insufficiency are important clinical predictors of perioperative cardiac risk for the patient undergoing noncardiac surgery (Fisher et al., 2010; Fleisher et al., 2014).

Preoperative evaluation includes an evaluation for myocardial infarction, heart failure, stable or unstable angina, arrhythmias and conduction disorders, cardiomyopathy, valvular heart disease, or stroke. Determine if the patient has undergone coronary interventions including coronary artery bypass grafting, angioplasty, or coronary stenting; valvular operations or procedures; or evaluation and management of cardiac rhythm disorders. Acquire all relevant data regarding the management interventions including the timing, the type and extent of the procedures, and if any devices are implanted. For a history of cardiomyopathy, ascertain the particular type including hypertrophic obstructive, restrictive, peripartum, or arrhythmogenic right ventricular. Obtain information about cardiology follow-up, the effectiveness of nonpharmacologic and pharmacologic therapies, and current functional capacity to provide optimum care during surgery.

When evaluating a patient with ischemic heart disease, the query should include a history of chest discomfort, precipitating factors, other symptoms, and interventions that relieve the discomfort. Shortness of breath or dyspnea can be associated with angina or heart failure, especially in the patient with risk factors or known cardiac disease (Fisher et al., 2010). Worsening symptoms should prompt further investigation and testing prior to elective surgery.

Heart failure can result as a consequence of reduced or preserved ventricular ejection fraction (EF), with ischemic heart disease being the most common culprit of reduced EF (systolic failure), and hypertension a frequent cause of heart failure with preserved EF (diastolic failure). Cardiomyopathies result from other conditions, including cardiotoxins, muscular dystrophies, alcohol abuse, and infectious diseases. Cancer patients who have received chemotherapy with doxorubicin can also develop cardiomyopathy (Fisher et al., 2010). Preoperatively, the focus is on the recognition of heart failure and any associated clinical complaints of shortness of breath, fatigue, orthopnea, cough, peripheral edema, or recent weight gain. Chest radiography is useful if pulmonary edema is suspected, whereas echocardiography will measure left ventricular EF, ventricular efficiency, and diastolic function. For patients with symptomatic heart failure, New York Heart Association Class III or IV, cardiology specialists should be consulted prior to surgery. Elective surgery for patients with decompensated heart failure is to be postponed until stability is achieved, due to the high risk this poses for the patient during surgery and anesthesia (Fisher et al., 2010).

Arrhythmias are common during the perioperative period, especially in the elderly population. If arrhythmia noted during the preoperative evaluation may complicate the operative course, further testing should be completed (Fisher et al., 2010; Fleisher et al., 2014). Uncontrolled atrial fibrillation, second- or third-degree heart block, symptomatic bradycardia, and ventricular tachycardia are considered high risk for anesthesia and warrant further investigation, postponement of elective surgical procedures, and referral to a cardiologist for evaluation and treatment. Newly discovered left bundle branch block is associated with coronary ischemic disease and also necessitates further testing and a cardiology consultation (Fisher et al., 2010).

Cardiac valvular stenotic lesions are poorly tolerated perioperatively. Aortic stenosis is a common valvular disorder in the United States and associated with the highest risk for perioperative complications (Fisher et al., 2010). Cardinal symptoms of aortic stenosis are angina, dyspnea, fatigue, palpitations, and lightheadedness. Patients with aortic stenosis are at high risk for sudden death from fatal arrhythmias, heart failure, and myocardial infarction; therefore, they require testing for coronary heart disease even with no other risk factors. Patients with severe disease are often not candidates for noncardiac surgery unless the benefits of surgery are a lifesaving event (Fisher et al., 2010). Preoperative evaluation for mitral stenosis should include history of dyspnea, orthopnea, pulmonary edema, or hemoptysis. With severe mitral stenosis, surgical repair or balloon valvuloplasty may be considered before high-risk surgery. However, surgical correction or intervention is generally not warranted for noncardiac surgery (Fleisher et al., 2014). Patients with chronic regurgitant aortic, mitral, and tricuspid lesions who have adequate functional status and ventricular function tolerate anesthesia better in comparison to those with stenotic lesions (Fisher et al., 2010).

Results of previous electrophysiology studies should be available and reviewed during the preoperative evaluation. Individuals with cardiovascular implantable electronic devices (CIEDs) such as pacemakers or automatic cardioverter defibrillators require evaluation, as these patients have known or are at risk for abnormal cardiac rhythms. The type of device should be determined by the manufacturer's identification card or through consultation with the patient's cardiology or electrophysiology team. The device should be interrogated prior to the day of surgery to facilitate proper intraoperative management of the patient. Evaluate if the patient is pacemaker dependent for a symptomatic bradyarrhythmia, a successful atrioventricular nodal ablation, or if the device interrogation reveals no evidence of innate ventricular activity when the device is programmed to VVI mode at the lowest programmable rate (American Society of Anesthesiologists Task Force, 2005). If the patient is pacemaker dependent, the device should be programmed to an asynchronous mode or converted to an asynchronous mode using a magnet over the chest during surgery (Fleisher et al., 2014). Automatic defibrillators should be programmed off prior to surgery to prevent unwarranted shocks from surgical artifact that may be interpreted as a tachyarrhythmia. The device should be interrogated and reprogrammed postoperatively, ideally in the PACU.

Ultimately, decompensated heart failure, severe stenotic valvular disease, unstable or severe angina, ventricular arrhythmias that are symptomatic, high-grade heart blocks, and supraventricular arrhythmia or atrial fibrillation with rapid ventricular response pose the highest risk for anesthesia and surgery. Patients with these conditions should undergo noncardiac surgery only for a life-threatening emergency situation (Fisher et al., 2010).

PREOPERATIVE PHYSICAL EXAMINATION

Preoperative cardiovascular physical examination includes inspection, palpation, and auscultation. Simple visual inspection of the patient during the medical history interview process can elicit a multitude of useful information. Body habitus, respiratory pattern, skin or mucous membrane color, presence of edema, and clubbing of digits can give clues to the overall health of the patient, particularly his or her cardiac health (Fleisher et al., 2014). During the physical examination, vital signs should be assessed with blood pressure measured in both arms. Height and weight should be recorded, and body mass index calculated. Obesity and a large neck circumference, greater than 17 inches for males and 16 inches for females, are important not only in predicting OSA but also in predicting difficulty with mask ventilation (Fisher et al., 2010).

Baseline oxygen saturation by pulse oximetry is useful to the anesthesia professional, as it provides information regarding the patient's baseline pulmonary status. In addition, chest wall deformities, scars indicative of implanted devices, and previous cardiac or vascular surgery should be noted (Fleisher et al., 2014). The lungs should be auscultated for wheezing, crackles, rhonchi, and diminished or abnormal breath sounds. Respiratory effort, use of accessory muscles, or cyanosis should be noted and may require further testing if these are new findings or if these are findings that have not been previously investigated.

Auscultation of heart tones with attention to the presence of murmurs can be a significant finding, and the practitioner must determine if the murmur warrants further testing. Diastolic murmurs are considered pathologic and require in-depth evaluation (Fisher et al., 2010). A systolic ejection murmur, in the right upper sternal border with radiation to the neck, could indicate aortic stenosis and requires investigation as well (Fisher et al., 2010). As mentioned, stenotic lesions, particularly aortic stenosis, create a high-risk situation for the noncardiac surgical patient. Alternatively, patients with significant regurgitant flows are at higher risk for perioperative heart failure (Fleisher et al., 2014). The presence of a third or fourth heart sound over the apical area could be indicative of a failing left ventricle, although absence of such a heart sound does not rule out this condition.

Pressures of the carotid contour and jugular vein should be evaluated. All peripheral pulses should be palpated, noting the presence of peripheral edema (Fleisher et al., 2014). The presence of arrhythmias or conduction pathology may also be detected by auscultation. If either is discovered during the preoperative physical, further testing is necessary, as these may be signs of underlying ischemia, cardiopulmonary disease, electrolyte abnormalities, or other derangements. Although atrial fibrillation is the most common arrhythmia in the elderly, it is poorly tolerated from a surgical standpoint, due to the increase in ventricular wall thickness and loss of elasticity, which promotes dependence on the "atrial kick" for complete ventricular filling (Hata & Hata, 2013). In addition, supraventricular tachyarrhythmias can cause ischemia in patients with coronary heart disease by increasing myocardial demand (Fleisher et al., 2014).

Neurologic physical exam should include any sensory or motor deficits or changes in mentation. These should be noted if preexisting, and further investigated if new in onset (Fisher et al., 2010).

PREOPERATIVE RISK EVALUATION

Risk stratification for perioperative and postoperative cardiovascular events and cardiac-related mortality is an integral component of the preoperative patient assessment. Clinical tools estimate a patient's risk of perioperative cardiac complications. These tools are derived by incorporating various patient-related cardiac risk factors—age, health history, co-morbidities, laboratory data—with the type of surgery to predict the risk of future cardiac complications. Factors with prognostic importance that define preoperative ischemic heart disease, which also correlate with major cardiac complications, are used as variables for these tools. The purpose of the preoperative evaluation is to provide a clinical risk profile that the patient, primary care practitioners, cardiovascular clinicians, anesthesia professionals, and surgeons can use in making treatment decisions that may influence short- and long-term cardiac outcomes.

Physical Status Classification

Since 1941, the American Society of Anesthesiologists (ASA) has used a Physical Status Classification, which stratifies risk based on patient health status, functional limits, and anticipated survival (Table 4.2). The classification ideally serves as a reflection of the patient's preoperative status and is not an estimate of anesthetic risk. This system is commonly utilized in preprocedural and preoperative evaluations to provide a general understanding of the patient's health condition.

TABLE 4.2 American Society of Anesthesiologists (ASA) Physical Status Classification System

ASA PS Classification	Definition	Examples Including (But not limited to . . .)
ASA I	A normal healthy patient	Healthy, non-smoking, no or minimal alcohol use
ASA II	A patient with mild systemic disease	Mild diseases only without substantive functional limitations. Examples include (but not limited to): current smoker, social alcohol drinker, pregnancy, obesity (30 < BMI < 40), well-controlled DM/HTN, mild lung disease
ASA III	A patient with severe systemic disease	Substantive functional limitations; One or more moderate to severe diseases. Examples include (but not limited to): poorly controlled DM or HTN, COPD, morbid obesity (BMI ≥ 40), active hepatitis, alcohol dependence or abuse, implanted pacemaker, moderate reduction of EF, ESRD undergoing regularly scheduled dialysis, premature infant PCA < 60 weeks, history (> 3 months) of MI, CVA, TIA, or CAD/stents.
ASA IV	A patient with severe systemic disease that is a constant threat to life	Recent (< 3 months) MI, CVA, TIA, or CAD/stents, ongoing cardiac ischemia or severe valve dysfunction, severe reduction of EF, sepsis, DIC, ARD, or ESRD not undergoing regularly scheduled dialysis
ASA V	A moribund patient who is not expected to survive without the operation	Ruptured abdominal/thoracic aneurysm, massive trauma, intracranial bleed with mass effect, ischemic bowel in the face of significant cardiac pathology, or multiple organ/system dysfunction

(continued)

TABLE 4.2 American Society of Anesthesiologists (ASA) Physical Status Classification System (*continued*)

ASA PS Classification	Definition	Examples Including (But not limited to . . .)
ASA VI	A declared brain-dead patient whose organs are being removed for donor purposes	

ARD, acute respiratory disease; BMI, body mass index; CAD, coronary artery disease; COPD, chronic obstructive pulmonary disease; CVA, cerebral vascular accident; DIC, disseminated intravascular coagulation; DM, diabetes mellitus; EF, ejection fraction; ESRD, end-stage renal disease; HTN, hypertension; MI, myocardial infarction; PCA, patient-controlled analgesia; TIA, transient ischemic attack.

Note: The addition of "E" to any one of these classification denotes emergency surgery: (An emergency is defined as existing when delay in treatment of the patient would lead to a significant increase in the threat to life or body part.)

Reprinted with permission from the American Society of Anesthesiologists.

Risk Stratification Models

Several cardiac risk stratification models have been developed and are currently used to identify those patients at increased risk of perioperative complications. The Revised Cardiac Risk Index (RCRI) was derived from the Original Cardiac Risk Index created by Lee Goldman in 1977 (Lee et al., 1999). The Goldman index used multivariate discriminant analysis to identify nine independent factors, listed in Table 4.3, with significant correlation to life-threatening and fatal cardiac complications (Lee et al., 1999).

The Goldman Index was derived from a study of 4,315 surgical patients in which the risk of major cardiac complications, which included myocardial infarction, cardiogenic pulmonary edema, cardiac arrest, and cardiac death, was analyzed. The RCRI is a modification of the Goldman Index consisting of six variables, as noted in Table 4.4 (Fleisher et al., 2014). In the RCRI, variables are either absent or present, and assigned one point each in a scoring system. Although a more complex index might achieve greater accuracy, the RCRI can be performed quickly with a simple calculation and readily available information. The index does not address specific types of surgery, although it differentiates between high-risk versus non-high-risk procedures. In addition, the RCRI was not applied to emergency surgeries; therefore, its generalizability to these procedures is unknown (Gupta et al., 2011).

TABLE 4.3 Risk Factors in the Goldman Index

Preoperative third heart sounds or jugular venous distention
Myocardial infarction in the preceding 6 months
More than five premature ventricular contractions per minute documented at any time before the operation
Rhythm other than sinus or presence of premature atrial contractions on preoperative electrocardiogram
Age older than 70
Intraperitoneal, intrathoracic, or aortic operation
Emergency surgery
Important valvular aortic stenosis
Poor general medical condition

Source: Lee et al. (1999).

TABLE 4.4 Components of the Revised Cardiac Risk Index (RCRI) Risk Factors

Condition	Definition	Points
Coronary artery disease	History of myocardial infarction Positive exercise stress test Chest pain secondary to myocardial infarction Pathologic Q waves on EKG	1
Heart failure	Pulmonary edema Paroxysmal nocturnal dyspnea Bibasilar rales S_3 gallop Pulmonary vascular congestion on chest x-ray	1
Cerebrovascular disease	Transient ischemic attack Cerebrovascular accident	1
Diabetes mellitus	On insulin therapy	1
Renal insufficiency	Serum creatinine > 2.0 mg/dL	1
High-risk surgery	Cardiac risk > 5%	1

Based on the presence of none, one, two, or three or more risk factors, the occurrence of major cardiac complications is estimated at 0.4%, 0.9%, 6.6%, and 11%, respectively. A patient's risk increases with the number of variables present with perioperative cardiac complications, defined as myocardial infarction, pulmonary edema, ventricular fibrillation, primary cardiac arrest, and complete heart block. The RCRI is used widely by health care clinicians managing presurgical patients and is incorporated into the 2014 preoperative cardiac risk evaluation guideline from the American College of Cardiology (ACC) and American Heart Association (AHA) (Fleisher et al., 2014; Goldman et al., 1977; Lee et al., 1999).

The predictive value of the RCRI is improved for risk assessment of cardiovascular mortality by adding the risk factor of age older than 70 and a more detailed classification of the type of surgical procedure (Boersma et al., 2005). Both age and surgery types are valuable determinants of adverse cardiovascular outcome. Cardiovascular mortality increases progressively with age (Boersma et al., 2005). Additionally, identification of the inherent risk of the surgical procedure adds detail to the patient's clinical surgical stressors and, therefore, to the factors leading to alterations in well-being. Table 4.5 provides a general classification of low, intermediate, and high risk by anatomic types of surgery (Flu, Van Kuijk, Hoeks, Bax, & Poldermans, 2010).

TABLE 4.5 Cardiac Risk Associated With Noncardiac Surgery

Low Risk, < 1%	Intermediate Risk, 1%–5%	High Risk, > 5%
Breast Dental Endocrine Eye Gynecology Knee Urologic (minor)	Abdominal Carotid, PTA, and EVAR Hip and spine Head and neck Neurologic Transplantation Urologic (major)	Open aortic Peripheral vascular

EVAR, endovascular aneurysm repair; PTA, percutaneous transluminal angioplasty.

Reprinted from Flu, van Kuijk, Hoeks, Bax, and Poldermans (2010, pp. 286–294), with kind permission from Springer Science and Business Media.

Another clinically useful model is the Gupta Perioperative Cardiac Risk Calculator, from the American College of Surgeons National Surgical Quality Improvement Program (NSQIP), Myocardial Infarction and Cardiac Arrest (MICA) risk prediction rule, which predicts risk specifically for perioperative myocardial infarction or cardiac arrest within 30 days of surgery (Gupta et al., 2011). The variables in this risk calculator are detailed in Table 4.6 and include surgical type, functional status, creatinine level, ASA class, and age.

This model provides an exact model-based estimate of the probability of cardiac complications. The online calculator can be found under Gupta Perioperative Cardiac Risk Calculator at www.qxmd.com/calculate-online/cardiology/gupta-perioperative-cardiac-risk. Once the required data are entered into this calculator, a model-based percent estimate of risk is provided. This approach is more precise than a point system, although it is more difficult to implement without

TABLE 4.6 Gupta Perioperative Risk Calculator Variables, American Society of Surgeons National Surgical Quality Improvement Program (NSQIP), Myocardial Infarction and Cardiac Arrest (MICA) Risk Prediction Rule

Type of surgery—defined by anatomical or systemic areas
  Anorectal
  Aortic
  Bariatric
  Brain
  Breast
  Cardiac
  ENT
  Foregut/Hepatopancreatobiliary
  Gallbladder, appendix, adrenal, and spleen
  Hernia (ventral, inguinal, femoral)
  Intestinal
  Neck (thyroid and parathyroid)
  Obstetrical/Gynecologic
  Orthopedic and non-vascular extremity
  Other abdominal
  Peripheral vascular
  Skin
  Spine
  Thoracic
  Non-esophageal
  Vein
  Urology

Functional status
  Totally independent
  Partially dependent
  Totally dependent

Creatnine level
  < 1.5 mg/dL
  > 1.5 mg/dL

American Society of Anesthesiologists (ASA) class

Age

ENT, ear, nose, throat.
Source: Gupta et al. (2011).

readily available technology (Boersma et al., 2005). The calculator adds components to the scoring not found in other models, including functional capacity, which has been correlated to postoperative complication rates (Gupta et al., 2011).

Johns Hopkins Surgical Criteria

An additional risk stratification tool is the Modified Johns Hopkins Surgical Criteria, which characterizes cardiac risk into three categories, Grade I, II, and III, based on the invasiveness of the planned procedure, risk to the patient, and potential blood loss (Table 4.7).

TABLE 4.7 The Modified Johns Hopkins Surgical Criteria

Grade	General	Includes	Excludes
I	Minimal to mild risk independent to anesthesia Minimal to moderately invasive procedure Potential blood loss less than 500 mL	Breast biopsy Removal of minor skin or subcutaneous lesions Myringotomy tubes Hysteroscopy Cystoscopy Vasectomy Circumcision Fiberoptic bronchoscopy Diagnostic laparoscopy Dilatation and curettage Fallopian tube ligation Arthroscopy Inguinal hernia repair Laparoscopic lysis of adhesion Tonsillectomy/Rhinoplasty	Open exposure of internal body organs Repair of vascular or neurologic structures Placement of prosthetic devices Postoperative monitored care setting Open exposure of abdomen, thorax, neck, cranium Resection of major body organs
II	Moderately to significantly invasive procedures Potential blood loss 500–1,500 mL Moderate risk to patient independent of anesthesia	Thyroidectomy Hysterectomy Myomectomy Cystectomy Cholecystectomy Laminectomy Hip/knee replacement Nephrectomy Major laparoscopic procedures Resection/reconstructive surgery of the digestive tract	Open thoracic or intracranial procedure Major vascular repair (e.g., aortofemoral bypass) Planned postoperative monitored care setting (ICU, ACU)
III	Highly invasive procedure Potential blood loss greater than 1,500 mL Major to critical risk to patient independent of anesthesia Usual postoperative ICU stay with invasive monitoring	Major orthopaedic-spinal reconstruction Major reconstruction of the gastro-intestinal tract Major genitourinary surgery (e.g., radical retropubic prostatectomy) Major vascular repair without post-operative ICU stay Cardiothoracic procedure Intracranial procedure Major procedure on the oropharynx Major vascular, skeletal, neurologic repair	

ACU, acute care unit; ICU, intensive care unit.

Source: Donati et al. (2004).

ACC/AHA Guidelines

A detailed and well-explained guideline for practitioners evaluating patients pre-operatively for noncardiac surgery is published periodically and reviewed annually by the ACC and the AHA (Fleisher et al., 2014). The current guidelines, the ACC/AHA 2014 Guidelines on Perioperative Cardiovascular Evaluation and Care for Noncardiac Surgery, are also intended as a model to assist health care providers in the perioperative clinical decision making (Figure 4.1) by describing a range of generally acceptable approaches for the diagnosis, management, and prevention of specific diseases or conditions, and to provide a framework for considering preoperative cardiac risk. The guidelines indicate that a basic clinical evaluation obtained by history, physical examination, and review of the ECG usually provides the clinician with sufficient data to estimate cardiac surgical risk. It is recommended that the risk assessment be conducted in a systematic, methodical, step-wise fashion.

- Step 1—Urgency of surgery
- Step 2—If urgent or elective, determine acute cardiac condition
- Step 3—Perioperative risk of major adverse cardiac event (MACE), clinical/surgical risk
- Step 4—MACE less than 1%, no further testing
- Step 5—MACE equal to or greater than 1%, evaluate functional capacity
- Step 6—Less than 4 METs or unknown functional capacity, evaluate further testing
- Step 7—Testing does not impact surgical decision or alternative treatment strategy (Fleisher et al., 2014)

Step 1—Surgical Urgency

First consider the urgency of surgery, as emergency surgery increases the risk of cardiac morbidity and mortality two- to fivefold (Mangano, 1990). Thus, if the procedure is elective, and active cardiac conditions are identified, surgery should be delayed for further testing, additional therapeutic interventions, or improvement of health status. If the surgery is an emergency and must proceed without delay, attempts at medical optimization are necessary, including pharmacologic management or specialized intraoperative invasive monitoring. The 2014 ACC/AHA guidelines provide guidance on the definition of surgical procedure categorization into four categories: emergency, urgent, time sensitive, and elective (Table 4.8; Fleisher et al., 2014).

TABLE 4.8 Surgical Procedure Categories

Type	Life or Limb Threatened	Time Requirement for Procedure	Clinical Evaluation
Emergency	Yes	<6 hours	Very limited or minimal
Urgent	Yes	6–24 hours	Limited
Time sensitive	No	>1–6 weeks	Partially limited
Elective	No	Up to 1 year	Unlimited

Adapted from Fleisher et al. (2014).

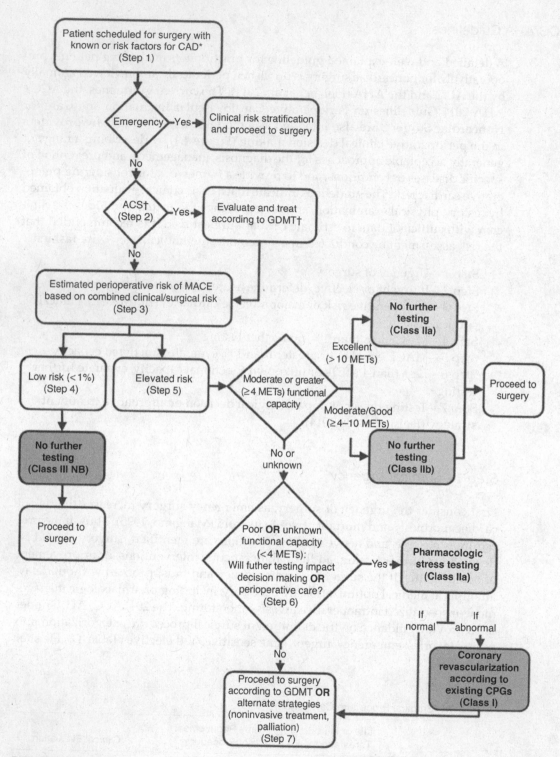

FIGURE 4.1 Stepwise approach to perioperative cardiac assessment for CAD.

ACS, acute coronary syndrome; CAD, coronary artery disease; GDMT, guideline-directed medical therapy; MACE, major adverse cardiac event; MET, metabolic equivalent.

Reprinted from Fleisher et al. (2014), with permission from Elsevier.

Step 2—Active Cardiac Condition

Consider if the patient is exhibiting signs or symptoms of an active cardiac condition. Examples of active cardiac conditions are listed in Table 4.9. Such conditions would warrant cancelation or delay of surgery to provide further investigation with the goal to optimize the cardiovascular status to prepare for the stress of surgery. In particular, evaluate for acute coronary syndrome (ACS) and if the patient is experiencing an ACS, then refer to cardiology for further management.

TABLE 4.9 Active Cardiac Conditions for Which the Patient Should Undergo Evaluation and Treatment Before Noncardiac Surgery (Class I, Level of Evidence: B)

Condition	Examples
Unstable coronary syndromes	Unstable or severe angina* (CCS Class III or IV)[†]
	Recent MI[‡]
Decompensated HF (NYHA functional Class IV; worsening or new-onset HF)	
Significant arrhythmias	High-grade atrioventricular block
	Mobitz II atrioventricular block
	Third-degree atrioventricular heart block
	Symptomatic ventricular arrhythmias
	Supraventricular arrhythmias (including atrial fibrillation) with uncontrolled ventricular rate (HR greater than 100 bpm at rest)
	Symptomatic bradycardia
	Newly recognized ventricular tachycardia
Severe valvular disease	Severe aortic stenosis (mean pressure gradient greater than 40 mmHg, aortic valve area less than 1.0 cm², or symptomatic)
	Symptomatic mitral stenosis (progressive dyspnea on exertion, exertional presyncope, or HF)

CCS, Canadian Cardiovascular Society; HF, heart failure; HR, heart rate; MI, myocardial infarction; NYHA, New York Heart Association.

*According to Campeau.

[†]May include "stable" angina in patients who are unusually sedentary.

[‡]The American College of Cardiology National Database Library defines recent MI as more than 7 days but less than or equal to 1 month (within 30 days).

Reprinted from Fleisher et al. (2007), with permission from Wolters Kluwer Health.

Step 3—Perioperative Risk of MACE—Clinical and Surgical Risk

Estimate the perioperative risk of MACE utilizing a risk estimator that combines both surgical and clinical risk parameters. Clinical risk factors associated with cardiac disease must be identified and assessed. A review of systems with attention to the cardiovascular system will identify associated conditions that can heighten the risk of anesthesia and may complicate cardiac management. The prevalence and adverse consequences of cardiovascular disease make it a prime consideration in the overview of systems. The most common clinical risk predictors associated with increased perioperative cardiovascular risk are listed in Table 4.10

TABLE 4.10 Clinical Predictors of Increased Perioperative Cardiovascular Risk

Mild angina pectoris
Prior myocardial infarction by history or pathologic Q waves
Compensated or prior congestive heart failure
Diabetes mellitus
Advanced age
Abnormal ECG
   Left ventricular hypertrophy
   Left bundle branch block
   ST-T abnormalities
Rhythm other than sinus
History of stroke
Uncontrolled systemic hypertension
Renal insufficiency

(Freeman & Gibbons, 2009). The probability of coronary heart disease varies with the type and number of risk factors present, the duration of the disease, and other associated end-stage organ dysfunction.

Cardiac risk is correlated to the surgical interventions depending on the magnitude, duration, location, blood loss, and intravascular fluid shifts related to the specific procedure (Mangano, 1990). Surgical procedures are classified low risk, intermediate risk, or high risk for the development of 30-day adverse cardiac outcome (Gupta et al., 2011). Large-scale studies have demonstrated low morbidity and mortality rates in superficial procedures performed on an ambulatory basis (Fleisher et al., 2014). In addition, studies have demonstrated that perioperative cardiac morbidity increases among patients who undergo major thoracic, abdominal, or vascular surgery. Therefore, to stratify cardiac risk in patients undergoing noncardiac surgery, knowledge of the risk related to particular surgical characteristics is important. A surgical procedure is considered low risk if the risk of a perioperative cardiac event is less than 1%, intermediate risk if the risk of a perioperative cardiac event is 1% to 5%, and high risk if the risk of a perioperative cardiac event is greater than 5% (Table 4.5). However, the most recent ACC/AHA 2014 guidelines acknowledge two risk categories for surgical procedures, low risk less than 1% and elevated risk equal to or greater than 1% for MACE (Fleisher et al., 2014).

Step 4—MACE Less Than 1%

If a determination is made that the patient has a low risk of MACE, then further testing in not indicated. As long as there are no further concerns, then the patient may proceed for the surgical procedure.

Step 5—MACE Equal to or Greater Than 1%, Evaluation of Functional Capacity

Cardiopulmonary fitness is determined by ascertaining exercise or work activity levels. An excellent exercise tolerance is defined as the ability to perform moderate exertion or exercise without symptoms of oxygen deprivation—dyspnea, chest pain, or fatigue. An excellent exercise tolerance suggests that the myocardium can be stressed without compromise. A poor exercise tolerance is defined as the reduced capacity for exercise or activity, due to symptomatic limitations. If a patient cannot walk a mile without becoming short of breath, the probability of critical coronary heart disease is high. Poor reported exercise tolerance, inability to walk four blocks or climb two flights of stairs, independently predicts an increased complication rate (Barash et al., 2013). Indeed, the likelihood of a serious adverse event has been inversely related to the number of blocks that can be walked. Estimated energy requirements for various activities can also be determined by ascertaining the METs of a task (Table 4.11). METs refer to a measure of the volume of oxygen consumed during an activity, and it has been demonstrated that the inability to perform average levels of exercise (4 to 5 METs) identifies a patient at risk for perioperative complications (Fisher et al., 2010). Functional capacity can be characterized as excellent, good, moderate, and poor at values greater than 10, 7 to 10, 4 to 6, or less than 4 METs, respectively (Fleisher et al., 2014).

TABLE 4.11 Estimated Energy Requirements for Various Activities

1 MET	Can you . . .	4 METs	Can you . . .
	Take care of yourself?		Climb a flight of stairs or walk up a hill?
	Eat, dress, or use the toilet?		Walk on level ground at 4 mph (6.4 kph)?
	Walk indoors around the house?		Run a short distance?
	Walk a block or two on level ground at 2 to 3 mph (3.2 to 4.8 kph)?		Do heavy work around the house such as scrubbing floors or lifting or moving heavy furniture?
4 METs	Do light work around the house such as dusting or washing dishes?		Participate in moderate recreational activities like golf, bowling, dancing, doubles tennis, or throwing a baseball or football?
		Greater than 10 METs	Participate in strenuous sports like swimming, singles tennis, football, basketball, or skiing?

kph, kilometers per hour; MET, metabolic equivalent; mph, miles per hour.

Reprinted from Fleisher et al. (2007), with permission from Wolters Kluwer Health.

Step 6—Less Than 4 METs or Unknown Functional Capacity, Evaluate Further Testing

For patients with poor or unknown functional capacity, determine if further testing is indicated, and how management strategies may change. Changes to the preoperative management strategy may include pharmaceutical management, coronary revascularization with coronary artery bypass surgery or percutaneous coronary intervention, or a decision to forgo the surgical intervention. Surgery may be replaced with alternative treatments including radiation or palliative care. In general, if further cardiac testing reveals a normal study, then the surgical process can move forward.

Step 7—Testing Does Not Impact Surgical Decision or Alternative Treatment Strategy

In other situations, further cardiac evaluation and testing do not impact the management decision. Therefore, the decision to proceed with surgery or an alternative treatments strategy, radiation or palliative services, can be determined without further diagnostic testing or interventions.

As discussed earlier, the best determinants of cardiac-related risk of mortality and morbidity for patients undergoing noncardiac surgery are the physical condition and risk factors of the patient, the risk associated with the planned surgical procedure, and the patient's functional capacity (Freeman & Gibbons, 2009). These models and strategies of preoperative evaluation are used to guide the clinician to initiate either medical treatments—such as statins, nitrates, and beta blockers—or preoperative stress or electrical testing and more invasive treatments—such as coronary revascularization—to reduce the risk for cardiac events. The risk profile may also address if surgery should be postponed to optimize medical treatment, perform coronary revascularization surgery, or recommend percutaneous coronary interventions.

CARDIOPULMONARY DIAGNOSTIC TESTING

Preoperative testing is dependent upon revelations discovered during the history and physical examination. Diagnostic testing is valuable in identifying coronary heart disease and the associated level of severity; however, testing must accompany a defined purpose by determining surgical risks and benefits or impacting patient management throughout the perioperative period. There are three primary categories of diagnostic testing for preoperative cardiac evaluation: cardiac testing, pulmonary testing, and laboratory tests.

Electrocardiography

When performed in conjunction with the history and physical examination, the ECG is valuable in detecting cardiac risk. The 12-lead ECG is noninvasive, rapid, inexpensive, and allows for longitudinal comparison of cardiac conduction over time. Q waves, S-T or T wave changes, and arrhythmias are suggestive of underlying cardiac disease. The ACC/AHA Task Force Committee on Electrocardiography has identified patient groups for which the ECG is indicated, including patients with: (1) known cardiovascular disease, (2) increased risk of developing cardiac dysfunction (diabetes mellitus, hypertension, males older than 45, females older than 55), and (3) no suspected heart disease, although the patient receives cardiotoxic medications (chemotherapeutics), or is employed in special occupations (fire fighter, police, pilot), or is a competitive athlete (Schlant et al., 1992). For patients who have no risk factors, and are scheduled for low-risk surgery, preoperative ECG is not indicated (Poldermans et al., 2009).

Echocardiogram

The anesthesia provider relies on the echocardiogram report completed within the last 12 months for information about valvular function, ventricular function, and the EF in patients with known cardiovascular abnormalities or those who are symptomatic. The echocardiogram is instrumental in identifying valvular abnormalities, valvular dimensions, ventricular thickness, cardiac structure, and left ventricular function. Patients with a new murmur, a murmur with worsening symptoms, moderate to severe aortic stenosis, documented cardiomyopathy, and prior valve replacement or repair with worsening symptoms should complete an echocardiogram prior to the scheduled surgery. Assessment of the ventricular wall motion at baseline and following exercise or pharmacologic stress (dobutamine) is useful to identify ischemic conditions (Kertai et al., 2003). Although these tests are not recommended for routine preoperative evaluation of left ventricular function for all patients, individuals scheduled for high-risk surgery, such as open abdominal aortic aneurysm repair, may benefit from this testing even when asymptomatic (Poldermans et al., 2009). Others who may benefit are those with a prior valve replacement who have not had testing within the past 5 years, or those with a murmur who have not had testing in the past 2 years (Freeman & Gibbons, 2009). When the echocardiogram results indicate an EF of less than 35%, there is a higher occurrence of myocardial infarction and death during the perioperative period (Kertai et al., 2003). The anesthesia provider will refer these patients to the cardiovascular team for evaluation before the scheduled surgical procedure. Also, patients diagnosed with severe aortic stenosis, an aortic valve area less than 1 cm², have a significantly increased risk of intraoperative death, and a cardiac consultation is sought prior to surgery (Goldman, 2013).

Exercise Stress Testing

During the preoperative patient interview and assessment, the anesthesia provider asks questions related to the patient's exercise ability and tolerance, and dyspnea or chest pain with minimal exertion raises a suspicion of coronary heart disease and ischemia. A significant determinant of perioperative risk is the inability to climb stairs, walk a mile, and do mild exercise without experiencing ischemic symptoms; these conditions are indicators for further testing. The exercise stress test is a cost-effective, noninvasive method of detecting coronary ischemia in patients with a suspicion of coronary heart disease. The test offers 70% to 80% sensitivity and 60% to 75% specificity for identification of ischemic heart disease (Kertai et al., 2003). Treadmill or bicycle exercise stress testing, along with blood pressure, heart rate, and ECG data analysis, is useful to identify the functional capacity for patients who are able to perform the test. For those who cannot (due to prior stroke, physical limitations, severe aortic stenosis, severe hypertension, heart failure, or endocarditis), pharmacologic echocardiography or radionuclide myocardial perfusion imaging may be appropriate. Both the ACC/AHA and the European Society of Cardiology (ESC) agree that stress testing is not useful for low-risk surgeries and in those who demonstrate high levels of exercise tolerance. In general, stress testing is considered when there are three or more risk factors in patients undergoing intermediate- to high-risk surgeries (Flu et al., 2010).

Cardiovascular Imaging

Magnetic resonance imaging, cardiac computed tomography, positron emission tomography, and single photon emission computed tomography are all indicated for the detection and characterization of coronary heart disease. These diagnostic tests are useful only if management strategies throughout the perioperative period are anticipated to change based on findings from the studies. Given that management is not likely to change for cardiac-stable patients undergoing low-risk surgeries, these tests are not indicated in this situation (Flu et al., 2010). Additionally, no conclusive data exists for intermediate-risk surgeries and testing must be individualized based on the patient status. In general, obtaining these diagnostic studies for those undergoing high-risk surgeries should be considered only if two or more risk factors are present (Poldermans et al., 2009).

Cardiac Catheterization—Coronary Angiogram

The coronary angiogram provides very detailed and accurate information about the coronary artery anatomy, ventricular function, and valvular function. This highly invasive test is generally reserved for patients with prior inconclusive noninvasive studies or those undergoing cardiac surgery. Evaluation for extensive left main coronary artery disease is important, as a 50% or greater occlusion in this vessel yields an intraoperative mortality rate of 15% (Kerati et al., 2013). Cardiac catheterization is valuable for patients undergoing coronary artery bypass graft or valvular surgery, although for noncardiac surgery, alternative tests that provide additional functional information are recommended initially (Kertai et al., 2003).

Chest Radiograph

In general, routine preoperative chest radiographs are not indicated unless there is an indication or suspicion of underlying lung disease. A meta-analysis of the value of routine preoperative chest x-rays was conducted for a 26-year span, and it was concluded that abnormalities were reported in 10% of routine x-rays, although only 1.3% of the x-rays revealed unexpected abnormalities (Archer, Levy, & McGregor, 1993). Signs such as shortness of breath, continuous cough, abnormal findings on auscultation, or values of 90% or below on pulse oximetry are indicators for chest x-rays. In conjunction with symptoms, the chest x-ray may be useful for care-management decisions when pneumonia, pulmonary masses, or pulmonary edema are identified. Also, there is some benefit to obtaining the information provided from a chest x-ray in patients with chronic obstructive lung disease or heart failure; in patients who have a history of smoking; and in those older than 50 years of age scheduled for upper abdominal, thoracic, or aneurysm repair (Qaseem et al., 2006).

Pulmonary-Function Testing

The current standard anesthesia monitoring of pulse oximetry and end-tidal carbon dioxide waveform used throughout the intraoperative phase have almost eliminated the necessity for routine pulmonary-function testing. There is no evidence to support pulmonary-function testing in asymptomatic patients, and thus it is reserved only for those with preexisting pulmonary disease. Spirometry may be indicated in the presence of chronic obstructive lung diseases, difficulty breathing, or productive cough (Johansson et al., 2013). Forced expiratory volume in 1 second (FEV_1) values equal to or less than 1 are indicative of a potential for postoperative complications and warrant further evaluation. Overall, the single best strategy to reduce the perioperative pulmonary risks for the patient is to advise discontinuation of smoking. A meta-analysis of smoking cessation was conducted and the authors confirmed that terms of cessation longer than 4 weeks resulted in a relative risk decrease of postoperative complications by 20% (Mills et al., 2011).

Laboratory Testing

A review of the evidence indicates that there is no rationale to support routine laboratory testing in asymptomatic patients, particularly those patients undergoing low-risk surgical procedures (Johansson et al., 2013). Therefore, laboratory testing is indicated only in patients with known or suspected disease processes, and to determine pregnancy status in women of childbearing age.

Complete Blood Count

A complete blood count (CBC) is recommended for patients with conditions that are associated with high probabilities of infection or anemia, and those scheduled for surgery with a significant anticipated blood loss. Anemia results in decreased oxygen delivery to the tissues as a result of associated reductions in arterial oxygen content. There have been many attempts to define anemia, and most rely on the World Health Organization's 40-year-old definition. More recently, in an effort to identify the lower limit of acceptable hemoglobin, Beutler and Waalen (2006) based suggestions on improved laboratory practices. These authors suggest the lower limits of 13.7 g/dL for White males ages 20 to 59, 13.2 g/dL for White males age 60 and older, 12.9 g/dL for Black males ages 20 to 59, 12.7 g/dL for Black males 60 and older, 12.2 g/dL for all White females, and 11.5 g/dL for all Black females.

Chronic conditions associated with anemia include renal, hematologic, hepatic, and inflammatory diseases. Additionally, anemia may result from treatment of malignancies with chemotherapeutic agents and radiation. In high blood-loss surgery, the CBC can guide the calculation of acceptable blood loss and the determination of transfusion requirements, and should accompany a type and cross (Feely et al., 2013). The American Association of Blood Banks developed a guideline in 2012 to provide recommendations for red blood cell transfusion (Carson et al., 2012). Recommendations from this guideline include the adherence of a restrictive strategy for transfusion with preexisting cardiovascular disease, and to consider transfusion for symptoms or for a hemoglobin level equal to or less than 8 g/dL (Carson et al., 2012).

The physiologic compensatory mechanisms associated with anemia include a right shift of the oxygen-hemoglobin dissociation curve and increased cardiac output. For elective procedures, the anesthesia provider prefers the values to be above the lower limits of acceptable hemoglobin levels to facilitate appropriate oxygen delivery, as drug-induced effects may interfere with these compensatory mechanisms. Wu et al. (2007) reported mild levels of anemia to be associated with postoperative morbidity and mortality in older adults undergoing noncardiac surgery.

Serum Chemistry

Preoperative alterations of fluid and electrolyte homeostasis are associated with neurologic, cardiac, and muscular disturbances; therefore, it is essential to identify and evaluate any alterations. Patients with a history of diabetes, or renal or hepatic diseases, are candidates for evaluation of electrolytes, renal function, liver function, albumin, and glucose measurement. Another indicator for performing serum chemistry testing is medication administration that may alter homeostasis, for example, diuretics, corticosteroids, digoxin, and angiotensin-acting medications.

Sodium is the ion with the highest concentration (135–145 mEq/L) in the extracellular fluid, which makes up one third (15 liters) of the total body fluid (Grocott, Mythen, & Gan, 2005; Lobo, Macafee, & Allison, 2006). When the condition of hyponatremia exists, there is movement of water into the cerebrospinal fluid, and cerebral edema occurs. These events are often a result of hypotonicity; thus, in this condition, the anesthesia provider avoids routine fluid replacement with an isotonic solution of D_5W, as the glucose is rapidly metabolized and free water is distributed.

Alterations in potassium levels are often related to changes in renal function and diuretic administration. Potassium is mostly an intracellular ion with a primary role in cell polarization and electrical impulse transmission. Wahr et al. (1999) reported that hypokalemia (< 3.5 mmol/L) is a predictor of perioperative arrhythmias, and suggest that surgery be delayed until low potassium levels are reversed. Hyperkalemia has been associated with life-threatening cardiac arrhythmias when the potassium level is greater than 7.0 mmol/L (Wahr et al., 1999). Therefore, the use of potassium containing intravenous fluids, such as Ringer's lactate, is avoided in conditions of hyperkalemia. Also, anesthesia providers prefer to anesthetize patients with renal failure–induced hyperkalemia after dialysis to avoid serum potassium levels above 6.0 mmol/L.

A decrease in ionized calcium is a matter of concern, as this condition has the potential to lead to neuromuscular and cardiovascular alterations. These alterations include seizures, laryngospasm, ECG changes (prolonged Q-T interval), and hypotension. Hypocalcemia is further exacerbated by metabolic or respiratory alkalosis; thus, administration of a bicarbonate or hyperventilation will aggravate the condition and is avoided. Often low calcium levels are associated with reduced albumin and magnesium levels; therefore, it is important to assess albumin levels, as many anesthetic drugs are protein bound, and increased amounts of free drug are available with low albumin values (<3.9 g/dL).

Frisch et al. (2010) reported that hyperglycemia is associated with poor clinical outcomes in patients who undergo noncardiac surgery. Diabetic patients should be managed to optimize serum glucose and glycated hemoglobin values to ensure the best outcomes. The anesthesia provider routinely evaluates blood glucose levels in all diabetics preoperatively, throughout the anesthetic, and in the postoperative phase. Insulin is administered in cases of hyperglycemia, with a glucose-containing solution initiated as an intravenous infusion; this is done as a precaution against hypoglycemia.

Urinalysis

Urinalysis has little benefit for the preparation of patient management for anesthetics and surgery. A urinalysis identifies protein, glucose, leukocytes, or blood in the urine for the purpose of identifying urinary tract or renal disease. Serum electrolytes, creatinine clearance, and serum glucose values are more informative for the evaluation of renal function, fluid and electrolyte balance, and diabetes. Therefore, urinalysis is primarily indicated for patients undergoing prosthetic joint replacement, cardiac valve replacement, or urologic procedures (Feely et al., 2013).

Liver Function Tests/Coagulation Studies

Liver enzyme tests are indicated in the presence of alcoholism, hepatitis exposure, statin medications, and chronic liver disease. Additionally, the international normalized ratio (INR), prothrombin time (PT), albumin, and bilirubin levels should be assessed in these conditions. In addition to patients with liver disease, those patients on anticoagulant medications, or who have a history of bleeding, coagulation disorder, or family history of coagulopathy, should have coagulation-related testing such as PT, partial thromboplastin time (PTT), and platelet count. The goals of testing are to avoid any further injury to the liver with anesthetic agents and to correct any abnormalities that can be addressed by administering colloid solutions and blood products (Grocott et al., 2005).

B-Type Natriuretic Peptide

B-type natriuretic peptide (BNP) levels are useful in identifying individuals with heart failure and in evaluating patients at low risk for cardiac morbidity and mortality after major surgery with heart failure symptoms. Currently, BNP equal to or greater than 108.5 pg/mL has been deemed the optimal cutoff for prediction of cardiac events with 87% sensitivity, 87% specificity, 42% positive predictive value, and 98% negative predictive value (Goldman, 2013).

PERIOPERATIVE MANAGEMENT

There are four main classifications of anesthesia: (1) local; (2) regional, including peripheral nerve and neuraxial blockade, spinal, and epidural; (3) monitored, intravenous sedation with or without local anesthesia; and (4) general with volatile agents, total intravenous, or a combination of both. The selection of anesthesia agents is highly dependent on the surgical procedure, length of the procedure, and individual patient factors, including previous anesthesia experience, overall health, functional status, medications, and the presence of chronic disease.

Beta adrenergic receptor blockers (beta blockers), nitrates, statin agents, alpha-2 agonists, calcium channel blockers, and anticoagulants are commonly prescribed pharmacologic agents in patients with cardiovascular disease, and are often employed during the perioperative period. The 2014 ACC/AHA recommendations (Class IB) include the continuation of beta blockers preoperatively in patients who are chronically prescribed those medications. In addition, beta blockers are recommended preoperatively for patients scheduled for vascular surgery in which ischemic heart disease was discovered with preoperative testing. Class IIb recommendations included those patients identified with intermediate or high-risk preoperative testing, equal to or greater than three RCRI factors, or long-term indications for beta blockade therapy (Fleisher et al., 2014). This practice was proposed to decrease the incidence of perioperative myocardial ischemia and mortality associated with myocardial infarction in high-risk patients (Fleischmann et al., 2009). However, in 2008, the Poise trial demonstrated that while beta blockade did afford some myocardial protection, there were other risks associated with perioperative administration of a long-acting beta blocker, metoprolol. The metoprolol group experienced a significant incidence of stroke and increased risk of death (Devereaux et al., 2008). The current recommendation for beta blockade is to continue treatment in the perioperative period for patients receiving therapy for angina, symptomatic arrhythmia, or hypertension. Otherwise, risk factors, surgical procedure, and clinical judgment should be used when determining if beta blockade is appropriate, and if so, should be titrated to heart rate and blood pressure (Fleischmann et al., 2009). In general, beta blockers should not be started on the day of surgery (Fleisher et al., 2014).

Alpha-2 agonists have also demonstrated some myocardial protection during the perioperative period (Wijeysundera, Naik, & Beattie, 2003). Clonidine administered during the perioperative period in patients at risk for or who have coronary heart disease resulted in a decrease in myocardial ischemia and postoperative mortality related to heart disease. However, for the prevention of cardiac events, alpha-2 agonists are not currently recommended (Fleisher et al., 2014).

A published meta-analysis of perioperative calcium channel blockers in noncardiac surgery indicated a significant reduction in ischemia and supraventricular tachycardia as well as reduced myocardial infarct and death (Stevens et al., 2003). The calcium channel blocker diltiazem demonstrated the most impressive results, although large-scale trials were recommended to reinforce the findings (Fleisher et al., 2014).

The current recommendation for statin therapy is for continuation throughout the perioperative period for patients who are chronically prescribed a statin (IB), and to consider prescribing a statin for vascular surgery patients (IIA) or for patients with one clinical risk factor scheduled for an intermediate-risk surgery (Fleisher et al., 2014; Lindenauer, Pekow, Wang, Gutierrez, & Benjamin, 2004). The pharmacologic actions of these drugs indicate they may reduce the incidence of cardiovascular events (Fleisher et al., 2014).

The management of antiplatelet therapy requires consideration from the entire team of clinicians, with the challenges of recent coronary stenting particularly difficult. Low-dose aspirin therapy for patients undergoing elective noncardiac surgery does not require discontinuation prior to surgery (Burger, Chemnitius, Kneissl, & Rucker, 2005). The current recommendation is to evaluate if the continuation of aspirin carries an associated surgical bleeding risk similar to or worse than the cardiovascular risks of discontinuing use; if so, consideration is made for withholding aspirin prior to surgery. For noncardiac vascular surgery, preoperative aspirin is a drug of choice and has demonstrated improved peripheral bypass graft patency (Fleisher et al., 2014). Aspirin use prior to cardiac surgery is associated with more blood loss and risk for reoperation, but not an increase in mortality. However, the benefit of aspirin therapy is improved saphenous vein-graft patency and the prevention of early thrombotic closure (Fleisher et al., 2014). Conversely, there is currently minimal data available for the risk or benefit of using aspirin perioperatively in patients scheduled for other types of noncardiovascular surgical procedures (Burger, Chemnitius, Kneissl, & Rucker, 2005). Mono antiplatelet therapy with a thienopyridine, such as clopidogrel, may be continued prior to elective noncardiac surgery; however, there are no conclusive studies to determine the bleeding risk associated with its preoperative use. Indeed, according to ACC/AHA recommendations, clopidogrel should be discontinued 7 days prior to elective coronary bypass surgery (Fleisher et al., 2014). In all instances, the risk–benefit ratio of withholding the antiplatelet therapy should be considered in light of the surgical procedure and the patient's medical condition.

Information amassed during the preoperative evaluation, combined with the physical assessment, diagnostic testing, and pharmacologic regimen, is vital to ensure the best patient outcomes. These evaluations provide a foundation for targeted interview questions about the patient's current state of health or illness and assist the health care team in the development of the presurgical and surgical plan of care. Anesthesia technique, fluid therapy, and choice of anesthetic agents are based on the patient's condition as explored during the preoperative phase. Examples of decisions based on preoperative evaluations include the patient on anticoagulant therapy or aortic stenosis that precludes the administration of a subarachnoid block, or a patient receiving ACEI that may require vasoactive infusions to manage hypotension intraoperatively. Further, potential complications can be anticipated as a direct result of the preoperative evaluation and prevented by appropriate intraoperative and postoperative management.

Anesthesia providers collaborate with clinicians, cardiovascular specialists, and surgeons to determine the best approach to safely care for the patients undergoing surgery. Perioperative management of the cardiac patient for noncardiac surgery requires a collaborative approach in directing assessment and optimizing care. These evaluations also allow for case management discussions to occur between the anesthesia practitioner and the surgeon to consider decreasing the need for opioids through the use of nonsteroidal anti-inflammatory agents, utilizing local anesthesia or a regional anesthetic, as well as evaluating the safety of performing surgeries as an outpatient. Patient outcomes can be vastly improved by utilizing appropriate tools to achieve an understanding of surgical risk and by developing a balance between preoperative testing and prudent decision making. The goal of this chapter was to set forth some parameters that practitioners may utilize in assessing the cardiac status of a patient undergoing noncardiac surgical procedures.

For full reference citations to this chapter, please see "Section References" in the back of the book, under the heading "Section I."

Chronic Cardiovascular Conditions

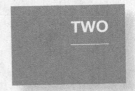
TWO

Hypertension

JOHN N. MERIWETHER AND DOROTHY L. MURPHY

Hypertension is a disease of vascular tone that has been identified as a significant risk factor for many diseases, including atherosclerosis, nonischemic cardiomyopathies, and cerebrovascular disease (Go et al., 2013). Hypertension occurs in approximately 28% of all Americans (Go et al., 2013) with a prevalence pattern that increases by age—with few individuals younger than 30 years affected by the disease, compared with 67% of all people older than 60 years with hypertension (Go et al., 2013). Men are affected slightly more than women (29.4%:27.5%). Ethnicity plays a significant role in hypertension in the United States. People who describe themselves as of African American descent have a prevalence rate of hypertension of 40.4%, whereas the rate is approximately 27% for White and Hispanic identifying people (Go et al., 2014). Unfortunately, even after identification of hypertension, a majority of the hypertensive population remain without adequate blood pressure (BP) control. For those individuals older than 40 years, only 50% of hypertension is controlled. Control is better among women than men, and White than Black or Hispanic patients (Go et al., 2013). Given the prevalence of hypertension and adverse outcomes from lack of control, the magnitude of effect in controlling hypertension may be great.

CLASSIFICATIONS

Hypertension may be of primary or secondary etiology. Primary hypertension, which may also be termed essential hypertension, is the most common etiology of hypertension, accounting for 90% of all hypertension diagnoses (Go et al., 2013). Historically, there has been no single identifiable cause of primary hypertension; however, a genetic basis is accepted. The search for a genetic etiology is fueled by studies indicating trends for hypertension both within families as well as between identical twins as compared with other siblings (Cui, Hopper, & Harrap, 2002). Many alleles have been discovered to date that contribute to hypertension. Individually, the alleles contribute little to hypertension, though multiple alleles together have a more prominent effect (Franceschini & Le, 2014). In the future, antihypertensive treatment may be tailored to an individual's genetic profile. Secondary hypertension occurs in approximately 10% of all hypertension diagnoses, with 3% to 5% attributed to renal disease (Go et al., 2013). Secondary causes are often correctable and are the result of disorders such as chronic kidney disease, renovascular disease, primary aldosteronism, coarctation of the aorta, Cushing's syndrome, pheochromocytoma, hyperthyroidism, and obstructive sleep apnea.

STAGES OF HYPERTENSION

The American Heart Association (AHA) defines normal BP as arterial pressure less than 119/79 mmHg (Pickering et al., 2005). Prehypertension is the range of BP between 120 and 139 mmHg systolic and 80 to 90 mmHg diastolic. Stage 1 hypertension is 140 to 159 mmHg systolic and 90 to 99 mmHg diastolic. Stage 2 hypertension is greater than 160 mmHg systolic and greater than 100 mmHg diastolic. Emergency or urgent treatment is generally recommended for BP greater than 180 mmHg systolic or diastolic greater than 110 mmHg. The distinctions just mentioned are relevant in the discussion of treatment for hypertension.

In the setting of severe elevations in BP over 180/110 mmHg, hypertensive urgency and hypertension emergency will be diagnosed. Without signs of end organ damage, blood pressures in this range constitute hypertensive urgency. Hypertensive emergency occurs when elevated blood pressures cause end organ damage, chest pain, cardiac protein elevation, acute renal failure, or neurologic disturbance. While hypertensive urgency may be managed in the clinic, referral to an emergency department or hospital admission is the best management for hypertensive emergencies.

PATHOPHYSIOLOGY

BP is regulated through systematic mechanisms that vary in location of action and duration of effect. Understanding these mechanisms is necessary to understand the evaluation and treatment of hypertension. Disruptions or overactivation of any pathway may result in BP dysregulation. Chronic hypertension results in end organ damage, causing increased morbidity and mortality.

Chemoreceptors and baroreceptors located in vasculature and the midbrain can regulate BP within seconds. Chemoreceptors monitor oxygen and carbon dioxide. When arterial O_2 content decreases and CO_2 content increases, chemoreceptors increase ventilation and sympathetic activation. Baroreceptors monitor BP. When BP changes, baroreceptors respond with the sympathetic nervous system and vagal tone, resulting in BP and heart rate adjustments.

The kidneys regulate BP more slowly, through sodium and water regulation, which occurs over days or weeks. Water is reabsorbed due to increased solute gradients, increasing intravascular volume. Chronic elevated sodium levels will also cause fluid retention to preserve serum osmolality at 275 to 295 mOsm/kg. The renin-angiotensin system is a significant regulator of systemic BP. Renal perfusion and arterial sodium concentration signals the juxtaglomerular apparatus to release renin. Renin cleaves angiotensin I, mainly from the lungs, enabling angiotensin-converting enzyme (ACE) to create angiotensin II. Angiotensin II has direct effects on vasculature and indirect effects through the release of vasoactive proteins, resulting in vasoconstriction. Sodium retention is increased through the effects of angiotensin II and adrenal steroids, cortisol, and aldosterone, among other pathways.

The adrenergic system affects the heart and vasculature. Beta-1 receptor stimulation results in increased cardiac inotropy and chronotropy. Beta-2 activation results in smooth muscle relaxation, notably bronchial and arterial. Alpha-2 activation results in vasoconstriction.

Age has a significant effect on BP. With increasing age, arteries lose elasticity. Central loss of elasticity results in an elevated systolic pressure; loss of elasticity in central and peripheral arteries results in systolic and diastolic hypertension. Drugs affecting the nitric oxide pathway may help improve arterial compliance and reduce BP.

COMPLICATIONS OF HYPERTENSION

Long-standing, uncontrolled hypertension can cause system-wide end organ damage. The direct consequences of uncontrolled hypertension on the cardiac system include left ventricular hypertrophy, diastolic dysfunction, accelerated coronary heart disease (CHD), myocardial ischemia, and heart failure. Hypertension may also cause cerebrovascular, ophthalmologic, and renal disease.

CLINICAL PRESENTATION

Hypertension is known as the "silent killer" because there are often no signs or symptoms. Any symptoms are usually due to effects of hypertension on target end organs, including renal disease, heart failure, or stroke. In times of acutely elevated BP, the presenting complaint may include headache, chest pain, or fatigue.

PHYSICAL EXAMINATION

Individuals with hypertension presenting for the initial office visit should have a thorough physical examination. Findings will both direct the etiology of elevated BP and identify sequelae of elevated BP over time. BP measurement should be obtained a minimum of twice, taken at least 1 minute apart (Pickering et al., 2005). BP should be checked with an appropriately sized, manual calibrated sphygmomanometer in both arms to detect discrepancy, which may be related to aortic coarctation or dissection. The patient should be seated with uncrossed legs for 5 minutes before obtaining BP readings. Ophthalmoscopy may detect thickening of the retinal arteries, causing a red-brown discoloration, "copper-wiring," and compression of veins where crossed by arteries, "arteriovenous (AV) nicking." The delicate arteries may break under elevated systemic pressure, resulting in "flame hemorrhages." The neck should be examined for elevated jugular venous pressure resulting in a distended internal jugular vein noticeable above the clavicle, known as JVD (jugular venous distention). As hypertension is a known risk factor for atherosclerosis, the carotid arteries should be auscultated for carotid bruits. Chest examination includes palpation of the chest wall for a precordial heave associated with an enlarged right ventricle, as well as the point of maximal impulse (PMI). A wide or inferolaterally displaced PMI may indicate a dilated left ventricle. An S_4 gallop would indicate a poorly compliant left ventricle due to a thickened left ventricular wall. Peripheral pulses should be checked in all extremities; as with BP measurement, discrepancy of the pulses may be related to aortic coarctation, subclavian steal, or dissection. Additionally diminished pulses may be a result of peripheral atherosclerotic disease (PAD). PAD is most notable in the lower extremities and may be associated with loss of hair and a history of claudication.

DIAGNOSTIC TESTING

Laboratory

Initial laboratory evaluation for an individual with hypertension aims to assess for sequelae of hypertension, co-morbidities that may guide management, and, if suspected, secondary causes. For individuals with benign essential hypertension, laboratory evaluation may include electrolytes, renal function, magnesium, thyroid-stimulating hormone (TSH), glycated hemoglobin, and lipid profile. A basic metabolic profile will provide information on renal function, as well as electrolyte abnormalities that may suggest chronic kidney disease, hyperaldosteronism, or hypercortisolism. A TSH evaluates for hyperthyroidism, a common secondary cause of hypertension. Evaluating for diabetes is important, as management of hypertension may be influenced by this co-morbidity. As hypertension is a risk factor for atherosclerosis, measuring lipids allows for risk stratification and prevention.

Ambulatory Monitoring

Ambulatory BP monitoring may be indicated for suspected "white coat" hypertension when there is a discrepancy between self-measurement and clinical examination. Ambulatory monitoring is also useful for the evaluation of episodic hypotension, refractory hypertension, or for monitoring treatment.

Self-Measurement

Electronic home self-measurement and recording may provide helpful assistance for the cardiovascular clinician when determining an antihypertensive treatment plan. BP home monitors should be validated. Patients should be instructed on the proper position and timing to obtain an accurate reading.

SECONDARY HYPERTENSION

Should secondary sources of hypertension be suspected, additional laboratory or imaging modalities will be required. Table 5.1 provides an overview of common secondary causes of hypertension, along with clinical clues and diagnostic testing that may be appropriate.

TABLE 5.1 Common Causes of Secondary Hypertension, Clinical Findings, and Diagnostic Testing

Suspected Diagnosis	Clinical Findings	Diagnostic Testing
Chronic kidney disease	Estimated GFR < 60 mL/min/1.73 m^2 Urine albumin-to-creatinine ratio ≥ 30 mg/g	Renal sonography
Renovascular disease	New elevation in serum creatinine, marked elevation in serum creatinine with ACEI or ARB, drug-resistant hypertension, flash pulmonary edema, abdominal or flank bruit	Renal sonography (atrophic kidney), CT or MR angiography, invasive angiography
Coarctation of the aorta	Arm pulses > leg pulses, arm BP > leg BP, chest bruits, rib notching on chest radiography	MR angiography, TEE, invasive angiography
Primary aldosteronism	Hypokalemia, drug-resistant hypertension	Plasma renin and aldosterone, 24-hr urine aldosterone and potassium after oral salt loading, adrenal vein sampling
Cushing's syndrome	Truncal obesity, wide and blanching purple striae, muscle weakness	1 mg dexamethasone-suppression test, urinary cortisol after dexamethasone, adrenal CT
Pheochromocytoma	Paroxysms of hypertension, palpitations, perspiration, and pallor; diabetes	Plasma metanephrines, 24-hr urinary metanephrines and catecholamines, abdominal CT or MR imaging
Obstructive sleep apnea	Loud snoring, large neck, obesity, somnolence	Polysonography

ACEI, angiotensin-converting enzyme inhibitors; ARB, angiotensin receptor blockers; BP, blood pressure; CT, computed tomography; GFR, glomerular filtration rate; MR, magnetic resonance; TEE, transesophageal echocardiogram.

Source: Victor (2012).

DIAGNOSIS OF HYPERTENSION

The diagnosis of hypertension is commonly established upon the results of two BP recordings equal to or greater than 140/90 mmHg on two separate visits. The European Society of Hypertension and the European Society of Cardiology (ESH/ESC) recommend that at least two interval BP readings on two separate visits be used to accurately diagnose hypertension (Mancia et al., 2013). If an individual presents with hypertensive urgency or emergency, diagnosis is confirmed.

THERAPEUTIC MANAGEMENT OF HYPERTENSION

The Eighth Joint National Commission recently revised the guidelines regarding medical therapy for hypertension (James et al., 2014). Initiation of an antihypertensive regimen is dictated by both age and comorbid illness. Goals for generally healthy patients younger than the age of 60 have been established on the basis of expert opinion. For patients younger than 60 years, treatment should be initiated at 140 mmHg systolic or 90 mmHg diastolic; for patients older than 60 the systolic is higher at 150/90 mmHg, as these values are consistent with the reduction of cardio- and cerebrovascular disease (James et al., 2014). Should a patient older than the age of 60 have BP controlled to below 140/90 mmHg without any adverse effect, then treatment may continue without changes (James et al., 2014).

Lifestyle Modifications

Therapeutic diet and lifestyle changes can significantly lower BP. A 1- to 2-month trial of dietary and lifestyle modification should be the initial choice of management in newly diagnosed Stage 1 hypertension. Lifestyle modification will include dietary changes, exercise, tobacco cessation, and alcohol moderation. Reduction in dietary sodium has repeatedly been validated with improvements in BP.

The PREMIER Trial demonstrated that diet and lifestyle changes as described earlier are attainable and result in continued BP reduction over 18 months (Appel et al., 2003). Reduction was most marked in patients that made diet and exercise modifications over exercise alone. These results signify the imperative nature of addressing diet and lifestyle modification early in hypertension management and readdressing at each clinic visit.

Dietary Modifications

Major sources of sodium in the American diet include canned foods, preprepared meals, foods from most restaurants, and salt added to meals. A meta-analysis of randomized trials evaluating the effects of daily sodium intake showed that reducing salt intake reduced BP by an average of 3.39/1.54 mmHg (He, Li, & Macgregor, 2013). The Cochrane Review further validated a diet under 2 gm compared with over 2 gm reduced BP by 3.47/1.81 mmHg. The effect of salt reduction on hypertension has a greater effect for the elderly and those of African American heritage.

The Dietary Approaches to Stop Hypertension (DASH) eating plan to reduce BP recommends low salt consumption. This diet recommends, in specified weekly amounts for either 1,600 or 2,000 kCal diets and the following changes over the average American diet: increased fruits, vegetables, nuts, and grains; limiting red meats while increasing fish and poultry; and limiting sweets. The main difference between the DASH and Mediterranean diet is in the recommendations for the latter to include olive oil and a moderate consumption of red wine. Importantly, the effects of the DASH diet are independent of a low-salt diet and are augmented by a low-salt diet—though the effects are not fully additive.

Physical Activity

In addition to diet changes, exercise is key to improving hypertension. Aerobic exercise may reduce BP by 3.84/2.58 mmHg as shown in a meta-analysis of 54 trials (Whelton, Chin, Xin, & He, 2002). The magnitude of BP reduction increased with total weekly exercise duration. Interestingly, there was no difference in BP reduction between exercise vigor (low, moderate, or intense). One effect of diet and exercise changes is weight loss. The reduction in BP with weight loss is independent of the weight loss strategy pursued. Obesity may lead to obstructive sleep apnea, another well-known cause of hypertension.

Tobacco Cessation

Smoking raises BP and heart rate, reduces the effect of beta blockers, and is an independent risk factor for cardiovascular disease beyond hypertensive effects. Smoking increases all-cause mortality in the hypertensive patient (Huynh et al., 2014). Patients should be counseled on cessation at every patient encounter.

Alcohol Moderation

Alcohol abuse should be assessed at every visit. The JNC-7 guidelines allow for two drinks per day in men and one drink per day for women. A drink is classified as 12 ounces of beer, 1.5 ounces of distilled liquor (at 80 proof), or 4 to 5 ounces of wine. Alcohol consumption raises BP immediately, and daily alcohol use raises BP chronically.

PHARMACOLOGIC THERAPY

The medication choice will depend on age and comorbid illness; additionally, patient ethnicity is a factor in medication selection. Chapter 29 details the pharmacotherapeutics of hypertension. Previous guidelines dictated initiation with a one-drug regimen for reductions in BP of 20/10 mmHg or less. With a requirement for greater reduction, BP at or over 160/100 mmHg, a two-drug regimen is necessary, as it is unlikely a single medication will achieve the required reduction.

First-line treatment of hypertension in the non-Black population may include thiazide diuretics, calcium channel blockers (CCBs), angiotensin-converting enzyme inhibitors (ACEI), or angiotensin receptor blockers (ARB). Beta adrenergic blocking agents (beta blockers) are listed as second line, as a randomized controlled trial demonstrated a reduction in stroke with an ARB compared with a beta-blocking medication. For Black patients, thiazide diuretics and CCBs are first-line therapy, not ACEI, as per the Antihypertensive and Lipid-Lowering Treatment to Prevent Heart Attack (ALLHAT), ACEI in Black patients are both less effective and carry a higher risk of stroke (ALLHAT, 2002). The current JNC-8 recommendations did change first-line therapy for diabetic patients, as outcomes in relation to cerebral and cardiovascular diseases were similar to nondiabetic patients. Note, however, the American Diabetes Association recommends initiation of BP-lowering medications with ACEI for the renal protective effects.

Thiazide Diuretics

Thiazide diuretics include both hydrochlorothiazide (HCTZ) and chlorthalidone. The ALLHAT trial that demonstrated benefit with thiazide diuretics used chlorthalidone (2002). Currently, there is a movement to switch to chlorthalidone over HCTZ in clinical practice, as chlorthalidone has a more potent antihypertensive effect than HCTZ.

Calcium Channel Blockers

For CCBs, the distinction between dihydropyridines and nondihydropyridines is important. The dihydropyridines, amlodipine, and nifedipine, have more potent antihypertensive effects and less arteriovenous nodal blocking agents than the non-dihydropyridines, verapamil and diltiazem. The former are primarily prescribed for BP, and the latter are mainly for tachyarrhythmias. An important common side effect of CCBs is peripheral edema, which may be severe enough to require cessation of the medication.

Beta Adrenergic Blockers

There are many beta adrenergic blocking medications, and this class of medications is heterogeneous with variable effects on beta receptors and alpha receptors. This distinction is important when selecting medications based upon the antihypertensive and the nodal blocking effects. Two commonly prescribed beta blockers are carvedilol and metoprolol. Carvedilol has alpha blocking capability and is an appropriate selection with concomitant heart failure. Metoprolol has minimal alpha blocking effect and more consequence as a nodal blocking agent; therefore, it is prescribed for supraventricular arrhythmias frequently. Beta blockers should be used cautiously in patients with chronic lung diseases such as chronic obstructive lung disease and asthma, because they may induce exacerbations or counteract treatment with beta-agonist bronchodilators.

Angiotensin-Converting Enzyme Inhibitors

ACEI reduce the conversion of angiotensin I to angiotensin II. Angiotensin II is a potent vasoconstrictor and, by blocking the conversion to angiotensin II, vasoconstriction is prevented, thereby lowering BP. ACEI are used especially in patients with diabetes to reduce diabetic nephropathy. Core measures also dictate all patients with heart failure with reduced systolic function are prescribed ACEI for effects on remodeling. A class side effect is cough and angioedema, which will necessitate the immediate discontinuation of the medication. Patients may be trialed on an ARB as only 0.9% to 2% of patients with ACE-induced angioedema will have recurrence with ARB.

Angiotensin Receptor Blockers

ARBs prevent vasoconstriction by blocking the binding of angiotensin II to the angiotensin II receptors in the blood vessels. Reducing the activity of angiotensin II on the blood vessels allows for vasodilation and reduces BP. Individuals who are intolerant of ACEI due to cough are likely to tolerate ARBs without adverse effects. Individuals with a history of angioedema with an ACEI may be safely switched to an ARB.

FOLLOW-UP

The JNC-7 recommends that individuals with hypertension be evaluated for adequate control every month until the BP is at goal. Once BP is at goal, follow-up typically occurs every 6 months. Individuals prescribed diuretics, ACEI, and/or ARBs should have BUN, creatinine, and GFR checked upon follow-up. If a diuretic, ACEI, or ARB is selected for hypertension management for individuals with renal dysfunction, a basic metabolic panel should be obtained within 1 week of initiating the medication (Joint National Committee [JNC], 2003).

REFERRAL

Despite the best efforts, hypertension may not be easily controlled. Hypertension uncontrolled by three medications is termed resistant hypertension. Referral is necessary once a patient has been maximized on three medications without attaining control. Referral is also warranted for patients with secondary causes of hypertension; these may be to nephrology, endocrinology, or surgery as indicated.

For full reference citations to this chapter, please see "Section References" in the back of the book, under the heading "Section II."

6

Lipid Metabolism Disorders

JOHN N. MERIWETHER AND DOROTHY L. MURPHY

The prevalence of hypercholesterolemia, defined by a total cholesterol value of over 240 mg/dL, among adults in the United States is almost 14% (Go et al., 2014). Prevalence of elevated low-density lipoproteins (LDL) greater than 190 mg/dL is even more excessive at 38% of U.S. adults (Muntner et al., 2013). More significantly, patients most at risk for cardiovascular disease (CVD) often have poor control of hypercholesterolemia. In examining National Health and Nutrition Examination Survey (NHANES) results, Egan, Qanugo, and Wolfman (2014) report 60% of hypertensive patients have concomitant hypercholesterolemia of LDL by ATP (Adult Treatment Panel) III guidelines; however, only half of these patients are undergoing treatment. Furthermore, control was attained in only half of these patients. In updating the Million Hearts initiative, Ritchy, Wall, Gillespie, George, and Jamal (2014) also reviewed the NHANES. These researchers noted that patients younger than 45 years are less likely to control CVD risk factors, including high cholesterol. Individuals with two or more CVD risk factors by the age of 50 have a tenfold higher risk for atherosclerosis (Ritchy et al., 2014).

High total cholesterol and LDL cholesterol levels are contributors to atherosclerosis. In addition to protein and triglyceride, lipoproteins are more than 50% cholesterol, containing approximately 70% of total body cholesterol (Nauck, Warnick, & Rifai, 2002). LDL transports cholesterol from the liver to the peripheral tissue, including the coronary vasculature. As LDL delivers cholesterol to the tissue, LDL has become a target of screening and a biomarker for treatment efficacy.

Often the terms "dyslipidemia" and "hypercholesterolemia" are used interchangeably. However, hypercholesterolemia is defined as a higher than normal level of total plasma cholesterol, whereas dyslipidemia may be an elevation of plasma cholesterol, triglycerides, LDL, or a reduction of high-density lipoproteins (HDL), or a combination of these abnormalities. Dyslipidemia is not associated with a true numerical value. By ATP III guidelines, total cholesterol over 200 mg/dL is borderline high and over 240 mg/dL is high; LDL levels in the range 160 to 189 mg/dL are high, and over 190 mg/dL very high; triglycerides over 150 mg/dL are elevated; and HDL less than 40 mg/dL is low. The newest guidelines on the management of cholesterol provide less emphasis on these values, although they recommend pharmacologic therapy for LDL greater than 190 mg/dL and the use of the pooled risk equation, which incorporates total cholesterol and HDL.

PATHOPHYSIOLOGY

Cholesterol and triglycerides are vital components for daily functioning. Both are necessary components of the human cell membrane. Triglycerides may also be catabolized for fuel in the fasting state. Cholesterol is a building block for steroid hormones and vitamin D. One factor that may provide an overabundance of these lipid molecules is a diet rich in fats and cholesterol, and another factor is abnormalities in genetically influenced cholesterol transport pathways. In overabundance, cholesterol can deposit within the arterial intima-media, leading to atherosclerosis.

Cholesterol, triglycerides, and free fatty acids are hydrophobic. Therefore, to move in an aqueous environment these molecules must be either packaged into lipoproteins or micelles, or bound to proteins. Free fatty acids and some fat-soluble vitamins may travel through the serum bound to protein. Micelles, composed of bile salts with a hydrophobic core, form in the intestinal lumen. Lipoproteins are large heterogeneous molecules with a phospholipid outer wall. The phospholipid has a hydrophilic head on the outer aspect of the molecule to allow mobility through the aqueous environment. The inner portion of the phospholipid contains lipophilic tails that create a lipid inner environment, which sequesters esterified cholesterol and triglyceride molecules as well as some fat-soluble vitamins. Proteins along the outer aspect of the lipoprotein wall, such as Apo-B100, Apo-B48, and Apo-CII, among others, allow the lipoproteins to bind at various tissues and organs as well as activate enzymes. These apolipoproteins (Apo-proteins) distinguish the types of lipoproteins and are used to quantify lipid levels. These three carriers transport lipids through the intestines and the circulatory system.

In the intestinal lumen, bile salts form micelles to allow cholesterol, triglycerides, free fatty acids, and fat-soluble vitamins to approximate the brush border. At the brush border, cholesterol is transported via the Niemann-Pick C1-Like1 (NPC1L1) transporter. The NPC1L1 transporter is the site of action of ezetimibe. Triglycerides are broken down into glycerol and free fatty acids at the brush border and are reassembled within the enterocyte. Cholesterol and triglycerides are packaged by the enterocyte into chylomicrons, Apo-B48 and Apo-CII containing lipoprotein. Chylomicrons deliver triglycerides to fat cells where Apo-CII activates lipase, an enzyme. Lipase breaks triglycerides into the glycerol and free fatty-acid components for transport into the fat cell. The resulting fatty acid–depleted chylomicron remnants deliver dietary cholesterol to the liver.

The liver performs three main functions for cholesterol: production, circulation, and excretion. Cholesterol is manufactured by the liver through the mevalonate or cholesterol synthesis pathway. The rate-limiting step is conversion of 3-hydroxy-3-methylglutaryl-coenzyme A (HMG-CoA) to mevalonate. This is catalyzed by the enzyme HMG-CoA reductase. HMG-CoA-reductase inhibitors, "statins," inhibit this rate-limiting cholesterol production step, thereby reducing cholesterol levels. HMG-CoA reductase also has feedback inhibition through increased dietary cholesterol. Once either produced or absorbed through the gastro-intestinal system, the liver performs one of the two other major functions: excretion into the biliary system or release to systemic circulation.

Excretion of cholesterol is achieved through the biliary system. Bile is produced mainly by the liver through the metabolism of cholesterol. The bile salts are then further saturated with cholesterol and emptied either directly into the duodenum or indirectly after storage in the gallbladder. The intestinal tract recycles approximately 98% of bile, recovering and recirculating the cholesterol in the same process. Approximately 1 gm of cholesterol is excreted daily. Cholestyramine is a bile acid binding resin that prevents the reabsorption of bile and increases the amount of cholesterol excreted. The human body unfortunately does not have a method of catabolizing cholesterol. Cholesterol is utilized, stored, or excreted.

If not excreted, cholesterol is circulated via the liver through small lipoproteins called LDL. These lipoproteins are considerably smaller than chylomicrons. There are three types of LDL; all contain Apo-B100, which binds to the LDL receptor. These lipoproteins bring esterified cholesterol and triglycerides to the tissue from the liver. Very low-density lipoprotein (VLDL) is the largest of the three and contains ~60% triglycerides. VLDL, like chylomicrons, has Apo-CII in the wall to deliver triglycerides to muscle for use as an energy source. As the lipoprotein decreases in size, it becomes an intermediate-density lipoprotein (IDL), then an LDL. LDL contains ~60% cholesterol, which is delivered to the tissue; Apo-B100 remains bound to LDL, although Apo-CII does not. Cells, such as those of the muscles or liver, take up the LDL though endocytosis. The three types of LDL deliver lipids from the liver to the peripheral tissue. Several genetic abnormalities affect this pathway leading to high LDL, and are the targets of novel lipid-lowering therapies.

Circulating LDL binds to the LDL receptor on the hepatocyte. The LDL receptor-LDL complex is endocytosed, where the LDL-receptor is cleaved and returns to the cell surface. The LDL molecule is then delivered to lysosomes. A protein, proprotein convertase subtilisin/kexin type 9 (PCSK9), binds to the LDL-receptor while on the cell surface. Binding of PCSK9 to LDL-R marks the receptor for degradation. Increase in activity of PCSK9 results in increased circulating LDL as well as in increased incidence of CVD. Loss-of-function mutations in PCSK9 result in decreased LDL, increased HDL, and decreased cardiovascular events. Recently, medications have been created inhibiting PCSK9 function. These PCSK9 inhibitors are showing promising results in LDL reduction.

Another lipoprotein, similar to LDL, is lipoprotein (a) or LP(a). This particular lipoprotein has a similar composition as LDL and also has Apo-B100. LP(a) is unique due to the apolipoprotein (a) attached to the outer membrane. LP(a) is variable in size, which is determined by individual genetic makeup. Interestingly, LP(a), especially the smaller variants of LP(a), may have a greater role in atherogenicity through the inhibition of fibrinolysis. Current research is being conducted to elucidate the role of this VLDL-like particle in atherosclerosis and coronary thrombosis.

HDL are the smallest of the lipoproteins and function to return cholesterol to the liver. HDL contains Apo-A2, and this apolipoprotein activates the enzyme lecithin-cholesterol acyltransferase (LCAT). LCAT esterifies cholesterol, allowing storage in the lipoprotein. HDL will also remove free cholesterol from VLDL particles. The cholesterol esters are returned to the liver for recirculation or excretion. HDL is known as the "good cholesterol" because the lipoprotein scavenges cholesterol from the body and returns it to the liver. The liver will then either excrete or repackage the cholesterol.

Cholesterol becomes pathologic in overabundance. In the gallbladder, cholesterol-saturated bile acids may result in the formation of gallstones. In the circulatory system, cholesterol-laden LDL molecules are deposited under the endothelium. These molecules are oxidized by enzymes in the intima. Oxidized LDL particles (LDL-P) attract macrophages and T-cells. These immune cells activate the inflammatory cascade by releasing proinflammatory cytokines and chemokines. Macrophages endocytose the oxidized LDL-P. As the cholesterol builds up inside macrophages, they become foam cells. Eventually the lipid-laden macrophages will change and become the lipid core of a growing atherosclerotic plaque.

CLASSIFICATION SYSTEMS

Initially, hyperlipidemia was classified according to the type of lipoprotein elevated. Though infrequently used in current day-to-day practice, this classification should be recognized. Table 6.1 details lipoprotein disorder types and provides a description of each type.

TABLE 6.1 Classification of Lipoprotein Disorders

Type		Description
I	Familial hyperchylomicronemia	Rare; LPL or Apo-C2 deficiency that results in elevated chylomicrons
IIa	Heterozygous familial hyper-cholesterolemia	Common; autosomal dominant LDL receptor deficiency that results in elevated LDL
IIb	Familial combined hypercholesterolemia	Results from reduced LPL receptor and increased Apo-B and results in increased LDL and VLDL
III	Familial hyperlipidemia	Rare dyslipidemia in which Apo-E2 is defective and LDL is elevated.
IV	Familial hyperlipidemia	Elevation in VLDL only due to increased VLDL production
V	Lipoproteinemia (endogenous hypertriglyceridemia)	Rare; results of increased VLDL production and decreased LPL resulting in elevated VLDL and chylomicrons

LDL, low-density lipoproteins; LPL, lipoprotein lipase; VLDL, very low-density lipoprotein.

SECONDARY CAUSES OF LIPOPROTEIN ABNORMALITIES

Diabetes mellitus and hypothyroidism are two processes that may cause lipoprotein abnormalities. Diabetes mellitus, type 1 and type 2, is associated with hyperlipoproteinemia and, more importantly, increased incidence of atherosclerosis and associated disease, myocardial infarction, stroke, and claudication. Lipoprotein lipase (LPL) activity is insulin dependent, reduced by both lack of insulin and insulin insensitivity. Furthermore, insulin insufficiency and absence result in increased fatty acid release from adipocytes, which causes an elevation in hepatic VLDL synthesis. Thus, diabetes is associated as a causative factor for hypertriglyceridemia. Elevated VLDL and LDL are also common in diabetics, though HDL is usually reduced. Another metabolic disorder, hypothyroidism, results in increased triglycerides, total cholesterol, and LDL, due to multiple pathways. New research in mice suggests a potential effect of thyroid hormones on reducing Apo-B (Rizos, Elisaf, & Liberopoulos, 2011).

CLINICAL PRESENTATION

Individuals with hyperlipidemia frequently do not have symptoms related to their high lipid levels. Symptoms may arise from collection of lipids in subcutaneous tissue, arteries, or effects on the pancreas. Possibly more than half of patients with xanthelasma, which is a collection of lipid-laden macrophages in subcutaneous tissue, will have elevated levels of cholesterol. Lipid collection beneath the arterial intima causes plaque formation and obstruction. Presenting symptoms are generally related to cerebrovascular disease, coronary vascular disease, or peripheral arterial disease. Symptoms may include weakness, sensory deficits, anginal chest pain, shortness of breath, syncope, claudication, and abdominal discomfort. Abdominal pain etiology may not be ischemic, but rather due to pancreatitis should triglyceride levels exceed 500 mg/dL. The asymptomatic nature of hyperlipidemia, until the manifestation of associated severe disease, compels screening and management imperatives for those at risk.

PHYSICAL EXAMINATION

The physical examination for the hyperlipidemic patient should evaluate for the end organ damage described earlier. Cardiovascular exam is paramount and may disclose bruits in the carotid arteries, abdominal aorta, renal arteries, or femoral arteries. Cardiac examination may reveal mitral regurgitation from papillary muscle damage, as well as S_3 from left ventricular failure or S_4 from left ventricular wall poor compliance. Weakness, paresthesia, or facial asymmetry may be noted on neurologic exam from cerebral ischemia. A thorough skin examination may note xanthelasma, or yellow/orange dermal plaques or nodules over the metacarpophalangeal and proximal interphalangeal joints, tendons, or the periorbital area. Lower extremities may have hair loss, asymmetric pulses, cyanosis, or be cool to cold due to poor perfusion.

SCREENING

Due to the lack of consistent symptoms and signs, screening is the first step in identification of both hyperlipidemia as well as comorbid conditions. In June 2008, the U.S. Preventive Services Task Force (USPSTF) recommended screening for hyperlipidemia includes LDL and HDL. Triglyceride screening is neither recommended nor discouraged. Screening is recommended to start as early as age 20 in male and female patients at risk for coronary artery disease. All males older than 35 and females older than 45 are recommended for screening regardless of coronary heart disease (CHD) risk. A recommended frequency of 5 years is stated, though frequency should be tailored to the patient's cholesterol level and risk. The American Heart Association (AHA) and American College of Cardiology (ACC) are less specific in recommending screening. In the 2013 Guidelines on the Assessment of Cardiovascular Risk, the AHA and ACC suggest measuring lipid levels in patients 20 to 79 years of age every 4 to 6 years in order to calculate the risk for atherosclerotic cardiovascular disease (ASCVD) as reasonable (Goff et al., 2013). The USPSTF, however, makes no recommendation as to the age at which to discontinue measurement (2014).

DIAGNOSTIC LABORATORY EVALUATION

Lipoproteins are measured directly in the serum, usually through a basic lipid panel. Preferably the patient is fasting at the time of lab draw—without eating or drinking for 8 hours prior to obtaining the sample. Cholesterol information is reported as triglycerides, total cholesterol, LDL cholesterol, HDL cholesterol, and non-HDL cholesterol.

When evaluating for lipid metabolism disorders, a comprehensive evaluation including contributing causes and co-morbidities is essential. Thyroid-stimulating hormone (TSH) should be a component of routine screening for patients with newly discovered hyperlipidemia to evaluate for hypothyroidism, which may increase lipid levels. In addition, evaluate a basic metabolic panel and urinalysis to evaluate renal function. Significantly elevated cholesterol levels, urine protein, and creatinine may indicate nephrotic syndrome. A glycated hemoglobin may be checked as well to evaluate for diabetes, which is a metabolic disease associated with insulin absence or resistance that results in an increased release of fatty acids and plasma LDL levels.

Initial laboratory evaluation prior to beginning a statin regimen should include an evaluation for liver and muscle injury. Specifically, evaluate transaminase with a liver panel or liver function test (LFT). The risk for statin-induced hepatotoxicity increases with active viral hepatitis and other forms of liver inflammation. An exception is nonalcoholic fatty liver disease where a statin may be beneficial. In most situations, a statin may safely be prescribed if the transaminases are within three times the normal upper limit. If the transaminase levels are within normal laboratory-specified limits at initiation, routine evaluation of the liver panel is not required, as the risk for statin-induced liver injury is rare. A creatine kinase (CK) level, creatine phosphokinase (CPK), evaluates for the presence of muscle injury. If the CK is normal, routine reevaluation is not required. However, for both liver transaminase and CK levels, reevaluation should occur if symptoms or signs arise for statin-induced liver injury or myopathy, respectively.

In patients prescribed a statin, symptoms such as abdominal pain, jaundice, or hepatomegaly are concerning for statin-induced liver injury. Typically, statin-induced liver injury has a hepatocellular injury pattern on the liver panel with elevations in alanine aminotransferase (ALT) and aspartate aminotransferase (AST). Should the transaminases be elevated, the statin should be discontinued and the liver panel repeated between 2 and 6 weeks later to evaluate for a decrease in transaminases off statin therapy. If the transaminases normalize, a different statin may be initiated with close monitoring for recurrence of liver injury. Also, review the patient's medication list for possible drug interactions that may increase statin drug levels, as well as other causes of hepatocellular injury.

Statin-induced myopathy is characterized by diffuse or group-specific muscle aches, general malaise, or muscle weakness. Statins may exacerbate exercise-induced myopathy, and women and older patients have a higher incidence of this symptom. Myopathy also occurs in a dose-dependent fashion, and the adverse reaction is varied, from mild to severe. Rhabdomyolysis, the most severe form, may result in renal failure. For patients in whom statin-induced myopathy is suspected, laboratory data should examine muscle injury with serum CK level and renal function. A urinalysis may be added to evaluate for myoglobinura; the results will be positive for blood, without red blood cells in the sample. The statin should be stopped and the medication list evaluated for drug interaction. In severe cases with CK levels significantly elevated, such as over 1,000, the patient should be admitted and hydrated with IV normal saline to preserve renal function. With resolution of statin-induced myopathy, the statin may be reduced in dose or another statin may be started with close monitoring for recurrence.

The vertical auto profile (VAP) and ion mobility analysis directly measure the number of LDL-P. Additionally, as the LDL-P vary in size, these tests sub-fractionate LDL and HDL by particle size (Caulfield et al., 2008). As there is a variety of sizes of LDL-P, calculated LDL levels may not adequately represent cholesterol levels and risk of atherosclerosis. Studies evaluating these laboratory tests indicate that higher numbers of smaller and more dense cholesterol particles are associated with higher atherosclerotic CVD risk (Mackey et al., 2012; Musunuru et al., 2009; Otvos et al., 2011). A possible explanation is the diffusion of LDL-P across the endothelium along a concentration gradient. At this time, there is not conclusive evidence to base treatment thresholds and goals for subfractions of LDL. In the VAP results, the protein Apo-B measurement provides an estimate of the number of circulating LDL-P. One Apo-B is present per LDL, IDL, VLDL, and chylomicron, with 90% of Apo-B on the LDL-P. The Apo-B provides a precise measurement of LDL cholesterol rather than the Friedewald Equation (Caulfield et al., 2008).

In 2011, the National Lipid Association (NLA) created guidelines for the use of these nonroutine cholesterol measurements (Davidson et al., 2011). For LDL-P, Apo-B, and LP(a), the consensus states that for patients with 5% to 20% risk for coronary heart disease, known coronary heart disease, or an equivalent to CHD, checking any of the three markers is reasonable. Practitioners should consider testing in patients with significant family history of CHD, as elevated LDL-P number is discordant with measured LDL cholesterol (LDL-C) in approximately 50% of patients. When elevated LDL-P is discordant with the LDL-C in patients treated for hyperlipidemia, the NLA guidelines recommend increasing lipid-lowering therapy. Similarly for Apo-B, discordance may exist with statin therapy between LDL-C and Apo-B. If Apo-B is elevated above the level of LDL-C, the risk for CHD may still be elevated, as the number of LDL-P is higher than the number estimated by LDL-C. The elevated Apo-B also suggests that therapy should be intensified. Lp(a) may prove additive in risk to the traditional Framingham Score. The NLA recommends consideration for testing those patients with a strong family history for early CHD, especially if the LDL cholesterol levels are not significantly elevated (Davidson et al., 2011).

RISK STRATIFICATION

The 2013 ACC/AHA Guidelines on the Assessment of Cardiovascular Risk do not continue to recommend the Framingham 10-year risk score for CHD (Goff et al., 2013). This decision was based on two shortcomings of the Framingham score:

ethnicity of the cohort and assessment of risk for coronary heart disease only. The 2013 guidelines created a new calculator of risk, the Pooled Cohort Equation, based on findings of the most current evidence. The Framingham cohort represents a predominantly Caucasian population, leading to questions concerning applicability to other ethnicities. African Americans are represented in the new risk equation score; however, there was insufficient evidence to include other ethnicities. The second significant change is the focus of the risk equation that evaluates for risk of CHD, as well as additional ASCVD. ASCVD is defined as CHD death, non-fatal myocardial infarction, or stroke. The new algorithm provides an updated evaluation of 10-year risk for ASCVD in patients age 40 to 79 and lifetime risk in 20- to 79-year-old patients, including African American patients, who have never had an event.

Components of the Pooled Cohort Equation include:

- Gender—Male or female
- Age in years
- Race—White/Other or African American
- Total Cholesterol mg/dL
- HDL Cholesterol mg/dL
- Systolic blood pressure mmHg
- Treatment for high blood pressure—Yes or no
- Diabetes—Yes or no
- Smoker—Yes or no

Hyperlipidemia is a component of metabolic syndrome, which is a disorder of energy utilization and storage. This syndrome consists of five possible signs: hypertension (> 130/85), hypertriglyceridemia (> 150 mg/dL), low HDL (< 35 mg/dL), insulin resistance, and increased abdominal girth (> 40 in men, > 35 in women). Presence of any three signs is necessary for diagnosis. Current treatment for a condition, for example, treatment for hypertension, constitutes positivity for the specific criterion. Metabolic syndrome is significant, as it conveys a risk for developing many serious diseases, including ASCVD. Patients with metabolic syndrome should be treated with both lifestyle changes and medications as indicated for each associated condition.

THERAPEUTIC LIFESTYLE MODIFICATIONS

A healthy lifestyle is imperative in improving the lipid profile. A diet should limit high fat and red meats, and include plant sterols, nuts, and high dietary fiber. The dietary approaches to stop hypertension (DASH) diet and Mediterranean diets fulfill these requirements. Exercise should be aerobic in nature and moderate in intensity. Overweight or obese patients should seek to lose weight with these interventions. Weight loss in the obese patient, a body mass index (BMI) greater than 20% over ideal, and exercise result in increased HDL and reduced LDL. The goal is a multidisciplinary approach to lifestyle change that addresses all risk factors—mental, physical, and dietary—for ASCVD.

An essential dietary change is reducing "bad fats" and increasing the intake of "good fats." So-called good fats are unsaturated fats or unsaturated fatty acids. These fatty acids do not have two hydrogen ions per carbon. They exist in a liquid form at room temperature and are found in natural plant and animal products such as avocado, olive oil, tree nuts, and fish. "Bad fats" include saturated fats and trans-fats. These fats are found in a solid state at room temperature. Saturated fats occur naturally and are found in pork and red meats. Trans-fats are created through "partial hydrogenation" of unsaturated fats such as vegetable oil, found in processed foods, as they have the benefit of increasing the shelf life of food. Both saturated fats and trans-fats are associated with increased LDL and reduced HDL cholesterol levels, as well as ASCVD.

There are two widely discussed types of fiber—soluble and insoluble fiber. Fiber is not digested or absorbed in the gastrointestinal system. Soluble fiber creates a gel in the gastric lumen and results in slowed gastric emptying, creating a sensation of fullness. This sensation may result in less overall dietary intake and in slower glucose uptake. Soluble fiber is in many vegetables, beans, fruits, seeds, and nuts. Insoluble fiber adds bulk to stool and improves bowel transit and is a component of wheat, grains, and most vegetables. Increasing dietary fiber alone may reduce cholesterol by 5% to 10% (Bruckert & Rosenbaum, 2011). People with high dietary intake of soluble and insoluble fiber have reduced risk of developing atherosclerotic coronary disease (Anderson, Hanna, Peng, & Kryscio, 2000; Pereira et al., 2004; Threapleton et al., 2013). This reduction in risk is an association; the exact mechanism is unknown, though it is likely related to a more healthful diet.

Plant sterols inhibit intestinal cholesterol absorption through competing for uptake by the NPC1L1 transporter. A 2 gm/day consumption can reduce cholesterol by 10% (Varady & Jones, 2005). Plant stanols reduce serum cholesterol modestly. Plant stanols significantly reduce LDL-C and at a greater level than sterols. Stanols also are transported from the gut lumen via the NPL1C1 transporter; however, they are returned by the enterocyte to the gut lumen. Hallika-inen, Sinonen, and Gylling (2014) noted in a review of 13 trials with approximately 850 patients that plant stanols reduced LDL cholesterol in a dose-dependent fashion. Reductions of close to 20% were achieved with a supplement of 9 gm/day of stanols, and LDL-C reductions of 10% were achieved with a daily stanol supplement of 2 to 3 gm/day. The amount of plant stanols required to significantly reduce cholesterol is greater than what a healthy diet of fruits and vegetables can provide, requiring fortified foods or supplements. Stanols do not interact with statins and may be a useful addition to more traditional therapies (Gylling et al., 2014).

Smoking increases LDL and lowers HDL cholesterol mildly (Campbell, Moffatt, & Stamford, 2008). More importantly, however, tobacco smoke increases arterial plaque formation through endothelial dysfunction (Henderson et al., 2008). The exact mechanism is still unknown, but includes effects of carbon monoxide, complement activation, endothelial injury, and cell cycle arrest (Henderson et al., 2008; Weber, Al-Dissi, Marit, German, & Terletski, 2011). Diet, exercise, and weight loss will reduce cholesterol, and the addition of tobacco cessation will reduce the risk of myocardial infarction, stroke, and peripheral arterial disease.

PHARMACOLOGIC THERAPY

The 2013 AHA Guidelines to Reduce Cardiovascular Risk recommend lipid-lowering medication for use in preventing ASCVD but no longer focus on specific levels of LDL and non-HDL cholesterol. The LDL cholesterol level is, however, a component of risk stratification (Goff et al., 2013). This change is a reflection of the clinical trial data available, which used fixed doses of medication and did not treat to a lipid goal. The guidelines do not recommend the use of nonstatin lipid-lowering medications as primary agents, as their effectiveness for lipid lowering and prevention of atherosclerotic disease is not as compelling (Stone et al., 2013). The guidelines are applicable for the primary and secondary prevention of ASCVD events in patients 21 years of age or older who do not have New York Heart Association (NYHA) Class II–IV heart failure.

HMG-CoA Reductase Inhibitors (Statin)

Statin therapy offers cardiovascular risk reduction across the spectrum of LDL cholesterol levels above 70 mg/dL. For prevention of ASCVD, four patient groups were identified in which the benefits of lipid-lowering therapy with statins outweighed the possible adverse effects (Stone et al., 2013).

- The benefits of statin therapy outweigh the possible risks in individuals with known clinical ASCVD. For individuals who are 21 to 74 years old, a high-intensity statin dose is recommended; for individuals 75 years or older, a moderate-intensity statin dose is recommended.
- For individuals with LDL greater than 190 mg/dL, a high-intensity statin dose is recommended.
- For individuals with diabetes mellitus who are in the age range of 40 to 75 and have an LDL in the range 70 mg/dL to 189 mg/dL without ASCVD, the recommendation is a moderate-intensity dose statin. However, the individual who has had diabetes for 10 years or longer has a cardiovascular-event rate equal to or greater than 7.5%; hence, high-intensity statin therapy is recommended.
- For individuals with a 10-year risk of cardiac event equal to or greater than 7.5% and an LDL greater than 70 mg/dL to 189 mg/dL are recommended moderate- to high-intensity statin therapy (Stone et al., 2013).

Statin intensity refers to the medication and dose required to produce a level of LDL reduction. A reduction in LDL cholesterol of greater than or equal to 50% may be expected from a high-intensity statin (Stone et al., 2013). A medium-intensity statin is expected to achieve a 30% to 50% reduction in LDL cholesterol (Stone et al., 2013). A medication and dose that result in under 30% reduction is referred to as a low-intensity statin therapy (Goff et al., 2013). Figure 6.1, from the 2013 ACC/AHA guidelines on cholesterol, provides an evidence-based algorithm for the treatment of hypercholesterolemia.

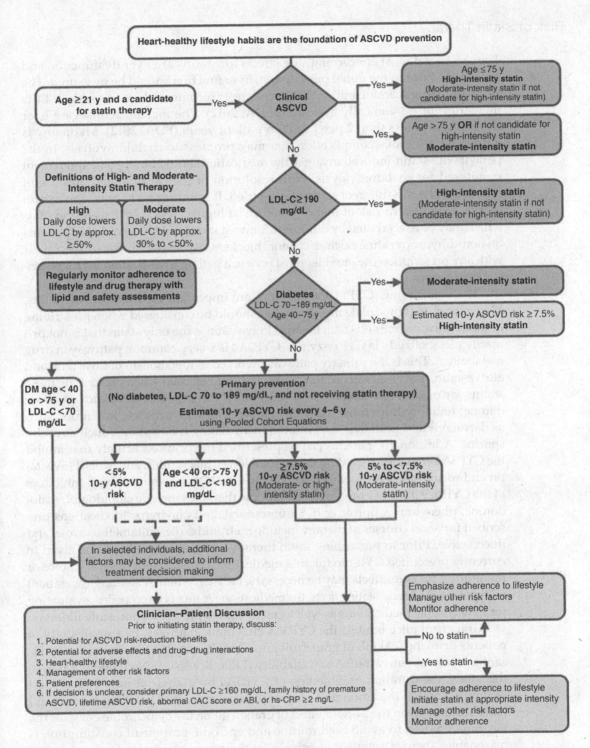

FIGURE 6.1 Summary of statin initiation recommendations for the treatment of blood cholesterol to reduce ASCVD risk in adults.

ASCVD, atherosclerotic cardiovascular disease; CAC, coronary artery calcium; hs-CRP, high-sensitivity C-reactive protein.

Reprinted from Stone et al. (2013, p. S9), with permission from Wolters Kluwer.

Risk of Statin Therapy

The major and most concerning side effects for statins are liver dysfunction and myopathy. Prior to the initial prescription, liver function should be measured. The Food and Drug Administration (FDA) no longer recommends monitoring of LFTs thereafter unless clinically indicated (FDA, 2012). The incidence of severe liver dysfunction is less than 2 per 1 million patient years (FDA, 2012). Myopathy is a potentially serious complication that may progress to rhabdomyolysis. In the patient with statin-induced myalgia, the medication should be stopped and patient monitored for rhabdomyolysis. With resolution of the myalgia and absence of rhabdomyolysis, a different statin may be tried. It is important to note simvastatin carries a significant risk of rhabdomyolysis at higher doses, such as 80 mg/day, which may be exacerbated by diltiazem. Simvastatin should be avoided in patients on non-dihydropyridine calcium channel blockers, especially diltiazem. Of course, with any prescription the provider must review a patient's medication list for potential interactions.

The cytochrome (CYP) P450 enzymes are important metabolizers of statins. Medications that modulate these enzymes should be considered when prescribing or monitoring patients on statin therapy. Pravastatin is the only statin that is not primarily metabolized via CYP enzymes. CYP3A4 is a very common pathway in drug metabolism. This is the primary pathway involved in metabolism of lovastatin and atorvastatin, as well as simvastatin. Caution should be used when prescribing these statins for patients chronically on CYP3A4-inhibiting medications, such as amiodarone; nondihydropyridine calcium channel blockers; protease inhibitors, such as darunavir and indinavir; and immunomodulating medications, such as cyclosporine. Additionally, patients can be prescribed medications acutely that inhibit the CYP3A4 enzymes, including fluoroquinolones, macrolides, and azols. Fluvastatin and rosuvastatin are metabolized via the CYP2C9 enzyme pathway. Inhibitors of the CYP2C9 pathway prescribed for chronic therapies include clopidogrel, amiodarone, phenytoin, valproic acid, 5-fluorouracil, and efavirenz. Medications prescribed for short courses of therapy include metronidazole, sulfamethoxazole, and fluconazole. Prior to prescribing statin therapy, consideration should be given to currently prescribed CYP-modulating medications. Adjustment of statin choice or monitoring for side effects may be necessary. Further, when evaluating the patient with potential adverse statin effects, the medication list must be reconciled, evaluating for new chronic medications as well as medications prescribed for acute illnesses.

Grapefruit juice inhibits the CYP3A4 enzymatic pathway. In a small study of patients drinking 200 mL of grapefruit juice three times daily, there was a significant increase in simvastatin bioavailability (Lilja, Kivisto, & Neuvonen, 2000). In this study, the duration of inhibition of CYP3A4 by grapefruit juice was at least 24 hours. Though the amount of grapefruit juice consumed was large in this and other studies, given the 24-hour effect of grapefruit on the cytochrome enzyme, the recommendation to avoid both routine and episodic grapefruit consumption is reasonable. There is a variety of opinion on the recommendation to avoid grapefruit juice; some providers allow small daily grapefruit consumption.

Statins are associated with an increased risk for diabetes mellitus, although there is a trend for the development of diabetes with increasing age. However, the risk is low for statin-associated diabetes mellitus, as more than 250 patients are required to be treated for 4 years each to account for one additional case of diabetes

(Sattar et al., 2010). Given this meta-analysis, and as the study authors conclude, the overarching benefit of statins in improving ASCVD outweighs the risk of developing diabetes mellitus.

Nicotinic Acid (Niacin)

Recently there has been a great deal of controversy surrounding niacin (vitamin B_3). HDL is increased significantly and LDL is decreased modestly with nicotinic acid. Niacin, however, carries significant flushing and pruritis as side effects, making it poorly tolerable at therapeutic levels. These side effects are more common with higher doses and the immediate release formulations. More severe adverse effects include hepatitis or hepatic necrosis, which occur more frequently at higher doses and with extended release formulations. Niacin confers an increase in insulin resistance regardless of the preparation chosen. Blood glucose must be monitored in the diabetic or prediabetic patient. Two trials, AIM-HIGH and HPS2-THRIVE, failed to demonstrate a morbidity or mortality benefit with the addition of niacin therapy to patients already treated to goal LDL levels (AIM-HIGH Investigators, 2011; HPS2-THRIVE Collaborative Group, 2014). The risk-benefit profile for niacin may not be beneficial to patients with well-controlled LDL and prior history of a vascular event, which were excluded in these studies.

Bile Acid Sequestrants

The use of bile acid sequestrants was one of the original options to reduce serum cholesterol levels. The liver uses cholesterol to produce bile acids; bile is saturated with cholesterol. These bile acid sequestrants prevent the formation of micelles in the intestinal lumen and prevent absorption of lipid-soluble material, including cholesterol. This results in the elimination of excreted cholesterol. Bile acid sequestrants cause significant intestinal upset and may decrease absorption of other oral medications.

Fibrates

Fibrates primarily reduce triglyceride levels and should be the first class of medication chosen when triglyceride levels are over 500 mg/dL. A trygliceride level elevated to more than 500 mg/dL is a risk factor for pancreatitis. These medications, though not the first choice for prevention of ASCVD per the ACC/AHA Guidelines, should not be discounted (Goff et al., 2013). They may be options in patients intolerant of statins or additive to statins in patients with familial hyperlipidemia; however, side effects increase with the combination.

Cholesterol Absorption Inhibitor (Ezetimibe)

Ezetimibe also inhibits cholesterol absorption in the gastrointestinal tract. Ezetimibe has demonstrated a decrease in total and LDL cholesterol in association with a statin. However, the ENHANCE trial failed to show a reduction in carotid arterial intima-media thickness with ezetimibe compared with simvastatin, despite significant reduction in LDL cholesterol (Kastelein, Sager, de Groot, & Veltri, 2005). A proposed explanation for the lack of reduction in morbidity and mortality with ezetimibe therapy, despite achieving lower LDL goals, is lack of anti-inflammatory effects in addition to lowering LDL.

Omega-3 Fatty Acids (Fish Oil)

Omega-3 polyunsaturated fatty acids (PUFAs) are commonly prescribed and consumed without physician guidance as over-the-counter (OTC) products. These are usually found as eicosapentaenoic acid (EPA) and docosapentaenoic acid (DHA) combinations. Omega-3 PUFAs increase HDL, have variable effects on LDL, and reduce triglycerides. Additional effects include a blood pressure reduction via increased arterial elasticity, reduced inflammation, and reduced platelet aggregation. Omega-3 PUFAs may be consumed as seafood, OTC preparations, and a prescription-only preparation. More recent trials and meta-analysis fail to show either a morbidity or mortality benefit of omega-3 PUFAs in primary or secondary prevention of ASCVD (Kwak, Myung, Lee, & Seo, 2012; Rauch et al., 2010; Risk and Prevention Study Collaborative Group, 2013). These medications are not without side effects; most are mild and include dyspepsia, dysgeusia, nausea and vomiting, and pruritus. More serious and uncommon adverse effects include elevation of transaminases, bleeding diathesis, and anaphylaxis. A variety of opinions exist on the recommendation of PUFAs for the prevention of ASCVD; further study is planned to evaluate which population may benefit the most from these medications.

Emerging Therapies

Two new medications in phase 3 clinical trials at the time of writing are the PCSK9 inhibiting monoclonal antibodies, evolocumab and alirocumab. Both agents are proving to significantly lower cholesterol as well as other lipoproteins associated with coronary atherosclerosis and adverse coronary events. LDL was reduced by 31% in homozygous familial hypercholesterolemia patients (Raal et al., 2014a) and by 60% in heterozygous familial hypercholesterolemia patients treated with evolocumab and taking baseline statin therapy (Raal et al., 2014a). Evolocumab also significantly reduced Apo-B and a nonsignificant trend was noted in Lp(a) reduction (Raal et al., 2014b). A 47% reduction in LDL-C was achieved by alirocumab monotherapy, which was significantly greater than the 16% reduction by ezetimibe (Roth et al., 2014). Alirocumab does significantly reduce Lp(a) by approximately 30% (Gaudet et al., 2014). Additionally, data from mice models suggest alirocumab improves plaque morphology, decreases atherosclerotic plaque necrotic core, and reduces inflammation (Kühnast et al., 2014). These effects are increased with concomitant atorvastatin therapy (Kühnast et al., 2014). As promising as these medications are in reduction of LDL, more studies are required to demonstrate improvement in morbidity and mortality as well as adverse effects.

SPECIAL CONSIDERATIONS

Clinicians may find controlling the patient with homozygous familial hypercholesterolemia difficult, as the presenting LDL level is often greater than 300 mg/dL and may be as high as 600 mg/dL. These patients require an approach combining lipid-lowering pharmacotherapies and may require newer agents including LDL apheresis or newer medications. Individuals who continue to experience uncontrolled hyperlipidemia with maximally tolerated medical therapy with statin, fibrate, cholesterol binder, and/or ezitimibe should be considered for these advanced therapies. LDL apheresis may reduce cholesterol by over 50%. The effect, however transient, provides a lower LDL mean over time. A prospective study of 120 familial hyperlipidemia patients treated over a mean of 6 years showed a statistically significant 87% decrease in major atherosclerotic coronary events with LDL apheresis that may not be fully explained by reduction in LDL alone (Jaeger et al., 2009).

Lomitapide and mipomersen decrease circulating LDL by reducing the Apo-B lipoproteins, VLDLs, and chylomicrons. Lomitapide is an oral agent available only through certified pharmacies and by certified prescribers enrolled in the JUXTAPID REMS program; mipomersen is available as an injection through a restricted prescribing and distribution program, the KYNAMRO REMS. Lomitapide inhibits microsomal triglyceride transport protein (MTP), which catalyzes transfer of triglycerides, diacylglycerols, and cholesterol esthers across membranes (Jamil et al., 1995). The MTP is a key protein in the formation of lipoproteins in the intestines and liver (Cuchel et al., 2013), which introduce cholesterol to the systemic circulation. A multinational open-label study with 29 familial hypercholesterolemia patients showed a 50% reduction of LDL with lomitapide. This medication is an oligosaccharide that binds to Apo-B mRNA, inhibiting Apo-B production. Collection is predominately hepatic, resulting in the decrease of Apo-B100 and VLDL. A mean 25% reduction in baseline cholesterol was achieved with mipomersen in a multinational randomized controlled trial (Raal et al., 2011). No cardiovascular effects were evaluated in either of the two latter clinical trials.

FOLLOW-UP AND REFERRALS

In general, patients with pharmacologically controlled hypercholesterolemia should follow up every 6 to 12 months, depending on individual patient co-morbidities or risk factors. Patients with heterozygous familial hypercholesterolemia, either uncontrolled with maximum statin therapy or intolerant of statin therapy, should be referred to a lipid specialist for management and close follow-up. Additionally, families with genetic causes for significant hyperlipidemia, such as homozygous familial hyperlipidemia, and families with strong family history of early myocardial infarction may benefit from management by a cardiovascular lipid specialist.

Proper adherence to dietary advice is a key aspect of therapy. All patients with high cholesterols should be given dietary advice in the office by a qualified professional, who may be a physician, advanced practice provider, or dietician. In 2000, a clinical trial found a significant reduction in LDL in the initial 3 months among patients who were given dietary advice from a dietician compared with a physician

(Henkin et al., 2000). LDL reduction decreased by half in both groups, as did the beneficial effects of dietician-supplied counseling over physician counseling. Non-familial hypercholesterolemia patients who experience difficulty understanding or initiating a proper low-saturated fat diet after an initial office appointment, or who are not achieving LDL cholesterol goals, may benefit from consultation from a registered dietician or a nutritionist to dedicate additional time solely to patient-centered dietary changes. Patients with familial hypercholesterolemia should receive advisement from a certified dietician as part of an interdisciplinary approach to reducing elevated cholesterol and thus CHD risk. The 2013 ACC/AHA Guideline on Lifestyle Management to Reduce Cardiovascular Risk recommends correct intensity levels and weekly duration of exercise (Eckel et al., 2013). There is little evidence to support referring specific patient groups to exercise specialists. High-risk cardiovascular risk groups such as familial hyperlipidemia patients should be referred as a part of an aggressive multidisciplinary team approach. Obese patients and patients with joint ailments such as arthritis may benefit from a tailored exercise regimen. Patients who are having difficulty adhering to an exercise regimen may derive benefits from referral as well. EXERT, a British randomized trial comparing the effectiveness of exercise programs versus exercise advice only, found improved adherence to an exercise regimen when participants were in a group; however, there was no difference in LDL cholesterol reduction (Isaacs et al., 2007).

For full reference citations to this chapter, please see "Section References" in the back of the book, under the heading "Section II."

Diabetes and the Metabolic Syndrome

JOHN N. MERIWETHER

Diabetes mellitus is a chronic disease characterized by increased circulation of glucose in the serum accompanied by changes in fatty acid utilization and serum lipoprotein composition. The increased glucose is caused either by the total absence of insulin or by the lack of sufficient insulin production. Lack of sufficient insulin production may be the effect of a failing pancreas or a byproduct of insulin insensitivity. Due to a shift in energy utilization and storage, diabetics have increased circulating cholesterol and fatty acids. Type 2 diabetes may also induce inflammation and result in increased atherosclerosis as compared with type 1 diabetes. Diabetes mellitus is a known risk factor for the development of atherosclerotic vascular disease and should be treated through a multimodality approach including proper diet, exercise, weight loss, and, if needed, pharmacotherapy.

Diabetes mellitus affects an estimated 8% of the U.S. population, or almost 26 million people. Of those 26 million people, the Centers for Disease Control and Prevention (CDC) estimates that 7 million, or 27%, are undiagnosed (CDC, 2011). Diabetes prevalence increases with age (11.3% of adults older than 20: 26.9% of adults older than 65). Women are approximately equally affected as men (10.8%: 11.8%). African Americans are considerably more affected than non-Hispanic Caucasians (18.7%:10.2%). Additionally, the CDC estimates that 35% of the U.S. adult population over 20, and half of the elderly population, are prediabetics (CDC, 2011). Unfortunately, many of the prediabetics will progress to overt diabetes unknowingly. The duration of poor glycemic control increases the chance of diabetic complication.

These percentages are alarming given the increased risk for complications, including cardiovascular complications, in the diabetic patient. In 2011, almost 22% of all diabetics are reported to have coronary heart disease (CHD). Though the percentage of diabetics reporting CHD has remained stable over the past 10 years, the number of diabetics has increased by greater than 60% in this time frame (CDC, 2011, 2013). Diabetics are at a two- to four-times increased risk for myocardial infarction (MI) and stroke, as reported on the National Diabetes Fact Sheet published by the CDC in 2011. Further, 68% of diabetes-related deaths have cardiovascular disease listed as an additional causative diagnosis (CDC, 2011). The Framingham data establish that the contribution of diabetes to CHD is increasing as diabetes becomes more prevalent (Fox et al., 2007). It is imperative that diagnosis and glucose control be improved to further prevent CHD and cardiovascular events.

PATHOPHYSIOLOGY

Lack of insulin at onset of disease defines type 1 diabetes mellitus. Initially considered juvenile diabetes, type 1 is known to occur in the young adult population and elderly population as well. Etiology for type 1a diabetes is considered to be autoimmune with the inciting event likely a viral infection in the genetically predisposed individual. Also, lack of sufficient insulin may occur by decreased beta-islet function in the elderly or longstanding type 2 diabetics. Early onset type 1 diabetes is important, as these patients are at significant risk for early cardiovascular events. McVeigh, Gibson, and Hamilton (2013) recommend that additional research should be devoted to screening for cardiovascular disease in type 1 diabetes.

Type 2 diabetes mellitus is the result of insensitivity to insulin, the result of genetic predisposition, and associated with lifelong glucose excess, obesity, and sessile lifestyle. Importantly, in contrast to type 1 diabetes, type 2 diabetes has a more insidious onset. There may be years between actual hyperglycemia and diagnosis, especially in the patient who is without routine primary care follow-up.

Type 2 diabetes shifts energy utilization and storage, resulting in increased circulating low-density lipoproteins (LDL). Type 2 diabetics have higher LDL and lower high-density lipoprotein (HDL) levels. In addition to dyslipidemia as a source of increased cardiovascular risk, type 2 diabetes mellitus is associated with increased inflammation, which may result in atherosclerosis (Brownlee et al., 2011; Festa, Hanley, Tracy, D'Agostino, & Haffner, 2003). New evidence is demonstrating type 2 diabetes to result in a higher cardiovascular disease burden compared with type 1 diabetes. A small observational study of juvenile to young adult type 1 and type 2 patients showed, as compared with type 1, that type 2 diabetics carry the same risk of retinopathy and nephropathy, and a significantly higher risk for cardiovascular disease (Constantino et al., 2013). This new evidence lends credence to the prior assessment that type 2 diabetes carries a significantly higher cardiovascular risk than type 1.

THE METABOLIC SYNDROME

This group of cardiovascular risk factors—insulin resistance, obesity, hypertension, and hyperlipidemia—are together termed "metabolic syndrome." In order to confirm this diagnosis, the patient must have three or more of the following diagnostic criteria:

- Fasting serum glucose equal to or greater than 100 mg/dL or medications for diabetes mellitus
- Waist circumference equal to or greater than 40 cm (men) and equal to or greater than 35 cm (women)
- Triglycerides equal to or greater than 150 mg/dL or medications to treat high triglycerides
- HDL less than 40 mg/dL (men) or less than 50 mg/dL (women)
- Blood pressure equal to or greater than 130/85 mmHg or treatment for hypertension

The etiology of the metabolic syndrome is likely multifactorial from diet, lifestyle, and genetic predisposition. One pathway that illustrates the interdependent nature of these conditions is the relationship of metabolic syndrome to hypertriglyceridemia: obesity reduces sensitivity to insulin. Insulin-insensitive adipocytes will release more fatty acids, which the liver packages into triglycerides and releases as very-low-density lipoproteins (VLDL). Again, the circulating fatty acids may result in increased inflammation. To reduce the risk for cardiovascular events, each manifestation of the metabolic syndrome must be addressed.

CLINICAL PRESENTATION

Individuals, or their families, can usually report a specific time of onset for type 1a diabetes mellitus. As the pancreas ceases to produce insulin, blood glucose rapidly accumulates. The body has no time to adjust to the "starvation" condition. Individuals may present with signs of diabetic ketoacidosis (DKA) including malaise, tachypnea, orthostasis, lethargy, confusion, and/or coma. Early in the course, the patient or family may note the three Ps of diabetes: polyuria, polydipsia, and polyphagia. The Ps arise from the osmolar diuresis caused by glucosuria, dehydration related to osmolar diuresis, and the body's response to "starvation" as the cells respond to the inability to utilize glucose.

Type 2 diabetics are generally unable to report the time of diabetes onset, unless they have good primary care provider follow-up and are aware of the progression from prediabetes to overt diabetes. Type 2 diabetics may report the three Ps (polydipsia, polyuria, and polyphagia) of diabetes mellitus, may present with symptoms of complications from diabetes mellitus such as neuropathy, or may present acutely in a hyperosmolar hyperglycemic nonketotic state with malaise, vomiting, high fever, visual changes, confusion, delirium, or coma. These complaints usually arise over several days; however, they may develop quickly. Routine medical follow-up and attempts at controlling diabetes in the prediabetic state are preferable from a perspective of management and the prevention of complications.

PHYSICAL EXAMINATION

The physical examination will evaluate for the sequelae of diabetes, noting that these complications may occur regardless of the degree of diabetic control. Ophthalmoscopy should be performed to evaluate for cotton wool spots, flame hemorrhages, or neovascularization, as these are signs of potential visual impairment risk. All pulses—carotid, femoral, radial, dorsalis pedis, and posterior tibial—should be palpated for briskness and symmetry. The carotid arteries should be auscultated for bruits, a sign of possible atherosclerosis. Atherosclerosis may also result in decreased extremity perfusion, which manifests as hair loss, ulcers, cyanosis, and/or coolness of the poorly perfused extremity. Cardiac examination may reveal murmurs or gallops, which may arise from poorly perfused or scarred myocardium as a result of atherosclerosis. All new murmurs and gallops should be fully investigated.

The neurologic examination focuses on decreased and altered nerve conduction as a result of microvascular disease. A 10-gram monofilament provides consistent force to evaluate pressure sensation, the lack of which is implicated in the formation of diabetic ulcers. Testing the sensation to light touch, temperature distinction, vibration, and proprioception, especially in the lower extremities, completes the neurologic sensory examination. The lower extremities are particularly susceptible to neurologic change as a result of diabetic microvascular alterations due to the length of the nerve fibers and subsequent cumulative nature of the insult.

DIAGNOSTIC TESTING

A hemoglobin A1C, or a percentage of glycosylated hemoglobin, provides a 3-month estimate of overall blood glucose control. In addition, diabetic patients should evaluate their blood glucose at home. Early morning pre-meal blood glucose values reveal baseline control, whereas pre-prandial and bedtime blood glucose values are representative of the post-prandial status. These values and the timing of the values guide the tailoring of anti-diabetic medications.

Diabetic renal disease is a serious and common effect of hyperglycemia. Microalbuminuria is a sign of diabetic renal disease and should be evaluated at least annually in the diabetic patient. Positive results should be repeated in 2 or more weeks to evaluate for a false positive. If the value is confirmed, patients benefit from angiotensin-converting enzyme (ACE) inhibitor therapy and annual monitoring for progression.

Due to changes in nerve innervations, diabetic patients may not present with typical anginal symptoms during cardiac ischemia. MI may be silent in this patient population. An ECG should be performed with the initial visit to obtain a baseline value as well as to evaluate for the possibility of prior silent ischemic disease.

As diabetes is a coronary equivalent and often reveals atypical or no symptoms, an exercise stress test to evaluate the safety of exercise is warranted if a sessile diabetic patient older than 35 years of age desires initiation of an exercise regimen.

NONPHARMACOLOGICAL MANAGEMENT

A proper diet should be low in simple carbohydrates, including sugar, and consistent in energy content with each meal. Complex carbohydrates reduce blood glucose spikes and require more energy for metabolism. Snacks of complex carbohydrates, vegetables, or fruits between meals and prior to bedtime will reduce hypoglycemic events. A consistent carbohydrate diet improves the likelihood that an antidiabetic regimen will control postprandial blood glucose spikes while avoiding hypoglycemic episodes. Further information and meal planning guides can be obtained from a registered dietician and information for diabetic diets can be found at www.diabetes.org/food-and-fitness/food/planning-meals/diabetes-meal-plans-and-a-healthy-diet.html.

Exercise is a necessary addition for all individuals, especially those with diabetes mellitus, hyperlipidemia, and hypertension. Diabetic patients should be counseled to begin at a level of exercise that is individualized for their level of fitness and slowly increase, reporting anginal chest pain or palpitations. An exercise stress test may be appropriate to evaluate the safety of exercise. An exercise regimen is as simple as 30 to 60 minutes of aerobic exercise, including brisk walking, 4 to 7 days per week. Patients should be monitored for safety and encouraged at every visit to continue their new routine.

Proper diet and exercise with resultant weight loss should improve insulin resistance as well as lipid profile and hypertension. Though intensive glycemic control alone may not reduce macrovascular complications, glycemic control with aggressive risk factor modification are cornerstones of preventing major atherosclerotic cardiac events. Healthy diet, tobacco cessation, exercise, and weight loss are the initial therapies for risk-factor modification and are accompanied by pharmacotherapy as needed.

PHARMACOLOGICAL THERAPY

The goal of diabetic control from a cardiac risk prevention aspect is multifaceted. Along with hyperglycemic control, risk factors must be aggressively controlled. Aspirin may additionally be added for primary prevention of macrovascular adverse cardiac events. Lifestyle changes are the initial therapies for controlling blood glucose, blood pressure, and hyperlipidemia via exercise, nutrition, weight loss, and tobacco cessation.

Proper glucose control is a reduction of the A1C to a value less than 7%. This may reduce microvascular complications in both type 1 and 2 diabetics; however, it has not been proven to reduce macrovascular complications, such as atherosclerosis and MI, as revealed in the Action to Control Cardiovascular Risk in Diabetes (ACCORD), Action in Diabetes and Vascular Disease (ADVANCE), and Veterans Affairs Diabetes Trial (VADT) studies (Duckworth et al., 2009; Gerstein et al., 2008; Patel et al., 2008; Tandon, Ali, & Narayan, 2012). However, the American Heart Association (AHA), American College of Cardiology (ACC), and American Diabetes Association (ADA) continue to recommend treating hyperglycemia to an A1C less than 7% to continue to reduce microvascular disease (Dailey, 2011; Skyler et al., 2009).

In regard to the type of medication to prescribe, no medication has been shown to specifically reduce macrovascular complications, although metformin and insulin have been most studied. The ADA recommends starting with metformin but tailoring specific therapy to individual patient factors and co-morbidities (ADA, 2014). In a meta-analysis of trials evaluating macrovascular complications in diabetes, neither metformin with insulin or insulin alone was shown to be superior (Hemmingsen et al., 2012). Metformin has the added benefits of weight loss and low risk for hypoglycemia. Rosiglitazone reduces LDL and has been shown in the Rosiglitazone Evaluated for Cardiovascular Outcomes in Oral Agent Combination Therapy for Type 2 Diabetes (RECORD) Trial to be noninferior to sulfonylureas or metformin when given in combination with either; however, rosiglitazone carries a twofold increased risk for heart failure (Home et al., 2009). Pioglitazone may reduce risk for MI and death; the Prospective Pioglitazone Clinical Trial in

Macrovascular Events (PROactive) demonstrated a reduction of all-cause mortality, stroke, and nonfatal MI in patients with type 2 diabetes on pioglitazone (Dormandy et al., 2005). GLIP-1 analogs have a similar profile in serum glucose reduction, weight loss, and low risk for hypoglycemia, improving weight loss and glycemic control when added to metformin (Nauck et al., 2009). Metformin with or without the addition of GLIP-1 analogs may be especially beneficial in the metabolic syndrome patient.

In the diabetic patient with concomitant hypertension, blood pressure control should include an ACE inhibitor or angiotensin receptor blockers (ARB) unless otherwise contraindicated (ADA, 2014). ACE inhibitors reduce the progression of diabetic nephropathy as noted by proteinuria. After the addition of an ACE inhibitor, other antihypertensives should be added as per the hypertension section to reduce blood pressure to a goal of under 140/90 mmHg (ADA, 2014; James et al., 2014). The 2013 AHA guidelines have raised the blood pressure goals for individuals with diabetes mellitus, compared with the JNC-7 guidelines, due to lack of benefit of a lower blood pressure in this population (James et al., 2014). If a patient's blood pressure is controlled under goal without adverse effect, a change in therapy is unnecessary. Attention should focus on renal function in order to properly titrate doses over time. Pharmacotherapy must be accompanied by a low-sodium, low-alcohol diet (per 2014 ADA Standards of medical care for diabetes), which includes a less than 2,300 mg salt per day diet, exercise, weight loss, and tobacco cessation.

The ACC/AHA Guideline on the Treatment of Blood Cholesterol to Reduce Atherosclerotic Cardiovascular Risk in Adults (Stone et al., 2013) primarily recommends statin therapy in the prevention of atherosclerotic cardiovascular disease. The algorithm devised is based on comorbid conditions, including diabetes mellitus, and the associated risk of atherosclerotic vascular disease. The recommendations are a reflection of the most recent trials, where LDL goals were not the primary target of therapy, and fixed-intensity doses of statins were recommended. Diabetic patients 40 to 75 years old with an LDL 70 mg/dL to 189 mg/dL who are without atherosclerotic cardiovascular disease (ASCVD) are recommended to be on moderate intensity dose statin. If the patient has a 10-year risk for major atherosclerotic cardiovascular event equal to or greater than 7.5%, LDL equal to or greater than 190 mg/dL, or known ASCVD, a high-dose statin should be used. Control of lipids should be a component of a general approach that includes lifestyle interventions, including a low-fat, high-vegetable diet, weight loss, and exercise.

Though aspirin does not modify a risk factor, the ADA, ACC, and AHA recommend its addition in select patients for primary prevention of atherosclerotic vascular disease. The Antithrombotic Trialists' meta-analysis of trials, including diabetic and nondiabetic patients, reported a significant reduction in all primary vascular events with aspirin therapy, most markedly in initial nonfatal MI. Aspirin was also significantly beneficial for secondary prevention of vascular disease (Antithrombotic Trialists' Collaboration, 2002). Three trials examined aspirin for primary prevention in diabetic patients: Japanese Primary Prevention of Atherosclerosis With Aspirin for Diabetes (JPAD), the Prevention of Progression of Arterial Disease and Diabetes (POPDAD), and Early Treatment Diabetic Retinopathy Study (EDTRS) (Ogawa et al., 2008). These trials revealed insignificant trends in reduction of ASCVD events, with a meta-analysis of these trials reporting an insignificant 9% decrease in CHD (Pignone et al., 2010). Two further meta-analyses have reached similar conclusions (Butalia, Leung, Ghali, & Rabi, 2011). The adverse events for aspirin are related to bleeding, especially gastrointestinal and cerebrovascular bleeding. Though the results are inconclusive, the AHA, ACC, and ADA continue to recommend low-dose, 81 to 162 mg, aspirin for primary prevention of vascular disease in the diabetic patient without prior bleeding complications, including gastrointestinal bleeding (Pignone et al., 2010). The ADA Standards of Care specifically recommends low-dose aspirin to be prescribed in the diabetic with a risk greater than 10% for coronary vascular events (ADA, 2014).

FOLLOW-UP AND REFERRALS

Patients on a stable diabetic regimen should be evaluated biannually with an A1C for continued control. Cholesterol and renal function should be measured at least annually. Symptoms, blood pressure, weight, diet, exercise, and tobacco should be assessed at every visit and recommendations and referrals provided as necessary. Referral to an endocrinologist should be sought for poorly controlled diabetics, despite primary care management, or if the patient is a candidate for and considering use of a continuous insulin infusion pump.

For full reference citations to this chapter, please see "Section References" in the back of the book, under the heading "Section II."

Chest Pain

JOHN N. MERIWETHER AND DOROTHY L. MURPHY

Chest pain is a common clinical condition that results in individuals seeking care across the health care continuum. The etiology of chest pain can arise from many different causes and encompass multiple systems, from cutaneous to vascular; therefore, the cardiovascular clinician must maintain suspicion for all causes of chest pain. The cardiovascular clinician's first priority in the evaluation of chest pain is to identify any urgent or acute life-threatening cardiovascular causes of chest pain and refer as appropriate. The next step is to distinguish between cardiac and noncardiac causes of chest pain. A comprehensive history will clarify potential etiologies and direct the focus of the physical examination and diagnostic evaluation. The purpose of this section is to inform the cardiovascular clinician in the evaluation and management of the syndrome of chest pain.

ETIOLOGIES OF CARDIAC CHEST PAIN

Estimates predict that cardiac chest pain constitutes 50% of all chest pain syndromes that contribute to individuals seeking health care (Kontos, Diercks, & Kirk, 2010). Chest pain from angina is the most common cardiac chest pain and may be stable or unstable. Less commonly, nonischemic etiologies of chest pain occur, such as myocarditis or pericarditis.

Angina

Angina is classified as typical, atypical, or non-anginal. Typical angina meets all three of the following criteria: (1) substernal chest discomfort, (2) provoked by exertion or emotional stress, and (3) relieved by rest or nitroglycerin. Atypical angina meets two of the typical angina characteristics. Non-anginal chest pain meets only one or none of the typical angina characteristics. Individuals may experience discomfort in other locations, associated symptoms, or anginal equivalents that are particular for that individual. With angina, these symptoms signal that the myocardium is not receiving an adequate oxygen supply due to reduced blood flow. The discomfort may be elicited with exertion, physical or psychological stress, or an acute occlusion of an artery by thrombus. Tools such as the Canadian Cardiovascular Society Angina Classification assist in classifying the degree of angina (Campeasu, 1976). The Canadian Cardiovascular Society Angina classification categorizes the degree of angina into four categories, Class I–IV (Campeasu, 1976). Class I angina is described as angina occurring only during strenuous prolonged exertion (Campeasu, 1976). Class II angina is described as angina occurring only during vigorous exertion and results only in slight physical limitation (Campeasu, 1976). Class III angina is described as angina that occurs with normal activities of daily activity and results in moderate physical limitation (Campeasu, 1976). Class IV angina is described as angina that occurs with any activity or at rest, causing the individual severe limitations (Campeasu, 1976).

Angina is caused by a mismatch in the myocardial oxygen requirement versus the oxygen supply. The ultimate underlying mechanism may be the lack of supply or an increase in demand for blood flow. Blood flow to the myocardium may be reduced through intraluminal obstruction, arterial vasospasm, arterial dissection, and vascular compression. Atherosclerotic plaque, intraluminal thrombosis, and thromboembolism are sources of intraluminal obstruction. In the hypertrophied myocardium, compression of prearterioles and arterioles during systole may not allow adequate perfusion. As blood flow is reduced, oxygen supply to the myocardium is reduced, resulting in pain or discomfort.

Cardiac oxygen demand refers to the amount of oxygen needed for cardiac performance. Oxygen demand varies depending upon ventricular wall tension, heart rate, and myocardial contractility. An acute increase in cardiac demand for oxygen that exceeds oxygen supply leads to myocardial ischemia, resulting in angina.

Chronic stable angina is defined as typical angina that occurs predictably after a consistent quantity of exertion or the same quality and severity of stress, and resolves after minutes of rest or use of nitroglycerin. Atherosclerotic plaques slowly enlarge, causing intraluminal obstruction. In the resting state, the obstructed artery still provides adequate blood flow. Heart rate and contractility increase during exertion; therefore, the myocardium requires more oxygen. Local factors such as adenosine cause arterial vasodilatation to increase blood flow. Sections of artery occluded by atherosclerotic plaque cannot dilate appropriately in response to the increased demand, thus reducing blood flow distal to the obstruction. The myocardial oxygen demand is not met, resulting in anginal symptoms that occur predictably with equivalent levels of exertion. As the patient stops to rest, the myocardial oxygen demand is reduced, and angina resolves.

Unstable angina, non-ST-segment elevation myocardial infarction (NSTEMI), and ST-segment elevation myocardial infarction (STEMI) are together classified as acute coronary syndromes (ACS). *Unstable angina* is angina that becomes increasingly severe or is triggered with lower levels of exertional activity, occurs at rest, or awakens a patient from sleep. The chest pain may continue for greater than 15 minutes and exhibits little to no response to nitrates. Cardiac biomarkers are normal to mildly elevated. NSTEMI is defined as unstable angina with elevated cardiac biomarkers, although without definite signs of ischemia (ST-segment elevations) on the ECG. Symptoms of an NSTEMI are acute onset of anginal chest pain, and the etiology is due to partial or total occlusion of a coronary artery. Atherosclerotic plaque may enlarge and cause significant intraluminal obstruction resulting in symptoms with less exertion or at rest.

STEMI is unstable angina accompanied by elevated cardiac biomarkers and pathologic ST-segment elevation of 1 mm or greater in two contiguous leads on the ECG leads. ECG demonstrates ST-segment elevations signifying transmural ischemia that may progress to Q-waves denoting infarction. Total occlusion of an artery without collateral blood flow may result in myocardial infarction and requires immediate reperfusion. Symptoms may range from typical anginal symptoms to anginal equivalents: epigastric pain, neck or jaw pain, nausea, vomiting, diaphoresis, fatigue, and weakness, among others. Guidelines highly recommend that patients with STEMI receive proper medical management in the emergency department and then progress to a coronary reperfusion therapy in time-specific manner.

Not all patients experience the typical pain of myocardial ischemia or infarction. Notably, typical myocardial infarction symptomatology decreases with age and is less common in women and individuals with diabetes. The diabetic patient may experience no symptoms due to neuropathy. Diabetic patients at most risk for silent infarction have demonstrated autonomic dysfunction as a manifestation of neuropathy. Older patients and female patients may have atypical symptoms of infarction such as fatigue or abdominal pain (Mann, Zipes, Libby, & Bonow, 2015).

Microvascular angina is due to dysfunction of the prearterioles. Local vasoactive agents and neurohumoral factors regulate the prearterioles. These vessels arise from the pericardial coronary arteries and supply consistent blood flow to arterioles. Patients with microvascular angina may have typical or atypical symptoms usually with exertion; however, symptom resolution with rest is delayed and inadequate with nitrates. Microvascular angina predominantly affects females.

Symptoms of *Prinzmetal's* or *variant angina* manifest as typical angina pain in quality and severity with onset occurring at rest, usually at late night or early morning hours, and are typical for cardiac ischemia. The onset, however, is unrelated to exercise, and exertional capacity is unaffected. Vasospasm or severe vasoconstriction leads to subtotal to total luminal occlusion of a coronary artery and causes the interruption of blood flow. Unfortunately, the pathogenesis of coronary artery vasospasm is not well understood. Variant angina is associated with cold weather exposure; illicit drugs, including cocaine; prescription drugs, including triptans and ergotamine; tobacco use; hypomagnesemia; and aspirin-induced asthma (Mann et al., 2015). Patients with variant angina may have transient ST-segment elevation on the ECG. During cardiac catheterization, the vasospastic segment is identifiable and generally responds to intra-arterial nitrates.

Pericarditis

Pericarditis commonly manifests as a severe pleuritic chest pain, often described as sharp, and may radiate to one or both shoulders. The pain is worsened with lying down and deep breaths, reduced with leaning forward, and may be accompanied by early symptoms of fever, malaise, and muscle aches.

Myocarditis

Myocarditis may occur concurrently with pericarditis and often after a viral illness. The heart failure symptoms of dyspnea with exertion, orthopnea, paroxysmal nocturnal dyspnea, or fatigue are the hallmark clinical findings, in addition to chest pain. Myocarditis may cause symptoms typical of the pain of acute myocardial infarction or acute decompensation of heart failure.

ETIOLOGIES OF NON-CARDIAC CHEST PAIN

The cardiovascular clinician is often confronted with the responsibility to consider etiologies of noncardiac chest pain. Noncardiac chest pain may result from various etiologies across bodily systems. The following text describes, though not comprehensively, etiologies of noncardiac chest pain.

Aortic Dissection

Individuals with aortic dissection typically present with a sudden onset of severe chest pain that may be described as tearing, sharp, ripping, or stabbing that radiates to the mid-back and/or left shoulder. Individuals with aortic dissection may present with symptoms of heart failure, myocardial infarction, tamponade, or shock.

Aortic Aneurysm

Aortic aneurysms are generally asymptomatic. However, individuals with an aortic aneurysm dissection may present with sharp chest pain, back pain, syncope, or presyncope. A physical exam may reveal tachycardia, hypotension, engorged jugular veins from jugular venous congestion, pulsating abdominal mass, or hoarseness from recurrent laryngeal compression, if the aortic arch structures are compromised.

Pulmonary Embolism

Pulmonary emboli clinically manifest as sudden pleuritic chest pain that is worsened with deep respirations and may be associated with dyspnea and tachypnea. Suspicion of pulmonary embolism should be elevated in individuals who have a history of hypercoagulable states, recent prolonged immobilization or surgery, or cancer.

Pneumonia

Pneumonia, especially associated with effusion or empyema, may cause pleuritic chest pain that worsens with cough and deep inspiration. Pulmonary infections are usually associated with fever, chills, and productive cough.

Bronchitis

Substernal chest pain may be a presenting symptom if bronchitis involves the trachea. Individuals experience chest pain symptoms associated with recent or ongoing viral upper respiratory tract infection with dry to scantly productive cough.

Pneumothorax

Individuals with a tension pneumothorax often present with an acute onset of pleurisy, chest pain, dyspnea, tachycardia, tachypnea, and hypoxia. Pneumothorax may be associated with trauma or a history of prior spontaneous pneumothorax.

Esophageal Spasm

An esophageal spasm is often described as a sharp retrosternal chest pain that radiates to the back. The patient may have a history of dysphagia, globus, heartburn, and regurgitation of non-digested food. Note that patients with esophageal spasm may report improvement with nitroglycerin.

Esophageal Reflux

Esophageal reflux often presents as an epigastric or retrosternal burning to sharp chest pain that is worse at night or when lying, associated with the ingestion of food. Reflux is associated with water brash, hoarseness, and nocturnal cough.

Gastric or Duodenal Ulcer

Gastrointestinal ulcerations typically present as a gnawing, epigastric pain that is aggravated by an empty stomach, relieved with eating, and recurs 30 minutes after completion of a meal.

Gastritis

Gastritis is described as a burning epigastric pain associated with nausea or vomiting. Eating may either improve or worsen the pain.

Costochondritis

Costochondritis is classically described as a pinpoint, sharp chest-wall pain that is worsened with movement of the thorax or arms, and on palpation of the chest wall. Generally, costochondritis is not accompanied by dyspnea, nor aggravated by cardiopulmonary exertion, and not relieved with rest. Minor traumas, viral respiratory infections, and overuse of chest muscles are events that predispose individuals to costochondritis.

Herpes Zoster

Herpes zoster, also known as shingles, is described as a sharp, severe pain cutaneous to the chest wall and localized along a thoracic unilateral dermatome that is a prodrome or accompanied by a vesicular rash. A history of varicella is significant for herpes zoster.

Panic Disorder

The pain associated with panic disorder is of any form, usually squeezing discomfort, associated with anxiety or stress and with patients feeling the sensation of walls close in around them. Shortness of breath and tachycardia may also be associated with panic disorder and panic attacks.

Unknown, Idiopathic

At times, the etiology of chest pain remains unknown, even after extensive evaluation and testing.

For full reference citations to this chapter, please see "Section References" in the back of the book, under the heading "Section II."

Stable Ischemic Heart Disease

DOROTHY L. MURPHY AND JOHN N. MERIWETHER

The heart has a high metabolic demand and must receive a continuous supply of well-oxygenated blood. Any pathology that interrupts the oxygen supply can cause transient or permanent loss of cardiac function and myocardial cell death. The most common etiology of myocardial oxygen deprivation is coronary atherosclerosis. Coronary heart disease (CHD) occurs in approximately 83 million U.S. adults and accounts for 48.2% of all cardiovascular deaths (Go et al., 2013; Kochanek, Xu, Murphy, Minino, & Kung, 2011). While atherosclerosis is the most prevalent cause of CHD and the focus of this section, nonatherosclerotic coronary abnormalities occur, including congenitally abnormal coronary vessels (anomalous coronary artery), myocardial bridging, and coronary vasospasm in the absence of atherosclerosis (Corrado, Thiene, Cocco, & Frescura, 1992).

PATHOPHYSIOLOGY

There has been significant advancement in the understanding of the pathogenesis of atherosclerosis and the pathophysiology of CHD over the past two decades. The complex genesis of atherosclerosis, initially thought to be primarily a result of lipid accumulation in the intima, is now known to be a complex, multifactorial interaction of cardiovascular incursion of known risk factors, the arterial wall, and blood and molecule messages.

Normal arteries have a trilaminar, three-layer structure consisting of the tunica intima, tunica media, and the adventitia. The tunica intima consists of remarkable endothelial cells possessing mechanisms of vascular homeostasis. Aging results in thickening of the tunica intima. The tunica media consists of smooth muscle cells, and in normal arteries it maintains homeostasis of the extracellular matrix. The adventitia consists of fibroblasts and mast cells.

When the arterial endothelium encounters incursions, oxidative stress induces cytokine development that promotes the attraction and adherence of leukocytes. The leukocytes may then become interconnected with macrophage colony stimulating factor and, as a result, promote the expression of scavenger receptors. Scavenger receptors stimulate the uptake of modified lipoprotein and the promotion of macrophage foam cell development. Smooth muscle cells from the tunica media migrate into the intima and develop an extracellular matrix that promotes atherosclerotic plaque growth—a fatty streak. Immune and inflammatory cells play a significant and complex role in the transformation of a fatty streak into atherosclerosis (Hansson, 2005). Immune cells infiltrate the fatty streak, consequently producing inflammatory cytokines (Hansson, 2005). The fatty streak develops into a fibro fatty lesion and, if fibrosis continues, results in smooth muscle cell death, calcification, and plaque mineralization of the artery.

The conditions of coronary atherosclerosis, including the location, degree, and disease burden, impact the extent of myocardial consequence. Chronic obstructive coronary atherosclerosis may result in myocardial ischemia or infarct. Chapter 8 describes acute consequences of coronary atherosclerosis; this section focuses on the evaluation and management of chronic stable ischemic heart disease (SIHD).

CLINICAL PRESENTATION

The most common presenting symptoms for SIHD are chest pain and dyspnea. In approximately 50% of individuals with SIHD, chest pain or discomfort is the presenting symptom (Roger et al., 2012). Individuals may present with angina equivalents such as dyspnea; diaphoresis; fatigue; nausea or vomiting; indigestion; and neck, jaw, or arm pain. The symptoms are further evaluated to elicit onset, quality, severity, radiation, progression, exacerbating factors, alleviating factors, and associated symptoms. Additionally, the clinician should inquire of previous cardiac events and whether the current symptoms are similar to a previous experience. Typical anginal pain associated with SIHD is severe substernal pressure, and may radiate to one or both shoulders, the left neck, and the left arm. Angina is generally associated with dyspnea, nausea, vomiting, diaphoresis, and fatigue. Chronic stable angina is a recurrent and predictable chest pain that has an onset with exertion or emotional stress and is alleviated with rest or nitroglycerin. Unstable angina develops a pattern of escalating severity and a decrease in duration of exertion prior to the onset of pain.

HEALTH HISTORY

The health history should survey for known coronary, peripheral vascular, and cerebrovascular disease, cardiovascular events, prior cardiac evaluations, and disease risk factors. Prior myocardial infarctions (MIs), coronary artery bypass surgery, coronary artery percutaneous interventions, and cardiovascular diagnostic testing identify the level of atherosclerotic burden. Similar etiologies cause many vascular diseases; thus, a history of prior transient ischemic attacks (TIAs), ischemic cerebrovascular accidents (CVAs), peripheral arterial disease (PAD), mesenteric ischemia, and erectile dysfunction are important elements in the evaluation of ischemic heart disease (IHD). Important risk factors for IHD are listed in Table 9.1. These co-morbidities and hereditary predisposition contribute to endothelial dysfunction (Haffner, Lehto, Ronnemaa, Pyorala, & Laakso, 1998), which are key contributors to the development of coronary atherosclerosis.

Social and behavioral factors have been identified as significant risk factors for SIHD. A detailed social history, including a 24-hour diet recall; type, duration, and frequency of physical activity; and assessment of substance abuse that includes the type, amount, frequency and duration of tobacco, alcohol, illicit drugs, and/or caffeine, should be obtained.

TABLE 9.1 Risk Factors for Ischemic Heart Disease (IHD)

History of smoking
Dyslipidemia
Hypertension
Diabetes mellitus
Obesity
Metabolic syndrome
Physical inactivity
Family history of premature IHD
Peripheral artery disease
Rheumatologic illnesses
Chronic infectious diseases
Ischemic cerebrovascular disease

Family history of premature atherosclerosis, defined as a first-degree male younger than 55 or a female younger than 65 with premature MI, is an independent risk factor for cardiovascular disease (Sesso et al., 2001), and the identification of a positive family history improves risk-stratification accuracy (Goff et al., 2013). A strong family history of risk factors for IHD including diabetes, hypertension, and hyperlipidemia is a component of the health history. In the review of systems, the clinician should explore for the presence of conditions that inform SIHD diagnosis and management.

PHYSICAL EXAMINATION

Individuals with IHD may have a normal physical exam or may demonstrate significant physical abnormalities that are suggestive of advanced cardiovascular disease. The physical exam should focus on the cardiovascular, peripheral vascular, respiratory, and body systems related to IHD risk factors.

CARDIAC RISK ASSESSMENT IN THE ASYMPTOMATIC ADULT

Several risk stratification modalities have been proposed for cardiac risk assessment for asymptomatic adults. These risk assessment tools, based upon large cohort studies, are used to predict cardiac risk in order to provide recommendations for cardiac risk reduction, particularly for the use of cardiovascular protective agents such as statins. The widely known risk stratification assessment, the Framingham Risk Score, projects 10-year risk of MI or death based on the following variables: age, gender, total cholesterol, high-density lipoproteins (HDL), smoking, systolic blood pressure (SBP), and the use of antihypertensive medications. The 2013 American College of Cardiology Foundation (ACCF)/American Heart Association (AHA) Guidelines on the Assessment of Cardiovascular Risk recommended a new risk stratification tool, the Pooled Cohort Equation, for the prediction of 10-year risk of atherosclerotic cardiovascular disease (ASCVD) events, which includes nonfatal MI, CHD death, or stroke. The following variables are used to project ASCVD events: gender, age, race, total cholesterol, HDL, SBP, antihypertensive treatment, presence of diabetes, and smoking status. An ASCVD risk score greater than 7.5% represents elevated cardiovascular risk, and reduction with moderate or high-intensity statin therapy is recommended.

NONINVASIVE DIAGNOSTIC TESTING

There are multiple clinical and noninvasive testing mechanisms available that provide clinicians a framework for cardiovascular risk stratification and modification strategies for individuals with CHD or who are at risk for CHD. Selection of the appropriate diagnostic testing is dependent upon cardiovascular risk factors, clinical presentation, and functional capacity. Individuals often present for evaluation due to a suspected cardiac symptom such as chest pain, shortness of breath, or activity intolerance in which interpretation is based upon the presence or absence of CHD or the suspected degree of cardiovascular risk factors.

The initial step in the newly symptomatic patient with previously undiagnosed IHD is diagnosis. A resting 12-lead electrocardiogram (ECG) is recommended in all individuals who present with chest pain, unless the pain is distinctly not of cardiac etiology (Fihn et al., 2012). Acute ischemia may manifest as T-wave inversion or ST elevation in at least two contiguous leads of at least 1 mm, and may be accompanied with reciprocal ST depression. For example, should the lateral wall have ischemic ST elevations apparent in leads V4 to V6 of at least 1 mm, then leads V1 and AvR may display ST depressions. T-wave flattening and nonspecific ST changes are less precise markers for ischemic cardiac disease. Q-waves in any two contiguous leads may represent prior infarction. Significant Q-waves are those at least one third the height of the following R-wave.

CARDIAC RISK ASSESSMENT IN THE SYMPTOMATIC ADULT

The ACCF/AHA 2012 Guidelines for the Diagnosis and Management of Patients with SIHD provide evidence-based risk assessment modalities aimed at predicting risk and selecting the most appropriate cardiac evaluation method for individuals with newly diagnosed angina who have suspected or known IHD. Table 9.2 stratifies cardiovascular risk based upon history, chest pain, clinical findings, ECG, and cardiac biomarkers. It is important to note at this time that the evaluation and management of individuals with high-risk features is beyond the scope of this chapter.

DIAGNOSTIC EVALUATION

Diagnostic evaluation with cardiac stress testing or imaging modalities should be reserved for symptomatic patients. An exception to this rule is the sessile diabetic patient seeking a new exercise program, in which exercise testing will provide information regarding the safety of the new exercise routine. In the initial evaluation

TABLE 9.2 Assessment of Short-Term Risk of Death or Nonfatal MI in Patients With UA/STEMI

Feature	High Risk (*1 or more features*)	Intermediate Risk (*No high-risk feature 1 or more features*)	Low Risk (*No high- or intermediate risk features May have any of the following*)
History	Accelerating tempo in preceding 48 hr	Prior MI or CABG, PVC, CVD	-
Chest pain	Prolonged ongoing (>20 min) or at rest	Prolonged (>20 min) rest angina, now resolved, with moderate or high likelihood of CHD Rest angina (>20 min) relieved with rest Nocturnal angina New onset or progressive CCS Class III or IV angina in previous 2 weeks without prolonged rest pain Intermediate or high likelihood of CHD	Increased frequency, severity, or duration Provoked at a lower level of activity New onset within 2 weeks or 2 months before presentation
Clinical findings	Pulmonary edema New/worsening MR S_3 New/worsening rales Hypotension, bradycardia, or tachycardia Age >75	Age >70	-
ECG	Angina at rest with transient ST-segment changes >0.5 mm New bundle branch block Sustained VT	T-wave changes Pathologic Q waves or resting ST-depression <1 mm in multiple leads	Normal/unchanged
Biomarkers troponin	Elevated Tn>0.1 ng/mL	Slight elevation 0.01>Tn<0.1 ng/mL	Normal

CABG, coronary artery bypass graft; CCS, Canadian Cardiovascular Society; CHD, coronary heart disease; CVD, cardiovascular disease; MI, myocardial infarction; PVC, premature ventricular contraction; STEMI, ST-elevation myocardial infarction; UA, unstable angina; VT, ventricular tachycardia.

Modified from Fihn et al. (2012).

of chest pain, for patients with low-risk characteristics who can exercise, standard treadmill testing is advised for the evaluation of IHD. If baseline ECG is abnormal, then the addition of myocardial imaging with echocardiography or nuclear myocardial perfusion imaging (MPI) improves sensitivity. Pharmacologic cardiac stress testing should be reserved for those patients unable to exercise. Recommendations (Fihn et al., 2012) support intermediate risk patients undergoing exercise treadmill testing; however, exercise echocardiography or nuclear MPI are reasonable substitutes, and should be considered for underlying ECG changes limiting ECG interpretation. Figure 9.1 provides an evidence-based algorithm and summarizes diagnostic evaluation for individuals with suspected SIHD (Fihn et al., 2012).

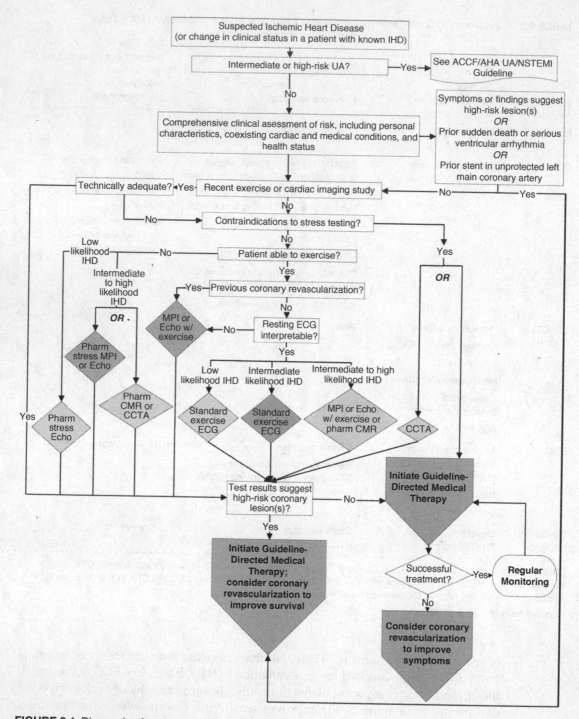

FIGURE 9.1 Diagnosis of patients with suspected IHD.

ACCF, American College of Cardiology Foundation; AHA, American Heart Association; CCTA, coronary computed tomographic angiogram; CMR, cardiac magnetic resonance; IHD, ischemic heart disease; MPI, myocardial perfusion imaging; UA, unstable angina.

Reprinted from Fihn et al. (2012), with permission from the American Heart Association.

Laboratory Evaluation

Laboratory assessment useful in initial risk stratification for SIHD includes serum fasting glucose, glycated hemoglobin, lipid profile, hemoglobin and hematocrit, electrolytes, thyroid panel, liver function tests, and renal function. Yearly surveillance of these values, or sooner if clinical presentation warrants, is recommended for individuals who are at risk for or have been diagnosed with CHD (Fihn et al., 2012).

Coronary Angiography

Coronary angiography may be considered for individuals with suspected SIHD when coronary angiography would change therapeutic management or in candidates for coronary revascularization (Fihn et al., 2014). Coronary angiography is reasonable for coronary definition in patients who have suspected IHD and are unable to undergo noninvasive evaluation. Angiography is also reasonable for individuals who have inconclusive noninvasive diagnostic tests or for patients who would be candidates for coronary revascularization due to clinical presentation or results of noninvasive testing that indicate a high likelihood of severe SIHD (Fihn et al., 2014). Cardiac coronary angiography may reasonably be substituted in patients with underlying wall motion abnormalities and who are unable to undergo evaluation by an MRI.

THERAPEUTIC MANAGEMENT OF SIHD

The goals of SIHD management are to reduce premature cardiovascular morbidity and cardiovascular mortality; to maintain, restore, or improve functional capacity and health-related quality of life; to minimize symptoms of SIHD; and to minimize the burden of health care resources. Table 9.3 details the indication of evidence-based therapeutic management of SIHD aimed at reducing mortality and/or symptoms. While therapeutic management options may achieve all of these objectives, certain therapeutic options may be indicated only for one of the objectives. For example, physical activity is indicated for all the objectives, whereas antiplatelet therapy is indicated for the reduction of mortality and does not offer any improvement in functional capacity. The clinician will also be confronted with situations in which therapeutic management goals conflict, and, as reasonably appropriate, reduction of mortality is the priority objective. While there is a plethora of evidence that supports multiple therapeutic management options, the clinician must consider the multifactorial circumstances that present in the cardiovascular care of each individual with CHD. There must be a partnership between the cardiovascular clinician and an informed patient who actively participates in diagnostic evaluation and therapeutic management decisions. Therapeutic management involves controlling co-morbid illnesses and risk factors as previously discussed in this chapter, incorporating pharmacologic and lifestyle changes.

TABLE 9.3 Indications for Therapeutic Management of SIHD

Therapy	Reduce Mortality	Reduce Symptoms
Anti-platelet	✓	
Statin	✓	
Beta blocker	✓	✓
ACEI/ARB	✓	
Nitrates		✓
Ranolazine		✓
PCI		✓
CABG		✓
EECP		✓
Spinal stimulation		✓

ACEI, angiotensin-converting enzyme inhibitors; ARB, angiotensin receptor blockers; CABG, coronary artery bypass graft; EECP, enhanced external counterpulsation; PCI, percutaneous coronary intervention; SIHD, stable ischemic heart disease.

Source: Fihn et al. (2012).

NONPHARMACOLOGIC MANAGEMENT

Education

It is vitally important that clinicians provide individuals with CHD straightforward education regarding the etiology, clinical manifestation, diagnostic and therapeutic treatment options, and their prognosis. Recommended communication with patients includes:

- Explanation of therapeutic options, pharmacologic and nonpharmacologic management, and cardiovascular risk reduction strategies
- Promotion of the recommended exercise regimen, nutrition, and weight control
- Instruction on self-monitoring skills and recognizing worsening cardiovascular symptoms and appropriate actions
- Information about targeted blood pressure and lipid management, smoking cessation, avoiding secondhand smoke, stress management, and alcohol moderation (Fihn et al., 2012)

Lifestyle Modification

Lifestyle changes include enhancing a healthy weight, physical activity, proper nutrition, and smoking cessation. Weight loss should be directed to achieve two goals: normal body mass index (BMI) and waist size. A normal BMI is 18.5 to 24.9 kg/m^2; with the exception of patients with high muscle mass, this is consistent with a decrease in total body fat. Waistline goal is less than 40 inches for men and 35 inches for women.

Exercise and an overall increase in daily activity level will improve weight control as well as improve other atherosclerosis-related diseases. Sessile patients can engage in periodic, short breaks in tasks that require sedentary behavior for activities that require more movement, including walking, cleaning, or yard work. In addition to increasing basal activity level, patients should exercise at minimum 5 days per week and preferably every day for 30 to 60 minutes. The exercise should be aerobic and moderate in intensity, for example, walking at a brisk pace.

In addition to dietary modification as a tool for weight loss, it can also be used to modulate comorbid illnesses. As discussed previously, diets should be low in cholesterol. The guidelines recommend saturated fats for less than 7% of calories, and total cholesterol intake restricted to less than 200 mg/day. A reduction in cholesterol is a pathway to decreasing progression of atherosclerosis. Daily salt-intake reductions will assist in the reduction of hypertension. In general, dietary modification should include multiple daily servings of fresh vegetables and fruits, lean protein, and whole grains.

Tobacco Cessation

Tobacco use is a significant modifiable risk factor. The cardiovascular clinician must be versed in assessing the use of tobacco, the patient's readiness to quit and quit-attempt history, and viable cessation options. The health care team role is to provide education and support to individuals who use tobacco, while assisting the smoker to discontinue.

Glycemic Control

Though the role of an A1C under 7% has not demonstrated improvement in macrovascular disease, it will improve lipid levels and decrease the progression of renal disease and neuropathy (American Diabetes Association [ADA], 2012). Nevertheless, the ADA and the ACCF/AHA continue to recommend treating to an HbA1c under 7%, unless the patient is experiencing hypoglycemic episodes.

Clinical Surveillance

Clinical surveillance is dependent upon individual patient factors, though the patient with chronic SIHD should be evaluated at least annually. At visits, the clinician should evaluate the patient's progress in attaining therapeutic management goals, assess for the presence of modifiable risk factors and new or worsening symptoms, and monitor for signs of adverse outcomes related to IHD, including heart failure and dysrhythmias. The routine use of echocardiography is discouraged unless a structural change in the heart is suspected and the testing may change management. Also, routine stress testing is not indicated per the ACCF/AHA Guidelines unless the patient has a change in condition or symptoms (Fihn et al., 2012).

PHARMACOLOGIC THERAPY

Antiplatelet Therapy

Platelet aggregation is a significant contributor of the thrombotic development in response to plaque disruption. Antiplatelet therapy has indications for primary, secondary, and tertiary treatment of SIHD. Primary prevention of cardiovascular events is considered reasonable for men 45 years and older and women 55 years and older when the treatment benefit outweighs the risks (USPSTF, 2009). The risk of a cardiovascular event may be calculated based upon the presence or absence of specific cardiovascular risks with a global cardiovascular risk assessment instrument. In a meta-analysis of randomized controlled trials evaluating antiplatelet therapy with aspirin in high-risk individuals, low-dose aspirin was associated with a 46% reduction in the risk for unstable angina and a 53% reduction in the need for coronary angioplasty (Antithrombotic Trialists' Collaboration, 2002; Fihn et al., 2012). Therefore, antiplatelet therapy with low-dose aspirin (75–162 mg) daily is recommended in all individuals with known SIHD unless contraindicated.

Aspirin is contraindicated in individuals with known allergic reaction to non-steroidal anti-inflammatory drugs (NSAIDs), asthma if exacerbated by NSAIDs, or in the presence of gastrointestinal pathology causing gastrointestinal bleeding. Clopidogrel 75 mg daily, a thienopyridine-derived platelet inhibitor, is considered a reasonable and equally efficacious approach to antiplatelet therapy when aspirin is contraindicated due to allergy or asthma.

Clopidogrel is recommended in conjunction with aspirin in high-risk individuals or for the reduction of mortality and for the prevention of thrombosis after percutaneous coronary angioplasty (CAPRIE Steering Committee, 1996; Fihn et al., 2012). The Clopidogrel in Unstable Angina to Prevent Recurrent Events (CURE) trial demonstrated that clopidogrel plus aspirin is superior to aspirin alone in the reduction of cardiovascular death, MI, and stroke in individuals with recent non-ST-elevation myocardial infarction (NSTEMI) (2001). Therefore, unless contraindicated, individuals who are post-NSTEMI are commonly protected with dual antiplatelet therapy (DAPT) for 12 months. The risk of stent thrombosis after bare metal stent (BMS) is highest within 30 days of placement. Therefore, DAPT is recommended for a minimum of 30 days post-BMS, unless placed during an acute coronary syndrome in which DAPT is recommended for 12 months (Fihn et al., 2012; Grines et al., 2007). Late stent thrombosis has been reported after drug-eluting stent (DES) placement; therefore, DAPT is recommended for at least 12 months post-percutaneous coronary intervention (PCI) with DES (Fihn et al., 2012). Another thienopyridine-derived antiplatelet, ticlopidine, compares less favorably to clopidogrel in the reduction of mortality (Fihn et al., 2012).

A follow-on study to the CAPRIE trial, the CHARISMA (Clopidogrel for High Atherothrombotic Risk Ischemic Stabilization, Management, and Avoidance) trial, evaluated clopidogrel and aspirin versus aspirin alone for prevention of atherothrombotic events, revealing that the combination of clopidogrel and aspirin did not reduce the rate of MI, stroke, or cardiovascular death among individuals with SIHD or individuals with multiple cardiovascular risk factors (Bhatt et al., 2006). Therefore, DAPT with clopidogrel and aspirin is not recommended for individuals with multiple cardiovascular risk factors for the prevention of acute coronary syndromes.

Newer antiplatelet agents, prasugrel and ticagrelor, have been compared with clopidogrel in conjunction with aspirin for initiation during an acute coronary syndrome (Wallentin et al., 2009; Wiviott et al., 2007). The TRITON-TIMI (Trial to Assess Improvement in Therapeutic Outcomes by Optimizing Platelet Inhibition with Prasugrel-Thrombolysis in Myocardial Infarction) demonstrated a 19% relative risk reduction of cardiovascular death, nonfatal MI, or nonfatal stroke with the use of prasugrel compared with clopidogrel in acute coronary syndrome (ACS) patients scheduled for percutaneous revascularization (Wiviott et al., 2007). However, there was an associated increased risk of bleeding with prasugrel compared with clopidogrel (Wiviott et al., 2007). Prasugrel has not been tested in stable SIHD. Individuals who have experienced a recent ACS may remain on these newer agents for risk reduction as detailed or may be prescribed clopidogrel if indicated. Ticagrelor was compared with clopidogrel in individuals who experienced an acute coronary syndrome, regardless of ST-segment elevation, with ticagrelor demonstrating a significant reduction in vascular death, MI, and CVA without an increased risk of major bleeding (Wallentin et al., 2009). Ticagrelor has not been studied in patients with SIHD (Fihn et al., 2012).

Statin Therapy

The association between low-density lipoproteins (LDL) cholesterol and risk for SIHD is well established, and there is convincing evidence supporting the efficacy of statin therapy for the primary and secondary prevention of ischemic events (Cholesterol Treatment Trialists' Collaboration, 2010). LDL–targeted treatment for SIHD has been informed by multiple trials, including the Heart Protection Study Collaborative Group (2002), the Treating to New Targets (TNT Steering Committee Members & Investigators, 2004) trial, and the Incremental Decrease in Endpoint Through Aggressive Lipid Lowering (IDEAL; IDEAL Study Group, 2005) trial.

Furthermore, there is strong evidence that statin therapy lowers LDL, and, perhaps more importantly, improves endothelial function, reduces vascular inflammation, and stabilizes coronary plaque (Blake & Ridker, 2000; Ridker et al., 2008). The landmark JUPITER trial, which evaluated the anti-inflammatory mechanisms of statin (rosuvastatin) therapy for reduction of high sensitivity C-reactive protein (hs-CRP) and cardiovascular risk in individuals with normal lipid values, was stopped prematurely after midterm analysis suggested significant cardiovascular risk reduction. Subsequently, the JUPITER (Justification for Use of Statins in Primary Prevention: An Intervention Trial Evaluating Rosuvastatin) trial led to the Food and Drug Administration approval of rosuvastatin for the reduction of cardiovascular risk in individuals with elevated hs-CRP and one additional cardiovascular risk factor (Ridker et al., 2008).

Recently, discrepancy surfaced between guidelines and recommendations regarding lipid-target treatment. The National Cholesterol Education Program (NCEP) Adult Treatment Panel III recommended an LDL goal less than 100 mg/dL for secondary prevention in individuals with CHD, with the option of further reduction to less than 70 for individuals at very high risk (NCEP, 2002). Lipid treatment goals were often left unrealized, requiring high-dose statins and/or second-line cholesterol-lowering pharmacologic therapy, thereby increasing the risk of adverse reactions. Furthermore, nonstatin therapies compared with statins were not found to reduce atherosclerotic cardiovascular risk (Stone et al., 2013). The paradigm has now shifted toward a "tailored-treatment approach," emphasizing treatment based upon cardiovascular risk despite LDL levels.

The 2013 ACC/AHA Guideline on the Treatment of Blood Cholesterol to Reduce Atherosclerotic Cardiovascular Risk in Adults recommends a new perspective on treatment goals, recommending moderate- or high-intensity statin therapy for primary and secondary prevention of atherosclerotic cardiovascular risks (Stone et al., 2013). The newest guideline recommends using the Pooled Cohort Equation to estimate 10-year atherosclerotic cardiovascular risk for accurate identification of higher risk individuals most likely to benefit from statin therapy. However, it should be noted that the ACCF/AHA Guideline for the Diagnosis and Management of Patients With Stable Ischemic Heart Disease now recommends moderate or high doses of statin for secondary prevention in individuals with SIHD (Fihn et al., 2012).

Beta Blocker Therapy

Beta blocker therapy is indicated for reduction of mortality in all individuals with normal left ventricular (LV) function for 3 years after MI or ACS and may be considered for chronic therapy for all individuals with other cardiovascular diseases (Fihn et al., 2012). Beta blocker therapy is indicated as an ACCF/AHA Class I initial treatment to relieve symptoms of angina. Beta blocker therapy reduces myocardial oxygen demand by mechanisms of heart rate and blood pressure reduction, atrioventricular (AV) nodal inhibition, and decreasing myocardial contractility. The lower oxygen demand not only improves the ischemic threshold for symptoms but also reduces angina during exercise and significantly reduces exercise-related deaths and recurrent MI in individuals who have prior MI, recurrent ischemia, or tachyarrhythmias (Kernis et al., 2004). Because all-cause mortality is associated with higher heart rates, beta blocker therapy is dose-adjusted to maintain resting heart rate to 55 to 60 bpm (Diaz, Bourassa, Guertin, & Tardif, 2005; Jouven et al., 2005).

Calcium Channel Blockers

If beta blockers are contraindicated or if an individual with SIHD has breakthrough angina, calcium channel blockers may be substituted or used in addition to beta blockers for the relief of symptoms (Fihn et al., 2012). Calcium channel blockers regulate calcium ion transport through the calcium channels and produce a negative inotropic effect and smooth muscle relaxation. All calcium channel blockers decrease coronary vascular resistance and improve arterial blood flow, resulting in decreased myocardial demand to provide similar anginal relief. Therefore, pharmaceutical agent selection should be individualized, considering class differentials such as compelling indications and potential for adverse event or drug interactions. Calcium channel blockers are not recommended for individuals with LV dysfunction, due to depression of myocardial contractility (Elkayam et al., 1990).

Renin-Angiotensin-Aldosterone Blocker Therapy

Angiotensin-converting enzyme inhibitors (ACEI) reduce angiotensin II and increase bradykinin, promoting beneficial cardiac hemodynamics and improved myocardial oxygen supply, thereby decreasing cardiac remodeling and the progression of atherosclerosis, plaque disruption, and thrombosis. Unless contraindicated, ACEI therapy is recommended to reduce mortality for all individuals with CHD and comorbid hypertension, diabetes, left ventricular ejection fraction (LVEF) less than 40%, or chronic kidney disease (Fihn et al., 2012). In the event that an ACEI is not tolerated, angiotensin receptor blockers (ARBs) may be substituted.

Short-Acting Nitrates

Sublingual nitroglycerin or spray is an ACCF/AHA Class I recommendation for immediate relief of angina in individuals with SIHD. Nitrates relax arterial smooth muscle, resulting in arterial dilation, coronary blood flow redistribution through collaterals, and reduction of preload, diminishing myocardial ischemia. Nitrates improve functional capacity, increase the duration before the development of ST depression, and delay the onset of angina in individuals with SIHD (Fihn et al., 2012; Heidenreich et al., 1999). Short-acting nitrates may be used to treat angina or to prevent angina prior to exertional activity. While short-acting nitrates are commonly prescribed for individuals with SIHD, clinicians should ensure that patients understand how and when to administer, as the consequences of failing to take the medication as prescribed may dismiss the potential benefit and increase the risk of these agents. Patients should be advised about the potential adverse reaction of hypotension and headaches and to seek treatment if angina persists.

Long-Acting Nitrates

If beta-adrenergic blockers or calcium channel blockers are contraindicated, or if an individual with SIHD experiences breakthrough angina, long-acting nitrates may be substituted for or prescribed adjunctively with other pharmaceuticals (Fihn et al., 2012). Nitrates should be avoided in individuals with hypertrophic cardiomyopathy and severe aortic valve stenosis. Phosphodiesterase inhibitors such as sildenafil are strictly contraindicated within 24 to 48 hours of taking a long-acting nitrate due to the risk of significant hypotension.

Ranolazine

Ranolazine reduces sodium-induced calcium excess in myocytes that results in ventricular diastolic relaxation and oxygen utilization (Fihn et al., 2012). Ranolazine is an ACCF/AHA Class IIa recommendation for the treatment of stable angina as monotherapy or in addition to beta blockers (Fihn et al., 2012). Studies have demonstrated that ranolazine successfully reduces angina and recurrent ischemia after infarction; however there is limited data to indicate a reduction in MI or death (Morrow et al., 2007). Dose-related QTc prolongation has been identified; therefore, contraindications include use in combination with potent cytochrome CYP3A4 inhibitors and with significant hepatic impairment, because increased concentrations may result in further QT prolongation (Morrow et al., 2007). Caution should be exercised in treatment of individuals with creatinine clearance less than 30 mL/min, which may result in an increase in plasma concentrations, up to 50% (Fihn et al., 2012; Jerling & Abdallah, 2005).

ADVANCED THERAPEUTIC MANAGEMENT OF SIHD

Coronary Revascularization

Coronary revascularization with either PCI or coronary artery bypass grafting meets evidence-based criteria for improving survival and symptoms in select patients. Angiography is reserved for those carefully selected patients in whom revascularization would be beneficial. Notably, meta-analysis of clinical trials has repeatedly demonstrated that PCI does not improve mortality in patients with stable ischemic coronary disease, or stable angina. Chapter 36 further details the indications for coronary angiography and revascularization.

Enhanced External Counterpulsation (EECP) Therapy

EECP therapy is a noninvasive, mechanical procedure in which pressure cuffs, distributed on the lower extremities, cycle inflation and deflation in a cardiac-timed rhythm to increase circulation from the lower extremities to the heart. EECP is a painless therapy that consists of 35, 1-hour therapy sessions over 7 weeks. EECP therapy may be considered for the treatment of refractory angina in individuals with SIHD (Fihn et al., 2012). EECP is associated with improved LV diastolic filling and endothelial function and recruitment of coronary collaterals. EECP therapy increases exercise time to equal to or greater than 1 mm ST-segment depression, improves perfusion images, and reduces angina (Fihn et al., 2012; Shah, Shapiro, Mehta, & Snyder, 2012). EECP is contraindicated for individuals with decompensated heart failure, severe aortic regurgitation, and severe peripheral artery disease.

Spinal Cord Stimulation

Spinal cord stimulation therapy involves electrode placement into the epidural space to stimulate the spinal cord by modifying central nervous system anti-ischemic channels (Foreman et al., 2000). Spinal cord stimulation therapy may be considered for the treatment of refractory angina in individuals with SIHD (Fihn et al., 2012). There is limited evidence to evaluate long-term risks and benefits of spinal cord stimulation therapy (Fihn et al., 2012). Spinal cord stimulator placement is contraindicated in certain spine anatomical conditions, and in the presence of demand-type cardiac pacemakers, coagulopathy, or immunosuppression. Caution is advised when considering spinal stimulator therapy for individuals with implanted cardiac pacemakers (demand pacemakers are contraindicated), anticoagulation, or antiplatelet therapy.

SPECIAL CONSIDERATIONS FOR SIHD

Women with SIHD may present with stable atypical angina or with an angina equivalent symptom that occurs in a typical pattern, duration, and frequency. This may be because microvascular disease is more prevalent in women than obstructive epicardial coronary atherosclerosis. When considering ischemic evaluation, it is important to consider that the diagnostic accuracy of noninvasive cardiac stress testing is increased with the addition of imaging (Fihn et al., 2012). When considering coronary revascularization, it should be noted that women have a higher risk of procedural complications and in-hospital death after PCI and coronary artery bypass grafting compared with men (Fihn et al., 2012; Hannan et al., 2006).

For full reference citations to this chapter, please see "Section References" in the back of the book, under the heading "Section II."

Valvular Heart Disease

DOROTHY L. MURPHY

The multifaceted issues associated with valvular heart disease (VHD) require an individualized approach to management. Individuals with VHD present in the outpatient setting with different etiologies, severity, and coinciding cardiac conditions. This chapter provides an overview of common mitral, aortic, tricuspid, pulmonic, and prosthetic valve disorders.

THE MITRAL VALVE

The primary components of the mitral valve (MV) are the anterior and posterior leaflets, chordae tendineae, papillary muscle bundles, the annulus, and the right and left ventricular walls. Disorders of any of these components can result in dysfunction of the MV. This section explains common MV diseases, including mitral valve prolapse (MVP), mitral regurgitation (MR), and mitral stenosis (MS).

MITRAL VALVE PROLAPSE

MVP is a common and often benign condition characterized by abnormally thick MV leaflets that billow into the left atrium (LA) during systole. Diagnostic criteria for MVP have been refined since first recognized in the 1960s, and were widely overdiagnosed in the 1980s, due to lack of understanding of normal MV structure. Since the 1980s, improved knowledge of MV anatomy and subsequent echocardiogram criteria redefined MVP diagnosis to ensure the accuracy and uniformity of diagnoses (Freed et al., 1999). MVP, which occurs in approximately 2.5% of the population, is usually asymptomatic and generally does not affect life expectancy (Freed et al., 1999). MVP is more frequently diagnosed in women than men, though it has been detected in men of all ages (Freed et al., 1999).

Pathophysiology of MVP

MVP may be a result of excessive valve tissue or left-heart structural abnormalities and is associated with connective tissue disorders. The most common cause of MVP is myxomatous degeneration. Features of myxomatous degeneration are abnormal leaflet thickening and elongated, redundant chordae resulting in an abnormally pliable MV. Endothelial disruption is typical, and these structural abnormalities predispose patients to endocarditis and thrombus formation. Mechanical alterations of the chordae and the stress of redundant leaflets can cause atypical chest pain, and, in isolated but severe cases, may result in chordal rupture. MVP is the most common cause of MR. The severity of MR depends on the degree of prolapse, and may range from absent to severe. Left atrial dilation and left ventricle (LV) enlargement may result from severe MR, with left-heart remodeling resulting in LV dysfunction.

While myxomatous degeneration is the most frequent primary cause of MVP, other primary causes of valve prolapse may be excessive valve tissue, chordal extension, or a disproportionately undersized LV cavity. MVP is also associated with connective tissue disorders, including Marfan and Ehlers-Danlos syndromes. Secondary causes of MVP include papillary muscle dysfunction, myocardial ischemia or infarction, or mitral valvotomy for the treatment of MS. MVP is also associated with musculoskeletal malformations such as pectus excavatum and straight thoracic spine.

Clinical Presentation

MVP is often asymptomatic and may be incidentally identified during cardiac evaluation. Common symptoms that warrant suspicion for MVP include atypical sharp chest pain, palpitations, syncopal events, and anxiety. MVP associated with severe MR with diminished cardiac reserve may present with symptoms of fatigue, dyspnea with exertion, and functional limitation.

Physical Examination

General physical findings that should elicit suspicion for MVP include thoracic malformation. The physical findings of MVP may be normal if the prolapse is mild and MR is absent. The classic cardiac examination finding of MVP is a mid-systolic click that is best auscultated with the diaphragm of the stethoscope at the apex or the left lower sternal border. The mid-systolic click results from the MV apparatus as the leaflet prolapses into the LA during systole and may be followed by a late systolic medium- to high-pitched murmur. If MR is present, a mid- to late-systolic crescendo murmur is a common finding and is best auscultated at the apex. Maneuvers that decrease the LV volume produce an early-systolic click or murmur. Alternatively, maneuvers that increase LV pressure produce a late-systolic click or murmur.

12-Lead Electrocardiogram

The electrocardiogram (ECG) is usually normal when MVP is asymptomatic. Many individuals with symptomatic MVP have an abnormal ECG and may demonstrate cardiac arrhythmias. Common ECG changes associated with MVP include inverted or biphasic T waves and nonspecific ST-segment changes. A less common ECG finding is prolonged QT interval that is associated with ventricular arrhythmias. If MR is severe and the LA is dilated, it is common to see P wave abnormalities that suggest left atrial enlargement. Atrial and ventricular arrhythmias have been documented in MVP, including premature contractions, supraventricular tachy-cardia (SVT) and ventricular tachyarrhythmia, various degrees of atrioventricular (AV) block, and bradyarrhythmias. Paroxysmal SVT is the most common arrhythmia in individuals with MVP. Ambulatory electrocardiography monitoring is warranted in individuals with MVP who are symptomatic for cardiac arrhythmias (Nishimura et al., 2014).

Transthoracic Echocardiogram

Echocardiographic criteria for MVP diagnosis require visualization of one or both MV leaflets with prolapse of more than or equal to 2 mm above the mitral annulus into the LA with or without leaflet thickening or MR. Echocardiogram is indicated for the initial evaluation and surveillance of MVP; degree of MR; and for cardiac structure, function, and hemodynamic measurements (Bonow et al., 2008). Frequency of surveillance is dependent upon the degree of prolapse, regurgitant flow, and symptoms.

Therapeutic Management of MVP

Therapeutic management of MVP depends on the degree of valve thickening and prolapse, the presence of MR, cardiac arrhythmias, or symptoms. For asymptomatic individuals with benign MVP without MR, patients should be reassured of the favorable prognosis, encouraged to engage in a healthy lifestyle, continue monitoring with a cardiology specialist, and obtain echocardiogram surveillance every 3 to 5 years (Bonow et al., 2008). Individuals with mild MVP with or without mild MR may experience atypical, sharp left-sided chest pain and palpitations that may be relieved by cessation of cardiovascular stimulants such as caffeine and tobacco.

Predictors associated with significant MVP include MV leaflet thickness more than 5 mm, moderate to severe MR, and left ventricular ejection fraction (LVEF) less than 50% (Marks, Choong, Sanfilippo, Ferre, & Weyman, 1985). MV leaflet thickness greater than 5 mm is associated with increased risk of ventricular arrhythmias, sudden death, endocarditis, ruptured chordae, and cerebral embolus (Marks et al., 1985; Nishimura et al., 1985). Therefore, these individuals should undergo surveillance more frequently, receive patient-centered therapeutic management, and be evaluated for surgical repair. Surgical repair or replacement of the MV may be necessary in the case of a flail mitral leaflet that results from chordae tendineae rupture or elongation, severe MR, symptoms of heart failure, LV dysfunction, and severe pulmonary hypertension (Bonow et al., 2008).

Surgical Intervention

Individuals with MVP associated with severe MR and symptoms or LV dysfunction require surgical repair or replacement of the MV. MV repair for MVP associated with MR has demonstrated excellent long-term survival, particularly in posterior leaflet disorders (Bonow et al., 2008). There is a higher risk of reoperation associated with anterior MV leaflet repair (Bonow et al., 2008).

Complications of MVP

Infective Endocarditis

Infective endocarditis (IE) has long been considered a rare but serious complication of MVP. MVP is the leading predisposing cardiovascular diagnosis in individuals with IE (Hayek, Gring, & Griffin, 2005). Perhaps the most notable clinical conundrum in the everyday management of MVP is the issue of antibiotic prophylaxis of IE. For decades, IE prophylaxis with antibiotics for individuals with MVP undergoing dental or various invasive procedures was commonplace. While there remain clinical indications and prescribing practices for antibiotic prophylaxis, recent evidence has warranted reevaluation of prophylaxis. Current evidence suggests individuals are at no higher risk of IE associated with dental or invasive procedures compared with day-to-day exposure to random bacteremia (Hayek et al., 2005). Furthermore, prophylaxis may not prevent IE, and the risks of antibiotics' adverse effects outweigh the benefits (Hayek et al., 2005). Oral hygiene may play a more important role in preventing IE than prophylactic antibiotics (Hayek et al., 2005). Antibiotic prophylaxis for IE is considered reasonable for individuals with underlying cardiac conditions at highest risk of adverse outcomes from IE (Hayek et al., 2005). Individuals with MVP who are at the highest risk of IE are those who have a past history of IE or prior valve repair with prosthetic material, or individuals with a prosthetic valve who are undergoing dental procedures in which gingival tissue is manipulated (Bonow et al., 2008).

MR Associated With MVP

MR in MVP occurs and progresses in varying degrees. MR may result as part of myxomatous degeneration or from chordal rupture. The presence and degree of MR are predictors of cardiovascular risk and are important in determining therapeutic management of MVP. Mild MR is often asymptomatic, and annual surveillance to assess for progressive regurgitation is reasonable (Bonow et al., 2008). MR should be evaluated at regular intervals with an echocardiogram, as moderate or severe regurgitation may result in dilation of the LA and ventricle. Moderate to severe MR may ultimately result in LV dysfunction, heart failure, right-ventricular dysfunction, and pulmonary hypertension. Currently, there is no evidence to support primary pharmacological treatment to improve the structure or function of MVP with MR. MR is discussed later in this chapter.

Cerebral Emboli

MVP increases the incidence of thromboembolic disorders including cerebral emboli resulting in transient ischemic attack (TIA) or stroke (Bonow et al., 2008). It is postulated that cerebral emboli associated with MVP are platelet-fibrin thrombi from the myxomatous mitral leaf or enhanced platelet activation associated with high-degree MR (Bonow et al., 2008). There is an increased risk of cerebral emboli in MVP when MV leaflet thickness is more than 5 mm, or if there is associated valve redundancy, atrial fibrillation, hypertension, heart failure, left atrial thrombus, advanced age, or history of prior stroke (Bonow et al., 2008). For individuals with MVP who have risk factors for embolic event, the ACC/AHA (American College of Cardiology/American Heart Association) 2008 guidelines recommend antiplatelet therapy with aspirin (Table 10.1) or anticoagulation (Table 10.2) with warfarin, with a target international normalized ratio (INR) of two to three.

TABLE 10.1 Aspirin Therapy for MVP Thromboembolic Risk Reduction

- Individuals with MVP who have a history of TIA
- Individuals with high-risk MVP predictors
  - MV leaflet thickness >5 mm or leaflet redundancy
  - Moderate to severe MR who are in sinus rhythm
- Individuals with MVP and a history of CVA who have contraindications to anticoagulation
- Individuals with MVP who have atrial fibrillation who are <65 years and do not have MR, hypertension, or heart failure

CVA, cerebrovascular accident; MR, mitral regurgitation; MV, mitral valve; MVP, mitral valve prolapse; TIA, transient ischemic attack.

Source: Bonow et al. (2008).

TABLE 10.2 Anticoagulation for MVP Thromboembolic Risk Reduction

- Individuals with MVP with a history of recurrent TIA on aspirin
- Individuals with MVP and atrial fibrillation who are >65 years
- MVP with AF and have MR, left atrial thrombus, or heart failure
- Individuals with high-risk features of MVP with a history of CVA despite age, presence of atrial fibrillation, MR, heart failure, or left atrial thrombus
- Individuals with MVP who have a history of CVA, MR, atrial fibrillation, or left atrial thrombus

AF, atrial fibrillation; CVA, cerebrovascular accident; MR, mitral regurgitation; MV, mitral valve; MVP, mitral valve prolapse; TIA, transient ischemic attack.

Source: Bonow et al. (2008).

Cardiac Arrhythmias and Sudden Cardiac Death

Individuals with MVP may experience palpitations with or without identified arrhythmia (Bonow et al., 2008). Patients with MVP who have palpitations or syncopal episodes should undergo ambulatory electrocardiography monitoring. In patients who experience mild symptomatic arrhythmias, cessation of stimulants may reduce symptoms. When symptoms or tachyarrhythmias are not reduced by lifestyle changes, beta blockers have demonstrated effectiveness in relieving palpitations and reducing tachyarrhythmias (Bonow et al., 2008). In moderate to severe MR, left atrial dilation may result in electrical remodeling in the atrium and possibly result in atrial fibrillation. Sudden cardiac death (SCD) is a rare complication of MVP, likely a consequence of ventricular tachyarrhythmia, which occurs in less than 2% of individuals with MVP and has an associated annual mortality rate less than 1% (Bonow et al., 2008). Risk factors for SCD include the familial forms of MVP, severe MR, redundant chordae, flail leaflet, LV dysfunction, QT prolongation, and the presence of ventricular ectopy (Bonow et al., 2008).

CHRONIC MR

MR is the retrograde flow through the MV from the LV into the LA during systole. While trivial MR is routinely identified in healthy individuals, moderate to severe MR is the most prevalent valve disorder, affecting 2.0 to 2.5 million people in the United States (Singh et al., 1999). MR is classified as either primary or functional. Primary MR, also known as degenerative MR, is a result of MV apparatus abnormality and most frequently occurs as a result of MVP (Bonow et al., 2008). Less commonly, primary MVP may result due to chordal rupture, IE, rheumatic heart disease, or connective tissue disease. Functional, or secondary, MR is due to dysfunction or scarring of the LV or a dilated LV, resulting in abnormal MV leaflet coaptation. Coaptation is the complete closure and symmetrical overlap of the valve leaflets with correct apposition.

Pathophysiology of MR

Abnormalities in any part of the MV structural framework can cause MR. Regardless of etiology, the primary deficit is the reduction or elimination of coaptation between the anterior and posterior MV leaflets. The pathophysiology and disease progress of MR are multifactorial and influenced by etiology, structural framework of the MV, significance of regurgitation, and cardiac chamber structure and function.

Individuals with mild to moderate MR in the absence of primary valve abnormality may remain asymptomatic without hemodynamic consequence. MR that is caused by abnormal valve or cardiac structure tends to be more progressive and associated with hemodynamic compromise (Nishimura et al., 2014). In the presence of chronic severe MR, a cascade of compensatory mechanisms ensues. If the cardiac structure and function remain well compensated, individuals with severe MR may be seemingly asymptomatic. Compensated severe MR may last many years (Bonow et al., 2008); however, protracted volume overload may result in LV remodeling, dysfunction, dilation, and increased filling pressure. Ultimately, LV remodeling and hemodynamic abnormalities can progress to systolic dysfunction and heart failure. Surgical correction of MR should be performed before the progression of LV decompensation (Nishimura et al., 2014).

Clinical Presentation

Individuals with chronic MR may be asymptomatic for decades, although with disease progression, symptoms of dyspnea on exertion, fatigue, and palpitations are common. Late signs and symptoms of severe MR include dyspnea, fatigue, edema, postural nocturnal dyspnea, orthopnea, arrhythmias, or systemic embolization.

Physical Examination

Cardiac examination of an individual with chronic MR often reveals a pansystolic, soft-blowing murmur best heard at the apex that may radiate to the axilla or back. Maneuvers that decrease the LV volume, such as sudden standing, will decrease the regurgitation and murmur. Maneuvers that increase the LV volume, such as handgrip, will increase the regurgitation and murmur. Chronic MR may reveal a soft S_1, and hemodynamically significant MR may produce an S_3. A loud P2 suggests the presence of pulmonary artery hypertension.

12-Lead ECG

ECG in chronic MR may demonstrate normal sinus rhythm, P wave abnormality suggestive of left atrial enlargement, or atrial fibrillation. Left ventricular hypertrophy may be evident in secondary, functional MR from primary LV disease.

Transthoracic Echocardiogram

Echocardiogram is recommended for individuals with signs or symptoms of MR for initial diagnosis and evaluation of valve structure, etiology and severity of regurgitation, myocardial structure, function, and hemodynamics for assessing clinical outcomes and determining the need for valve surgery. Valve structure is evaluated for abnormalities or valve thickening, calcification, and prolapse. Echocardiogram allows for detection and quantification of MR, which is estimated by the distance of high-velocity jet(s) flowing into the LA. There are multiple echocardiographic parameters to assist in the categorization of MR severity as mild, moderate, or severe. See Table 10.3 for echocardiographic hemodynamic categorization of MR. The presence of MR is associated with an increased LV preload and normal afterload that increases LVEF; therefore, the "normal" LVEF may be 70% (Nishimura et al., 2014). Left ventricular end-systolic volume offers prognostic value in surgical outcomes (Bonow et al., 2008). Individuals with LV dimensions 40 mm or greater are associated with better outcomes than those with dimensions greater than 50 mm (Bonow et al., 2008).

TABLE 10.3 Categorization of MR by Echocardiogram Hemodynamics

MR Severity	Central Jet	Vena Contracta (cm)	Regurgitant Fraction (%)	Regurgitant Volume (mL)	Effective Regurgitant Orifice (cm²)	Equivalent Angiographic Grade
Mild	<20% of LA	<0.3	-	-	-	-
Moderate	20%–40% of LA or late systolic eccentric jet MR	<0.7	<50	<60	<0.4	1–2+
Severe	>40% of LA or holosystolic eccentric jet MR	≥0.7	≥50	≥60	≥0.4	3–4+

LA, left atrium; MR, mitral regurgitation.

Source: Nishimura et al. (2014).

Cardiac Magnetic Resonance (CMR) Imaging

Although transthoracic echocardiogram (TTE) is the primary diagnostic technique for the evaluation of MR, CMR may be useful if transthoracic echocardiography image quality is poor (Nishimura et al., 2014).

Transesophageal Echocardiogram

Transesophageal echocardiogram (TEE) is indicated if the transthoracic image quality is poor in order to obtain diagnostic information of the MV including the severity of MR, LV function, or endocarditis (Nishimura et al., 2014). TEE is not recommended for routine surveillance of MR.

Exercise Testing

Exercise treadmill testing (ETT) may be used to evaluate exertional symptoms in chronic primary MR. Exercise hemodynamic evaluation via echocardiogram (exercise stress echocardiogram) or cardiac catheterization with exercise may be beneficial in the evaluation of individuals with chronic MR who experience dyspnea on exertion (Nishimura et al., 2014). Exercise hemodynamic evaluation allows for assessment of pulmonary artery and LV diastolic pressure, with elevations suggestive that MR is responsible for exertional symptoms.

Cardiac Catheterization

Cardiac catheterization has an ACC/AHA Class I (Level of Evidence C) indication for hemodynamic assessment in individuals with symptomatic VHD when noninvasive evaluation is inconclusive, or if there is a discrepancy between the noninvasive diagnostic examination and the clinical presentation (Nishimura et al., 2014). Because stable ischemic heart disease (SIHD) worsens the prognosis of VHD, coronary evaluation with angiography is recommended (ACC/AHA Class I) prior to valve surgery for individuals who have a high pretest likelihood of SIHD, a history of SIHD, symptomatic angina, evidence of ischemia, LV systolic dysfunction, or functional MR (Nishimura et al., 2008).

Therapeutic Management of MR

Therapeutic management of MR is dependent on patient-specific etiology, valve structure and function, symptoms, left ventricular function, and the presence of cardiac co-morbidities (Figure 10.1). Individuals with mild to moderate MR without LV remodeling or dysfunction who are asymptomatic should have annual evaluation by a cardiovascular clinician. Patients should be educated about the signs and symptoms of progressive MR and instructed to notify a clinician if signs or symptoms develop.

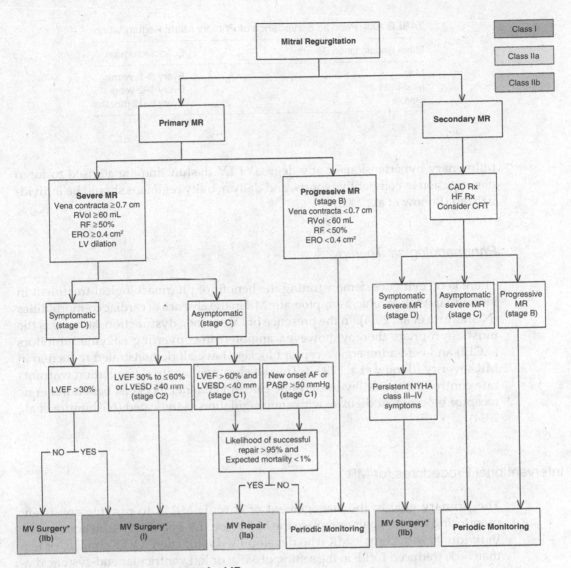

FIGURE 10.1 Indications for surgery for MR.

AF, atrial fibrillation; CAD, coronary artery disease; CRT, cardiac resynchronization therapy; ERO, effective regurgitant orifice; HF, heart failure; LVEF, left ventricular ejection fraction; LVESD, left ventricular end-systolic diameter; MR, mitral regurgitation; MV, mitral valve; NYHA, New York Heart Association; PASP, pulmonary artery systolic pressure; RF, regurgitant fraction; Rx, prescription therapy.

*Mitral valve repair is preferred over mitral valve replacement when possible.

Reprinted from Nishimura et al. (2014, p. 95), with permission from Elsevier.

An echocardiogram is recommended for periodic monitoring (Table 10.4) and if there is clinical evidence of progressive MR, including change in symptoms or physical examination findings.

Physical Activity

Individuals with MR of any severity, who are asymptomatic, have normal cardiac structure and function, and have normal pulmonary artery pressure (PAP), may exercise without restriction (Bonow et al., 2008). Individuals with LV enlargement,

TABLE 10.4 Periodic Surveillance of Primary Mitral Regurgitation

Mitral Regurgitation Severity	Echocardiogram
Mild	Every 3–5 years
Moderate	Every 1–2 years
Severe	Every 6–12 months

pulmonary hypertension, or any degree of LV dysfunction are advised to forgo participation in competitive sports, and daily activity regimens should be individualized (Bonow et al., 2008).

Pharmacological Therapy

There is no evidence demonstrating the benefit of pharmacological treatment in individuals with chronic, asymptomatic MR in the absence of cardiac co-morbidities (Nishimura et al., 2014). In the presence of LV systolic dysfunction, surgery is the most appropriate therapy; however, angiotensin-converting enzyme inhibitors (ACEI) and beta-adrenergic receptor blockers have all demonstrated reduction in MR severity (Bonow et al., 2008). The development of atrial fibrillation warrants rate control with nondihydropyridine calcium channel blockers, beta-adrenergic receptor blockers, or digoxin, with anticoagulation as indicated (Nishimura et al., 2014).

Interventional Procedures for MR

The primary goal in the management of chronic MR is to provide consistent monitoring and to repair or replace the MV before LV systolic dysfunction ensues. Individuals with chronic MR who develop LV dysfunction, LVEF equal to or less than 60% (reduced LVEF in the setting of MR), or left ventricular end-systolic diameter (LVESD) equal to or greater than 40 mm, have poorer postoperative prognosis (Nishimura et al., 2014). MV repair has demonstrated superior long-term outcomes compared with MV replacement (Bonow et al., 2008).

Surgical MV Repair

MV repair is an ACC/AHA Class I recommendation for the management of chronic severe primary MR, limited to the posterior leaflet (Nishimura et al., 2014). If the anterior or both leaflets are involved, MV repair is more complex, though it is the preferred surgical strategy if feasible (Nishimura et al., 2014). Surgical repair of the MV is considered the safest, most effective, clinically approved interventional treatment of severe degenerative or functional MR (Bonow et al., 2008; Nishimura et al., 2014). MV repair is considered first-line treatment for individuals with functional MR when the MV structure is anatomically suitable. MV repair preserves the native valve, leading to improved postoperative LV function and survival (Bonow et al., 2008). Furthermore, for individuals with severe MR who are in a sinus rhythm, repair of the MV avoids the risk of lifetime anticoagulation, which is generally required with MV replacement.

MV Replacement

Mitral valve replacement (MVR) is an ACC/AHA Class I recommendation for symptomatic individuals with chronic severe primary MR and LVEF greater than 30%, asymptomatic individuals with chronic severe primary MR and LV dysfunction, or in conjunction to cardiac surgery for other indications (Nishimura et al., 2014). MVR may include partial or full removal of the MV apparatus. Full removal of the MV apparatus is performed only when the native valve and apparatus are severely diseased and cannot be spared (Bonow et al., 2008). MV competence, LV function, and postoperative survival outcomes are superior when the MV apparatus remains intact (Bonow et al., 2008). Biological prosthetic valves or mechanical prosthetic valves are available for MVR. Important considerations in determining the best option for individuals who require MVR are patient's preference, life expectancy, indications or contraindications for warfarin therapy, and co-morbidities. Bioprosthetic valves degenerate more rapidly, although they are preferable when lifetime anticoagulation is not in the patient's interest, life expectancy is limited, the patient is a female of childbearing years, or the patient states a preference. Mechanical valves require lifelong anticoagulation; however, they are more durable and may be preferred in individuals who already require anticoagulation therapy for a comorbid condition, are at higher risk of bioprosthetic deterioration, or are anticipated to have a long life expectancy. Individuals who undergo MVR transition their native valve condition to "prosthetic valve disease," which is detailed later in this chapter.

Percutaneous Transcatheter MV Repair

The percutaneous transcatheter treatment option with the MitraClip® has demonstrated great promise as a less invasive, lower risk alternative to open MV repair or replacement (Lim et al., 2013). The U.S. Food and Drug Administration (FDA) approved the MitraClip in October 2013, although the credentialing of operators and institutions is pending (Feldman, 2014). The MitraClip is indicated for use in individuals with significant symptomatic primary (degenerative) MR, equal to or greater than 3+ abnormality angiographically; who are at prohibitively high risk for MV repair or replacement; and have no existing co-morbidities that would offset the expected benefit of reducing MR (Lim et al., 2013; Whitlow et al., 2012). The procedure is a transvenous-transseptal approach in which the MitraClip deploys one or more clips at the sites of leaflet mal-coaptation. The ACCESS-EU is a large, multicenter, prospective study evaluating safety and outcomes in the real-world setting at 30 days and 1 year postprocedure (Tamburino et al., 2010). The EVEREST II (Endovascular Valve Edge-to-Edge Repair Study II) and EVEREST II High Risk have demonstrated a low risk of procedural complication and significant improvement of MR (Feldman et al., 2005; Lim et al., 2013; Whitlow et al., 2012). The use of MitraClip for the treatment of secondary (functional) MR is currently being evaluated in the COAPT (Clinical Outcomes Assessment of MitraClip Percutaneous Therapy for Extremely High-Surgical-Risk Patients) and RESHAPE-HF (A Randomized Study of the MitraClip Device of Heart Failure Patients With Clinically Significant Functional Mitral Regurgitation) trials (Feldman, 2014).

MITRAL STENOSIS

MS is commonly a result of rheumatic carditis, although this is currently less prevalent in Westernized nations (Bonow et al., 2008). Degenerative (senile MS), congenital, and inflammatory diseases are responsible for less than 1% of MS (Bonow et al., 2008).

Pathophysiology of MS

MS is a structural abnormality of the valve apparatus that results in valve narrowing and left ventricular inflow obstruction during diastole. MS is predominantly (99%) caused by rheumatic carditis characterized by MV leaflet thickening, calcification, and fusion of the valve apparatus and/or chordae (Carapetis, Steer, Mulholland, & Weber, 2005). Degenerative MS results from mitral calcification that begins at the annulus, extends to the leaflets, and is not accompanied by leaflet fusion.

MS left untreated is typically a slowly progressive disease that remains stable for many years. Symptoms of dyspnea on exertion may be present in mild MS. Symptoms at rest typically do not occur until the mitral valve area (MVA) is less than 1.5 cm^2 (Bonow et al., 2008). As MS becomes more severe, cardiac output becomes abnormal. These changes result in an increase in left atrial pressure, decreased pulmonary venous compliance, increased pulmonary venous pressure, and pulmonary vein and capillary distention that may lead to pulmonary edema. In the setting of chronic severe MS, pulmonary edema may not occur due to the decrease in microvascular permeability (Bonow et al., 2008).

Clinical Presentation

Individuals with MS experience a spectrum of clinical manifestations, although symptoms are generally associated with valvular disease severity, and mild MS may be asymptomatic. Individuals with moderate to severe MS may be asymptomatic or experience dyspnea, fatigue, and palpitations. Individuals with severe MS may present with symptoms of angina, heart failure, pulmonary hypertension, or cardiac arrhythmias.

Physical Examination

In MS, cardiac auscultation may reveal a loud S_1 with an opening snap that results from the thickened MV. The best location to detect a diastolic rumble associated with MS is by auscultating the apex with the bell of the stethoscope. Mild MS may be best auscultated in the left lateral decubitus position.

12-Lead ECG

ECG in individuals with MS in sinus rhythm may reveal left atrial abnormalities. Atrial fibrillation is a common finding when stenosis results in left atrial structural and electrical remodeling.

Transthoracic Echocardiogram

TTE is the primary diagnostic evaluation of MS to assess the valve structure, area, mean gradient, PAP, and cardiac chamber size and function. TTE is indicated for initial evaluation of suspected MS and periodic reevaluation for surveillance and clinical changes or symptoms. When individuals have asymptomatic, clinically stable MS, TTE for surveillance of MVA, PAP, and valve gradient is recommended based on MS severity (Table 10.5) (Bonow et al., 2008).

TABLE 10.5 Periodic Surveillance of Primary Mitral Stenosis

Mitral Stenosis Severity	Mitral Valve Area (cm²)	Echocardiogram
Mild	>1.5	Every 3–5 years
Moderate	1.0–1.5	Every 1–2 years
Severe	<1.0	Every 6–12 months

Transesophageal Echocardiogram

TEE is indicated if TTE imaging is suboptimal or not consistent with the clinical presentation. TEE is useful for the evaluation of the severity of MS, the presence of left atrial thrombus, and in individuals undergoing evaluation for percutaneous mitral balloon valvotomy or surgical repair (Bonow et al., 2008).

Cardiac Catheterization

Cardiac catheterization may be indicated to evaluate the MV and hemodynamics for echocardiographic findings inconsistent with the clinical presentation and evaluation prior to valve repair or replacement.

Therapeutic Management of MS

All individuals with MS from rheumatic endocarditis should receive treatment for group A *beta-hemolytic Streptococcus* bacteria and subacute bacterial endocarditis prophylaxis (Bonow et al., 2008). Mild asymptomatic MS does not require additional therapy. Individuals who experience dyspnea associated with exertional tachycardia may benefit from pharmacological agents with negative chronotropic properties (Monmeneu et al., 2002; Stoll, Ashcom, Johns, Johnson, & Rubal, 1995). Medical therapy for volume control is indicated in the presence of pulmonary congestion.

Anticoagulation

Anticoagulation therapy with a vitamin K antagonist (VKA) or heparin is an ACC/AHA Class I recommendation for protection from arterial embolization in the presence of MS and atrial fibrillation, prior embolic event, or left atrial thrombus (Nishimura et al., 2014). There are currently no studies that support the efficacy of newer oral anticoagulants in preventing arterial embolic events in individuals with MS.

Heart Rate Control

The control of heart rate should be considered in individuals with MS. MS is associated with atrial tachyarrhythmias, such as atrial fibrillation with rapid ventricular response. Acute episodes of rapid atrial fibrillation may cause hemodynamic instability and require emergent electrical or chemical cardioversion with anticoagulation. Heart rate control may also be considered for individuals with MS in normal sinus rhythm in which exertional activities result in symptomatic tachycardia (Monmeneu et al., 2002). Pharmacotherapeutic agents that control ventricular response by slowing AV node conduction include digoxin, beta-adrenergic receptor blockers, and nondihydropyridine calcium channel blockers.

Interventional Procedures for the Treatment of MS

Interventional procedures for rheumatic MS are based on MS severity, symptoms, and clinical factors (Figure 10.2).

Percutaneous Mitral Balloon Commissurotomy

Percutaneous mitral balloon commissurotomy (PMBC) is a catheter-based approach in which one or more large balloons are inflated across the MV to open the fused commissures. MV morphology is a pivotal consideration to determine the appropriateness for the procedure. Best outcomes are achieved with PMBC when the MV is pliable, noncalcified, and associated with minimal subvalvular-apparatus fusion (Ben Farhat et al., 1998; Nishimura et al., 2014). PMBC is not indicated in

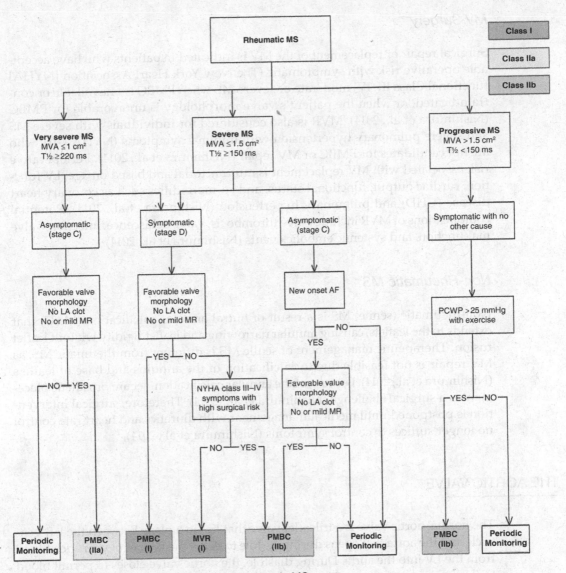

FIGURE 10.2 Indications for intervention of rheumatic MS.

AF, atrial fibrillation; LA, left atrium; MR, mitral regurgitation; MS, mitral stenosis; MVA, mitral valve area; MVR, mitral valve replacement; NHYA, New York Heart Association; PCWP, pulmonary capillary wedge pressure; PMBC, percutaneous mitral balloon commissurotomy.

Reprinted from Nishimura et al. (2014, p. 73), with permission from Elsevier.

mild MS, and the approach is contraindicated in moderate to severe MR or left atrial thrombus (Nishimura et al., 2014). PMBC achieves success in 80% to 95% of patients, resulting in an MVA greater than 1.5 cm², LA pressure less than 18 mmHg, the absence of complications, and immediate clinical-symptom improvement (Nishimura et al., 2014). Common complications include acute severe MR (2%–10%), large atrial septal defect with double balloon technique (<12%) and Inoue balloon technique (<5%), small atrial septal defect, perforation of left ventricle (0.5%–4.0%), embolic events (0.5%–3%); and myocardial infarction (0.3%–0.5%; Ben Farhat et al., 1998; Bonow et al., 2008). Mortality with PMBC is 1% to 2% (Ben Farhat et al., 1998; Bonow et al., 2008).

MV Surgery

Surgical repair or replacement of the MV is indicated in patients who have acceptable operative risk with symptomatic (The New York Heart Association [NYHA] functional Class III–IV) moderate or severe MS when PMBC is unavailable or contraindicated, or when the patient's valve morphology is unfavorable for PMBC (Nishimura et al., 2014). MVR is also considered for individuals with severe MS and severe pulmonary hypertension with minimal symptoms (NYHA I–II), who are not candidates for PMBC or MV repair (Nishimura et al., 2014). Perioperative risk associated with MV replacement is multifactorial and based on age, LV function, cardiac output, functional status, and co-morbidities such as coronary heart disease (CHD) and pulmonary hypertension (Nishimura et al., 2014). Potential complications of MVR include valve thrombosis, valve dehiscence, infection, valve malfunction, and systemic embolic events (Nishimura et al., 2014).

Non-Rheumatic MS

Non-rheumatic (senile) MS is a result of mitral annulus calcification (MAC) that extends to the leaflets, causing annular narrowing and leaflet rigidity without leaflet fusion. Therapeutic management of senile MS is different from rheumatic MS, as MV repair is not feasible due to calcification of the annulus and base of leaflets (Nishimura et al., 2014). Because of the annular calcification, secure prosthetic placement is a surgical challenge (Nishimura et al., 2014). Therefore, surgical intervention is postponed until medical management with diuretics and heart rate control no longer suffices to control symptoms (Nishimura et al., 2014).

THE AORTIC VALVE

The normal aortic valve is a trileaflet valve that lies in a plane between the left ventricle and the aorta that opens during systole to allow the flow of oxygen-rich blood from the LV into the aorta. During diastole, the aortic valve closes to permit blood to flow through the aorta. This section will detail common disorders of the aortic valve including aortic regurgitation (AR) and aortic stenosis (AS).

AORTIC VALVE REGURGITATION

Chronic aortic valve regurgitation (AR), also known as aortic insufficiency (AI) or incompetence, occurs in less than 1% of all adults and less than 2% of adults 75 years and older in the United States (Nkomo et al., 2006). AR may result from disease of the aortic valve or the aortic root. In the United States, the most prevalent causes of AR are congenital bicuspid aortic valve and aortic valve calcification (Nishimura et al., 2014). A bicuspid aortic valve occurs in 1% to 2% of live births (Carabello & Paulus, 2009). While aortic valve stenosis (AS) is the most common complication of a bicuspid aortic valve, incomplete coaptation or leaflet prolapse may cause AR. In addition, AR may develop as a result of rheumatic fever, IE, or rheumatic arthritis. Chronic AR may also result from disease processes that cause aortic root dilation, including age-related degeneration, chronic systemic hypertension, and Marfan's syndrome. A dilated aortic root results in aortic leaflet separation, thickening, or retraction, causing AR to develop. Chronic AR can progress and lead to LV volume overload, chamber dilation, and hypertrophy.

Pathophysiology of AR

AR occurs as a result of incompetent closure of the aortic valve during diastole. Incompetent closure may be a result of abnormalities of the leaflets and/or aortic root. Pathophysiology of AR depends on the etiology of the AR. The degree of hemodynamic consequence of chronic AR depends on the degree of regurgitation. During systole, the LV ejects blood through the aortic valve to the aorta. During diastole, depending on the significance of the AR, blood from the aorta regurgitates into the LV. In the setting of chronic AR, LV volume overload occurs, causing an increased end-diastolic volume. As LV pressures exceed left atrial pressure, the MV closes prematurely during diastole. In the event of high ventriculoatrial gradient pressure, the MV may open late in diastole or early systole, causing MR. Over time, the LV volume overload causes myocardial fiber stretching. LV wall thickness and stroke volume increase as a compensatory mechanism. The LV eventually ceases to compensate for AR, and LV dysfunction ensues.

Clinical Presentation

Chronic AR develops gradually and is commonly asymptomatic in the early stages; therefore, assessment should focus on common risk factors (Table 10.6). Individuals with a family history of bicuspid aortic valve may undergo screening echocardiogram, and AR is discovered prior to symptom development. A newly identified diastolic cardiac murmur may result in further evaluation in individuals with aortic valve thickening or mild valvular AR. Significant AR frequently manifests with symptoms of angina, exertional dyspnea, orthopnea, postural nocturnal dyspnea, palpitations, or tachycardia.

TABLE 10.6 Risk Factors for Chronic Aortic Regurgitation

- Bicuspid aortic valve
- Aortic valve sclerosis
- Disease of the aortic sinuses
- Disease of the ascending aorta
- History of rheumatic fever
- Known rheumatic heart disease
- History of infective endocarditis

Source: Nishimura et al. (2014).

Physical Examination

In AR, palpation of the point of maximum impulse (PMI) may be prominent and laterally displaced if LV overload, hypertrophy, or dilation is present. Auscultation of an early diastolic low-pitched, rumbling murmur is highly predictive of AR.

Individuals with chronic severe AR may demonstrate *de Musset sign* (bobbing of the head during systole), *Corrigan's pulse* (rapid rise and fall of the carotid pulse), or *Hill's sign* (leg systolic blood pressure [SBP] > 20 mmHg higher than arm SBP).

12-Lead ECG

12-lead ECG findings associated with AR may reveal left-axis deviation, voltage criteria for left ventricular hypertrophy (LVH), left bundle branch block (LBBB), or left atrial enlargement. Severe AR with uncompensated LV overload may demonstrate prominent Q waves in leads I, aVL, V3-6, or a left ventricular strain pattern.

Radiography

Chest radiograph findings associated with AR may reveal cardiomegaly, aortic calcification, and aortic root dilation.

Transthoracic Echocardiogram

TTE is recommended for individuals with signs or symptoms of AR for initial diagnosis and evaluation of valve structure, etiology and severity of regurgitation, ascending aorta structure, LV size, and function. These findings are utilized for assessing clinical outcomes and evaluating indications for valve surgery (Nishimura et al., 2014). Table 10.7 describes the hemodynamic assessment of AR severity and provides an overview of echocardiographic and angiographic grading of AR severity.

TABLE 10.7 Hemodynamic Assessment of Aortic Regurgitation (AR) Severity

AR Severity	Jet Width	Vena Contracta (cm)	Regurgitant Fraction (%)	Regurgitant Volume (mL/beat)	Effective Regurgitant Orifice (cm^2)	Equivalent Angiographic Grade
Mild	<25% of LVOT	<0.3	<30	<30	<0.10	1+
Moderate	25%–64% of LVOT	0.3–0.6	30–49	30–59	0.10–0.29	2+
Severe	≥65% of LVOT*	>0.6	≥50	≥60	≥0.3	3–4+

LVOT, left ventricular outflow tract.

*Presence of left ventricle dilation required for diagnosis.

Source: Nishimura et al. (2014).

Advanced Cardiac Imaging

CMR imaging is useful in evaluating AR severity, aortic valve and aortic morphology, LV volume, and systolic function when TTE is suboptimal or there is a discrepancy between clinical assessment and AR severity by echocardiogram.

Cardiac Catheterization

Cardiac catheterization is recommended for evaluating AR severity when there is discrepancy between clinical assessment and AR severity by echocardiogram and when CMR is unavailable or contraindicated (Nishimura et al., 2014). Cardiac catheterization is indicated for preoperative evaluation of aortic valve replacement (AVR) to assess the valve condition and to define coronary anatomy prior to AVR (Nishimura et al., 2014). In individuals who have significant CHD in whom AVR is indicated, concomitant coronary artery bypass graft (CABG) and AVR decrease the risk of perioperative myocardial infarction, mortality, late mortality, and morbidity compared with AVR alone (Wijns et al., 2010).

Exercise Testing

Exercise stress testing may be useful for assessment of functional capacity and symptom status in individuals with AR who have equivocal or no symptoms from AR (Nishimura et al., 2014).

Therapeutic Management of AR

Clinical Surveillance

Clinical surveillance frequency of individuals with chronic AR is dependent upon severity and clinical presentation of the regurgitation, LV structure and function, co-morbidities, and patient circumstances. Clinical surveillance includes assessment for new symptoms associated with AR such as dyspnea or angina. The clinician should assess functional capacity, eliciting accurate current functional capacity compared to functional capacity from 6 months prior, in order to distinguish symptoms of disease deterioration. Individuals with mild to moderate AR with normal LV structure and function are commonly evaluated in the clinical setting for disease progression annually. Individuals with severe asymptomatic AR should be evaluated every 6 months for new onset symptoms (Nishimura et al., 2014).

Patient Education

Individuals with asymptomatic mild to moderate AR should receive individually appropriate education regarding the etiology, typical clinical and pathological progression, treatment, and prognosis of AR at every clinical visit. Individuals with mild to moderate asymptomatic AR should be reassured that it is not necessary to restrict physical activity; however, they must be observant for new symptoms of clinical progression. Individuals with symptomatic or severe AR should maintain their current activities but avoid competitive sports and monitor for and report symptoms of decreased functional capacity, dyspnea, angina, palpitations, dizziness, lightheadedness, near-syncope, syncope, orthopnea, and postural nocturnal dyspnea.

TTE Surveillance

TTE surveillance is recommended in the event of new onset symptoms or for changes in cardiac symptoms. Periodic surveillance frequency is dependent upon AR severity, with more frequent evaluation conducted with more severe disease (Table 10.8). Individuals with severe AR and LV dilation will require frequent clinical and echocardiogram evaluations.

TABLE 10.8 Periodic Surveillance of Primary Aortic Regurgitation

Aortic Regurgitation Severity	Echocardiogram
Mild	Every 3–5 years
Moderate	Every 1–2 years
Severe	Every 6–12 months

Source: Nishimura et al. (2014).

Symptom Management

Individuals with chronic severe AR who develop cardiac symptoms have a high risk of mortality if AVR is not performed. Pharmacological therapy, although not a replacement for AVR, may improve symptoms in individuals with symptomatic severe AR and LV dysfunction who are awaiting AVR. Symptoms may be improved with low-sodium diet, diuretics, ACEI/angiotensin receptor blockers (ARBs), digitalis, and vasodilators (Nishimura et al., 2014). Long-term vasodilators are not associated with decreased disease progression in asymptomatic severe AR (Evangelista, Tornos, Sambola, Permanyer-Miralda, & Soler-Soler, 2005).

Hypertension Management

Hypertension treatment with dihydropyridine calcium channel blockers or ACEI/ARBs is recommended for individuals with chronic AR to maintain SBP less than 140 mmHg. While vasodilators are effective in reducing SBP, long-term therapy is not associated with halting AR progression in asymptomatic individuals with severe AR and normal LV function (Nishimura et al., 2014). Because of the reduction in heart rate and associated higher stroke volume, beta blockers are less effective in SBP control in individuals with chronic severe AR.

Physical Activity

There are no restrictions in physical activity for individuals with asymptomatic mild to moderate AR. Individuals with symptomatic or severe AR should avoid vigorous activity, and discuss individualized activity recommendations based on the patient's status.

Surgical AVR

AVR is an ACC/AHA Class I recommendation for individuals with severe symptomatic AR regardless of LV function, and for asymptomatic individuals with chronic severe AR and LV systolic dysfunction (LVEF < 50%; Nishimura et al., 2014). Figure 10.3 provides current guidance for the indication of AVR for chronic AR in symptomatic and asymptomatic individuals. Variables that impact the consideration of AVR include the severity, symptomatology, and LVEF and LVESD.

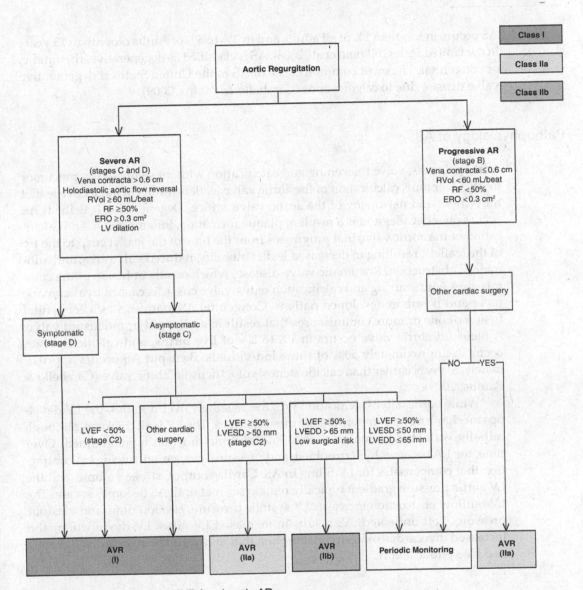

FIGURE 10.3 Indications for AVR for chronic AR.

AR, aortic regurgitation; AVR, aortic valve replacement; LVEF, left ventricular ejection fraction; LVEDD, left ventricular end-diastolic diameter; LVESD, left ventricular end-systolic diameter.

Reprinted from Nishimura et al. (2014, p. 58), with permission from Elsevier.

Surgical Repair or Replacement of Aortic Root or Ascending Aorta

Individuals with chronic AR caused by aortic root dilation in the absence of aortic valve thickening, deformation, or calcification may be eligible for a valve-sparing replacement of the aortic sinuses and ascending aorta (Nishimura et al., 2014).

AORTIC VALVE STENOSIS

AS occurs in less than 1% of all adults and in 3% to 5% of adults older than 75 years in the United States (Nkomo et al., 2006). AS is classified as degenerative, rheumatic, or congenital. The most common cause of AS in the United States is degenerative valve disease due to calcifications (Carabello & Paulus, 2009).

Pathophysiology of AS

Aortic sclerosis, valve thickening and calcification without stenosis, is a precursor to AS. Over time, calcification of the aortic valve leaflets results in ineffective leaflet movement and narrowing of the aortic valve orifice. Degenerative (calcified) AS occurs over decades and is a result of plaque formation, inflammation, and calcification of the aortic valve that progresses from the base of the leaflet cusp to the tip of the leaflets, resulting in decreased leaflet mobility, reduced valve area, and, ultimately, obstruction. Rheumatic valve disease, which results in fusion of the commissures with scarring and calcification of the valve cusps, is caused by rheumatic fever and is rare in developed nations. Congenital AS manifests as a congenital fusion of one or more commissures that result in a bicuspid or unicuspid valve. A bicuspid aortic valve occurs in 1% to 2% of live births, and calcific changes occur in approximately 50% of these individuals. Bicuspid AS occurs approximately 20 years earlier than calcific stenosis of a tricuspid aortic valve (Carabello & Paulus, 2009).

While aortic valve calcification progresses slowly over decades, the LV develops mechanisms to compensate for these changes. The LV wall thickens, although initially wall stress remains normal and systolic function is maintained. Over time, the LA becomes hypertrophied, and pressures elevate, enhancing LA contraction that compensates for LV filling in AS. Cardiac output, stroke volume, and the LV aortic pressure gradient typically remain normal until AS becomes severe. The LV outflow obstruction increases LV systolic pressure, ejection time, and diastolic pressure. Left untreated, AS results in increased LV mass, LV dysfunction, and increased myocardial oxygen consumption that may result in myocardial ischemia and LV systolic failure.

Clinical Presentation

Chronic valvular AS develops gradually and progressively over decades. Individuals with a family history of bicuspid aortic valve may undergo screening echocardiogram, and AS is discovered prior to symptom development. A newly identified systolic cardiac murmur may result in further evaluation in individuals with aortic valve thickening or mild valvular AS. Severe valvular AS frequently presents with symptoms of typical angina, exertional dyspnea, syncope, or heart failure.

Physical Examination

Palpation of the PMI may demonstrate lateral and posterior displacement in the presence of severe AS and LV failure. Concurrent palpation of the PMI and the carotid artery may demonstrate a delay in carotid pulsation in severe AS. A harsh (Grade 3/6), crescendo–decrescendo, late-peaking systolic murmur may be present. The murmur is best auscultated at the base and may radiate to the carotid arteries. Auscultation may also reveal a single or paradoxically split S_2. A thrill is highly specific for severe AS, and is often palpable in the right- and/or left-second intercostal space.

12-Lead ECG

In AS, the ECG may be normal or demonstrate nonspecific abnormalities in the presence of mild to moderate AS. Electrocardiographic evidence of disease progression includes left axis deviation, voltage criteria for LVH, or left atrial enlargement.

Transthoracic Echocardiogram

TTE is an essential tool for the diagnosis, surveillance, and management of valvular AS. Echocardiogram is used to identify the number of aortic valve leaflets (bicuspid or tricuspid), leaflet calcification, valve motion, aortic valve area, transvalvular velocity, mean pressure gradient, and LV structure and function, and to evaluate coinciding MR. Table 10.9 classifies valvular AS severity based upon echocardiographic findings. The normal aortic valve has an orifice area of 3.0 to 4.0 cm², jet velocity of less than 2.0 m/s, and a pressure gradient of a few mmHg (Saikrishnan, Kumar, Sawaya, Lerakis, & Yoganathan, 2014).

TABLE 10.9 Classification of Aortic Stenosis

Severity	Aortic Valve Area (cm²)	Pressure Gradient (mmHg)	Jet Velocity (m/sec)
Sclerosis	–	–	2.6–2.9
Mild	1.5	<25	<3.0
Moderate	1.0–1.5	25–40	3.0–4.0
Severe	<1.0	>40	>4.0
Very severe	<0.6	>60	>5.0

Source: Baumgartner et al. (2009).

Exercise Testing

Exercise testing may be considered in severe *asymptomatic* AS, with a calcified aortic valve and an aortic velocity of greater than or equal to 4.0 m/sec or mean pressure gradient 40 mmHg or higher to evaluate for the presence of exercise-induced symptoms or abnormal blood pressure responses (Nishimura et al., 2014). Exercise stress is contraindicated in symptomatic severe AS but is recommended for prognostic evaluation and surgical timing if a patient is historically asymptomatic with severe AS. Echocardiogram imaging *during* exercise stress testing is recommended versus post-exercise imaging. Symptom development, abnormal BP response, an increase in mean pressure gradient greater than 18 mmHg, blunted LVEF, and/or a systolic pulmonary arterial pressure greater than 60 mmHg during exercise is associated with poor prognosis and considered an indication for surgical treatment.

Because of the risk of complications such as syncope, ventricular tachyarrhythmias, and death, exercise testing is contraindicated in *symptomatic* individuals with AS in which echocardiogram demonstrates aortic velocity more than or equal to 4.0 m/sec or mean pressure gradient more than or equal to 40 mmHg.

Radiography

In AS, chest radiography may be normal or reveal nonspecific findings of cardiomegaly from an enlarged LV, calcification of the aortic valve cusps, or post-stenotic dilation of the aorta.

Advanced Cardiac Imaging

Cardiac computed tomography (CT), MRI, and TEE provide accurate aortic valve area definition and may be useful in the evaluation of AS, especially when a discrepancy exists between clinical presentation and echocardiographic findings.

Cardiac Catheterization

Cardiac catheterization is useful to confirm diagnosis of valvular AS when there is a discrepancy among clinical presentation and noninvasive imaging studies. Cardiac catheterization is recommended before aortic valve surgery to assess for coronary artery disease, to obtain measurements of AS severity, and to evaluate hemodynamic pressures and gradients. Cardiac catheterization is not recommended in asymptomatic valvular AS.

Therapeutic Management of AS

Clinical Surveillance

The frequency of clinical surveillance of individuals with AS is dependent upon AS severity and clinical presentation, LV structure and function, co-morbidities, and patient circumstances. Clinical surveillance includes assessment for new symptoms associated with AS such as dyspnea, angina, palpitations, and syncope. The clinician should assess the functional capacity, eliciting accurate current functional capacity compared with functional capacity from 6 months prior, in order to distinguish symptoms of disease deterioration. Individuals with mild to moderate AS should be evaluated for disease progression in the clinical setting at least annually. Individuals with moderate to severe asymptomatic AS should be evaluated every 6 months for new onset symptoms.

Patient Education

Individuals with asymptomatic mild to moderate AS should receive individually appropriate education regarding the etiology, typical clinical and pathological progression, treatment, and prognosis at every clinical visit. Individuals with mild to moderate asymptomatic AS should be reassured that it is not necessary to restrict physical activity; however, they must be observant for new symptoms of clinical progression. Individuals with symptomatic or severe AS should maintain their current activities but avoid competitive sports and monitor for and report symptoms of decreased functional capacity, dyspnea, angina, palpitations, dizziness, light-headedness, near-syncope, syncope, orthopnea, and postural nocturnal dyspnea.

TTE Surveillance

TTE surveillance is recommended for asymptomatic individuals with AS for assessment of valve area, pressure gradients, LV structure and function, and MV assessment. TTE is recommended for reevaluation if there is a change in cardiac symptoms or signs, or during pregnancy. Surveillance TTE is recommended based on AS severity, as is shown in Table 10.10 (Nishimura et al., 2014). Routine annual TTE is not indicated in the absence of clinical status change in mild to moderate AS (Nishimura et al., 2014).

TABLE 10.10 Periodic Surveillance of Primary Aortic Stenosis

Aortic Stenosis Severity	Aortic Valve Area (cm²)	Echocardiogram
Mild stenosis	1.5	Every 3–5 years
Moderate stenosis	1.0–1.5	Every 1–2 years
Severe stenosis	< 1.0	Every 6–12 months
Very severe stenosis	< 0.6	Frequently, as needed

Source: Nishimura et al. (2014).

Hypertension Management

Individuals with asymptomatic AS should receive standard therapy for blood pressure reduction, starting at low doses of pharmaceuticals with gradual upward titration and frequent monitoring. Concentric left ventricular hypertrophy and dysfunction are common complications of AS (Carabello & Paulus, 2009). There is concern that antihypertensive medications may result in decreased cardiac output in individuals with AS; however, in asymptomatic AS, hypertension is associated with a higher rate of cardiovascular events compared with normotensive individuals with AS (Rossebo et al., 2008). Diuretics should be avoided in AS if the LV chamber is small, to prevent a fall in filling pressures and cardiac output.

Hyperlipidemia

Individuals with hyperlipidemia and AS should receive standard therapy for lipid reduction. Statin therapy has not been shown to slow hemodynamic progression of calcific AS (Nishimura et al., 2014).

Bleeding Risks

Type 2A von Willebrand syndrome and gastrointestinal angiodysplasia (Heyde's syndrome) are associated with severe AS (Vincentelli et al., 2003). The von Willebrand factor proteolysis is a common result of the "high shear forces" as blood is ejected through a severely stenotic aortic valve (Vincentelli et al., 2003). According to Vincentelli et al. (2003), bleeding was present in approximately 20% of individuals with severe AS and most commonly manifested as spontaneous epistaxis, ecchymosis, gastrointestinal hemorrhage, or gingivorrhagia. Furthermore, the degree of von Willebrand factor abnormalities is directly related to the severity of AS. AVR improves von Willebrand abnormalities and associated bleeding risk. There are no current recommendations for AVR based upon a history of major bleeding events; however, the bleeding risk associated with AS has clinical relevance. Clinicians should consider bleeding risk in therapeutic management of AS, particularly in perioperative cardiac evaluation.

Antibiotic Prophylaxis

Individuals with VHD and specific co-morbidities are at risk for IE. Antibiotic prophylaxis prior to dental procedures is recommended for individuals with VHD with a history of prosthetic cardiac valve; IE; cardiac transplant with abnormal valve structure or function; or congenital heart defect repaired with prosthetic material or device for the first 6 months after the procedure, or indefinitely if residual defects remain at the site of the prosthesis (Nishimura et al., 2014). The use of antibiotic prophylaxis for AS is unwarranted otherwise.

Physical Activity

There are no physical activity restrictions for individuals with asymptomatic mild AS. Individuals with moderate to severe AS should avoid competitive sports and undergo evaluation and exercise testing prior to beginning an exercise program.

Percutaneous Aortic Balloon Dilation

Percutaneous aortic balloon dilation (valvuloplasty or valvotomy) may be considered in severely symptomatic individuals with severe AS as a bridge to AVR, or for palliative care for individuals who have contraindications for AVR (Nishimura et al., 2014). In most situations, percutaneous valvuloplasty is not an alternative to AVR in adults with AS, due to high mortality, repeat procedures, and the frequency of AVR post-valvuloplasty (Lieberman et al., 1995).

Aortic Valve Replacement

AVR with either mechanical or bioprosthetic valve is the primary treatment of severe, symptomatic AS. AVR may be accomplished with either a surgical or transcatheter approach, depending on multiple criteria, including surgical risk and co-morbidities. AVR timing is dependent upon AS severity, symptoms, and LV structure and function (Table 10.11). Surgical AVR is recommended for individuals with low to intermediate surgical risk. The PARTNER trial provided support for transcatheter aortic valve replacement (TAVR) for individuals with severe symptomatic AS with a post-TAVR survival estimate of more than 12 months who are at prohibitively high surgical risk, or for individuals for whom co-morbidities would preclude the expected benefit of surgical AVR (Leon et al., 2010).

AVR with a mechanical valve is associated with fewer reoperations and is recommended for individuals with a mechanical valve in the mitral or tricuspid location, in the absence of contraindications to anticoagulation (Nishimura et al.,

TABLE 10.11 Indications for Aortic Valve Replacement in Chronic Aortic Stenosis

Indication	Symptomatic	Asymptomatic
Recommended	Severe high-gradient AS Severe AS when undergoing other cardiac surgery	Severe AS with LVEF <50%
Reasonable	Low-flow/low-gradient severe AS with reduced LVEF and low-dose dobutamine stress study revealing aortic velocity ≥4.0 ms with valve area <1.0 cm² at any dobutamine dose	Very severe AS and low surgical risk Severe AS and decreased exercise tolerance or systolic BP drop with exercise Moderate AS when undergoing other cardiac surgery Severe AS with rapid disease progression and low surgical risk

AS, aortic valve stenosis; BP, blood pressure; LVEF, left ventricular ejection fraction.

Source: Nishimura et al. (2014).

2014). A bioprosthetic valve is recommended for individuals who decline warfarin or for whom warfarin is contraindicated, individuals younger than 65 years who prefer bioprosthesis, individuals older than 65 years who are without risk for thromboembolism, and women of childbearing age (Nishimura et al., 2014). Bioprosthetic valves carry a higher risk for valve failure, reoperation, and reduction in long-term survival (Stassano et al., 2009). Figure 10.4 provides a guideline-driven decision tree of indications for AVR due to AS.

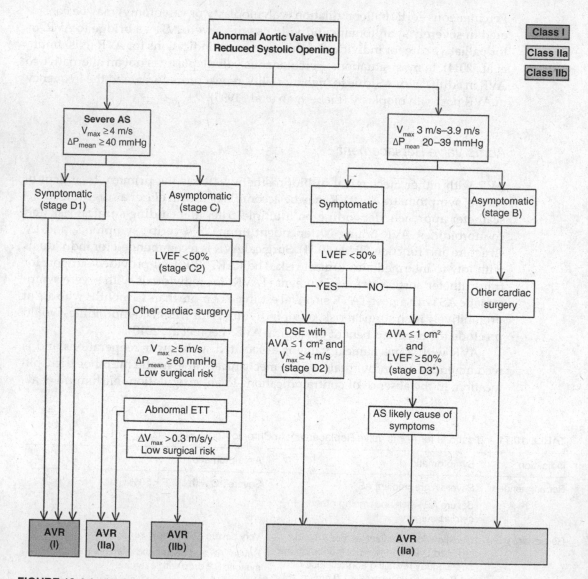

FIGURE 10.4 Indications for AVR in patients with AS.

AS, aortic valve stenosis/aortic stenosis; AVR, aortic valve replacement; LVEF, left ventricular ejection fraction.

Reprinted from Nishimura et al. (2014, p. 41), with permission from Elsevier.

THE TRICUSPID VALVE

The tricuspid valve lies in a plane between the right atrium and right ventricle. The primary components of the tricuspid valve apparatus include three triangular-shaped leaflets, chordae tendineae, papillary muscle bundles, the annulus, and the right and left ventricular walls. The three cusps, named by their respective anatomical location, are the anterosuperior (largest), posterior cusps, and the septal cusp (smallest). Disorders of any of these components can result in dysfunction of the tricuspid valve. This section details the most common tricuspid valve disorder, tricuspid regurgitation (TR).

TRICUSPID VALVE REGURGITATION

Trace to mild TR is a clinically benign finding on TTE in individuals with an anatomically normal tricuspid valve and is not associated with long-term physiological consequence (Nishimura et al., 2014). Primary disorders of the tricuspid apparatus that may cause varying degrees of TR include rheumatic disease, leaflet prolapse, Epstein's anomaly, infective endocarditis, carcinoid, radiation, blunt chest wall trauma, and RV intra-annular pacemaker or defibrillator leads. Functional tricuspid valve disorders account for 80% of all tricuspid disorders and commonly result from RV dilation, RV remodeling, elevated RV pressures, or volume overload (Nishimura et al., 2014). Functional TR may be mild, moderate, or severe. Even patients with severe TR may be clinically asymptomatic with normal physical examination findings. Functional TR may be transient in the setting of acute heart failure; however, in the setting of prolonged or recurrent RV dilation or overload the tricuspid valve apparatus may acquire permanent damage and dysfunction.

Clinical Presentation

Unless pulmonary hypertension or congestion is present, the individual with TR is often asymptomatic. In the setting of pulmonary hypertension and severe TR, cardiac output is diminished and pulmonary congestion may occur. If pulmonary congestion coincides with TR, symptoms of right-sided heart failure manifest. Presenting symptoms include dyspnea, peripheral edema, abdominal distention and pain (congestive hepatomegaly), fatigue, and weakness.

Physical Examination

Often there are no physical exam findings suggestive of TR, even severe TR (Nishimura et al., 2014). However, TR may produce a short, medium-pitch, blowing, systolic murmur, best audible at the left lower sternal border (Bickley, 2013). The cardiac murmur of TR may vary in intensity and increases with inspiration (Bickley, 2013). In individuals with severe TR that coincides with pulmonary hypertension, physical examination often reveals jugular venous distention, jugular venous systolic thrill and murmur, hyperdynamic right ventricular impulse upon palpitation of the chest wall, ascites, and peripheral edema (Mann, Zipes, Libby, & Bonow, 2015).

12-Lead ECG

ECG may be normal or reveal nonspecific abnormalities, incomplete right bundle branch block, Q waves in lead V1, and atrial fibrillation (Mann et al., 2015).

Radiography

In the setting of functional severe TR, chest x-ray may reveal cardiomegaly, prominent right atrium, pleural effusion, and superior diaphragm displacement in the presence of ascites (Mann et al., 2015).

Transthoracic Echocardiogram

TTE is an ACC/AHA Class I recommendation for evaluation of suspected TR (Nishimura et al., 2014). TTE is useful in evaluating severity and etiology, primary or functional, of TR. TTE assists in the further definition of TR and provides assessment of right-heart wall chamber size and thickness, RV systolic function, associated left-sided chamber or valve disorders, and PAP (Table 10.12).

TABLE 10.12 Echocardiographic Hemodynamic Evaluation of Triscuspid Regurgitation

Severity of Tricuspid Regurgitation	Central Jet Area (cm²)	Vena Contracta Width	Hepatic Vein Flow
Mild	<5.0	Not defined	Systolic
Moderate	5.0–10.0	Not defined but <0.7 cm	Systolic blunting
Severe	>10.0	>0.7 cm	Systolic reversal

Source: Nishimura et al. (2014).

Cardiac Catheterization

During evaluation of TR, a right-heart catheterization may be appropriate for measurement of PAPs and pulmonary vascular resistance in individuals with TR when there is a discrepancy between clinical and noninvasive diagnostic findings (Nishimura et al., 2014). Right-heart catheterization with vasodilator challenge may be useful in determining the appropriateness of pharmacological management with pulmonary vasodilator therapy. Coronary angiogram may also be appropriate in cases in which ischemia is suspected or prior to valve repair or replacement (Nishimura et al., 2014).

Therapeutic Management of TR

Therapeutic management of TR is dependent upon TR etiology (primary or functional), degree of TR, RV structure and function, presence and degree of pulmonary hypertension, presence of symptoms, and presence of coinciding left-sided VHD requiring surgical intervention. Individuals with severe TR who are symptomatic with right-sided failure and pulmonary congestion may benefit from loop diuretic therapy to reduce volume overload. In individuals who present with hepatic congestion and optimized on loop diuretic therapy, aldosterone antagonist may provide additional benefit (Nishimura et al., 2014). Pulmonary vasodilators may be indicated in the setting of pulmonary hypertension to reduce RV afterload (Nishimura et al., 2014).

Otherwise healthy individuals with severe or symptomatic primary and functional TR should undergo evaluation with a cardiologist who has VHD experience, with a heart valve team, or at a heart valve center of excellence. Individuals who have undergone invasive hemodynamic evaluation and pulmonary vasodilator challenge may benefit from pulmonary artery vasodilator therapy with epoprostenol, sildenafil, or bosentan. Tricuspid valve repair is indicated for mild, moderate, or severe functional TR during left-sided valve surgery for individuals with either tricuspid annular dilation or history of right-heart failure (Nishimura et al., 2014). While tricuspid valve repair is preferred to prosthetic replacement, replacement is indicated for primary, uncorrectable tricuspid valve disease.

THE PULMONARY VALVE

The pulmonary semilunar, trileaflet valve lies in plane within the central fibrous body and is a conduit of deoxygenated blood between the right ventricle and the pulmonary artery. The pulmonary valve is the least likely cardiac valve to be diseased in otherwise healthy adults. While disorders of the pulmonary valve are rare, severe or chronic pulmonary valve disease threatens the right-heart structure and function and may result in right-sided heart failure.

PULMONARY VALVE REGURGITATION

Asymptomatic mild to moderate pulmonary regurgitation (PR) is a clinically benign finding on TTE in individuals with an anatomically normal pulmonary valve; it has no long-term physiological consequence and requires no clinical surveillance or intervention (Nishimura et al., 2014). Primary PR may occur after surgical correction of tetralogy of Fallot or other congenital defects. Secondary PR may occur as a result of chronic pulmonary hypertension and pulmonary valve annular dilation. Severe PR may cause RV dilation and dysfunction and present as right-sided heart failure. Pulmonary valve replacement may be considered in symptomatic individuals with severe PR (Bonow et al., 2006). Individuals with severe or symptomatic PR should undergo evaluation with a cardiologist with congenital heart or VHD experience (Nishimura et al., 2014).

PULMONARY VALVE STENOSIS

Pulmonary valve stenosis (PS) is a rare disorder primarily associated with congenital heart disease; it is less commonly caused by carcinoid, tumors, or vegetation (Nishimura et al., 2014). Most often, individuals in Westernized countries with PS and/or congenital heart disease are identified and treated in childhood or adolescence. Adults with chronic severe PS may present with dyspnea and fatigue secondary to decreased cardiac output, lightheadedness, or syncope in the presence of dehydration. Left untreated, severe PS may result in TR and right ventricular failure (Bonow et al., 2006). As with other valvular disorders, TTE is the diagnostic standard for evaluation of PS (Bonow et al., 2006). Echocardiogram may reveal evidence of pulmonary valve thickening, calcification, distortion, decreased excursion, right ventricular outflow tract narrowing, right ventricle or right atrium enlargement, or enlargement of the main branch of the pulmonary artery (Nishimura et al., 2014). Individuals with severe or symptomatic PS should undergo evaluation with a cardiologist having congenital heart or VHD experience. Balloon valvotomy is the primary standard treatment of severe and/or symptomatic PS; after pulmonary balloon valvotomy, PR is often a clinically benign consequence (Bonow et al., 2006).

THE PROSTHETIC VALVE

Since the first prosthetic cardiac valve was placed in the 1960s, issues surrounding the evaluation and management of the prosthetic valve have evolved significantly. In most situations, individuals who have indications for a prosthetic valve and who undergo valve replacement have an improved quality of life and longer life expectancy; however, there are additional lifelong issues such as anticoagulation and the lingering possibility of prosthetic disorder or failure. The clinical course of individuals who have received a prosthetic valve varies based upon the presence of coinciding cardiac disease.

Diagnostic Surveillance

Individuals who undergo prosthetic valve replacement should have echocardiographic examination 6 weeks to 3 months after valve implant. In the asymptomatic and stable individual after prosthetic valve replacement, annual evaluation with history and physical examination is recommended. Echocardiogram is recommended if there are clinical symptoms or signs suggestive of valve dysfunction. Given that bioprosthetic valve degeneration markedly increases after the 10-year point, annual echocardiogram surveillance is considered a reasonable approach to surveillance of a bioprosthetic valve older than 10 years.

Anticoagulation for the Prevention of Thromboembolic Events

Prosthetic valve thrombosis and thromboembolic events are associated with prosthetic cardiac valves; therefore individuals with mechanical prosthetic valves must
be protected from thromboembolism with VKA anticoagulation. Current evidence
suggests that hospital-based anticoagulation clinic monitoring is associated with
lower complications and is a cost-effective strategy given the reduction of bleeding and hemorrhagic complications (Metlay et al., 2008). Home self-monitoring
may be considered for engaged, educated, and motivated individuals (Nishimura
et al., 2014).

The most recent ACC/AHA 2014 Guidelines for Management of VHD (Nishimura et al., 2014) recommends that individuals with aortic mechanical valves
including an aortic bileaflet or "current generation single tilting disc" who have no
additional risk factors for thromboembolism be maintained on VKA with a target
INR of 2.5 (INR range 2–3). Individuals with mechanical AVRs who have additional risk factors for thromboembolic events including atrial fibrillation, history of thromboembolism, LV dysfunction, hypercoagulability, or older generation
mechanical valves (ball-in-cage) should be maintained at a target INR of 3 (INR
range 2.5–3.5).

Mechanical MVR is associated with a higher incidence of thrombosis compared to mechanical AVR prosthesis; therefore, the recommended goal of VKA
anticoagulation is an INR of 3.0 (INR range 2.5–3.0; Nishimura et al., 2014). Furthermore, ASA (aspirin) 75 to 100 mg is recommended in addition to VKA anticoagulation in individuals with mechanical prosthesis for improved reduction of the
incidence of embolism or death (Nishimura et al., 2014). Despite the slight increase
in minor bleeding with combination VKA and ASA, the combination significantly
decreases the incidence of major embolism, death, stroke, and mortality (Nishimura
et al., 2014).

VKA anticoagulation is reasonable for the first 3 months after bioprosthetic
MVR, AVR, or MV repair. In individuals without additional risk factors for thromboembolism, mitral bioprosthesis carries a higher annual incidence of thromboembolism compared to aortic bioprosthesis, 2.4% and 1.9%, respectively. The overall
risk of ischemic CVA after all MV surgery is elevated. Anticoagulation with VKA
is considered reasonable for the first 3 months post-bioprosthetic MVR or repair
with goal INR of 2.5 (Nishimura et al., 2014). Lifelong aspirin therapy (75–100 mg)
is considered reasonable in all individuals with a bioprosthetic aortic valve or MV
(Nishimura et al., 2014).

Anticoagulation with oral direct thrombin inhibitors or anti-Xa is not approved
or recommended in individuals with mechanical valves. The RE-Align trial
was stopped due to increased thrombolytic complications in the dabigatran arm
(Nishimura et al., 2014). While not the current standard of care, in 2006 the FDA-
approved randomized testing of lower anticoagulation for the newer generation
aortic mechanical prosthetic valve, from On-X Life Technologies, Inc.™ (Kumbhani,
2011). Reduced anticoagulation after mechanical AVR is currently being evaluated
for thromboembolic protection and reduced incidence of bleeding in the PROACT
Trial (Puskas et al., 2014). There is evidence that supports the use of reduced anticoagulation among individuals enrolled in the high-risk AVR arm of the PROACT
Trial; however, full analysis of reduced anticoagulation for mechanical valves continues (Puskas et al., 2014).

Prosthetic Valve Disorders

Prosthetic valve disorders are not a frequent occurrence. However, the possibility of prosthetic stenosis, regurgitation, degeneration, or paravalvular leak should be considered with consistent clinical cardiac signs or symptoms. Prosthetic valve stenosis is rare; however, it may occur in the mechanical valve as a result of chronic valve thrombus, pannus (granulation tissue) formation, or a combination of both. On rare occasions, patient–prosthesis mismatch may occur, when the size of the implanted prosthetic valve is unable to maintain the requirement for blood flow (Nishimura et al., 2014). Prosthetic valve replacement is indicated for severe symptomatic prosthetic stenosis (Nishimura et al., 2014). Prosthetic valve regurgitation with a bioprosthetic valve may occur as a result of valve tissue calcification and degeneration. Paravalvular leak is a potential complication of mechanical and bioprosthetic valve implant as a result of inadequate surgical suturing, infectious endocarditis, or significant scarring (Nishimura et al., 2014; Smolka & Wojakowski, 2010). Structural valve deterioration (SVD) is rare in mechanical prosthetic valves. SVD rates increase 7 years post–prosthetic valve placement. Risk factors for SVD include young age at the time of implant, valve positioning, hypertension, LV hypertrophy or dysfunction, and renal insufficiency.

Infective Endocarditis

Individuals who have a prosthetic valve or intracardiac device are at a significantly greater risk of IE. Prevention of IE with antibiotic prophylaxis against IE is recommended for individuals with prosthetic cardiac valves (Nishimura et al., 2014).

For full reference citations to this chapter, please see "Section References" in the back of the book, under the heading "Section II."

Chronic Heart Failure

DOROTHY L. MURPHY AND KELLEY M. ANDERSON

Heart failure (HF) is a complex, hemodynamic, and neurohormonal-mediated clinical syndrome resulting from conditions that alter cardiac output, increase venous pressure, and cause progressive deterioration of the heart, with a composite of ensuing symptoms. According to the American Heart Association (AHA), almost 6 million adults in the United States are diagnosed with HF, and predictions are that from 2013 to 2030 the prevalence will increase by 25% (Go et al., 2013). HF currently affects approximately 2% to 3% of adults 45 years and older (Davies, 2001), with 650,000 new cases diagnosed annually in this age group (Go et al., 2013).

The burdens of HF include high mortality, frequent hospitalizations, and significant financial costs. At the time of diagnosis, 5-year mortality for HF with reduced ejection fraction (HFrEF) is approximately 50% (Go et al., 2013). In the United States, HF is one of the most frequent causes of hospitalization in those 65 years and older, accounting for more than 70% of the estimated 1 million hospitalizations in 2010 (Roger et al., 2012). Approximately 50% of all hospital admissions for clinically decompensated HF occur in individuals with normal left ventricular ejection fraction (LVEF; Bursi et al., 2006). The economic cost in the United States exceeds $40 billion annually and is projected to increase to $70 billion by 2030 (Go et al., 2013; Roger et al., 2012). Although the implications of HF are significant in all the clinical settings, the purpose of this section is to provide guidance on the evaluation and management of chronic stable left-sided HF with preserved and reduced LVEF.

PATHOPHYSIOLOGY

HF With Reduced Ejection Fraction

HFrEF is defined as an LVEF less than or equal to 40% and cardiac incapacity to produce sufficient cardiac output for the perfusion of vital organs. Cardiac output is dependent upon stroke volume and heart rate (HR). Stroke volume is determined by three interrelated components: cardiac contractility, preload, and afterload. Cardiac contractility, defined as the degree of myocardial fiber shortening, is regulated by myocardial stretch, oxygenation, and sympathetic nerve supply. Cardiac contractility may be decreased in the event of ventricular remodeling, myocardial ischemia or infarction, cardiomyopathies, and myocarditis. In the state of decreased cardiac contractility, the stroke volume is decreased and left ventricular end-diastolic volume (LVEDV) increases, causing ventricular dilation and an increase in preload. Left ventricular preload, or left ventricular end-diastolic pressure (LVEDP), is the pressure produced at the end of diastole. The volume of venous return to the ventricle and the ventricular end-systolic volume regulate ventricular preload. Afterload is the force against the ejection of blood from the left ventricle, and it is consistent with the aortic systolic pressure.

According to Laplace's Law, wall tension is directly correlated to the effect of intraventricular pressure and internal radius. Thus, wall tension is inversely related to ventricular wall thickness. During HFrEF, the decrease in cardiac output activates compensatory mechanisms purposed to maintain hemodynamic stability. In response to suboptimal cardiac output, the sympathetic nervous system (SNS) activates the release of epinephrine and norepinephrine that bind to adrenergic receptors, increasing cardiac output by increasing cardiac contractility and rate. However, when chronic HF ensues, incessant neurohormonal activation has deleterious effects on the cardiac structure and function. Protracted SNS response increases myocardial oxygen consumption, resulting in myocyte cell death, ventricular hypertrophy, and arrhythmias.

A decrease in cardiac output and SNS activation stimulates the renin-angiotensin-aldosterone system (RAAS). Renin is released and precipitates the conversion of angiotensinogen to angiotensin I (AI); subsequently, angiotensin-converting enzyme (ACE) converts AI to angiotensin II (AII). AII is a powerful peripheral vasoconstrictor that increases afterload, ventricular wall stress, and myocardial oxygen requirements. AII also increases sodium reabsorption in the proximal tubule of the nephron, SNS activation, aldosterone release from the adrenal cortex, and myocardial fibrosis. Aldosterone, a mineralocorticoid hormone, stimulates sodium reabsorption in the distal tubules of the nephrons and contributes to volume overload and escalation of myocardial fibrosis. Furthermore, SNS and RAAS activate the production of endothelin-1. This potent vasoconstrictor, which is produced by the vascular endothelial cells, regulates sodium retention and myocardial contractility.

Further neurohormonal cascades include the release of arginine vasopressin (AVP) from the hypothalamus, impairment of the nitric oxide (NO) system, and release of natriuretic peptides. AVP release promotes water reabsorption in the nephron, increases peripheral vasoconstriction, and decreases cardiac contractility. NO is an endothelium-derived potent vasodilator that results in relaxation of the vascular smooth muscle, as well as in a reduction in afterload. An impaired NO system is associated with decreased cardiac contractility and ventricular remodeling. The structural and mechanical impairment and neurohormonal-mediated response is a perpetual cycle, which compounds the HF pathology. Natriuretic peptides, atrial natriuretic peptide (ANP) and B-type natriuretic peptide (BNP), are released from the atrial and ventricular walls, respectively, in response to wall stress. These natriuretic peptides counteract the SNS and RAAS, resulting in peripheral vasodilation and sodium excretion to delay myocardial fibrosis and hypertrophy.

HF With Preserved Ejection Fraction (HFpEF)

Integral processes occur during diastole in the normal heart. After left ventricular systolic ejection, isovolumetric relaxation occurs and results in a rapid decrease in left ventricular pressure. Subsequently, when the left ventricular pressure decreases and becomes less than the left atrial pressure, rapid left ventricular filling begins. Filling ceases when the pressure between the left ventricle (LV) and left atrium (LA)

TABLE 11.1 Risk Factors for Heart Failure (HF)

HF With Reduced Ejection Fraction (HFrEF)	HF With Preserved Ejection Fraction (HFpEF)
Coronary heart disease	Hypertension
Hypertension	75 years or older
Valvular heart disease	Female gender
Severe renal failure	Obesity
Diabetes mellitus/metabolic syndrome	Atrial fibrillation
Constrictive pericarditis	Valvular heart disease
Cardiomyopathies	
Tachyarrhythmias	
Human immunodeficiency virus	
Muscular dystrophy	
Cardiotoxins	
Chemotherapy, alcohol, cocaine	
Obesity	

are approximately equal, termed diastasis. During diastasis, the LV pressure depends on ventricular compliance and influences atrial systole. Diastolic dysfunction results from delayed myocardial relaxation, impaired LV filling, and LV stiffness. Diastolic dysfunction causes an increase and leftward shift in the end-diastolic pressure volume relationship. HFpEF is purported to be a manifestation of diastolic dysfunction resulting in increased systemic venous return.

Many cardiac and chronic diseases can be a precursor to HF (Table 11.1); however, the most common causes of HF are coronary heart disease (CHD) and hypertensive heart disease (Yancy et al., 2013).

CARDIOMYOPATHY

Cardiomyopathies are diseases of the heart muscle. There are primarily three distinct types: dilated, hypertrophic, and restrictive. Although the risk factors, etiologies, and management strategies differ, the cardiomyopathies have a common element of potentially provoking clinical manifestations of HF.

Dilated Cardiomyopathy

Dilated cardiomyopathy (DCM) refers to diseases of the myocardium that result in left- and/or right-ventricular dilation and systolic dysfunction. DCM is commonly a result of CHD, HF, stenotic or regurgitant valvular disease, metabolic disorders, renal failure, cardiotoxins, infections, inflammation, or idiopathic or genetic disorders. Ischemic cardiomyopathy is the most common DCM. Systemic disorders associated with DCM include obesity, obstructive sleep apnea, diabetes mellitus, hyperthyroidism, and excess or deficiency of growth hormones. Cardiotoxins that may result in DCM include alcohol, cocaine, chemotherapeutic agents, anthracyclines, and trastuzumab.

Symptoms of DCM include HF, dyspnea, fatigue, and/or nonanginal chest pain. Physical examination may reveal cardiomegaly, S_3 or S_4 gallop, and a murmur of tricuspid or mitral regurgitation. Chest x-ray (CXR) may reveal moderate to severe cardiomegaly or pulmonary venous hypertension. Echocardiogram findings associated with DCM include left ventricular dilation, often with systolic dysfunction. Cardiac catheterization findings consistent with DCM are left ventricular enlargement and dysfunction, elevated left- and/or right-sided filling pressures, tricuspid and/or mitral regurgitation, and diminished cardiac output. Therapeutic management consists of treating reversible causes, as well as standard HF therapeutic management.

Depending on the etiology, reversible causes of DCM can potentially reverse the cardiomyopathy through revascularization, withdrawal of cardiotoxins, treatment of obstructive sleep apnea, or control of metabolic disorders.

Hypertrophic Cardiomyopathy

Hypertrophic cardiomyopathy (HCM) refers to diseases that result in left and/or right ventricular thickening, commonly asymmetrical and involving the interventricular septum. HCM is a genetic heart defect in which the septal wall hypertrophies and the enlargement may result in a left ventricular outflow tract obstruction. Patients with HCM may be asymptomatic or present with dyspnea, syncope, myocardial ischemia, HF, cardiac arrhythmia, or sudden cardiac death (SCD). Physical examination findings consistent with HCM may reveal apical systolic thrill and heave, S_4 gallop, systolic murmur that increases with Valsalva, and brisk carotid upstroke. Echocardiogram assessment may reveal mild to moderate cardiac enlargement, asymmetrical septal hypertrophy, or small or normal-sized LV with a narrow LV outflow tract. Cardiac catheterization findings consistent with HCM include diminished LV compliance, mitral regurgitation (MR), vigorous systolic function, and dynamic LV outflow gradient. Therapeutic management of HCM with outflow tract obstruction may require invasive or surgical treatment to reduce septal hypertrophy, such as alcohol septal ablation or myotomy-myectomy.

Restrictive Cardiomyopathy

Restrictive cardiomyopathy is characterized by a decreased left and/or right ventricular diastolic size, rigid and noncompliant myocardium that results in restrictive filling, and normal or near-normal systolic function. Restrictive cardiomyopathy may be idiopathic or a result of systemic diseases, including scleroderma, sarcoidosis, amyloidosis, and hemochromatosis. Physical examination may reveal findings consistent with cardiomegaly, including an S_3 or S_4 gallop, murmur of tricuspid or mitral regurgitation, and Kussmaul sign. Echocardiogram may reveal increased LV wall thickness and mass, small or normal-sized LV with normal systolic function, and pericardial effusion. Cardiac catheterization findings consistent with restrictive cardiomyopathy include diminished LV compliance, normal systolic function, and elevated left- and right-sided filling pressures. Restrictive cardiomyopathy treatment is dependent upon the etiology and includes treatment aimed at reversing systemic causes and managing cardiac manifestations, such as HF and cardiac arrhythmias.

HF CLASSIFICATION

HF classification provides an evidence-based structure for assessing disease progression, symptoms, and prognosis, and guiding therapeutic management. There are three predominant classification systems utilized in HF: HF based on LVEF, the American College of Cardiology Foundation/American Heart Association (ACCF/AHA) Stages, and the New York Heart Association (NYHA) system. HFrEF, systolic HF, presents with increased left ventricular cavity volume and reduced LVEF, defined as LVEF equal to or less than 40% (Yancy et al., 2013). HFpEF, diastolic HF, is characterized by the clinical presentation of HF with normal systolic function and impaired left ventricular relaxation (diastolic dysfunction). HFpEF is defined as clinical HF with LVEF 50% or greater (Yancy et al., 2013). The ACCF/AHA classifies HF according to four stages, A to D (Table 11.2) based on identified risk factors, cardiac structure, cardiac function, and symptoms (Yancy et al., 2013).

TABLE 11.2 ACCF/AHA Stages of Heart Failure (HF)

HF Stage	A	B	C	D
HF risk factors	Yes	Yes	Yes	Yes
Structural heart disease	No	Yes	Yes	Yes
Symptoms	No	No	Yes	Yes
HF	No, at risk	No, at risk	Yes	Yes

ACCF, American College of Cardiology Foundation; AHA, American Heart Association.

The NYHA Classification (Table 11.3) is a subjective assessment that provides a guide for evaluating HF symptom severity, graded I to IV, with Class I representing less severe symptoms to Class IV with the most severe symptoms.

TABLE 11.3 New York Heart Association (NYHA) Functional Classification

NYHA Class	Severity	Symptom Characteristics
I	Mild	No symptoms or limitations with ordinary physical activity
II	Mild	Symptoms of HF on ordinary exertion
III	Moderate	Symptoms of HF on less-than-ordinary exertion
IV	Severe	Symptoms of HF at rest

HF, heart failure.

DIAGNOSIS

HF is a clinical syndrome in which a diagnosis is confirmed on the simultaneous presence of compelling past medical history, physical examination findings, and clinical symptoms. The Framingham Criteria for Congestive Heart Failure (McKee, Casteilli, McNamara, & Kannel, 1971) is 100% sensitive and 78% specific for correctly diagnosing an individual with HF. The Framingham Criteria for Congestive Heart Failure include major and minor criteria suggestive of HF. For a clinical diagnosis of HF, at least two major criteria or one major criterion in conjunction with two minor criteria not attributed to another health condition must be present. Major criteria include paroxysmal nocturnal dyspnea, neck vein distention, rales, acute pulmonary edema, S_3 gallop, hepatojugular reflux, weight loss more than 4.5 kg in 5 days in response to treatment, and radiographic evidence of cardiomegaly. Minor criteria include bilateral ankle edema, nocturnal cough, dyspnea on ordinary exertion, hepatomegaly, pleural effusion, decrease in vital capacity (one third from maximum recorded), and tachycardia with heart rate higher than 120 beats/minute.

Clinical Presentation

Individuals with chronic HF may present with mild to severe clinical findings of dyspnea, fatigue, orthopnea, paroxysmal nocturnal dyspnea, cough, peripheral edema, ascites, rapid weight gain, nausea, and/or early satiety. While not a sensitive predictor, dyspnea is the most specific indicator for detecting HF. In end-stage HF, patients may present with significant weight loss associated with cardiac cachexia.

Health History

Obtaining a thorough health history is the single most important tool available for identifying cardiac or noncardiac disorders, family history, or behaviors that contribute to the evaluation and management of chronic HF. Past health history that has been associated with HF includes CHD, systemic hypertension, diabetes mellitus, sleep apnea, alcohol use, chest irradiation, HIV, thyroid disease, connective tissue disease, or cardiotoxic chemotherapeutic agents. The presence of prior cardiac disease, including valvular disease, should be evaluated. The frequency and timing of HF hospital admissions are prognostic and may signal a need for optimizing therapeutic management.

Medication History

Important to assess is the patient's medication history and adherence habits. Inadvertent or intentional medication nonadherence to HF regimens is a common precipitator of decompensated HF and is associated with an adverse prognosis. Intentional discontinuation of HF medication may reflect intolerance, adverse reaction, or no perceived value by the patient. Assess medication history for pharmacotherapeutics that may exacerbate HF, including glitazones, nonsteroidal anti-inflammatory drugs (NSAIDs), rofecoxib, calcium channel blockers, Class I and III antiarrhythmics, metformin, cilostazol, and amphetamines (Amabile & Spencer, 2004).

Family History

Three-generation family history is recommended in patients with idiopathic DCM to support the diagnosis of familial cardiomyopathy (Lindenfeld et al., 2010; Yancy et al., 2013). Family history should explore for the presence of first-degree relatives with an unexplained sudden death when younger than 35 years, conduction defects that result in bradycardia and syncopal or pre-syncopal episodes, and cardiac arrhythmias that are associated with SCD (Mestroni et al., 1999).

Social History

Social history should include assessment for tobacco, alcohol, or illicit drug use. Smoking is associated with a twofold increased risk for multiple HF hospitalizations, and alcohol use is associated with fivefold higher risk (Evangelista, Doering, & Dracup, 2000).

Review of Systems

Review of systems should attempt to elicit the following symptoms: weight gain or loss, fatigue, headaches, weakness, visual changes, dizziness, syncope or near-syncope, numbness, dry mouth, shortness of breath at rest or with activity, cough—noting if productive or nonproductive, hemoptysis, chest pain, tightness, or pressure, palpitations, orthopnea, postural orthostatic dyspnea, edema, change in appetite, early satiety, abdominal distention, urinary frequency, scrotal edema in males, and leg pain or edema. Individuals with chronic HF should be asked to describe their level of activity and ability to complete the usual activities of daily living, noting and documenting cardiac symptoms according to the NYHA Classification. Assessment of mental health, sleep patterns, and social support also assists in identifying factors that contribute to HF outcomes.

DIAGNOSTIC EVALUATION

Physical Examination

Clinicians must be vigilant for physical signs identifying HF status. The constitutional or general assessment may include fatigue and weight changes. Individuals with chronic HF should be evaluated for signs of volume status at every clinical encounter. Serial assessment of the following is absolutely essential: vital signs (weight, blood pressure [BP], respiratory rate [RR], heart rate [HR]), estimates of jugular venous distention (JVD), evaluation for the presence of cardiac (S_3 or S_4) or pulmonary auscultatory abnormalities, hepatomegaly, hepatojugular reflux, peripheral edema, and orthopnea. According to a systematic review (Mant et al., 2009), the most specific indicators of clinical HF are additional heart sounds (99%), hepatomegaly (97%), pulmonary rales (81%), peripheral edema (72%), and elevated JVD (70%). Skin should be assessed for color, temperature, and moisture.

Hemodynamic Profile

Hemodynamic profiling described by Nohria, Mielniczuk, and Stevenson (2005) is a quick, evidence-based method to estimate LV filling pressures and degree of perfusion. LV filling pressures are the closest hemodynamic parameter associated with HF decompensation and clinical outcomes. LV filling pressures correlate with B-type natriuretic peptide (BNP) levels, as BNP is released from the ventricles in response to elevated ventricular volume or pressure. The degree of congestion at rest, "wet" or "dry," indicates that the LV filling pressure is elevated or not, respectively. Highly predictive signs and symptoms of elevated LV filling pressures include orthopnea, JVD, and hepatojugular reflux. The adequacy of peripheral perfusion, "warm" or "cold," refers to adequate or reduced perfusion, respectively. Narrow pulse pressure, pulsus alternans, impaired mental status, and cool extremities are indicative of inadequate peripheral perfusion. Figure 11.1 is a useful resource for classifying hemodynamic profiles of individuals with HF into four categories. These profiles provide risk stratification of early or late mortality (Nohria et al., 2005).

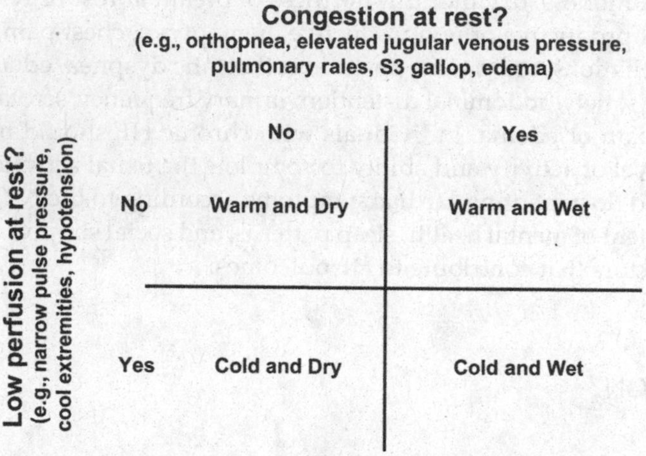

Congestion at rest?
(e.g., orthopnea, elevated jugular venous pressure, pulmonary rales, S3 gallop, edema)

	No	Yes
No	Warm and Dry	Warm and Wet
Yes	Cold and Dry	Cold and Wet

Low perfusion at rest? (e.g., narrow pulse pressure, cool extremities, hypotension)

FIGURE 11.1 Rapid clinical assessment of acute heart failure syndromes.
Reprinted from Nohria et al. (2005, p. 35), with permission from Elsevier.

12-Lead Electrocardiogram

Electrocardiogram (ECG) evidence of prior myocardial infarction, myocardial ischemia, left bundle branch block, and left ventricular hypertrophy with or without ST or T wave abnormalities are identified as high-risk features for HF (Okin et al., 2006).

Laboratory

Initial laboratory assessment in the evaluation of stable LV dysfunction includes a complete blood count, basic metabolic panel of electrolytes and renal function, magnesium, calcium, fasting lipids, liver function test, thyroid panel, and urinalysis. Serum creatinine and potassium is indicated on a regular basis given the risk for renal injury and hyperkalemia with ACE inhibitor (ACEI), angiotensin receptor blocker (ARB), and aldosterone antagonist pharmacotherapy. With significant systemic congestion, liver enzymes may be elevated in patients with right-sided HF. If dyspnea is present, BNP is useful to differentiate dyspnea of cardiac or pulmonary origin. BNP value–guided therapeutic management may be useful to achieve optimal dosing in clinically stable euvolemic individuals; however, there is little evidence that serial measurement of BNP reduces mortality or risk of hospitalization in individuals with chronic stable HF (Yancy et al., 2013). Etiologic evaluation may include screening for hemochromatosis, HIV, rheumatologic disease, amyloidosis, and pheochromocytoma.

Cardiac troponin is a specific marker of myocardial cell injury and may be elevated in the presence of LV strain due to HF. Novel serum biomarkers of myocardial stress, ST2 and galectin-3, correlate with ventricular hypertrophy, dysfunction, and fibrosis (Shah et al., 2014). Cystatin-c is an early marker of renal injury that is presumed to provide additional information in chronic or acute HF (Moran et al., 2008). Each of these new biomarkers has been evaluated and may prove useful for additional prognostic determination of acute and chronic HF in the future (Yancy et al., 2013).

Chest X-Ray

CXR is an ACCF/AHA Class I recommendation for individuals suspected of having new-onset or acute decompensated HF to assess cardiac size and pulmonary congestion, and to evaluate for potential alternative cardiac or pulmonary abnormalities that may contribute to the patient presentation (Yancy et al., 2013). CXR may reveal cardiac enlargement, increased pulmonary venous pressure, pulmonary edema, and/or valvular or pericardial abnormalities.

Cardiac Catheterization

Left-heart catheterization is reasonable if ischemia is considered as an etiology to HF when individuals are eligible for coronary revascularization. Right-heart catheterization is typically reserved for individuals in acute decompensated HF whose hemodynamic status remains unclear or is unresponsive to therapy.

HF RISK STRATIFICATION

Several risk assessment models have been validated and may be useful in the evaluation of mortality risk in chronic HF. Risk assessment is recommended to assess for adverse outcomes and to guide therapeutic management (Yancy et al., 2013). The Seattle Heart Failure Model (SHFM) is a well-validated, multivariate risk model derived from the PRAISE 1 database and substantiated prospectively in the ELITE 1, UW, RENAISSANCE, Val-HeFT, and IN-CHF trials (Latini et al., 2004; Levy et al., 2006; Mann et al., 2004; Mozaffarian, Nye, & Levy, 2003; Packer et al., 1996; Pitt et al., 1999). The SHFM integrates common clinical and laboratory factors, as well

TABLE 11.4 Components of the Interactive Seattle Heart Failure Model

Characteristics	Medications	Diuretics	Lab Data	Devices	Interventions
Age	ACEI	Lasix	Hemoglobin	None	ACEI
Gender	Beta blocker	Bumex	Lymphocytes	BiV pacemaker	ARB
NYHA class	ARB	Demadex	Uric acid	ICD	Beta blocker
Weight	Statin	Metolazone	Total cholesterol	Biv/ICD	Statin
EF	Allopurinol	HCTZ	Sodium		Aldosterone
Systolic BP	Aldosterone				blocker
Ischemic etiology	blocker				Device therapy
QRS > 120 msec					

ACEI, angiotensin-converting enzyme inhibitors; ARB, angiotensin receptor blockers; BP, blood pressure; EF, ejection fraction; HCTZ, hydrochlorothiazide; ICD, implantable cardioverter defibrillator; NYHA, New York Heart Association.

Source: Levy et al. (2006).

as pharmacologic and device therapy, to estimate survival (Table 11.4). An online calculator is available at www.SeattleHeartFailureModel.org that provides baseline survival, mortality, and mean life expectancy at 1, 2, and 5 years. The SHFM provides clinicians with an ability to calculate risk reduction with the use of recommended pharmacologic and device therapies.

NONPHARMACOLOGIC MANAGEMENT

Self-Care Education

Patient self-care education, an ACCF/AHA Class I recommendation, improves patient knowledge, self-monitoring, and medication adherence (Yancy et al., 2013). Furthermore, patient self-care educational interventions have been shown to decrease unplanned hospitalizations, emergency room visits, hospitalized days, costs, and mortality rates (Yancy et al., 2013). Unfortunately, according to data from the IMPROVE HF registry, only 61% of adults with HF receive self-care education within a 12-month period (Fonarow et al., 2010).

Self-care education for individuals with chronic HF should be included in every clinical encounter. Individuals with HF need to comprehend the following: the basic pathophysiology of HF and basic pharmacologic and nonpharmacologic therapeutic mechanisms, monitoring volume status, scheduling and taking their medications, and when and who to notify if signs or symptoms of volume overload are identified.

Sodium Restriction

Dietary sodium restriction has been at the core of therapeutic management of HF for decades. Recently, this basic therapeutic management guideline has been questioned and challenged (Institute of Medicine, 2013). After a systematic review of randomized controlled trials, the Institute of Medicine concluded that low-sodium diet may lead to higher risk of adverse events in individuals with mid to late stage

HFrEF who are concurrently on aggressive therapeutic regimens. The ACCF/AHA recommends a 1,500-mg sodium limitation for individuals with Stage A and B HF. The Heart Failure Society of America recommends a 2- to 3-g sodium restriction for individuals with HF regardless of ejection fraction (EF) and less than 2 g daily for individuals with moderate to severe HF (Lindenfeld et al., 2010).

Fluid Restriction

Fluid restriction is considered a reasonable therapeutic approach for individuals in Stage D HF with hyponatremia (Yancy et al., 2013). Hyponatremia occurs in individuals with advanced HF due to the inability to eliminate fluid volume. Fluid restriction to less than 2 L per day may improve hyponatremia, a common electrolyte imbalance in advanced HF that is associated with poorer outcomes.

Sleep Hygiene

Sleep apnea is a common co-morbidity of chronic HF, with studies demonstrating that 61% of individuals with HF are affected (Bradley et al., 2005). Therefore, the cardiovascular clinician should have a high level of suspicion for sleep apnea. Furthermore, studies have documented that individuals with sleep disorders report experiencing daytime sleepiness (Arzt et al., 2006). If clinically supported, the clinician should consider referring individuals with HF with suspicion of sleep disturbance for a sleep study. Studies have demonstrated that continuous positive airway pressure (CPAP) significantly decreases the apnea-hypopnea index and improves nocturnal oxygenation, LVEF, functional capacity, and health-related quality of life in individuals with HF and sleep apnea (Bradley et al., 2005; Kaneko et al., 2003; Mansfield et al., 2004).

Exercise

According to the HF-ACTION trial, a 3-month exercise-training program in individuals with HFrEF (mean LVEF 25%) significantly reduced all-cause mortality, cardiovascular mortality, and hospitalizations compared with usual care (O'Connor et al., 2009). An individualized approach based on HF stage, NYHA classification, and current functional capacity, as well as clinical judgment, should be applied when making therapeutic recommendations for exercise in individuals with HF. Furthermore, a functional stress test is useful in determining appropriate activity recommendations. For individuals with stable (Stage A or B) HF who have NYHA Class I–II symptoms, a simple daily walking regimen may be sufficient. Cardiac rehabilitation may also be useful in individuals with stable HF to improve functional capacity, enhance health-related quality of life, and reduce mortality (O'Connor et al., 2009). Medicare recently approved cardiac rehabilitation for individuals with stable HFrEF with LVEF 35% or less and NYHA Class II to IV symptoms despite optimal therapy for at least 6 weeks (Centers for Medicare & Medicaid Services [CMS], 2013).

PHARMACOLOGIC THERAPY

HF With Reduced Ejection Fraction

There is a significant quantity of evidence supporting pharmacologic management of chronic stable HFrEF. Therapeutic management recommendations are based upon the HF Stage and NYHA Classification. Unless contraindicated, all individuals with chronic HFrEF should be prescribed ACEI or ARBs, one of three proven beta blockers (metoprolol succinate, carvedilol, or bisoprolol), and diuretics in the presence of volume overload. Abrupt withdrawal of ACEI or ARBs, beta blockers, or a diuretic may result in clinical deterioration and is a common cause of decompensated HF. Appropriate pharmacologic management principles are determined based on the stages of the development of HF (Figure 11.2) and the NYHA Classification.

HF With Preserved Ejection Fraction

The objectives of managing HFpEF include systolic and diastolic blood pressure (DBP) control, balancing intravascular volume with diuretics and/or low-sodium diet, and maintaining sinus rhythm. LV wall thickness regression is associated with improved diastolic filling, active relaxation, and decreased chamber stiffness. ACEI, ARBs, or calcium channel blocker (CCB) may regress LV thickness more than beta blockers (Klingbeil, Schneider, Martus, Messerli, & Schmieder, 2003). Diuretics are recommended for volume control in individuals with HFpEF who have symptoms of volume overload. Maintenance of sinus rhythm with rate control may improve symptomatic HF. Unlike the benefits associated with renin-aldosterone system inhibition in HFrEF, there is not an associated decrease in mortality or hospitalizations for clinical HF in individuals with HFpEF (Komajda et al., 2011; Yusuf et al., 2003).

Angiotensin-Converting Enzyme Inhibitors

Treatment with ACEI is an ACCF/AHA Class I recommendation for reduction of morbidity and mortality in individuals with HFrEF (Yancy et al., 2013). ACEI should be initiated at a low dose and gradually titrated to the targeted dose, unless contraindicated or not tolerated. Renal function and serum potassium should be assessed prior to and within 2 weeks of initiating an ACEI, particularly in individuals with renal insufficiency, hypotension, hyponatremia, or diabetes, and with concomitant administration of potassium supplements, aldosterone antagonists, and diuretics. ACEI are typically well tolerated among individuals with HFrEF; however, some individuals will experience angioedema, which requires immediate discontinuation, and an ACEI–induced cough (recurrent, nonproductive cough) that will resolve once the ACEI is discontinued. There is no evidence suggesting superiority in symptoms or survival among ACEI, as each ACEI has a similar class effect.

Heart Failure

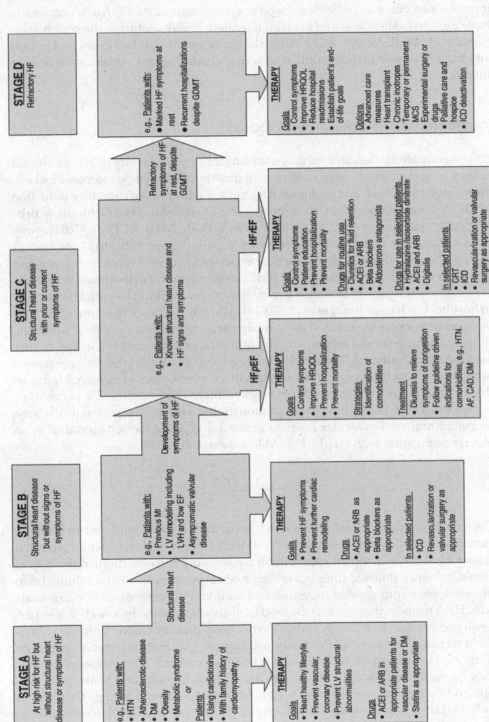

FIGURE 11.2 Stages in the development of HF and recommended therapy by stage.

ACEI, angiotensin-converting enzyme inhibitors; ARB, angiotensin receptor blockers; CAD, coronary artery disease; CRT, cardiac resynchronization therapy; DM, diabetes mellitus; EF, ejection fraction; GDMT, guideline-directed medical therapy; HF, heart failure; HRQOL, health-related quality of life; HTN, hypertension; ICD, implantable cardioverter defibrillator; LV, left ventricle; LVH, left ventricular hypertrophy; MCS, mechanical circulatory support; MI, myocardial infarct.

Reprinted from Yancy et al. (2013, pp. e240–e327), with permission from Wolters Kluwer Health.

Angiotensin Receptor Blockers

ARBs are considered to be as efficacious as ACEI. ARBs are commonly utilized to improve outcomes in individuals who are intolerant of ACEI. ARBs commonly have minimal side effects and are well tolerated, and do not have the cough associated with ACEI. As with ACEI, ARBs should be initiated at low doses and gradually titrated upward while monitoring serum creatinine and potassium at regular intervals.

Beta-Adrenergic Receptor Blockers (Beta Blockers)

Unless contraindicated, individuals with current or prior history of HFrEF should receive pharmacologic therapy with one of three beta-adrenergic receptor blockers, bisoprolol, carvedilol, and metoprolol succinate, with proven mortality reduction (CIBIS-II Investigators and Committees, 1999; Domanski, 2000; Eichhorn & Bristow, 2001; Hialmarson et al., 2000; Poole-Wilson et al., 2003). ACEI or ARB therapy does not need to be fully optimized prior to initiating an indicated beta blocker therapy, because the mortality reduction associated with beta blockers recommend initiation as soon as a diagnosis of HFrEF is established. Furthermore, safety has been demonstrated with initiation in clinically stable individuals with HFrEF prior to hospital discharge (Yancy et al., 2013). Initially, low doses are recommended with upward titration as tolerated. If there is current or recent history of fluid overload, diuretic therapy should accompany the initiation of beta blocker therapy to prevent the exacerbation of fluid overload. A high level of caution should be exercised in the use of beta blockers in individuals with co-morbidities of asthma, bradycardia, or second- or third-degree heart block without the presence of a pacemaker. Nebivolol, a beta-1 selective blocker, demonstrated a modest reduction in all-cause mortality and cardiovascular hospitalization but did not reduce mortality in an elderly population with HFpEF (van Veldhuisen et al., 2009).

Diuretics

Diuretic therapy combined with sodium restriction is often indicated to improve clinical signs and symptoms in individuals with HF and evidence of fluid retention (Yancy et al., 2013). Loop diuretics inhibit the reabsorption of sodium at the loop of Henle, whereas thiazide diuretics inhibit reabsorption in the distal tubule. Loop diuretics are recommended to restore and maintain volume status in individuals with HF. Thiazide diuretics may be used in individuals with chronic HF for hypertension control or to intensify diuresis when loop diuretics alone produce suboptimal results. Once signs of fluid overload improve, diuretic maintenance may be continued to prevent the reoccurrence of volume overload. A fixed dose of diuretic may be prescribed for individuals who are attuned to their fluid status and comprehend therapeutic use of diuretics. Individuals who consume a high-sodium diet or NSAIDs, or who have significant renal impairment, may develop resistance to diuretic therapy. HF decompensation may occur, in which case diuretic therapy will need to be adjusted. The most common risks associated with diuretic therapy include electrolyte imbalance (depletion of sodium and/or magnesium), hypotension, and azotemia. Serum creatinine, potassium, and magnesium should be evaluated within 5 to 7 days of initiating diuretic therapy, and regular surveillance should be individualized for each patient's history and presentation.

Aldosterone Receptor Antagonist

Aldosterone receptor antagonists significantly reduce all-cause mortality, SCD, and HF hospitalizations (Pitt et al., 1999; Zannad et al., 2011) in individuals with HFrEF. Spironolactone or eplerenone is recommended for individuals with HFrEF with LVEF less than 35%, NYHA Class II to IV symptoms, serum creatinine less than 2 mg/dL (female) or 2.5 mg/dL (male), and potassium less than 5 mEq/dL, who are already optimized on ACEI and beta blocker therapy. Eplerenone has demonstrated favorable outcomes when compared to spironolactone for the reduction of death and risk of HF hospitalization in individuals with HFrEF (Zannad et al., 2011). Serum creatinine and potassium should be evaluated within 3 days and again at 7 days of initiating aldosterone receptor antagonist. Monthly monitoring of serum creatinine and potassium is recommended every month for 3 months, then every 3 months thereafter. This monitoring schedule should be restarted if there is an increase in aldosterone receptor antagonist, ACEI, or ARB therapy. Potassium supplements should be discontinued upon initiation of an aldosterone receptor antagonist, because there is major risk of hyperkalemia secondary to decreased potassium excretion. Furthermore, the combination of an ACEI, ARB, and aldosterone receptor antagonist is hazardous and should be avoided. Individuals treated with an aldosterone receptor antagonist should be advised to avoid high-potassium foods and NSAIDs.

Vasodilators

Vasodilator therapy reduces preload and afterload and may improve cardiac output. In particular, the combination of hydralazine and isosorbide dinitrate has demonstrated significant reduction in morbidity and mortality in Black individuals with HFrEF with NYHA Class III to IV, receiving optimal therapeutic management with ACEI and beta blockers (Taylor et al., 2004). Therefore, the combination of hydralazine and isosorbide dinitrate is recommended as standard therapy in addition to ACEI and beta blocker for African Americans with HFrEF, NYHA II to IV (Lindenfeld et al., 2010). For non–African American individuals with HFrEF who remain symptomatic despite optimized standard therapy, the combination of hydralazine and isosorbide dinitrate may be considered (Yancy et al., 2013). Hydralazine and isosorbide dinitrate are available separately or in a combination single form. Dosages of hydralazine 20 mg and isosorbide dinitrate 37.5 mg are scheduled three times daily as a fixed dose or separately in low doses and titrated upward until therapy is optimized. Common side effects include headache, hypotension, dizziness, and gastrointestinal upset.

Digoxin

Digoxin may be considered for symptom management, to improve functional capacity, and to reduce hospitalizations in individuals with Class II to IV HFrEF, unless contraindicated (Yancy et al., 2013). Digoxin is contraindicated for individuals who have sinus or atrioventricular block in the absence of permanent pacing, and it should be used cautiously in individuals who also take medications that can depress sinus or atrioventricular nodal functions, or that may potentiate digoxin levels. Clinicians may consider low dose (0.125 mg) every other day for individuals older than 70 years or who have renal insufficiency or low body mass index. The recommended maintenance plasma concentration of digoxin for HF is between 0.5 and 0.9 ng/mL. Due to the narrow therapeutic index, individuals receiving digoxin therapy should be evaluated for signs and symptoms of digoxin toxicity.

Anticoagulation

It is well recognized that individuals with chronic HFrEF are at a 1% to 3% annual increased risk of thromboembolic events secondary to blood stasis in a dilated hypokinetic left ventricle, even when there is no echocardiographic evidence of LV thrombus (Yancy et al., 2013). However, in the absence of additional risk factors for cardioembolic stroke (atrial fibrillation, prior stroke, pulmonary embolism, or cardioembolic source), anticoagulation is not recommended, as there is no evidence of benefit and it increases the risk of major bleeding events (Yancy et al., 2013). Chronic anticoagulation is indicated in individuals with chronic HF who have atrial fibrillation and an additional cardioembolic risk factor. Chronic anticoagulation is considered reasonable in individuals with chronic HF who have atrial fibrillation without additional cardioembolic risk factors. However, chronic anticoagulation is not recommended in HFrEF in the absence of atrial fibrillation, a prior thromboembolic event, or a cardioembolic source (Yancy et al., 2013).

Antiplatelet Therapy

There are conflicting data to support the benefit of low-dose aspirin in individuals with chronic HF without CHD, prior myocardial infarction (MI), or additional cardiovascular risk factors (Yancy et al., 2013). Therefore, currently aspirin therapy for empiric primary prevention in individuals with HF without additional cardiovascular risk factors is not supported (Yancy et al., 2013).

Statin Therapy

Several studies have evaluated the benefit of statin therapy in individuals with chronic HF; however, there is insufficient evidence to support statin therapy in the absence of other indications for treatment such as cardiovascular or peripheral atherosclerosis, hyperlipidemia, or diabetes mellitus (Yancy et al., 2013).

CARDIOVASCULAR IMPLANTABLE ELECTRONIC DEVICE THERAPY

There are strong indications and recommendations for cardiovascular implantable electronic device (CIED) therapy in the management of HF (Yancy et al., 2013). Implantable cardiac devices, including implantable cardioverter defibrillators (ICD) and biventricular pacemakers, have improved cardiovascular outcomes of individuals with HF (Yancy et al., 2013). The cardiovascular clinician should educate individuals with HF about the risk of complications, as sudden and non-sudden death may result from HF. Furthermore, the cardiovascular clinician provides an essential role in the referral of patients to electrophysiology services and in assisting patient understanding of device therapy, including safety, efficacy, and possible complications of cardiac device therapy.

Implantable Cardioverter Defibrillator

Individuals with HFrEF are at high risk of ventricular tachyarrhythmia that may lead to SCD (Singh, Carson, & Fisher, 1997). Furthermore, individuals with HFrEF who have experienced sustained ventricular tachycardia, ventricular fibrillation, cardiac arrest, or syncopal episodes are at even higher risk for reoccurrence of these disorders (Lane, Cowie, & Chow, 2005). ICD implantation is associated with 23% to 30% reduction in mortality individuals with HFrEF less than or equal to 35% (Moss et al., 1996).

Primary prevention for SCD with ICD therapy is recommended for individuals with LVEF less than or equal to 35% with NYHA Class II or III, with HF of ischemic etiology, and after at least 40 days post-MI, who have received optimal therapeutic management on appropriate pharmacologic therapy for a minimum of 3 to 6 months without LV function recovery (Yancy et al., 2013). The landmark trials, MADIT and MADIT-II, provided substantial evidence supporting ICD for primary prevention of SCD in the absence of patient-experienced or documented life-threatening cardiac arrhythmias (MADIT Executive Committee, 1991; Moss et al., 1996).

The cardiovascular clinician must recognize that despite the strong evidence supporting the use of ICD, the decision for individuals is complex and a difficult one. The clinician must educate individuals and their families regarding the statistical risk of ventricular arrhythmias and SCD, benefits and risks associated with ICD placement, and long-term device management. After implant, cardiac devices are regularly interrogated to assess the burden of cardiac arrhythmias and to ensure optimal device functioning.

Common tachyarrhythmias in this patient population include atrial fibrillation and nonsustained ventricular tachycardia. According to the MADIT-RIT trial, ICD device programing such as antitachycardia pacing can be optimized to reduce the incidence of inappropriate shocks. Elevated burden of cardiac arrhythmias places an individual at risk for frequent ICD shocks. Alternatively, cardiac electrophysiology treatment with antiarrhythmic pharmacotherapeutic and/or catheter ablation can decrease the incidence of tachyarrhythmia and hence the risk of ICD shock. It should be noted that frequent ICD shocks may decrease quality of life and cause psychological distress (Sears & Conti, 2002).

Cardiac Resynchronization Therapy

Individuals with HFrEF accompanied by ventricular dyssynchronous contraction manifested as a QRS prolongation greater than 120 ms have poorer outcomes than individuals with normal ventricular conduction (Young et al., 2003). Ventricular dyssynchrony reduces cardiac output and worsens valvular function. Cardiac resynchronization therapy (CRT) restores ventricular synchrony through pacing of both ventricles almost simultaneously, called biventricular pacing. Two large trials, the COMPANION and CARE-HF, have demonstrated that CRT in combination with optimal medical management improves LVEF, HF symptoms, and health-related quality of life, and reduces HF hospitalization and mortality in individuals with HFrEF with QRS duration 120 ms or more with NYHA Class II/IV symptoms (Bristow et al., 2004; Cleland et al., 2005; Yancy et al., 2013).

CLINICAL CHALLENGES

Optimizing Therapeutic Management

According to analysis from the IMPROVE HF trial, only 27% of individuals with chronic HF received all recommended therapies in which they were eligible. Health care quality measures evaluate LVEF assessment, symptom and activity assessment, symptom management, self-care education, pharmacologic therapy with beta blocker and ACEI or ARB, and ICD therapy counseling (Fonarow et al., 2010). Given the burden of chronic HF, significant resources are allocated to improve optimal therapeutic management. An effective system of care coordination is an ACCF/AHA Class I Level of Evidence B indication. Cardiovascular clinicians must work within the care team and with the individual/family to develop a clear, detailed, and evidence-based plan of care to optimize therapeutic management of chronic HF and co-morbidities. Strategies to improve successful care management and therapeutic regimens are outlined by the ACCF/AHA Guidelines for management of HF (Yancy et al., 2013).

Adherence to Therapeutic Regimen

Adherence to therapeutic management is a significant challenge in the management of chronic diseases. Nonadherence is a precipitating factor for HF decompensation and hospitalization in up to 40% of individuals with chronic HF (Michalsen, Konig, & Thimme, 1998). Multiple causes of nonadherence have been identified, including therapeutic regimen intolerance; adverse effects; individually perceived lack of benefit or contraindication; access to medications or resources; social support; educational deficits; or transportation to health care appointments (Hauptman, 2008; Sayers, Riegel, Pawlowski, Coyne, & Samaha, 2008; van der Wal et al., 2006). It is important to assess for therapeutic regimen adherence at each clinical encounter and provide supportive services to assist the individual and family to overcome barriers to adherence.

HF self-care patient education and support interventions have demonstrated notable improvement in self-care behaviors and have significantly decreased the deleterious outcomes of HF (Jaarsma, Stromberg, Martensson, & Dracup, 2003; Krumholz et al., 2002; McAlister, Stewart, Ferrua, & McMurray, 2004; Stromberg et al., 2003). Additional solutions to adherence barriers may be to provide alternative approaches to pharmacologic therapies that reduce adverse effects, prescribe more cost-effective pharmacotherapeutics, involve concerned and proactive family members in the plan of care, plan for follow-up visits that are conducive with the individual and/or family activities of daily living, or referring the individual who needs outside social support to appropriate community agencies.

Decompensated HF

The cardiovascular clinician must maintain vigilance in evaluating for precipitating factors of HF decompensation and proactively implement primary and secondary interventions to attempt to manage factors that place individuals at risk of decompensation. Factors that have been associated with HF decompensation are detailed in Table 11.5.

TABLE 11.5 Factors That Precipitate HF Decompensation

Precipitating Factors
Nonadherence with therapeutic regimen
Uncontrolled hypertension
Acute cardiovascular disorders (ACS, endocarditis, myopericarditis)
Cardiac arrhythmias
Negative inotropic drugs (nifedipine, diltiazem, verapamil)
Excessive alcohol
Illicit drug use
Uncontrolled endocrine disorders
Infections (influenza, pneumonia)
Educational deficits

ACS, acute coronary syndrome.

Transitions of Care

Individuals with HF have the highest risk of mortality and hospital readmission within the first 30 days and 1 year of a hospital discharge for HF, and transitions of care are a vulnerable period of time (Yancy et al., 2013). It is recommended that individuals hospitalized with HF have hospital discharge follow-up within 7 to 10 days of discharge. Common clinical issues that must be addressed at discharge follow-up include evaluating volume status and medication regimen, reevaluating appropriate optimization of therapeutic regimen, assessing for nonadherence and troubleshooting to improve therapeutic regimen adherence, and surveying serum basic metabolic panel. The hospital follow-up visit typically requires extensive therapeutic management and self-care education. Depending on the patient status, it may be necessary for frequent, even weekly, follow-up visits until therapeutic regimen is optimized and clinical status is determined stable.

ADVANCED HF

Individuals with symptomatic advanced HF who are optimized on therapeutic management require a coordinated team-based approach to advanced care planning. Advanced or refractory HF, HF Stage D, or NYHA Class IV is HF refractory to optimized therapeutic regimen and these patients may be eligible for advanced treatment options, such as mechanical circulatory support (MCS), ultrafiltration, continuous inotropic infusions, cardiac transplantation, or those with end-stage HF who would benefit from palliative or hospice care (Yancy et al., 2013). Individuals with a recent HF hospitalization or other high risk factors for decompensation may benefit from coordinated care services offered by specialty HF clinics. Individuals at high risk for decompensation include those with NYHA Class III to IV symptoms despite optimal therapeutic management, history of frequent hospitalizations, renal disease, chronic obstructive pulmonary disease, and persistent nonadherence to treatment regimens (Lindenfeld et al., 2010).

REFERRALS AND CONSULTATIONS

The cardiovascular clinician has a vast range of expert resources available for collaboration to improve outcomes. A dietary consult is useful in supplementing patient education regarding cardiac diet, dietary modifications of low-sodium or fluid restriction, and to promote healthy weight in those overweight or with cachexia. Nephrology can provide assistance when titrating ACEI/ARBs in the presence of chronic kidney disease. Cardiac rehabilitation is recommended in clinically stable individuals with HF to improve quality of life, functional capacity, and mortality and reduce hospitalizations (Yancy et al., 2013). Electrophysiology specialists assist in determining appropriateness of device therapy and management of the devices. Advanced HF management programs offer coordinated care to individuals at high risk. Selected patients with Stage D HF and poor prognosis despite optimal medical devices and/or surgical treatment should be referred to a cardiac transplant center for heart transplant (HT) evaluation (Yancy et al., 2013). Patient selection for HT is a multidisciplinary approach undertaken by experienced advanced HF and HT health care providers. The International Society for Heart and Lung Transplantation provides detailed listing criteria.

Individuals with end-stage HF, despite the decision to refer for MCS or HT evaluation, should be considered for referral to palliative care (Yancy et al., 2013). Palliative care services provide patient and family guidance related to advanced HF treatment modalities and/or end-of-life issues. Palliative care services also provide timely patient referral to hospice care when indicated.

ADVANCED HF MANAGEMENT PROGRAMS

Advanced HF management programs have become prevalent over the past decade in an attempt to reduce HF hospital admissions and costs. Advanced HF management programs vary in services offered but generally should provide a systematic approach to patient surveillance, care coordination, treatment, risk modification, and education. Multiple studies have demonstrated positive health care outcomes, including reduced HF re-hospitalization rates and emergency room visits, fewer hospital days, reduced cost of care, and improved patient functional status and quality of life (Fonarow et al., 1997; Yancy et al., 2013).

LEFT VENTRICULAR ASSIST DEVICE

There has been significant progress in MCS over the past decade. Before 2008, all MCS devices implanted in the United States were either pneumatically driven volume displacement pumps or pulsatile flow pumps (Stewart, 2012). Since the advent of the continuous-flow ventricular assist device (VAD), survival after implant has improved, associated complications have decreased, and the use of VADs has been expanded (Stewart, 2012).

The left ventricular assist device (LVAD), originally FDA approved in the 1990s as a short-term bridge to transplant, has become a mainstream treatment for individuals as a bridge to transplant (BTT), bridge to candidacy (BTC), bridge to recovery (BTR), or as destination therapy (DT) (Stewart, 2012). Individuals who are actively listed for HT with refractory congestion, progressive end-organ damage, anticipated long waitlist time, or who seek improved quality of life while awaiting transplant may be eligible for BTT MCS. Individuals who may be eligible but not actively listed for HT and have no absolute contraindication to HT may be eligible for BTC MCS. Individuals ineligible for HT who need long-term MCS with only LV support may be candidates for DT. Individuals with reversible cardiac insult who require temporary MCS and are expected to recover may be candidates for BTR MCS. In general, individuals with LVEF less than 25%, NYHA Class III to IV despite optimal medical and device therapy with either high predicted 1- to 2-year mortality or dependence on continuous inotropic support should be referred to HT centers for evaluation for MCS (Yancy et al., 2013).

Despite significant advancements in continuous-flow MCS devices that have improved patient outcomes, serious complications may occur. Complications include the risk for thromboembolic events, bleeding, and infection. The REMATCH trial reported that 24% of individuals with LVADs experience a significant neurologic event, including stroke (Lietz et al., 2007). Inadequate anticoagulation therapy is the strongest risk factor for thromboembolic event. Postoperative hemorrhage occurs in approximately 60% of individuals undergoing VAD implant. MCS device infection is less common in continuous-flow devices, but may involve the percutaneous driveline and/or pump pocket. Device infection carries significant risk of mortality and is challenging to eradicate. RV failure is another risk associated with LVAD implant (Deng et al., 2005). Careful patient selection for MCS is undertaken by experienced HF MCS health professionals.

HEART TRANSPLANT

Individuals with end-stage HF have a dire prognosis. One-year average survival for HT-eligible patients is 39%. HT is the gold standard therapy for qualifying individuals with end-stage HF. HT alone is associated with an 8.5-year life expectancy increase and significant cost savings (Long, Swain, & Mangi, 2014). However, there is a critical shortage of donor hearts, often resulting in a median list wait time of 5.6 months. HT evaluation is indicated for select individuals with Stage D HF despite optimal medical, device, and/or surgical treatment (Yancy et al., 2013).

HF is a prevalent, complex disease process requiring multifaceted care. Significant advancements in HF treatment modalities have been made over the past 20 years that have demonstrated improved patient outcomes, including increased quality of life, reduced mortality, and decreased health care–associated cost. Despite these advancements, HF is the only cardiovascular disease that continues to increase in prevalence and remains a significant burden upon patients, families, and the health care system. Cardiovascular clinicians must be astute in the care, evaluation, and management of individuals with HF.

For full reference citations to this chapter, please see "Section References" in the back of the book, under the heading "Section II."

Cardiac Electrophysiology

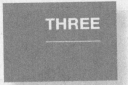
THREE

Common Electrophysiology Presentations

ROBERT L. McSWAIN

Given that electrophysiology (EP) is a subspecialty of cardiology, it is more likely that patients are referred after an initial evaluation by a general cardiologist or a primary care clinician. The reason for the referral may be to determine whether a patient's symptoms are related to EP condition for the purposes of establishing a diagnosis or for consultation in the management of known EP conditions. Nonetheless, patients do occasionally self-refer, sometimes because a friend or family member suffered similar symptoms and received benefit from an EP specialist. Common reasons for EP referral include the evaluation of symptoms of palpitations, syncope and near syncope, chest pain, fatigue, dyspnea, and concerns regarding genetic syndromes.

Besides finding a solution for the symptoms, it is important to make a prompt and proper diagnosis, because some arrhythmias can be harmful or even lethal. For example, atrial fibrillation (AF) predisposes individuals to cerebrovascular accidents, and ventricular tachycardia potentially places the patient at risk for sudden cardiac death. However, the significance of an arrhythmia depends on the underlying health of the heart in question, as predominantly determined by the left ventricular function and the status of the coronary arteries. With occasional exception, including genetic syndromes, tachyarrhythmias of both atrial and ventricular origin tend to be a nuisance rather than a danger in patients with a structurally normal heart. The term "nuisance" does not depreciate the importance of symptoms or the arrhythmia itself, but it is meant to contrast with the potentially poor prognosis of patients with untreated ventricular arrhythmias in the setting of cardiomyopathy or coronary heart disease. As an example of the prognostic importance of overall heart health, documented wide-complex tachyarrhythmias in patients with known coronary heart disease can be presumed to be malignant ventricular arrhythmia unless proved to be otherwise. Therefore, symptom evaluation may require further diagnostic testing, including 12-lead electrocardiogram (ECG), ambulatory ECG monitoring, orthostatic vital signs, tilt table testing, echocardiogram, ischemic evaluations, and electrophysiology studies (EPS).

PALPITATIONS

Palpitations are the most common reason for patients to directly seek an EP evaluation. The focus of the evaluation is the determination of whether the symptoms are due to an arrhythmia, and, if so, its type and significance. When a patient reports palpitations, it indicates an experience of a sensation from time to time that the heartbeat is rapid, erratic, or pounding. The patient may not verbalize these specific terms, instead describing the symptoms as skipped beats or a "racing" heart; sometimes, the symptoms are very subtle, with the patient simply uncomfortably aware of the heartbeat.

Regardless of the particular description, the focus is on translating the symptoms of palpitations into a precise medical diagnosis that can be further evaluated or treated. Toward that goal, a careful history is crucial, often suggesting a diagnosis based on the nature of the symptoms. For further clues, the patient should be asked about the onset, location, duration, associated findings, characteristics, aggravating and alleviating factors, frequency, timing, and severity of symptoms, as well as potentially interacting conditions. Extremely brief symptoms, often described as "skipped beats," may represent premature atrial contractions (PACs) or premature ventricular contractions (PVCs). Symptoms lasting a few seconds may represent brief runs of atrial arrhythmia or nonsustained ventricular tachycardia (NSVT); symptoms with a longer duration can be due to sustained arrhythmias. In the setting of arrhythmias, palpitations will be related to some form of atrial or ventricular tachyarrhythmia.

The frequency of symptoms may not support the primary diagnosis, because there is variability from mild to severe cases of almost all arrhythmic syndromes. However, the frequency can be extremely important for decisions regarding therapy; occasionally, there is an indication for "watchful waiting" when symptoms occur rarely. Especially for benign conditions, clinicians avoid initiating a situation in which side effects of the treatment may be more bothersome to the patient than the disease itself. For example, a patient might prefer to suffer 10 minutes of debilitating palpitations once a year rather than experience the daily side effects of an antiarrhythmic agent.

Triggers and timing of palpitations may not provide a firm diagnosis in and of themselves, but these factors can provide meaningful information. Patients with supraventricular tachycardia (SVT) commonly report episodes that begin after bending to obtain an object from the floor and then returning to an upright position. Both AF and ventricular arrhythmias can be triggered by exercise. Palpitations that occur at night or after heavy meals may suggest AF. Caffeine, fatigue, over-the-counter cold medications containing stimulant decongestants, beta-agonist therapy for allergic and pulmonary disorders, and alcohol can serve as triggers for most of these arrhythmic syndromes; thus, these triggers do not particularly discriminate.

Symptom severity correlates with heart rate more than the chamber of origin, and it cannot reliably differentiate between atrial and ventricular arrhythmias. Nonetheless, rapid ventricular arrhythmias tend to be the most symptomatic of all, and, more commonly, lead to loss of consciousness and adverse events than atrial arrhythmias. Symptom severity can vary greatly in individuals presenting with palpitations, even for the same condition. Occasionally, symptoms will be disproportionate to the extent of the objective arrhythmic disease identified. Some patients are practically incapacitated by occasional PVCs or AF, while others are entirely asymptomatic and somewhat blissfully unaware. Symptoms may be a double-edged sword, causing the patient to suffer, for example, in AF that is highly symptomatic but prompting the patient to seek evaluation and therapy, and serving as a direct long-term gauge of the success of therapy. On the other extreme, asymptomatic patients with AF do not suffer from palpitations, but occasionally will present with a cerebrovascular accident, with the subsequent diagnosis of AF determined to be the etiology.

The presence of interacting co-morbid conditions can provide important causes for the etiology of palpitations. Hyperthyroidism, or overly treated hypothyroidism, is a risk factor for AF. There is also a well-established association between obstructive sleep apnea and AF. The presence of cardiomyopathy or coronary heart disease requires that ventricular arrhythmias are considered a cause for palpitations, although atrial arrhythmias are commonly associated with these co-morbidities as well.

Even with a carefully obtained, accurate history, there is substantial symptom overlap between the various identifiable arrhythmias, and thus further testing is often required, usually in the form of ambulatory ECG monitoring. Historically, this has existed in the form of noninvasive Holter or event monitoring, though, if necessary, implantable loop recorders are available. Additional testing may include an echocardiogram, ischemic evaluations, and EPS, although even with further testing, a specific arrhythmia may not be identified. However preferred and ideal it is to know a specific diagnosis, occasionally it is reasonable and common to treat palpitations empirically with beta blockers or calcium channel blockers, presuming that a structurally normal heart exists based on the assessment, including echocardiogram and ischemic evaluation.

SYNCOPE

Syncope is a transient loss of consciousness; presyncope is a constellation of symptoms that indicate a loss of consciousness is imminent, although it does not occur. Patients experiencing recurrent and especially unexplained syncope are often referred for EP. The possible causes for syncope are myriad, and 30% to 40% of cases remain unexplained. In many instances, syncope is not rhythm or even cardiac related. As such, a parallel evaluation with neurology often coincides with the cardiac workup. The etiology of syncope is also related to the patient's age, for example, a younger patient is more likely to have a vasovagal reaction and an older adult is more likely to have aortic valve disease. However, in the overall population, the primary established causes of syncope are neurally mediated or vasovagal, followed by primary arrhythmias (Strickberger et al., 2006). Sometimes, EP becomes involved because the diagnosis has been established, and therapy involving an EP specialist is needed; for example, a pacemaker implantation for complete heart block. But often, patients are referred, because the diagnosis is elusive despite a fairly extensive cardiac and neurologic workup. In this case, the history and diagnostic testing are valuable to determine the possible causes of syncope.

Prior history of any known cardiac disease must be determined, as syncope in the setting of coronary heart disease, structural heart disease, accessory pathways, genetic ion-channel disorders, or cardiomyopathy increases the probability of arrhythmia as the origin of syncope (Strickberger et al., 2006). Arrhythmias associated with syncope include pauses from sick sinus syndrome, atrioventricular block, or ventricular tachycardia. The mechanism of syncope due to these arrhythmias is a decreased cardiac output leading to hypotension and cerebral hypoperfusion.

The patient history and report of symptoms is important to differentiate causes of syncope, and neurologic conditions are more likely to present with prodrome, auras, focal neurologic deficits, and syncope followed by amnesia or confusion.

Cardiac arrhythmias often present suddenly: Pauses can lead to syncope without unheralded warning, whereas ventricular tachyarrhythmias might cause transient palpitations before loss of consciousness. The observations of the patient by witnesses of the syncopal event are particularly helpful, as the patient is often unaware of events that occur during the syncopal episode.

An evaluation of pharmaceuticals, over-the-counter medications, and supplements is important in the evaluation of syncope. Many medications are associated with syncope, with the primary classes including antihypertensives, antiarrhythmics, tricyclic antidepressants, nitrates, and antiparkinsonian medications (Strickberger et al., 2006). Other pharmacologic agents are associated with QT prolongation and may increase the risk for torsades de pointes (TdP), a form of polymorphic ventricular tachycardia (Table 12.1).

EP can offer syncope testing based on the presenting symptoms and findings of the history and physical examination, including orthostatic vital signs. The EP testing for syncope involves event monitoring, implanted loop recorders (ILR), tilt table testing, and a diagnostic (invasive) EP study (Figure 12.1). If neurocardiogenic syncope is suspected, then the evaluation may begin with a tilt table test. If structural heart disease is involved, a diagnostic EP study may be a component of the initial evaluation to exclude potentially malignant bradyrhythmia or tachyarrhythmias. In cases in which the diagnosis remains elusive, an ILR may be the best option and it improves the diagnostic yield in a significant number of patients with unexplained syncope (Strickberger et al., 2006). The ILR can record the rhythm at the time of syncope even if episodes occur infrequently, limited only by ILR battery life, which is approximately 2 to 3 years. The size of the ILR has recently decreased substantially, and over time the ILR may shift to an earlier position in the diagnostic algorithm for syncope. An EP study is conducted in select situations, because in individuals with no known heart disease, the diagnostic yield is low, and in the normal evaluation of syncope, it is approximately 3% (Strickberger et al., 2006).

The management of syncope is highly dependent on the etiology, and there is a range of approaches, including increased salt intake; mineralcorticoids; support stockings; hydration; pharmaceuticals; and device therapies, including pacemakers and implantable cardioverter defibrillators. Syncope is not associated with increased mortality in the absence of underlying heart disease, yet the patient may be at risk for physical injury or falls due to the loss of consciousness and postural tone (Strickberger et al., 2006).

TABLE 12.1 Medications With Potential QT Prolongation Properties and Risk for TdP

Amiodarone	Disopyramide	Haloperidol	Procainamide
Anagrelide	Dofetilide	Ibutilide	Quinidine
Arsenic trioxide	Dronedarone	Levofloxacin	Sevoflurane
Azithromycin	Droperidol	Methadone	Sotalol
Chloroquine	Erythromycin	Moxifloxacin	Thioridazine
Chlorpromazine	Escitalopram	Ondansetron	Vandetanib
Citalopram	Flecainide	Pentamidine	
Clarithromycin	Halofantrine	Pimozide	

TdP, torsades de pointes.

Adapted from www.QTdrugs.org.

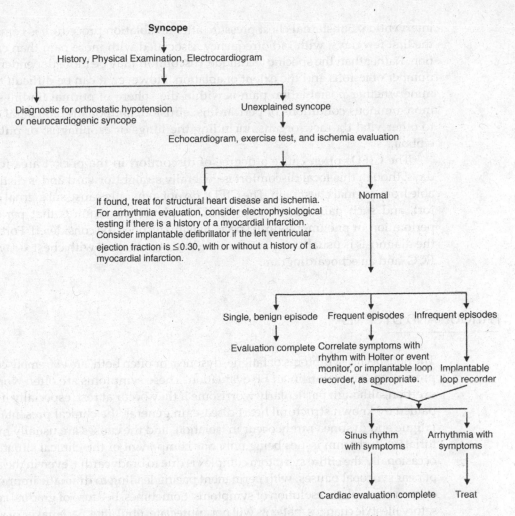

FIGURE 12.1 Flow chart for the diagnostic approach to the patient with syncope.
Reprinted with permission from the American Heart Association.

CHEST PAIN

Although chest pain is a common symptom in general cardiology—often assessed in conjunction with an ischemic evaluation—pain of any type is an unusual presentation for EP and generally a less important symptom. Arrhythmias, whether fast or slow, do not usually cause pain, though one exception is tachyarrhythmias, which can lead to a vague feeling of chest discomfort. If the pain is truly from the fast rhythm, then once the arrhythmia terminates, the pain will subside almost immediately. Occasionally, a fast rhythm will uncover an underlying cardiac condition, including coronary heart disease, which may be unknown until the tachycardia and chest pain develop.

Chest pain might correlate to an EP procedure or a cardiovascular implantable electronic device (CIED). Shortly after an ablation or device implant, chest discomfort can range from an anticipated, self-limited condition to a serious issue requiring intervention. Substernal chest pressure after an ablation procedure is common for the first few days, with radiofrequency associated with more pain than cryoablation. Rather than the specific technique, discomfort may be more dependent on the number of lesions and the extent of ablation. However, it can be difficult to determine whether postablation pain is within the sphere of normal findings versus more ominous conditions of pericarditis; effusion; tamponade; collateral damage to other vital thoracic organs, including the lungs or esophagus; or pulmonary emboli.

The CIEDs often cause a degree of discomfort in the pocket area for a few days, though this local discomfort is generally straightforward and is distinguishable from anginal chest pain. The CIEDs do not generally cause substernal discomfort, and such pain shortly after CIED implantation requires that pericarditis, perforation, or pneumothorax (especially with dyspnea) be considered. Fortunately, the diagnosis is usually apparent after a basic evaluation with chest x-ray (CXR), ECG, and an echocardiogram.

FATIGUE AND DYSPNEA

The nonspecific symptoms of fatigue, dyspnea, or often both, are extremely common presenting complaints in an EP evaluation. These symptoms are often worse with exertion, although particularly worrisome if they occur at rest, especially if accompanied by known structural heart disease. In general, the clinical presentations of fatigue and dyspnea rarely occur in isolation, and the causes are usually multifactorial, with rhythm issues being only one component of the clinical situation. But occasionally, the entire symptom complex is due to bradycardia, even in the absence of near syncopal pauses, with permanent pacing leading to dramatic improvement or even a complete resolution of symptoms. Sometimes, because of gradual compensatory lifestyle changes, patients will not appreciate, until after pacemaker placement, the degree to which they were symptomatic. Antihypertensives and antiarrhythmics can contribute to symptoms of fatigue directly, or do so indirectly by causing bradycardia, especially beta blockers or calcium channel blockers. Therefore, in the symptomatic patient, these side effects must be balanced against the benefits of the medications.

Patients with dyspnea are referred to an EP specialist when the cause of dyspnea is likely due to an EP-related condition, most commonly symptomatic heart failure. In this situation, the heart failure or cardiomyopathy is already known, and the referring clinician is seeking consultation for device therapy. When the cardiomyopathy is combined with evidence of electrical dyssynchrony, the primary device therapy for dyspnea related to heart failure is biventricular pacing.

GENETIC SYNDROMES

Patients will occasionally present directly for EP evaluation, because a family member has been diagnosed with a particular genetic syndrome, most commonly long-QT syndrome, and was instructed to encourage other family members to be evaluated even if asymptomatic. In these individuals, a basic evaluation will consist of a history, with a focus on family history; a physical examination; a 12-lead ECG; and perhaps echocardiography with exercise treadmill testing. Cardiovascular genetic testing is rapidly evolving, and further subspecialty referral is occasionally appropriate. If through genetic testing there is no specific gene mutation in question, reassurance can be provided. In general, treatment decisions should not rely on genetic testing alone but rather on the results of a comprehensive clinical evaluation (Priori et al., 2013).

For full reference citations to this chapter, please see "Section References" in the back of the book, under the heading "Section III."

Common Conditions for Electrophysiology Referral

ROBERT L. McSWAIN

In electrophysiology (EP) practice, it is common to receive referrals from primary-care or general cardiology clinicians. Consultation may be sought after a new rhythm-related diagnosis; for EP assistance with a known refractory condition; or for advanced, usually invasive, EP therapies. For example, a primary care clinician may initially manage a patient with atrial fibrillation (AF) with the aid of rate control and oral anticoagulation; then, a general cardiologist might become involved and perform a cardioversion (CV) to restore normal rhythm. If these efforts are unsatisfactory, EP assistance may be sought for consideration of antiarrhythmic-drug therapy, ablation, or device-related therapy.

ATRIAL FIBRILLATION

AF is a supraventricular tachyarrhythmia in which nearly continuous chaotic electrical signals cause ineffective atrial contraction, resulting in an irregular ventricular response and a heart rate (HR) that may be fast, slow, or even normal. On electrocardiogram (ECG), the normal P wave is replaced by a fibrillatory baseline, and on auscultation, the rhythm is classically "irregularly irregular." The most common contemporary reason for an EP referral, AF affects 1% to 2% of the general population and increases in prevalence with age (Wadke, 2013). The risk also increases with underlying hypertension, coronary heart disease (CHD), heart failure (HF), valvular heart disease, recent surgery, obesity, diabetes mellitus, alcohol, obstructive sleep apnea, hyperthyroidism, and many other disorders (American Heart Association [AHA], 2014).

AF is an area where treatment modalities and expectations have risen tremendously over the past decade. Once believed to be a diffuse atrial disease that did not lend itself to curative ablation therapy—as compared with focal conditions such as Wolf–Parkinson–White (WPW) or atrial flutter (AFL)—the pendulum has swung to the point that successful results are expected, even in situations of substantial co-morbidities related to advanced age, obesity, valvular disease, and atrial enlargement. The truth lies somewhere in between, and in properly selected patients, ablation can offer life-changing benefits in terms of symptom control and quality of life. The field continues to evolve rapidly, and potential survival benefits and optimal techniques remain under active investigation (CABANA Investigators, 2015). Given their extensive knowledge of the treatment options and the disease trajectory, electrophysiologists have alternatives for most patients with AF, even if that includes the control of symptoms without the elimination of the arrhythmia.

Even with the older adult patient on a simple rate-control and anticoagulation strategy, the electrophysiologist can optimize adequate rate control while avoiding symptomatic bradycardia and, ultimately, implant a pacemaker for tachycardia-bradycardia syndrome if necessary.

AF Classification

AF can be classified as paroxysmal, persistent, persistent long-standing, or permanent. These classifications may change over time for an individual patient, as AF tends to be slowly progressive.

- Paroxysmal AF—terminates spontaneously or with medical intervention, duration of approximately 7 days but usually less than 48 hours
- Persistent AF—sustained AF for more than 7 days
- Persistent long-standing—sustained AF for more than 12 months
- Permanent AF—acceptance of AF, without plans to intervene and change the rhythm
- Nonvalvular AF—AF without mechanical or bioprosthetic heart valve, mitral valve repair, or rheumatic mitral stenosis (January et al., 2014; NHLBI, 2014)

Clinical Manifestations

Patients with AF may be asymptomatic and diagnosed incidentally by physical examination or ECG. Unfortunately, the diagnosis is occasionally made retrospectively when patients present with symptoms of a cerebrovascular accident. Palpitations are the most common presenting symptom, though dyspnea, weakness, exercise intolerance, chest discomfort, or dizziness is often reported.

Diagnostic Evaluation

The initial evaluation includes an ECG and common blood tests that include electrolytes and thyroid-hormone levels. Liver and renal blood profiles also guide which antiarrhythmics could be administered safely for management. Holter monitoring can assess the adequacy of rate control and help determine whether or not episodes are paroxysmal in nature. Echocardiography and stress testing are indicated, in part to help exclude secondary causes for the arrhythmia and also to provide prognostic information, including marked left atrial enlargement in the setting of mitral valve disease, which may portend a relatively refractory situation.

AF MANAGEMENT

Three issues must be adequately addressed for each AF patient as part of a comprehensive management strategy: stroke prevention, symptom relief, and occasionally the prevention of tachycardia-related cardiomyopathy (CM). Most providers are comfortable in utilizing starter medications for AF, including beta blockers, calcium channel blockers, or digoxin. However, even general cardiologists often request EP assistance when membrane-active antiarrhythmic drugs (AADs) are required. These specialty medications may require inpatient initiation and a thorough understanding of contraindications to increase the probability that benefits will outweigh the potential risks. These risks include not only end-organ toxicity but also potential proarrhythmia effects. For example, dofetilide causes QT prolongation and carries a known risk of torsades de pointes (TdP); not only is a 3-day hospitalization mandated by the Food and Drug Administration (FDA) but also prescribers are required to obtain additional training and certification. Through a process of medication trial, the electrophysiology specialist can often achieve adequate AF control; however, if necessary, therapy can be escalated to invasive options if pharmacologic therapy alone is inadequate. Still somewhat in evolution, left-atrial ablation therapy now offers hope of symptom relief, if not a cure, for many sufferers of AF. Even for those who have exhausted available pharmacologic or ablative approaches, electrophysiologists can offer permanent pacing to expand the options for AF control. A pacemaker cannot directly prevent AF or lower rapid rates; nonetheless, this approach allows uptitration of rate- or rhythm-controlling agents without concern for bradycardia. The rhythm data collected by the pacemaker can also help guide management over time. When all else fails, pacemakers allow ablation of the atrioventricular (AV) junction to achieve somewhat "perfect" rate control even without the need for negative chronotropic agents, although with the obvious requirement of pacemaker dependence. Electrophysiologists can also assist in determining when AF is refractory, that a cardiac surgery evaluation is appropriate, and the patient should be referred for consideration of a surgical MAZE.

Stroke Prevention

The most significant risk of AF is a potentially devastating cerebrovascular accident (Ezekowitz, Aikens, Nagarakanti, & Shapiro, 2011), although simultaneously it is also the most straightforward issue and is generally prevented with oral anticoagulation. All humans have a nonzero risk of stroke, but certain conditions, including AF, are associated with an increased statistical risk, such that the potential benefits of long-term anticoagulation outweigh the potential risks for most patients. Although other methods—such as left-atrial appendage (LAA) closure devices—are under investigation, generally the only way to lower the risk for stroke in patients with AF is by anticoagulation, to prevent clots that may form in the LAA and embolize unpredictably to the brain. A risk versus benefit analysis must always be employed, and strategies must be individualized based on a comprehensive approach. For some patients, the risk of bleeding may be substantially higher than the risk of stroke, but AF in the setting of mitral stenosis is associated with a risk of stroke that is 20 times that of an individual with a normal heart structure in normal sinus rhythm (Anderson et al., 2013).

Patients tend to fear the risk of stroke when in AF, but they perceive the risk to disappear once normal rhythm has been restored. The mechanisms remain somewhat poorly understood, but they are certainly more complex than mechanical theories of stagnant flow within the appendage. The true stroke risk is perhaps best viewed over the long term, such that the risk remains elevated compared with controls even during sinus rhythm.

TABLE 13.1 CHA2DS2VASc

Congestive heart failure/left ventricular	1
Hypertension or hypertension treatment	1
Age > 75	2
Diabetes mellitus	1
CVA/TIA/thromboembolism	2
Vascular disease	1
Age 65–74	1
Sex category (female gender)	1
Maximum score	9

The CHADS2 scoring system estimates the risk of stroke in patients with AF with the identified factors of congestive HF, hypertension, age more than 75 years, diabetes, or a prior stroke (Gage et al., 2001). A CHADS2 score of 0 is a condition sometimes known as "lone AF," with a stroke risk sufficiently low that anticoagulation is generally not warranted from a risk-to-benefit standpoint. A CHADS2 score of 1 places a patient squarely "on the fence," such that it is reasonable to individualize the decision regarding anticoagulation. A score of 2 or higher generally warrants long-term oral anticoagulation. A revised risk stratification scheme, known as CHA2DS2VASc, also accounts for vascular disease, an intermediate age of 65 to 74 years, and female gender (Table 13.1). With this newer scheme, the lowest score a woman can achieve is 1.

AF type and overall arrhythmia burden are not included in the scoring systems, such that the decision regarding anticoagulant therapy should be made independent of the AF pattern classification of paroxysmal, persistent, or permanent. In addition, risk stratification schemes are imperfect models, such that patients with low CHADS2 or CHA2DS2VASc will, nonetheless, occasionally suffer strokes.

Bleeding Risk

A system that predicts the risk of bleeding has been developed as well. The HAS-BLED score incorporates hypertension, renal disease, liver disease, stroke, prior major bleeding or predisposition to bleeding, labile international normalized ratio (INR), older than 65 years, medication usage that predisposes to bleeding, and alcohol use history. This scoring system has not gained widespread acceptance compared with the CHADS2-based scoring system, partly because of relatively poor predictive accuracy. Bleeding risk, from a clinical standpoint, is most often approached subjectively, combining a perception regarding fall risk and a somewhat more objective history regarding prior gastrointestinal bleeding. In all cases, it remains critical to approach each patient individually, taking into account risks, benefits, and patient preferences. In terms of risk, bleeding is often, though not always, treatable, compared with stroke, where therapy often remains supportive.

Anticoagulants

Previously, the only effective anticoagulant for those with AF and risk of stroke was warfarin. Several novel oral anticoagulants (NOACs) have subsequently become available, starting with dabigatran, which obtained FDA approval in 2010, followed by rivaroxaban and apixaban. The following discussion pertains to nonvalvular AF, as patients with valvular AF warrant anticoagulation regardless of CHADS2 score, and NOACs have not been studied in these patients. Warfarin remains the standard of care for anticoagulation for patients with valvular AF and mechanical valves.

Perhaps the main advantage of the novel agents is that the daily dosage is fixed, eliminating the need for frequent phlebotomy to maintain the INR within the therapeutic range, and eliminating the confusion caused by the ever-changing dose of warfarin. The main disadvantages of the NOACs are cost and lack of an available reversal agent; with widespread adoption, cost may become less of an issue, and antidotes are actively under development. The main advantages of warfarin are reversibility with vitamin K or plasma, the many years of accrued experience, and the flexibility to use the medication in most cases of AF regardless of valvular status.

For well-selected patients with an acceptable bleeding risk, both warfarin and the NOACs offer superior protection from stroke compared with no anticoagulation. Generally speaking, warfarin and the NOACs offer similar protection from stroke when compared with each other, and bleeding risks are likewise similar. When selecting between warfarin and the novel agents, quality of life must also be considered, as the dietary restrictions associated with warfarin and the time required to manage it are not inconsequential. For these various reasons, use of the NOACs is increasing. Nonetheless, it is important to individualize therapy, and involve patients in the decision, based on a thorough understanding of the risks and benefits as it applies to them. For patients who are well controlled on warfarin, it is reasonable to continue the status quo.

Although anticoagulation is important at all times, it can be especially critical around the time of CV. To reasonably ensure the absence of a LAA thrombus, 3 weeks of adequate anticoagulation or a negative transesophageal echocardiogram are required before elective CV of AF over 48 hours. An advantage of therapy with one of the NOACs is that adequate anticoagulation can be reasonably presumed as long as the patient does not miss a dose. With warfarin, serial INRs greater than 2 are required during the 3-week period, and a single subtherapeutic INR requires restarting the time period. Because a CV in a warfarin-treated patient can be delayed for weeks due to a subtherapeutic INR, the NOACs have a distinct advantage compared with warfarin.

Patients on long-term anticoagulation will occasionally require surgical interventions. Collaboration between the surgeon and the team managing anticoagulation is required to ensure the best patient outcomes, taking into consideration both bleeding and clotting risks. A trend in electrophysiology is to perform device implants without interruption of warfarin, again after a consideration of risks and benefits.

Previous guidelines recommended that low-risk patients could be prescribed aspirin for stroke prevention. This recommendation was recently changed based on aspirin risks and the weakness of data linking aspirin to a reduction in stroke risk (January et al., 2014). The decision of aspirin versus warfarin has increasingly become a decision of warfarin versus NOAC versus no anticoagulation. Clopidogrel plays a minor role in AF stroke prevention.

Additional Anticoagulation Considerations

It is not known whether a successful AF ablation reduces the long-term risk of stroke, though studies are ongoing (CABANA Investigators, 2015). Therefore, AF ablation is currently viewed as a strategy to control symptoms, rather than a mechanism to eliminate the need for long-term anticoagulation. All patients generally require anticoagulation in the early recovery period; the need beyond that period is dictated by the long-term stroke risk as evaluated by the CHA2DS2VASc score, rather than by the success or failure of the procedure. For example, risk–benefit analysis would indicate that a young patient with lone AF would not require indefinite anticoagulation even after unsuccessful ablation, whereas an elderly diabetic with a prior stroke would require it, even if the procedure were successful.

Symptom Relief

Besides anticoagulation, the vast majority of AF management efforts are directed toward the control of symptoms. Indeed, the primary goal of most available AF therapies is to control symptoms and improve quality of life, and the issues related to anticoagulation and stroke risk are largely independent of those regarding symptom control. The general treatment options (Table 13.2) consist of HR control, AADs, AF ablation, CV, pacemaker approaches with or without AV node ablation, and open-heart surgery using the robotically assisted MAZE approach. One or more approaches may be required over time, sometimes in combination; for example, a pacemaker with AAD. A step-by-step approach is appropriate, starting with simpler, less-invasive treatment strategies, escalating over time as necessary. First-line efforts usually involve beta blockers or calcium channel blockers. If these measures are inadequate, the next step would be AADs that can be initiated on an outpatient basis for appropriate candidates, followed by AF ablation(s) or further trials of AADs, some with significant long-term risk and others requiring inpatient initiation. One or more cardioversions may be required along the trajectory of treatment. If symptoms remain inadequately controlled despite these efforts, a surgical MAZE or a pace and ablate strategy can be considered.

TABLE 13.2 General Step-by-Step Approach to AF Management

Beta-adrenergic blockers (beta blockers)
Calcium channel blockers
Antiarrhythmics
Cardioversions—electrical or pharmacological
Antiarrhythmics requiring hospitalization or amiodarone
Ablation
Pacemaker and ablation
Surgical MAZE

AF, atrial fibrillation.

The fight against AF is often a struggle comprising many battles. There will be periods when the treatment is temporarily successful, but AF can be tenacious and will sometimes recur despite the best of efforts. An understanding of this concept can enhance the ability to properly set and manage expectations. The AADs do not purport to cure AF, but rather lessen the AF burden over time compared with what might be expected if the disease were allowed to run its course.

Cardioversion

Electrical or chemical CV is a tool used in conjunction with other AF treatment strategies. For patients with relatively rare episodes of AF, CV can be a stand-alone strategy. Patients will occasionally opt for an as-needed pharmacologic approach, with no daily therapy until an episode of AF occurs, at which time they would take a relatively large single dose of AAD, hoping to effect a chemical CV. The need for emergent CV of AF associated with hemodynamic compromise is often discussed, but this scenario is rare in clinical practice except in the case of preexcited AF.

HR Control

A stand-alone strategy that allows AF but controls symptoms through HR control is often termed rate control and anticoagulation, though anticoagulation is not unique to the rate-control strategy and, indeed, must be considered independently regardless of the overall approach. In addition, rate-control considerations are important even during a rhythm-control strategy, as a backup control of symptoms when rhythm efforts fail.

For persistent states of AF, HR and symptoms must remain under control for the approach to be successful. Rate control is generally achieved through the use of beta blockers and calcium channel blockers, alone or in combination. Digoxin is still prescribed, although its role is increasingly limited. Co-morbidities affect the selection of rate-controlling medications (Table 13.3). Rate control is easily achieved in some patients, whereas in others it is difficult to titrate to the dose required to control the rate, and it is limited by hypotension or symptomatic bradycardia. This

TABLE 13.3 Pharmaceutical Considerations for AF Rate Control in Selected Cardiovascular Conditions

	Beta Adrenergic Blockers	Diltiazem/ Verapamil	Digoxin	Amiodarone
No cardiovascular diseases	×	×		×
Hypertension	×	×		×
Heart failure, preserved EF (HFpEF)	×	×		×
Heart failure, reduced EF (HFrEF)	×		×	×
Left ventricular dysfunction	×		×	×
Chronic obstructive pulmonary disease		×		

AF, atrial fibrillation; EF, ejection fraction.

Adapted from Anderson et al. (2013).

tachycardia–bradycardia syndrome is difficult to manage without a pacemaker, though after pacemaker implantation, rate-controlling medications can be further titrated without concern for bradycardia.

Rate control has been validated as a reasonable long-term treatment strategy, so long as symptoms are adequately controlled and stroke prevention by way of anticoagulation is addressed (AFFIRM Investigators, 2002). Recent studies have suggested that more lenient HR control may be adequate (resting HR < 110 versus < 80), though overall the required degree of rate control remains controversial (January et al., 2014; Van Gelder et al., 2010). In general, the severity of AF symptoms correlates with increasing HR, although some patients are asymptomatic despite rapid rates, and others are highly symptomatic even when rates are well controlled. The latter patients are poor candidates for a rate-control strategy.

Before presuming a rhythm-control strategy is superior to one involving rate control alone, the potential downsides of permanent AF must be balanced against the challenges of rhythm control, which generally include more medical encounters, invasive procedures, and AADs with side effects. An elderly, asymptomatic patient, stable on warfarin, may be better served with a rate-control and anticoagulation strategy, whereas a younger patient with bothersome symptoms despite rate control might require rhythm-control efforts. When encountering a newly diagnosed patient, regardless of the degree of symptoms, it should be considered that almost everyone deserves at least one attempt at achieving a normal rhythm.

Antiarrhythmic Medications

The primary medications in AF rhythm control efforts consist of "membrane active" AAD therapy. For the purposes of this text, six oral AADs are in common use these days: sotalol, dronedarone, flecainide, propafenone, amiodarone, and dofetilide (Table 13.4). In addition, beta blockers have weak antiarrhythmic properties and are primarily considered rate-control agents. Although patients often seem to convert to a normal rhythm after an intravenous injection of diltiazem, this drug is considered only for its rate control. None of the AADs represent a cure, and, thus, it is important to set proper patient expectations. The goal is that the AAD will, on a relative scale, lower the AF burden compared with a similar patient not prescribed the medication, and, on an absolute scale, limit the recurrences of AF such that quality of life is improved. Rhythm control strategies based on structural heart disease are presented in Figure 13.1.

Sotalol is considered a "beta blocker plus." At lower doses, it exhibits only beta-adrenergic blocking properties, although at higher doses significant Class III antiarrhythmic effects are exhibited (Table 13.4). Some experts will initiate sotalol in selected low-risk patients starting in normal sinus rhythm on an outpatient basis, though hospitalization is usually required. Hospitalization is required primarily to monitor for potential QT prolonging effects that could predispose to TdP. This medication must be administered cautiously in patients with renal insufficiency or CM, although CHD is not a contraindication.

Despite FDA approval in 2009, dronedarone, which controls HR through AV nodal blockade, remains the newest available AAD in the United States. After eagerly awaiting this drug for several years, with a promise of most of the benefits

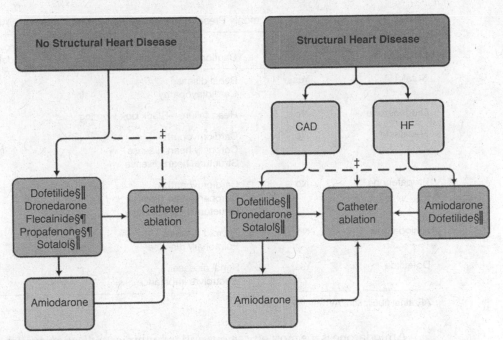

FIGURE 13.1 Strategies for rhythm control in patients with paroxysmal and persistent AF.

AF, atrial fibrillation; AV, atrioventricular; CAD, coronary artery disease; HF, heart failure; LVH, left ventricular hypertrophy.

Notes: Catheter ablation is recommended only as first-line therapy for patients with paroxysmal AF (Class IIa recommendation). Drugs are listed alphabetically. Depending on patient preference when performed in experienced centers.

§Not recommended with severe LVH (wall thickness >1.5 cm).

‖Should be used with caution in patients at risk for torsades de pointes ventricular tachycardia.

¶Should be combined with AV nodal blocking agents.

Reprinted from January et al. (2014), with permission from Elsevier.

of amiodarone without the potential side effects, the EP community has been somewhat disappointed with the drug in terms of efficacy. However, there remains a role for dronedarone. For those for whom it works, it is well tolerated. It can be initiated safely as an outpatient and used in patients with CHD. The medication is contraindicated for use in patients with permanent AF or HF; the PALLAS study was stopped early for safety reasons due to elevated rates of HF, stroke, and cardiovascular mortality in patients with permanent AF who were at risk for major cardiovascular events (Connolly et al., 2011).

Flecainide and propafenone are similar antiarrhythmic Class IC drugs, and they are also considered safe to initiate on an outpatient basis. Both medications are contraindicated in the presence of structural heart disease, including CM or CHD; therefore, a well-suited candidate for these medications will have a structurally normal heart. Both flecainide and propafenone require a "helper" medication, generally a calcium channel blocker or beta blocker, for concomitant AV nodal blockade. Without the combination of medications, there is a risk of a 1:1 slow AFL with paradoxically rapid rates and a risk of hemodynamic collapse.

TABLE 13.4 Comparison of Commonly Prescribed Antiarrhythmic Medications for AF

Medication	Inpatient Initiation	Cautions and Contraindications	Concomittant AV Nodal Blockade
Sotalol	Yes	Renal disease Cardiomyopathy	No
Dronedarone	No	Heart failure—Black box warning	No
Flecainide	No	Cardiomyopathy Coronary heart disease Structural heart disease	Yes
Propafenone	No	Cardiomyopathy Coronary heart disease Structural heart disease	Yes
Amiodarone	No	Thyroid disease Pulmonary disease	No
Dofetilide	Yes	Renal disease Electrolyte imbalance	No

AF, atrial fibrillation; AV, atrioventricular.

Amiodarone is the most efficacious antiarrhythmic medication available, sometimes succeeding in maintaining normal sinus rhythm when other antiarrhythmics fail. Amiodarone can be initiated as an outpatient medication and is administered in patients with CHD or HF. The use of amiodarone is limited primarily because of the well-known long-term risks of significant end-organ toxicity, potentially affecting the eyes, thyroid, lungs, liver, and skin.

Dofetilide is not only used to maintain normal sinus rhythm in patients with a history of AF but also indicated for the chemical conversion of AF to NSR. The main risk of this Class III antiarrhythmic is the risk of TdP, because dofetilide has QT-prolonging effects. As such, the FDA requires a 3-day hospitalization to initiate the drug with serial ECG, QT, electrolyte, and telemetry monitoring, plus special training for prescribers. For patients who present to the hospital with AF, an electrical CV is usually planned toward the end of the admission but is often unnecessary because the dofetilide accomplishes the task. Dofetilide is contraindicated in renal failure, but it is generally well tolerated and can be safely used in patients with CM or CHD.

AF Ablation

Perhaps the most exciting area in EP these days, AF ablation offers many patients the hope of long-term rhythm control and, therefore, symptom control. The term *cure* is used with reticence. Not long ago, AF was not considered amenable to ablation, given the diffuse nature of the disease. However, a 1998 seminal observation that the pulmonary veins are an important source of ectopic beats that initiate AF, as well as the experimental determination that these ectopic foci respond to ablation, has transformed AF management and EP itself. The discovery has spurred technological innovation in mapping and ablation technologies, with crossover benefits to other areas of EP, and led to an ever-increasing number of patients ablated over the past decade. The cornerstone of the ablation procedure is termed pulmonary vein isolation (PVI), wherein the veins are electrically disconnected from the remainder of the heart by creating a line of scar tissue at the interface between the vein and the atrium. Currently, the most common energy sources that create the scar are radiofrequency, which is ablation with heat, or cryoablation, which is ablation by freezing the pertinent tissue. Point-by-point lesions can be achieved with catheters using either energy source to create somewhat of a "string of pearls" lesion set around the pulmonary venous ostia; a cryoballoon is also available to broadly isolate an entire vein with a single application of energy. Transseptal puncture is required, and intracardiac ultrasound and three-dimensional mapping technologies are often employed to monitor the locations of catheters within the heart and to record the location of ablation lesions. In paroxysmal AF, PVI alone is often adequate, whereas more persistent forms of AF often require additional lesion sets—lines, rotors, or areas of complex fractionation. There is tremendous variability in the quoted success rate, with 70% being perhaps the most frequently cited rate. The success rate is influenced by a number of factors, primarily with the extent of left atrial enlargement factoring prominently; the rate of success is also affected by the intensity of surveillance for recurrences. Major complications of AF ablation include cardiac tamponade; stroke; or damage to surrounding organs, including atrio-esophageal fistula, pulmonary vein stenosis, or phrenic nerve palsy. The rate of each of these complications is approximately 1% (January et al., 2014). According to the latest guidelines, AF ablation receives a Class I indication for symptomatic paroxysmal AF patients who have trialed at least one AAD without benefit; other indications are Class II.

Tachycardia-Induced Cardiomyopathy

The third area of concern regarding AF is the risk of tachycardia-induced cardiomyopathy (TIC). Though somewhat poorly understood, TIC must be considered in patients who develop or are found to have a significant CM in the setting of poorly controlled AF (Ellis & Josephson, 2013; Khasnis et al., 2005). Nonetheless, many patients will not develop this condition despite uncontrolled heart rates for months or years. If the entity did not exist, rate control would lose significance in patients who were otherwise asymptomatic and anticoagulated. But it is important to intervene early when TIC is suspected, as rhythm or improved rate control can lead to reversal of CM in a subset of patients. The dilemma in patients with poorly controlled AF and CM is about whether the cause of the rapid rates led to the CM or vice versa. The TIC can be suspected ahead of time but is somewhat confirmed only in hindsight; if AF control leads to the resolution of CM, a diagnosis of TIC is likely. If average rates in AF are reasonably known to be less than 100, the diagnosis of AF-induced CM is unlikely.

BRADYCARDIA

Another common reason for EP referral is bradycardia, usually for consideration and evaluation for permanent pacemaker (PPM) placement. Often, patients are referred after a bradyarrhythmia is discovered on a routine ECG, regardless of whether or not symptoms are present. Conversely, patients may be referred for symptoms that are suspicious for bradycardia, including fatigue, exercise intolerance, or syncope, though documentation of bradycardia is elusive. In either situation, EP correlates the symptoms with objective findings to determine whether permanent pacing is, ultimately, warranted. Sometimes, the decision is straightforward, for example, a patient with recurrent syncope who presents with complete heart block (CHB) and profound bradycardia. However, in many situations, the documented bradyarrhythmia is relatively mild and sporadic, and the symptoms may have alternative explanations. In these cases, the difficult risk-and-benefit decision is often balanced on whether to err on the side of withholding therapy and risking injury in the event of syncope or committing the patient to permanent pacing with its attendant risks. The downsides of permanent pacing are not limited to the risks of the initial implant, as a lifetime of monitoring and further procedures for generator exchanges and possible lead revision may be required.

Before the decision for PPM placement is made, further evaluation is sometimes required. Comprehensive health history may reveal that the bradycardia is related to beta blocker pharmacologic therapy that is required to manage chronic angina, in which case permanent pacing may be warranted. Reversible causes for bradycardia or CHB must be considered, for example, Lyme disease or right coronary ischemia. Ambulatory ECG monitoring in its various forms is often utilized to assist in the diagnosis. Echocardiography can identify alternative explanations for syncope, including aortic stenosis or ventricular tachycardia (VT) in the setting of CM, and guide the most appropriate type of pacemaker for the patient, perhaps biventricular or a pacemaker with an implantable cardioverter defibrillator (ICD) component. Exercise treadmill testing can establish the presence of chronotropic incompetence. An invasive EP study is rarely a component of the bradycardia evaluation, as the implant decision is usually based on clinical judgment grounded in the history and results of noninvasive testing.

What is important is that PPMs are indicated for *symptomatic* bradycardia, with the one exception being CHB (Epstein et al., 2012). Mild or nocturnal bradycardia without attributable symptoms does not require permanent pacing. Even numerically significant resting sinus bradycardia may not require permanent pacing if, for example, the patient is a well-conditioned athlete. This area of medicine is certainly one in which the adage "Treat the patient, not the numbers" could be applied.

Bradycardia symptoms can be grouped into two primary categories of fatigue, including low energy levels and exercise intolerance, or syncope, including near syncope, dizziness, and lightheadedness. The bradycardia itself can be grouped into disorders of the sinoatrial node, sick sinus syndrome with failure to initiate an electrical impulse, and disorders of the AV node, including AV block with failure to propagate the electrical signal from the atrium to the ventricle. The AV block can be partial or complete, and it can be fixed or occur intermittently. The Wenckebach pattern of block is generally considered a benign conduction disorder; however, it warrants permanent pacing if accompanied by symptoms. Tachycardia–bradycardia syndrome is another entity, with periods of tachycardia, which is usually AF, punctuated by periods of symptomatic sinus bradycardia or the more ominous offset pause with risk of syncope. In this syndrome, medications that treat the tachyarrhythmia tend to exacerbate the bradycardia, and permanent pacing can enable treatment of the former without further concern for the latter.

Overall, permanent pacing is an established and reliable therapy used to increase the HR as instructed. In well-selected patients suffering from symptomatic bradycardia, a PPM can improve the patient's quality of life. However, it is difficult for the PPM to make a difference if the symptoms are due to something else or if the symptoms are entirely absent.

SUPRAVENTRICULAR TACHYCARDIA

Patients are often referred to EP for the evaluation and management of supraventricular tachycardia (SVT), either with symptoms suspicious for this arrhythmia or with an established diagnosis. Fortunately, SVT generally does not adversely affect overall prognosis or lead to serious sequelae such as stroke or MI, with symptoms consisting of a combination of palpitations, dyspnea, chest discomfort, lightheadedness, and rarely syncope. Nonetheless, SVT can considerably reduce quality of life because of the severity of symptoms during episodes, and because of anxiety about when the next episode might occur without warning. The condition can negatively impact emotional well-being and force an altered lifestyle, with some patients limiting travel far from home.

There are three general treatment options for SVT: watchful waiting, medications, and ablation. If episodes are short lived or infrequent, no specific therapy may be required. Some patients are able to reliably terminate SVT with vagal maneuvers, another valid strategy. If more intervention is required, a beta blocker or calcium channel blocker may be initiated, and if the medications fail or the side effects are burdensome, therapy can be escalated to ablation. It is also appropriate to adopt an early ablation strategy, if preferred. Clinicians can reasonably involve EP at any time to establish a relationship and prepare the patient for ablation if the SVT is intolerable to the patient.

There are many different SVTs, but most true reentrant SVTs are due to either atrioventricular node reentry tachycardia (AVNRT) or an accessory pathway (AP)-mediated tachycardia. If the AP is conducted in an antegrade direction with the classic delta wave on ECG, it is termed WPW syndrome. In WPW treatment of symptomatic patients, ablation is considered earlier in the treatment algorithm, as AV node blocking agents are contraindicated, and there is a small risk of sudden death in the event of preexcitation AF. If the baseline ECG is normal without preexcitation, then the SVT may be due to either AVNRT or an AP that is conducted in a retrograde manner, the concealed bypass tract.

Each of these arrhythmias can be successfully ablated in the order of 90% to 95%, though the specific diagnosis is often not known until clarification at the time of diagnostic electrophysiology study (EPS). If the patient has AVNRT, the main risk from ablation is CHB, which occurs in approximately 1% of cases and requires PPM implantation. The ablation risk of an AP-mediated tachycardia, whether manifest or concealed, depends on the AP location. If the AP is located near the AV node, the risk for CHB is similar to that for AVNRT. The APs located along the mitral valve, a common situation, present a small risk of stroke from working within the arterial bloodstream, and a small risk of pericardial tamponade if the transseptal approach is used. Patients often select ablation—with its high success rate and low risks—as a first-line opportunity of an SVT cure; this is one of the few areas in all of medicine where use of the term is appropriate.

ATRIAL FLUTTER

Falling somewhere between AF and SVT, AFL is commonly encountered in clinical practice. Well known for its sawtooth pattern on ECG, AFL carries a risk of stroke similar to AF, but it can be ablated curatively with a success and risk rate similar to that for SVT. In its typical form, AFL is due to reentrant counterclockwise conduction around the entirety of the right atrium and through the cavotricuspid isthmus (CVTI) at the base of the tricuspid valve. This ridge of tissue serves as a bridge, and ablation to interrupt conduction across the CVTI can reliably result in a cure of the arrhythmia (O'Neill et al., 2006).

CARDIOMYOPATHY AND HEART FAILURE

CM patients are at an increased risk for cardiac arrest (CA) and sudden cardiac death (SCD). An EP evaluation is often warranted for consideration of an ICD as the primary prevention for SCD, sometimes combining this therapy with cardiac resynchronization therapy (CRT). Since the first ICD was implanted in 1980 (Mirowski, 1985), enormous strides in knowledge and technology have led to the annual implantation of thousands of ICDs worldwide, and the device is now as commonplace as a PPM. Another determination that must be made during the EP evaluation is whether a single, dual, or biventricular system is warranted. Recently, the decision has become even more complex, as entirely subcutaneous approaches with no transvenous lead have become available. Establishment of the EP relationship facilitates many ICD-related issues that may arise over time, including appropriateness of shocks, refinement in settings, generator changes and upgrades, recalls, lead fractures, discovery of atrial arrhythmias, and infections.

Numerous large trials have demonstrated a mortality reduction with ICD implantation, providing data for guideline development (Buxton et al., 1999; Yancy et al., 2013) to stratify which patients are the most likely to benefit from this therapy. It is important to note that patients often do not fit neatly within the guidelines, and clinical judgment is required (Kusumoto et al., 2014). The device guidelines are complex and ever evolving, though a few key points are important. The single most important risk factor for SCD and thus primary prevention ICD consideration is the left ventricular ejection fraction (LVEF). The EP referral is appropriate for patients with an LVEF less than 35%. Reversible CM from ischemic heart disease should be ruled out first, with revascularization obtained, if indicated. There are relevant waiting periods and pharmacologic treatment options after diagnosis of CM to ensure the LVEF does not improve before committing the patient to potentially lifelong

ICD therapy. The waiting periods are 3 months if the CM is nonischemic or after revascularization, or 40 days after a myocardial infarction (MI). It is presumed that during this waiting period, all patients are concomitantly receiving guideline-directed medical therapy (GDMT).

Multiple clinical trials have contributed to the body of evidence to prove that ICDs can prevent mortality, but two landmark studies have perhaps influenced clinical practice more than any others. The MADIT-2 trial established that patients with an ischemic CM with an LVEF less than 30% after suffering an MI benefit from an ICD (Moss et al., 2002). The SCD-HeFT trial extended the mortality reduction benefit to nonischemic patients with an LVEF less than 35% and NYHA Class II to III HF (Bardy et al., 2005). In addition, SCD-HeFT demonstrated that, at least for this patient population, amiodarone was no more effective at preventing death than placebo.

A subset of these ICD candidates, in addition, suffer from impaired electromechanical coupling, known as electrical dyssynchrony, which contributes to poor cardiac output in the failing heart. For these patients, the benefits of biventricular pacing, known as CRT, have also been established in multiple clinical trials (Yancy et al., 2013). Figure 13.2 provides an algorithm for CRT indications. Dyssynchrony is diagnosed based on a wide QRS morphology on ECG; efforts to identify potential

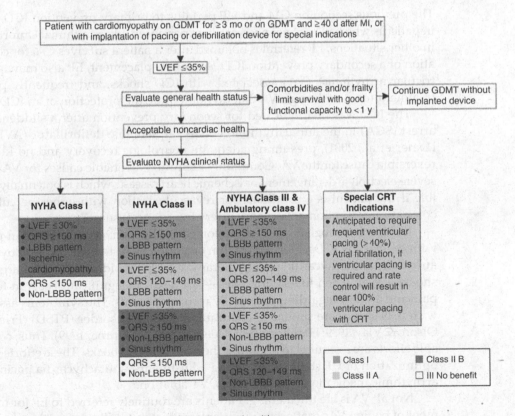

FIGURE 13.2 Indications for CRT therapy algorithm.

CRT, cardiac resynchronization therapy; GDMT, guideline-directed medical therapy; LBBB, left bundle branch block; LVEF, left ventricular ejection fraction; NYHA, New York Heart Association.

Reprinted from Yancy et al. (2013, pp. e240–e327), with permission from Elsevier.

responders to CRT based on echocardiographic indices of dyssynchrony have thus far failed. Based on the initial trials validating CRT, the traditional QRS cutoff width has been greater than 120 ms, although clinically it appears that the wider the QRS segment, the greater the potential expected benefit. Recent guideline updates have codified this understanding to reserve a Class I CRT indication only for patients with QRS greater than 150 ms and a left bundle branch block (LBBB) morphology, as opposed to the right bundle branch block (RBBB) or intraventricular conduction delay (IVCD) pattern (Tracy et al., 2013). The CRT has demonstrated improvement in functional status along with objective measures, including mortality and EF in these patients. By adding a pacing lead to the left ventricle by way of the coronary sinus to pace the right and left sides of the ventricle somewhat simultaneously, the efficiency of cardiac contraction can be improved. It is important to recognize that CRT is not a therapy for HF per se, but rather for electrical dyssynchrony, such that patients with a narrow QRS are not expected to benefit. The CRT is also not a replacement for GDMT, but rather an adjunctive measure.

VENTRICULAR ARRHYTHMIAS

The previous section on CM and HF pertains to primary prevention ICD therapy in patients who have not yet necessarily experienced an arrhythmia. Unfortunately in other situations, EP referral is obtained after a patient survives CA, for consideration of a secondary prevention ICD. After ICD placement, EP also manages ventricular arrhythmias (VA) associated with ICD shocks, and frequently provides treatment for more benign VA that do not require the protection of an ICD.

The ICD was first indicated for secondary prevention after a sudden cardiac arrest (SCA) in the antiarrhythmic versus implantable defibrillator (AVID) trial (Exner et al., 2001), presuming adequate neurologic recovery and no identified reversible cause for the VA. Commonly identified reversible causes for VA include severe electrolyte derangement or ischemic heart disease, which is potentially reversible if the patient is a candidate for revascularization with either percutaneous coronary intervention or coronary artery bypass graft surgery.

Electrophysiologists are often involved in the management of VA in patients with preexisting ICDs. Normal rhythm can often be restored painlessly by way of automatic antitachycardia pacing therapy, thereby avoiding ICD discharges. ICD shocks—even when life-saving ones—can result in significant costs in terms of pain and anxiety regarding potentially recurrent events. The symptoms associated with ICD shocks are similar to posttraumatic stress disorder (PTSD) (Fricchoine, Olson, & Vlay, 1989; Hamner, Hunt, Gee, Garrell, & Monroe, 1999). Thus, considerable efforts are instituted to minimize the need for ICD shocks. These efforts include optimization of HF status, ICD setting adjustments, antitachycardia pacing, antiarrhythmic medications, and, at times, VT ablation.

Not all VA is life threatening. Patients are routinely referred to EP for management of benign VAs that occur in patients with structurally normal hearts, including right ventricular outflow tract (RVOT) and fascicular VT. These normal heart VTs are comparable with SVT, as CA is not a concern, and the focus is on the control of symptoms. Therapies include beta blockers or calcium channel blockers to prevent palpitations or near syncope; at times, ablation can be curative. Conversely, some patients are at risk for malignant VA, and thus CA, even in the setting of preserved left ventricular systolic function. Patients at risk for malignant VA include those with long-QT syndrome, Brugada syndrome, and hypertrophic cardiomyopathy (HCM). Treatment for those patients may include the use of AADs and, at times, ICD therapy. Although "normal heart" premature ventricular contractions (PVCs) are generally benign, a high PVC burden may result in a form of TIC (Baman et al., 2010); this condition is fortunately often reversible if the arrhythmia can be adequately controlled, usually necessitating medications or ablation.

For full reference citations to this chapter, please see "Section References" at the back of the book, under the heading "Section III."

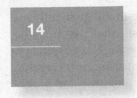

Electrophysiology Diagnostic Studies and Cardiovascular Implanted Electronic Devices

ROBERT L. McSWAIN

ELECTROPHYSIOLOGY DIAGNOSTIC STUDIES AND TESTS

12-Lead Electrocardiogram

The value of the basic 12-lead electrocardiogram (ECG) is not to be overlooked as a baseline measurement and for the evaluations of arrhythmia over time. Even if an arrhythmia in question is not detected, much can be learned from the tracing. For example, mild sinus bradycardia might suggest sick sinus syndrome as a cause for fatigue; bundle branch block or QT prolongation may provide an etiology for syncope; or Q waves can elicit a search for ischemic heart disease and its potentially associated arrhythmias. Even an entirely normal ECG can be helpful; although a normal baseline tracing cannot entirely exclude the possibility of intermittent arrhythmias, it might require an expansion of the differential diagnosis to include conditions that are not rhythm related. In other situations, the ECG might provide the diagnosis without the need for any further testing—cryptogenic stroke patients may have underlying atrial fibrillation (AF); patients with palpitations might present with supraventricular tachycardia (SVT); or the tracing of those with syncope or profound fatigue may uncover high-grade atrioventricular (AV) block.

Orthostatic Vital Signs

This simple test is often performed before electrophysiology (EP) referral. Combined with a suggestive history, a positive test defined as a systolic drop in blood pressure (BP) equal to or greater than 20 mmHg or a diastolic drop equal to or greater than 10 mmHg when changing from the supine to standing position may be all that is required to secure a diagnosis of orthostatic intolerance. If the result is nondiagnostic, but the condition is still suspected, tilt table testing can be considered to reassess the patient's response to gravitational stress in a more controlled environment.

Tilt Table Testing

Although its utility has been questioned, the somewhat barbaric tilt table test has, nonetheless, stood the test of time as part of the evaluation of syncope and dizziness (Saklani, Krahn, & Klein, 2013; Strickberger et al., 2006). It is helpful in establishing the diagnosis of neurocardiogenic syncope and can play a role in the evaluation of postural orthostatic tachycardia syndrome (POTS), orthostasis, and psychogenic pseudosyncope (Raj et al., 2014). The test is commonly performed in the hospital on a specialized motorized table, along with ECG and BP monitoring, intravenous access, and resuscitation equipment. Depending on the patient response and protocol used, the test may be very brief or last up to 40 minutes.

The patient is secured to the tilt table for safety in case of loss of consciousness (LOC), and baseline vital signs are recorded in the supine position. Though specific protocols vary, the table is then slowly rotated into the head upright position at varying degrees, 60, 70, or 90. The upright position is maintained until the patient experiences syncope or symptoms, or the test is otherwise concluded by returning the asymptomatic patient to the supine position after a specified time period. Provocative agents such as isoproterenol or nitroglycerin are sometimes used.

A negative test does not exclude a diagnosis of neurocardiogenic syncope. If an otherwise healthy young patient faints at the sight of blood, the diagnosis is likely neurocardiogenic even if the tilt is negative on a given day. A classically positive result will yield the patient's prodromal symptoms, often accompanied by sinus tachycardia, followed by an abrupt drop in heart rate and BP at the time of syncope. Bradycardia is often due to a junctional rhythm, though asystolic pauses, occasionally dramatically long, are often noted. Syncope may be accompanied by seizure-like activity from cerebral hypoperfusion, which sometimes contributes to a misdiagnosis of epilepsy. The symptoms typically resolve quickly and spontaneously once the patient is returned to the supine position.

With orthostatic intolerance, symptomatic hypotension will often develop quickly once the patient is upright. An inadequate heart rate response to hypotension might suggest concomitant chronotropic incompetence. Patients with POTS will typically have a normal heart rate and BP when supine; once upright, the BP will remain relatively normal while the heart rate increases to more than 140 beats per minute. Psychogenic pseudosyncope is occasionally encountered, with normal vital signs at the time of apparent LOC.

Cardiac Stress Testing

Besides the prominent role that cardiac stress testing has in the general cardiology evaluation of ischemic heart disease, the results from this modality may have additional specific implications for patient management from an EP perspective. Exercise treadmill testing can uncover a predilection to tachyarrhythmias, especially AF, SVT, long-QT syndrome (LQTS), or ventricular tachycardia (VT). Similarly, some patients with poor exercise tolerance will demonstrate chronotropic incompetence or exercise-induced AV block. By knowing whether or not ischemic heart disease is present through stress testing, along with left ventricular ejection fraction (LVEF), if provided, EP is able to ensure accuracy in risk-stratifying patients and in prioritizing potential arrhythmia diagnoses. Some arrhythmic conditions will become self-limited or resolve entirely when significant structural heart disease has been addressed, including valvular disease or coronary insufficiency.

Transthoracic and Transesophageal Echocardiogram

Within the purview of general cardiology, transthoracic and transesophageal echocardiography (TEE) also provide valuable data to help the practicing electrophysiologist care for patients. The two most important predictors of prognosis in EP are the ejection fraction (EF), as usually determined by echocardiography, and the status of the coronary arteries. When determining the potential need for an implantable cardioverter defibrillator (ICD), the EF is almost always the starting point. In patients already undergoing a cardiovascular implantable electronic device (CIED)-related procedure, the EF guides the selection of the most appropriate device.

The TEE can specifically evaluate the left atrial appendage for thrombus prior to cardioversion or AF ablation, and identify valvular or lead-related vegetations in patients with potential CIED infections. Left atrial size and the potential severity of associated mitral valve disease, as assessed by either imaging modality, can contribute to the prediction of the likelihood of success when an AF rhythm control strategy is considered. Finally, echocardiography will occasionally uncover an alternative treatable diagnosis that is essentially not rhythm related, for example, critical aortic stenosis in a patient with syncope.

Ambulatory ECG Monitoring

With advances in technology, an assortment of ambulatory ECG monitoring options has been developed; however, the 24-hour holter maintains its place as the initial test of choice for many arrhythmia evaluation indications. If longer monitoring periods are required to capture the potential arrhythmia in question, event monitors can add value. The advantages of the holter include the relatively short and thus convenient recording period, and the storage of all heart beats for the day in question. This latter feature provides snapshots of the best and worst rhythms of the day, along with valuable trend data. The trend data are particularly useful when assessing AF rate control and for quantifying premature ventricular contraction (PVC) burden. The main disadvantage of the holter is that any arrhythmia outside the short 24-hour monitoring window will be missed out.

The event monitor allows for longer monitoring periods, though at the expense of a loss of trend data. However, the latest products by several competing mobile telemetry companies offer the best of both worlds. Another exciting innovation allows patients to record a single-lead tracing on a smartphone and then later to present the information to the treating provider either electronically or in person.

Implantable Loop Recorder

When noninvasive ambulatory ECG monitoring fails to capture a highly suspected symptomatic arrhythmia, an implantable loop recorder (ILR) may be indicated. Although the device has been available for several years, recent further miniaturization and the addition of wireless transmission capabilities will likely lead to an earlier position in the diagnostic algorithm for several conditions, including syncope; cryptogenic stroke, possibly from undiagnosed AF; and palpitations. As with all of the ambulatory monitoring systems, artifact can be an issue, though the ILR generally can record a high-quality, single-lead ECG tracing either manually, if the patient activates for symptoms, or automatically, if prespecified criteria for brady- or tachyarrhythmias are met. The latest ILR is minimally invasive to the extent that cost may be the only significant downside; the device may be, nonetheless, cost effective by eliminating the need for other expensive, low-yield tests. Compliance with the ILR is good, because the system is self-contained beneath the skin with no exposed wires, and monitoring can last for up to 2 to 4 years. Lastly, it goes without saying that the ILRs are for monitoring purposes only, and they do not provide any form of therapy.

Electrophysiology Study

The diagnostic electrophysiology study (EPS) represents the gold standard for arrhythmia evaluation. Although the test is safe and minimally invasive, its role is, nonetheless, somewhat limited. For example, decisions regarding the need for permanent pacing are often based on symptoms and noninvasive diagnostic studies. Similarly, primary prevention ICD therapy is determined based on clinical variables of health history, EF, QRS width, and heart failure class, rather than on the results of an EPS. Even VT and SVT are often diagnosed noninvasively, though the EPS can be confirmatory and guide therapy. Frequently, the EPS clarifies the mechanism of an arrhythmia previously discovered by noninvasive means, although at times the EPS establishes the diagnosis of a suspected though previously undocumented arrhythmia. Thus, the test is most beneficial when the pretest probability of uncovering a significant arrhythmia is relatively high.

The EPS procedure is comparable with the more familiar coronary angiography, with the latter involving arterial puncture and dye injection, whereas the former uses the more forgiving venous system and temporary pacing. Arterial access is rarely required unless left ventricular mapping and ablation are planned. Generally performed with sedation, the EPS begins with the placement of fluoroscopically guided temporary pacing and recording catheters into the heart via the femoral vein(s). Catheters are generally placed in the right atrium and ventricle, at the His bundle recording site near the AV node, and often in the coronary sinus. Left atrial access, if required, can be achieved by way of transseptal puncture, which is commonly facilitated by the use of intracardiac echocardiography (ICE). Once the catheters are in place, baseline electrical parameters are recorded. Atrial pacing and extra stimulation—for example, pacing-induced premature contractions—is then performed to assess the health of the sinoatrial and AV nodes and to predict the potential for bradycardia. To rule out the presence of inducible atrial or ventricular tachyarrhythmias, rapid pacing and extra stimulation is generally performed from both chambers as well. Some arrhythmias can be induced reliably, including atrioventricular node reentry tachycardia (AVNRT) or atrial flutter, although other arrhythmias—such as PVCs or atrial tachycardia—are less predictable. Isoproterenol is often used to facilitate arrhythmia induction.

If ablation is performed, a waiting period, generally about 30 minutes, will often follow initial success to ensure the result is lasting. The basic EPS can be completed within an hour, although mapping and ablation can potentially add hours to the procedure. Resuscitation equipment, including transcutaneous patches that allow defibrillation or emergency pacing, is immediately available, although tachyarrhythmias in the EP lab can often be terminated with overdrive pacing. Sophisticated three-dimensional computerized mapping systems improve the overall efficiency and safety of the process. If the study is performed on an outpatient basis, the patient is typically discharged after several hours of bed rest, monitoring, and observation. Patients are asked to avoid exertional activity for several days, mainly to enable the venous access sites to heal.

The chance of complications from an EPS is low, but risks include vascular injury, including hematoma, pseudoaneurysm, or fistula; anesthesia complications; or—rarely—cardiac perforation with tamponade. Generally, stroke or MI are not direct risks unless the arterial system is entered. There are additional risks if ablation is performed, as previously discussed. An inferior vena cava (IVC) filter is at least a relative contraindication to performance of the EPS via the femoral approach.

CARDIOVASCULAR IMPLANTED ELECTRONIC DEVICES

Once typically placed by a surgeon or cardiologist in the operating room with portable C-arm fluoroscopy, CIEDs are currently more likely implanted by an electrophysiologist in a dedicated EP laboratory. Except for the difference in size, the implant procedure is similar for permanent pacemakers (PPMs) and ICDs, especially now that defibrillation threshold testing is performed less routinely than in the past. Device improvements, including higher maximal shock strengths, combined with the enormous wealth of collective clinical experience, have led to the current perception—validated in a recent clinical trial—that an ICD will reasonably detect and successfully treat future life-threatening ventricular arrhythmias (VA) even if not tested at the time of implant. The numerical risk is small, but, nonetheless, there remains the risk that the rare patient cannot be successfully resuscitated from intentional iatrogenic ventricular fibrillation (VF).

Single, dual, and biventricular lead systems are available, depending on specific patient factors and requirements. Systems can be, and frequently are, upgraded, either at the time of generator exchange or earlier, if warranted. Most patients receive dual chamber systems, unless permanent AF is present, in which case there is no requirement for the atrial lead. If the chronicity of AF is uncertain, implanters will often include the atrial lead to provide the option of a future rhythm-control strategy. Various algorithms are utilized to minimize the need for ventricular pacing, given its potentially deleterious long-term impact on ventricular function; patients frequently receive PPMs for a complete heart block (CHB), in which chronic ventricular pacing is mandatory. For pacemaker settings, the North American Society of Pacing and Electrophysiology (NASPE) and the British Pacing and Electrophysiology Group (BPEG) published a generic code for antibradycardia pacing, as shown in Table 14.1 (Bernstein et al., 2002). All PPMs currently manufactured operate in a demand mode and most are fairly automated in offering rate responsivity, a faster pacing rate when one or more sensors detects patient activity and thus a potential need for additional heart rate support. Most are capable of mode switching to a nontracking mode in the event of AF, to prevent rapid ventricular pacing that would ensue if the PPM otherwise attempted to track the rapid atrial rates.

TABLE 14.1 The Revised NASPE/BPEG Generic Code for Antibradycardia Pacing

Position	I	II	III	IV	V
	Chamber(s) paced	Chamber(s) sensed	Response to sensing	Rate modulation	Multisite pacing
Category	O = None A = Atrium V = Ventricle D = Dual (A + V)	O = None A = Atrium V = Ventricle D = Dual (A + V)	O = None T = Triggered I = Inhibited D = Dual (T + I)	O = None R = Rate modulation	O = None A = Atrium V = Ventricle D = Dual (A + V)
Manufacturers' designation only	S = Single (A or V)	S = Single (A or V)			

BPEG, British Pacing and Electrophysiology Group; NASPE, North American Society of Pacing and Electrophysiology.
Reprinted from Bernstein et al. (2002), with permission from John Wiley and Sons.

The PPMs are not capable of regulating all rates and rhythms, and medications may continue to be necessary. In particular, the primary capability of PPMs is to increase heart rates or prevent a low heart rate; however, they are ineffective in lowering a rate that is too fast, such as rapid AF. Nonetheless, with a PPM, problems involving rapid rhythms can be better managed by allowing the use of rhythm- and rate-controlling medications without further concern for bradycardia.

All ICDs are PPMs, but not all PPMs are ICDs. Single-chamber ICDs are preferred, unless an atrial lead is warranted in, for example, a patient who has an additional intermittent history of either bradycardia or an atrial tachyarrhythmia, commonly AF. In the former scenario, the atrial lead can provide atrial-based rate support when needed and can prevent only ventricular-based pacing that is not coordinated with atrial activity. In the latter, the atrial lead can allow the use of dual-chamber discriminators, for example, algorithms to minimize unnecessary ICD shocks for relatively benign rapid AF by utilizing the data from both channels. As previously discussed, an additional left ventricular lead that constitutes a biventricular system is warranted in the setting of a wide QRS, especially left bundle branch block (LBBB).

The implant procedure time for a PPM or an ICD lasts approximately 1 to 1.5 hours. The variation is considerably higher for biventricular systems, depending on patient anatomy; a difficult case may require several hours. In all cases, a pocket is formed either above the pectoralis major muscle—preprectoral—or below the muscle—subpectoral. There are advantages and disadvantages to either location. The subpectoral approach yields a more esthetically pleasing result and carries a lower risk of device erosion in thin patients; however, this location requires more extensive dissection and thus more postoperative pain both initially and at the time of subsequent generator exchanges. Given the reductions in generator size over the past several years, the vast majority of implants are placed in a prepectoral location. The CIEDs can be implanted on either side in the upper chest below the lateral aspect of the clavicle; the left side is generally preferred, both because it represents the nondominant side for most patients and because leads from this location form a gentle "C" curve to reach the heart, as opposed to the "S" curve from the right.

Venous access is achieved by a combination of subclavian and axillary puncture, and occasionally direct cephalic vein cutdown. The latter approach adds minimally to the complexity of the procedure but eliminates the risk of pneumothorax. Initially placed j-tipped guidewires are exchanged for hollow sheaths that allow the passage of the lead(s) to the heart with fluoroscopic guidance. Leads are occasionally tunneled subcutaneously from one side to the other, typically if venous occlusion prevents the addition of a lead on the existing side. Low-dose contrast-dye injection is occasionally required, with its well-known attendant risks of allergic reactions and contrast nephropathy; common uses for contrast include venography to locate or determine the patency of the subclavian venous system and to delineate the coronary venous anatomy for left ventricular lead placement. Passive, tined, and fixation leads are still occasionally used, especially the left ventricular leads of biventricular systems. However, the majority of implants currently utilize active fixation leads, with a tiny metal "corkscrew" that embeds the tip of the lead within the myocardium. The proximal ends of the leads are anchored to the floor of the pocket and the incision is closed after the leads and attached generator are tucked within the pocket. Implant cases are occasionally challenging. Hemodialysis patients may have limited venous access options because of current or previous externalized catheters or surgical arteriovenous fistulas, and it is generally advisable to avoid placing a CIED on the side of either. The rare patient will have a persistent left superior vena cava; rarer still will be the patient with dextrocardia.

The CIED technology is mature, and the device can be safely implanted in the vast majority of cases. Relatively uncommon serious risks include pneumothorax, which requires chest-tube insertion, and cardiac perforation with tamponade, which requires percutaneous or surgical drainage. Leads can dislodge and require surgical repositioning, although typically if the leads remain in place the first night they will remain in place indefinitely. Ipsilateral subclavian venous thrombosis after the CIED implant may require oral anticoagulation for a matter of months. Infection is an ever-present risk and generally requires device explant and eventual reimplant. A pocket hematoma is another risk, which is generally exacerbated by the need for postoperative anticoagulation or in patients with acquired clotting disorders. Hematomas also increase the risk of infection. The best treatment is prevention; without that option, conservative monitoring usually suffices, as most wounds eventually heal as the body resorbs the blood. Needle drainage is generally ineffective, and surgical hematoma evacuation, though occasionally required, also leads to an increased infection risk due to increased pocket manipulation. There is an emerging trend to perform CIED implant procedures on patients who remain therapeutically anticoagulated with warfarin (Ghanbari et al., 2012). This approach limits the thromboembolic risks incurred when anticoagulation is interrupted, and it reduces the risks related to postoperative hematomas in patients requiring short-term anticoagulation, especially with low-molecular-weight heparin.

After the CIED implant, patients are typically monitored overnight and discharged the next morning, unless other issues require ongoing hospitalization. One or more chest x-rays are obtained to exclude pneumothorax and confirm lead positioning. Postoperative antibiotics are commonly prescribed. The wound is evaluated and monitored to ensure it is intact and free of significant bleeding or hematoma. Though not mandatory, patients are commonly provided with a sling to limit shoulder movement on the first night. Device interrogation is commonly performed before discharge, mostly to confirm the integrity of the lead tip to the tissue interface, as assessed by the pacing threshold, impedance, and sensing parameters of each lead.

The EP community is learning the value of simplicity regarding CIEDs, and single-lead systems often suffice. Single-coil ICD leads are similar in efficacy to their dual-coil cousins, and they are easier and safer to extract if necessary. A lead never placed cannot fracture or require removal. A lesson learned from pacing programming includes the principle to minimize ventricular pacing as able. For ICD programming, it is beneficial to minimize shocks through higher VT cutoffs and longer detection times. Besides the pain involved, ICD shocks are not entirely benign, and VA will often resolve spontaneously if the ICD is programmed appropriately.

Common CIED manufacturers' 24-hour technical support include:

- Medtronic: 800-633-8766
- St. Jude: 800-722-3774
- Boston Scientific: 800-227-3422
- Biotronik: 800-547-0394

Temporary Pacing

Temporary pacing is frequently required, often on an emergency basis. The most common scenario involves a patient with CHB and a bradycardic escape rhythm with hemodynamic instability. Transcutaneous pacing can be utilized to keep the patient alive, but the current requirement is uncomfortable, often requiring intubation to allow adequate sedation. Temporary transvenous pacing eliminates the significant discomfort of transcutaneous pacing, but it requires successful placement of the lead within the right ventricle, accomplished with either the guidance of fluoroscopy or the use of a balloon-tipped pacing catheter via the internal jugular, subclavian, or femoral vein. Passive-fixation catheters are vulnerable to lead dislodgement, which can recreate the emergency in the pacemaker-dependent patient. This issue can be overcome somewhat with the use of an active-fixation temporary pacing catheter. If the requirement for a temporary pacing is expected to last beyond a few days, a temporary-permanent system can be created, with a PPM generator and lead temporarily implanted and affixed to the skin externally. A typical scenario where this solution might prove useful would involve a pacemaker-dependent patient awaiting resolution of a significant systemic infection prior to permanent CIED implantation, often after the patient's prior device was removed because it was involved in the infection.

CIED Follow-Up and Monitoring

Regardless of who implants a CIED, the managing provider must be knowledgeable of the related issues that may need to be addressed from time to time. Some of these issues are predominantly patient related, whereas others are predominantly device related, although there is considerable overlap. As an illustration of the former, the patient's cardiac status may change over time, and new or worsening arrhythmias may be identified. A common example would be a new diagnosis of AF as detected by the device, requiring the clinician to address issues related to anticoagulation and potentially antiarrhythmic therapy. Similarly, documentation of nonsustained VT by a PPM might require a review of the patient's EF and coronary status, as well as potential consideration of an echocardiogram, ischemic evaluation, or a device upgrade. A patient with a PPM and previously normal left ventricular systolic function might develop a cardiomyopathy (CM), leading to a discussion of a device upgrade to include ICD and/or cardiac resynchronization therapy (CRT) components. An occasional pacemaker-dependent patient with compliance issues might present for a PPM interrogation, and the energy required for the interrogation itself might lead to pacemaker failure and emergent bradycardia in the doctor's office.

Device-related issues include leads that may fracture, resulting in a pacemaker failure, or, in the case of an ICD, potentially multiple painful or even dangerous shocks. Pacing thresholds may increase, requiring device reprogramming or lead replacement. Electrical "noise" may be intermittently captured on one or more leads, such that troubleshooting must determine whether lead failure is imminent, or whether the noise originated from an external source and the CIED is functioning normally.

Despite the issues outlined earlier, CIEDs are, nonetheless, reliable and interrogations are usually routine. As technology evolves, these routine checks are increasingly occurring remotely. Remote checks from the patient's home do not eliminate the need for in-office checks but can reduce their required frequency. Older and basic transtelephonic pacemaker monitoring systems are still in use, though the latest home monitoring solutions provide a more robust interrogation report, similar to the information provided in an in-office check. In an ideal although common scenario, after the patient goes to sleep, the patient's home monitor, which has been set up to the phone line, will wake at the appointed time, interrogate the patient's device wirelessly, and transmit the findings to the host web server. The provider can log in to the website the next morning to review a PDF-formatted report of the findings. One of the few remaining limitations to in-home checks at this point is that data flow is unidirectional, from the patient's home to the clinician's office. Iterative programming to check thresholds cannot be performed remotely—unless the device has autocapture capabilities—and device settings cannot be changed remotely. This limitation is less a shortcoming of the available technology and more an intentionally imposed safety restriction.

Magnets and CIEDs

Historically, magnets assisted with the interrogation of devices and the determination of battery life. Nowadays, the main function of the magnet response is to simply and temporarily alter CIED function in the operating room without the need for a programmer. The general rule is that a magnet placed over a PPM will place the device in an asynchronous pacing mode, such that electrocautery would not potentially lead to pacing inhibition and to intraoperative symptomatic bradycardia. When the magnet is removed, normal PPM function will resume. If the device is an ICD, the general rule is that magnet application will temporarily disable tachyarrhythmia detection and therapy, such that electrocautery would not potentially lead to inappropriate shocks. Once the magnet is removed, normal ICD function will resume. It is important to note that magnet application over an ICD will not affect pacing function; thus, it would be possible for electrocautery to temporarily cause pacing inhibition and potentially symptomatic bradycardia in this situation.

Therefore, pacemaker-dependent patients with an ICD may require interrogation and reprogramming perioperatively if electrocautery is used. A consensus statement is available to address the perioperative complexities (Crossley et al., 2011).

CIED Revision and Extraction

Patients with previously implanted CIEDs occasionally require that leads be added or removed for various reasons. Lead management is becoming increasingly important when evaluating infected systems, recalled or malfunctioning leads, and upgrade scenarios. Transvenous leads scar into place over time, and simple traction techniques are generally not adequate to remove leads that have been in place beyond a year or two. Fortunately, laser-powered extraction sheaths are available to facilitate lead removal by breaking up scar tissue, which binds the lead to the vasculature, the heart, or other adjacent leads. With proper precautions, the risk of serious complications from extraction is low, but a venous tear or cardiac perforation may require emergent open heart surgery (Wazni et al., 2010).

If a CIED becomes infected, the general rule is that the infection cannot be eliminated until the hardware is removed, including both generator and lead(s). Infections involving the pocket are often obvious with erosion, erythema, or purulent drainage, but in occult infections, recurrent unexplained gram-positive bacteremia may be the only clue to the correct diagnosis. In either case, complete system removal is required.

When a lead malfunctions or is recalled because of a tendency to do so, a complex discussion between the patient and electrophysiologist is required regarding the risks and benefits of extraction versus abandonment of the lead at the time of replacement. Sometimes, it is reasonable to continue using the affected lead and monitoring it over time. A similar lead management discussion is also warranted at the time of device upgrade—for example, a PPM to ICD—especially if the subclavian venous system is known or determined to be occluded. The difficult decision is to determine whether to assume the current risks of extraction, or potentially face a riskier extraction scenario at a later date, when the leads have scarred further and the patient is older and potentially sicker.

Withdrawal of CIED Therapy

In 2010, the Heart Rhythm Society (HRS) published a consensus statement on the management of CIEDs in patients nearing the end of life or requesting device deactivation (Lampert et al., 2010). The CIEDs can be life saving, but all patients will eventually die. Up to 20% of patients with ICDs receive shocks in the last few weeks of life (Lampert et al., 2010). In situations where life-prolonging measures are no longer the priority, the painful shocks reduce quality of life and cause suffering for patients and families. A relationship with the EP team is imperative as the relevant medicolegal and ethical issues regarding potential device deactivation are discussed and considered. These conversations are best initiated even prior to implantation of the CIED.

For full reference citations to this chapter, please see "Section References" in the back of the book, under the heading "Section III."

Vascular Disorders

FOUR

Peripheral Arterial Disease

CONSTANCE RYJEWSKI

Although there are many conditions that may interfere with the vitally important ability to ambulate, peripheral arterial disease (PAD) remains one of the most common causes, affecting an estimated 8 to 12 million Americans and carrying with it an inordinately high socioeconomic burden (Criqui et al., 1985; Selvin & Erlinger, 2004). The economic burden arises from the decreased capacity of the individual to function and also from the associated high cardiovascular risk. PAD is a well-recognized predictor of increased risk for cardiovascular events (Leng et al., 1996; Ness & Aronow, 1999).

Incidence is a measure used to describe the calculated risk that PAD will develop in a specific population over an expressed period of time; it is helpful in understanding the etiology of disease. Prevalence refers to the proportion of total number of patients with PAD to a total population in a given period of time. Prevalence, therefore, is more indicative of the pervasiveness of PAD and generally a better descriptor of socioeconomic burden. As incidence increases, so does prevalence; therefore, both are important to our understanding of the significance of PAD.

PAD is universally one of the most profoundly underdiagnosed and undertreated diseases—until symptoms of severe limb ischemia become evident. The incidence of PAD has been studied worldwide and in a large number of subpopulations, including the elderly, women, diabetics, various income groups, and inhabitants of specific geographic locations. Prevalence has similarly been studied and found to be steeply rising, especially in the aged. An often-cited study conducted by investigators Selvin and Erlinger (2004) involved the analysis of 2,174 participants in the National Health and Nutrition Survey 1999 to 2000. These investigators evaluated the prevalence of PAD by age and gender, and it concluded that in 2000 there were an estimated 5 million adults with PAD. In individuals older than the age of 70, the prevalence was estimated to be 14.5% (Selvin & Erlinger, 2004). In an additional study, PAD prevalence was evaluated in people 60 years of age and older in the United States. Data from 3,947 men and women who had undergone an ankle-brachial index (ABI) assessment for PAD were evaluated. The PAD prevalence was reported to be 12.2% overall and 23.2% in adults who were 70 years of age and older (Ostchega, Paulose-Ram, Dillon, Gu, & Hughes, 2007).

More recently, Fowkes et al. (2013) compared global estimates of prevalence and risk factors for PAD in 2000 and 2010. In high-income countries, including the United States, the prevalence of PAD in men and women between 45 and 49 years of age was greater than 5%. Prevalence rose sharply with age in both men and women, and by the age of 85 to 89, PAD prevalence exceeded 18%. Due largely to advancing age, the number of people with PAD increased globally by an estimated 23.5%, with the investigators concluding that as many as 202 million people were afflicted with PAD in 2010 (Fowkes et al., 2013).

According to the Centers for Disease Control Executive Summary on the State of Aging and Health in America (2013), the population of Americans aged 65 years and older is expected to double in the next 20 years. Given the chronicity of PAD and its increased prevalence among the elderly, these numbers have far-reaching implications and pose unprecedented opportunities for clinicians in the early detection and management of PAD. The predictive link of PAD to cardiovascular events increases the importance of early detection, aggressive risk-factor modification, diagnostic evaluation, appropriate and timely intervention, and patient education. The clinician's challenges, therefore, rest in understanding the significance of PAD and the methods and benefits of early recognition, valuing a thorough history and physical examination, identifying patient-appropriate treatment and risk reduction strategies, and performing clinical assessment and care activities.

PATHOPHYSIOLOGY

The formation and growth of atherosclerotic plaque leading to the compromise of luminal cross-sectional areas, as well as the restriction of blood flow during times of increased metabolic need, are the basic processes contributing to the development of PAD. These processes cause the characteristic changes in skin, muscles, and bones of the leg and foot, as well as the development of the clinical symptoms of PAD. Atherosclerosis represents abnormal healing of the intimal layer of the arterial wall in response to endothelial injury (Munro & Cotran, 1988). The endothelial injury, which may be caused by low- or very-low-density lipoproteins, leads to the migration of inflammatory cells into the intima and the ingestion of these lipoproteins within the wall in a cyclic and ongoing manner. Thus, the lipid atheroma is formed. Over time, these atheroma calcify, producing the characteristic atherosclerotic plaque (Faxon et al., 2004; Libby, Ridker, & Maseri, 2002).

Flow-limiting stenosis occurs as the plaque burden increases and encroaches on the arterial lumen, impairing blood flow to vascular beds distal to the site. The body's initial response is to vasodilate, whereas the continued growth of the plaque exceeds the ability of the vessel to dilate, and the flow through the vessel is compromised (Glagov, Zarins, Bassiouny, & Giddens, 1995). When the narrowing exceeds 50%, the lesion is deemed hemodynamically significant. From this point, continued loss of the cross-sectional area correlates with a decrease in distal flow and perfusion, and generally, the onset of symptoms. Rupture or ulceration of the plaque may activate platelets and clotting factors on the surface that can break free and move downstream as embolic debris, causing more significant tissue ischemia. As might be expected from a slowly progressive process, atherosclerosis and luminal narrowing of lower extremity vessels initially cause muscle fatigue during periods of increased muscle activity, such as running or walking fast. As blood flow is further decreased, a patient may experience muscle fatigue while walking only short distances or even at rest.

RISK FACTORS

Although atherosclerosis seems to be a fundamental aspect of the human condition, there are several known risk factors that accelerate the process and increase the likelihood of PAD. These risk factors include smoking, elevated cholesterol, hypertension, diabetes mellitus, chronic kidney disease, hyperhomocysteinemia, and a sedentary lifestyle. Not surprisingly, the relationship between smoking and PAD has been recognized for more than 100 years (Erb, 1911). It is perhaps the most modifiable of risk factors, and the reduction or cessation of smoking is a mainstay of therapeutic interventions. Cigarette smoking not only confers a markedly increased risk for the development of PAD but also, based on the number of cigarettes smoked, is associated with increased disease severity and progression to amputation. The prevalence of PAD increases more than twofold in active smokers (Willigendael et al., 2004). A recent meta-analysis of active smoking and PAD has demonstrated this association to be greater than that between smoking and heart disease, and although PAD risk decreases with smoking cessation, the risk remains significantly higher when compared with individuals who never smoked (Lu, Mackay, & Pell, 2014).

Elevated serum cholesterol is also firmly established as a risk factor for atherosclerosis and PAD. Aggressive cholesterol management, especially with 3-hydroxy-3-methylglutaryl-coenzyme A (HMG-CoA) reductase inhibitors (statin therapy), imparts a similar benefit to patients with symptomatic PAD as it does in patients with symptomatic coronary heart disease (Heart Protection Study Collaboration Group, 2002). Statin therapy has also been associated with reductions in perioperative mortality in PAD patients undergoing major vascular surgery (Poldermans et al., 2003). The benefit of lipid-lowering therapies is not found in their ability to cause regression of existing stenosis, but rather in their ability to stabilize the atherosclerotic lesion (Grundy et al., 2004; Hirsch et al., 2006). In 2013, the American College of Cardiology, in conjunction with the American Heart Association, released guidelines on the management of high cholesterol to prevent atherosclerotic cardiovascular disease (ASCVD) (Stone et al., 2013). In the recommendations, four primary statin benefit groups were defined. The first group was those individuals with clinical ASCVD, as defined as coronary, cerebral, and peripheral vascular diseases. Specifically, regarding PAD, ASCVD is characterized by previous arterial revascularization or PAD of atherosclerotic origin. In the absence of contraindications, it is recommended that individuals with these PAD characteristics receive high-intensity statin therapy (Stone et al., 2013).

Based on the Framington Heart Study data, hypertension is associated with a two and a half to fourfold increased risk for developing PAD, a risk proportional to the severity of the elevated blood pressure (Kannel & McGee, 1985). The mechanisms by which hypertension exerts its effect are not clearly elucidated, but they appear to be mainly due to mechanical stress, endothelial damage, and the release of vasoactive substances that contribute to smooth-muscle cell proliferation (Raij, 1991). The Eighth Joint National Committee (JNC-8) guidelines for the management of hypertension recommend a blood pressure (BP) goal less than 150/90 mmHg in people 60 years of age and older, and less than 140/90 mmHg in people 30 through 59 years of age, including those with diabetes or chronic kidney disease (James et al., 2014).

Diabetes mellitus is a systemic disease with far-reaching, long-term complications that are accelerated by poor glycemic control. Due largely to the aging population and rampant obesity, the number of persons in the United States diagnosed with diabetes was estimated at 20.9 million in 2011, rising sharply from 5.6 million in 1980 (CDC, 2013). Atherosclerosis and its sequelae are considered the most common cause of death in the diabetic patient. Diabetes correlates to an increased risk between twofold and fourfold for PAD (Criqui, Denenberg, Langer, & Fronek, 1997), and to an increased risk of death in people with PAD. A recent study of 487 hospitalized patients with symptomatic PAD showed a 5-year mortality rate of 23% in diabetic patients younger than 75 years of age, and 52% in diabetic patients equal to or older than 75 years of age (Mueller et al., 2014). This was statistically significant compared with nondiabetic controls. Treatment goals are directed toward strict blood glucose control and a glycated hemoglobin less than 7.0% or as close to normal (< 6.0%) as possible.

Chronic kidney disease is also independently associated with an increased prevalence of PAD (O'Hare, Glidden, Fox, & Hsu, 2004) and with the future risk of developing clinically significant PAD (Wattanakit et al., 2007). The development of strategies both to screen for subclinical PAD and to prevent progression of PAD in this population is clinically warranted.

Hyperhomocysteinemia and elevations in the inflammatory markers C-reactive protein (CRP) and fibrinogen are predictors of risk for PAD. Their association with PAD is not as strong as smoking, hypertension, diabetes, and dyslipidemia, whereas their validity as biomarkers for PAD risk is well established in the literature (Fowkes, 1995; Khandanpour, Loke, Meyer, Jennings, & Armon, 2009; Ridker, Cushman, Stampfer, Tracy, & Hennekens, 2004). Treatment of homocysteine levels, however, has not demonstrated a reduction in atherosclerosis development or vessel patency after PAD intervention (Andras, Stansby, & Hansrani, 2013). Similarly, although CRP and fibrinogen are important inflammatory markers in which increased levels may contribute to the early diagnosis of PAD, no clinical trials have demonstrated that inhibiting or lowering these levels will improve PAD outcomes.

Finally, a history of a sedentary lifestyle is associated with a significantly higher risk of developing PAD (Wilson et al., 2011). Physical inactivity is predictive of all-cause mortality in patients with intermittent claudication (IC). Gardner, Montgomery, and Parker (2008) performed a retrospective review of survival status in 434 patients with stable IC with a mean follow-up of 5.33 years. They concluded that weekly physical activity was associated with a reduced rate of mortality, even when adjusting for other predictors such as age, ABI, and body mass index (Gardner, Montgomery, & Parker, 2008). Independently, and in concert, modifiable risk factors are predictive of PAD. The greater the number of modifiable risk factors and risk factor burden, the higher the likelihood that PAD will be present (Berger et al., 2013). Risk factor modification is critical to PAD development, slowing disease progression and enhancing the benefits of invasive surgical interventions.

DIAGNOSIS

There are two major forms of PAD. The more common and more benign form is IC, and the more severe form is critical limb ischemia (CLI). Many believe that these forms of PAD may simply represent a trajectory of progression of PAD in the lower extremity. However, some vascular specialists acknowledge that these forms may be distinct manifestations of PAD, based on the findings that only 10% of those with IC progress to CLI, and many who present with CLI deny a history of IC.

Clinical Presentation

Aching pain, fatigue, or muscle cramping in the lower extremities induced by walking and rapidly relieved by rest characterizes IC. The presence and severity of these symptoms are largely dependent on the size and location of the diseased artery, the metabolic demands of muscle tissue during activity, and the formation of collateral vessels. The symptom distribution of the affected muscle group is generally distal to the culprit lesion (Table 15.1).

TABLE 15.1 Intermittent Claudication Symptoms and Corresponding Artery

Symptom Distribution	Diseased Artery
Buttocks	Aortoiliac
Thigh	Iliofemoral
Upper calf	Superficial femoral
Lower calf	Popliteal
Foot	Tibial or peroneal

Principles of oxygen supply and demand provide the underpinnings for ischemic muscle pain. The development of collateral vessels that circumvent the occlusive lesion and permit delivery of blood and nutrients to distal tissues will also influence tissue perfusion and the distance of claudication discomfort (Hills, Shalhoub, Shepherd, & Davies, 2009; Wessler & Silberg, 1953). The ambulation distance that elicits discomfort and the location and severity of the pain are usually consistent for most patients. These distinguishing characteristics help differentiate IC from other less common etiologies that cause similar symptoms (White, 2010). Table 15.2 describes differential diagnosis for IC from the TransAtlantic Inter-Society Consensus (TASC II) Working Group (Norgren et al., 2007).

Chronic CLI is characterized by either ischemic rest pain or the presence of ischemic ulceration or ischemic gangrene of the foot or toes. In the setting of arterial occlusions throughout the lower extremity, tissue perfusion may drop below the level required to maintain viability. Rest pain, characterized by disturbing coldness or aching pain, usually of the forefoot or toes, occurs when the patient is lying supine with legs on the bed. In the absence of gravity, the toes and forefoot become severely ischemic, triggering pain receptors. This pain can quickly resolve by

TABLE 15.2 Differential Diagnosis of Intermittent Claudication

Condition	Prevalence	Location	Characteristics	Effect of Exercise	Effect of Rest	Effect of Position	Other Characteristics
Calf IC	3%–5% of adult population	Calf muscles	Cramping, aching discomfort	Reproducible onset	Quickly relieved	None	May have atypical limb symptoms on exercise
Thigh and buttock IC	Rare	Buttocks, hip, thigh	Cramping aching discomfort	Reproducible onset	Quickly relieved	None	Impotence may have normal pedal pulses with isolated iliac artery disease
Foot IC	Rare	Foot arch	Severe pain on exercise	Reproducible onset	Quickly relieved	None	Also may present as numbness
Chronic compartment syndrome	Rare	Calf muscles	Tight, bursting pain	After much exercise (jogging)	Subsides very slowly	Relief with elevation	Typically heavy muscled athletes
Venous claudication	Rare	Entire leg, worse in calf	Tight, bursting pain	After walking	Subsides slowly	Relief speeded by elevation	History of iliofemoral deep vein thrombosis, signs of venous congestion, edema
Nerve root compression	Common	Radiates down leg	Sharp lancinating pain	Induced by sitting, standing, or walking	Often present at rest	Improved by change in position	History of back problems worse with sitting; relief when supine or sitting
Symptomatic Baker's cyst	Rare	Behind knee, down calf	Swelling, tenderness	With exercise	Present at rest	None	Not intermittent
Hip arthritis	Common	Lateral hip, thigh	Aching discomfort	After variable degree of exercise	Not quickly relieved	Improved when not weight bearing	Symptoms variable History of degenerative arthritis
Spinal stenosis	Common	Often bilateral buttocks, posterior leg	Pain and weakness	May mimic IC	Variable relief but can take a long time to recover	Relief by lumbar spine flexion	Worse with standing and extending spine
Foot/ankle arthritis	Common	Ankle, foot arch	Aching pain	After variable degree of exercise	Not quickly relieved	May be relieved by not bearing weight	Variable, may relate to activity level and present at rest

IC, intermittent claudication.

Reprinted from Norgren et al. (2007, S5–S67), with permission from Elsevier.

placing the feet in a dependent position; symptoms abate as a result of gravitational forces that pull blood to distal tissues. Patients become accustomed to the reduction of pain in this position and will dangle their foot over the side of the bed during the night.

As ischemia worsens, the skin loses its ability to regenerate, becoming thin and friable so that minor trauma to the foot may result in the development of small, painful ulcers of the foot or toes. If perfusion worsens, ischemic gangrene may develop with necrotic skin covering areas of the foot or toes. Although the documentation of ischemic rest pain, ulceration, or gangrene strongly suggests the presence of CLI, their absence does not exclude this problem. Approximately 20% of patients with PAD may be completely asymptomatic (Fowkes et al., 1991). This is especially true in the elderly or in patients who do not walk significant distances due to other chronic conditions such as lung disease or arthritis. In this group of sedentary patients, chronic CLI is most readily identified by the coolness and general pallor of the foot and toes; the presence of thin, friable skin; and thickened toenails.

Health History

An accurate and comprehensive health history and a systematic physical examination are essential to evaluate the patient with PAD, and possibly the most important elements in determining disease significance. The history and physical are invaluable tools whose importance cannot be overestimated, despite an environment of ever-increasing technological advances. A detailed patient history provides the clinician with an appreciation of the impact of the disease and an understanding of those factors that may contribute to disease onset and progression. Armed with this information, the clinician can begin formulating a plan for patient education and care. Similarly, the basic concepts of inspection, palpation, and auscultation yield much and provide the underpinnings for clinical decision making.

The patient history should begin with the chief complaint. Because the most common presenting symptom in PAD is limb pain, a problem-oriented approach is frequently the most useful. Assessment of the symptomatic limb, therefore, should be directed at understanding and documenting the character of pain; its onset, duration, and frequency; precipitating or aggravating factors; and activities that provide relief or symptom resolution.

Additional historical information should include a thorough assessment of significant risk factors, including hypertension, dyslipidemia, and diabetes mellitus; prior surgical procedures, including open, minimally invasive, and percutaneous interventions; and ongoing or past medical problems, especially disease affecting the vasculature. The likelihood that a patient may have significant peripheral disease is increased when there is vascular pathology of the coronary or cerebrovascular systems (Hirsch et al., 2001). A review of current medications also yields important information, especially in patients who may be poor historians or who are uncertain about their co-morbidities.

Physical Examination

The techniques of physical assessment include inspection, palpation, and auscultation. Each of these techniques provides unique but complementary information and should be applied in total for an accurate clinical impression. Developing patient rapport and providing a nonthreatening, comfortable, and private environment will aid in the examination process.

The vascular examination should begin with a general observation of the patient and then progress to a focused assessment. Much can be garnered about the patient's overall health status, nutritional state, hygiene practices, and anxiety level using a keen eye at the time of introduction.

Both lower extremities should be thoroughly inspected for size, symmetry, muscle mass or wasting, edema, and ischemic changes even when the presenting symptoms are unilateral. Positioning the patient with the legs dependent and with the legs elevated 30 to 45 degrees while observing color changes may help define arterial compromise. Pallor of the foot and toes with elevation indicates that there are proximal arterial blockages, and blood cannot flow against gravity through narrow collateral pathways. Dependent rubor, which is defined as deep redness of the foot when in the dependent position, is suggestive of severe peripheral vascular disease and it occurs when blood pools in the small arterioles and capillaries at the skin surface (Figure 15.1).

Trophic changes are those affecting the skin and nailbeds. In patients with chronic peripheral vascular disease and ischemia, the skin of the distal lower extremity may be pale, hairless, cool, and shiny, with thickened nails and changes in foot or toe structure. These changes occur as a result of decreased blood flow and impaired delivery of oxygen and other nutrients that are vital to maintaining healthy tissue.

Actual or impending skin breakdown resulting from minor trauma or an ischemic process should also be noted. Ulcerations may occur from activities as seemingly innocuous as trimming a toenail too closely or the development of a blister. Injuries such as these may result in wounds that fail to heal despite attentive local care. Ischemic ulcerations have distinguishing features and frequently develop in areas of prolonged contact or pressure such as the heels, tips of the toes, between the toes where they rub against one another, and bony prominences that are in contact with other surfaces such as bed linen, shoes, or socks. Arterial ulcers generally have irregular edges with poor granulation tissue, and they are often deep with a round or punched-out appearance and sharp demarcation. In the presence of infection, there may be swelling or redness around the ulcer base. These ulcers may involve muscle, tendon, or bone. Ischemic ulcers are typically very

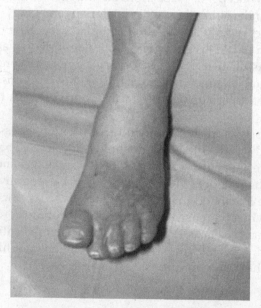

FIGURE 15.1 Dependent rubor of the lower extremity. See color insert.

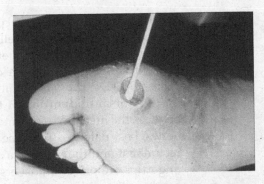

FIGURE 15.2 Plantar ischemic ulceration.

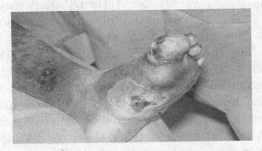

FIGURE 15.3 Ischemic ulceration with gangrene.

painful, regardless of size, and especially at night (rest pain). Documented assessment of these ulcers should include onset and duration, size, location, depth, and the presence of any odor or drainage (Figure 15.2).

Gangrene results from critically insufficient blood flow to distal tissues and resultant cell death (Figure 15.3). Dry gangrene frequently begins in the toes. There is limited putrefication and even bacteria fail to survive. The affected tissue is dry, shrunken, and a dark-reddish color. Wet gangrene is suggestive of infection and carries a poorer prognosis. Thriving bacteria cause the affected tissue to swell, become soft and putrid, and emit a foul odor. Septicemia may result in the absence of intervention.

The location of arterial occlusive lesions may be determined by palpation of peripheral pulses. An examination should be conducted with the patient supine and in a comfortably warm environment to avoid temperature-induced peripheral vasoconstriction. Pulse assessment should include the presence and nature of the femoral, popliteal, posterior tibialis, and dorsalis pedis (DP) pulses. Palpation is conducted using the fingertips and applying gentle pressure over the artery. The intensity of the pulse is graded on a scale of 0 to 4+, with 0 indicating no palpable pulse; 1+ a faintly detectable pulse; 2+ a normal pulse; 3+ an increased pulse; and 4+ a bounding pulse. Pulses should also be assessed for symmetry, rate, and rhythm.

The common femoral artery is an extension of the external iliac artery and begins at the inguinal ligament. Here, it emerges into the upper thigh. It is best palpated by standing on the ipsilateral side of the patient and pressing deeply in the midgroin, approximately one and a half to two fingerbreadths lateral to the pubic tubercle. It may be difficult to palpate in the obese or muscular patient (Figure 15.4).

The popliteal artery passes through the popliteal space deep behind the knee joint, slightly lateral to the midplane. Even the experienced examiner may find the popliteal pulse difficult to palpate. To evaluate the popliteal pulse, we need to ensure that the patient is supine, with the knees partially flexed, and the calf muscles relaxed. The hands encircle and support the knee from each side with the thumbs resting on the patella. The pulse is detected by allowing the supporting fingertips to sink deeply into the middle of the popliteal space. Relaxation of the muscles is essential to this examination, but even then, the popliteal pulse may not be palpable. Alternatively, the patient may lie prone with the knee flexed 45 degrees. A nonpalpable popliteal pulse may not be clinically important when distal pulses are identified. Conversely, an easily palpable and bounding popliteal pulse may suggest aneurysmal dilation.

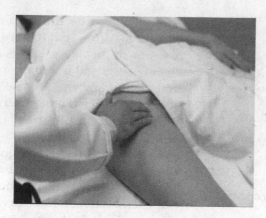

FIGURE 15.4 Palpation of the femoral pulse.

The palpation of the distal pulses of the foot is a common and well-known practice. Again, obesity or edema may prevent successful detection of these pulses. The DP artery is usually found on the dorsal midportion of the foot between the first and second metatarsal bones, best palpated with the patient recumbent and the ankle relaxed. The fingertips are placed transversely and gently on the middle portion of the dorsum of the forefoot near the ankle (Figure 15.5A). The DP artery may require some searching and may be nondetectable in the presence of edema. This pulse is congenitally absent in approximately 10% of the population (Dean, Yao, Thompson, & Bergan, 1975). Figure 15.5B provides a radiographic image displaying both pedal pulses. The posterior tibial artery lies in the hollow behind the medial malleolus and is most easily palpated by gently grasping the ankle between the thumb and fingertips. The fingertips curl around the dorsum of the foot anteriorly and apply pressure to the soft tissues in the space between the medial malleolus and the Achilles tendon, above the calcaneus, with the thumb providing stability on the opposite side (Figure 15.5C).

Briefly compressing the tips of the toes or nailbeds and then releasing pressure assesses capillary refill. The application of pressure will cause blanching; the rapidity with which pink color returns is then measured in time. A prolonged capillary refill time, defined as greater than 3 seconds, may indicate decreased distal perfusion. Because capillary refill may be affected by a variety of external sources, it is generally considered an unrefined measure of distal blood flow.

Sensory and motor function may be diminished in patients with an acutely ischemic limb. Decreased perfusion of distal nerve fibers and muscle may be assessed by touch or pressure and by having the patient flex and extend the toes. Sensory loss and muscle weakness may suggest loss of viable tissue (Dormandy & Rutherford, 2000).

The femoral artery should be auscultated for the presence of a bruit. The vessel should be auscultated with the bell of the stethoscope, applying light pressure. Pressing too firmly may yield misleading information by either intensifying the

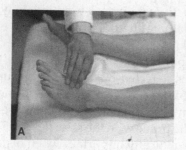
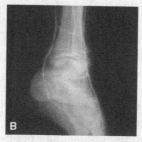
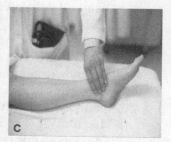

FIGURE 15.5. Evaluation of pedal pulses.

(A) Dorsalis pedis (DP), (B) angiographic image of DP, and (C) posterior tibialis.

sound or preventing its detection. A bruit is an unusual, rushing sound resulting from vibrations within the vessel wall caused by turbulent blood flow. The sound may indicate a local narrowing or obstruction, or it may be transmitted along the artery from a more proximal lesion. In general, bruits are not audible until an artery is approximately 50% occluded (Hill & Smith, 1990).

Diagnostic Testing

Ankle-Brachial Indices

The ABI remains the most effective, objective, low-cost, noninvasive measure for the detection of PAD and should be considered in all individuals 65 years of age and older. This recommendation is based largely on The German Epidemiologic Trial on Ankle Brachial Index Study Group, which studied 6,880 patients, 21% of whom had either asymptomatic or symptomatic PAD (Diehm et al., 2009). The ABI is a simple, clinically useful, noninvasive test that examines the ratio of the systolic blood pressure measured at the level of the ankle to that of the brachial artery (Figure 15.6). Originally described as a diagnostic tool for lower-extremity PAD

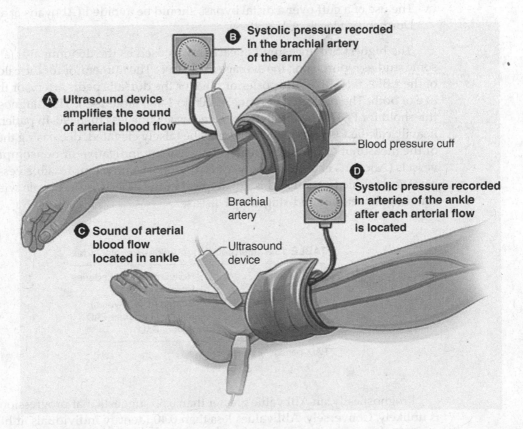

FIGURES 15.6 Measurement of the ankle-brachial index.
Source: commons.wikimedia.org.

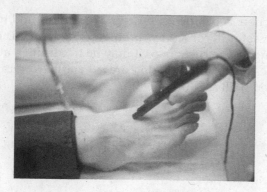

FIGURE 15.7 Doppler measurement of ankle-brachial index.

(Yao, Hobbs, & Irvine, 1969), it was later shown to be an indicator of vascular disease in other beds and a marker for cardiovascular events (Criqui et al., 1992; Fowkes et al., 2008).

Measurement of the ABI should be done with the patient supine and after resting for 15 minutes (Figure 15.7). The recommendations for ABI assessment techniques as reported by Aboyans et al. (2012) in the American Heart Association Scientific Statement on measurement and interpretation of the ABI are given next.

- The Doppler method should be used to measure the systolic blood pressure (SBP) in each arm and each ankle.
- The cuff size should be appropriate, with a width of at least 40% of the limb circumference.
- The ankle cuff should be placed just above the malleoli.
- Any open lesion with the potential for contamination should be covered with an impermeable dressing.
- The use of a cuff over a distal bypass should be avoided (Aboyans et al., 2012; Dormandy, Heeck, & Vig, 1999).

The highest SBP measured in each arm is used as the denominator, although some studies report using the average of the two. The numerator for the calculation of the ABI is the SBP of the posterior tibial or the dorsalis pedis artery, or the average of both. The normal ABI range is 1.00 to 1.40 (Table 15.3). The diagnostic ABI threshold for PAD is generally recognized as a value less than .90. In patients with heavily calcified vessels, ABI values may be falsely elevated, decreasing the utility of the measurement. Values greater than 1.40 are indicative of noncompressible vessels (Aboyans et al., 2012; Fowkes et al., 2008). A noncompressible vessel suggests severe calcification and is not atypical in the elderly or in people with long-standing diabetes or end-stage renal disease.

TABLE 15.3 Interpretation of Ankle-Brachial Index

>1.4	Noncompressible arteries
1.00–1.40	Normal
0.91–0.99	Borderline (equivocal)
0.41–0.90	Mild-to-moderate PAD
00.00–0.40	Severe PAD

PAD, peripheral arterial disease.

Prognostically, an ABI value greater than 0.50 suggests that progression to CLI is unlikely. Conversely, ABI values less than 0.40 identify individuals at high risk for CLI and are an indicator for ineffective healing of ischemic ulcers. An ABI of less than 0.4 carries a 5-year survival probability of only 44% (Dormandy et al., 1999;

McKenna, Wolfson, & Kuller, 1991). In addition to the utility of ABI for PAD diagnosis and prognosis, ABI is also routinely used to monitor disease progression as well as the efficacy of therapeutic interventions.

In circumstances when the suspicion and risk of PAD are high but resting ABIs are normal, arterial stress testing of ABIs may provide clinically useful information. In arterial stress testing, a baseline ABI is obtained; then, the patient engages in leg exercise by walking on a treadmill or by a series of tip-toe maneuvers until claudication symptoms occur, after which the ABI is again measured. A positive diagnosis is made if the ABI decreases by 15% to 20% from the baseline measurement (Hirsch et al., 2006; Norgren et al., 2007).

Segmental Arterial Pressure Measurements

This noninvasive study is analogous to the ABI, although it requires the sequential placement of blood pressure cuffs on the lower extremity. Generally, a three-cuff system is used, with systolic blood pressure measurements at the level of the thigh, calf, and ankle. Pressure gradients between adjacent segments, generally greater than 20 mmHg, can identify the location of an arterial stenosis. For example, a pressure gradient between the thigh and calf would signify a stenosis of the superficial femoral or popliteal artery (Rutherford, Lowenstein, & Klein, 1979). Importantly, noncompressible vessels, as in the ABI measurement, may yield uninterpretable results.

Toe Pressures (Toe-Brachial Indices)

In individuals with noncompressible vessels, ABI and segmental arterial pressure measurements may be less sensitive, and the diagnosis and severity of PAD may be determined by calculating the toe-brachial index. This test is a sensitive marker for PAD, largely because the small digital arteries are generally spared from the calcification process that affects the more proximal vessels. A small cuff is placed on the great or second toe and inflated until pulsatility is occluded. Values are recorded at the point at which pulsatility returns. Toe-brachial indices less than 0.70 are considered diagnostic for PAD, whereas values between 0.00 and 0.19 confer a severe risk for ischemia (Vincent, Salles-Cunha, Bernhard, & Towne, 1983).

In most vascular labs, ABIs, segmental pressure measurements, and toe pressures are typically performed in conjunction with pulse-volume recordings. Doppler waveforms or tracings depict the amplitude and magnitude of systolic and diastolic pressures at each measured segment, and they are useful in assessing vessel patency and blood flow. Sequential reductions in waveform measurements are diagnostic for a proximal flow-limiting lesion. Pulse-volume recordings are also useful in evaluating small-vessel disease of the feet.

Arterial Duplex Ultrasound

Arterial duplex ultrasound is useful for detecting the anatomic location and degree of stenosis of the studied vessel. Ultrasound is extensively used to evaluate vessel patency after both open and endovascular revascularization, and more broadly to evaluate for the presence of aneurysmal dilation, arterial dissection, pseudoaneurysms, or lymphocele (Hirsch et al., 2006). Hemodynamically significant stenoses are diagnosed based on the ratio between peak systolic velocities within or beyond the diseased artery, compared with an upstream, presumably healthy arterial segment. Turbulent blood flow and pulselessness are indicative of high-grade stenosis or occlusion (Moneta, Yeager, Lee, & Porter, 1993; Sacks, Robinson, Marinelli, & Perlmutter, 1992). Degree of stenosis is frequently reported in ranges, including less than 50%, 50% to 69%, 70% to 99%, or occlusion. The utility of duplex scanning, however, may be limited when multiple stenotic segments are present (Allard, Cloutier, Durand, Roederer, & Langlois, 1994).

Computed Tomographic Angiography

Multidetector computed tomographic angiography (CTA) of the abdominal aorta, iliac vessels, and legs utilizes the rapid succession of thin-sliced cross-sectional CT images, which are then reformatted to depict a three-dimensional anatomical image similar to conventional digital subtraction arteriography (Figure 15.8A). The CTA is a rapidly evolving imaging modality that is both highly sensitive and specific in diagnosing both the location and severity of PAD, and it is especially useful in evaluating patients who are candidates for intervention (Met, Bipat, Legemate, Reekers, & Koelemay, 2009). Key advantages of CTA are its relatively short study duration and the ability to rotate images 360 degrees to allow the visualization of eccentric lesions. The CTA is an excellent alternative to magnetic resonance angiography, especially in the presence of a pacemaker or metallic implants that may obscure images or be contraindicated with magnetic imaging techniques. A disadvantage of CTA is the requirement of the administration of intravenous iodinated contrast, and is, therefore, contraindicated in people with known sensitivity to contrast agents, renal disease, or elevated serum creatinine levels.

Magnetic Resonance Angiography

Gadolinium-enhanced magnetic resonance angiography (MRA) of the distal aorta, iliac arteries, and lower-extremity arterial tree is an effective tool in the evaluation of patients with PAD (Figure 15.8B). The MRA is a radiation-free imaging modality that employs the use of a powerful magnetic tube and radio-wave pulsations to visualize the blood vessels with a proven high degree of accuracy (Koelemay, Lijmer, Stoker, Legemate, & Bossuyt, 2001; Menke & Larsen, 2010). Unlike CTA, which requires contrast for visualization, MRA requires only flowing blood. The administration of nonionic contrast (gadolinium), however, markedly enhances the quality of the images. The MRA is highly sensitive and specific, and it has been considered by some investigators as superior to conventional angiography when assessing the vessels of the distal calf and foot (Dorweiler, Neufang, Krietner, Schmiedt, & Oelert, 2002; Kreitner et al., 2000). One of the principal advantages of MRA is the minimal risk of gadolinium-induced nephrotoxicity. More recently, however, nephrogenic systemic fibrosis has gained attention and been found to be related to the administration of gadolinium. Patients considered at the greatest risk are those with glomerular filtration rates less than 30 mLs/min/1.73 m^2 and

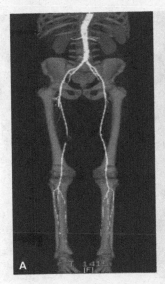
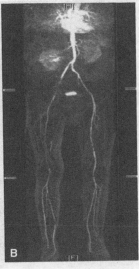

FIGURE 15.8 (A) Computed tomographic angiography and (B) magnetic resonance angiography imaging of abdominal aorta with runoff.

those with chronic kidney disease on hemodialysis. Though not an absolute contraindication to MRA, benefit versus risk should be thoughtfully assessed in this subpopulation of patients, and careful consideration should be given to noncontrast enhanced imaging or the use of less toxic and lower doses of gadolinium-based contrast (Hellman, 2011; Kaewlai & Abujudeh, 2012). The MRA may also pose problems for the severely claustrophobic patient or for those who cannot be supine for an extended period due to cardiac, pulmonary, or orthopedic pathologies. The MRA is generally contraindicated in patients with implantable electronic devices such as pacemakers or cardiac defibrillators, insulin pumps, neurostimulators, cochlear implants, and certain mechanical prosthetic heart valves. Most coronary, peripheral vascular, and aortic stent grafts have been tested and are labeled "MR-safe" (Hirsch et al., 2006).

Contrast Angiography

Contrast angiography has long been the gold standard and universally accepted method for the evaluation of peripheral arterial anatomy (Figure 15.9A). Conventional angiography is used diagnostically for strategizing open revascularization procedures, and therapeutically for guiding percutaneous endovascular interventions. The use of complementary imaging modalities such as ultrasound, CTA, and MRA can frequently enable the interventionalist to selectively image a vessel, thereby reducing the contrast load and radiation exposure. Although there are many advantages of contrast angiography, there are also inherent risks, including bleeding, infection, arterial injury, contrast allergy, and renal toxicity. However, appropriate patient selection, careful planning, and vigilant post-procedural observation can mitigate many of these risks.

Carbon dioxide (CO_2) is an alternative and reliable angiographic contrast agent that is gaining broader acceptance (Figure 15.9B). This is particularly noteworthy, given our aging population and the stepwise increase in diabetes and renal insufficiency, because of the known risks associated with the use of contrast agents in

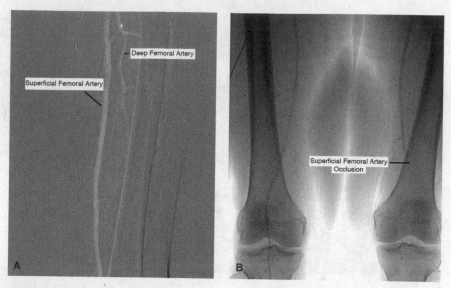

FIGURE 15.9 (A) Conventional angiography and (B) CO_2 angiography of femoral arteries.

these populations. CO_2 has the advantage of eliminating allergic risk; due to the pulmonary clearance, it does not reenter the circulation, eliminating the risk of contrast-induced nephrotoxicity (Shaw & Kessel, 2006). Advances in technological imaging and improved delivery systems have, in the opinion of some investigators, rendered CO_2 angiography nearly comparable to an iodinated contrast media equivalent (Hawkins, Cho, & Caridi, 2009). As with all imaging modalities, the utility of CO_2 angiography is largely dependent on operator skill and experience, and it should be reserved for appropriately selected patient populations.

NATURAL HISTORY

Several landmark studies have documented the link between an abnormal ABI and coronary or cerebrovascular disease. The PARTNERS Study evaluated 6,979 patients in primary-care practices throughout the United States (Hirsch et al., 2001). Of those studied, 29% had PAD as defined by an ABI equal to or less than 0.90; within this group, 16% had PAD and cardiovascular disease (Hirsch et al., 2001). The Edinburgh Artery Study evaluated 1,592 subjects from 10 general practices over a 5-year period and described the prevalence of asymptomatic and symptomatic PAD with respect to ischemic heart disease. These investigators concluded that the risk for cardiovascular death in subjects with PAD was significantly greater when compared with normal controls (Fowkes et al., 1991). More recently, 2,777 male patients with documented claudication were followed over 15 years at a Veterans Administration Hospital (Muluk et al., 2001). In this study, the mortality rate was 12% per year; of those deaths with a known cause, 66% were due to cardiac disease. Significant independent mortality predictors were age, cerebrovascular accident, diabetes mellitus, and lower ABI (Muluk et al., 2001).

THERAPEUTIC INTERVENTIONS

IC seldom progresses to the limb-threatening stage and, therefore, infrequently requires surgical intervention. Treatment strategies are directed at risk factor control and reduction, symptom management, and structured walking exercises to increase exercise tolerance and to promote development of collateral vessels. Previously discussed in greater detail, smoking, hypertension, diabetes mellitus, and lipid metabolism disorders are factors known to increase the likelihood of developing PAD; therefore, they are the primary targets for risk-reduction strategies. Treatment goals (Table 15.4) include smoking cessation, blood pressure and serum glucose control, and cholesterol management. Lifestyle changes, a healthy diet, and exercise further increase the likelihood of a positive outcome.

Exercise Rehabilitation

The benefits of a supervised treadmill walking exercise program are well supported. A structured exercise regimen of 3 months' duration or longer performed thrice weekly for 60 minutes improves walking distance and efficiency, endothelial function, and skeletal muscle adaptation (Stewart, Hiatt, Regensteiner, & Hirsch, 2002). During exercise sessions, the patient walks on a treadmill at a speed and grade that induces claudication; then, the patient stops exercising to rest until symptoms abate.

TABLE 15.4 Therapeutic Risk Factor Modification for PAD

Risk Factor	Treatment Recommendations
Smoking	Advise cessation Provider and/or group counseling Antidepressant therapies Nicotine replacement
Diabetes mellitus	Hgb A1c < 7.0%

Hypertension	< 150/90 in patients ≥ 60 years of age
	< 140/90 in patients 30–59 years of age
	Antihypertensive agents
	  Thiazide diuretics
	  Angiotensin-converting enzyme inhibitors
	  Calcium channel blockers

Hypercholesterolemia	LDL < 100 if asymptomatic PAD LDL < 70 if symptomatic or disease in other vascular beds Treatment increased triglycerides and low HDL patterns Dietary modification Statin therapy Fibrates or niacin to ↓TG or ↑HDL
Sedentary lifestyle	Increase activity Rehabilitation program
Hyperhomocysteinemia	Use of folate supplementation is not recommended

HDL, high-density lipoproteins; LDL, low-density lipoproteins; PAD, peripheral arterial disease.

Adapted from James et al. (2014); Norgren et al. (2007).

The exercise–rest–exercise cycle is repeated over a total period of 50 minutes. During the course of the program, the speed or grade of treadmill exercise is gradually increased, determined by the patient's ability to tolerate a given setting for 10 minutes or longer without stopping. The patient is encouraged to walk independently on nonsupervised days. Outcome assessment includes measuring the time to onset of claudication and the time to absolute claudication necessitating cessation of walking exercise and a period of rest. Such programs, unfortunately, are not widely available and are unlikely to be covered by insurance providers. Home-based programs can be equally as effective as supervised/exercise if exercise activity is quantified and monitored (Gardner, Parker, Montgomery, Scott, & Blevins, 2011). Alternatively, all patients with symptoms of IC, non-limb-threatening disease, and the absence of contraindications should be encouraged to walk 1 or more hours, three or more times per week, stopping as needed and resuming when claudication symptoms resolve. Consistent exercise in this manner for a period of at least 3 to 6 months elicits the greatest improvement. The functional improvements associated with structured exercise have been extensively studied and are well supported by the literature. Additional benefits for exercise include improved blood pressure, enhanced glycemic control, weight loss, and reductions in serum lipid levels.

Pharmacotherapeutics

Antithrombotic Medications

All individuals with diagnosed PAD should be on antiplatelet therapy with aspirin, unless contraindicated (Rooke et al., 2011). Aspirin has long been the antiplatelet agent of choice for reducing the risk of serious cardiovascular events, including myocardial infarction, cerebrovascular accidents, and vascular death. Dosing recommendations for PAD range from 75 mg to 325 mg daily. The Antithrombotic Trialists' Collaboration (2002) conducted a meta-analysis of randomized trials of antiplatelet therapy and concluded that 81 mg of aspirin conferred the greatest proportional reduction in vascular events (Antithrombotic Trialists' Collaboration, 2002). More recent studies evaluating aspirin use (100 mg daily versus placebo) were found to have mixed results and limited generalizability to patients with clinical PAD (Rooke et al., 2011).

Clopidogrel, 75 mg per day, has demonstrated significantly reduced risk of thrombosis and has, therefore, been recommended as a safe and effective alternative to aspirin therapy in patients with PAD (Hirsch et al., 2006; Rooke et al., 2011). Clopidogrel may be used in isolation or in combination with aspirin therapy in patients at an exceptionally high cardiovascular risk who are not at high risk for bleeding. Prasugrel and ticagrelor are newer antiplatelet agents that have gained increasing attention as possibly more effective platelet inhibitors. The superiority of these agents, however, compared with the current lower-cost generic clopidogrel is yet to be determined in patients with PAD.

The addition of the oral anticoagulant warfarin, without concomitant clinical indication, to antiplatelet therapies in patients with PAD who are at risk for cardiovascular events is without benefit and potentially harmful due to the increased risk of major bleeding (Hirsch et al., 2006; Rooke et al., 2011).

Cilostazol, a phosphodiesterase III inhibitor with vasodilatory and antiplatelet activity, has demonstrated improvement in symptoms, exercise performance, and quality-of-life measures in patients with IC. Headache, diarrhea, and palpitations are reported side effects, and these are contraindicated in patients with heart failure (Beebe et al., 1999; Regensteiner et al., 2002; Strandness et al., 2002).

Pentoxifylline is a hemorheologic agent whose benefits have been extensively studied compared with placebo and other agents. Findings, however, remain variable and unclear. Early trials demonstrated modest increases in treadmill walking distance. Later studies questioned the overall clinical benefit, largely because of inconsistencies in study design. Consequently, the role of pentoxifylline in IC remains uncertain (Salhiyyah, Senanayake, Abdel-Hadi, Booth, & Michaels, 2012).

Statin Therapy

Secondary prevention and the initiation of high-intensity statin therapy is recommended in patients equal to or younger than 75 years of age with clinical PAD who are not already on statin therapy, unless contraindicated. In individuals with clinical PAD who have already been prescribed a low- or moderate-intensity statin agent, increasing the intensity of their statin dosage may be of benefit (Stone et al., 2013).

Antihypertensive Agents

Beta blockers, as well as all other classes of antihypertensive medications, are considered appropriate treatment for hypertension in patients with PAD. Although there is overwhelming evidence regarding the benefits of blood pressure control in terms of cardiovascular risk reduction, it is unknown whether the use of antihypertensive agents in individuals with PAD confers any specific or significant additional outcome benefit (Lane & Lip, 2013).

Foot Care

Attentive foot care is paramount to avoiding complications in patients with PAD. Proper-fitting shoes that prevent chafing and pressure on bony prominences and digits, and careful nail care with the avoidance of injury from clipping, protect the patient with PAD from adverse sequelae. Patients should be instructed to examine their feet with a mirror, allowing complete viewing of the plantar portion of the foot. These measures are especially important in patients with diabetes and peripheral neuropathies when the foot is insensate and the risk for injury is high. If, despite attentive personal care, a foot ulcer develops, the patient should be referred to a specialist in foot care to improve rapid healing. A team of specialists, including wound care, diabetes management, plastic surgery, and podiatry, may each have a role in evaluating and managing foot wounds.

Surgical Intervention

There are patients who do not improve with structured exercise and pharmaco-therapy, and for whom claudication symptoms significantly compromise their work and daily activities. In addition, claudication symptoms may prevent successful completion of a cardiac rehabilitation program and therefore warrant a more aggressive approach. In these cases, patients may derive significant benefit from revascularization (Hirsch et al., 2006; Spronk et al., 2009; Whitehall, 1997). For the majority of individuals with claudication, symptoms may curtail activity, result in functional impairment, and negatively impact quality of life, but the disease process remains stable and the limb threat is minimal. Approximately 20% of those individuals with claudication symptoms, however, may deteriorate to the point that their symptoms become incapacitating and surgical intervention is necessary (Whitmore & Belkin, 2000). Treatment goals for patients with PAD manifesting as IC are symptom relief, improved exercise performance, and greater functional capacity. Structured exercise and pharmacotherapy, therefore, remain the therapeutic mainstay. In general, revascularization procedures are considered when noninvasive measures fail.

Patients with IC should be referred for evaluation by a vascular specialist if they have failed an initial therapeutic vascular regimen or have symptoms that significantly interfere with employment or quality of life. Patients with limb-threatening lower extremity ischemia, either acute or chronic, should be referred as soon as these urgent diagnoses are established. Treatment of the occlusive disease should be based on the expertise of the vascular specialists for optimal outcomes. If there is sufficient expertise to support either an endovascular or an open approach to treatment, an endovascular approach is generally considered a better first option, especially in the elderly or in those at high risk for complications due to co-morbidities. Conversely the longer-term patency associated with reconstructive procedures may be a better option for the younger and healthier patient (Alhara et al., 2014; Antoniou et al., 2013).

Technology is rapidly evolving to reduce the common failure modes of endovascular therapy, such as in-stent restenosis, with the development of bioresorbable stents, local drug delivery systems, and antithrombotic medications. However, these advanced technologies will remain palliative treatment unless a vigorous effort is made to identify and control all cardiovascular risk factors and to slow the development of atherosclerosis.

Early diagnosis, risk factor modification, and secondary prevention improve prognosis and reduce complication risk. The mainstay of diagnosis remains the thorough patient assessment with a comprehensive health history and physical examination. For these reasons, advanced practice nurse cardiovascular clinicians are uniquely positioned to positively impact the development, progression, and risk for complication in patients with PAD.

For full reference citations to this chapter, please see "Section References" in the back of the book, under the heading "Section IV."

Abdominal Aortic Aneurysm

KELLEY M. ANDERSON

Aneurysm is derived from the 15th-century Greek word "aneurusma," meaning to widen, dilate, or stretch. An abdominal aortic aneurysm (AAA) is an abnormal, irreversible, localized dilation of the descending aorta. AAAs are most commonly located in the infrarenal position of the aorta. By convention, an AAA is defined as an enlargement of the abdominal aorta with a diameter greater than 3 cm or 1.5 times the expected normal aortic diameter. The normal diameter varies by age, gender, and height, with an average infrarenal aortic diameter of 1.5 to 2.5 cm in elderly men (Liddington & Heather, 1992). A true aneurysm affects all three layers of the vasculature, the intima, media, and adventitia; a false aneurysm or pseudo-aneurysm contains blood between layers of the arterial wall.

The incidence of aneurysm rupture has not improved significantly over the past 20 years and is associated with significant mortality (Kent et al., 2004). Approximately 15,000 occurrences of AAA rupture occur in the United States each year, with a mortality of 65% to 85% (Sakalihasan, Limet, & Defawe, 2005). Similarly, the RESCAN investigators reported a 20% survival after AAA rupture (Bown, Sweeting, Brown, Powell, & Thompson, 2013). However, there is notable improvement in mortality in individuals screened and with early repair before rupture (Sakalihasan et al., 2005). Therefore, current clinical practice focuses on the identification of those at risk, as well as appropriate screening, monitoring, referral, management, and the avoidance of aneurysm rupture.

AAA is the most prevalent form of aneurysm, estimated at 1.3% to 8.9% in men and 1% to 2.2% in women (Sakalihasan et al., 2005), varying based on modifiable and non-modifiable risk factors (Newman, Arnold, Burke, O'Leary, & Manolio, 2001). The major risk factors clearly linked to the development of an AAA include male gender, age greater than 65 years, first-degree relative with AAA, and history of smoking more than 100 cigarettes. Less significant risk factors include hypertension; connective tissue disease; dyslipidemia; increased height; obesity; and the cardiovascular disorders of coronary heart disease, peripheral vascular disease, and cerebrovascular accident (Kent et al., 2010). The prevalence of AAA is greater in Caucasians and Native American ethnicities, with lower prevalence in African Americans, Hispanics, and Asian populations (Kent et al., 2010).

PATHOPHYSIOLOGY

The pathophysiology of AAA is dependent on the etiology of the aneurysm, with an atherosclerotic-type disorder as a common precipitating factor. In this process, connective tissue changes, particularly in the media of the vascular wall, exhibit a reduction of elasticity through the loss of elastin fibers and degradation of collagen (Sakalihasan et al., 2005). The area of aneurysm experiences thinning of the aortic wall, plaque deposits, calcification, and subsequent arterial enlargement (Xu, Zarins, & Glagov, 2001). Over time, there is substantial atrophy of the media with loss of lamellar architecture with apoptosis. The alteration of elastin and collagen is related to the overproduction of inflammatory cells and proteolytic enzymes, including matrix metalloproteinase and plasmin (Sakalihasan et al., 2005). These proteolytic enzymes are released and increase medial erosion (Xu et al., 2001) with a reduction of smooth-muscle cell density (Sakalihasan et al., 2005). In addition, many patients have an associated mural thrombus with AAA (Sakalihasan et al., 2005).

Less frequently, aneurysms occur due to congenital, inflammatory, traumatic, or infectious processes. Congenital aneurysms may develop in individuals with genetic risks of connective tissue disorders, such as Ehlers-Danlos syndrome and Marfan syndrome. In Marfan syndrome, the thoracic aorta is the usual area of aneurysm, although the lesion may extend to the abdominal aorta. Inflammatory aneurysms are related to the atherosclerotic type and associated with peri-aneurysmal fibrosis and adhesions in the abdominal cavity, including the retroperitoneum (Hellmann, Grand, & Freischlag, 2007; Sakalihasan et al., 2005). Infectious processes with subsequent inflammatory changes can contribute to the etiology and pathophysiology of aneurysm development. Staphylococcus or Salmonella are the primary infectious agents of the aorta, with a few case reports of fungal infections (Ortmann, Wüllenweber, Brinkmann, & Fracasso, 2010), brucellosis, and tuberculosis.

Based on recent molecular and animal studies, the mechanism of the development of AAA likely differs from the usual atherosclerotic process. Traditional risk factors for most atherosclerotic diseases include an elevated blood pressure (BP) and dyslipidemia, but those conditions appear less important for the development of AAA. There is also an inverse relationship with diabetes for development of AAA, indicating differences in the pathophysiologic processes for occlusive atherosclerotic disease and AAA.

RISK FACTORS

Modifiable and non-modifiable risk factors are associated with AAA; the most important predictors of AAA are age, gender, smoking history, and family history of AAA. Kent et al. (2010) conducted an analysis of risk factors in more than 3 million men and women for AAA and describe these predictors as age older than 65 years; male gender; family history of AAA, particularly in siblings; and smoking duration and frequency (Kent et al., 2010). The genetic transmission of AAA risk appears in both an autosomal recessive (72%) and autosomal dominant (25%) pattern with familial clustering around a combination of genetic and environmental factors (Kuivaniemi et al., 2003). A study by Kuivaniemi et al. (2003) investigated 233 families encompassing 653 individuals with AAA spanning nine nations with an all-White cohort. This study revealed that first-degree relatives, especially male relatives, were associated with increased risk for AAA.

Although the mechanism is unclear, there is a strong association between tobacco smoking and AAA, with smokers four times more likely to develop AAA, and continued smoking is associated with progression of AAA size (Sakalihasan et al., 2005). The relationship is fairly linear with increasing years of smoking and number of cigarettes smoked, resulting in increased risk for the development of AAA and AAA rupture (Kent et al., 2010). This associated risk of smoking for the manifestation and clinical progression of AAA decreases over time after the individual ceases smoking.

Additional risk factors are associated with AAA, including a history of hypertension, dyslipidemia, and a previous AAA. Physical characteristics associated with AAA include obesity with BMI greater than 25 kg/m² and increased height (Liddington & Heather, 1992). Co-morbidities associated with an increased susceptibility of AAA are Marfan syndrome, Ehlers-Danlos syndrome, connective tissue disease, and infectious processes. Caucasians and Native Americans are at higher risk for AAA than African Americans, Hispanics, and Asians (Kent et al., 2010).

An analysis was conducted to evaluate antihypertensive medications and risk of AAA in 438 patients with aneurysms and 5,373 case controls. Secondary measures evaluated aortic characteristics in relationship to antihypertensive therapies. Calcium channel blockers (CCBs) were independently related to an increase in aortic wall stiffness and the presence of AAA (Wilmink et al., 2002).

Several characteristics are consistent with lower risk for AAA, although individuals with these findings are not free of risk. Reduced risk for AAA is associated with specific ethnic groups (African American, Hispanic, and Asian), female gender, and diabetes mellitus. Regular exercise and a healthy diet with fruits, vegetables, and nuts are related to reduced risk of AAA. Smoking cessation is linked with a reduced likelihood of the development of AAA with longer duration of cessation associated with lower risk (Kent et al., 2010).

Specific risk factors increase an individual's risk for AAA. Similarly, having an AAA is associated with increased risk of other cardiovascular diseases (Freiberg et al., 2008), including coronary heart disease (CHD), myocardial infarction (MI), and cerebral vascular accident (Eldrup, Budtz-Lilly, Laustsen, Bibby, & Paaske, 2012) or cholesterol embolization (Kronzon & Saric, 2010). After surgical repair of AAA, individuals are at risk for disseminated intravascular coagulation and abdominal hernia.

DIAGNOSIS

The diagnosis of AAA is the result of a combination of stratification of individuals at risk, clinical presentation, health history, physical examination findings, and diagnostic testing.

Clinical Presentation

The vast majority of patients with stable AAA are asymptomatic. Individuals with symptoms may describe a generalized lower back discomfort or a vague midabdominal or flank discomfort with associated radiation to the back or groin, unaffected

TABLE 16.1 Immediate Surgical Evaluation for AAA

Hypotension
Abdominal or back pain
Pulsatile abdominal mass

AAA, abdominal aortic aneurysm.

by movement. Common misdiagnosis for AAA includes genitourinary, vertebral, gastrointestinal, and cardiac causes (Banerjee, 1993). Individuals with leaking AAA and impending or progressive rupture may present with acute, significant back, abdominal, or flank pain associated with systemic symptoms of shock (hypotension or syncope) and pulsatile abdominal mass (Hirsch et al., 2006). Patients with this combination of findings require immediate surgical evaluation (Table 16.1).

Physical Examination

A comprehensive physical examination is required of all individuals with suspected cardiovascular disease (Chapter 3). Physical examination findings associated with AAA are often nonspecific and difficult to detect. BP readings may be consistent with hypertension, hypotension, widened pulse pressure, or differences of more than 20 mmHg between the arms. Cardiac sounds may include a new diastolic murmur or muffled heart sounds. Carotid, femoral, and brachial pulses may be asymmetric or bounding. Abdominal bruits may develop or progress in intensity. Neurologic changes may include syncope, altered mental status, or peripheral paresthesias.

Abdominal palpation is the only physical examination technique that demonstrates specific correlation for the detection of AAA. Palpation may reveal a palpable, pulsatile abdominal mass that may be a result of clinically important AAA; however, these findings are marred with wide ranges of sensitivity, specificity, and clinical predictive value. The abdominal palpation technique has improved diagnostic value for large AAA, with an estimated sensitivity of 61% for AAA, which are 3 to 3.9 cm in size, 69% for 4 to 4.9 cm, and 82% for greater than 5-cm diameter (Sakalihasan et al., 2005), bringing the overall positive predictive value to 43% for AAA greater than 3 cm (Lederle & Simel, 1999). In addition to AAA size, the findings of the abdominal palpation are limited and dependent on the individual's body habitus (Lynch, 2004). Abdominal palpation is regarded as a safe technique without reports of associated rupture.

The following technique is used to perform a bimanual abdominal assessment that is specific for the evaluation for AAA:

- Ensure that there is good lighting in the examination room
- Position the patient supine with the legs bent, knees raised, and abdomen relaxed
- Align your eyes with the patient's abdomen and inspect the abdomen for aortic pulsations above and to the left of the umbilicus
- Auscultate the abdomen for any abdominal bruits
- Evaluate the width of the aorta by placing both palms on the patient's abdomen with an index finger on each side of the abdominal aorta

- Evaluate the pulsation of the aorta with the cardiac cycle, noting a pulsation with systole that may move the fingers apart
- Evaluate the distance between the two index fingers to estimate the width of the abdominal aorta

A complication of AAA is thrombosis with distal embolization, and clinical examination findings may be consistent with these pathologic processes. Cholesterol embolization, or thromboembolism, results in microvascular narrowing and ischemia with resultant purple and blue toes, referred to as "blue toe syndrome" (Reis, 2005), and livedo reticularis, which are lacy patterns of reddish blue areas in the lower extremities (Kronzon & Saric, 2010). These findings are not specific for AAA, although they prompt an elective evaluation for aneurysm in patients with AAA-consistent risk factors. Clinical examination findings related to AAA dissection include pulsus paradoxus, distention of the jugular veins, and Kussmaul sign. Individuals with leaking or ruptured AAA may present with evidence of hemoperitoneum with ecchymosis of the trunk, Cullen sign (periumbilical), or Turner sign (flank), although these findings may be evident in other pathologic conditions, including acute pancreatitis.

Diagnostic Testing

The AAA diagnostic testing and screening is important because the majority of patients are asymptomatic, clinical examination findings are often unremarkable, and the complications of AAA are significant (Table 16.2).

TABLE 16.2 Complications of AAA

Rupture of AAA
Deaths due to rupture generally occur in
men older than 65 years
women older than 80 years
Strongest predictor of rupture is maximal aortic diameter
20% survival rate after AAA rupture
Development of thrombosis, with potential for embolization
Erosion of surrounding tissues and structures

AAA, abdominal aortic aneurysm.

Sources: Bown et al. (2013); Hirsch et al. (2006).

AAAs are discovered inadvertently during diagnostic studies for other conditions or purposefully with screening evaluations. Incidental findings on chest or abdominal radiographs consistent with AAA may be an enlarged silhouette, representing a tortuous aorta or the presence of aneurysm, or stippled calcifications in the aortic wall. During vertebral fracture assessment with dual-energy x-ray absorptiometry, abdominal aortic calcifications that are consistent with atherosclerosis may be appreciated (Schousboe, Wilson, & Kiel, 2006). Ultrasounds for other purposes, such as genitourinary, gastrointestinal, or pelvic evaluations, may reveal AAA (Hirsch et al., 2006).

Ultrasound Imaging

Ultrasound for the measurement of AAA is utilized for evaluation, surveillance, and screening in high-risk groups. Measurement of the abdominal aorta is obtained by evaluating the anteroposterior diameter in a plane that is perpendicular to the aorta (Hirsch et al., 2006). Ultrasound is the preferred screening methodology for 95% of individuals (Hirsch et al., 2006), due to the rapid evaluation time, safety, availability, low patient burden, and overall accuracy. Abdominal ultrasound achieves nearly 100% sensitivity and specificity for the presence of AAA (Hirsch et al., 2006; Silverstein, Pitts, Chaikof, & Ballard, 2005). In addition, portable ultrasound techniques are accurate and can be completed in 3 to 5 minutes (Lin et al., 2003), achieving 99% sensitivity and 98% specificity in the detection of AAA equal to or greater than 3 cm (Rubano, Mehta, Caputo, Paladino, & Sinert, 2013). There is minimal test preparation, although pretest fasting improves visualization.

Additional Diagnostic Imaging

CT and MRI are specific diagnostic imaging techniques used for the evaluation of AAA and can be combined with angiography. Computed topography is the preferred imaging for suspected AAA rupture. Computed tomography angiography (CTA) and magnetic resonance angiography (MRA) are currently the gold standard diagnostic evaluation techniques for pre- and postsurgical intervention, open or endovascular, of AAA (Hirsch et al., 2006). Abdominal CTA allows visualization of the transition zone of the aorta from normal to aneurysm, visceral and iliac arteries, thickness of thrombus, blood in thrombus, and retroperitoneal bleeding. The estimation of AAA size is larger with CT than ultrasound. Sprouse et al. (2003) evaluated 334 individuals post endovascular repair and reported mean sizes of AAA by ultrasound and CT as 4.74 cm and 5.69 cm, respectively. Disadvantages of CT include ionizing radiation and intravenous contrast agent, requiring the monitoring of renal function. MRA uses gadolinium, which is less nephrotoxic than the imaging agents for CTA. Limitations of MRA include a slower scan and difficulties in patients with implanted devices or claustrophobia. Direct arteriography has become less common, although it is used in conjunction with endovascular repair. The value of arteriography is the ability to evaluate arterial anatomy in the aorta and surrounding vessel to determine arterial characteristics and anatomic features (Hirsch et al., 2006).

Laboratory Evaluations

Few laboratory tests are helpful for the evaluation of AAA, although an increased prevalence of AAA has been associated with thrombosis and associated levels of fibrinogen degradation products, specifically D-dimer. An elevated plasma D-dimer greater than 400 ng/mL has been reported to correlate with a 12-fold increased risk for AAA (Golledge, Muller, Clancy, McCann, & Norman, 2011). D-dimer levels also demonstrate prognostic value in the evaluation of increasing AAA size over time (Golledge et al., 2011).

General diagnostic evaluation includes an assessment of BP, serum lipid levels, electrolytes, creatinine, and complete blood count. Diagnostic imaging that is used to evaluate for the presence and extent of aneurysm is primarily completed by ultrasound. CT, MRA, CTA, and conventional angiography are reserved to answer specific anatomic questions and for evaluation pre- and postrepair.

SCREENING

Abdominal ultrasound screening is an important component of AAA identification and the subsequent reduction of AAA rupture and AAA-related mortality in men aged 65 years or older (Guirguis-Blake, Beil, Senger, & Whitlock, 2014). In men, screening for AAA has resulted in a reduction in the number of aneurysm ruptures, with an associated decrease in mortality from both rupture and aneurysm repair (Cosford, Leng, & Thomas, 2007). The AAA screening has resulted in an increase in elective aneurysm surgery, with fewer emergency repairs and a reduction in 30-day mortality (Guirguis-Blake et al., 2014). Screening guidelines are available from health care societies and governmental organizations (Table 16.3). Ferket et al. (2012) evaluated seven screening guidelines in the United States and Canada. The one consistent recommendation throughout the various guidelines is a one-time

TABLE 16.3 One-Time Abdominal Ultrasound Screening Recommendations

Consensus statement cosponsored by the Society for Vascular Surgery, the American Association of Vascular Surgery, and the Society for Vascular Medicine and Biology
    All men aged 60 to 85 years
    Women aged 60 to 85 years with cardiovascular risk factors
    Men and women older than 50 years with a family history of AAA

Source: Kent et al. (2004).

U.S. Preventive Services Task Force (USPSTF)
    Men aged 65 to 75 years who have ever smoked
    In January (2014), the USPSTF published proposed draft recommendations for public comment. The recommendations suggest the selective screening for AAA in all men aged 65 to 75 years, regardless of smoking history. For women, the USPSTF suggests that the current evidence is insufficient to assess the balance of benefits and harms of screening for AAA in women aged 65 to 75 years who have ever smoked and recommends against routine screening for AAA in women who have never smoked.

Source: USPSTF (2005, 2014); LeFevre (2014).

ACC/AHA—American College of Cardiology/American Heart Association
    Men older than age 60 with first-degree relative with AAA
    Men aged 65 to 75 years who have ever smoked

Source: Hirsch et al. (2006).

Medicare
    Men aged 65 to 75 years who have smoked 100+cigarettes in their lifetime
    Men and women with family history of AAA

Source: DHHS/CMS (2014).

AAA, abdominal aortic aneurysm.

screening for the detection of AAA equal to or greater than 5.5 cm in elderly men. Guidelines varied on the recommendations for women and younger men, and risk factor criteria for screening.

Periodic screening surveillance is generally not recommended if no aneurysm is detected on the initial evaluation. The majority of aneurysms detected by ultrasound are small. From 1992 to 1993, Newman et al. (2001) evaluated 4,734 men and women for AAA, and they reported that 87.7% of aneurysms were equal to or less than 3.5 cm. For individuals with AAA below the surgical threshold, continuous reevaluation is recommended; some aneurysms may remain stable for months to years, whereas others increase more rapidly with individual variability in expansion rates (Table 16.4). For smaller aneurysms, surveillance is preferable, because early surgical intervention is not associated with improved long-term survival (Sakalihasan et al., 2005).

TABLE 16.4 Recommended Surveillance for AAA

Society of Vascular Surgery Practice Guidelines
   Maximum external aortic diameter
   2.6–2.9 cm every 5 years
   3.0–3.4 cm every 3 years
   3.5–4.4 cm every 12 months
   4.5–5.4 cm every 6 months

Source: Chaikof et al. (2009).

Consensus statement cosponsored by the Society for Vascular Surgery, the American Association of Vascular Surgery, and the Society for Vascular Medicine and Biology
   <3.0 cm no further testing
   3–4 cm yearly
   4–4.5 cm every 6 months
   >4.5 cm refer to vascular surgery

Source: Kent et al. (2004).

AAA, abdominal aortic aneurysm.

In general, the larger the baseline aneurysm size, the more quickly it increases in size and the higher likelihood of rupture. The strongest predictor of AAA rupture is the size of the aneurysm, with a low risk of rupture in aneurysms less than 5 cm (Table 16.5). Estimated annual risk of AAA rupture is 0% for less than 4 cm, 0.5% to 5% for 4 to 4.9 cm, 3% to 15% for 5 to 5.9 cm, 10% to 20% for 6 to 6.9 cm, 20% to 40% for 7 to 7.9 cm, and 30% to 50% for equal to or greater than 8 cm (Brewster et al., 2003).

TABLE 16.5 Baseline AAA and Average Duration to Reach Surgical Criteria by Gender

Baseline	3-cm Diameter	4-cm Diameter	5-cm Diameter
Men	Mean 7.4 years	Mean 3.2 years	Mean 0.7 years
Women	Mean 6.9 years	Mean 3.1 years	Mean 0.7 years

AAA, abdominal aortic aneurysm.
Source: Bown et al. (2013).

Sweeting, Thompson, Brown, and Powell (2012) conducted an analysis of characteristics of aneurysm growth and rupture in 15,475 individuals in 18 studies with a follow-up of small aneurysms. Aneurysm growth rate was increased in smokers and decreased in patients with diabetes; aneurysm rupture was significantly increased in smokers, women, and individuals with higher BP. Notably, women experience a higher mean rate of rupture for aneurysms of the same size, as depicted in Table 16.6 (Bown et al., 2013).

TABLE 16.6 Mean Rate of Rupture per 1,000 Person-Years by Gender

	3 cm at Baseline	4 cm	5 cm
Men	0.5	1.7	6.4
Women	2.2	7.9	29.7

THERAPEUTIC INTERVENTIONS

The cornerstone of therapy for all individuals with AAA is a healthy lifestyle and modification of cardiovascular risk factors (Chapter 28). Therapeutic management for AAA includes interventions to reduce atherosclerosis, management of hypertension, and smoking cessation (Kent et al., 2010). These measures are the mainstay of treatment for patients with small asymptomatic aneurysms (< 4 cm), with moderate aneurysms (4–6 cm) and limited life expectancy, and with high operative mortality risk.

Pharmacotherapeutics

Based on systematic reviews without clinical outcomes, there is insufficient evidence to support any antihypertensive medication that reduces expansion rates of AAA, including the beta-adrenergic blockers (beta blockers), CCBs, diuretics, and angiotensin-converting enzyme inhibitors (Guessous, Periard, Lorenzetti, Cornuz, & Ghali, 2008). The beta blockers atenolol, metoprolol, and propranolol have been evaluated most extensively, indicating that propranolol has a very small, nonsignificant effect on AAA growth (Rughani, Robertson, & Clarke, 2012). Nevertheless, the prescribing of oral beta blocker therapy is common in outpatient clinical practice, and the utilization of intravenous beta blocker therapy is common for inpatient acute presentations.

Antibiotics with anti-inflammatory properties, roxithromycin, azithromycin, and doxycycline, have been evaluated for the treatment of AAA. There is some indication that roxithromycin has a small, significant effect on AAA expansion rates (Rughani et al., 2012); however, studies of beneficial effect on clinical outcomes and surgical rates are not robust, and their use in this context remains controversial. Doxycycline has demonstrated inhibition of protease-mediated growth of AAA in animal models (Sakalihasan et al., 2005).

Nonsteroidal anti-inflammatory drugs have not demonstrated a reduction in AAA expansion rates (Guessous et al., 2008). Evidence is developing that 3-hydroxy-3-methylglutaryl-coenzyme A (HMG-CoA) reductase inhibitors may reduce AAA expansion rates, although this is based on a systematic review of observational studies without clinical outcomes (Guessous et al., 2008; Kent et al., 2010).

Surgical Intervention

There is no compelling indication to repair smaller asymptomatic aneurysms (Ballard, Filardo, Fowkes, & Powell, 2008; Santilli et al., 2002). Systematic reviews of large trials establish no difference in patient mortality between early surgery and ultrasound surveillance of asymptomatic aneurysms that are 4 to 5.5 cm in diameter (Filardo, Powell, Martinez, & Ballard, 2012; UK Small Aneurysm Trial Participants, 1998). The Aneurysm Detection and Management (ADAM) study was a prospective, randomized Veterans Affairs study of individuals aged 50 to 79 years with AAA between 4.0 and 5.4 cm who were assigned to early intervention ($n = 569$) versus ultrasound surveillance ($n = 567$). All-cause mortality was the primary outcome, and despite an overall low operative mortality (2.7%), early open aneurysm repair did not confer a survival benefit over a mean of 4.9 years (range 3.5–8.0 years) (Lederle et al., 2002).

Patients with symptomatic AAAs of any size and AAAs that are greater than 5.5 cm are candidates for evaluation of aneurysm repair. A retrospective analysis was conducted to evaluate short- and long-term mortality of 8,663 individuals with intact AAA and of 4,171 individuals with AAA rupture from 1987 to 2005 (Mani, Björck, Lundkvist, & Wanhainen, 2009). The analysis of almost 20 years of data demonstrated an improved 90-day and 5-year survival after repair of intact AAA and improved short-term, 90-day survival in ruptured AAA (Mani et al., 2009).

Surgical Evaluation

Evaluation for AAA repair includes an understanding of the relative risk of aneurysm rupture in association with the risk of the procedure, the eligibility for specific procedures, and patient factors, including overall health status and patient preferences. Individuals with coexisting diseases that reduce life expectancy to less than 2 years may not be candidates for AAA repair. Individuals with AAA require referral to a vascular surgical specialty team for evaluation of repair. The surgical team will evaluate the individual for the indication of repair and determine an appropriate approach and techniques, as warranted. Referrals should be provided to a high-volume center, as there is an association between low annual hospital number of AAA repairs and increased mortality (Holt, Poloniecki, Gerrard, Loftus, & Thompson, 2007).

Consider referrals and consultation to the vascular surgery team in:

- AAA greater than 4 cm
- Rapidly expanding AAA, an aneurysm with documented enlargement beyond 0.5 cm in less than 6 months
- Thromboembolism—clot from aneurysm with embolization to lower extremities
- Complicated aneurysm morphology

Urgent consultation to the vascular surgery team is necessary in:

■ Suspected or confirmed AAA rupture
■ Symptomatic AAA

For stable aneurysms, presurgical evaluation for major surgery is essential to determine the appropriateness of AAA repair. Operative complications and mortality associated with AAA repair are commonly attributable to CHD. Most individuals who will undergo nonemergency surgery or stent graft placement for an AAA will likely receive preoperative cardiac stress testing (see Chapter 4). Relative contraindications to AAA repair include advanced age, unstable angina, left ventricular ejection fraction below 30%, heart failure (HF), CHD, serum creatinine above 3 mg/dL, or significant pulmonary disease. If repair becomes necessary, individuals with these high-risk characteristics will require intensified preoperative and perioperative monitoring.

Preoperative risk scores assist in predicting mortality after open or endovascular repair. Giles et al. (2009) evaluated 45,660 individuals from a Medicare database by dividing the sample into a derivation and validation cohort to determine predictors of perioperative mortality after AAA repair (Giles et al., 2009). The open repair procedure was associated with increased mortality (Giles et al., 2009) in female-gender patients older than 71 years of age with co-morbidities of renal insufficiency with and without dialysis, HF, and vascular disease. A high-risk group of patients older than 80 years and with all the co-morbidities experienced a 38% mortality rate, versus a low-risk group aged 70 years and older with no co-morbidities and a mortality rate of 0.7%. Similarly, Egorova et al. (2009) evaluated a Medicare database to identify predictors of mortality with endovascular repair. Aged 70 years and older, female gender, and co-morbidities of renal insufficiency with and without dialysis, heart failure, lower-extremity ischemia, chronic liver disease, neurologic disorders, and chronic pulmonary disease were associated with increased mortality (Egorova et al., 2009). Institutional factors of hospital endovascular repair volume of less than seven procedures and surgeon experience less than three procedures correlated with higher mortality (Egorova et al., 2009). Endovascular repair was not recommended for high-risk patients, defined as predicted mortality greater than 10% based on the scoring system to identify preoperative risk (Egorova et al., 2009). Older predictive models of mortality, including the Glasgow Aneurysm Score, Hardman Index, and Leiden Score, originated for open repair only and are the most applicable with this technique; however, there are established risk predictors for both open and endovascular repair (Table 16.7).

Surgical Approaches

The two primary surgical approaches for the repair of AAA in appropriate surgical candidates are an open surgical repair (OSR) and endovascular aneurysm repair (EVAR) (Figure 16.1). The OSR is the traditional method for aneurysm repair, utilizing a transabdominal incision, which is generally a long midline or wide transverse incision or a retroperitoneal incision, with cross clamping of the aorta above the renal arteries and positioning a knitted synthetic graft in the diseased portion of the aortic aneurysm. Synthetic grafts are knitted gelatin-coated

TABLE 16.7 Preoperative Risk Predictors of Perioperative Mortality for AAA Repair

Age > 70
  Increased risk with increased age 70–74, 75–80, > 80
Female gender
Renal insufficiency
  Increased risk with dialysis
Heart failure
Vascular disease
  Peripheral vascular
  Cerebrovascular
Chronic liver disease
Neurologic disorders
Chronic pulmonary disease
Institutional volume
  Operator < 3 procedures
  Hospital annual < 7 procedures

AAA, abdominal aortic aneurysm.

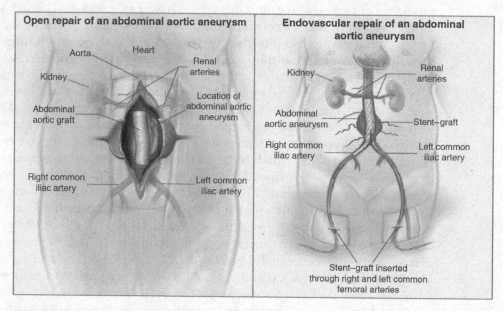

FIGURE 16.1 Open repair and endovascular repair of an infrarenal abdominal aortic aneurysm. See color insert.

Reprinted from Schermerhorn et al. (2008, p. 465), with permission from Massachusetts Medical Society.

Dacron bifurcation grafts, knitted collagen-coated Dacron grafts, and stretch polytetrafluoroethylene grafts. The EVAR was introduced in the early 1990s for AAA repair by utilizing a stent graft placed through the femoral or iliac arteries either via a cut-down or through percutaneous placement of an intra-aortic graft, an endovascular stent graft. The AAA morphology and size requires an evaluation to determine whether the aneurysm is amenable to endograft repair. The endograft comprises fabric and stents and is positioned both above and below the aneurysmal section.

There are advantages and limitations with both repair techniques, with the decision based on the overall health status, patient preferences, experience of the operator and setting, and aneurysm characteristics weighing both short- and long-term outcomes. The OSR is associated with an increase in 30-day complications, mortality, and longer hospitalization, whereas EVAR is associated with more late complications, including further AAA repair and increased risk of rupture (Becquemin et al., 2011; Stather et al., 2013). Overall, the long-term outcomes are similar with both approaches for elective repair of AAA.

The UK EVAR 1 trial was a large, randomized study that compared EVAR with OSR in 1,082 patients aged 60 years or older with aneurysms of at least 5.5 cm in diameter for elective AAA repair (Greenhalgh et al., 2004). The primary study outcome was all-cause mortality. The EVAR demonstrated a significantly lower 30-day postprocedure mortality and length of hospitalization with an increased risk for additional surgical intervention (Greenhalgh et al., 2004). In a subsequent EVAR Trial of 1,252 participants with a median follow-up of 6 years, endovascular repair of AAA was associated with a significantly lower operative mortality than OSR. However, no differences were seen in total mortality or aneurysm-related mortality in the long term. Endovascular repair was associated with increased rates of graft-related complications and reinterventions (Greenhalgh et al., 2010).

The Dutch Randomised Endovascular Aneurysm Management (DREAM) trial was a multicenter, randomized trial comparing OSR with EVAR in 345 patients with AAA equal to or greater than 5 cm and who were candidates for either technique (Prinssen et al., 2004). The primary outcomes were 30-day mortality, operative mortality, and moderate or severe complications. The EVAR demonstrated a reduction in perioperative mortality and an improvement in perioperative outcomes, including lower rates of systemic complications, reduced blood loss, shorter duration of surgery, reduced mechanical ventilation, and shorter length of hospital stays. However, the improved early survival of EVAR was not sustained after the first postoperative year (Blankensteijn et al., 2005). In the 6-year follow-up, both techniques demonstrated similar survival, with significantly higher secondary interventions for the EVAR group (De Bruin et al., 2010).

The Open Versus Endovascular Repair (OVER) trial randomized 881 veterans equal to or older than 49 years of age with AAA to OSR or EVAR to evaluate mortality, and to characterize hospitalization and secondary procedures. The EVAR group demonstrated reductions in 30-day mortality, procedure time, blood loss, transfusion requirements, mechanical ventilation, length of stay, and intensive care unit care. The EVAR group experienced higher exposure to contrast agents and fluoroscopy. There was no significant difference in secondary procedures, procedure failure, health-related quality of life, or erectile dysfunction (Lederle et al., 2009). Secondary procedures were broadly defined and included endovascular repairs, conversion to open repair, repairs to groin wounds and incisional hernias, amputations, and laparotomies for bowel obstruction or hematoma. Also encompassed as a secondary procedure were aortic graft and other arterial procedures, and procedures for wound complications or to relieve claudication, among others. Nine-year (mean 5.2 years) follow-up analysis indicated improved mortality with EVAR at 2 years that was reduced at 3 years and not sustained for more than 3 years (Lederle et al., 2012). There was a reduction in mortality in patients younger than 70 years of age who were initially randomized to the EVAR group.

A matched cohort study evaluated 45,660 Medicare beneficiaries with a mean age of 76 years who underwent EVAR ($n = 22,830$) with OSR ($n = 22,830$) in the United States from 2001 to 2004 (Schermerhorn et al., 2008). The EVAR was associated with lower perioperative morbidity and mortality, including a significant reduction in length of hospitalizations and complications of MI, pneumonia, acute renal failure, deep vein thrombosis, or pulmonary embolism. Survival after 3 years was similar for both groups. Reinterventions related to AAA were more common after EVAR, whereas laparotomy-related reinterventions and hospitalizations were associated with OSR.

For AAA equal to or greater than 5.5 cm, EVAR has not been shown to improve long-term survival or health status compared with OSR or as an alternative to OSR in patients who are medically unfit for open repair (Wilt et al., 2006). Currently, evidence suggests that EVAR does not improve all-cause mortality in individuals who may not be candidates for open surgical interventions; therefore, it is not considered an alternative in high-risk patients. In the EVAR 2 trial, 338 patients aged 60 years and older with AAA equal to or greater than 5.5 cm who were not appropriate candidates for OSR were randomized to EVAR or no intervention and followed for a mean of 3.3 years (Greenhalgh et al., 2005a, 2005b). There was no significant difference between EVAR and the control group in aneurysm-related mortality, all-cause mortality, or quality of life (Greenhalgh et al., 2005a, 2005b). A long-term analysis was reported in 2010, including all 338 original patients as well as 66 patients added after the 2005 midstudy report (Greenhalgh et al., 2010). The median follow-up was 3.1 years with an analysis of survival at 6 years, due to high attrition; the 8-year survival was not reported. Both EVAR and control groups experienced limited life expectancy beyond 8 years. Overall, EVAR demonstrated a reduction in aneurysm-related mortality, although similar all-cause mortality was consistent in both groups.

Research is continuing in the management of urgent AAA repair with EVAR. A systematic review and meta-analysis of 23 studies was conducted in individuals who required emergent AAA repair for ruptured or symptomatic AAA (Sadat et al., 2008). The analysis suggests EVAR is associated with reduced mortality and morbidity compared with OSR for emergent AAA repair, although due to limitations in the secondary data, caution is required with interpretation of these results (Sadat et al., 2008). In this analysis, there was a statistically significant reduction in 30-day mortality with EVAR and improved morbidity characteristics associated with hospitalization. The EVAR was associated with a significantly reduced length of intensive care unit duration, blood loss, procedure time, and length of overall hospitalization.

Post-EVAR Surveillance

After EVAR, the vascular surgery team or an endovascular specialist will supervise the initial follow-up period. Periodic surveillance with imaging, for the detection of endoleak, is important to confirm graft position, document stability of the aneurysm sac, and to evaluate the need for further intervention. An endoleak is often asymptomatic and occurs in up to 25% of patients post-EVAR (Stavropoulos & Charagundla, 2007). Endoleaks are classified into five types (Table 16.8), with Type II occurring most commonly, accounting for approximately 80% of cases (Stavropoulos & Charagundla, 2007).

TABLE 16.8 Types of Endoleaks After EVAR

Type	Description	Usual Treatment
I	Leak at graft site, inadequate seal	Extension of graft or open repair

II	Aneurysm sac filled by collateral blood flow
	    Lumbar arteries
	    Inferior mesenteric artery
	    Internal iliac artery
		Watchful waiting or embolization

III	Mechanical defect in graft	Additional graft
IV	Leak through graft fabric, graft porosity	Resolves in few days
V	Endotension, expansion of aneurysm sac without clear leak	Continued-growth extension graft or open repair

EVAR, endovascular aneurysm repair.

Post-EVAR surveillance is standardly conducted by CTA with alternative imaging, including MRA, digital subtraction angiography, and ultrasound (Stavropoulos & Charagundla, 2007). Due to the constraints of cost, time, contrast agents, and radiation, ultrasound has been studied as an alternative to CTA imaging. Wolf et al. (2000) compared 166 scan pairs in 76 patients who underwent duplex ultrasound scanning and CTA after EVAR. Ultrasound and CTA had a high correlation in the measurement of maximal transverse aneurysm sac diameter and the diagnosis of an endoleak (Wolf et al., 2000). Eight patients experienced endoleaks that required further evaluation, which was discovered by both methodologies. Employing contrast-enhanced CT as a reference standard, a systematic review of 31 studies evaluated duplex ultrasonography or contrast-enhanced ultrasonography after EVAR for the detection of types I and III endoleaks (Karthikesalingam et al., 2012). Both ultrasound techniques were specific for the detection of types I and III endoleaks, with duplex ultrasonography maintaining sufficient accuracy for surveillance after EVAR, without the associated implications of the contrast agent (Karthikesalingam et al., 2012).

SPECIAL POPULATIONS

Women

The incidence and natural history of AAA differs by gender, with the prevalence of AAA six times lower in women than in men (Guirguis-Blake et al., 2014). Opportunistic screening has resulted in an improvement in the incidence of aneurysm rupture and aneurysm-related death in men; however, this has not been reported in women (Cosford et al., 2007). Currently, there are no screening recommendations for AAA in women from Medicare, the American College of Cardiology, the AHA, or the U.S. Preventive Services Task Force (USPSTF). Currently, the USPSTF recommends against routine screening in women. The Society for Vascular Surgery recommends a one-time screening in women at 65 years who have ever smoked or have a family history of AAA.

Women with AAA experience aneurysm rupture four times more commonly than men at the same aneurysm size. In an analysis of systematic reviews and observational studies, the mean rate of rupture, per 1,000 person-years of AAAs with the same baseline diameter, occurred more frequently in women than in men

(Table 16.6). The higher occurrence of aneurysm rupture has led to the suggestion that evaluation for surgical intervention should be considered at a smaller aneurysm size in women (Bown et al., 2013). However, women experience an increased mortality associated with aneurysm repair, which complicates this decision. Giles et al. (2009) evaluated 45,660 individuals from a Medicare database to determine predictors of perioperative mortality after AAA repair, and approximately 20% of the cohort were women (Giles et al., 2009). Female gender was significantly associated with perioperative mortality with both OSR and EVAR. In addition, after AAA repair, 5-year survival is less in women compared with men for both open and endovascular repair. Comparisons on survival were evaluated for elective AAA, elective AAA excluding 90-day mortality, ruptured AAA, and ruptured AAA excluding 90-day mortality. Mortality related to AAA generally occurs in women aged 80 years and older. Therefore, specific recommendations for aneurysm screening, evaluation, and repair are difficult to determine based on female gender alone.

Elderly

Consideration for the elderly patient includes the upper age limit for screening, which is generally accepted at 75 years. Older individuals with small AAAs (3.0–5.4 cm) have an increased risk of AAA rupture (Guirguis-Blake et al., 2014). Advanced age is also linearly associated with increased risk of postrepair mortality, with individuals older than 80 years at the highest risk.

PATIENT EDUCATION

Patient education should focus on overall cardiovascular risk reduction, the management of high BP and dyslipidemia, and smoking cessation. Cigarette smoking significantly adds to the risk of aneurysm development, growth, and rupture. All patients should be advised to discontinue smoking and smoking cessation recommendations and interventions should be provided, including behavior modification, nicotine replacement, and pharmacotherapeutics. There is an association of fewer AAAs in individuals with a healthy lifestyle, which includes exercise and diets with vegetables, fruits, and nuts (Kent et al., 2010).

Evaluation and screening for AAA is essential to prevent aneurysm rupture and complications. Clinicians must routinely screen eligible and appropriate individuals to determine the presence and severity of abdominal aneurysms. If an AAA is detected, surveillance monitoring or referral for repair to a vascular specialty team is indicated. Aneurysm repair with an open or endovascular approach is an option for select individuals. The AAA is an important marker of cardiovascular disease and overall patient status.

For full reference citations to this chapter, please see "Section References" in the back of the book, under the heading "Section IV."

Acute Cardiovascular Conditions

Hypertensive Emergencies

HELEN F. BROWN AND LINDA BRIGGS

Approximately, 1% to 2% of individuals diagnosed with hypertension will experience an episode of hypertensive crisis in their lifetime. The incidence of hypertensive crisis is higher in the elderly and females, with more African Americans hospitalized than other demographic groups (Deshmukh et al., 2011). Inadequate blood pressure (BP) control, poor compliance with prescribed drug regimes, limited access to or no primary care provider, and significant changes in clinical status (Table 17.1) are frequently encountered risk factors among patients presenting to the emergency department experiencing a hypertensive crisis (Johnson, Nguyen, & Patel, 2012).

It is essential that practitioners recognize the difference between hypertensive crisis and hypertensive urgency, because they are managed differently. Hypertensive urgency is defined as a BP greater than 180/120 mmHg without symptoms or with mild symptoms of headache or shortness of breath (Chobanian et al., 2003). The asymptomatic patient with hypertensive urgency is managed as an outpatient with a gradual reduction of the BP with combination oral therapy (Wolf, Lo, Shih, Smith, & Fesmire, 2013).

Hypertensive crisis is an acute elevation in BP, a systolic pressure greater than 180 mmHg or a diastolic pressure greater than 120 mmHg, with evidence of end-organ damage (Aggarwal & Khan, 2006; Chobanian et al., 2003). Organs at greatest risk of injury from this sudden sustained elevation in BP are the heart, aorta, brain, kidneys, and eyes (Chobanian et al., 2003). Clinical manifestations indicative of a patient in hypertensive crisis with end-organ involvement include hypertensive encephalopathy, intracranial hemorrhage, stroke, acute coronary syndrome, acute heart failure, pulmonary edema with respiratory failure, aortic dissection, acute kidney injury, eclampsia, and hypertensive retinopathy. Emergent intervention to reduce the diastolic BP by 10% to 15% is recommended to prevent or limit target organ damage (Marik & Varon, 2007).

PATHOPHYSIOLOGY

Hypertensive crisis is caused by an abrupt rise in BP. This escalation in BP is caused by the sudden release of vasoactive substances, renin, angiotensin, vasopressin, or catecholamines, which produces a sustained increase in systemic vascular resistance. In an effort to compensate, the endothelium secretes the vasodilator, nitric oxide, and arterial smooth muscles contract to protect downstream tissues from the damaging forces of the elevated pressure. The purpose of these compensatory mechanisms is to limit end-organ injury. However, with sustained arteriolar constriction, endothelial dysfunction occurs, leading to a reduction in nitric oxide

TABLE 17.1 Precipitating Factors for Hypertensive Emergencies

Precipitating Factors	Clinical Signs and Symptoms
Catecholaminergic	
Sudden cessation of antihypertensive	Clinical diagnosis: Preexisting hypertension, lack of medication compliance, beta blocker withdrawal, clonidine withdrawal
Sympathomimetic drug use	Clinical diagnosis: Suspected drug abuse/misuse: cocaine, amphetamines, PCP, pseudoephedrine, caffeine, or appetite suppressants, +/– altered mental status Physical findings: Tachycardia, diaphoresis, pupillary dilation, nystagmus (PCP use only)
Pheochromocytoma	Clinical diagnosis: Severe headache, tachycardia, diaphoresis, anxiety, flushed skin, symptoms present with marked hypertension marked by asymptomatic period with normal BP Lab: 24-hour urine for catecholamine and metanephrines
Food or drug interaction with MAOI	Clinical diagnosis: Current use of an MAOI, such as isocarboxazid (Marplan), phenelzine (Nardil), selegiline (Emsam), tranylcypromine (Parnate), and ingestion of a trigger food or drug
Autonomic dysreflexia after SCI	Clinical diagnosis: SCI above T6, headache, blurred vision, nasal congestion, anxiety, and nausea Precipitating event: Bladder distention, bowel impaction, pressure sores, bone fracture, or occult visceral disturbances causing noxious stimuli Physical findings: Diaphoresis, marked hypertension, bradycardia, flushing, piloerection
Pregnancy	
Eclampsia/ Preeclampsia	Clinical diagnosis: > 20 weeks gestation, postpartum typically occurs in first 48 hours Eclampsia occurs with onset of seizure activity Headache, visual disturbance, upper abdominal pain, nausea, vomiting, chest pain, dyspnea, or altered mental status Lab: Proteinuria
Surgical	
Postoperative hypertension	Clinical diagnosis: Occurs within 2 hours following surgery and lasts for up to 6 hours Assess for cause prior to administering antihypertensive agents. Precipitating event: Pain, hypoxia, volume overload, shivering, hypothermia, anxiety, urinary retention, medication withdrawal due to NPO status

BP, blood pressure; MAOI, monamine oxidase inhibitor; NPO, nothing by mouth; PCP, phencyclidine; SCI, spinal cord injury.

Sources: Guttentag (2005); Johnson et al. (2012).

production. As a result, more vasoconstriction occurs, increasing pressure in the small arterioles. As the compensatory mechanisms fail, the arterioles may rupture or leak and are unable to maintain constriction, furthering endothelial damage. Endothelial injury initiates platelet activation via exposed tissue collagen and von Willebrand factor. Activated platelets promote intravascular thrombosis and inflammatory cytokines contribute to further tissue damage. End-organ ischemia increases the release of vasoactive mediators, and this cascade of events repeats, further elevating the BP (Johnson et al., 2012; Marik & Varon, 2007).

CLINICAL PRESENTATION

The clinical manifestations of a hypertensive crisis will reflect the target organ involved. Neurologic and cardiovascular symptomology are most prevalent. In patients demonstrating neurologic complications, 24% are due to cerebral infarction,

4% results from intracerebral or subarachnoid hemorrhage, and 16% reflects hypertensive encephalopathy. Cardiovascular complication rates include acute heart failure in 36% of patients, myocardial infarction or unstable angina in 12%, and aortic dissection in 2% (Zampaglione, Pascale, Marchisio, & Cavalle-Perin, 1996). Preeclampsia rates rose from 3.4% in 1980 to 3.8% in 2010. This increase was due to a rise in rates of severe preeclampsia—from 0.3% in 1980 to 1.4% in 2010, a relative increase of 322% (Ananth, Keyes, & Wapner, 2013).

TABLE 17.2 Medications That Induce Hypertension

Appetite suppressants
Cold medications containing pseudoephedrine
Monoamine oxidase inhibitors
Neosynephrine (nasal decongestants)
Nonsteroidal anti-inflammatory drugs
Oral contraceptives
Steroids
Tricyclic antidepressants

HEALTH HISTORY

In eliciting the history, the practitioner should evaluate the presenting symptoms, time of onset, progression, and any self-treatment. The past medical history including prescribed medications, medication compliance, and use of over-the-counter medications and herbal products is essential information (Table 17.2). Failure to take antihypertensive medications regularly can result in uncontrolled or rebound hypertension. Over-the-counter medication, such as decongestants, can exacerbate high BP and interactions between prescription medications can be problematic. Asking direct questions regarding substance abuse may reveal a potential cause for the hypertensive crisis, as substance abuse has been identified as a significant cause for hypertensive crisis in the emergency department population (Johnson et al., 2012; Marik & Varon, 2007).

PHYSICAL EXAMINATION

The focus of the physical assessment should be on the nervous, cardiovascular, ophthalmologic, and renal systems (Table 17.3). Determining the patient's level of consciousness and executive function provides initial clues to the effects of the current level of hypertension on the nervous system. A fundoscopic examination of the eyes is important in determining the presence of papilledema—a sign of possible increased intracranial pressure. Cotton-wool spots—white, wispy lesions—indicate recent severe hypertension. Other retinal changes, such as arteriovenous nicking and copper wiring, indicate longstanding hypertension (Oh, 2014). A new diastolic murmur may indicate aortic valve incompetence due to aortic dissection. Crackles in the lung fields indicate potential heart failure. Poor urine output signals possible renal failure.

TABLE 17.3 Hypertensive Emergencies—Complications and Diagnostic Findings

Target Organ Damage	Diagnostic Finding
Cerebrovascular	
Hypertensive encephalopathy	Clinical diagnosis: Altered mental status, headache, vomiting, seizures, and visual disturbance Associated physical findings that may occur: Papilledema, retinal hemorrhages, cardiomegaly, hematuria TRIAD: Severe hypertension, altered mental status, and papilledema MRI: Cerebral edema
Stroke	Clinical diagnosis: Focal neurologic deficit after other causes eliminated CT brain may demonstrate hypodense area but 60% are normal in first 6 hours post-onset of symptoms
Intracranial hemorrhage	Clinical diagnosis: Headache, altered mental status, focal neurologic deficit CT brain abnormal with evidence of intraparenchymal bleeding
Subarachnoid hemorrhage	Clinical diagnosis: Sudden onset maximal headache, nuchal rigidity, neurologic deficit CT brain abnormal blood in subarachnoid space and cisterns Lumbar puncture: RBC, xanthochromic
Cardiovascular	
Acute coronary syndrome	Clinical diagnosis: Chest pain, dyspnea, nausea, lightheadedness ECG: Evidence of STEMI or acute ST-T wave changes of ischemia
Acute aortic dissection	Clinical diagnosis: Sudden onset of severe chest pain radiating to the midthoracic region, may be described as ripping or tearing pain Associated physical findings: Pulse deficit, new diastolic murmur, neurologic deficits Chest x-ray: Abnormal aortic contour, mediastinal widening, pleural effusion CT scan contrasted: Identifies dissection as to location and Type A or B Transesophageal echocardiogram: Identifies location of dissection
Acute left ventricular failure	Clinical diagnosis: Dyspnea, orthopnea, activity intolerance Physical findings: Tachycardia, abnormal heart sounds, tachypnea, adventitious breath sounds, jugular venous distention Chest x-ray: Cardiomegaly, pulmonary vascular congestion, interstitial edema
Renovascular	
Acute kidney injury	Clinical diagnosis: Peripheral edema, loss of appetite, nausea, vomiting, confusion, hematuria, oliguria; often minimal to no symptoms Lab data: Elevated BUN/creatinine ratio, proteinuria, hypokalemic metabolic alkalosis, hemolytic anemia, hematuria, elevated urine fractionated sodium (FeNa)
Opthalmologic	
Hypertensive retinopathy	Clinical diagnosis: Headache, visual disturbance Physical finding: Retinal splinter hemorrhages, cotton-wool spots

BUN, blood urea nitrogen; ECG, electrocardiogram; RBC, red blood cell; STEMI, ST-elevation myocardial infarction.
Sources: Guttentag (2005); Johnson et al. (2012).

DIAGNOSTIC TESTING

The ordering of diagnostic studies is determined by the clinical signs and symptoms experienced by the patient. It is reasonable to obtain an ECG to assess for ventricular hypertrophy; a chest radiograph to evaluate for cardiomegaly, aortic pathology, or heart failure; a CT of the brain to assess for intracranial hemorrhage if neurologic symptoms are present; and laboratory studies, such as creatinine, electrolytes, and urinalysis if renal impairment is suspected. Cardiac biomarkers should be obtained if there are symptoms of acute coronary syndrome or heart failure (Johnson et al., 2012).

Prior to initiating therapy in the severely hypertensive patient, laboratory testing—including an ECG, chest radiograph, serum creatinine, and urinalysis—is recommended (Chobanian et al., 2003; Wolf et al., 2013). These recommendations were developed to guide safe practice for primary care providers and were not intended for use in the emergency department. If extensive testing or immediate results are desired, the patient should be evaluated in the emergency department.

MANAGEMENT

Routine initiation of antihypertensive medication for patients presenting to an emergency department with asymptomatic hypertensive urgency is not recommended (Wolf et al., 2013). These patients typically have no end-organ damage and do not require hospitalization. Normalization of this population's BP urgently can result in postdischarge pathology, such as hypotension-mediated syncope and neurologic injury due to cerebral hypoperfusion. Best practice advocates a gradual reduction of the BP using combination oral therapy under the surveillance of the primary care provider (Wolf et al., 2013). In addition, treatment of hypertensive urgency in the emergency department population is controversial because it is unclear that treatment is cost-effective or improves long-term outcomes (Johnson, Nguyen, & Patel, 2012).

There are several situations in the hypertensive urgency population that do warrant urgent evaluation and intervention. In select populations, such as individuals with limited access to care, lack of financial resources for testing, or concerns for outpatient follow-up, a serum creatinine may identify previously undiagnosed renal disease. Recognition of kidney injury may alter the practitioner's decision regarding disposition of the patient (Wolf et al., 2013). A decision to initiate or alter antihypertensive therapy may be appropriate in an asymptomatic severely hypertensive patient previously diagnosed with hypertension, individuals that have stopped their medications, or those who are poorly controlled on their current therapy (Slovis & Reddi, 2008). In these situations the BP should be gradually reduced over a 24- to 48-hour period, with oral medications (Marik & Varon, 2007; Slovis & Reddi, 2008). The BP should not be normalized during the initial emergency department evaluation (Wolf et al., 2013). Rather, the goal is a small reduction that will continue into the outpatient setting. The practitioner initiating or altering the pharmacologic regimen in the emergency department or outpatient setting should ensure that there is a follow-up assessment within 48 hours.

The development of signs and symptoms of organ dysfunction distinguishes hypertensive crisis from hypertension urgency. For patients with hypertensive crisis, the goal of therapy is to safely lower BP in an expedient, but not precipitous, manner to reduce morbidity and mortality. The objective of pharmacologic management is to reduce the mean arterial pressure (MAP) by no more than 25% within 1 to 2 hours, with a 10% to 15% reduction in 30 to 60 minutes (Chobanian et al.,

2003). In patients with ischemic stroke, treatment should be avoided unless the systolic BP is greater than 220 mmHg or the diastolic BP is greater than 120 mmHg; however, if a patient is a candidate for thrombolytic agents, the BP should be treated to achieve a systolic less than 185 mmHg or a diastolic less than 110 mmHg (Jauch et al., 2013). The challenge confronting the practitioner is to correctly identify the patient with true hypertensive crisis that requires emergent intervention, and carefully avoid "normalizing" the BP. In the patient experiencing a hypertensive crisis, the loss of vascular autoregulation can lead to exaggerated swings in pressure. The risk of reducing the MAP too quickly or returning it to "normal limits" is the development of end-organ ischemia due to hypoperfusion. Normalization of the BP in this patient population can result in myocardial, cerebral, or renal ischemia (Marik & Varon, 2007). One exception to the avoidance of normalization recommendation is the patient who has an aortic dissection. In this situation, the goal is to reduce the BP to "normal" to limit the shearing force against the intimal lesion and lower the heart rate. This should help to slow or prevent further dissection.

Safe practice in caring for all patients with hypertensive crisis warrants careful monitoring in the intensive care setting, use of appropriate monitoring, and the discussion of BP goals with the nursing staff to avoid even brief periods of hypotension or rapid reductions of the BP. A rapid reduction in BP can cause a drop in cerebral perfusion pressure, leading to cerebrovascular ischemia (Johnson et al., 2012).

Pharmacologic interventions depend on the patient's presentation and associated symptoms (Table 17.4). When selecting a medication to treat a patient in hypertensive crisis, consider the patient's history, presentation, and organ involvement to determine a medication that will have the greatest impact on the pathophysiology causing the emergent situation (Jois, 2012). For example, patients suffering from cocaine-induced hypertension should not receive beta blockers; instead, they should receive benzodiazapines as initial therapy, followed by nitroglycerin and nitroprusside (McCord et al., 2008). Regardless of the treatment, once reasonable BP control has been achieved, the patient should be transitioned to oral medication.

Nonpharmacologic interventions focus on patient education, as outlined in the discussion of lifestyle changes in Chapter 5 on hypertension, encouraging compliance with medication regimes, and ensuring follow-up. It is important to

TABLE 17.4 Pharmacologic Therapy in Hypertensive Crisis

Clinical Presentation	Preferred Agent
Hypertensive encephalopathy	Nicardipine, esmolol, labetalol, or fenoldopam
Acute ischemic stroke	Labetalol or nicardipine
Intracerebral or subarachnoid hemorrhage	Labetalol, nicardipine, esmolol, or oral nimodipine
Acute coronary syndrome	Nitroglycerin, beta blockers (metoprolol, esmolol), labetalol
Acute heart failure	Nitroglycerin, enalapril, or fenoldopam, and loop diuretic
Aortic dissection	Esmolol, labetalol, nitroprusside, nicardipine
Eclampsia	Magnesium sulfate, labetalol, hydralazine
Sympathetic crisis	Benzodiazepine, nitroglycerin, nicardipine, phentolamine

Source: Jois (2012); Yeo and Burrell (2010).

communicate with other clinicians as patients transition from one care setting to another, so that the plan of care is clearly communicated and the patient has a follow-up examination in an expedient manner.

For full reference citations to this chapter, please see "Section References" in the back of the book, under the heading "Section V."

Acute Coronary Syndrome

LINDA BRIGGS

The term *acute coronary syndrome* (ACS) refers to a group of cardiac conditions that involve acute myocardial ischemia. The conditions under this umbrella include ST-elevation myocardial infarction (STEMI), non-ST-elevation myocardial infarction (NSTEMI), and unstable angina (UA). In addition, due to the similarities in the initial presentations of NSTEMI and UA, these conditions are considered together as non-ST elevation ACS (NSTE-ACS; Amsterdam et al., 2014). Some experts also classify sudden cardiac death (SCD) as an ACS (Virmani, Burke, Farb, & Kolodgie, 2006). Research confirms that, in most cases, acute ischemia is caused by the rupture of an atherosclerotic lesion and subsequent thrombosis in a coronary artery (Fuster, Moreno, Fayad, Corti, & Badimon, 2005; Libby, 2013). The duration and degree of coronary occlusion, in addition to its location, determine the extent of myocardial injury (Arbab-Zadeh, Nakano, Virmani, & Fuster, 2012).

PATHOPHYSIOLOGY

Research conducted over the past 20 or so years has led to the discovery that inflammation and thrombosis play significant roles in acute coronary events. These processes are also involved, at a lower level of intensity, in the development and progression of atheromatous plaque (Finn, Nakano, Narula, Kolodgie, & Virmani, 2010; Mann & Davies, 1999). Interestingly, most myocardial infarctions (MIs) are not caused by the gradual complete or nearly complete occlusion of a coronary vessel, but rather, they are due to the rupture of smaller, nonflow-limiting atheromas and subsequent thrombosis (Arbab-Zadeh et al., 2012; Falk, Nakano, Betzon, Finn, & Virmani, 2013; Libby, 2013). This fact is corroborated by the observation that only 18% of ACS events occurred among patients with a long-standing history of angina (Roger et al., 2012). Another cause of ACS, plaque erosion, is frequently responsible for acute myocardial infarction (AMI) among women younger than the age of 50, while plaque rupture is more common among older women and men of all ages (Falk et al., 2013; Virmani et al., 2006). Calcified nodules that protrude into the artery lumen are an infrequent cause of MI or UA. These lesions usually occur in older adults with heavily calcified arteries (Falk et al., 2013). On occasion, ACS can be due to non-atherosclerotic processes, such as cocaine abuse, coronary dissection, and coronary arteritis (Hamm et al., 2011).

Plaque rupture, the most common cause of ACS, usually occurs in atheromatous lesions with thin fibrous caps (Arbab-Zadeh et al., 2012; Falk et al., 2013; Libby, 2013; Virmani et al., 2006). Some researchers have indicated that plaques with cap thicknesses less than 65 μm are at risk for rupture (Burke et al., 1997; Narula et al., 2013). Another important feature of thin-cap fibroatheromas (TCFA) is that they affect the major coronary vessels more frequently than smaller branches, and affect proximal segments more often than the midsections or distal portions. This has significant clinical implications, as plaque rupture in strategic regions can jeopardize large areas of the myocardium, and more importantly, left ventricular function. It is important to note that the most commonly involved coronary vessel is the left anterior descending (LAD) artery, and the right coronary artery (RCA) is the least likely to be affected by TCFAs (Finn et al., 2010).

Thinning of an atheroma's fibrous cap occurs due to an imbalance between processes that build and strengthen the fibrotic cap and those that break it down. Inflammatory processes are key actors in this interplay. Arterial smooth muscle cells produce the collagen responsible for the supporting structure of the fibrous cap. Activated T cells produce interferon-γ, which can interfere with collagen synthesis. Other inflammatory cells, macrophages, produce matrix-metalloproteinases (MMPs) that can break down collagen (Libby, 2013). Macrophages have been found in high concentrations in lesions that have caused fatal ACS events (Shah et al., 1995). The involvement of inflammatory processes in the development and destruction of plaques provides a possible target for therapies such as aspirin and statins.

The rupture of a TCFA is postulated to occur due to the combined effects of a friable cap, vasospasm, and punctate calcifications (Libby, 2013). Plaque rupture allows interaction between the blood and substances within the lipid-rich core of the atheroma. This lipid core contains tissue factor, a procoagulant produced by the macrophages within the core. Contact between tissue factor and inactive coagulation factors in the blood triggers thrombin formation and platelet activation, leading to clot development (Libby, 2013). Thrombosis at the site of plaque rupture then occludes, or partially occludes, the lumen of the coronary artery, leading to downstream ischemia and potential necrosis. The prevention and destruction of thrombi through the administration of antithrombotic, antiplatelet aggregation, and thrombolytic medications have become important interventions in the prevention and treatment of ACS.

UNIVERSAL CLASSIFICATION OF MI

While plaque-associated events account for the majority of ACS cases, there are other mechanisms that can cause MI. Recently, the development of newer, more sensitive serum biomarkers and imaging techniques have challenged traditional definitions of infarction. Based on the current knowledge of myocardial physiology and diagnostic testing, a *universal classification of MI* was developed by an international task force. The new classification system consists of five types of MIs, each with a specific cause or causes. The task force also designated specific criteria for the diagnosis of MIs based on the etiology and clinical circumstances (Thygesen et al., 2012).

Type 1: Spontaneous MIs are those caused primarily by plaque-related events and thrombus formation in a coronary artery or arteries. In most cases, there is angiographic evidence of coronary heart disease (CHD). However, in some instances, especially in women, there may be no evidence of CHD seen at the time of catheterization (Thygesen et al., 2012).

Type 2: Infarctions due to an ischemic imbalance are caused by a mismatch between oxygen supply and demand created by a variety of conditions other than CHD (Thygesen et al., 2012). Tachycardia or bradyarrhythmias may lead to myocardial ischemia and necrosis. The majority of coronary perfusion of the left ventricle (LV) occurs during diastole; tachycardia increases myocardial oxygen demand, decreasing the duration of diastole and reducing coronary blood flow when it is most needed. Normally, the physiologic response of coronary dilation will adequately compensate for the potential mismatch. However, at extremely high heart rates (HRs), compensatory mechanisms can be overwhelmed (Butterworth, Mackey, & Wasnick, 2013). In both tachy- and bradyarrhythmias, cardiac output can be decreased, which in turn affects blood pressure (BP) and coronary circulation.

Coronary artery blood flow is most dependent on aortic diastolic BP and is autoregulated over a range from 60 to 140 mmHg (Hoit & Walsh, 2011). When hypotension results in lower pressures, myocardial ischemia can occur. In contrast, during episodes of severe hypertension, due to the microcirculation characteristics of the different layers of the ventricular walls, the subendocardial tissue is more susceptible to ischemia (Hoit & Walsh, 2011).

Anemia and respiratory failure can also cause MI (Thygesen et al., 2012). Both of these conditions can decrease the oxygen content of the blood, creating increased cardiac workload leading to increased oxygen demands and imbalances between supply and requirements.

Restrictions of coronary blood flow caused by processes other than CHD are also responsible for MIs classified as Type 2 (Figure 18.1). These processes include mechanisms such as coronary endothelial dysfunction, coronary artery spasm, and coronary artery embolism (Thygesen et al., 2012). Coronary artery spasm may occur spontaneously, as in Prinzmetal angina (Amsterdam et al., 2014; de Lemos, O'Rourke, & Harrington, 2011) or as a result of drugs such as cocaine and methamphetamine (Hollander & Diercks, 2011).

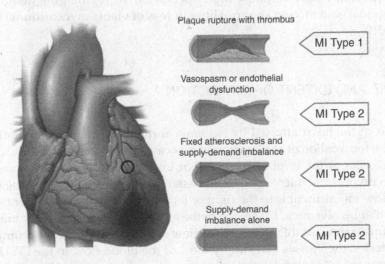

Plaque rupture with thrombus

MI Type 1

Vasospasm or endothelial dysfunction

MI Type 2

Fixed atherosclerosis and supply-demand imbalance

MI Type 2

Supply-demand imbalance alone

MI Type 2

FIGURE 18.1 Differentiation between myocardial infarction (MI) Type 1 and Type 2 according to condition of the coronary artery. See color insert.

Source: Thygesen et al. (2012).

Other clinical situations or conditions can lead to Type 2 infarctions, such as administration of catecholamines, including epinephrine or norepinephrine, stress responses related to major noncardiac surgery, and critical illness. In these situations, serum cardiac biomarkers may be elevated due to the direct toxic effects of high circulating catecholamine levels (Thygesen et al., 2012).

Type 3: MIs that result in cardiac death in patients with symptoms of ACS and ischemic electrocardiogram (ECG) changes or new left bundle branch block (LBBB) but for whom serum biomarkers are not available (Thygesen et al., 2012).

Type 4: MIs that occur in relation to a percutaneous coronary intervention (PCI). There are two subcategories, the first (4a) requires demonstration of several criteria, while the second (4b) stipulates evidence of stent thrombosis with a change in serum biomarkers so that at least one measurement is above the 99th percentile of the upper reference limit (URL) of normal. A Type 4a diagnosis requires cardiac troponin (cTn) changes *and* at least one of four additional characteristics. For Type 4a to be determined, cTn changes must either exceed five times the 99th percentile URL, in patients with baseline normal values, or rise more than 20% if the patient's baseline cTn levels were elevated but stable or falling. The additional criteria required for a Type 4a classification includes at least one of the following: (a) ischemic type symptoms, (b) ECG changes indicating ischemia or LBBB that are new, (c) angiographic evidence of decreased or no flow in a major coronary artery or side branch, or (d) imaging with findings of new regional wall motion abnormalities or loss of viable myocardium (Thygesen et al., 2012).

Type 5: MIs that occur in the setting of coronary artery bypass grafting (CABG). This classification also requires both cTn changes and other evidence of infarction. The cTn criterion for diagnosing an MI in the setting of CABG is 10 times the 99th percentile URL if the patient has a normal baseline cTn value. The additional requirement for Type 5 diagnosis is at least one of the following: (a) ECG changes of pathological Q waves or LBBB that are new, (b) angiographic evidence of new graft or native coronary artery occlusion, or (c) imaging demonstrating new regional wall motion abnormalities or loss of viable myocardium (Thygesen et al., 2012).

LOCATION, TYPE, AND EXTENT OF INFARCTION

The area of the heart affected by ischemia and necrosis is predominantly determined by the location of any changes in myocardial blood supply. Most often these changes occur at the level of epicardial or intramyocardial coronary vessels, but can also involve the microcirculation. Generally, the more proximal the source of blood flow impairment is to the right or left coronary ostia, the larger the area of myocardial involvement. Occlusion of the left main coronary artery can be particularly devastating, as this affects blood flow to both the LAD and circumflex coronary arteries, the vessels that supply most of the blood flow to the LV. Decreased or interrupted LAD circulation leads to injury and infarction of the anterior wall of the LV and interventricular septum. Stenosis or thrombosis of the circumflex affects the left ventricular lateral wall. Impaired blood flow to the RCA affects the oxygen supply to the right ventricle, the A-V node, and in 80% to 90% of people, the posterior wall of the LV. The extent of infarction is sometimes ameliorated by

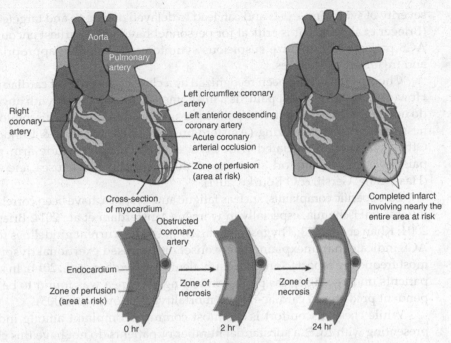

FIGURE 18.2 Progression of myocardial necrosis after coronary artery occlusion.
See color insert.

Reprinted from Schoen and Mitchell (2015, pp. 540–550), with permission from Elsevier.

the presence of collateral vessels that communicate between areas of adequate and inadequate blood flow and dilate in response to occlusion of one of the larger arteries (Hall, 2011b).

As mentioned previously, the subendocardial portion of the myocardium is more susceptible to ischemic insults because it is significantly compressed during systole. As a result, injury often occurs in this layer first and extends toward the epicardium (Figure 18.2), depending on the location and extent of the coronary artery occlusion (Hall, 2011b). If the resulting infarction extends through the full thickness of the ventricular wall, it is referred to as a transmural infarction. Areas of necrosis that do not involve the full thickness are called nontransmural or subendocardial infarctions (Antman, 2012). While the distinction between transmural and subendocardial infarction has important implications for overall heart function and potential complications following the event, contemporary diagnosis and therapy focus on the ECG presentation of the ACS patient—STEMI versus NSTEMI.

CLINICAL RECOGNITION AND PRESENTATION

The prompt recognition and treatment of ACS has significant impact on patient morbidity and mortality. Patient history, clinical presentation, physical examination, an ECG, and serum biomarkers are the keys to timely diagnosis. While there are some common signs and symptoms, significant variation in the type and severity of symptoms exists and can lead to delayed diagnosis and targeted therapy (Brieger et al., 2004). It is critical for personnel having the earliest encounter with ACS patients to recognize suspicious symptoms and initiate appropriate triage and treatment procedures.

Chest pain has long been recognized as a classic symptom of cardiac ischemia. However, the term "chest pain" is a misnomer, as most patients with angina or MI do not describe the sensation as pain. Instead, they describe it as discomfort, heaviness, tightness, or squeezing (Amsterdam et al., 2014; Sabatine & Cannon, 2012). Other symptoms associated with myocardial ischemia include arm pain, jaw pain, epigastric discomfort, shortness of breath, diaphoresis, nausea, and weakness (Hass, Yang, Gersh, & O'Rourke, 2011).

Less specific complaints, such as fatigue and dyspnea, have been correlated with myocardial ischemia, especially in women (Amsterdam et al., 2014; Brieger et al., 2004; Khan et al., 2013; Thygesen et al., 2012). In fact, current guidelines for NSTE-ACS indicate that unexplained new onset or increased exertional dyspnea is the most frequently reported anginal equivalent (Amsterdam et al., 2014). In a study of patients undergoing stress perfusion testing, dyspnea was found to be an independent predictor of cardiac-related mortality (Abidov et al., 2005).

While chest discomfort is the most common complaint among individuals presenting with ACS, a substantial number of patients do not have this characteristic. In 2007, Canto et al. conducted a systematic review of 69 studies of ACS presentations. They found that 37.5% of women and 27.4% of men presented without chest complaints. In a more recently published observational study of the National Registry of Myocardial Infarction (1994–2006), Canto et al. (2012) noted that more younger women than men with MI reported having no chest complaints, and even more remarkably, almost 50% of elderly MI patients (≥ 75 years) of both sexes denied chest discomfort. Analysis of the Global Registry of Acute Coronary Events (GRACE), a large international database of ACS patients, revealed that patients without chest pain experienced dyspnea, diaphoresis, nausea and vomiting, and presyncope or syncope as their most common symptoms (Brieger et al., 2004). An international study by Khan et al. (2013) reported that the most common non-chest pain complaints were weakness, dyspnea, cold sweats, flushing, and left arm or shoulder discomfort. Elderly patients may present with unexplained fatigue, diaphoresis, and/or nausea and vomiting (Anderson et al., 2013).

The duration of symptoms, particularly of chest pain, has been advocated as a determinant of the likelihood of acute MI (AMI). Classic teaching suggests that chest pain lasting more than 20 to 30 minutes is indicative of AMI (Sabatine & Cannon, 2012). However, a recent study using cardiac troponin-I (cTnI) as a marker of necrosis indicated that 15.8% of the patients with a documented AMI had chest pain for less than 20 minutes. This same study noted that no patients with chest pain less than 5 minutes were found to have AMI (Assaad et al., 2013).

The association of symptoms with activity, cold, or emotional stress is another factor in determining their clinical significance. Chest discomfort or other suspected ischemic symptoms that are associated with activity, stress, or cold temperatures and relieved by nitroglycerin or the removal of the inciting factor are considered indicative of angina. If these same symptoms are more severe than previously experienced, or occur at rest with more frequency or with less provocation, UA is suspected (Amsterdam et al., 2014; Sabatine & Cannon, 2012).

Symptoms that are more severe (Gimenez et al., 2014; Sabatine & Cannon, 2012) or appear suddenly (Sabatine & Cannon, 2012) are more often associated with MI. By contrast, patients with symptoms characteristic for cardiac ischemia but with normal biomarkers are classified as having UA (Thygesen et al., 2012). UA symptoms have also been defined as those that (a) occur at rest or with minimal exertion, (b) have a recent history of onset (within the past month), or (c) increase in frequency, severity, or duration (Anderson et al., 2013; Betriu, Heras, Cohen, & Fuster, 1992). Still, it is critical to note that a substantial number of MI patients do not experience any symptoms. Asymptomatic patients are more likely to be female, elderly, or diabetic (Brieger et al., 2004; Canto et al., 2012; Thygesen, Alpert, & White, 2007).

In addition to physical symptoms, anxiety is also frequently associated with ACS. Khan et al. (2013) found that among 1,015 men and women study participants, 76.9% reported anxiety. Anxiety was significantly more prevalent among those patients with chest pain (44.4% versus 32.5%; $p = 0.005$).

There are clinical tools for the evaluation of ACS symptoms. The McSweeney Acute and Prodromal Myocardial Infarction Symptom Survey (MAPMISS) was developed specifically to evaluate MI symptoms among women. It consists of 37 acute and 33 prodromal MI symptoms (McSweeney, O'Sullivan, Cody, & Crane, 2004). This tool was used to evaluate both men and women in an international study on sex and gender differences in an ACS presentation conducted by Khan et al. (2013).

Gimenez et al. (2014) developed a bedside evaluation tool for use in their study of sex differences in ACS presentation. Their tool consisted of 34 predetermined items. Of those items, the symptoms most likely to be associated with MI in both men and women were discomfort aggravated by exertion or relieved by nitrates, the severity of the pain, chest discomfort, pain area larger than 3 cm, and radiation to the arms and/or shoulders.

Women and ACS Symptoms

There is significant controversy over whether women's symptoms are different from those of men. The most common symptom of ACS for both men and women is chest pain (Amsterdam et al., 2014; Gimenez et al., 2014; Khan et al., 2013). That being said, women present without chest pain more frequently than men, especially women younger than the age of 45 (Canto et al., 2012; Khan et al., 2013). However, there is no discernable pattern of other symptoms that would assist providers in identifying ACS in women without chest pain (Gimenez et al., 2014; Khan et al., 2013). Khan et al. (2013) did find that verified ACS patients presenting without chest pain were more likely to be women (OR 1.95; 95% CI 1.23–3.11; $p = 0.005$) and to have tachycardia (OR 2.07; 95% CI 1.20–3.56; $p = 0.009$).

In an older, smaller study of women who sustained MIs ($n = 40$), McSweeney et al. (2004) found that the most frequent prodromal symptoms were unusual fatigue, shortness of breath, indigestion, discomfort in the shoulder blade area, dizziness, headache, and chest sensations, such as mild discomfort. The symptoms most commonly occurring at the time of the MI were chest sensations (65%), arm sensations (40%), and discomfort between or under the shoulder blades (35%). Severe chest pain occurred only in 28% of the women interviewed. Importantly, another 23% reported no pain or only mild discomfort. Dyspnea or feeling flushed occurred in more than 50% of those interviewed (McSweeney et al., 2004).

EVALUATION AND RISK STRATIFICATION

Symptoms are usually the initial drivers for additional evaluation of patients suspected of having ACS. For patients with atypical or no symptoms, other components of patient evaluation, such as past medical history, risk factors, the ECG, and/or biomarkers are important in determining the etiology of patients' problems. For anyone suspected of having ACS, a prehospital or early admission ECG is critical for determining the next steps in care. Optimally, an ECG should be obtained and interpreted by a qualified provider within 10 minutes of a patient's first contact with medical care. According to current guidelines, the appropriate provider to analyze the ECG is a physician with specialized training in emergency medicine or cardiology. This does not preclude the performance and evaluation of ECGs at the first point of medical contact with the emergency medical system (EMS) providers (Amsterdam et al., 2014) or other qualified personnel. ECG characteristics that are common in STEMI and NSTE-ACS are discussed in the following sections.

Based on the history (especially presenting symptoms), ECG findings, and serum biomarker results, patients typically fall into three diagnostic categories: low likelihood, intermediate likelihood, and high likelihood of ACS (Amsterdam et al., 2014). Of those patients with intermediate or high likelihood of ACS, presentation features consistent with NSTE-ACS versus possible STEMI must be delineated. Patients demonstrating ECG ST-segment elevation need to be considered for PCI or fibrinolytic therapy, preferably within 10 minutes of the ECG interpretation (O'Gara et al., 2013). Treatment should not be delayed while awaiting serum biomarker results for probable STEMI patients. Individuals considered eligible for PCI need to be transported to medical centers with this capability in such a manner as to achieve a first medical contact (FMC) to PCI balloon inflation time of 90 minutes at EMS to PCI-capable hospital and 120 minutes at non-PCI facility to PCI-capable hospital (O'Gara et al., 2013).

There are several tools that may be helpful in determining patient prognosis and risk of complications after ACS. These include the GRACE score, the Thrombolysis in Myocardial Infarction (TIMI) score, and the Platelet Glycoprotein IIb/IIIa in UA: Receptor Suppression Using Integrilin Therapy (PURSUIT) risk model (Amsterdam et al., 2014). Estimation of ongoing risk and prognosis help to determine the therapies that will be used to treat the patient and the appropriate setting for their delivery. All of the most widely used tools incorporate patient age in the calculation of risk. Indeed, age—older than 55 for men and 65 for women—has been found to be the most important historical risk factor (Ho, Miller, Hodge, Bailey, & Gibbons, 2002; Morise, Haddad, & Beckner, 1997).

The GRACE risk score was developed from a multinational registry and it uses readily available data from admission to determine the chances of death and/or MI while hospitalized and within 6 months. The data required on admission are patient age, systolic blood pressure (SBP), HR, serum creatinine, cardiac biomarkers, ST-segment deviation, signs of heart failure (HF), and presence or absence of cardiac arrest on admission (Fox et al., 2010). The TIMI risk score calculator, also derived from clinical trial data, uses slightly different factors to determine risk: (a) age older than 65; (b) more than three risk factors including hypertension, diabetes mellitus (DM), family history, lipid disorder, or smoking; (c) known coronary stenosis greater than 50%; (d) recent aspirin use; (e) more than two episodes of severe angina in the previous 24 hours; (f) greater than 0.5 mm ST-segment deviation; and (g) elevated serum cardiac biomarkers (TIMI Study Group, 2011). The patient's TIMI score is calculated by adding 1 point for each of the previously named factors. A score of 0 to 1 is correlated with a 4.7% risk of death, MI, or recurrent ischemia requiring revascularization within 14 days of the assessment. In contrast, a TIMI score of 6 to 7 is associated with a 40.9% risk of adverse outcomes within 2 weeks (Antman, 2000). The PURSUIT risk model uses five factors: (a) age, (b) sex, (c) Canadian Cardiovascular Society angina classification within the previous 6 weeks, (d) signs of HF, and (e) ST-segment depression (Boersma et al., 2000). The PURSUIT model is rarely used in clinical practice (Bawamia, Mehran, Qiu, & Kunadian, 2013). The GRACE risk tool and the TIMI risk calculator are both available online (TIMI Study Group, 2011; University of Massachusetts Medical School, 2014) and cited as being helpful in the setting of NSTE-ACS (Amsterdam et al., 2014).

The aforementioned models were designed primarily to determine continued risk among patients already identified as having ACS. In contrast, the HEART score was designed specifically for use in emergency department (ED) settings to predict the likelihood of ACS and potential outcomes within 6 weeks. It was developed using expert opinion concerning key decision-making factors for diagnosing ACS, rather than information from multivariate analysis of large registries or trial data. The tool was then retrospectively validated in a multicenter trial. The HEART score has four chief components: (a) presentation history, (b) patient age, (c) risk factors, and (d) ECG characteristics. Scores range from 0 to 10 and are used to divide patients into low-, intermediate-, and high-risk groups for developing MI, requiring PCI or CABG, or dying within 6 weeks of evaluation (Backus et al., 2011). A HEART score of 3 or less has been found to predict with greater than 98% certainty that the patient will not experience a major coronary event within 6 weeks (Backus et al., 2013).

HEALTH HISTORY

Beyond determining a patient's acute and prodromal symptoms, providers must assess other aspects of the patient history that increase the likelihood of ACS. Chest discomfort may result from a variety of noncardiac problems. In order to more accurately determine whether the patient's symptoms are due to ACS, it is important to obtain the defining characteristics of his or her complaints including onset, location, duration, quality, radiation, associated symptoms, triggers, aggravating factors, timing, and alleviating factors (Fang & O'Gara, 2012). Obviously, a history of angina or previous MI increases the likelihood that a patient might be experiencing

ACS. A history of other atherosclerotic diseases, such as stroke or peripheral arterial disease, also increases the risk of coronary events (Amsterdam et al., 2014). Older patients presenting with ACS are likely to be hypertensive or diabetic. Younger patients are likely to have hyperlipidemia, a smoking history, a family history of premature CHD, and other risk factors for CHD (Woo & Schneider, 2009). In multiple studies, the combined factors of age and gender were more important to determining the likelihood of ACS than all other historical factors including chest discomfort features. Age older than 55 in men and 65 in women is the critical history feature (Anderson et al., 2013). The use of cocaine or methamphetamines is also a risk factor for ACS (Amsterdam et al., 2014).

Co-morbid conditions such as hypertension, diabetes, and peripheral arterial disease (PAD) not only increase the likelihood that the patient with ischemic symptoms has ACS, they also indicate higher risk for poor outcomes. Diabetes and PAD are associated with increased rates of HF and death among patients with either STEMI or NSTE-ACS. A history of renal disease increases the risk of poor outcomes, especially for those with more severe kidney dysfunction. Obesity is associated with a lower short-term but higher longer-term mortality among ACS patients (Amsterdam et al., 2014).

A history of previous or current aspirin use is associated with an increased risk of cardiovascular events. This relationship was documented during the development of the TIMI risk score and may reflect a history of previous CHD or PAD (Antman et al., 2000).

PHYSICAL EXAMINATION

As a clinician first approaches a patient suspected of having ACS, it is vitally important to determine his or her stability. The ABCs—airway, breathing, and circulation—must be evaluated. If any of these factors are significantly impaired, actions must be taken to support the patient prior to further assessment. Depending on the level of cardiovascular impairment, neurologic function might also be affected. Patient presentation can vary from hyperactivity to unconsciousness. Hyperactivity, severe anxiety, and decreased level of consciousness can all interfere with accurate history-taking and physical assessment.

General Appearance

Patients with ACS may appear pale and diaphoretic (Ferri, 2014). If they are experiencing discomfort at the time of the examination, patients may appear anxious (Khan et al., 2013; Michaels, 2010). Occasionally patients with squeezing or tightness sensations will demonstrate the *Levine Sign*—a clenched fist positioned on the chest. Marcus et al. (2007) found the prevalence of the Levine Sign to be 11%, with a sensitivity of only 9%, but a specificity of 84% for abnormal cardiac testing. Therefore, if patients do exhibit the Levine Sign, there is a relatively high likelihood that they are experiencing a cardiac event, but the absence of the gesture does not rule out ACS.

Neurologic

Depending on the BP and circulatory status of the patient with ACS, there can be a variety of neurologic presentations, predominantly affecting the patient's mental status and level of consciousness. If the patient is severely hypotensive or severely hypertensive, cerebral perfusion can be affected, leading to decreased mentation. The elderly and those with cerebrovascular disease are especially susceptible to neurological problems. An abrupt decrease in cardiac output due to HF or arrhythmia can cause frank syncope (Litwin & Benjamin, 2010).

Head, Eyes, Ears, Nose, and Throat (HEENT)

There are no HEENT findings specific to ACS or MI. Due to increased sympathetic discharge arising from anxiety and from the physiologic stresses being placed on the heart, the pupils may appear dilated; however, administration of opiates for pain relief can lead to pupillary constriction.

Neck

Patients with ACS may develop HF due to decreased myocardial contractility as a result of ischemia (Depre, Vatner, & Gross, 2011). If HF is present, the patient may have jugular venous distention. Kussmaul sign, a rise in jugular vein height with inspiration, can occur with right ventricular infarction (Hass et al., 2011).

Heart and Blood Vessels

During the assessment of the basic ABCs, vital signs are assessed as part of determining the patient's stability. The BP of patients with ACS may be low, normal, or high. Patients may have hypotension due to circulatory failure or as a result of medications, including beta-adrenergic blockers (beta blockers), nitrates, and opiates used to relieve symptoms. Hypotension or bradycardia is often associated with inferior STEMI, due to excess parasympathetic stimulation (Antman, 2012). Hypertension may be due to pain, anxiety, or illicit drug use such as methamphetamines. Patients with anterior STEMI may have hypertension and tachycardia related to excess sympathetic nervous system discharge (Antman, 2012). The hypertension or hypotension might also be the cause of the patient's myocardial ischemia, especially if there is a preexisting history of CHD (Thygesen et al., 2012). A difference in the SBP of 15 mmHg or more between left and right arm measurements is suspicious for aortic dissection. This finding may be associated with unequal pulse amplitude (Amsterdam et al., 2014). Pulse strength is affected by the BP, any preexisting peripheral arterial disease, and the amount of vasoconstriction. Patients with hypotension are likely to have faint or "thready" pulses. An irregular pulse rhythm indicates the possibility of arrhythmia. Ventricular arrhythmias—especially premature ventricular contractions (PVCs)—are common in ACS (Antman, 2012); therefore, continuous cardiac monitoring is extremely important.

Assessing the heart sounds of patients with ACS is very important for the detection of HF, incompetent valves, potential ventricular septal rupture (VSR), pericardial tamponade, and pericarditis. It is important to document baseline findings carefully and accurately so that any subsequent changes can be thoroughly investigated. An S_3 in adult patients is a sign of HF. An S_4 may indicate left ventricular hypertrophy due to longstanding hypertension, or decreased left ventricular compliance related to wall motion abnormalities associated with STEMI (Antman, 2012). The rupture or dysfunction of papillary muscles due to infarction can lead to tricuspid or mitral regurgitation (Michaels, 2010). Both tricuspid and mitral regurgitation are systolic murmurs. Tricuspid regurgitation due to MI is rare and is associated with right ventricular infarction and sometimes caused by infarction of the right ventricular papillary muscle. This murmur is heard best at the lower-left sternal border during inspiration (Antman, 2012; Mancini, 2012). Mitral regurgitation occurs in approximately 1% of all MIs and is usually associated with inferior infarctions. The posteriomedial papillary muscle may rupture, leading to valvular incompetence (Ren, 2014). Mitral regurgitation may also occur due to acute dilation of the LV as part of the heart's early attempts at compensation post-MI (Reynolds & Hochman, 2008). Mitral regurgitation is best heard with the diaphragm at the apex with radiation to the axilla (Bickley & Szilagyi, 2013). If there is posterior leaflet involvement, the murmur will be displaced to the left sternal border. Mitral regurgitation often leads to HF in the setting of AMI and can be life threatening (Grasso & Brener, 2013).

VSR occurs very rarely, but can have life-threatening consequences. Initially, the patient may have no other symptoms, but there is a potential risk for hypotension, cardiogenic shock, and pulmonary edema. As blood moves from the higher-pressure LV, through the ruptured septum and into the lower-pressure right ventricle, it creates a harsh holosystolic murmur that is best heard at the lower-left sternal border. Often, this murmur is accompanied by a thrill (Antman, 2012; Ren, 2014). If this murmur develops, immediate evaluation by a cardiologist, and potentially a cardiac surgeon, is necessary. Color-flow echocardiography is the best method for determining the size of the defect, and the amount of left-to-right shunting (Grasso & Brener, 2013). Emergent surgical repair may be necessary for significant shunt findings.

The presence of a crescendo–decrescendo systolic murmur may indicate aortic stenosis, a non-CHD cause of chest pain. Significant aortic stenosis can cause myocardial ischemia by increasing ventricular workload and oxygen demand. In some instances, the patency of the coronary ostia can be affected by the calcification associated with aortic stenosis (Conti, 2011).

Pericardial tamponade can accompany pericarditis or ventricular free wall rupture (VFWR). Acute ventricular rupture leads to sudden death. In subacute VFWR, or pericardial tamponade due to pericarditis, the heart sounds are very diminished. This is accompanied by hypotension, jugular venous distention, and pulsus paradoxus (Grasso & Brener, 2013).

A pericardial friction rub is associated with pericarditis, which is thought to be an inflammatory reaction to myocardial tissue necrosis. The rub is often described as scratchy, or "creaking leather," and is best heard with the diaphragm placed at the lower-left sternal border. Classically, a pericardial rub has three components: (a) atrial systole, (b) ventricular systole, and (c) ventricular diastole (Bickley & Szilagy, 2013; Grasso & Brener, 2013), but rubs with only one or two components have also been documented (Grasso & Brener, 2013). Pericardial friction rubs are often fleeting in nature—heard often by one provider but not the next, even when there is a short period of time between assessments. Pericardial friction rubs can be heard as early as 24 hours post-STEMI. Most commonly, they are heard on the second or third day post-infarction but can be heard up to 2 weeks post-MI (Antman, 2012). Friction rubs occurring much later, approximately 2 to 3 weeks following a transmural MI, are associated with Dressler's syndrome, which has become somewhat rare in the age of PCI and fibrinolytics. Symptoms of Dressler's syndrome include fever, malaise, and an elevated sedimentation rate (Little & Oh, 2012; O'Gara et al., 2013).

Chest and Lungs

Myocardial ischemia and infarction can both lead to ventricular dysfunction. Impaired left-ventricular function leads to increased left atrial and pulmonary venous pressures, and ultimately to pulmonary edema. The most prominent pulmonary finding in acute HF and the resultant pulmonary edema is inspiratory crackles. Usually crackles are gravity-dependent and are first noted in the bases of one or both lungs. More severe pulmonary edema is manifested by more extensive crackles, tachypnea, and respiratory distress. Pink frothy sputum is sometimes associated with severe pulmonary edema. Rhonchi and wheezing may also be present (Sovari, 2012).

The Killip Classification for Patients with STEMI is a prognostic tool based on physical examination findings. The presence or absence of crackles, an S_3, and signs of cardiogenic shock determine the level of classification (Killip & Kimbal, 1967). The more extensive the crackles, the higher the Killip class and the worse the patient's prognosis (Table 18.1). This tool was first developed in the 1960s but continues to have clinical utility today.

Tachypnea without adventitious breath sounds can occur due to anxiety and increased sympathetic nervous system discharge. Use of accessory muscles, such as the scalene and sternocleidomastoid muscles, indicate more significant respiratory distress (Bickley & Szilagyi, 2013). The paradoxical movement of the abdominal

TABLE 18.1 Killip Classification of Heart Failure With STEMI

Killip Class	Clinical Findings
I	No clinical signs of heart failure
II	S_3 Crackles lower half of lung fields Pulmonary venous hypertension
III	Crackles throughout lung fields Pulmonary edema
IV	Cardiogenic shock Hypotension, SBP ≤90 mmHg Peripheral vasoconstriction

SBP, systolic blood pressure; STEMI, ST-elevation myocardial infarction.

Source: Nieminen et al. (2005).

muscles, outward with expiration, is a sign of respiratory fatigue. It can be due to a chronic obstructive pulmonary disease (COPD) exacerbation or other causes of respiratory failure (Williams, 2009).

Abdomen

The abdominal examination of a patient with ACS may be benign. However, patients with cardiogenic shock may have hypoactive to absent bowel sounds due to impaired mesenteric circulation. Patients with longstanding HF may have hepatomegaly. Hepatojugular reflux (HJR) occurs earlier in HF, with an increase of more than 3 cm being considered positive for HF (Pinsky & Wipf, 2014).

Genitourinary

Urine output can be affected by any fall in cardiac output. Oliguria—less than 0.5 mL/kg/h—can occur (Eachempati, 2013), but may not be readily apparent. For most patients presenting with ACS, insertion of a urinary catheter to monitor urinary output is unnecessary. However, for patients with hypotension, or signs of HF, close monitoring of urinary output is essential.

Extremities

The limbs of patients with ACS may appear normal, pale, or cyanotic. Pallor and cyanosis may indicate decreased circulation and impending or current shock state (Antman, 2012; de Moya, 2013). Edema may indicate the presence of HF; however, peripheral edema is not an early sign of new onset acute HF (Antman, 2012).

Skin, Hair, and Nails

As mentioned previously, among patients with suspected ACS, pallor is suspicious for decreased circulation. Of course, pallor could also be the result of anemia that is provoking an ACS event due to decreased oxygen delivery to the myocardium. Cyanosis can be an indicator of the decreased oxygen saturation of the blood supplying an affected area. Diaphoresis leading to cold, clammy skin can occur, especially in patients experiencing acute HF. Cold, clammy skin, mottling, and poor capillary refill can be signs of impending cardiogenic shock (Ren, 2014).

DIAGNOSTIC TESTING

The ECG and serum cardiac biomarkers are the cornerstones of diagnostic testing in ACS. Other testing that should be done during the initial evaluation include a prothrombin time (PT) and activated partial thromboplastin time (aPTT), complete blood count (CBC), a basic metabolic panel, and a chest x-ray. The primary purpose for obtaining coagulation studies, a CBC, and blood chemistries is to establish the patient's baseline and determine any abnormalities that might be contraindications for potential testing or therapies. For example, a patient with an abnormally high baseline PT and aPTT might not be a candidate for fibrinolytic therapy. Similarly, a patient with a significantly elevated serum creatinine might not be a good candidate for a coronary computed tomographic angiogram (CCTA).

Echocardiography can be a useful adjunctive test when the ACS diagnosis is in doubt. In addition, echocardiography is extremely useful in determining LV function, which in turn may influence decisions regarding medications and other therapies (Amsterdam et al., 2014). Coronary angiography is the gold standard for determining the degree of coronary artery disease and occlusion, but it is an invasive procedure with risks of arrhythmia, bleeding, renal failure, stroke, and death. Coronary computed tomography angiography is a promising noninvasive technique; its current utility is primarily related to its high negative predictive value.

12-Lead ECG

The ECG serves as the first and most immediately available diagnostic test in determining the likelihood of myocardial ischemia. As mentioned previously, the task of obtaining and interpreting the ECG as soon as possible following the patient's first contact with either prehospital or hospital personnel is critical. Optimally, the time interval from first contact to ECG interpretation should be 10 minutes or less (Amsterdam et al., 2014; Thygesen et al., 2012). Prehospital ECG interpretation is preferable, so that patients with ACS symptoms and ST-elevation can be sent directly to a PCI-capable hospital if feasible. The goal is PCI delivery for eligible patients within 90 minutes of FMC (O'Gara et al., 2013). In 2008, this goal was achieved for more than 75% of nontransferred patients by hospitals participating in the Door to Balloon (D2B) Alliance (Bradley et al., 2009).

In addition to obtaining an initial ECG, situational ECGs performed during symptoms can be helpful in determining the patient's diagnosis. ST-segment changes of at least 0.05 mV that occur with symptoms and resolve with symptom relief are strongly suggestive of acute ischemia and underlying CHD. Further, ECG patterns such as bundle branch block, left-ventricular hypertrophy, and paced rhythm are associated with a higher risk of death among ACS patients (Amsterdam et al., 2014). Performing serial ECGs at 15- to 30-minute intervals for the first hour post admission is also recommended if no significant abnormalities are noted on the initial tracing (Amsterdam et al., 2014; Thygesen et al., 2012). Having ECGs from previous medical encounters for comparison improves the accuracy of diagnosis, especially when the admitting or initial ECG demonstrates LBBB (O'Gara et al., 2013). Continuous 12-lead computer-assisted ECG recordings should be performed if available (Thygesen et al., 2012).

Serum Biomarkers

Over the years, a variety of serum biomarkers have been used to aid in the diagnosis of MI. Creatine kinase and its MB isoenzyme (CK-MB) have been used to detect myocardial necrosis for many, many years. While CK-MB is more concentrated in the myocardium, it can also be found in the skeletal muscle. Therefore, conditions such as trauma, myopathy, and significant exercise can cause false positive results. CK-MB rises 3 to 12 hours after a cardiac insult and peaks in 24 hours (Antman, 2012). Because levels return to normal within 48 to 72 hours, it can be helpful in differentiating reinfarction (Schreiber, 2013). CK-MB is also helpful in determining the diagnosis and prognosis of periprocedural MI (Anderson et al., 2013); however, due to the extreme sensitivity of newer cardiac troponin assays, CK-MB is no longer considered the primary biomarker in diagnosing ACS (Amsterdam et al., 2014).

Today, cardiac troponins (cTns) are the preferred biomarkers for the diagnosis of MI (Thygesen et al., 2012). Cardiac troponin I (cTnI) and cardiac troponin T (cTnT) are proteins found in the contractile structure of cardiac muscle. They are released during myocardial cell injury and enter the cardiac interstitial fluid, ultimately disseminating into the peripheral circulation. They can sometimes be detected as early as 2 to 4 hours following the onset of symptoms (Amsterdam et al., 2014). Peak concentrations of cTnI occur at about 24 hours following the insult, and return to normal within 5 to 10 days. cTnT peaks between 12 hours and 2 days. It remains elevated slightly longer and returns to normal in 5 to 14 days (Antman, 2012). Because cTns remain elevated for longer periods, they are helpful in diagnosing ACS patients who may have sustained their MIs days before their medical assessment. The degree of cTn elevation is valuable in determining patient prognosis (Amsterdam et al., 2014).

According to the National Academy of Clinical Biochemistry recommendations, cTn samples should be obtained on admission and 6 to 9 hours later (Morrow et al., 2007). The American College of Cardiology Foundation and the American Heart Association (ACCF/AHA) stress that the timing of samples should be determined based on the time since the onset of symptoms. According to the guidelines for NSTE-ACS, cTnI or cTnT should be drawn from all ACS patients at the time of presentation, and at 3 to 6 hours from symptom onset. Additional samples should be obtained at 3- to 6-hour intervals if the initial results are negative but the patient has an intermediate or high likelihood of having ACS. Repeat levels may also be obtained once on day three or four postinfarction to determine infarct size (Amsterdam et al., 2014).

There are a variety of immunoassays used to detect cTnI, but only one assay for cTnT. Clinicians must be knowledgeable of which troponin and corresponding URL of normal is used by the laboratory to apply the universal definition of MI criteria. Troponin I assays are considered less precise at the 99th percentile URL than cTnT (Schreiber, 2013); however, the ACCF and the European Cardiology Society have not recommended cTnT over cTnI (Schreiber, 2013; Thygesen et al., 2012).

Another important concept related to cTns is that they can detect as little as 1 gm of necrotic cardiac tissue. Because of this sensitivity, cTns can detect myocyte necrosis from causes other than AMI. Some conditions that can lead to cTn elevations include chest trauma, tachyarrhythmia, HF, left-ventricular hypertrophy, sepsis, burns, and renal insufficiency (Galvani et al., 1997). For patients with end-stage renal disease, cTnI elevation appears to be more specific to myocardial necrosis (Freda, Tang, Van Lente, Peacock, & Francis, 2002).

High-sensitivity cTns are becoming more available. A single sample hs-cTn has 90% sensitivity and specificity. The negative predictive value is 97% to 99% (Sabatine & Cannon, 2012). Cullen et al. (2013) paired hs-cTnI with TIMI scoring to determine which patients could be safely discharged from the ED within 2 hours. They found that a TIMI score of less than 1, an hs-cTnI less than the 99th percentile of URL, and no ischemic ECG changes had less than 0.8% chance of a major adverse cardiac event in 30 days.

Myogloblin, another protein found in both cardiac and skeletal muscle cells, has been used in EDs to speed the determination of potential MI patients. Myoglobin can be detected as soon as 1 hour after cardiac cell necrosis (Morrow et al., 2007). Because this marker is not cardiac-specific, elevated levels should be confirmed with another more specific serum marker, such as cTn. Current guidelines do not recommend the use of myoglobin in diagnosing NSTE-ACS (Amsterdam et al., 2014).

B-Type Natriuretic Peptides

This neurohormone is released when there is overstretching of ventricular myocytes. In addition to indicating HF, B-type natriuretic peptide (BNP) levels are strong independent predictors of short- and long-term mortality in ACS patients (Galvani et al., 2004). ACCF/AHA guidelines for NSTE-ACS state that BNP or NT-pro-BNP may be helpful in determining prognosis (Amsterdam et al., 2014).

Inflammatory Markers

The white blood cell (WBC) count of patients with AMI is elevated and the degree of elevation has implications for prognosis. During ACS, WBC counts generally range from 12 to 15 × 10³/mL. Elevations of C-reactive protein (CRP) on admission also signal an increased risk of poor outcome (Morrow et al., 1998), although current guidelines do not advocate obtaining CRP levels during initial ACS patient evaluations (Anderson et al., 2013; O'Gara et al., 2013).

Chest X-Ray

While there are no radiographic changes in chest x-rays that are definitive for MI, this diagnostic tool is valuable in ruling out other important causes of chest pain such as aortic dissection, pneumonia, and pneumothorax (Sabatine & Cannon, 2012). Signs of pulmonary vascular congestion may indicate HF associated with some MIs.

DIAGNOSIS OF ACS

As mentioned previously, the ECG and cardiac biomarkers are critical to the diagnosis of ACS. When combined with the patient's history and physical examination findings, a diagnostic pattern begins to emerge. Because the ECG requires relatively little time to obtain and interpret, it is often the key initial indicator. A normal ECG has a negative predictive value of 80% to 90% regardless of the presence of chest pain during the recording (Turnipseed et al., 2009). Still, myocardial damage due to left circumflex and RCA occlusions may not be noted on a standard ECG. In these cases, posterior chest leads V_7 to V_9 may provide evidence of the problem (Amsterdam et al., 2014). Key ECG abnormalities that determine the direction of treatment for ACS patients include ST-elevation, LBBB, ST-segment depression, and T-wave inversion. While other abnormalities are also important in determining the age of MI and prognosis, these four types of ECG changes provide guidance for initial therapy.

ST-ELEVATION MYOCARDIAL INFARCTION

The primary criterion for STEMI is ECG evidence of greater than 1 mm (0.1 mV) of ST-segment elevation in at least two leads associated with the same or adjacent regions of the heart (contiguous leads). When this type of ECG change is present, 90% of patients will also have significant elevations in cardiac biomarkers (Anderson et al., 2013). The development of LBBB either during observation, or when compared with an older ECG, is considered to be an indicator of possible AMI, but should be corroborated by additional signs and symptoms (Jain et al., 2011).

The Task Force for the Universal Definition of Myocardial Infarction employs more stringent ECG criteria, placing particular emphasis on the amount of ST-elevation in leads V_2 and V_3 when diagnosing an anterior MI. According to these criteria, new ST-elevation must be at least 2 mm (0.2 mV) in men or at least 1.5 mm (0.15 mV) in women in leads V_2 and V_3. Using the *Universal Definition of MI* criteria, other areas of myocardial involvement require at least 1 mm (0.1 mV) in other contiguous chest leads or the limb leads to be significant for STEMI (Thygesen et al., 2012).

Special ECG Presentations of MI

It is important to note that the ECG presentation for transmural posterior STEMI is ST-depression in two or more precordial leads (V_1–V_4), accompanied by ST-elevation in V_7–V_9. Another unusual presentation is ST-elevation in aVR, associated with ST depression in multiple additional leads. This occurs with left main or proximal LAD artery occlusion (O'Gara et al., 2013). Right ventricular infarction presents as ST-elevation in the right precordial leads V_1, and V_3R to V_6R (Antman, 2012). ST-elevations of 1 mm or more in V_1 and V_4R are the findings most sensitive for acute right ventricular infarction (Robalino, Whitlow, Underwood, & Salcedo, 1989). Because the blood supply to the inferior wall of the LV and the right ventricle both originate from the RCA, the ECG presentation of a right ventricular infarction may share ECG characteristics of an acute inferior STEMI and also ST-elevation in the right precordial leads. For this reason, all patients demonstrating ST-elevation in leads II, III, and AVF should also have right-sided chest leads recorded to assess for right ventricular involvement (Michaels, 2010).

Because STEMI patients have the highest risk of death during the early period of their illness, careful cardiac monitoring and aggressive therapy, such as PCI or fibrinolytics, are warranted (Amsterdam et al., 2014). Definitive care for these patients should not be delayed while awaiting cardiac biomarker results. Positive biomarker results are considered confirmatory and have prognostic value, but are not the key initial indicator of therapy.

TAKOTSUBO CARDIOMYOPATHY

Takotsubo cardiomyopathy, or broken heart syndrome, mimics STEMI. This disorder is precipitated by severe emotional or physical stress, and is likely mediated by catecholamine release (Antman, 2012; Tomich, 2012). ST-elevation occurs without evidence of coronary artery occlusion. However, cardiac biomarkers are elevated. A key feature of this problem is transient left-ventricular wall motion abnormalities. Apical bulging is a "classic" finding, but is not required for the diagnosis. The most common presenting symptoms are virtually indistinguishable from ACS and include chest pain and dyspnea (Tomich, 2012). For this reason, patients should initially receive the same treatment as STEMI patients, up to and including cardiac catheterization. The absence of thrombosis or significant coronary occlusion, determined by coronary angiography, is used to confirm the diagnosis (Tomich, 2012).

The disorder occurs predominantly among Asian and Caucasian postmenopausal women. Usually these patients do not have cardiac risk factors. Interestingly, nearly all victims will recover completely within 4 to 8 weeks, and at that time will have normal ventricular wall motion and ejection fractions. Despite the excellent prognosis, significant complications can occur, including HF, ventricular arrhythmias, cardiogenic shock, and death (Tomich, 2012).

NON-ST-SEGMENT ELEVATION MYOCARDIAL INFARCTION

The criteria for NSTEMI include a combination of positive biomarkers and ST-segment depression or T-wave inversion. In NSTEMI, the ST-depressions must be greater than or equal to 0.5 mm (0.05 mV) in two or more contiguous leads. The depth of ST-depressions and the number of leads involved increase the likelihood of non-Q-wave MI as opposed to UA (Lloyd-Jones, Camargo, Lapuerta, Giugliano, & O'Donnell, 1998). ST-depressions that are horizontal or downsloping are very suspicious for NSTE-ACS (Thygesen et al., 2012). Symmetrical T-wave inversions greater than or equal to 2 mm (0.2 mV) in depth indicate acute ischemia, and if present in V_2 and V_3, often represent critical proximal LAD stenosis (de Zwaan et al., 1989). Patients with ECG changes but without significant elevations of cardiac biomarkers are considered to have UA.

Because the criteria for diagnosing NSTE-ACS are more subtle than those for STEMI, additional information from the patient's history and physical examination can assist in determining the likelihood that the patient has cardiac ischemia and/or necrosis. Most notably, women present more frequently with UA than with NSTEMI or STEMI (Grady, Chaput, & Kristof, 2003). Despite a less severe presentation, women have an overall higher risk of poor outcomes (Antman & Morrow, 2012). In both sexes, a history of previous CHD or PAD increases the chances that the current presentation represents ACS. Other cardiac risk factors such as a history of hyperlipidemia, hypertension, or diabetes are also important. Any physical examination findings that are congruent with any of these disease processes increase the likelihood of NSTE-ACS. Signs of HF, such as crackles, an S_3, or a mitral regurgitation murmur, are indicators of high risk and poorer prognosis (Amsterdam et al., 2014). While much attention is placed on the higher early risk of death among STEMI patients, it must be emphasized that NSTE-ACS is associated with a higher incidence of later cardiac events and morbidity. In addition, it is important to note that cardiogenic shock can occur in NSTEMI as well as STEMI (Amsterdam et al., 2014).

NEGATIVE PROGNOSTIC INDICATORS

There are a number of patient characteristics that predict poor outcomes. Many of them have been discussed previously in relationship to risk-stratification tools. One of the most obvious indicators of possible poor prognosis is an initial presentation with cardiac arrest. Median survival to discharge in this group is only 22% but can be improved to 60% with successful PCI (Nichol et al., 2008). The presence of ECG abnormalities such as LBBB, paced rhythm, and left-ventricular hypertrophy are also among the characteristics with significantly negative outcomes (Amsterdam et al., 2014). In addition, diabetes and kidney disease increase the risk of death post-MI (O'Gara et al., 2013). Other high-risk indicators include female gender, an anterior MI, a history of previous MI, a history of smoking, hypotension, tachycardia, high Killip class, and prolonged time to reperfusion (Antman & Morrow, 2012; O'Gara et al., 2013). Not unexpectedly, a history of current or previous aspirin use is associated with increased cardiovascular risk (Antman et al., 2000). Finally, age has been used as an indicator of risk in prediction tools; however, the authors of the 2013 STEMI guidelines state that even the very elderly can benefit from aggressive therapy, and that data from the past has reflected the reluctance to provide these therapies to patients of advanced age (O'Gara et al., 2013).

THERAPEUTIC MANAGEMENT

There is a critical distinction in the management of patients with ACS based on ECG findings. Those patients who exhibit ST-elevation or probable new LBBB are treated with immediate reperfusion therapy—either primary PCI or fibrinolytics. The preferred method of reperfusion is primary PCI. Patients with definite NSTE-ACS should be stratified by risk (see Risk Stratification section). NSTE-ACS patients with medium to high risk may be considered for an early invasive strategy consisting of coronary angiography and possible PCI (Table 18.2). Lower-risk NSTE-ACS patients should be treated medically with a conservative, ischemia-guided strategy, unless they develop recurrent chest pain or demonstrate high-risk ischemia based on subsequent noninvasive testing (Amsterdam et al., 2014). Very detailed and specific evidence-based guidelines for the identification and management of both STEMI and NSTE-ACS have been published (Amsterdam et al.,

TABLE 18.2 Factors Associated With Appropriate Selection of Early Invasive Strategy or Ischemia-Guided Strategy in Patients With NSTE-ACS

Immediate invasive (within 2 hr)	Refractory angina Signs or symptoms of HF or new or worsening mitral regurgitation Hemodynamic instability Recurrent angina or ischemia at rest or with low-level activities despite intensive medical therapy Sustained VT or VF
Ischemia-guided strategy	Low-risk score (e.g., TIMI [0 or 1], GRACE [<109]) Low-risk Tn-negative female patients Patient or clinician preference in the absence of high-risk features
Early invasive (within 24 hr)	None of the above, but GRACE risk score >140 Temporal change in Tn New or presumably new ST depression
Delayed invasive (within 25–72 hr)	None of the above but diabetes mellitus Renal insufficiency (GFR <60 mL/min/1.73 m^2) Reduced LV systolic function (EF <0.40) Early postinfarction angina PCI within 6 months Prior CABG GRACE risk score 109–140; TIMI score ≥2

CABG, coronary artery bypass graft; EF, ejection fraction; GFR, glomerular filtration rate; GRACE, Global Registry of Acute Coronary Events; HF, heart failure; hr, hour(s); LV, left ventricular; NSTE-ACS, non–ST-elevation acute coronary syndrome; PCI, percutaneous coronary intervention; TIMI, Thrombolysis In Myocardial Infarction; Tn, troponin; VF, ventricular fibrillation; VT, ventricular tachycardia.

Source: Amsterdam et al. (2014).

2014; O'Gara et al., 2013). The major features of the guidelines are discussed in the following sections. For additional information, please refer to the individual guidelines.

STEMI MANAGEMENT

As mentioned previously, the ECG is central to the decisions regarding management of patients with ACS. Patients should have a prehospitalization 12-lead ECG or an ECG within 10 minutes of first contact with medical personnel (O'Gara et al., 2013). Patients demonstrating ST-elevations should be evaluated to determine the appropriateness of reperfusion therapy based on time since symptom onset, co-morbid conditions, and life expectancy, among other considerations. Choices for reperfusion include primary PCI, fibrinolytic therapy, or CABG, with primary PCI the preferred intervention for most. Bypass surgery is not recommended in the acute phase of STEMI, unless the patient's coronary anatomy is not conducive to PCI, or the patient is experiencing continued ischemia, severe HF, or cardiogenic shock. Optimally, reperfusion therapy should be delivered within 12 hours of symptom onset; however, it is reasonable to consider reperfusion for patients up to 24 hours after symptom onset, when there is evidence of ongoing ischemia (O'Gara et al., 2013). Once eligibility for reperfusion is determined, the circumstances of reperfusion—either at the admission facility or another institution—must be decided and the appropriate arrangements made. If PCI is the selected intervention, the goal is to achieve an in-facility FMC to device time of 90 minutes or less, or transfer facility FMC to device time of 120 minutes or less (Figure 18.3). If it is impossible to achieve either of these timeframes, fibrinolytic therapy should be initiated within 30 minutes of FMC, provided the patient has no absolute contraindications of prior intracranial hemorrhage; cerebral vascular lesion; malignant intracranial neoplasm; ischemic stroke in the prior 3 months, except acute ischemic stroke within 4.5 hours; suspected aortic dissection; active bleeding or bleeding diathesis; closed head or facial trauma in the prior 3 months; intracranial or intraspinal surgery in the prior 2 months; severe, uncontrolled hypertension; or prior treatment with streptokinase in the prior 6 months (O'Gara et al., 2013). There are relative contraindications to fibrinolytic therapy for STEMI that must be evaluated prior to administration, including chronic, severe, or poorly controlled hypertension or current hypertension, systolic blood pressure (SBP) greater than 180 mmHg, or diastolic

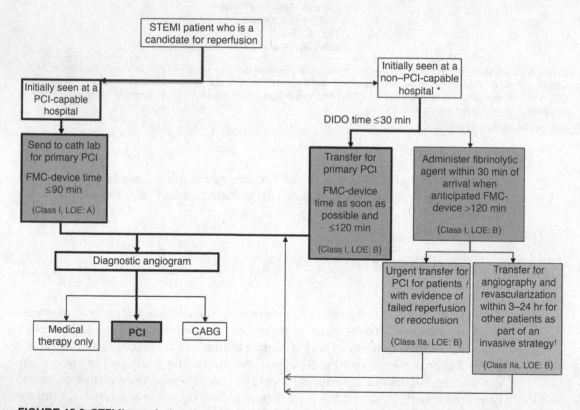

FIGURE 18.3 STEMI reperfusion algorithm.

CABG, coronary artery bypass graft; DIDO, door-in-door-out; FMC, first medical contact; LOE, level of evidence; MI, myocardial infarction; PCI, percutaneous coronary intervention; STEMI, ST-elevation myocardial infarction.

Reperfusion therapy for patients with STEMI. The bold arrows and boxes are the preferred strategies. Performance of PCI is dictated by an anatomically appropriate culprit stenosis.

*Patients with cardiogenic shock or severe heart failure initially seen at a non-PCI-capable hospital should be transferred for cardiac catheterization and revascularization as soon as possible, irrespective of time delay from MI onset (Class I, LOE: B).

†Angiography and revascularization should not be performed within the first 2 to 3 hours after administration of fibrinolytic therapy.

Source: O'Gara et al. (2013).

blood pressure (DBP) greater than 110 mmHg; history of prior ischemic stroke; dementia; intracranial pathology; prolonged or traumatic resuscitation; major surgery in the prior 3 weeks; internal bleeding in the prior 4 weeks; noncompressible vascular punctures; pregnancy; active peptic ulcer; or anticoagulant therapy (O'Gara et al., 2013).

Primary PCI Techniques

In most situations, either bare-metal stents (BMS) or drug-eluting stents (DES) are placed at the time of primary PCI for STEMI. DES improve the likelihood of long-term vessel patency but require a longer duration of antiplatelet therapy. BMS are recommended for patients who may not be able to complete a 12-month course of $P2Y_{12}$ receptor inhibitors due to compliance issues or bleeding risk. Another technique that may be useful to improve coronary artery perfusion in the immediate term is manual aspiration thrombectomy (O'Gara et al., 2013).

STEMI and Cardiogenic Shock

Patients demonstrating STEMI or new LBBB MI and cardiogenic shock should undergo cardiac catheterization and emergency revascularization via PCI or CABG as soon as possible (O'Gara et al., 2013). Results of the Should We Emergently Revascularize Occluded Coronaries for Cardiogenic Shock (SHOCK) trial demonstrated improved outcomes when revascularization was performed up to 54 hours post-MI and 18 hours following the onset of shock (Hochman et al., 2001).

Antithrombotic Therapy for Use With Primary PCI

Dual antiplatelet therapy (DAPT) is important for successful outcomes in STEMI patients receiving PCI. Non-enteric-coated aspirin 162 to 325 mg should be administered as soon as possible, preferably at FMC or in the ED. Following PCI, aspirin 81 to 325 mg should be continued indefinitely; aspirin 81 mg daily is the preferred maintenance dose. The second agent should be a $P2Y_{12}$ receptor inhibitor: clopidogrel, prasugrel, or ticagrelor. An appropriate loading dose of one of these agents should be administered as early as possible prior to the PCI. A drug-specific maintenance dose should be continued for at least 1 year following the placement of either BMS or DES (O'Gara et al., 2013). Of note, prasugrel is contraindicated in STEMI patients who have had a prior transient ischemic attack (TIA) or stroke (Lilly/Daiichi Sankyo, 2013; O'Gara et al., 2013).

Glycoprotein IIb/IIIa receptor antagonists (GP IIb/IIIa), such as abciximab, tirofiban, and eptifibatide are appropriate to use with unfractionated heparin (UHF) or the direct thrombin inhibitor, bivalirudin, in selected STEMI patients undergoing PCI who have a large thrombus burden or inadequate $P2Y_{12}$ receptor inhibitor loading. If a GP IIb/IIIa agent is used, an adjustment to the target activated clotting time (ACT) during the PCI should be made, with the new target being 200 to 250 seconds (O'Gara et al., 2013).

Anticoagulant Therapy for Patients With Primary PCI

Patients undergoing primary PCI should be anticoagulated with either unfractionated heparin (UFH) or bivalirudin. If a GP IIb/IIIa receptor antagonist is also used, adjustments to the target ACT should be made as previously noted. If no GP IIb/IIIa receptor antagonist is used, the target ACT should be 250 to 300 seconds for the HemoTec device and 300 to 350 seconds for the Hemochron device (O'Gara et al., 2013). For specific bolus and dosage recommendations for UHF, enoxaparin, and fondaparinux, please refer to the 2013 ACCF/AHA Guideline for the Management of ST-Elevation Myocardial Infarction (O'Gara et al., 2013, p. e97).

Fibrinolytic Therapy—Necessary Adjunctive Medications

STEMI patients receiving fibrinolytic agents should also receive anticoagulation with UFH, enoxaparin, or fondaparinux for at least 48 hours, and preferably for the duration of the index hospitalization, up to 8 days, or until revascularization is performed (O'Gara et al., 2013, p. e96). If UFH is used, a weight-adjusted bolus should be given to initiate therapy, followed by an infusion to maintain an aPTT of 1.5 to 2.0 times control. Close monitoring of the aPTT and platelet counts is recommended.

STEMI patients receiving a fibrinolytic medication should also receive DAPT with aspirin and clopidogrel. The loading doses for these medications should be aspirin 162 to 325 mg and clopidogrel 300 mg. If the patient is more than 75 years of age, the clopidogrel loading dose should be decreased to 75 mg. Maintenance therapy should be aspirin 81 mg daily indefinitely, and clopidogrel 75 mg daily for a minimum of 14 days and up to 1 year (O'Gara et al., 2013).

Assessing Reperfusion After Fibrinolysis

The *gold standard* for assessing patency of an infarct-related artery is coronary angiography. Other less direct, less precise indicators of restored blood flow include (a) a decrease in, or relief of, symptoms; (b) a decrease in ST elevation; and (c) reperfusion arrhythmias, such as accelerated idioventricular rhythm (O'Gara et al., 2013). If ST segment elevation has not decreased by at least 50% in the initially most elevated lead within 60 to 90 minutes following fibrinolytic therapy, immediate coronary angiography and possible PCI should be considered (O'Gara et al., 2013). It is also reasonable to transfer hemodynamically stable patients who experience successful reperfusion for coronary angiography and possible PCI. The intervention should occur at least 3 hours following completion of the fibrinolytic agent and preferably within the first 24 hours (O'Gara et al., 2013).

NSTE-ACS MANAGEMENT

Patients with a moderate or high likelihood of having NSTE-ACS (Table 18.3) should be managed in a closely monitored environment with defibrillation capability. Those with ongoing ischemic symptoms, hemodynamic instability, or definite ACS should be admitted to a critical care unit and considered for an early invasive

TABLE 18.3 Likelihood of Presentation Being CAD-Related

Feature	High Likelihood (*Any of the following*)	Intermediate Likelihood (*Absence of High Likelihood features and presence of any of the following*)	Low Likelihood (*Absence of High or Intermediate Likelihood features but may have*)
History	Chest or left arm pain or discomfort as chief symptom reproducing prior documented angina Known history of CAD	Chest or left arm pain or discomfort as chief symptom Age older than 70 Male sex Diabetes mellitus	Probable ischemic symptoms in absence of any of the intermediate likelihood characteristics Recent cocaine use
Examination	Transient MR murmur Hypotension, diaphoresis, pulmonary edema, or crackles (rales)	Extracardiac vascular disease	Chest discomfort reproduced
ECG	New, or presumably new, transient ST-segment deviation (≥1 mm) or T-wave inversion in multiple precordial leads	Fixed waves ST depression 0.5 to 1 mm or T-wave inversion >1 mm	T-wave flattening or inversion <1 mm in leads with dominant waves Normal ECG
Cardiac markers	Elevated cardiac TnI, TnT	Normal	Normal

ACS, acute coronary syndrome; CAD, coronary artery disease; ECG, electrocardiogram; MI, myocardial infarction; MR, mitral regurgitation; TnI, troponin I; TnT, troponin T.

Reprinted from Braunwald et al. (2000), with permission from Elsevier.

strategy (Amsterdam et al., 2014). Because the initial presentation of NSTE-ACS may not be as obvious or dramatic as the ECG changes that accompany STEMI, a high degree of suspicion should be maintained, and diagnostic measures should be repeated if normal or borderline on admission. ECG should be repeated with any symptom recurrence, as well as at 15- to 30-minute intervals for at least the first hour. Serum biomarkers should be obtained upon presentation, and every 3 to 6 hours following initial symptom onset for at least two to three sets. Additional samples may be warranted if the initial levels are normal but the ECG and/or symptoms are at least moderately suspicious for ACS (Amsterdam et al., 2014). Several recent studies have indicated that shorter diagnostic protocols may be safe and effective (Cullen et al., 2013; Than et al., 2012). Obviously, patients with recurrent symptoms, ischemic ECG changes, or positive cTns should remain hospitalized and monitoring of these parameters continued until the patient is stabilized. Stable patients can be cared for in intermediate care units, but patients with recurrent pain, hemodynamic instability, large MIs, or uncontrolled arrhythmias should be admitted to a coronary care unit (Amsterdam et al., 2014).

Clinicians caring for NSTE-ACS patients must consider which of two major treatment pathways—early invasive with angiography and possible PCI within 24 hours or ischemia guided with conservative medical management—is appropriate for each patient, based on his or her clinical features. Low-risk patients with negative cardiac biomarkers can receive additional diagnostic testing to determine the extent and severity of ischemia either during their current observational stay or very shortly after, within 72 hours, as an outpatient (Amsterdam et al., 2014). For moderate- and high-risk patients, the treatment pathway choice is between an invasive strategy, involving early coronary angiography and possible PCI, and an initially conservative strategy of optimizing guideline-directed medical therapy (GDMT) and performing a noninvasive assessment of ischemic territory. For those patients with significant ST-segment depression and positive cTnTs, an early invasive strategy has demonstrated benefit in numerous trials, including the Fragmin and Fast Revascularization during InStability in Coronary Artery Disease—II (FRISC-II; FRISC-II Investigators, 1999), and Treat Angina with Aggrastat and Determine Cost of Therapy with Invasive or Conservative Strategy (TACTICS TIMI-18) trials (TACTICS TIMI-18 Investigators, 2001). An ACS diagnostic strategy using the change in troponin levels (delta) over the first 2 hours of observation can facilitate the earlier identification of higher risk patients who would benefit from more aggressive management, such as GP IIb/IIIa inhibitors (Than et al., 2014). Others who should be considered for an early invasive strategy include the elderly (TACTICS TIMI-18 Investigators, 2001), patients who are unstable, or those who have refractory angina (Amsterdam et al., 2014). Patients with multiple or serious co-morbidities, such as liver failure or terminal cancer, should not receive early invasive therapy, as the risks outweigh the benefits (Amsterdam et al., 2014).

For patients who undergo either early or delayed angiography, those with significant left main coronary artery lesions, and those with left ventricular dysfunction in the setting of multi-vessel disease should be referred for CABG (Amsterdam et al., 2014). In addition, patients with diabetes should be referred for CABG. A recent meta-analysis of studies comparing the outcomes of CABG and PCI in this patient population revealed improved all-cause mortality rates among diabetics receiving CABG (Verma et al., 2013).

Antiplatelet Therapy in NSTE-ACS

As with STEMI patients, NSTE-ACS patients without contraindications should receive nonenteric coated, chewable aspirin (ASA) 162 to 325 mg as soon as possible and it should be continued indefinitely at 81 mg to 162 mg daily. If the patient is unable to tolerate aspirin, and provided that there are not any other contraindications, clopidogrel, a $P2Y_{12}$ inhibitor, should be initiated with a loading dose and continued with the recommended daily dosing. DAPT is recommended for non-aspirin allergic NSTE-ACS patients. Generally, either clopidogrel or ticagrelor can be prescribed along with ASA when the patient is initially evaluated and continued for at least 12 months. Ticagrelor is preferred for patients undergoing either early invasive or ischemia-guided interventions (Amsterdam et al., 2014). If ticagrelor is used, the recommended maintenance dose of aspirin is 81 mg, because ASA doses exceeding 100 mg have been linked to a decrease in the efficacy of ticagrelor (Amsterdam et al., 2014; Jneid et al., 2012). Another $P2Y_{12}$ inhibitor, prasugrel, should be initiated only after the determination to perform a PCI has been made. This stipulation for use is based on findings from the Trial to Assess Improvement in Therapeutic Outcomes by Optimizing Platelet Inhibition with Prasugrel—Thrombolysis in Myocardial Infarction—38 (TRITON TIMI-38) trial, in which prasugrel was associated with a significant decrease in death, or MI, but also increased the risk of major bleeding (Wiviott et al., 2007).

DAPT is recommended for up to 12 months in conservatively managed patients, based on findings from the Clopidogrel in Unstable Angina to Prevent Recurrent Events (CURE) trial (Amsterdam et al., 2014; Clopidogrel in Unstable Angina to

Prevent Recurrent Events Trial Investigators, 2001). Patients undergoing PCI with stent placement should receive a loading dose of a $P2Y_{12}$ inhibitor followed by at least 12 months of maintenance therapy.

GP IIb/IIIa Inhibitors in NSTE-ACS

NSTE-ACS patients undergoing coronary angiography and PCI as part of an early invasive strategy and who are at medium to high risk for complications may receive an intravenous GP IIb/IIIa inhibitor (epitfibatide or tirofiban) in addition to DAPT and anticoagulation (Amsterdam et al., 2014). It is important to note that the Acute Catheterization and Urgent Intervention Triage Strategy (ACUITY) trial results indicated that early (upstream) use of GP IIb/IIIa inhibitors was not superior to provisional use at the time of the PCI and was associated with more major bleeding (Stone et al., 2007). For patients receiving GP IIb/IIIa inhibitors and requiring urgent CABG, aspirin should be continued, but the GP IIb/IIIa should be discontinued at least 4 hours prior to surgery (eptifibatide and tirofiban). For low-risk patients or those with a high bleeding risk, the use of GP IIb/IIIa inhibitors in addition to ASA and a $P2Y_{12}$ inhibitor provides no additional benefit (Amsterdam et al., 2014).

Anticoagulation for NSTE-ACS

Patients receiving either invasive or ischemia-guided care should be anticoagulated with intravenous (IV) UFH, enoxaparin, or fondaparinux during or immediately after initial evaluation. UFH should be used if CABG is planned within the next 24 hours. UFH should be administered only for 48 hours or until a PCI is performed. Enoxaparin requires a downward dosage adjustment for patients with renal impairment (Cr Cl < 30 mL/min). Fondaparinux is the drug of choice for conservatively managed patients with higher risks of bleeding. Fondaparinux is contraindicated in patients with Cr Cl that is less than 30 mL/min (Amsterdam et al., 2014). Patients receiving fondaparinux and undergoing angiography and possible stenting should receive an anti-IIa agent in addition to fondaparinux at the time of the procedure to guard against catheter-associated thrombus formation (Steg et al., 2010). Bivalirudin is an additional anticoagulation option, although recommended for use only in patients anticipated to receive a PCI. This direct thrombin inhibitor can be initiated on admission and continued throughout the procedure. When bivalirudin is administered during the PCI, a GP IIb/IIIa agent can be used provisionally if the patient is receiving DAPT. Generally, anticoagulation should be continued for the duration of hospitalization or until the time of the PCI (Amsterdam et al., 2014).

For patients undergoing CABG, if they are receiving UFH, it should be continued up to the time of surgery. If the patient is receiving bivalirudin, it should be stopped 3 hours before the CABG. Enoxaparin should be terminated 12 to 24 hours prior to CABG and fondaparinux should be discontinued 24 hours preoperatively. Whenever any of these agents are discontinued, they should be replaced immediately by UFH (Anderson et al., 2013).

MEDICATION MANAGEMENT FOR ACS PATIENTS

During the first few hours following FMC, the most important goals of medication therapy are improving the myocardial oxygen supply to demand ratio with anti-ischemic therapies and pain relief. Prevention of further platelet aggregation with DAPT is also imperative and has been discussed previously.

Analgesics

The most important analgesic in caring for ACS patients is morphine sulfate. Intravenous morphine is usually administered when cardiac ischemic symptoms are not relieved by nitroglycerin. In addition to providing analgesia, morphine also acts as an anxiolytic agent, and a venodilator. Venodilation can be particularly useful in reducing preload in patients presenting with pulmonary edema. Data from the CRUSADE registry has raised some concerns about the use of morphine in NSTE-ACS patients (Meine et al., 2005). Morphine administration in this observational study population was associated with an increased risk of death. This finding has led to a call for a randomized trial and to a downgrading of the NSTE-ACS guideline recommendation for morphine from a Class I to a Class IIb (Amsterdam et al., 2014).

Anti-Ischemic Therapies

There are multiple medications used to improve the myocardial oxygen supply to demand ratio. Oxygen is usually supplied via nasal cannula to patients with arterial oxygen saturations less than 90% or who have any signs of hypoxemia (Amsterdam et al., 2014). Other methods of delivery may be necessary based on the patient's overall clinical status. Routine use of supplemental oxygen for normoxic patients may have adverse effects, such as reduced coronary blood flow and increased risk of mortality (Moradkhan & Sinoway, 2010).

Nitrates decrease ventricular preload and wall tension, leading to a decrease in oxygen demand. They also cause coronary artery vasodilation that improves coronary blood flow. Initial nitroglycerin therapy often begins with sublingual tablets or spray administered in the prehospital setting. If no symptom relief is obtained, intravenous nitroglycerin can be administered. Parenteral nitroglycerin is indicated to treat persistent ischemia, HF, or hypertension (Amsterdam et al., 2014). Any form of nitroglycerin is contraindicated when sildenafil or vardenafil have been used within the past 24 hours, or tadalafil has been taken within the past 48 hours. Oral or topical nitrates can be administered when symptoms have been controlled for 12 to 24 hours. Sublingual or spray nitroglycerin should be prescribed at discharge for all ACS patients (Amsterdam et al., 2014; O'Gara et al., 2013).

Beta adrenergic blockers decrease myocardial oxygen demand primarily via inhibition of catecholamine effects at beta receptor sites on the surfaces of myocardial muscle cells, sinus node tissue, and the atrioventricular (AV) node. By decreasing the HR, these medications not only reduce myocardial oxygen demand, they also increase the duration of diastole, which, in turn, leads to increased coronary artery and collateral vessel blood flow (Amsterdam et al., 2014; Anderson et al., 2013).

For all ACS patients without contraindications, oral beta blockers should be initiated within the first 24 hours (Amsterdam et al., 2014; O'Gara et al., 2013). Contraindications to beta blocker therapy include HF, P-R interval greater than 0.24 seconds, second- or third-degree heart block, acute asthma, reactive airway disease, low cardiac output states, or increased risk of cardiogenic shock as evidenced by SBP less than 120 mmHg, HR greater than 110 beats per minute, or age more than 70 (Anderson et al., 2013; O'Gara et al., 2013). The medications that have been most studied in the setting of AMI include metoprolol, propranolol, and atenolol. Selective beta-1 agents, such as sustained release metoprolol succinate and bisoprolol, or the beta-1, alpha-1 blocker carvedilol, are recommended for NSTE-ACS patients with stabilized HF and LV systolic dysfunction (Amsterdam et al., 2014). Drugs with sympathomimetic effects, such as acebutolol or pindolol, are less desirable. Intravenous beta blockers may be considered on admission for STEMI patients if they are hypertensive or are experiencing ongoing ischemia (O'Gara et al., 2013). In the setting of NSTE-ACS, parenteral beta blockers may increase the risk of developing shock in those patients predisposed to this complication (Amsterdam et al., 2014).

Ongoing therapy with beta blockers following hospitalization is recommended for secondary prevention of heart disease. This recommendation is particularly strong for patients with a left ventricular ejection fraction (LVEF) less than 40%. In addition to reducing long-term mortality, these medications decrease the frequency of ventricular dysrhythmias, as well as reduce ischemia and reinfarction (Amsterdam et al., 2014). If tolerated, beta blockers should be continued for at least 3 years in uncomplicated MI patients without HF or hypertension (Smith et al., 2011).

Calcium channel blockers (CCBs) may be beneficial in treating patients with contraindications to beta blockers or who fail to respond to them (Amsterdam et al., 2014). Some studies of nondihydropyridine CCBs, verapamil, and diltiazem demonstrate that these medications can decrease reinfarction rates among patients without LV dysfunction (Pepine, Faich, & Makuch, 1998). Nondihydropyridine CCBs should be considered for anti-ischemic therapy if patients have contraindications to beta blockers; however, patients with significant LV dysfunction, P-R intervals longer than 0.24 seconds, or higher-grade heart block should not receive these drugs. Patients with recurrent ischemia who are already receiving beta blockers and nitrates should receive verapamil or diltiazem, provided these individuals have no contraindications (Amsterdam et al., 2014; O'Gara et al., 2013). When these CCBs are added to beta blocker therapy, there is an increased risk for bradycardia and conduction disturbances. Immediate-release nifedipine should not be administered, as it may cause hypotension and tachycardia (Furberg, Psaty, & Meyer, 1995).

Renin-Angiotensin-Aldosterone System Inhibition

Angiotensin-converting enzyme inhibitors (ACEI) and angiotensin receptor blockers (ARBs) inhibit the multiple deleterious effects of renin-angiotensin-aldosterone system activation that may occur with AMI. ACEI are the preferred agents unless the patient is intolerant. These medications prevent vasoconstriction, fluid retention, and maladaptive ventricular remodeling. They also prevent future major cardiac events in STEMI patients, especially those with anterior MI, a history of prior MI, an EF less than 40%, HF, and tachycardia (O'Gara et al., 2013). Oral forms of ACEI or ARBs should be initiated within 24 hours of patient presentation and continued indefinitely in patients who have an EF less than 40%, HF, hypertension, DM, or an anterior STEMI (Amsterdam et al., 2014; O'Gara et al., 2013). While benefits in 30-day survival have been seen with ACEI started in the first 24 hours following AMI, they should be used cautiously in this early time period, as these medications can cause hypotension or renal dysfunction (ACE Inhibitor Myocardial Infarction Collaborative Group, 1998). These agents are also considered "reasonable therapy" for other cardiac or vascular disease patients without contraindications (Amsterdam et al., 2014; O'Gara et al., 2013).

In addition to an ACEI or ARB, patients with an EF less than 40%, and either symptomatic HF or DM, should receive an aldosterone antagonist, such as spirono-lactone or eplerenone (Amsterdam et al., 2014; O'Gara et al., 2013). To be effective in reducing mortality, an aldosterone antagonist should be initiated within the first 7 days post-MI (Adamopoulos et al., 2009). Aldosterone antagonists should be avoided in hyperkalemia with K+ greater than 5.0 mEq/L or with renal dysfunction, defined as a creatinine greater than 2.5 mg/dL in men or greater than 2.0 mg/dL in women (Amsterdam et al., 2014). Patients receiving both an ACEI/ARB and an aldosterone antagonist should be monitored closely for the potential development of hyperkalemia. If this occurs, dosage adjustment or discontinuation of one or both of these medications might be necessary.

Lipid-Lowering Medications

Statins (3-hydroxy-3-methyl-glutaryl-CoA reductase inhibitors) are an essential component of both preventative and post-ACS care. Use of statins following ACS decreases the risk of mortality, recurrent MI, and revascularization even among patients with low-density lipoprotein (LDL) levels less than 70 mg/dL (Cannon et al., 2004; Lee et al., 2011). Initiation or continuation of statins is recommended for all ACS patients regardless of admission lipid levels, provided that there are no contraindications, such as end-stage liver disease (Amsterdam et al., 2014; O'Gara et al., 2013). For all ACS patients without contraindications, high-intensity therapy is recommended: atorvastatin 40 to 80 mg or rosuvastatin 20 to 40 mg daily (Amsterdam et al., 2014; O'Gara et al., 2013; Stone et al., 2013).

Avoidance of Nonsteroidal Anti-Inflammatory (NSAID) Medications

Selective cyclooxygenase II inhibitor (COX-2) and other NSAID medication use have been associated with adverse events including death, MI, reinfarction, HF, and renal failure, particularly in patients with atherosclerotic cardiovascular disease (ASCVD; Coxib and Traditional NSAID Trialists' Collaboration, 2013; Varas-Lorenzo et al., 2013). These agents should be discontinued on admission and should be avoided both during hospitalization and in the future for patients with CHD, particularly those with STEMI and NSTE-ACS (Amsterdam et al., 2014). Of these drugs, naproxen sodium appears to have the best safety profile (Coxib and Traditional NSAID Trialists' Collaboration, 2013; Varas-Lorenzo et al., 2013). The Prospective Randomized Evaluation of Celexicob Integrated Safety Versus Ibuprofen or Naproxen (PRECISION) trial comparing the safety of selective COX-2 inhibitors to nonselective agents in patients with cardiovascular disease is currently under investigation.

When considering discharge medications, providers should evaluate the need for chronic analgesic therapy to treat musculoskeletal pain. A step-wise approach starting with acetaminophen, nonacetylated salicylates, tramadol, or small doses of narcotics should be considered. If the aforementioned medications are not effective, nonselective NSAIDs, for example, naproxen, can be administered. Nonsteroidal anti-inflammatory agents that are somewhat more selective for COX-2 should be prescribed only when other recommended therapies have failed (Amsterdam et al., 2014).

Interactions Between Proton Pump Inhibitors (PPIs) and P2Y$_{12}$ Receptor Inhibitors

Aspirin and P2Y$_{12}$ receptor inhibitors, taken alone or in combination, can increase the risk of gastrointestinal (GI) bleeding. Strategies to reduce this risk have been considered and implemented for several years but have been plagued by concerns about interactions between clopidogrel and proton pump inhibitors. The concern stems from the competitive inhibition of PPIs with cytochrome P-450 (CYP) enzymes CYP2C19 and CYP3A, which metabolize clopidogrel from its prodrug to its active metabolite state. Concomitant use of PPIs potentially competes for CYP2C19 and CYP3A binding sites, which could lead to a decrease in the conversion of clopidogrel from its prodrug to active drug state. Prasugrel is less susceptible to inhibition as it uses additional CYP-450 pathways for its activation. Ticagrelor is an active drug in its original form and is metabolized by CYP3A4. Studies examining the clinical importance of the clopidogrel-PPI interaction have had mixed results (Abraham et al., 2010; Agewall et al., 2013). For this reason, certain PPIs are recommended for the prevention of GI bleeding in patients at high risk for this problem, but are not recommended for low-risk patients. High-risk patients include patients receiving DAPT who have had previous GI bleeding, patients receiving DAPT and warfarin, and patients with other conditions that place them at high risk of bleeding (Amsterdam et al., 2014). While histamine-2 receptor antagonists (H2RAs) have not been implicated in reduced P2Y$_{12}$ receptor inhibitor activity, these drugs are less effective in decreasing GI bleeding in patients receiving DAPT and are not recommended for prophylaxis in the ACS population (Abraham et al., 2010).

MEDICATION ADJUSTMENTS IN WOMEN AND THE OLDER ADULT

Both women and the older adult tend to have less muscle mass, which affects drug distribution. Smaller doses may be required for some medications, including prasugrel, which is adjusted or contraindicated based on the patient's weight.

In addition, older patients often have diminished renal function, which may affect drug clearance, and therefore necessitate downward dosage adjustments. Two different formulas, the Cockcroft-Gault equation and the Modification of Diet in Renal Disease formula, are commonly used to estimate kidney function and guide dosage changes for renally cleared medication. The results of these two formulas are not equivalent (Nyman et al., 2011) and may result in differing recommendations for medication adjustments. It is important to note that most studies involving ACS patients have used the Cockcroft-Gault equation when determining dosage changes related to renal function. It is therefore recommended that this equation be used in determining dosages of medications such as bivalirudin (Medicines Company, 2013) and enoxaparin (Medscape Reference, 2014). The older adult is also at increased risk of major bleeding with anticoagulants, fibrinolytics, and $P2Y_{12}$ receptor inhibitors. Providers should refer to specific cautions and contraindications for these medications before prescribing them, especially for patients older than 75 years.

PRE-DISCHARGE RISK ASSESSMENT

For both STEMI and NSTE-ACS patients, an estimation of future risk for cardiovascular events should be conducted. Two critical factors in determining future risk are continued ischemia and LVEF. An ejection fraction of less than 35% increases the risk of adverse events, including increased mortality. Other high-risk features include large areas of stress-induced ischemia or wall motion abnormalities detected during stress imaging (Amsterdam et al., 2014). In-hospital events, such as ventricular tachycardia or ventricular fibrillation (VT/VF), also increase post-discharge mortality, especially if they occur more than 48 hours following STEMI (O'Gara et al., 2013). Patients with high-risk features may benefit from an invasive strategy if they have not already had their coronary anatomy and heart function delineated (Amsterdam et al., 2014).

Low- and intermediate-risk NSTE-ACS patients may receive stress testing prior to discharge if they have been free of ischemia at rest or low-level activity for at least 12 to 24 hours. In addition, they should undergo a noninvasive determination of their LV function to further delineate their current status and future prognosis (Amsterdam et al., 2014).

STEMI patients who have undergone angiography and PCI will already have anatomic data concerning the extent of CHD. Most will also have angiographic determinations of left-ventricular function. For STEMI patients who received fibrinolysis, a predischarge exercise or pharmacologic stress test with imaging offers the advantage of an earlier determination of individuals who may need revascularization as opposed to undergoing noninvasive testing 3 or more weeks following hospitalization. Predischarge stress testing also assists in determining the efficacy of medication regimens and the patients' functional capacity (O'Gara et al., 2013).

Post-ACS patients frequently undergo echocardiography before discharge to determine the global left ventricular function, as well as to assess for wall-motion abnormalities. Patients with a predischarge EF of 40% or lower should have a repeat echocardiogram at least 40 days after discharge to determine the appropriateness of implantable cardioverter defibrillator therapy (O'Gara et al., 2013).

POST-DISCHARGE MANAGEMENT OF ACS PATIENTS

Optimizing functional status and quality of life are two important goals of post-ACS therapy. Another equally important goal is the reduction of risk for future cardiovascular events. Patient and family education prior to and following discharge should include information addressing these topics as well as medications and follow-up appointments. Continuity of care is essential to ensure continued evidence-based treatment. Communication between hospital-based and community-based providers is key to maintaining the best medical therapy.

Functional Status

Post-ACS patients should be evaluated for and referred to cardiac rehabilitation (CR) programs (Amsterdam et al., 2014). In addition to structured exercise prescriptions, CR usually includes educational offerings regarding medications, nutrition, and risk-factor reduction. Participation in these programs has been associated with a 26% reduction in CV mortality (Taylor et al., 2004). Martin et al. (2013) found that CR resulted in an increase in cardiopulmonary fitness, and that for each one metabolic equivalent of functional improvement, all-cause mortality decreased by 25%. Further, Jolliffe et al. (2001) noted that CR led to improvements in ability to perform activities of daily living. The initial evaluation for such programs includes an exercise stress test, if one was not performed predischarge. Exercise can be safely undertaken 1 to 2 weeks post-ACS in patients treated with PCI or CABG (Thompson, 2005). Patients who are unwilling or unable to enter a CR program for financial, logistical, or other reasons should be encouraged to walk daily.

Quality of Life

Participation in CR programs has been associated with improvement in health-related quality of life (Heran et al., 2011). Patients benefit from both improved functional capacity and social interaction with others who have had similar experiences. Assessment and treatment of depression in post-MI patients are also important. Major depression is fairly common among post-MI patients and has been independently associated with future cardiac events (de Jonge, van den Brink, Spijkerman, & Ormel, 2006). Citalopram or sertraline have been shown to be safe and effective in treating major depression in cardiac patients (Lesperance et al., 2007).

Sexual concerns have a significant impact on quality of life; it is important for health care providers to discuss the resumption of sexual activity with patients and their partners. It is safe to resume sexual activity 1 week following an uncomplicated MI. For patients who undergo CABG via a median sternotomy, it is recommended to defer resumption of sexual activity until the sternum is healed—approximately 6 to 8 weeks after surgery (Levine et al., 2012). In general, for CHD patients who are able to perform mild to moderate exercise, three to five metabolic equivalents, without signs or symptoms of ischemia, the risk of developing ischemia during sexual activity is very low (Drory, 2002). In fact, regular exercise decreases the risk of MI during sexual activity (Muller, Mittleman, Maclure, Sherwood, & Tofler, 1996).

Phosphodiesterase type 5 (PDE5) inhibitors can be used in the treatment of stable CHD patients with erectile dysfunction; however, they should not be prescribed for patients receiving nitrates as part of their routine medications. For patients using PDE5 inhibitors, nitrates should not be given within 24 hours of administration of sildenafil or vardenafil, or within 48 hours of tadalafil dosing. These agents cause vasodilation, which can lead to an additional drop in BP in patients receiving nitrates (Levine et al., 2012).

Risk Factor Reduction

Secondary prevention includes not only medications and exercise; it encompasses interventions targeted at known risk factors for CHD. One extremely important issue is smoking cessation; upon cessation, future cardiovascular mortality is reduced by almost 50% (Wilson, Gibson, Willan, & Cook, 2000). Tobacco abstinence must be addressed while the patient is in the hospital, and interventions must be continued postdischarge to be effective. Telephone follow-up and counseling appear to be the most effective intervention methods after discharge. The addition of medications, such as bupropion or varenicline, has not been found to significantly improve quit rates for patients immediately after hospitalization (Rigotti, Clair, Munafo, & Stead, 2012). Avoiding second-hand smoke is also recommended (Anderson et al., 2013).

Controlling preexisting conditions, such as hypertension, hyperlipidemia, and diabetes, decreases the risk of future cardiovascular events. The STEMI guidelines were published prior to the introduction of the Joint National Committee (JNC)-8 guidelines and advocate tighter BP control based on the JNC-7 guidelines—BP less than 140/90 or less than 130/80 in patients with diabetes or chronic kidney disease (O'Gara et al., 2013). The NSTE-ACS guidelines were published following the dissemination of JNC-8 and advocate the use of JNC-8 recommendations to control BP as part of CHD secondary prevention. For patients younger than the age of 60 and diabetics of all ages, the JNC-8 target BP remains less than 140/90 (James et al., 2014). Patients diagnosed with hypertension prior to their ACS event might have their BP controlled within the goals of the JNC-8 guidelines by taking medications recommended for the treatment of ischemia and remodeling according to the STEMI and NSTE-ACS guidelines. In this case, there is no need to change medications; however, dosages may need to be titrated.

One significant change in the JNC-8 guidelines is that beta blockers are not recommended as first-line agents for the control of hypertension (James et al., 2014). However, this stance is based on studies that are not specific to post-ACS patients. For the post-ACS population, beta blockers continue to be an important part of GDMT (Amsterdam et al., 2014; O'Gara et al., 2013). These agents need to receive priority over other medications with antihypertensive properties in the post-MI population due to their effects in reducing post-MI mortality (Amsterdam et al., 2014). If a patient's BP is still above the JNC-8 goals, and the patient is already receiving a beta blocker and ACEI, a thiazide-type diuretic would be reasonable to add as the next agent in the patient's post-ACS drug regimen. Drugs recommended as the primary agents for controlling hypertension according to JNC-8 are thiazide-type diuretics, ACEI, ARB, and CCBs (James et al., 2014).

Lifestyle modifications, a healthy diet, weight loss, and regular exercise are essential ongoing components of BP, hyperlipidemia, and diabetes management. A diet high in whole grains and fruits and vegetables, and low in sodium and saturated fats, such as the DASH diet, is recommended for CVD risk reduction. Sodium intake should be reduced to between 1,500 and 2,400 mg daily. Saturated fats should comprise only 5% to 6% of total calories, and trans fats should be eliminated. Exercise recommendations for healthy individuals include engaging in moderate- to vigorous-intensity physical activity for 40 minutes three to four times per week (Eckel et al., 2014). Of course, exercise goals need to be modified based on the individual patient and post-MI stress test results. As mentioned previously, CR is an important method for assisting patients with lifestyle modifications, particularly for encouraging safe and regular exercise.

Control of diabetes is important during the acute and recovery phases following ACS. Patients with diabetes have significantly higher risk of poor outcomes following an ACS admission, particularly in the first 3 months (Fava, Azzopardi, & Aguis-Muscat, 1997). The degree of glucose control during critical illness has been controversial. The use of insulin and glucose infusions has been investigated in the setting of AMI but has not been found to be beneficial in improving morbidity or mortality (Malmberg et al., 2005). In a large randomized controlled trial, Normo-glycaemia in Intensive Care Evaluation-Survival Using Glucose Algorithm Regulation (NICE-SUGAR), medical and surgical critical care patients who received intensive insulin control (glucose 81 to 108 mg/dL) experienced more episodes of hypoglycemia and also higher 90-day mortality when compared with patients managed "conventionally" (glucose ≤ 180 mg/dL). There was no apparent link between the number of episodes of hypoglycemia and decreased 90-day survival (Finfer et al., 2009). Based on these results, and considering previous studies, blood glucose should be treated to maintain levels less than 180 mg/dL (Amsterdam et al., 2014). No specific recommendations regarding glucose control appear in the STEMI guidelines.

In general, diabetics have more extensive CHD than patients with normogly-cemia. Because of the more extensive nature of CHD in diabetics, these patients are frequently referred for CABG rather than PCI. The long-term outcomes for diabetic patients have been better with CABG than with PCI, especially when internal mammary arteries are used for grafts (Farkouh et al., 2012). However, the use of bilateral internal mammary arteries, especially in diabetics, is associated with an increased risk of sternal infection (Nakano et al., 2008). Maintaining glucose levels less than 180 mg/dL using a continuous insulin infusion protocol during the early postoperative period is advocated to reduce the risk of sternal infection in patients with diabetes (Hillis et al., 2011).

COMPLICATIONS OF ACS

Serious, life-threatening complications of MI most commonly occur in the STEMI population. These complications include cardiogenic shock, VFWR, VSR, severe HF, and arrhythmias. Complications can occur at any time during the acute phase of MI, but most commonly occur from the first 24 hours to the first week (O'Gara et al., 2013).

Cardiogenic shock in the setting of acute STEMI or NSTEMI should be treated with immediate revascularization, preferably via PCI or CABG (Amsterdam et al., 2014; O'Gara et al., 2013). Fibrinolytic therapy should be reserved for STEMI shock patients whose anatomy, comorbid conditions, or other individual circumstances are not amenable to more direct forms of revascularization (O'Gara et al., 2013). The presentation and treatment of cardiogenic shock is discussed in a separate chapter.

Ventricular Free Wall Rupture

VFWR is the most devastating complication of MI, as rupture may result in rapid hemodynamic collapse due to severe tamponade and electromechanical dissociation. If thrombus formation in the pericardial space is successful in occluding the rupture, pseudoaneurysm may occur (Antman & Morrow, 2012). Immediate surgical intervention should be performed for VFWR, but mortality remains extremely high. Fortunately, VFWR is fairly rare—0.8% to 6.2% (Birnbaum et al., 2003). VFWR occurs more frequently in women, the elderly, and those patients receiving thrombolytics more than 14 hours from symptom onset, steroids, or nonsteroidal anti-inflammatory agents. It is also more likely to occur with a first-time MI or an anterior MI (O'Gara et al., 2013). The first symptom in these patients may be hemodynamic collapse with accompanying electromechanical dissociation. Those patients with a subacute presentation might have prolonged or atypical chest pain, nausea, hypotension, bradycardia, or transient electromechanical dissociation (Birnbaum et al., 2003). A wide variety of ECG changes have been associated with VFWR, but ST elevation in AVL in a patient with an anterior MI increases the risk of VFWR by more than fivefold (Yoshino et al., 2000). An echocardiogram is the single best test to determine VFWR. Typically, the echocardiogram reveals a large pericardial effusion and signs of cardiac compression. Temporizing methods while preparing for emergent surgical repair may include rapid infusion of IV fluids, and a percutaneous pericardiocentesis (Birnbaum et al., 2003).

Ventricular Septal Rupture

Rupture of the ventricular septum is another rare complication of MI, occurring in approximately 1% to 2% of cases. It is associated most commonly with anterior or inferior infarctions (Bhimji, 2013; Menon et al., 2000). Data from the SHOCK (Should We Emergently Revascularize Occluded Coronaries for Cardiogenic Shock) Trial Registry indicated that septal ruptures occurred around 16 hours post-MI. Patients who experienced VSR tended to be female and/or elderly. The in-hospital survival rate was only 13% (Menon et al., 2000). Cardiogenic shock often occurs as a result of a severe drop in the LVEF due to left-to-right ventricular shunting. This shunting of blood across the compromised ventricular septum causes a loud, harsh holosystolic murmur best heard at the left sternal border, and is often associated with a thrill (Bhimji, 2013). The presence and degree of shunting can be evaluated with echocardiography and Doppler imaging. Emergent cardiac surgical consultation should be initiated.

Papillary Muscle Rupture

Rupture of a papillary muscle occurs rarely but may cause cardiogenic shock due to resultant valvular incompetence and regurgitation. The posteromedial papillary muscle of the mitral valve is affected more often than the anterolateral muscle. Involvement of the posteromedial papillary muscle can be associated with inferior MIs, while the anterolateral papillary muscle is sometimes affected by an anterolateral infarction. Physical examination may reveal a new holosystolic murmur. Echocardiography with color-flow Doppler is key to distinguishing mitral regurgitation from VSR and determining the degree of regurgitation. Due to the risk of rapid hemodynamic deterioration, urgent cardiac surgical consult should be initiated. Hemodynamic monitoring should be instituted to guide therapy. A nitroglycerin or nitroprusside infusion may be started, provided that the SBP is 90 mmHg or above. If these measures fail to stabilize the patient, intraaortic balloon pump (IABP) therapy can be initiated (Antman & Morrow, 2012). While the mortality from emergent mitral valve replacement is high, 20%, outcomes are better overall than medical therapy alone or delayed surgical intervention (O'Gara et al., 2013).

Heart Failure

Decreased myocardial contractility can occur via a variety of mechanisms in the AMI setting. Reduced right or left ventricular ejection may result directly from infarction of significant portions of the myocardium. Impaired cardiac function may also be due to ischemic wall motion abnormalities, myocardial stunning, valvular incompetence, or arrhythmias. An echocardiogram may help to determine the mechanism and extent of the inciting problem. STEMI patients exhibiting signs of HF should undergo cardiac cathetherization if they have not been studied previously. Revascularization should be performed if appropriate (O'Gara et al., 2013). Medical management of severe HF is discussed in the chapter on acute decompensated heart failure (ADHF). In general, HF should be treated with ACEI and beta blockers that are titrated according to the patient's BP. Diuretics may also be required to relieve pulmonary vascular congestion (Antman & Morrow, 2012; O'Gara et al., 2013). In mild HF, 10 to 40 mg doses of intravenous furosemide given every 3 to 4 hours as needed is often effective (Antman & Morrow, 2012).

Right-Ventricular Infarction

As previously discussed, right ventricular infarction is frequently associated with inferior STEMI (Antman & Morrow, 2012). ST-segment elevations in V1 and the right-sided chest lead V_4R are indicative of right ventricular involvement. Patients with these ECG changes should be monitored carefully for the potential development of hypotension. Drops in BP that seem disproportionate to therapies, such as morphine or nitrates, are clues that the right ventricle may be impaired (Antman & Morrow, 2012). Other physical clues include the simultaneous findings of hypotension, jugular venous distention, and clear lung fields. Echocardiography can be used to confirm the diagnosis. When right ventricular infarction is suspected, nitrates and diuretics are contraindicated. Measures that improve right ventricular preload, including

IV fluids, may be beneficial (Antman & Morrow, 2012; O'Gara et al., 2013). Inotropic support may also be required (O'Gara et al., 2013), but, in most cases, should not be initiated until the effects of a normal saline fluid bolus have been assessed.

Arrhythmias

Many types of arrhythmias can occur post-MI. Multiple conditions that are often present in MI patients may contribute to this problem. Some predisposing factors include ongoing ischemia, hypoxemia, increased sympathetic discharge, increased vagal tone, increased atrial or ventricular wall stretching due to volume overload, and electrolyte disturbances (Antman & Morrow, 2012; O'Gara et al., 2013). Interventions aimed at treating or preventing these factors decrease the risk of arrhythmias and their detrimental effects.

The most feared arrhythmias are VT and VF. Hreybe and Saba (2009) reported that ventricular tachycardia occurred in 7.6% of the 21,807 MI patients in their data analysis from the National Hospital Discharge Survey 1996 to 2003. The incidence of ventricular fibrillation was 8.5% in the same study population. Fortunately, the incidence of in-hospital VT/VF has been declining in the age of modern STEMI management. In addition to reperfusion therapies, administration of beta blockers within 24 hours of admission has been linked to decreasing the occurrence of VF (Antman & Morrow, 2012). The timing of the occurrence of VT/VF greatly affects long-term prognosis. In STEMI patients, sustained VT or VF that develops prior to PCI doubles 90-day mortality, whereas VT/VF that occurs after PCI increases mortality fivefold for the same time period (Mehta et al., 2009). Sustained VT/VF should be treated according to the Advanced Cardiac Life Support Guidelines (Neumar et al., 2010; O'Gara et al., 2013). If sustained VT/VF occurs beyond the first 48 hours post-MI, and is not associated with a correctable cause, consideration should be given to potential implantation of a cardioverter-defibrillator prior to discharge (O'Gara et al., 2013). Isolated ventricular premature complexes (VPCs), nonsustained VT, and accelerated idioventricular rhythm are not associated with increased risk, and should not be treated in the early post-MI period (O'Gara et al., 2013).

Supraventricular arrhythmias, especially atrial fibrillation, are common post-MI. Their effects should be assessed quickly, as they may cause increased myocardial oxygen demand, ischemia, and hemodynamic compromise. Treatment should be guided by the Advanced Cardiac Life Support Guidelines (Neumar et al., 2010). Anticoagulation to decrease the stroke risk associated with atrial fibrillation should still be initiated but with additional caution due to DAPT (O'Gara et al., 2013).

Bradycardia is most often seen in the setting of inferior and posterior MI and is caused by increased vagal tone (Antman & Morrow, 2012). Bradycardia should be treated only if hypotension or other signs of instability occur. Intravenous atropine or temporary pacing can be used in these circumstances (O'Gara et al., 2013).

All forms of AV block can occur post-MI but are relatively infrequent—occurring in approximately 4% of STEMI patients (Hreybe & Saba, 2009). First-degree AV block usually does not require specific treatment; however, careful rhythm monitoring should continue, as AV block may be associated with bradycardia. Reduction or discontinuation of beta blockers or CCBs is not recommended unless the P-R interval exceeds 0.24 seconds or a higher degree block develops (Antman & Morrow, 2012). Second degree, Type I AV block (Wenckebach) is caused by AV node ischemia and does not require treatment unless the ventricular response rate falls below 50 beats per minute or the patient becomes symptomatic. Type II AV block results from damage to the conduction system below the bundle of His (Antman & Morrow, 2012). Temporary pacing, transvenous or transcutaneous, should be initiated for patients with Type II AV block due to the potential for this conduction disturbance to advance to complete heart block (CHB).

CHB is associated with a large infarct size and can occur with both anterior and inferior infarctions. Surprisingly, patients with inferior or posterior MIs are nearly four times more likely to develop CHB than patients with lateral or anterior MIs. A high-grade block usually develops more slowly in the setting of inferior MI and is often preceded by first-degree or Type I second-degree AV block (Hreybe & Saba, 2009). In addition, CHB in patients with inferior or posterior MIs is usually transient, lasting only a few days. CHB may occur suddenly in patients with anterior MI and is usually associated with significant septal infarction. Patients with anterior or lateral MIs who develop CHB, new LBBB, or bifascicular block should receive temporary pacing (Amsterdam et al., 2014; O'Gara et al., 2103).

Intraventricular Block

Conduction disturbances can develop as a result of damage to the His-Purkinje system in AMI patients. The anterior fascicle of the left bundle branch is more susceptible to injury, as it receives blood flow only from the septal perforators, which arise from the LAD artery. By contrast, the right bundle branch and the left posterior fascicle are supplied by both the LAD and the RCA. Because the left posterior fascicle is larger, more diffuse, and has a dual blood supply, extensive ischemia and injury must occur before its conduction is affected. When this degree of damage is present, both fascicles are usually involved and result in complete LBBB. New right bundle branch block (RBBB) develops more often than complete LBBB (Hass et al., 2011) and is most often associated with an anteroseptal MI (Antman & Morrow, 2012). The incidence of either complete LBBB or RBBB is 10% to 15% (Hass et al., 2011), and both types of complete BBB are associated with higher in-hospital and long-term mortality (Brilakis et al., 2001). Temporary pacemaker placement is recommended for these patients, especially those with new LBBB or bifascicular block in the setting of anterior or lateral MI (O'Gara et al., 2013).

Ongoing Ischemia and Complications

If serum biomarkers—particularly CK-MB—do not fall within the first 18 to 24 hours post-MI, and ST-segment elevation persists or returns, the patient may be experiencing recurrent infarction (Antman & Morrow, 2012). A common cause of recurrent ischemia or infarction is reocclusion of the infarct-related artery. If the patient has symptoms congruent with ST-segment elevation, they should undergo urgent angiography and possible PCI. Based on the patient's clinical status, other treatments that may be considered include nitroglycerin, sublingual or intravenous; beta blockers; or the use of intraaortic balloon counterpulsation (Antman & Morrow, 2012).

Pericarditis

It is important to distinguish chest discomfort due to pericarditis from ischemic pain. Typically, the chest discomfort from pericarditis worsens with deep breathing or lying flat and is lessened or relieved by sitting up and leaning forward. The discomfort also classically radiates to the trapezius ridge (Antman & Morrow, 2012). A friction rub may be heard at the left lower sternal border, especially if the patient leans forward. The ST-elevation that occurs with pericarditis is more widespread—across virtually all leads of the ECG. Closer examination may reveal P-R segment depression (LeWinter & Hopkins, 2015). Pericarditis can occur during hospitalization, but may also occur up to 8 weeks post-MI. Late-occurring pericarditis is referred to as Dressler's syndrome and usually is associated with a low-grade fever, malaise, leukocytosis, and an elevated sedimentation rate (Antman & Morrow, 2012; O'Gara et al., 2013). Aspirin 650 mg three or four times daily is the recommended treatment. Other NSAIDs and glucocorticoids should be avoided because they may interfere with scar formation post-MI (LeWinter & Hopkins, 2015; O'Gara et al., 2013). If high-dose aspirin is not effective, acetaminophen, colchicine, or narcotic analgesics may be used (O'Gara et al., 2013).

Left Ventricular Aneurysm

True ventricular wall aneurysms occur in approximately 5% of all STEMI patients, most often in those with an anterior MI (Antman & Morrow, 2012). The cause is thought to be increased intraventricular wall tension that stretches the infarcted tissue and creates a thin, bulging area of necrotic muscle and fibrous tissue. The apex of the LV is the most common region that is affected. Diagnosis is confirmed with echocardiography or ventriculography as part of a cardiac catheterization procedure. Persistent ST-elevation does not reliably correlate with the presence of left ventricular aneurysm. Large ventricular aneurysms interfere with efficient ejection of blood and can lead to HF. Because of inefficient ejection and a prothrombotic state post-MI, mural thrombi may form, increasing the risk of stroke and other organ damage. Mural thrombi may also develop in patients who have extensive MIs without aneurysm (Antman & Morrow, 2012). Long-term anticoagulation with warfarin is recommended for patients who develop left ventricular aneurysm (Antman & Morrow, 2012), and for 3 months in patients with akinesis or dyskinesis and mural thrombi (O'Gara et al., 2013). Ventricular aneurysms are also associated with a high risk of ventricular arrhythmias and sudden death. Surgical resection is one form of treatment; however, if the aneurysm is very large, there may not be adequate remaining contractile tissue to maintain a reasonable stroke volume (Antman & Morrow, 2012).

For full reference citations to this chapter, please see "Section References" in the back of the book, under the heading "Section V."

Acute Decompensated Heart Failure

LINDA BRIGGS AND KELLEY M. ANDERSON

In the United States, the primary diagnosis for hospitalization in individuals 65 years or older is acute decompensated heart failure (ADHF). This incidence represents approximately one million hospital admissions annually, a rate that has climbed over the past 30 years (Go et al., 2014). ADHF increases in incidence and prevalence with age. In the coming years, the number of hospitalizations for heart failure (HF) will reflect our increasingly aging population demographic. Additionally, hospitalization for HF is a marker of clinical instability portending future hospitalization and mortality, which is estimated at 30% 1 year after hospitalization (Yancy et al., 2013).

ADHF is generally attributed to an exacerbation of symptoms of chronic HF, either HF with reduced ejection fraction (HFrEF) or HF with preserved ejection fraction (HFpEF). In these patients with longstanding impaired cardiac performance, small insults, such as medication or dietary nonadherence, may precipitate the development of ADHF. Other causes of ADHF include new onset HF or HF as a complication of other conditions, including uncontrolled hypertension, acute coronary syndrome (ACS), arrhythmias, renal disease, or pulmonary disorders (Table 19.1). The Acute Decompensated Heart Failure Registry (ADHERE) demonstrated that in almost 50% of HF hospitalizations, patients had an admission blood pressure greater than 140/90 mmHg (Adams et al., 2005). Data from the Organized Program to Initiate Lifesaving Treatment in Hospitalized Patients with Heart Failure (OPTIMIZE-HF) registry indicated that pulmonary ailments, myocardial ischemia, and arrhythmias were the most common causes of decompensation (Fonarow et al., 2007). Because the etiologies of acute HF are vast, Gheorghiade, Filippatos, and Felker (2012) prefer the term "acute heart failure syndromes" (AHFS).

Most patients with ADHF have preexisting heart disease including hypertension or coronary heart disease (CHD), and often additional medical co-morbidities of pulmonary disease, renal disorders, and metabolic abnormalities. In the OPTIMIZE-HF registry, more than 50% of ADHF patients had a history of CHD (Fonarow et al., 2007). For patients with no preexisting cardiac disease, inciting events, such as myocardial ischemia, are often associated with ADHF (Gheorghiade et al., 2012).

Due to the vast variability in causes of hospitalization for HF, it is important to evaluate the etiology. In addition to the known or suspected etiology, the severity of the HF presentation, and the chronicity of HF all have implications for determining appropriate interventions and management strategies. Further, determining the type and extent of any previous cardiac dysfunction can aid in selecting appropriate diagnostic tests and treatment for patients presenting with ADHF.

TABLE 19.1 Precipitants and Causes of Acute Heart Failure

Events usually leading to rapid deterioration
- ▪ Rapid arrhythmia or severe bradycardia/conduction disturbance
- ▪ Acute coronary syndrome
- ▪ Mechanical complication of acute coronary syndrome (e.g., rupture of interventricular septum, mitral valve chordal rupture, right ventricular infarction)
- ▪ Acute pulmonary embolism
- ▪ Hypertensive crisis
- ▪ Cardiac tamponade
- ▪ Aortic dissection
- ▪ Surgery and perioperative problems
- ▪ Peripartum cardiomyopathy

Events usually leading to less rapid deterioration
- ▪ Infection (including infective endocarditis)
- ▪ Exacerbation of COPD/asthma
- ▪ Anemia
- ▪ Kidney dysfunction
- ▪ Nonadherence to diet/drug therapy
- ▪ Iatrogenic causes (e.g., prescription of an NSAID or corticosteroid; drug interactions)
- ▪ Arrhythmias, bradycardia, and conduction disturbances not leading to sudden, severe change in heart rate
- ▪ Uncontrolled hypertension
- ▪ Hypothyroidism or hyperthyroidism
- ▪ Alcohol and drug abuse

COPD, chronic obstructive pulmonary disease; NSAID, nonsteroidal anti-inflammatory drug.
Adapted from McMurray et al. (2012).

PATHOPHYSIOLOGY

The pathophysiology of ADHF is grounded on the principles of: (a) hemodynamic dysfunction due to pressure or volume overload, (b) neurohormonal dysregulation, and (c) cardiac remodeling of hypertrophy, fibrosis, and apoptosis. In ADHF the left ventricular ejection fraction may either be preserved or reduced. Diastolic dysfunction due to passive ventricular stiffness, abnormal relaxation, or both, can occur, resulting in elevated ventricular diastolic pressure and volume. In general, left ventricular involvement affects right heart function. A small percentage of individuals have isolated right ventricular dysfunction—usually due to right ventricular myocardial infarction (Gheorghiade et al., 2012). Elevated diastolic ventricular pressure and volume in either ventricle stimulates neurohormonal responses from the renin-angiotensin-aldosterone system (RAAS) and the sympathetic nervous system, resulting in ventricular remodeling and peripheral vasoconstriction, as well as sodium and water retention (Gheorghiade et al., 2012). In addition, increased chamber pressures escalate myocardial wall stress, leading to cardiac remodeling and interfering with coronary artery perfusion, thus creating or exacerbating myocardial ischemia. As a result, ventricular geometry and myocardial performance may be altered, leading to alterations in stroke volume and valvular regurgitation (Gheorghiade et al., 2012).

CLINICAL PRESENTATION

A careful and complete history and physical examination is essential in determining the probable contributors of the patient's acute distress. Generally, patients presenting with ADHF tend to be older than 65 years of age, with men and women affected equally, although women constitute a higher percentage of HFpEF patients. Elevated ventricular diastolic pressures may or may not be clinically evident and patients with underlying chronic HF may not demonstrate radiographic or clinical signs of congestion, such as jugular venous distention (JVD), crackles, and edema (Gheorghiade et al., 2012). The clinical features of ADHF vary from patient to patient and depend to some degree on the inciting cause; however, data from the ADHERE indicate that dyspnea is the most common symptom, occurring in 89% of the patients in this cohort (Fonarow & ADHERE Scientific Advisory Committee, 2005). The symptom of dyspnea related to HF presents in many forms including orthopnea, paroxysmal dyspnea, dyspnea with exertion, and dyspnea at rest. Orthopnea, or shortness of breath precipitated by lying flat or at various degrees of head elevation, is quite common. Coughing that develops when a patient is in a recumbent position is considered an "orthopnea equivalent" (Dumitru, 2014). Paroxysmal nocturnal dyspnea—awakening with shortness of breath—is also frequently reported. Dyspnea with exertion may be insidious or occur acutely and limit exercise tolerance and activities of daily living. Dyspnea at rest suggests an increasingly severe level of HF, New York Heart Association (NYHA) Class IV, and often results in patients seeking care in the emergency department.

Other common symptoms of ADHF include fatigue, anxiety, chest pain, and palpitations (Dumitru, 2014). In the ADHERE, 31% of patients admitted with ADHF complained of fatigue (Fonarow & ADHERE Scientific Advisory Committee, 2005). Chest pain associated with ADHF requires further evaluation for ischemic etiologies. Patients may also report an increase in body weight. Palpitations or syncope may indicate an arrhythmogenic etiology for ADHF. Mental confusion, as reported by patients or family members, may be attributable to decreased cardiac output and hypoxemia. Frank pulmonary edema or cardiogenic shock represent severe manifestations of ADHF.

PHYSICAL EXAMINATION

General physical examination findings of patients with ADHF may include visible respiratory effort if the work of breathing is significant. Alterations may be discovered in basic vital signs of respiratory rate, blood pressure, heart rate, and the oxygen saturation obtained via pulse oximetry. Although some patients with ADHF present with hypotension, especially those with HFrEF, chronic hypertension is the most common etiology of HFpEF, and many patients are admitted either normotensive or hypertensive (Gheorghiade et al., 2012; Yancy et al., 2013). Data from the ADHERE indicate that 50% of the cohort were admitted with a systolic blood pressure (SBP) greater than 140 mmHg, and only 2% had an SBP less than 90 mmHg (Fonarow & ADHERE Scientific Advisory Committee 2005). Hypertension in ADHF may be a result of volume overload, RAAS activation, and sympathetic responses to impaired cardiac output, or it may be the precipitating factor for ADHF, as in hypertensive emergency (Gheorghiade et al., 2012). Other characteristics of the blood pressure may assist in identifying causative disorders with a low diastolic blood pressure (DBP) potentially indicative of aortic regurgitation, or vasodilation that can occur in high output states including sepsis or hyperthyroidism (Gheorghiade et al., 2012). A decreased pulse pressure (SBP-DBP) in the setting of AHFS is associated with a 2.5-fold increase in mortality (Aronson & Burger, 2004). Proportional pulse pressure, the pulse pressure/SBP, correlates with cardiac output and values less than 25% correspond to cardiac indices less than 2.2 L/min/m^2 (McGee, 2012).

Another common characteristic of ADHF patients is tachycardia. Similar to hypertension, tachycardia may be a precipitating factor for ADHF, or it may be a sequela. Many patients will have arrhythmias, with 20% to 30% presenting with atrial fibrillation (AF) (Fonarow & ADHERE Scientific Advisory Committee, 2005; Gheorghiade et al., 2006). Although identifying an irregular or rapid pulse is the first step in determining a potential problem, continuous monitoring and an electrocardiogram (ECG) are important for a definitive diagnosis of rhythm disorders. Identification of arrhythmias is important to determining appropriate therapy. Patients with AF will require evaluation for therapeutic anticoagulation (Yancy et al., 2013). Persistent tachyarrhythmias with evidence of decreased perfusion potentially will require chemical or electrical cardioversion.

Clinical indications of increased volume and elevated left ventricular diastolic pressure include JVD, crackles, and peripheral edema (Gheorghiade et al., 2012). JVD and peripheral edema are indicative of right-sided HF; however, right ventricular failure most commonly occurs as a result of left ventricular dysfunction. Therefore, JVD is commonly considered a sign of left-sided HF, particularly when it occurs as part of the triad of JVD, crackles, and peripheral edema. Elevated jugular venous pressure in patients with known HF is associated with an increased risk for HF hospitalization and death (Drazner, Rame, Stevenson, & Dries, 2001). Crackles or rales, especially when associated with JVD and/or an S_3, indicate a probable elevation in pulmonary artery occlusion pressure (PAOP) (Gheorghiade & Pang, 2009). In patients with a sudden onset of severe hypertension or severe left ventricular dysfunction, overt pulmonary edema with frothy sputum and respiratory distress may occur. Peripheral edema should only be considered an indicator of HF when it occurs in association with JVD. Peripheral edema may be evident on admission, but may migrate to less evident body regions, such as the abdomen and sacrum, due to prolonged bed rest (Gheorghiade et al., 2012).

Abnormal heart sounds may also be present. Murmurs may indicate new or chronic valvular disorders. An S_3 is commonly associated with HF and is an early indicator of ADHF, highly specific for left ventricular systolic dysfunction (Dumitru, 2014; Gheorghiade et al., 2012). Indications of chronic HF include a lateral displacement of the point of maximal impulse (Gheorghiade et al., 2012). A right ventricular heave is indicative of right ventricular dysfunction.

Abdominal findings of ADHF include hepatomegaly and ascites, which are indicators of right-sided HF (Gheorghiade et al., 2012). Hepatojugular reflux, when present, indicates elevated left ventricular filling pressures and left-sided HF (Dumitru, 2014).

The peripheral vasculature may be notable for diminished peripheral pulses when cardiac output is reduced. Integumentary changes may include cyanosis, pallor, or alterations in temperature and moisture.

DIAGNOSTIC TESTING

Although the diagnosis of HF is based upon clinical findings, diagnostic evaluations increase the clinical accuracy of diagnosing ADHF, as the signs and symptoms are similar to other cardiac and pulmonary disorders. The chest x-ray (CXR), and B-type natriuretic peptide (BNP) or NT-proBNP provide data to discriminate between cardiopulmonary disorders and are readily available in the emergency department, which is the usual point of entry for patients hospitalized for HF. The CXR of patients with severe chronic HF may not reflect volume overload, although findings of patients with ADHF may demonstrate cephalization, interstitial edema, and pleural effusions (Gheorghiade & Pang, 2009; Martinez-Rumayor, Vazquez, Rehman, & Januzzi, 2010).

Elevations in BNP or NT-proBNP are useful in confirming the clinical impression of ADHF, especially in situations of clinical uncertainty due to competing diagnoses or presentations that reflect multiple comorbid conditions. The Breathing Not Properly Multinational Study established the role of BNP testing in the emergency department, validating a cutoff of greater than 100 pg/mL for the diagnosis of HF in individuals with a primary complaint of dyspnea (Maisel et al., 2004). A systematic review was completed to evaluate BNP values in diagnosing HF in the emergency department setting (Korenstein et al., 2007). BNP levels less than 100 pg/mL had a sensitivity of 90% and specificity of 74% for excluding the diagnosis of HF, whereas BNP levels greater than 400 pg/mL were consistent with a HF diagnosis with a sensitivity and specificity of 81% and 90%, respectively (Korenstein et al., 2007). The negative predictive value of BNP values in the emergency department has strong clinical utility.

In addition, BNP levels are useful as prognostic indicators. In a systematic review of 19 studies that evaluated BNP levels in individuals with all stages of HF and those who were asymptomatic, BNP was predictive of cardiac events or mortality (Doust, Pietrzak, Dobson, & Glasziou, 2005). In a substudy of 1,197 patients from the Multicenter Automated Defibrillator Implantation Trial (MADIT-CRT-Cardiac Resynchronization Therapy), the risk of symptomatic HF or death was lowest in patients with low baseline BNP levels or with BNP levels that reduced from high to low (Brenyo et al., 2013). In this cohort, patients in the cardiac resynchronization therapy group experienced more reductions in BNP compared with the implantable cardioverter defibrillator group during the 1-year follow-up period. The use of these biomarkers to guide ongoing therapy remains controversial (Yancy et al., 2013). However, BNP levels predischarge and change of levels during admission are also predictive of clinical stability, with lower levels and greater reduction in levels associated with improved prognosis. A retrospective study of hospital therapies tailored according to BNP measurements to obtain levels less than 250 pg/mL with intensive acute care management strategies demonstrated lower event rates (Valle et al., 2008).

Because a significant number of ADHF patients develop HF as a result of myocardial ischemia, an ECG and serum biomarkers of troponin I or T assays are a component of the initial evaluation (Yancy et al., 2013). Confirming the presence or absence of ACS is critical to determining appropriate therapy; suitable patients with ST elevation myocardial infarction (STEMI) with ADHF should be evaluated for emergent percutaneous coronary intervention (O'Gara et al., 2013). In addition to evaluating ischemia, the ECG may reveal AF or other arrhythmias, which may indicate the etiology of the current ADHF episode, with implications to direct therapy. Ventricular dysynchrony, as noted by a prolonged QRS complex, may warrant consideration for cardiac resynchronization device therapy once the acute condition has stabilized (Gheorghiade & Pang, 2009; Yancy et al., 2013).

Cardiac troponin levels may be elevated in HF due to more subtle myocardial necrosis in the absence of acute myocardial infarction (AMI) (Yancy et al., 2013). Based on cohort data from the ADHERE registry, elevated cardiac troponin levels in ADHF are associated with poorer outcomes and increased mortality (Peacock et al., 2008).

ST2 is a marker of myocardial fibrosis and is less subject to changes associated with age, gender, obesity, and chronic renal disease than BNP. However, ST2 is a complementary biomarker with natriuretic peptides because ST2 is not a diagnostic marker, although it is considered the best predictor of 1-year HF mortality (Rehman, Martinez-Rumayor, Mueller, & Januzzi, 2008). The 2013 American College of Cardiology Foundation/American Heart Association (ACCF/AHA) HF guidelines provide a IIB recommendation for ST2 for risk stratification in acute and chronic HF for the evaluation of myocardial fibrosis (Yancy et al., 2013). ST2 is a relatively new biomarker in clinical practice; an international ST2 consensus panel published a report on ST2 for acutely decompensated HF in January 2015 (Januzzi, Mebazaa, & DiSomma, 2015). The consensus document details that in ADHF ST2 is a strong predictor of HF, HF severity, and HF complications (Januzzi et al., 2015). Galectin 3 is an additional emerging biomarker of myocardial remodeling and fibrosis. One study of 115 patients who presented with dyspnea to the emergency department were evaluated for galectin 3, which was correlated for mortality for a period of up to 4 years (Shah, Chen-Tournoux, Picard, van Kimmenade, & Januzzi, 2010). A comparison of ST2 and galectin 3 was conducted in 876 HF patients with a median follow-up of 4.2 years. In this study, ST2 demonstrated better predictive risk stratification (Bayes-Genis et al., 2014).

Other important serum laboratory tests in the initial assessment of ADHF include serum electrolytes including calcium and magnesium, as well as measures of renal function including blood urea nitrogen (BUN), creatinine, and estimated glomerular filtration rate. Renal dysfunction is frequently present at the time of admission (Heywood et al., 2007). Further, BUN and creatinine levels are important prognostic indicators in ADHF (Gheorghiade et al., 2012). Mild hyponatremia is present in approximately 25% of ADHF patients on admission (Gheorghiade et al., 2007). Baseline serum potassium and magnesium levels are important to guide replacement during diuretic therapy. Additional blood tests recommended for all initial HF evaluations include complete blood count, glucose, liver profile, fasting lipid panel, and thyroid-stimulating hormone (Yancy et al., 2013).

An echocardiogram should be a component of the initial evaluation of ADHF patients (Yancy et al., 2013), either in the emergency department setting or during the hospitalization, preferably at the earliest opportunity. Echocardiographic information for the assessment of ADHF includes ventricular ejection fraction, ventricular size, ventricular wall thickness, valvular function, diastolic function, filling pressures, and wall motion abnormalities.

Other noninvasive imaging, such as MRI and cardiac computed tomography (CCT), can determine myocardial viability and coronary atherosclerosis, which may provide additional information regarding the etiology of the ADHF. Disadvantages of MRI and CCT are the requirement to be supine in patients who often have orthopnea and the reduction of diagnostic accuracy with high heart rates, both common findings in ADHF (Yancy et al., 2013). When echocardiograhic images are not adequate, MRI can provide evaluation of left ventricular ejection fraction. Additionally, MRI is useful in the evaluation of infiltrative disorders.

Invasive diagnostic testing in ADHF is appropriate in specific circumstances. If myocardial ischemia is the suspected etiology, coronary arteriography is reasonable if the patient is otherwise a candidate for revascularization. Hemodynamic monitoring via a pulmonary artery (PA) catheter should be initiated for patients with acute respiratory distress or suspected cardiogenic shock, when clinical assessment is not adequate to determine therapy. PA catheters may also guide therapy in patients receiving vasoactive medications (Gheorghiade et al., 2012; Yancy et al., 2013).

RISK STRATIFICATION

There are several tools to predict the in-hospital mortality of patients with ADHF. These tools differ from those used to assess patients with chronic stable HF. The ADHERE Classification and Regression Tree (CART) is one method of determining risk for patients admitted with AHFS. The advantage of this tool is that it employs three commonly performed measurements—SBP, BUN, and serum creatinine—to determine low, intermediate, and high risk of in-hospital mortality. Critical values in this assessment are BUN equal to or greater than 43 mg/dL, SBP less than 115 mmHg, and serum creatinine equal to or greater than 2.75 mg/dL. A patient with none of these characteristics has a predicted mortality of less than 2.1%, while a patient with all three traits has a predicted mortality of 21.9% (Fonarow & the ADHERE Scientific Advisory Committee, 2005).

A similar but slightly more complex risk stratification tool is the Get With the Guidelines—HF Risk Score for in-hospital mortality. Variables used to predict risk include heart rate, SBP, BUN, serum sodium, age, race, and history of chronic obstructive pulmonary disecse (COPD). Risk is computed by the number of points accrued for each indicator, and ranges from less than 1% to greater than 50% (Peterson et al., 2010).

Using data from patients who are 65 years of age or older in the OPTIMIZE-HF registry, Kociol et al. (2011) determined that discharge BNP is a strong predictor of 1-year mortality and the combined outcome of 1-year mortality and hospitalization. This prediction model used a logarithmic transformation of BNP values rather than the actual laboratory value, making this tool less easily applied by clinicians. ST2 is an emerging biomarker of myocardial fibrosis with independent and additive predictive ability for 1-year mortality with BNP (Yancy et al., 2013).

MANAGEMENT

Two primary goals of treatment for ADHF are to: (1) identify and treat any correctable causes, such as hypertension, arrhythmia, and ischemia; and (2) optimize cardiac function while protecting the heart and kidneys (Gheorghiade et al., 2012). Patients with new onset HF are more likely to have correctable causes, such as acute MI. Therefore, determining whether the patient has worsening chronic HF or new-onset

TABLE 19.2 Initial Management for Acute Heart Failure Syndromes (AHFS)*

1. Treat immediate life-threatening conditions/stabilize patient	Life-saving measures may precede or parallel diagnostic evaluation (i.e., unstable arrhythmia, flash pulmonary edema, STEMI)
2. Establish the diagnosis	Based on medical history, signs (JVD, S_3, edema), symptoms (dyspnea), biomarkers (e.g., BNP), and CXR
3. Determine clinical profile and begin initial treatment	Key components include HR, BP, JVP, presence of pulmonary congestion, ECG, CXR, renal function, troponin, BNP, pulse oximetry, history of CAD
4. Determine and manage the cause or precipitant	Identifying the cause such as ischemia, hypertension, arrhythmias, acute valvular pathologies, worsening renal function, uncontrolled diabetes, and/or infectious etiologies is critical to ensure maximal benefits from HF management
5. Alleviate symptoms (e.g., dyspnea)	Usually a diuretic with or without other vasoactive agents. Morphine may also be used for pulmonary edema†
6. Protect/preserve myocardium and renal function	Avoid hypotension or increase in HR, particularly in patients with CAD. Use of inotropes should be restricted to those with low-output state (low BP with organ hypoperfusion)
7. Make disposition	Majority are admitted to telemetry, with a small number discharged home. Robust evidence to support risk stratification and disposition identifying the low-risk patient for safe discharge with close outpatient follow-up is lacking

BNP, B-type natriuretic peptide; BP, blood pressure; CAD, coronary artery disease; CXR, chest x-ray; ECG, electrocardiogram; HF, heart failure; HR, heart rate; JVD, jugular venous distention; JVP, jugular venous pressure; STEMI, ST-segment elevation myocardial infarction.

*These steps usually occur in parallel, not series.

†Retrospective data suggests morphine is associated with worse outcomes.

Reprinted from Gheorghiade and Pang (2009, p. 564), with permission from Elsevier.

HF is an important decision point in the emergency department. Initial management concerns are presented in Table 19.2. Continuing or initiating guideline-directed medical therapy (GDMT) is important, although it may require monitoring and titration during the acute phase. Reducing or discontinuing beta blocker therapy should only occur in special circumstances, such as low cardiac output, severe volume overload, or a history of recent beta blocker therapy changes. A beta blocker should be initiated for naïve patients once intravascular vasoactive and diuretic medications have been discontinued and volume status has been optimized. Aldosterone antagonists, angiotensin-converting enzyme inhibitors (ACEI), or angiotensin receptor blockers (ARBs) may be decreased or temporarily discontinued if renal function or hemodynamic status is compromised on admission (Yancy et al., 2013).

Based on the clinical presentation of ADHF, therapeutic targets and interventions are described in Table 19.3. In addition, there is an entire portfolio of resources available for the effective and evidence-based treatment of hospitalized HF patients based on data from the Get With the Guidelines Heart Failure registry. The clinical tools include order sets, pathways and algorithms, and patient-education materials (American Heart Association [AHA], 2014).

Oxygen Therapy

Supplemental oxygen should be initiated to achieve a PaO_2 greater than 60 mmHg or an oxygen saturation greater than 90%. For patients with SaO_2 values less than 90% or evidence of pulmonary edema on high-flow oxygen, noninvasive ventilation

TABLE 19.3 AHFS Presentation, Targets of Therapy, and Therapeutic Options

Clinical Presentation	Targets of Therapy	Therapeutic Options
Hypertension, SBP > 160 mmHg	Blood pressure control Volume management	Vasodilators Loop diuretics
Normal or moderately increased SBP	Volume management	Loop diuretic Consider vasodilator
Hypotension, SBP < 90 mmHg	Improve cardiac output	Inotropes with vasodilatory properties Consider digoxin Consider vasopressor Consider mechanical assist device
Cardiogenic shock	Improve cardiac contractility	Inotropes Consider vasoactive medications Consider mechanical assist device Consider corrective surgery
Acute pulmonary edema	Blood pressure control Volume management	Vasodilators Diuretics Invasive or noninvasive ventilation Consider morphine sulfate
Acute coronary syndrome	Coronary revascularization Improve ischemia	Reperfusion therapies

AHFS, acute heart failure syndromes; SBP, systolic blood pressure.
Source: Gheorghiade and Pang (2009).

may be necessary (Gheorghiade & Pang, 2009). Intubation and positive-pressure mechanical ventilation should be reserved for hypoxemic patients who are unable to tolerate noninvasive ventilation or are unable to maintain a patent airway (Gheorghiade et al., 2012).

Diuretics

Volume overload and congestion is treated with intravenous loop diuretics. For patients on chronic loop diuretic therapy, the initial intravenous dose should be equal to or more than the usual daily dose. Loop diuretics may be administered as intermittent boluses or a continuous infusion. The Diuretic Optimization Strategies Evaluation (DOSE) trial was a prospective, randomized trial of 308 participants with ADHF assigned to bolus every 12 hours or continuous infusion in high-dose and low-dose groups (Felker et al., 2011). The primary endpoints of this study were patient symptoms and change in serum creatinine. The study revealed no significant difference in renal function or patient symptom assessment between the modes of administration or dosing. A systematic review of eight trials compared the efficacy and adverse effects of continuous versus bolus loop diuretic therapy (Salvador, Rey, Ramos, & Punzalan, 2005). The review concluded that there was insufficient evidence for a conclusive recommendation, although the data suggests improved diuresis and safety with continuous diuretic infusion.

The maximum total furosemide dose for the first 6 hours of therapy should not exceed 100 mg. Twenty-four-hour total doses should be no more than 240 mg (Gheorghiade et al., 2012). In addition to loop diuretic therapy, a concurrent low-dose dopamine infusion may enhance renal perfusion and diuresis (Yancy et al., 2013). If the response to diuretics is inadequate, higher doses of the loop diuretic can be administered or an additional diuretic of a different class, a thiazide, can be prescribed (Yancy et al., 2013). For severe HF, metolazone may be prescribed 2.5 to 5.0 mg orally once or twice daily with a loop diuretic. Close monitoring of vital signs, urine output, and body weight should be conducted. Baseline, and at least daily, creatinine, BUN, and electrolyte monitoring and replacement should be performed (Gheorghiade et al., 2012; Yancy et al., 2013). There is no conclusive evidence that either serial BNP or hemodynamic monitoring improves outcomes. Symptomatic relief, negative fluid balance, and changes in physical findings are important indicators of clinical status (Yancy et al., 2013).

Vasodilator Infusions

When patients are not hypotensive, infusion of vasodilator medications such as nitroglycerin, nitroprusside, or nesiritide can be considered adjunctive therapy to relieve symptoms. Nitroprusside is advantageous in patients with severe hypertension or severe mitral regurgitation, but has the potential to cause marked hypotension. Accordingly, this medication should be used in the intensive care unit and BP monitoring should be via arterial line. Nesiritide, a recombinant BNP, may also cause significant hypotension (Yancy et al., 2013). Early studies suggested that nesiritide was associated with increased mortality, but more recent studies have not supported this conclusion. Still, it is not recommended for routine use in ADHF (O'Connor et al., 2011). Currently, there is no data to support that IV vasodilators improve outcomes; however, they can be prescribed for relief of dyspnea in selected patients (Yancy et al., 2013).

Vasopressin Antagonists

Patients who are hyponatremic and volume overloaded are at risk for cognitive impairment, with severe hyponatremia constituting a life-threatening situation. The etiology of the fluid and electrolyte imbalance should be ascertained and the underlying cause treated. Fluid restriction is usually the first intervention for volume overload and hyponatremia. If initial measures are not successful in correcting the imbalance, short-term treatment with tolvaptan, a V_2-selective vasopressin antagonist, or conivaptan, a non-selective vasopressin antagonist, can be considered (Yancy et al., 2013). The Efficacy of Vasopressin Antagonism in Heart Failure Outcome Study with Tolvaptan (EVEREST) trials were randomized controlled trials comparing tolvaptan versus placebo within 48 hours of ADHF admission (Gheorghiade et al., 2007; Konstam et al., 2007). Although tolvaptan did not demonstrate improvement in mortality or HF hospitalization, there was significant improvement in serum sodium, body weight, edema, and dyspnea without significant adverse effects. Long-term therapy with vasopressin antagonists is not recommended (Yancy et al., 2013).

Inotropic Support

The inotropic agents dopamine, dobutamine, and milrinone may be considered in the treatment of AHFS. Dopamine may encourage renal perfusion at low doses, and at slightly higher doses provide both blood pressure and inotropic support. Milrinone decreases both systemic and pulmonary vascular resistance and can cause hypotension. Low-dose dobutamine may also cause hypotension. The use of these agents should be for temporary support to preserve end-organ function and to maintain systemic perfusion until more definitive therapy, such as mechanical circulatory support (MCS) or cardiac transplant, can be initiated. Short-term use for prevention of hypotension and end-organ damage is reasonable for patients with impaired left ventricular function. Long-term intravenous inotropic support may be considered for symptom control in selected patients, particularly for palliative therapy; although in general, intermittent or long-term use is not recommended and may be harmful (Yancy et al., 2013).

Digoxin

Digoxin is not an appropriate medication for the initial treatment of ADHF. It is more commonly prescribed in the setting of relatively stable chronic HF, although its use has declined. Once GDMT has been instituted, digoxin may be added with the intent of reducing readmissions and improving quality of life for patients who remain symptomatic. However, a retrospective study of Medicare beneficiaries hospitalized with ADHF revealed that for patients with an ejection fraction less than 45%, a new prescription for digoxin was significantly associated with a decrease in 30-day and 1-year readmission, as well as mortality (Ahmed et al., 2014). Digoxin may also be used for rate control in AF following the initiation of a beta blocker, although beta blockers are considered first-line agents for rate control of AF in HF (Yancy et al., 2013). When HF results from AF, rhythm control should be attempted (Yancy et al., 2013). If the onset of AF is known to be less than 48 hours, the patient may be a candidate for electrical cardioversion. Patients with AF for more than 48 hours or of unknown duration should be prescribed medications for rate control and for the prevention of thromboembolism. Elective cardioversion should then be considered after 4 to 6 weeks of effective anticoagulation (Yancy et al., 2013).

Morphine Sulfate

In patients with dyspnea unrelieved with diuretics, morphine sulfate may relieve symptoms in some patients due to its properties as a venous dilator and weak arterial dilator. The opiate is usually administered in dosages of 2 to 4 mg intravenously. There are no randomized controlled trials with morphine in ADHF, and some studies suggest an increase in mortality associated with the administration of this medication, although its use is commonly associated with the combined conditions of ACS and ADHF.

Anticoagulants

Patients with ADHF are at risk for thromboembolism even if they do not experience AF. Conditions often associated with ADHF, such as reduced cardiac output and increased systemic venous pressure, increase the likelihood of thromboembolism. According to the 2013 HF guidelines from the ACCF/AHA, patients admitted for decompensated HF benefit from thromboembolism prophylaxis. Recommendations include enoxaparin 40 mg subcutaneously (SQ) daily or unfractionated heparin 5,000 units SQ every 8 hours provided the patient has adequate renal function, defined as a serum creatinine under 2.0 mg/dL (Yancy et al., 2013).

ULTRAFILTRATION

Ultrafiltration is an additional short-term mechanism to remove water and electrolytes by venous blood filtration. The Ultrafiltration versus Intravenous Diuretics for Patients Hospitalized for Acute Decompensated Congestive Heart Failure (UNLOAD) trial randomized 200 patients to intravenous diuretics or veno-venous ultrafiltration (Costanzo et al., 2007). Primary endpoints were weight loss, dyspnea, BUN, creatinine, electrolytes, and hypotension. Analysis of these factors demonstrated an improvement in weight loss with ultrafiltration. Additional benefits included decreased length of stay, a reduction in unscheduled medical visits for HF, and fewer rehospitalizations at 90 days (Costanzo et al., 2007). The Cardiorenal Rescue Study in Acute Decompensated Heart Failure (CARRESS-HF) trial randomized 188 patients admitted with ADHF with declining renal function and congestion to ultrafiltration versus a stepped diuretic strategy (Bart et al., 2012). Ultrafiltration was associated with an increase in adverse events including an increase in creatinine levels without a difference in weight loss (Bart et al., 2012). In patients unresponsive to diuretic therapy, ultrafiltration may be considered as an adjunctive strategy to decrease volume overload and to improve the symptoms of congestion. Benefits of ultrafiltration include sodium removal, increased diuretic responsiveness, and decreased neurohormone levels (Yancy et al., 2013). This therapy is most often provided in consultation with a nephrologist and requires specialized equipment and trained health care providers.

FLUID AND SODIUM RESTRICTION

ACCF/AHA guidelines suggest that fluid restriction to 1.5 to 2.0 liters per day may be considered for patients with ADHF, especially those with hyponatremia (Yancy et al., 2013). However, aggressive fluid and sodium restriction was not supported in a randomized trial of 75 patients assigned to either standard diet and liberal fluid intake or a fluid (800 mL/day) and sodium (800 mg/day) restricted diet (Aliti et al., 2013). In this study, the participants who were randomized to the aggressive fluid and sodium restriction experienced greater thirst, without effect of weight loss or clinical stability, at 3 days (Aliti et al., 2013).

MECHANICAL CIRCULATORY SUPPORT

Patients with HF who experience decompensation without improvement with medical management may benefit from short- or long-term MCS to improve cardiac output. MCS has three primary indications: as a bridge to recovery (BTR), bridge to transplantation (BTT), or as destination therapy (DT). Short-term MCS is indicated as a BTR after an acute cardiac event to optimize clinical function and to preserve neurologic status, or as a temporary measure until a long-term device can be implanted. General indications for long-term MCS include left ventricular ejection fraction less than 25%, NYHA functional Class III or IV on guideline-directed therapy, high predicted 1- to 2-year mortality, or chronic parenteral inotropic therapy. The Interagency Registry for Mechanically Assisted Circulatory Support (INTER-MACS) provided the 6th report of data from 2006 to 2013 with over 12,000 patients enrolled in the registry (Kirklin et al., 2014). DT represents the largest proportion of MCS implantations, with continuous flow device implantations increasing from 14.7% during the period 2006 to 2007 to 41.6% during 2011 to 2013, with a concurrent decline in listings for cardiac transplantations. The registry demonstrates that survival for continuous-flow left ventricular assist devices has improved to 80% for the first year (Kirklin et al., 2014).

TRANSITIONS IN CARE

The issues in HF are multifaceted and include the incorporation of patient factors, HF characteristics, and GDMT to ensure appropriate acute care management and successful discharge transitions (Table 19.4). A HF hospitalization is a clinical marker associated with adverse posthospitalization events including vulnerability for rehospitalizations and mortality. When ADHF patients are stabilized, they may be discharged to their homes or transferred to a lower acuity level of care. Prior to discharge or transfer, patients should reach their optimal volume status and be transitioned from intravenous to oral diuretics, with adequate blood pressure and heart rate control. GDMT should be instituted and optimized. The cause of the decompensation episode and current heart function should be determined either predischarge or during early follow-up visits (Yancy et al., 2013).

Patient and family education is a key component in maintaining quality of life and reducing rehospitalizations. An interdisciplinary educational approach facilitates delivery of guideline-directed recommendations for diet, exercise, and medications. Social services and care management assist the patient and family with financial issues, care providers, durable medical equipment, and rehabilitative placement as needed. Communication and coordination of care between hospital personnel and outside care providers is critical in optimizing care and preventing readmissions. For patients discharged home, a follow-up visit should be arranged within 7 to 14 days, and/or telephone conversation within 3 days (Yancy et al., 2013). The plan of care, including medication reconciliation, should be immediately available to the clinicians assuming care, regardless of setting. Essential information includes nutrition, dietary or fluid restrictions, medications, activity level, weight monitoring, and warning signs that require contacting their health care providers

TABLE 19.4 Multifaceted Issues in Heart Failure

Stable >>>>>>>>>>>>>>>>>>>>>>>>>>>>>>>>>>>>> Decompensated >>>>>

Patient Factors	HF Characteristics	Management	Hospitalization	Discharge
Demographics Age Gender Ethnicity	**Etiology** Ischemic disease Hypertension Valvular Arrhythmias	**Non-Pharmacological** Outpatient visits Multidisciplinary Telephone Education Sodium/fluid	**Symptoms** Dyspnea Fatigue Orthopnea PND	**Discharge Planning** Length of stay Comprehensive Follow-up Timing Specialist Outpatient care Education
Co-morbidities Ischemic disease Hypertension Valvular Arrhythmias Renal insufficiency Anemia Sodium Cognitive function Pulmonary disease	**HF Type** HFpEF HFrEF ALVD Mixed	**Pharmacological** ACEI/ARB BB Diuretics Digoxin Aldosterone agonist Statin	**Clinical Characteristics** VS - HR/BP Pulmonary congestion S_3 JVP Hepatojugular reflux Edema Ascites Oxygen saturation Ambulation	**Disposition** Home Home health Institutional Hospice
Psych Attributes Knowledge Anxiety Depression Substance abuse Adherence QOL Self-care	**HF Classification** NYHA I-II AHA A-D	**Devices/Surgery** Resynchronization ICD LVAD Transplant	**Diagnostic** Biomarkers Renal function Echocardiogram Electrocardiogram Chest X-ray PA catheter	
Social Attributes Support Financial			**Acute Treatment** Pharmacologic agents Diuretics Vasodilators Vasopression antagonists Inotropes Digoxin Oxygen Monitoring Weight Intake/output Education Ultrafiltration	

ACEI/ARBs, angiotensin-converting enzyme inhibitors/angiotensin receptor blockers; AHA A-D, American Heart Association A-D; ALVD, asymptomatic left ventricular dysfunction; BB, beta blocker; HF, heart failure; HFpEF, HF with preserved ejection fraction; HFrEF, HF with reduced ejection fraction; ICD, implantable cardioverter defibrillator; JVP, jugular venous pressure; LVAD, left ventricular assist device; NYHA I-II, New York Heart Association I-II; PA, pulmonary artery; PND, paroxysmal nocturnal dyspnea; QOL, quality of life; VS-HR/BF, vital signs-heart rate/blood pressure.

or seeking emergency care (Yancy et al., 2013). For chronic HF patients in particular, consideration should be given to the evaluation for referral to specialty HF disease management clinics; cardiac rehabilitation; electrophysiology services for cardiac electronic implantable devices; centers with advanced therapies of assist devices and cardiac transplantation; nutritional therapy for sodium, fluid recommendations, or for cardiac cachexia; and palliative or hospice care for end-of-life considerations. All patients should be evaluated for advanced directives.

For full reference citations to this chapter, please see "Section References" in the back of the book, under the heading "Section V."

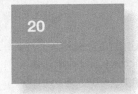

Shock States: Cardiogenic and Obstructive

LINDA BRIGGS

CARDIOGENIC SHOCK

Cardiogenic shock (CS) has many etiologies, some due to chronic disease processes and others due to acute problems. Irrespective of the etiology, CS is life threatening, with an overall in-hospital mortality of 57% (Ren, 2014). However, if providers are vigilant in monitoring for signs and symptoms suggesting its onset, interventions can be initiated to prevent progression to overt shock or to provide life-supporting therapies, such as ventricular-assist devices or cardiac transplantation.

Etiology

The most common cause of CS is acute myocardial infarction (MI). Still, there are other important etiologies that must be considered. Acute causes other than MI include heart failure (HF), myocardial contusion, cardiopulmonary bypass, arrhythmias, myocarditis, Takotsubo cardiomyopathy, endocarditis, chordae tendineae rupture, and aortic dissection (Ren, 2014; Reynolds & Hochman, 2008). Metabolic disturbances, such as acidosis, hypocalcemia, and hypophosphatemia, may cause or exacerbate CS (Ren, 2014). Medications with myocardial depressant effects, such as beta blockers, calcium channel blockers (CCBs), and antiarrhythmics, may impair left ventricular (LV) function and precipitate CS, particularly in the setting of MI (Ren, 2014). Medications with direct cardiotoxic effects—such as doxorubicin—do not usually abruptly precipitate CS, but can diminish LV function over time. Chronic disorders that can lead to CS include hypertrophic cardiomyopathy, aortic stenosis, and mitral stenosis. When these chronic disorders are present, acute stresses—such as severe hypertension or infection—can lead to decompensation, and ultimately to shock (Reynolds & Hochman, 2008).

Approximately 5% to 10% of acute MI patients develop CS, occurring more commonly in the setting of ST-segment elevation myocardial infarction (STEMI); however, approximately 2% of non-ST-segment elevation myocardial infarction (NSTEMI) patients develop CS. The most common type of MI associated with CS is an anterior MI. Further, CS due to ischemic causes is often precipitated by the loss of more than 40% of LV muscle (Ren, 2014). It is also important to note that women are more likely than men to develop CS in the setting of MI (Akhter et al., 2009; Ren, 2014). Further, ventricular septal rupture, papillary muscle rupture, and severe mitral regurgitation, all precipitants of CS, are more common in women (Wong et al., 2001). Individuals who are elderly, have diabetes, or have a history of a previous inferior MI are also at increased risk for CS following MI (Ren, 2014).

Pathophysiology

In CS related to myocardial ischemia, both systolic and diastolic functions can be adversely affected. Lack of adequate blood flow can affect contractility, not only in the region supplied by the occluded artery, but also in more remote regions. As systolic function declines, and stroke volume and aortic pressure decrease, there is an overall decrease in coronary perfusion that is exacerbated by any preexisting coronary heart disease (CHD), leading to further decreases in contractility. Diastolic function is impaired due to ischemia-related decreases in myocardial compliance (Ren, 2014; Reynolds & Hochman, 2008). Decreased ventricular compliance leads to increased LV end-diastolic pressure, wall strain, and increased oxygen demand, which can further exacerbate ischemia and decrease contractility. Increased filling pressures also lead to pulmonary vascular congestion and pulmonary edema (Ren, 2014).

In right ventricular (RV) infarction, the decrease in RV stroke volume ultimately leads to inadequate LV filling and reduced cardiac output. Additionally, high RV end-diastolic pressure may cause the interventricular septum to bow into the LV cavity, further compromising LV filling and contractility (Reynolds & Hochman, 2008). The use of nitrates and diuretics in patients with RV infarct can lead to unexpected and exaggerated drops in blood pressure (BP) due to their effects on preload (Antman & Morrow, 2012).

Decreased cardiac output, regardless of the initial cause, leads to the release of catecholamines that increase contractility and peripheral blood flow. Increased contractility increases myocardial oxygen demand, which may exceed the supply provided by the coronary arteries, leading to further increases in myocardial ischemia. Adding to the ischemic insult is the cardiotoxicity of catecholamines, which further exacerbates myocardial functional impairment (Reynolds & Hochman, 2008). Poor perfusion to peripheral vascular beds causes a switch to anaerobic metabolism and lactic acid production in the affected areas. Lactic acid is yet another substance that impairs ventricular contractile function, thus creating a downward decline of worsening cardiac performance (Ren, 2014).

Decreases in cardiac output and BP lead to increases in vasopressin, an antidiuretic hormone, and angiotensin II. These substances lead to vasoconstriction and increased afterload, and cause sodium and water retention. The combination of increased left-sided filling pressures—due to the failing left ventricle—and increased fluid retention results in pulmonary edema (Reynolds & Hochman, 2008).

Diagnosis

Because the majority of cases of CS occur in the setting of MI—especially STEMI—providers should monitor patients carefully for subtle changes that indicate worsening cardiac function. Not all patients will exhibit CS on initial presentation. Approximately 25% will develop CS within 6 hours of MI onset, and another 25% will exhibit CS signs and symptoms within the first 24 hours (Hochman & Ingbar, 2012). Tachycardia and low BP are two signs that may be indicative of impending shock (Reynolds & Hochman, 2008). Other signs of hypoperfusion increase the likelihood of this diagnosis. A systolic blood pressure (SBP) of less than 90 mmHg for more than 30 minutes or vasopressor therapy to maintain an SBP of greater than 90 mmHg are overt indicators of cardiogenic shock (Ren, 2014). A mean arterial BP 30 mmHg or more below a patient's baseline is another defining characteristic of CS (Reynolds & Hochman, 2008).

Clinical Presentation

In addition to sinus tachycardia and hypotension, patients in CS are often cool, pale, and clammy. Poor perfusion is evidenced by mottling of the extremities, and on occasion there is cyanosis as well as mental status changes (Michaels, 2010; Ren, 2014). Careful physical examination and testing will help determine the etiology of their signs and symptoms.

Physical Examination

Patients with hypoperfusion may have altered mental status that ranges from confusion to coma. As mentioned previously, the skin may be pale, cyanotic, or mottled (McNulty, 2014). Possible abnormal heart sounds include an S_3 of HF, an S_4 related to decreased ventricular compliance, or murmurs caused by valvular regurgitation or a ventricular septal defect. The harsh systolic murmur caused by ventricular septal rupture is usually associated with a left parasternal thrill (Ren, 2014). Peripheral pulses may be faint due to the hypotension and vasoconstriction. Patients with CS most often demonstrate signs of volume overload, such as jugular venous distention, edema, and pulmonary crackles. Concurrently, poor perfusion leads to oliguria and potentially acute renal failure (Michaels, 2010; Ren 2014). In cases of RV infarction, hypotension and jugular venous distention are present as in other cases of shock; however, the lungs are often clear to auscultation (O'Gara et al., 2013). Patients with RV infarct may also have hepatomegaly. In the setting of tricuspid regurgitation, the liver may be pulsatile (McNulty, 2014).

Diagnostic Testing

There is no single diagnostic test that will confirm CS. However, careful selection of tests coupled with a thorough physical examination can inform the diagnosis and intervention.

12-Lead ECG

Because CS is most commonly associated with acute STEMI, rapidly obtaining and interpreting an ECG is critically important. Patients with STEMI will benefit from prompt reperfusion either via percutaneous coronary intervention (PCI) or concomitant coronary artery bypass graft (CABG) (O'Gara et al., 2013). If inferior MI is present, RV lead recordings should be obtained to rule out RV infarction, as RV involvement is managed somewhat differently than LV-related shock. Patients with CS may also demonstrate ECG evidence of NSTEMI. When the ECG is normal, CS can still be present, but due to other less-common causes. The ECG can also help identify arrhythmias that might be contributing to the shock state.

Echocardiography

An echocardiogram provides a substantial amount of data in determining the etiology of CS. First, wall motion analysis of the LV and RV can localize and quantify the extent and severity of ischemic involvement or valvular abnormalities. Doppler color flow can be used to evaluate the degree of regurgitation if present. Color flow is also helpful in determining the presence of intraventricular septal rupture in the setting of acute MI. In addition, echocardiography can be used to estimate pulmonary artery pressures and ventricular end-diastolic pressures. Assessing the LV ejection fraction (EF) not only determines the severity of impairment but also indicates the patient's prognosis (Picard et al., 2003).

Chest X-Ray

A chest film helps to rule out other causes of cardiovascular compromise, such as aortic dissection, tension pneumothorax, and cardiac tamponade. Pulmonary edema can also be evaluated, but radiologic manifestations often lag behind clinical symptoms.

Laboratory Evaluations

Serum electrolytes, including calcium, magnesium, and phosphorus, are important to identify correctable causes of impaired contractility or arrhythmias.

Arterial blood gases should be obtained to assess the patient's oxygenation, adequacy of ventilation, and acid–base status. There should be a low threshold for intubation of CS patients, especially those with ischemia, as mechanical ventilation not only assists in optimizing oxygenation but is an adjunctive measure to correct acidosis and decrease the work of breathing. Continuous positive airway pressure (CPAP) and bilevel positive airway pressure can also be placed as noninvasive alternatives (Ren, 2014).

Lactate levels can indicate the severity of the shock and degree of anaerobic metabolism. Procalcitonin levels have been used to evaluate patients with septic shock. This biomarker's utility in evaluating CS remains controversial. However, at least one group of researchers has demonstrated that procalcitonin levels are elevated in CS, and that procalcitonin's dynamic rise over time is associated with poorer outcomes (Picariello, Lazzeri, Valente, Chiostri, & Gensini, 2011).

Pulmonary Artery Catheterization

Monitoring filling pressures and using the Fick method to obtain cardiac-output readings, as well as calculating the cardiac index, stroke work, and systemic vascular resistance, can help guide and tailor therapy for individual CS patients. In CS, the cardiac index is less than 1.8 L/min/m^2 without support or less than

2.0 to 2.2 L/min/m^2 with support (Ren, 2014; Reynolds & Hochman, 2008). The pulmonary capillary wedge pressure (PCWP) is usually greater than 15 mmHg (Ren, 2014). If the PCWP is low or normal, but the central venous pressure is high, one should suspect RV infarction, which should be confirmed by ECG. A "step up" in the mixed venous oxygen saturation levels from the right atrium to the right ventricle of more than 5% is diagnostic for left-to-right intracardiac shunting that occurs with a ventricular septal defect (McNulty, 2014; Ren, 2014).

Coronary Angiogram and PCI

As mentioned previously, patients with STEMI who demonstrate the signs and symptoms of CS should undergo immediate coronary angiography to determine the potential culprit lesion(s). An immediate PCI or CABG should be performed (O'Gara et al., 2014). While the most benefit occurs with very early intervention, the Should We Emergently Revascularize Occluded Coronaries for Cardiogenic Shock (SHOCK) trial demonstrated that patients could still benefit from intervention more than 12 hours after the onset of MI (Ren, 2014; Webb et al., 2003).

Management

Because the most common cause of CS is MI, revascularization is an important treatment for CS patients and the only therapy to demonstrate improved survival. Other interventions—such as inotropic agents, vasopressors, and ventricular-assist devices—help stabilize or improve hemodynamics, but only temporarily (Antman & Morrow, 2012; Reynolds & Hochman, 2008). These therapies are still important, because they help support the patient while the specific cause of CS is determined and appropriate interventions are initiated, such as PCI or cardiac surgery. In addition to revascularization, surgical procedures may be directed toward repair of the mechanical causes of CS, such as papillary muscle rupture or ventricular septal defect.

While it may seem counterintuitive to give IV fluid boluses to a patient in CS, it is important to rule out hypovolemia as the cause of the hypotension demonstrated in suspected CS. A central venous or pulmonary artery catheter may provide information to guide multiple CS therapies. An arterial line enables continuous BP monitoring. Initial fluid resuscitation should be considered, especially when a hypotensive patient has clear lung fields, as in some cases of RV infarction. When administered, saline boluses should be given in small increments of 200 to 300 mL, followed by a reassessment of hemodynamic performance (McNulty, 2014). Filling-pressure targets, in particular pulmonary artery occlusion pressure (PAOP), are slightly higher than normal values due to the decreased ventricular compliance associated with ischemia. A PAOP of 18 to 22 mmHg may be required to optimize contractility, but it should be based on the patient's response (McNulty, 2014).

Electrolyte imbalances and acidemia can exacerbate the cellular disturbances in CS and should be corrected (Ren, 2014). Mechanical ventilation may be required to normalize systemic pH, improve oxygenation, and decrease the work of breathing. The use of beta blockers and angiotensin-converting enzyme inhibitors (ACEI)/ angiotensin receptor blockers (ARBs) must be reassessed, but ACEI should be administered as long as they are tolerated (O'Gara et al., 2013).

Inotropic Agents

Dopamine and dobutamine are the preferred agents for improving contractility. These drugs may be administered alone or in combination. The lowest effective dose(s) should be used (Reynolds & Hochman, 2008). While these drugs increase contractility, they also increase myocardial oxygen demand and irritability. Supraventricular or ventricular tachyarrhythmias may occur with either medication, although dobutamine is considered to cause less tachycardia. Low-dose dopamine promotes coronary, renal, and splanchnic vasodilation (Overgaard & Dzavik, 2008); however, doses higher than 5 mcg/kg/min can cause systemic vasoconstriction (Antman & Morrow, 2012). In a predefined subgroup analysis of CS patients in a recent study comparing dopamine with norepinephrine in the treatment of shock, dopamine was found to be associated with increased 28-day mortality. In the same study, among all types of shock, dopamine was associated with a higher incidence of arrhythmias, especially atrial fibrillation. Dopamine was also more likely to be terminated due to "severe arrhythmias" (De Backer et al., 2010).

Dobutamine has less vasoconstrictor activity than dopamine (Overgaard & Dzavik, 2008). In patients with a low cardiac index but a normal or high systemic vascular resistance, dobutamine at doses less than 15 mcg/kg/min may have the combined beneficial effect of increasing contractility while decreasing afterload (McNulty, 2014; Overgaard & Dzavik, 2008; Ren, 2014). Because dobutamine at lower doses has a net effect of peripheral vasodilation (Overgaard & Dzavik, 2008), it should not be used as a single agent in patients with a SBP lower than 80 mmHg (Ren, 2014).

Phosphodiesterase inhibitors (PDIs), such as inamrinone and milrinone, increase contractility and decrease both peripheral and pulmonary vascular resistance (PVR). Because of their vasodilating effects, these agents usually require simultaneous administration of a vasopressor to support the patient's BP. While PDIs are less likely to cause increased myocardial oxygen demand, they are more likely than dobutamine to cause tachyarrhythmias (Ren, 2014).

Vasopressors

Of the many vasopressor agents, norepinephrine is the drug that has the least number of detrimental effects in the setting of CS. In a comparison with dopamine, norepinephrine use resulted in less adverse events (De Backer et al., 2010). The predominant effect of norepinephrine is vasoconstriction, which makes it effective in improving BP. Unlike epinephrine and isoproterenol, it has minimal effects on heart rate and therefore is less likely to cause cardiac ischemia (Overgaard & Dzavik, 2008). When systemic vascular resistance is less than 1,800 dynes/sec/cm^5, a norepinephrine infusion of 2 to 10 mcg/min may be beneficial (Antman & Morrow, 2012).

Epinephrine improves BP and contractility; however, it also increases heart rate and systemic vascular resistance. Epinephrine infusions have been associated with increased lactate levels. Other detrimental effects include potential myocardial ischemia and arrhythmias. Because of these characteristics, epinephrine should only be used in treating patients who are not responsive to dopamine, dobutamine, and/or norepinephrine (Ren, 2014).

Other Vasoactive Medications

Alpha adrenergic agents, such as phenylephrine, are contraindicated in CS (Antman & Morrow, 2012). The calcium-sensitizing agent levosimendan has not been approved for use in the United States. This medication improves contractility; however, it also causes significant vasodilation. Therefore, it can exacerbate hypotension. It has been used primarily in the treatment of acute and chronic HF in other countries (Antman & Morrow, 2012; Overgaard & Dzavik, 2008; Ren 2014).

Vasodilators, such as nitroglycerin, may be used to decrease preload and afterload in specific situations in CS (Ren, 2014). These agents are used in combination with other supportive medications, such as dopamine. Due to the potential to exacerbate hypotension, vasodilators must be used with caution in CS.

Ventricular Assistive Devices

The intra-aortic balloon pump (IABP) has been used to treat CS for more than 30 years. It consists of a pneumatic pump console and a large catheter onto which a long cylindrical balloon has been mounted. The catheter is inserted via the femoral artery, and the tip is advanced into the descending aorta just inferior to the takeoff of the left subclavian artery. Helium is shuttled back and forth from the console to inflate and deflate the balloon. Balloon inflation is timed to occur immediately after aortic valve closure, in diastole. The inflation of the balloon increases pressure in the aortic arch and improves coronary perfusion. The balloon is timed to deflate immediately prior to the next systole. Deflation at this time decreases the pressure in the aortic arch, therefore decreasing afterload and the work required to eject blood from the ventricle. This reduction in stroke work decreases the stress and oxygen demand on the heart.

Other more invasive circulatory support devices have been developed and utilized in the treatment of CS. These devices are employed most often when the etiology of CS is not acute ischemia and infarction. Usually, the primary intent is circulatory support as a bridge to transplantation. However, for patients who are not candidates for cardiac transplant, some devices may be used as long-term or lifetime therapy (Kirklin et al., 2011).

One such circulatory support device can be used for either left or right ventricular support. The system has a long catheter that is inserted percutaneously. An arterial approach from the femoral or right axillary artery can be used to advance the tip of the catheter to the left ventricle. A small rotating pump within the catheter pulls blood in from the LV cavity and discharges it into the ascending aorta. For RV support, the catheter is inserted via the femoral vein and advanced through the inferior vena cava (IVC) until the tip crosses the pulmonary valve. In this circumstance, blood is pulled into the catheter from the right ventricle and is discharged into the main pulmonary artery (Abiomed, 2014). There are other devices that can be inserted percutaneously; however, most require at least minor surgical procedures.

Follow-Up and Referral

In-hospital mortality rates for CS are poor but have improved in recent years. The ability to revascularize patients with acute MI-related CS has been credited with much of the improvement in survival (McNulty, 2014; Ren, 2014). Indicators of poor 1-year survival include EF less than 28%, moderate to severe mitral regurgitation, advanced age, and history of prior MI (Ren, 2014). Patients surviving CS regardless of the cause will require continued care under the supervision of a cardiovascular clinician for varying periods of time even if they are fortunate enough to be discharged to their homes. Many patients will experience extended hospitalization and rehabilitation. Collaboration among the multidisciplinary team of cardiologists, cardiac surgeons, physical therapists, nurse practitioners, physician assistants, social workers, and others is critical to ensuring the optimal recovery for CS patients.

OBSTRUCTIVE SHOCK

Obstructive shock is caused by the mechanical interference of ventricular preload, which, in turn, impairs stroke volume and cardiac output. The causes of obstructive shock include tension pneumothorax, massive pulmonary embolism, cardiac tamponade, constrictive pericarditis, and autopositive end expiratory pressure (auto-PEEP) (Young, 2011).

Pathophysiology

In tension pneumothorax, air enters the pleural cavity but is unable to escape. As a result, intrathoracic pressure rises. When the pressure in the thorax exceeds vena-caval and right-atrial pressures, these vessels collapse and RV filling and any further forward blood flow is impaired (Jones & Stearley, 2011). The increased pressure leads to the collapse of the lung on the affected side and a shifting of the trachea and mediastinum toward the normal lung. Shifting of these structures further increases the mechanical obstruction to blood flow, and the loss of ventilation in the collapsed lung leads to hypoxemia.

Tension pneumothorax most often occurs due to blunt or penetrating trauma, but can result from barotrauma to the lung during mechanical ventilation. During mechanical ventilation, increased airway pressure can lead to the rupture of alveoli and leaking of air into the perivascular sheath in the lung and then to the pleural space, the mediastinum, or the pericardium, where accumulating air compresses vital structures (Hoo, 2013).

Another complication of mechanical ventilation is auto-PEEP. This condition can result from inadequate expiratory time, bronchospasm, or ventilator circuit obstruction. As a result of any of these conditions, gases are trapped in the airways, leading to increased pleural and intrathoracic pressure. This can lead to compression of the superior vena cava and results in decreased venous return; compression can occur with airway pressure levels of 10 cm H_2O or more. Auto-PEEP or high levels of extrinsic PEEP can lead to overdistention of alveoli. These pressures are transmitted to the pulmonary vasculature and cause a rise in PVR. Elevated PVR increases RV workload and may lead to RV failure (Berlin, 2014).

Massive pulmonary embolism, especially in the form of a saddle embolus at the bifurcation of the main pulmonary artery, impedes blood flow to the left atrium and ventricle and leads to a loss of preload, stroke volume, and cardiac output. If multiple clots obstruct as much as 50% to 60% of the pulmonary vascular bed, pulmonary arterial pressure rises and increases the RV workload, ultimately causing RV failure (Fedullo, 2011). Lesser amounts of clot burden can still lead to RV failure as PVR increases due to pulmonary artery vasoconstriction (Goldhaber, 2015). As forward flow decreases, as a result of the failing right ventricle, preload for the left ventricle is decreased. In addition, high pressures in the right ventricle cause bowing of the intraventricular septum so that it decreases left ventricle cavity size (Reynolds & Hochman, 2008). This further decreases LV stroke volume and cardiac output, leading to hypotension, shock, and potential cardiac arrest. In addition to circulatory impairment, significant hypoxemia can occur due to the ventilation to perfusion mismatch (Goldhaber, 2015). Patients presenting in shock due to pulmonary embolism (PE) have an estimated mortality rate of 30%, with those presenting in cardiopulmonary arrest incurring a mortality rate of about 70% (Fedullo, 2011).

Cardiac tamponade occurs when blood or fluid accumulates in the potential space between the visceral and parietal layers of the pericardium and compresses the cardiac chambers, leading to impaired cardiac output. Normally only about 15 to 50 mL of serous fluid occupies this space (Imazio, 2014). Increasing fluid, in the form of a pericardial effusion, may have several etiologies including inflammation, HF, malignancies, and infections. Bleeding into the pericardial space can occur with trauma, free wall rupture of the left ventricle due to MI, or aortic dissection, or as a complication of cardiac surgery, cardiac catheterization, pacemaker insertion, or ablation procedures (Imazio, 2014; LeWinter & Hopkins, 2015). When fluid accumulates quickly, as in ventricular rupture or bleeding following cardiac surgery, a volume of 100 to 200 mL may lead to an abrupt rise in pericardial pressure to levels between 20 and 30 mmHg (Imazio, 2014). This pressure exceeds the pressure in the right atrium, right ventricle, and the vena cava and can lead to collapse of these structures and an obstruction of forward blood flow. When the fluid accumulates more slowly, as in metastatic disease or renal failure, changes occur in the parietal pericardium, allowing it to distend. In these situations, 1,000 to 2,000 mL can accumulate before overt tamponade occurs (Imazio, 2014).

Constrictive pericarditis is a relatively rare cause of cardiac tamponade and obstructive shock, occurring in 2% to 5% of patients who experience acute pericarditis following cardiac surgery (Imazio, 2014). Pericarditis from other causes, such as tuberculosis, radiation therapy, and renal failure, can also lead to thickening, scarring, and calcification of the parietal pericardium (Hoit, 2011). The thickened, stiff pericardium restricts the expansion of the ventricles during diastolic filling and limits the critical myocardial fibril stretching necessary to increase contractility in response to physiological demands.

Clinical Presentation

The clinical presentation of patients with obstructive shock varies according to the inciting cause. Patients with tension pneumothorax generally present in severe respiratory distress. The degree of respiratory distress seen in patients with moderate to severe PE or auto-PEEP may be somewhat variable. All forms of obstructive shock can potentially present as cardiopulmonary arrest or can rapidly deteriorate to this condition.

Physical Examination

The most common general finding in obstructive shock is hypotension, with additional findings dependent on the source of the circulatory obstruction. Timely and efficient assessment is key to determining the cause and initiating life-saving treatment. Rapid assessment of the level of consciousness, BP, respiratory rate and effort, heart and breath sounds, and jugular venous pressure are all important.

Tension Pneumothorax

In addition to respiratory distress, patients will have decreased or absent breath sounds on the affected side. Due to the collapse of the lung and the large amount of air in the intrapleural space, there is hyperresonance to percussion and, potentially, tracheal deviation toward the unaffected lung. If the patient is a trauma victim, a primary assessment might reveal a penetrating wound or multiple rib fractures.

Severe Auto-PEEP

Because mechanically ventilated patients are often sedated, development of life-threatening levels of auto-PEEP may occur without warning. The most effective way to avoid this problem is to routinely check for the development of auto-PEEP by assessing for ventilator dyssynchrony, observing ventilator flow-time curves for a return to zero flow prior to the inhalation phase, and measuring total or true PEEP during an expiratory pause (Berlin, 2014).

Pulmonary Embolism

Patients with PE typically present with tachypnea and tachycardia. Severe PE patients may also demonstrate jugular venous distention or sudden loss of consciousness (Fedullo, 2011). Other, nonpulmonary signs, such as unilateral lower-extremity edema, may suggest the source of the embolus.

Cardiac Tamponade

Depending on the rate of fluid accumulation in the pericardium, patients may present as restless, obtunded, or unconscious. Due to increased venous pressure, the neck veins are distended. Heart sounds may be distant or muffled. Pulsus paradoxus, a decrease of more than 10 mmHg in the SBP during inspiration, is most evident if the patient already has an arterial pressure monitoring line; however, it can be assessed noninvasively. In patients with palpable radial or brachial pulses, a decrease in the strength of the pulse during inspiration is suspicious for pulsus paradoxus. Using a BP cuff, the difference between the SBP during inspiration and exhalation can be determined by slowly deflating the cuff and noting the pressure at which Korotkoff sounds first occur but are intermittent (disappear during inspiration), as well as the pressure at which they are continuously present (Hoit, 2011).

Constrictive Pericarditis

Generally, constrictive pericarditis does not develop rapidly, and so physical signs develop slowly over time. Patients demonstrate signs of RV dysfunction including jugular venous distention, edema, ascites, and hepatosplenomegaly. Occasionally a pericardial knock will be heard (Hoit, 2011). This sound is best heard at the left sternal border or the left fifth intercostal space, along the midclavicular line. It occurs slightly earlier and has a higher pitch than an S_3 (LeWinter & Hopkins, 2015).

Diagnostic Testing

The diagnosis of obstructive shock begins with a clinical suspicion regarding the cause of hypotension, loss of consciousness, or cardiopulmonary arrest.

Tension Pneumothorax

Tension pneumothorax is considered to be a clinical diagnosis. Critical time can be wasted by attempting to verify physical findings with a chest x-ray (Young Jr., 2011).

Pulmonary Embolism

Multiple tests can be helpful in diagnosing PE; however, when PE results in shock, there may not be adequate time to perform these or obtain the results. The ECG may be the most readily available aid to diagnosis, but unfortunately, observed changes are not very definitive. Rodger et al. (2000) found that only tachycardia and incomplete right bundle branch block (RBBB) were more common in patients with PE than in control patients. The S1Q3T3 sign of acute cor pulmonale can be present in any patient with RV overload. This sign consists of an

S wave in lead I, and a Q wave, slight ST elevation, and inverted T wave in lead III (Chan, Vilke, Pollack, & Brady, 2001). Pulse oximetry may reveal a decreased oxygen saturation, but it may be difficult to obtain readings in a severely vasoconstricted, hypotensive patient.

Spiral CT angiography is the most conclusive diagnostic imaging study for diagnosing PE if the patient can be supported long enough for the test to be performed. The CT is useful both in ruling in PE and ruling out other potential causes of shock such as cardiac tamponade and overwhelming pulmonary infection. Tests such as the D-dimer are helpful for the negative predictive value, although not specific for PE, and do not help to quantify the extent of pulmonary vascular involvement.

Cardiac Tamponade

In cardiac tamponade, the ECG voltage in all leads is typically significantly diminished due to the fluid in the pericardial sac. Electrical alternans may also be present, which is caused by the anterior–posterior movement of the heart with each contraction (LeWinter & Hopkins, 2015). The chest x-ray of a patient with cardiac tamponade usually shows an enlarged cardiac silhouette and a widened mediastinum.

An ECG is the most definitive noninvasive test for determining the presence of cardiac tamponade. A dark, echo-free area surrounds the heart when there is a significant effusion. Compression of low-pressure chambers, such as the right atrium and ventricle in diastole, is a sensitive and specific indicator of tamponade. Distention of the superior and IVC that does not decrease with inspiration is another echocardiographic indicator (LeWinter & Hopkins, 2015).

In patients with pulmonary artery catheters, the central venous pressure, right atrial pressure, pulmonary artery diastolic, and PAOPs become equalized as the pressure in the pericardial space rises to 20 to 25 mmHg. This equalization is most evident during inspiration (LeWinter & Hopkins, 2015).

Constrictive Pericarditis

The most important imaging test for diagnosis of constrictive pericarditis is echocardiography. Using this modality, the pericardium is usually noted to be thickened. A *septal bounce* may also be observed; this finding is the unusual rapid movement of the intraventricular septum during early diastole (LeWinter & Hopkins, 2015).

Management

Obstructive shock requires immediate intervention targeted at the source of the problem. While other forms of shock may be life threatening, obstructive shock has a rapid progression to cardiopulmonary arrest.

Tension Pneumothorax

Whatever the initial inciting factor, if not recognized and treated in an emergent manner, tension pneumothorax can result in circulatory collapse. Rapid decompression with a chest tube or large-bore needle inserted at the second intercostal space midclavicular line is the treatment of choice (Jones & Stearley, 2011). If the patient is mechanically ventilated, settings will be adjusted to decrease peak inspiratory airway pressures and plateau pressures, usually by lowering tidal volumes (Hoo, 2013).

Auto-PEEP

Because patients are most often sedated during mechanical ventilation, hemodynamic collapse may be the first sign of severe auto-PEEP. The most rapid treatment is to remove the patient from the ventilator circuit to allow a brief period of apnea, and then manually ventilate the patient while other interventions are instituted to support circulation, treat bronchospasm, and correct ventilator settings. Manual breaths per minute should not exceed 8 to 10. If hemodynamic instability is less severe, adjustments in ventilator settings allow additional time for exhalation, usually by decreasing the ventilator rate. Lowering tidal volumes can prevent overinflating the lungs. Ventilator dyssynchrony may need to be managed by sedating the patient (Berlin, 2014).

Fluid resuscitation may help restore hemodynamic stability if hypotension persists; however, fluid administration can be deleterious if RV failure is present. The best method for assessing the effects of fluid bolus therapy in patients with auto-PEEP is echocardiography. Assessing for positive changes in stroke volume during passive leg lift can help predict the response to fluids. Conversely, if the intraventricular septum is flattened and the right ventricle is dilated, additional volume will not improve cardiac performance. In cases where fluid is not helpful, vasopressors may be useful in supporting the BP and circulation (Berlin, 2014).

Pulmonary Embolism

Extensive PE sufficient to cause shock symptoms should be treated with systemic thrombolytics, catheter-directed thrombolytics, surgical embolectomy, or IVC filter placement. Alteplase 100 mg delivered as a 2-hour infusion can be used for systemic thrombolysis if there are no contraindications. This therapy can be effective even if administered as late as 14 days after the onset of symptoms. Catheter-directed thrombolysis requires smaller doses of thrombolytic medications. Usually tissue-plasminogen activator (tPA) is used at a dose of 25 mg or less. Mechanical clot removal or aspiration can be performed with a variety of catheters. Surgical embolectomy is not usually recommended when there are symptoms of shock (Goldhaber, 2015).

Other supportive therapies include oxygen, mechanical ventilation, and vasopressors. Not all patients will require mechanical ventilation; however, most will require supplemental oxygen. Respiratory status should be carefully monitored. Retrievable or permanent IVC filter placement with or without thrombolytic therapy has been shown to decrease mortality rates (Stein, Matta, Keyes, & Willyerd, 2012). For patients without contraindications, anticoagulation should be instituted with initial therapy of unfractionated heparin, low molecular weight heparin, or fondaparinux. Long-term therapy is maintained with warfarin, factor Xa inhibitors, or direct thrombin inhibitors. The duration of therapy is usually 3 to 6 months. Newer medications, such as the factor Xa inhibitor rivaroxaban, are not indicated for the treatment for massive PE (Goldhaber, 2015).

Cardiac Tamponade

In patients demonstrating shock-like symptoms, immediate relief of the pressure caused by fluid in the pericardial space is required, especially if the cardiac tamponade has developed rapidly (e.g., following cardiac surgery). Most often a pericardiocentesis is performed. When bleeding is the suspected cause, performing an open pericardiocentesis (a surgical procedure) is favored unless the bleeding rate is thought to be fairly slow, such as that caused by a procedural puncture of a cardiac chamber. An open pericardiocentesis is also recommended for loculated pericardial effusions or those containing clots. A closed pericardiocentesis is most often performed in a cardiac catheterization laboratory under echocardiographic guidance. In a closed pericardiocentesis, a long, large-gauge needle is initially inserted via a subxiphoid approach. After some fluid is removed via syringe, a guidewire is used to replace the rigid needle with a flexible catheter for further drainage. This catheter is often left in place for several days so that additional drainage can occur. If the cause of the pericardial effusion is unknown, the fluid is often sent for culture and cytology. Hemodynamic monitoring of patients before, during, and after a pericardiocentesis can be helpful in assessing the effects of the procedure and determining any further interventions (LeWinter & Hopkins, 2015).

Constrictive Pericarditis

As mentioned previously, constrictive pericarditis develops over time and can be the result of radiation therapy or disease processes such as renal failure. Radiation-induced constrictive pericarditis is a relative contraindication for surgical treatment. Other patients with severe comorbid conditions or frailty may not be good surgical candidates. Removal of the parietal pericardium is the most effective treatment, although perioperative mortality ranges from 2.2% to 15% at major cardiac surgical centers (LeWinter & Hopkins, 2015). Timely diagnosis and referral of patients for pericardiectomy prior to the development of shock is an important strategy.

For full reference citations to this chapter, please see "Section References" in the back of the book, under the heading "Section V."

Aortic Dissection

HELEN F. BROWN AND LINDA BRIGGS

Acute aortic syndrome encompasses several life-threatening pathologies affecting the aorta. These diseases include aortic dissection, ruptured aortic aneurysm, penetrating atherosclerotic ulcer, and intramural hematoma (Tsai, Nienaber, & Eagle, 2005). The incidence of aortic dissection is approximately 3.5/100,000 persons per year. Acute aortic dissection is diagnosed in 3 out of every 1,000 patients presenting to the emergency department with acute chest, back, or abdominal pain (Diercks et al., 2015; Golledge & Engle 2008). This deadly disease is extremely challenging to diagnose due to its variable clinical presentation and the low frequency of cases; it is estimated that 50% of patients with aortic dissection are not diagnosed on initial evaluation (Diercks et al., 2015). The negative consequences of a delay in diagnosis are progression of the disease—including aortic rupture—or the inappropriate initiation of thrombolytic therapy or anticoagulation for a suspected myocardial infarction, cerebrovascular accident (CVA), or pulmonary embolism. Both situations can result in a devastating error, increasing the morbidity and mortality for the patient.

The International Registry of Acute Aortic Dissection (IRAD), started in 1996, is a prospective registry that collects data on patients diagnosed with aortic dissection. It currently has data of more than 2,000 patients from at least 26 clinical sites (Tsai, Trimarchi, & Nienaber, 2009). According to IRAD data, aortic dissection is more prevalent in males in the fifth and sixth decades (Hagan et al., 2000). There is a bimodal distribution based on age. Younger patients under the age of 40 are more likely to have a genetic disorder such as Marfan syndrome or bicuspid aortic valve—or to have had prior aortic surgery. For those older than the age of 50, the major risk factor is chronic hypertension (Tsai et al., 2005). Acute aortic dissections are more likely to occur during the cold, winter months and in the early morning between 6 and 10 (Lentini & Perrotta, 2011). Risk factors associated with acute aortic dissection are a history of hypertension, older age, atherosclerosis, and previous cardiovascular surgery, including prior repair of an aortic aneurysm or dissection (Tsai et al., 2009).

PATHOPHYSIOLOGY

Aortic dissection is a disruption of the tunica media of the aorta, producing a blood-filled channel that separates the intima from the medial or adventitial layers of the aorta (Lentini & Perrotta, 2011). Chronic hypertension and degeneration of the medial layer of the aortic wall are the common pathology. Acquired and genetic conditions weaken the medial layer of the aorta, increasing wall stress and causing dilation of the aorta with aneurysm formation and ensuing intramural hemorrhage, aortic dissection, and ultimately aortic rupture (Tsai et al., 2005). Genetic syndromes predisposing individuals to aortic syndromes are the bicuspid aortic valve, vascular Ehlers–Danlos syndrome, Marfan syndrome, annuloaortic ectasia, and familial aortic dissection (Hiratzka et al., 2010). Acquired disorders increasing the risk for developing aortic wall weakness are atherosclerosis, inflammatory disorders including vasculitis, Takayasu's arteritis, giant cell arteritis, Behçet disease, Ormond's disease, tertiary syphilis, decelerating trauma incurred in a motor vehicle collision or fall from a height, and sympathomimetic abuse with cocaine or methamphetamines (Hiratzka et al., 2010; Tsai et al., 2005).

There are two classification systems used to describe the location of the aortic dissection, the Stanford and the De Bakey (Figure 21.1). The most commonly used classification is the Stanford system, which identifies the dissection based on ascending aortic involvement. A lesion involving the ascending aorta and/or the arch is classified as a Type A. A defect encompassing only the descending aorta is considered to be a Type B (Hiratzka et al., 2010). Dissection involving the ascending aorta is the most common.

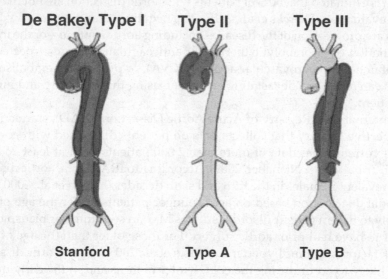

De Bakey

Type I   Originates in the ascending aorta, propagates at least to the aortic arch and often beyond it distally

Type II   Originates in and is confined to the ascending aorta.

Type III Originates in the descending aorta and extends distally down the aorta or, rarely, retrograde into the aortic arch and ascending aorta.

Stanford

Type A   All dissections involving the ascending aorta, regardless of the site of origin.

Type B   All dissections not involving the ascending aorta.

FIGURE 21.1 The most common classification systems of thoracic aortic dissection: Stanford and De Bakey. See color insert.

Reprinted from Nienaber and Eagle (2003, pp. 628–635), with permission from Wolters Kluwer Health.

DIAGNOSIS

The symptoms of aortic dissection are similar to other life-threatening cardiovascular pathology, including acute coronary syndromes and pulmonary embolus. As mentioned previously, diagnostic errors can lead to incorrect—and sometimes lethal—treatment decisions. Whenever aortic dissection is among the possible differential diagnoses, care should be taken to rule out this possibility. Historical features that are associated with a high risk of aortic dissection include Marfan syndrome, connective tissue disease, a family history of aortic disease, preexisting aortic valve disease, known thoracic aortic aneurysm, and a history of recent aortic manipulation (Hiratzka et al., 2010). Sympathomimetic abuse, such as chronic cocaine use, increases the risk of developing dissection of the descending aorta (Tsai et al., 2005).

CLINICAL PRESENTATION

The false channel, created by the abrupt disruption of the intimal layer of the aorta, typically produces a sudden onset of severe chest pain that radiates to the midscapular area of the back. According to the IRAD, the most common presenting symptom of acute aortic dissection was abrupt onset of severe pain, present in 84% of all patients with dissection (Tsai et al., 2009). The classical description is a ripping or tearing sensation of maximal intensity from the onset of discomfort. Another important feature is that the pain is accompanied by a feeling of impending doom (Lentini & Perrotta, 2011). If the dissection occurs in the ascending aorta (Type A) and involves the common carotid artery, the presentation may include syncope or a CVA (Hiratzka et al., 2010). A dissection involving the descending aorta (Type B) can result in abdominal pain and neurologic symptoms, including acute low back pain, lower extremity and perineal paresthesia, or lower extremity paresis (Hiratzka et al., 2010). Additional signs and symptoms include hypertension (49%), aortic regurgitation (32%), abdominal pain (30%), any pulse deficit (27%), migrating pain (19%), hypotension, shock, cardiac tamponade (18%), and any focal neurologic deficit (12%) (Golledge & Engle, 2008).

PHYSICAL EXAMINATION

In the majority of patients with an acute aortic dissection, the physical examination is normal. Physical findings that may occur as a result of an aortic dissection include a new aortic insufficiency murmur (32%) and pulse deficit between the right and left radial or femoral arteries (15%) (Hagan et al., 2000). Alterations in blood pressure (BP) are a common finding. In the IRAD, hypertension was seen in 49% of cases and occurred more frequently in Type B dissection. Hypotension was experienced by approximately 25% of patients with a Type A dissection (Golledge & Engle, 2008). A difference in systolic blood pressure of more than 20 mmHg between corresponding bilateral limbs is a high-risk indicator of dissection (Hiratzka et al., 2010). As the dissection progresses with the development of an aneurysmal wall, it can compress surrounding mediastinal structures, including the recurrent laryngeal nerve, superior cervical sympathetic ganglion, and the esophagus. These changes can produce a hoarse voice, Horner syndrome, and dysphagia (Mancini, 2014).

DIAGNOSTIC TESTING

There are several diagnostic tests that are important in determining the likelihood of aortic dissection. Some help to rule out alternative diagnoses; others are more helpful in demonstrating the presence of dissection. It may be difficult to differentiate between acute coronary syndrome and acute aortic dissection in the patient presenting with chest pain. ECG results may be within normal limits or demonstrate evidence of ischemia, injury, or infarction. Evidence of myocardial ischemia or infarction on ECG was noted in 17% of cases in the IRAD. Twenty-six percent showed left ventricular hypertrophy, and 30% of patients had normal ECGs (Golledge & Engle, 2008). A Type A dissection involving the ostia of a coronary artery can produce ECG changes of ST-segment elevation myocardial infarctions (STEMI) (Lentini & Perrotta, 2011; Tsai et al., 2005).

A chest x-ray (CXR) is also an important, although not very sensitive, diagnostic test. In the IRAD registry, mediastinal widening was noted on CXRs in 60% of cases (Figure 21.2). Abnormal aortic contours were observed in 48% of patients, and only 16% had normal films (Golledge & Engle, 2008). Klompas (2002) evaluated 21 studies to determine if clinical history, physical examination, and CXR findings could be used to detect aortic dissection. This author determined that the

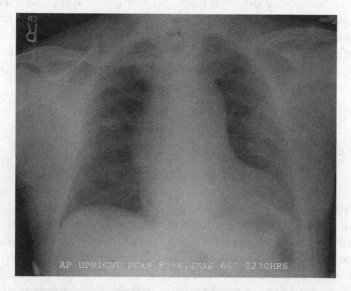

FIGURE 21.2 Chest x-ray with wide mediastinum. There is aortic dissection with aneurysmal formation in the descending aorta.

absence of three clinical features significantly decreased the likelihood of dissection: (1) sudden, tearing chest pain; (2) BP or pulse differential; and (3) mediastinal widening on CXR.

Echocardiography can be an important diagnostic tool; however, it has some limitations. Transthoracic echocardiography has limited use when the entire aorta requires evaluation. It is useful in evaluating the proximal ascending aorta for lesions (Tsai et al., 2005). The transesophageal echocardiogram (TEE) is both sensitive and specific for identification of a thoracic aneurysm. The one caveat to its use is that the quality of the study is operator dependent. A second consideration when obtaining a TEE is the need for procedural sedation. The American College of Emergency Physicians recommends that TEE not be relied upon for definitive diagnosis of aortic dissection; rather, the patient should be transferred to a facility capable of a full evaluation, including consultation with a cardiovascular surgeon (Diercks et al., 2015).

Both the American College of Emergency Physicians (Diercks et al., 2015) and the guidelines endorsed by multiple organizations for the diagnosis and management of thoracic aortic disease (Hiratzka et al., 2010) consider CT scanning to be a sensitive and reliable method for diagnosing aortic dissection. One advantage of CT scanning over transesophageal echocardiography is that with CT, the entire length of the aorta can be evaluated (Figures 21.3 and 21.4). Magnetic resonance angiography is also very sensitive and specific, although a disadvantage of MRI is the duration required for imaging (Hiratzka et al., 2010).

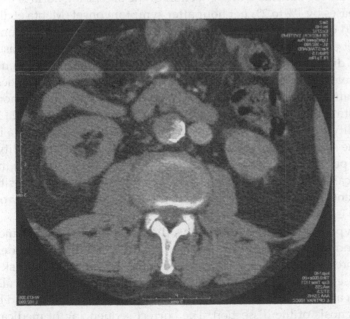

FIGURE 21.3 Contrasted CT of the abdomen with aortic dissection. Type B dissection at the level of the renal arteries. True and false lumens are visible.

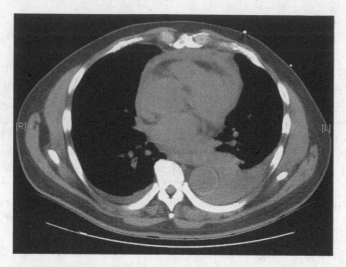

FIGURE 21.4 Noncontrasted CT image of a ruptured thoracic aortic aneurysm.

MANAGEMENT

The mortality rate for patients with dissection of the ascending aorta is extremely high, and increases by 1% to 2% per hour after symptom onset (Mehta et al., 2002). Therefore, rapid diagnosis and consultation with a cardiothoracic surgeon is critical (Hiratzka et al., 2010). Surgical repair is recommended to manage ascending thoracic aortic dissection and involves resection of the affected segment of the aorta. If extensive aortic root dissection is present, the aortic root is replaced with a composite graft or with a valve-sparing root replacement. In a partial aortic root dissection, treatment is with an aortic valve resuspension (Hiratzka et al., 2010).

The mortality rate for acute aortic dissection of the descending aorta is lower than that for the ascending aorta (Tsai et al., 2005). There is a 10% mortality rate at 30 days in this population (Mehta et al., 2002). The recommendation for this population is medical management of the dissection (Hiratzka et al., 2010). In situations where the patient develops organ compromise due to ischemia, surgery or endovascular repair is recommended (Hiratzka et al., 2010).

For both Type A and Type B dissections, the goal of initial management is to lower the BP and heart rate, limiting the shearing forces on the intimal defect. By reducing the force of left ventricular contraction and systemic BP, the risk of converting the dissecting aorta to an aneurysm is decreased (Hiratzka et al., 2010). Treatment with antihypertensives and vasodilators to manage BP should be initiated upon diagnosis of the dissection. The correct sequencing of medications is essential to avoid triggering a compensatory increase in heart rate and myocardial contractility, which could increase shearing forces. A negative inotropic and chronotropic agent should be initiated first to lower the heart rate and decrease myocardial contractility. Beta blockade, using esmolol, metoprolol, or labetolol, is appropriate therapy to achieve this goal. If beta blockers are contraindicated, nondihydropyridine calcium channel blockers can be used, including verapamil. Initial target BP is a systolic pressure of 100 to 120 mmHg and heart rate of 60 beats per minute (Hiratzka et al., 2010). If this target cannot be achieved with beta blockers, then a vasodilator, such as nitroprusside, or an angiotensin-converting enzyme inhibitor (ACEI) should be used to obtain optimal BP control (Hiratzka et al., 2010).

If the patient demonstrates hemodynamic instability with hypotension, then fluid resuscitation should be initiated. The hemodynamically unstable patient requires immediate evaluation by the cardiovascular surgeon to arrange for definitive management of the dissection. Patients with acute aortic dissection require admission to the intensive care unit for hemodynamic monitoring and medication titration until surgical or endovascular therapy can be initiated. Following surgery, patients will continue to need careful monitoring especially for bleeding and other complications, which is best accomplished in a surgical intensive care unit.

COMPLICATIONS OF AORTIC DISSECTION

Complications associated with dissections of the ascending aorta include: (a) retrograde involvement of the right coronary ostia, producing inferior wall myocardial infarction, (b) development of cardiac tamponade, (c) compromise of the aortic valve producing aortic insufficiency, and (d) involvement of the common carotid artery producing syncope or stroke (Lentini & Perrotta, 2011; Tsai et al., 2005). Complications of Type B aortic dissections are less common but include end-organ malperfusion, aneurysmal expansion, limb ischemia, and refractory pain. Poor perfusion can result in mesenteric, renal, or spinal cord ischemia. If prompt surgical or endovascular intervention for these complications does not occur, organ failure or paralysis can occur (Austin, 2005). Independent indicators for a poor outcome in both types of dissection are advanced age, rupture of the aorta, and malperfusion syndromes leading to renal failure, mesenteric ischemia, or infarction of the spinal cord (Tsai et al., 2005).

FOLLOW-UP

Patients with aortic dissection will need risk factor reduction postdischarge. Adequate BP control, equal to or less than 140/90 mmHg, is essential. Patients should continue oral beta blocker or calcium channel blocker medication long term. Smoking cessation and treatment of dyslipidemia are also important (Hiratzka et al., 2010). Continuing follow-up with the cardiovascular or vascular surgeon is also important to ensure that any repairs remain structurally intact and that there is no further progression of the disease. Reimaging via CT scanning can be performed at 1, 3, 6, and 12 months, and then yearly if the affected area remains stable (Hiratzka et al., 2010).

For full reference citations to this chapter, please see "Section References" in the back of the book, under the heading "Section V."

Pericarditis and Infective Endocarditis

LINDA BRIGGS

PERICARDITIS

Pericarditis is a common cause of chest pain among patients who present to emergency departments. The challenge for providers is to distinguish acute pericarditis from more serious, life-threatening conditions, such as acute ST-elevation myocardial infarction (MI) and aortic dissection. There are many causes of pericarditis; however, the vast majority of cases are *idiopathic*, with no identifiable etiology (Imazio & Adler, 2013). Inflammation of the pericardium can result from viral or bacterial infections, MI, radiation, cancer, medications, connective-tissue diseases, other inflammatory processes, renal failure, trauma, cardiac surgery, and numerous other disorders (Imazio & Adler, 2013; LeWinter & Hopkins, 2015).

Pathophysiology

The main pathologic process is inflammation of the pericardium, including infiltration of polymorphonuclear leukocytes (Spangler, 2013). In some cases, the acute inflammation can lead to an effusion (LeWinter & Hopkins, 2015; Spangler, 2013).

Diagnosis

The diagnosis of pericarditis depends on obtaining a careful history of the chest discomfort, frequent cardiac auscultation, echocardiogram, and a close examination of the ECG.

Clinical Presentation

The most common feature of acute pericarditis is chest pain. This pain is usually characterized as being sharp and increasing with inspiration or lying flat. Another key feature is that sitting up and leaning forward often relieves the discomfort. Radiation of the pain to the trapezius ridge is highly specific for pericarditis (Hoit, 2011; LeWinter & Hopkins, 2015). Also, the pain may radiate down the left arm, leading the patient and others to believe that the pain is due to an acute coronary syndrome (ACS), although it is not (Hoit, 2011; LeWinter & Hopkins, 2015; Spangler 2013). Associated symptoms include palpitations, dyspnea, and sometimes hiccups (Hoit, 2011; Spangler, 2013). Often patients will describe having a viral illness with fever and myalgias prior to the onset of the chest pain (Hoit, 2011; LeWinter & Hopkins, 2015).

Physical Examination

A low-grade fever and tachycardia are commonly associated with pericarditis. The most classic—although intermittent—finding is a pericardial friction rub. This creaking sound usually has three components and is best heard with the patient leaning forward. Auscultation should be performed with the diaphragm of the stethoscope positioned over the lower-left sternal border or at the cardiac apex (Hoit, 2011; LeWinter & Hopkins, 2015).

Diagnostic Testing

There are relatively few abnormal tests in idiopathic pericarditis. Generally, the ECGs of patients with pericarditis exhibit tachycardia and widespread ST elevations. Unlike MI, which produces regional ST elevation, the ST elevation associated with pericarditis usually involves all leads except AVR. Lead V_1 is also frequently unaffected. Often there is P-R segment depression (LeWinter & Hopkins, 2015). Usually the ECG returns to normal within 2 weeks (Hoit, 2011).

Because of the increased risk of arrhythmias in pericarditis, serum electrolytes should be obtained and corrective treatment initiated (Spangler, 2013). Blood urea nitrogen (BUN) and creatinine levels may offer clues regarding the likelihood of renal failure as an etiology for the inflammation. The assessment of renal function is also important in determining the appropriate treatment for pericarditis, because nonsteroidal anti-inflammatory drugs (NSAIDs) are often considered first-line therapy for patients with normal kidneys. Measuring serum troponin levels is reasonable to rule out MI and myocarditis. Up to 15% of patients with pericarditis also have myocarditis. Troponin levels are not elevated in pericarditis without myocarditis. A complete blood count can inform if bacterial infections are a potential etiology. In the absence of a severe bacterial infection, pericarditis usually causes a mild lymphocytosis. Serum high-sensitivity C-reactive protein (hs-CRP) is usually elevated, and serial hs-CRP can be used to help determine the length of therapy (LeWinter & Hopkins, 2015).

The chest x-ray (CXR) and echocardiogram are both normal in uncomplicated acute idiopathic pericarditis. Bacterial pericarditis can occur with severe pneumonia. An echocardiogram should be performed to assess for pericardial effusions and to determine left ventricular function. Moderate to large effusions are not usually associated with idiopathic pericarditis but can occur in pericarditis due to other disease processes such as cancer. Impaired left ventricular function in patients with no cardiac history is suspicious for myocarditis (LeWinter & Hopkins, 2015).

Additional testing is guided by the particular disease process(es) thought to be responsible for the pericarditis. For example, if a significant pericardial effusion is present and there are suspicious nodules on the CXR, a diagnostic pericardiocentesis to rule out malignancy would be appropriate.

Management

Acute idiopathic pericarditis usually resolves without serious complications or recurrences (LeWinter & Hopkins, 2015). Features associated with poor prognosis include fever above 38°C, gradual onset, large pericardial effusion, cardiac tamponade, and poor response to 1 week of aspirin or NSAID therapy (Imazio, 2014). The most common initial treatments are aspirin or NSAIDs. Aspirin 2 to 4 g divided into three or four doses daily, ibuprofen 600 to 800 mg every 8 hours, or indomethacin 50 mg every 8 hours should be administered until symptoms resolve and hs-CRP normalizes. A typical course of therapy is 10 to 14 days (Imazio, 2014; Imazio & Adler, 2013; LeWinter & Hopkins, 2015), and then treatment should be tapered. Usually, the chest pain resolves within 1 to 2 days in uncomplicated idiopathic pericarditis and treatment can be tapered in 3 or 4 days (Hoit, 2011). Recently, colchicine 0.5 mg twice daily has been demonstrated to be effective (0.5 mg daily in patients less than 70 kg and the elderly); however, it may not be tolerated due to gastrointestinal side effects (Imazio & Adler, 2013). All of the previously mentioned therapies are contraindicated or used with extreme caution in patients with renal impairment and the elderly.

When patients fail to respond to aspirin, NSAIDs, or colchicine, corticosteroids may be initiated. While corticosteroids are effective in reducing symptoms and indicators of inflammation, there is a higher rate of recurrence in patients receiving this therapy. A reasonable approach is 0.2 to 0.5 mg/kg/day with a slow taper following normalization of the hs-CRP. When therapy is continued for several weeks, patients should receive calcium and vitamin D supplementation (Imazio & Adler, 2013; LeWinter & Hopkins, 2015).

Patient Education

The suspected cause of pericarditis should be explained to patients, especially if it is associated with a chronic disease, such as systemic lupus erythematosus or renal failure. Education regarding medications, their duration, and possible side effects is imperative. Patients must also be instructed to report any recurrence of symptoms.

Follow-Up

A cardiologist should evaluate all patients with suspected pericarditis. Once the initial evaluation of pericarditis is completed, patients without high-risk features often can be managed at home. A follow-up visit should be scheduled for 7 to 10 days after the initial evaluation (Imazio, 2014). Additional follow-up is dependent on the resolution of symptoms and any identified cause.

INFECTIVE ENDOCARDITIS

Infective endocarditis (IE) occurs relatively infrequently; it is estimated to affect 2 to 6 people per 100,000 person-years (Keys, 2014). IE is most likely to occur in patients with valvular heart disease or valvular replacement, or in intravenous drug abusers. An increasing number of cases are found among elderly patients with degenerative changes in their native heart valves. The incidence of IE associated with rheumatic heart disease has decreased in developed countries. Regardless of the cause, this disorder can lead to significant complications such as stroke, limb ischemia, and death. In-hospital mortality is high at 17.7% (Murdoch et al., 2009).

Pathophysiology

Current theory suggests that minor endothelial injury due to instrumentation, such as pacemaker leads and central venous lines, and even mere repetitive valve closure can lead to the development of a microscopic thrombus, which becomes the nidus for the entrapment of any circulating bacteria (Crawford, 2014). Transient bacteremia commonly occurs during chewing and with toothbrushing in addition to more obvious causes, such as intravenous drug use or invasive procedure contamination (Habib et al., 2009).

Endocardial inflammation not caused by injury can lead to the expression of beta-1 integrins by the endothelial cells. These integrins bind fibronectin to the endothelium. Some bacteria, such as *Staphylococcus aureus*, have fibronectin-binding proteins on their surfaces. These proteins assist bacterial binding to the endothelial surface (Habib et al., 2009). In a recent multinational study, *S. aureus* was the most common cause of endocarditis, followed by coagulase negative staphylococcus, and then *viridans* group streptococci (Murdoch et al., 2009). Unfortunately, *S. aureus* IE is also the most deadly, with mortality rates reaching 50% in patients with prosthetic heart valves (Crawford, 2014).

Artificial heart valves and implanted material used for structural repairs may also be sites of bacterial attachment. In fact, the rate of infection for prosthetic valves is approximately 0.5% per patient-year, which is higher than the diseased native valve rate (Crawford, 2014). Once the bacteria are incorporated in the thrombus structure, they are fairly protected from the body's usual defense mechanisms and the colony or colonies continue to grow. These colonies can destroy underlying cardiac structures, leading to valvular incompetence, abscesses, and possible conduction disturbances (Crawford, 2014). Also, irregular structures can develop called *vegetations* that can embolize, leading to stroke or tissue ischemia and infarction in other organs or limbs.

Vegetations commonly begin on the edges of valve leaflets and progress toward the base of the valve. The mitral valve is most frequently affected, followed by the aortic, tricuspid, and the pulmonic valves. Regurgitation is caused by the irregularity created along the valve edges, erosion of the valve surface, or, in some cases, by involvement of the chordae tendineae. Abscesses and aneurysms of numerous cardiac structures can occur. Bacteremia, antibody production, and immune-complex formation lead to other problems, such as the development of glomerulonephritis. Septic emboli can cause brain abscesses (Crawford, 2014).

Fungi can also cause endocarditis, however, only among patients who are immunocompromised or who have undergone invasive procedures. *Candida, Histoplasma capsulatum,* and *Aspergillus* are the most commonly encountered organisms. Patients with fungal IE may have fewer signs and symptoms initially, but later embolization of vegetations can cause obstruction of large arteries and large anchored vegetations can sometimes obstruct valve openings (Crawford, 2014).

Endocarditis can be classified by its location and the involvement of intracardiac devices. These categories are left-sided native valve IE, left-sided prosthetic valve IE, right-sided IE, and device-related IE—which includes infection related to pacemaker and cardioverter-defibrillator leads (Habib et al., 2009). Left-sided IE can lead to severe stroke; right-sided IE may result in pulmonary embolism.

Heart failure (HF) is the most common cause of death from endocarditis and most often results from valvular regurgitation. Neurologic complications are the next most frequent negative consequence of IE. Neurologic sequelae include stroke, brain abscesses, meningitis, encephalopathy, and seizures. Renal complications can result from renal-vessel occlusion, immune complex–mediated glomerulonephritis, antibiotic-induced interstitial nephritis, and abscess formation (Habib et al., 2009; Paterick, Paterick, Nishimura, & Steckelberg, 2007).

Diagnosis

The primary methods of diagnosis for endocarditis are blood cultures and echocardiographic findings. Approximately 85% of patients have positive blood cultures, with the remainder having negative cultures due to previous antibiotic treatment, fastidious bacteria, or intracellular bacteria, such as *Chlamydia*. The European Society of Cardiology guidelines recommend three sets of blood cultures obtained from three different peripheral vein sites, approximately 30 minutes apart, and including at least one aerobic and one anaerobic media bottle. Each specimen should contain 10 mL of blood. It is extremely important to obtain these samples prior to the initiation of antibiotics; however, depending on the condition of the patient, it is reasonable to start empiric antibiotic therapy once the cultures are obtained. When culture results are known, therapy can be targeted to the identified organism (Crawford, 2014; Habib et al., 2009).

Either a transthoracic echocardiogram (TTE) or a transesophageal echocardiogram (TEE) may be used to assess for vegetations and other cardiac abnormalities, depending on the initial degree of clinical suspicion. Transesophageal echocardiography is able to detect vegetations as small as 1 to 2 millimeters. The diagnostic sensitivity and specificity of TEE for endocarditis is more than 90% (Crawford, 2014). Patients who are more likely to have IE, based on high-risk features—such as IV drug abuse, prosthetic heart valve, or previous history of IE—should undergo TEE (Baddour et al., 2005). Even though TEE may be more sensitive in detecting vegetations, useful information regarding chamber sizes, ventricular dysfunction, and pulmonary artery pressures can be obtained from a TTE. Thus, it is reasonable to perform both (Crawford, 2014; Habib et al., 2009).

The Modified Duke Criteria (MDC) for diagnosis of endocarditis incorporates the results of cultures and echocardiographic findings with other features, such as temperature elevation, patient history of predisposing factors, and physical findings, to determine the likelihood that a patient has endocarditis (Table 22.1). The MDC consists of a set of major and minor criteria. Various combinations of major and minor criteria determine the overall likelihood that endocarditis is present. Improving diagnostic certainty by applying the MDC to the patients' findings helps prevent the inappropriate use of long-term intravenous antibiotic therapy. In addition, the sensitivity of the MDC assists in finding cases that may not have classic presentations (Li et al., 2000).

Along with tests to confirm the diagnosis, other diagnostic studies should be performed to assess for complications, such as destruction of the conduction system, renal failure, or other organ failure. An ECG should be obtained to assess for rhythm or conduction disturbances and ACS. A basic metabolic panel is important in determining any renal involvement. In addition, a hepatic panel may be necessary to assess for hepatic infarction. A CXR may demonstrate multiple focal infiltrates if the patient has septic pulmonary emboli that can result from tricuspid valve endocarditis due to IV drug abuse (Paterick et al., 2007).

TABLE 22.1 Modified Duke Criteria for the Diagnosis of Infective Endocarditis (IE)

Major Criteria

Blood cultures positive for IE

■ Typical microorganisms consistent with IE from two separate blood cultures:
Viridans streptococci, *Streptococcus bovis*, HACEK group, *Staphylococcus aureus*; or
Community-acquired enterococci, in the absence of a primary focus;

or

■ Microorganisms consistent with IE from persistently positive blood cultures:
At least two positive blood cultures of blood samples drawn > 12 hours apart; or
All of three or a majority of ≥ 4 separate cultures of blood (with first and last sample drawn at least 1 hour apart)

or

■ Single positive blood culture for *Coxiella burnetii* or phase I IgG antibody titer > 1: 800

Evidence of endocardial involvement

■ Echocardiography positive for IE
Vegetation—Abscess—New partial dehiscence of prosthetic valve
■ New valvular regurgitation

Minor Criteria

■ Predisposition: predisposing heart condition, injection drug use
■ Fever: temperature > 38°C
■ Vascular phenomena: major arterial emboli, septic pulmonary infarcts, mycotic aneurysm, intracranial hemorrhages, conjunctival haemorrhages, Janeway lesions
■ Immunologic phenomena: glomerulonephritis, Osler's nodes, Roth's spots, rheumatoid factor
■ Microbiological evidence: positive blood culture but does not meet a major criterion or serological evidence of active infection with organism consistent with IE

Diagnosis of IE is definite in the presence of	Diagnosis of IE is possible in the presence of
2 major criteria, or	*1 major and 1 minor criteria, or*
1 major and 3 minor criteria, or	*3 minor criteria*
5 minor criteria	

Adapted from Li, Sexton, Mick, Nettles, Fowler, Ryan, Bashore, and Corey. Reprinted from Habib et al. (2009), with permission from Oxford University Press.

Risk Stratification

In 2002, Wallace and his colleagues reviewed 208 cases of IE retrospectively to determine predictors of poor outcome. They found that several readily attainable pieces of data were helpful in determining outcome. A white blood cell count less than 3,000 or greater than 11,000/mm³, an albumin less than 3 gm/dL, and serum creatinine equal to or greater than 1.5 mg/dL were each individually associated with increased in-hospital and 6-month mortality. Abnormal heart rhythm, presence of two major MDC criteria, and visible vegetations noted on admission were also indicators of poor prognosis (Wallace et al., 2002). Other predictors of poor outcome identified in the European Society of Cardiology IE guidelines (Habib et al., 2009) include advanced age, prosthetic valve IE, insulin-dependent diabetes, co-morbidities, *S. aureus*, fungi or gram-negative bacilli, large vegetations, and the development of complications of heart or renal failure, stroke, and septic shock (Habib et al., 2009).

Clinical Presentation

The signs and symptoms of endocarditis may vary depending on the organism and valve involved. Commonly patients complain of fever, fatigue, malaise, and arthralgias. They may also have chills or night sweats (Crawford, 2014).

Physical Examination

Most patients have fever, and usually their temperatures are greater than 38°C, but in subacute or chronic forms, patients may have low-grade fevers (Habib et al., 2009). If the causative agent is *S. aureus*, patients may have rigors. Reappearance of fever during the course of treatment is a significant finding that warrants reevaluation (Crawford, 2014).

Murmurs are often associated with endocarditis. The presence of new or worsening murmur, especially associated with fever, is suspicious for IE. Occasionally vegetations are very small or in locations where they do not cause significant regurgitation. In this case, the murmur may be too soft to be appreciated. The characteristics of the murmur may sometimes indicate which valve structure is involved. For example, a systolic murmur that radiates to the patient's back may be caused by the prolapse of the anterior mitral leaflet into the left atrium (Crawford, 2014).

A recent multinational study revealed that most patients, ~ 90% or more, did not exhibit classic findings (Murdoch et al., 2009). Classic findings include Osler's nodes and Janeway lesions. Osler's nodes are painful nodules found on the pads of the fingers and toes. These lesions are believed to be due to vasculitis or septic emboli. In contrast, Janeway lesions are painless, red macules found on the palms or soles of the feet and thought to be due to vasculitis. Splinter hemorrhages—brown streaks in the proximal portions of nailbeds—are another classic sign of endocarditis. It has been suggested that the absence of classic signs may be due to the rapid development of acute bacterial endocarditis and the decreased prevalence of chronic or subacute IE (Murdoch et al., 2009; Paterick et al., 2007).

Clinical signs of complications, such as HF, stroke, or shock, may be present in patients with severe valvular involvement. HF occurs in 50% to 60% of all IE cases, especially among patients with aortic valve involvement (Baddour et al., 2005). HF signs that are new or worsening may be an indication for urgent or emergent cardiac surgery to replace the defective valve (Habib et al., 2009).

Management

The two primary modalities of treatment for IE are long-term antibiotic (ABX) therapy and surgery. Consultation with an infectious-disease specialist, a cardiologist, and a cardiothoracic surgeon is essential. There may not be an immediate need for surgery; however, if the patient's condition deteriorates, having a surgeon who is already familiar with the case is extremely valuable. An evaluation of current management practices revealed that 44% to 56% of all IE patients undergo cardiac surgery during their initial hospital evaluation (Murdoch et al., 2009). The primary indications for surgery during the antibiotic-treatment phase are HF, uncontrolled infection, and the prevention of embolic events (Habib et al., 2009).

Because most patients with IE will receive intravenous antibiotics for extended periods of time, referral and collaboration with an infectious-disease specialist are essential. These practitioners have mechanisms in place for the delivery and monitoring of long-term outpatient intravenous ABX therapy. ABX therapy for native valve IE should be 2 to 6 weeks, while treatment for prosthetic valve endocarditis (PVE) should be for at least 6 weeks. The duration of therapy should always begin from the date of ABX initiation based on culture results that demonstrate efficacy for the cultured organism (Habib et al., 2009). Due to the ever-changing patterns of bacterial resistance, no specific antibiotic regimens will be recommended here. It should be noted that IE with negative blood cultures may be treated with oral antibiotics depending on the suspected organism (Habib et al., 2009). Therapy usually extends over many weeks to months and is best guided by a collaborative team of providers that includes an infectious-disease specialist.

Treatment of IE can be divided into two stages, the critical phase and the continuation phase. The critical phase includes the evaluation to establish the presence and extent of IE, continuous surveillance for complications, and the initiation of antibiotics. This phase usually lasts 2 weeks and is preferably conducted in an inpatient setting. When the patient is considered medically stable and an effective plan of continuing care has been formulated, the patient can move to the continuation phase of therapy (Habib et al., 2009).

Patient Education

From the time of diagnosis, patients and their families should be taught about the IE disease process, the anticipated plan of therapy, and possible complications. Patients and families must be included in discussions regarding outpatient antibiotic therapy so that an agreeable plan is developed. Patients should also be advised to contact their clinician if they develop fever or chills, as these symptoms may represent relapse or reinfection. Preventative strategies should also be discussed, including antibiotic prophylaxis, good oral hygiene, and regular dental care.

Care Coordination

Patients with IE have a significant need for effective multidisciplinary care. Social workers, pharmacists, nurses, advanced practice clinicians, and various physician specialists are required to assist patients and families to successfully navigate through the many aspects of the treatment plan. Social workers may need to determine the level of the patient's insurance coverage for inpatient as well as outpatient care. Insurance may not cover intravenous medications administered at home. Alternatively, patients may need transportation if they receive their antibiotics at an infusion center or to obtain scheduled follow-up appointments. Pharmacists may need to recommend or make antibiotic dosage adjustments based on the patient's renal function throughout the course of therapy. Advanced practice clinicians may coordinate care and ensure smooth transitions from the hospital to home or subacute-care facility.

Follow-Up

According to the European Society of Cardiology guidelines, there is no evidence to guide the optimal timing of IE follow-up; however, it is recommended that clinical evaluations, TTEs, and blood samples for white blood cells and CRP be performed at 1, 3, 6, and 12 months (Habib et al., 2009).

For full reference citations to this chapter, please see "Section References" in the back of the book, under the heading "Section V."

Syncope

HELEN F. BROWN AND LINDA BRIGGS

Syncope is a challenging chief complaint to evaluate, diagnose, and manage. Syncope is a transient loss of consciousness (TLOC) due to a brief "decrease in global cerebral perfusion characterized by rapid onset, short duration, and spontaneous complete recovery" (Moya et al., 2009, p. 2635). By incorporating the three key characteristics of onset, duration, and recovery of the episode, the definition excludes other causes for loss of consciousness, such as seizures or minor traumatic head injury (Moya et al., 2009). A common presentation to emergency departments (ED) and primary care settings, TLOC is responsible for 1% to 3% of ED visits. One third of these patients will be hospitalized (Sun, Emond, & Camargo, 2004; Thiruganasambandamoorthy et al., 2014). Of those patients seeking care for an episode of TLOC, 7% to 23% will experience a serious adverse event, such as myocardial infarction (MI), stroke, pulmonary embolism, or death, within 7 to 30 days of their initial presentation to the ED (Quinn et al., 2008; Quinn, McDermott, Stiell, Kohn, & Wells, 2006; Thiruganasambandamoorthy et al., 2014). Therein lies the challenge in managing the patient presenting with TLOC—differentiating between potentially life-altering pathology and a benign episode of syncope. TLOC can be a result of neurologic or cardiac events, metabolic disturbances, or the cause may be multifactorial. The "rule of 15s" for syncope states that TLOC is the initial presenting symptom in 15% of patients experiencing a subarachnoid hemorrhage, acute coronary syndrome, aortic dissection, ruptured aortic aneurysm, and ectopic pregnancy (Mattu, 2009). Due to the transient nature of the presenting episode, determining the underlying mechanism for the event can be difficult. In approximately one third of patients with TLOC, no cause for the episode is identified even following the completion of a thorough diagnostic evaluation (Arnar, 2013). When assessing a patient presenting with TLOC, a practical approach is to consider whether the event is due to stimulation of neurocardiogenic reflexes, an autonomic disorder, a primary cardiovascular event, or a combination of these pathologies (Juul-Moller, 2013).

PATHOPHYSIOLOGY

To sustain function, the brain requires at least 3 mL of oxygen per 100 g of tissue per minute; less than this will produce loss of consciousness (Moya et al., 2009). Mechanisms reducing oxygen delivery to the neuron result in impaired function. Situations that produce a decrease in oxygen available for extraction, such as severe hypoxia, may result in syncope. Additionally, TLOC can be caused by conditions that alter oxygen-carrying capacity, including severe anemia, carbon monoxide poisoning, methemoglobinemia, hypophosphatemia, hypothermia, hyperthermia, and acid–base disturbances (Wieling et al., 2009). However, the most common cause of TLOC is an alteration in cerebral perfusion pressure (CPP) that results in global cellular dysfunction and loss of consciousness (Moya et al., 2009).

Factors affecting CPP are the mean arterial pressure (MAP), intracranial pressure (ICP), and the partial pressures of oxygen and carbon dioxide. The primary factor influencing CPP is the MAP, which is a product of cardiac output and systemic vascular resistance. Any pathologic situation that decreases one of these parameters will produce syncope due to impaired cerebral perfusion. In response to a change in MAP, ICP, or a metabolic derangement such as hypoxia, hypercarbia or hypocarbia, the cerebral vasculature will autoregulate to maintain constant cerebral blood flow. Autoregulation can maintain cerebral blood flow over a wide range of CPPs (50–150 mmHg). However, at lower CPPs, the relationship between cerebral blood flow and CPP becomes linear. Therefore, as CPP falls below 50 mmHg, global perfusion pressure drops and loss of consciousness occurs. A reduction of CPP by 35% or complete cessation of perfusion for 5 to 10 seconds will produce TLOC (Ammirati et al., 1998).

ETIOLOGY

The causes of cardiovascular-related syncope can be placed into one of the following categories: neurocardiogenic, orthostatic hypotension, and cardiovascular (Table 23.1) (Kapoor, 2000; Soteriades et al., 2002).

Neurocardiogenic Syncope

The most common cause of TLOC—irrespective of age, gender, or co-morbidities—is reflexive or vasovagal syncope (Sheldon et al., 2006; Soteriades et al., 2002). Neurally or reflex-mediated syncope is an assortment of disorders that produce a final common pathway of vasodilation, causing hypotension and absolute or relative bradycardia resulting in TLOC (Saklani, Krahn, & Klein, 2013). The constellation of disorders that can produce neurocardiogenic TLOC includes vasovagal, situational, and carotid sinus syncope. Neurally mediated syncope is due to an abrupt withdrawal of sympathetic response and an increase in parasympathetic tone (Saklani et al., 2013). This form of TLOC can have a prodromal pattern of lightheadedness with diaphoresis, nausea, or a sensation of warmth. A patient report of a slowly progressing sensation of impending loss of consciousness and the presence of prodromal symptoms suggests vasovagal syncope. This form of TLOC rarely lasts longer than 20 seconds, followed by immediate recovery with appropriate mentation and orientation (Moya et al., 2009).

Carotid sinus syndrome is more common in men, the older adult, individuals with ischemic heart disease, and those with certain head and neck malignancies (Wieling et al., 2013). Carotid sinus syndrome is produced by hypersensitivity of the carotid sinus bodies located at the carotid bifurcation bilaterally. An external force stimulating a sensitive carotid body, producing either bradycardia with subsequent hypotension or vasodilation with hypotension, typically results in a total

TABLE 23.1 Etiologies and Mechanisms of Cardiovascular Syncope

Category	Etiology	Mechanism
Neurocardiogenic	Vasovagal	Emotional stress: fear, pain
	Situational	Cough, sneeze, gastrointestinal stimulation, micturition, neuralgia, post-exercise, post-prandial, laughing, weight lifting, playing an instrument (Trumpeter's syndrome)
	Carotid sinus syndrome	Tight collar, neck turning or manipulation, elder, hypersensitive carotid sinus body
	Atypical	No apparent trigger or atypical presentation
Orthostatic hypotension	Primary autonomic failure	Dysautonomies: Multiple system atrophy, Parkinson's disease, multiple sclerosis, postural orthostatic tachycardia syndrome, Shy-Drager syndrome, Lewy body dementia
	Secondary autonomic failure	Diabetes, amyloidosis, uremia, spinal cord injury, autoimmune diseases
	Drug induced	Alcohol, cocaine
	Medication induced	**Vasoactive**: Antihypertensives, nitrates, diuretics, phosphodiesterase type 5 inhibitors, anti-Parkinson drugs **Conduction System**: Cardiac glycosides, antiarrhythmics, beta blockers, calcium channel blockers **QT interval prolongation**: Antiarrhythmics, antiemetics, antipsychotics, antidepressants
	Volume depletion	Blood loss, vomiting, diarrhea, excessive sweating, volume shifts such as 3rd spacing, overdiuresis
	Deconditioning	Prolonged bedrest, lengthy illness, older adult
Cardiovascular	Bradycardia	SA node dysfunction (tachybrady syndrome), AV conduction system disease, pacemaker malfunction
	Tachycardia	Supraventricular Ventricular: idiopathic, second to structural heart disease, or channelopathies
	Medication induced	Bradycardia or tachycardia
	Structural heart disease	Valvular cardiac disease, prosthetic valve dysfunction, acute coronary syndrome or myocardial ischemia, hypertrophic cardiomyopathy, cardiac masses, pericardial disease, cardiac tamponade, congenital anomalies of the coronary arteries
	Other	Myocarditis, pulmonary embolus, acute aortic dissection, pulmonary hypertension

Source: Moya et al. (2009).

loss of consciousness. A bradycardic response is most common, with stimulation of the carotid body slowing heart rate and resulting in asystole for more than 3 seconds. The vasodepressor response is less common with a decrease in systolic blood pressure (SBP) to 50 mmHg (Wieling et al., 2013).

Orthostatic Hypotension

Orthostatic hypotension, a common cause of syncope, is estimated to be responsible for one fourth of syncopal episodes presenting to an ED (Lemonick, 2010). This form of syncope is most common in older adult patients (Calkins & Zipes, 2015).

Orthostatic hypotension is defined as a decrease in SBP of greater than 20 mmHg or a decrease in diastolic blood pressure (DBP) of 10 mmHg within 3 minutes of standing (Consensus Committee of the American Autonomic Society & American Academy of Neurology, 1996). Orthostatic hypotension represents the autonomic nervous system's inability to compensate for the physiologic changes that occur when an individual assumes an upright position. This decrease in cerebral perfusion with changing positions—from a lying to sitting or sitting to standing—can result in TLOC. The normal physiologic response to assuming an upright position is an increase in heart rate and peripheral-vascular resistance. This results in little or no change in the MAP, and thereby maintains CPP. If the physiologic response is insufficient to maintain an adequate CPP, the individual will become symptomatic, experiencing lightheadedness; visual disturbance of tunnel vision, blurring, or a brightness; hearing disturbance of hearing impairment, tinnitus, or crackles; or pain in the cervical, lumbar, or precordial areas (Moya et al., 2009). The prodrome may or may not include diaphoresis or nausea followed by loss of consciousness (Fedorowski & Melander, 2013). The signs and symptoms that are evidence of the body's inability to maintain adequate CPP due to an abnormality anywhere in the blood pressure (BP) regulation system are referred to as *orthostatic intolerance* (Calkins & Zipes, 2015).

Conditions that can result in an inability to maintain postural tone include primary and secondary dysautonomia, intravascular volume depletion, medication-induced orthostasis, and deconditioning. Primary dysautonomia refers to disorders in which abnormalities in the autonomic nervous system are the direct cause of the problem, for example, familial dysautonomia, or multiple system atrophy (Horwitz, Horwitz, & Noggle, 2012). Secondary dysautonomias are disorders in which the autonomic nervous system has been affected by aging or another disease state, including spinal cord lesions or autoimmune diseases (Calkins & Zipes, 2015). Secondary dysautonomia is frequently associated with advanced age or diabetes and is due to the decreased autonomic response to the gravitational volume shifts that occur with a change in position (Fedorowski & Melander, 2013). Serious causes of orthostatic hypotension including volume depletion due to hemorrhage or dehydration and adverse medication reactions can appear clinically in a similar manner as non-life-threatening causes such as primary dysautonomias, so it is imperative to evaluate this patient population judiciously.

Cardiovascular

Cardiovascular causes of syncope are potentially life-threatening disorders and associated with higher mortality rates than TLOC from other causes. A large cohort of 400 individuals experiencing syncope was followed for 60 months. Those experiencing cardiac-induced syncope had a mortality rate of 50%, compared with 34% for those with noncardiac TLOC and 24% in individuals experiencing syncope due to an unidentified cause (Kapoor, 1990). The three categories of cardiovascular causes are arrhythmias, structural disorders, and ischemic cardiac events (Arnar, 2013; Lemonick, 2010). Arrhythmia is the most frequent cause of cardiac-induced syncope (Moya et al., 2009). The presyncopal prodrome can include dizziness, palpitations, shortness of breath, chest pain, or a sudden onset of lightheadedness

(Arnar, 2013). Individuals experiencing TLOC related to an arrhythmia may experience minimal warning of an impending loss of consciousness. Particularly worrisome is syncope that occurs during exertion or while the individual is supine (Arnar, 2013). Electrocardiographic findings that confer an increased risk for sudden death in the setting of syncope include the following:

- Nonsustained ventricular tachycardia (VT)
- Bifascicular block or prolonged intraventricular conduction, QRS greater than 120 msec
- Preexcitation QRS, short P-R with delta wave as seen in Wolfe-Parkinson-White syndrome
- Abnormal short or prolonged QT interval, electrolyte or medication induced
- Brugada syndrome pattern in leads V_1 and V_2 with pseudo right bundle branch block plus ST-segment elevation in one right precordial lead, V_1 to V_3 plus one clinical criteria
- Bradycardias including second- and third-degree heart block (Arnar, 2013; Lemonick, 2010)

Structural or functional cardiac disorders associated with TLOC are ischemic heart disease, nonischemic-dilated cardiomyopathy, and severe aortic stenosis (Arnar, 2013). Structural or functional problems produce syncope when oxygen demand exceeds the ability of the heart to increase cardiac output (Arnar, 2013; Moya et al., 2009). Of concern is structural disease that impedes left ventricular outflow due to a fixed or dynamic obstruction (Moya et al., 2009). It is important to recognize that eliciting a reflex response, developing orthostatic hypotension, or experiencing a dysrhythmia—particularly atrial fibrillation—in the presence of a structural or functional lesion results in a multifactorial cause for the TLOC (Arnar, 2013; Moya et al., 2009). In these situations, it is necessary to recognize the relative contribution of each disorder to the syncope, so the underlying processes can be addressed if necessary (Arnar, 2013; Moya et al., 2009).

Structural heart disease and primary electrical disturbances are risk factors for sudden cardiac arrest and mortality in patients with TLOC (Moya et al., 2009). Orthostatic hypotension, in combination with structural heart disease, also conveys an increased risk for death. In these situations, the poor outcomes are related to the co-morbidities producing the TLOC, not the syncope itself (Moya et al., 2009).

DIAGNOSIS

The purpose of a diagnostic evaluation of individuals experiencing TLOC is to recognize persons who may experience sudden decompensation and those likely to experience a recurrent serious event, associated with morbidity or mortality (Huff et al., 2007). The cornerstone of the diagnostic evaluation is a thorough history, physical examination, and interpretation of the ECG. This initial evaluation leads to a confirmed or suspected diagnosis for the TLOC in 50% of cases (Brignole et al., 2006). Routine laboratory testing is not recommended, as the data obtained from testing of electrolytes, renal function, and blood counts typically do not yield information that identifies the cause of the TLOC (Huff et al., 2007; Kapoor, 2000; Moya et al., 2009). Any additional diagnostic interventions should be guided by the findings obtained from the initial evaluation.

CLINICAL PRESENTATION

Elucidating the history of the TLOC event is one of the defining factors in risk stratifying the patient (Table 23.2). An accurate account of prodromal events, the characteristics of the episode, and symptoms following the return of consciousness are obtained from the patient and any witness to the event (Huff et al., 2007). Important historical data to elicit includes body position, activity, and environmental factors prior to the episode of TLOC. Having the patient describe the events immediately prior to the syncopal event begins the risk factor stratification process, helping separate life-threatening causes for syncope from neurocardiogenic syncope or orthostatic hypotension–induced syncope.

TABLE 23.2 Historical Data to Obtain About the Syncopal Episode

Presyncope events
  Prodromal: Impending sense of fainting, aura
  Position: Standing, sitting, laying
  Activity: Rest, with or following excursion or exercise, position change, with micturition, defecation, coughing
  Environmental: Prolonged standing, hot or crowded room
  Situational: Pre- or post-prandial, head or neck movement, emotional stress, fear, anxious, severe pain

Events at the onset of syncope
  Symptoms: Palpitations, dyspnea, chest pain, dizziness, light-headedness, visual disturbance
  Associated with nausea, vomiting, cold clammy skin, excessive sweating
  Physical signs: (Provided by witness)
  General: Sudden loss of consciousness, duration of loss of consciousness, position of fall, slumped over, partial fall, or complete loss of postural tone
    Color change: Pale, cyanosis, flushing
    Respiratory pattern: Apnea, stentorious, labored
    Neurologic: Seizure activity, focal, generalized, or automatism, duration of seizure activity, onset of seizure activity in relation to the loss of postural tone, incontinence

Postsyncope events
  General: Evidence of injury, tongue biting, myalgia
  Neurologic: Spontaneous recovery versus delayed period of altered sensorium, postictal state, confusion
  Cardiovascular: Color change, diaphoresis, chest pain, palpitation
  Gastrointestinal: Nausea, vomiting

Past medical history
  Cardiac: Myocardial infarction, heart failure, valvular heart disease, structural defect
  Neurologic: Seizure disorder, Parkinson disease, multiple sclerosis, Lewy body dementia
  Metabolic: Diabetes, adrenal insufficiency, hypoglycemia
  Medications: Beta blockers, calcium channel blockers, antihypertensives, antidysrhythmics, diuretics, medications that can prolong the QT interval such as antipsychotics, antidepressants, antiemetics, over-the-counter medications, laxative, decongestants
  Social: Alcohol use, drug use
  Family: History of sudden death, dysrhythmias, syncope

Sources: Huff et al. (2007); Lemonick (2010); Moya et al. (2009).

In neurocardiogenic syncope, important clinical features include no history of cardiac disease and a prior history of multiple episodes of syncope; a sense of deja vu or impending feeling of faintness; loss of consciousness that occurs following noxious stimuli, an unpleasant sight, smell, or pain; prolonged standing, particularly in a warm and crowded environment; nausea and vomiting; carotid sinus pressure due to a tight collar or head turning; or syncope following strenuous activity (Moya et al., 2009). Historical features suggesting orthostatic hypotension include syncope with position change; prolonged standing, particularly in a warm crowded room; temporal relationship with medication ingestion or changes in medication dosage; and known autonomic neuropathy or Parkinson's disease (Moya et al., 2009). Clinical features associated with cardiovascular syncope include TLOC during exertion or lying supine, sudden loss of consciousness without warning, palpitations immediately prior to the TLOC, family history of sudden death, and presence of structural heart disease (Moya et al., 2009). TLOC without warning or occurring during exertion is highly suggestive of an arrhythmia or structural cardiac disease (Arnar, 2013).

PHYSICAL EXAMINATION

The physical examination is the second key component in the initial evaluation of an individual with TLOC. At the time the physical assessment is performed, the patient frequently is asymptomatic and the examination is normal. As the examination is performed, the clinician is assessing for subtle clues or physical findings that would indicate a cardiovascular or neurologic cause. Also, the provider should evaluate the patient for signs of trauma, noting the presence or absence of defensive injuries. A lack of defensive wounds or trauma to the hands, wrists, or knees is concerning for a sudden loss of consciousness occurring without a warning. In this situation, arrhythmia must be considered in the differential diagnosis for the TLOC (Arnar, 2013; Moya et al., 2009).

Assessment of the cardiovascular system should include vital signs, bilateral arm BPs, orthostatic vital signs, auscultation of the heart for location of the point of maximal impulse, and for the presence of a murmur. The peripheral vasculature is assessed for pulse strength and the major blood vessels for bruits. A decrease in BP is a transient feature in TLOC. Therefore, persistent hypotension suggests alternative pathology for the syncopal episode and requires a full diagnostic investigation (Huff et al., 2007). During the cardiopulmonary assessment, the practitioner should actively look for clinical features of heart failure, including an S_3, jugular vein distention (JVD), pulmonary crackles, and peripheral edema. In multiple studies assessing risk factors for TLOC, individuals with left ventricular dysfunction, low ejection fractions, and a history of heart failure are at greater risk for sudden death (Colivicchi et al., 2003; Martin, Hanusa, & Kapoor, 1997; Quinn et al., 2004; Sarasin et al., 2003; Thiruganasambandamoorthy et al., 2014).

A neurologic evaluation is necessary to assess for focal neurologic deficits or autonomic dysfunction, as evidenced in peripheral neuropathies. Gastrointestinal assessment is performed to evaluate blood loss by a rectal examination to assess for frank or occult blood loss. The oral cavity is evaluated for evidence of trauma, such as tongue or buccal-mucosal injury.

DIAGNOSTIC TESTING

The final component of the initial diagnostic evaluation for syncope is the 12-lead ECG. According to Moya et al. (2009), ECG findings that are suggestive of an arrhythmia-induced syncope include the following:

- Bifascicular block
- Interventricular conduction delay greater than 120 msec
- Asymptomatic "inappropriate" bradycardia
- Second-degree heart block, particularly Mobitz Type 2
- Ventricular tachycardia
- Preexcitation syndromes
- Altered QT interval
- Brugada criteria
- Presence of ischemic changes or Q waves indicating prior MI

Additional diagnostic testing is based on information obtained from the history, physical examination, and ECG. Carotid sinus massage is indicated in patients older than the age of 40 with syncope of unknown etiology after the initial evaluation and provided that no carotid bruit was auscultated on physical examination (Moya et al., 2009). Carotid sinus massage is diagnostic if syncope is produced with greater than 3 seconds of asystole or there is a decrease in SBP greater than 50 mmHg (Moya et al., 2009). Laboratory testing is ordered based upon data collected during the physical examination. The American College of Emergency Physicians' clinical policy statement on evaluation and management of syncope in adult patients states that laboratory testing rarely produces diagnostically relevant information and routine use is not recommended (Huff et al., 2007). Based on the history and physical, if a metabolic disturbance such as hypoglycemia, electrolyte imbalance, thyroid disorder, or anemia is suspected, testing is indicated. A pregnancy test for women of reproductive age is always indicated as part of the TLOC evaluation.

Cardiac monitoring is indicated when there is a high probability that the TLOC is associated with an arrhythmia. Individuals requiring hospitalization or intensive evaluation include those with severe structural heart disease, coronary heart disease, and clinical or ECG features suggesting arrhythmia-induced syncope. High-risk clinical features include syncope with exertion or lying supine, palpitations just prior to the TLOC episode, family history of sudden cardiac death, and concomitant severe anemia or electrolyte disturbance (Moya et al., 2009). High-risk ECG features are tachyarrhythmia, bradyarrhythmia, conduction defect or disease, and new ischemia or old infarct (Sheldon et al., 2011). The diagnostic yield of 24 to 48 hours of continuous monitoring is approximately 16%; however, admission is justified to diminish imminent risk to the patient (Huff et al., 2007; Moya et al., 2009). This period of time provides the primary provider with an opportunity to obtain additional studies and an expedited cardiology consultation with a goal of identifying additional management strategies. These interventions might include Holter monitoring, an external event recorder, an external loop recorder, or an internal loop recorder to assess for life-threatening arrhythmia. These monitoring devices will continue to evaluate the patient in the outpatient setting, increasing the yield for identifying an arrhythmia as cause of the TLOC. The advantages of an internal loop recorder are the long duration of recording, the absence of surface electrodes attached to the patient, and no requirement for patient participation in recording events (Saklani et al., 2013). The major disadvantage is the need for minor surgery to place the device. However, an implantable loop recording as a primary strategy to identify dysrhythmia as the cause of TLOC has demonstrated efficacy and cost-effectiveness when compared with conventional investigative methods (Krahn, Klein, Yee, Hoch, & Skanes, 2003). If arrhythmia is highly suspicious for the cause of syncope, referral to an electrophysiologist specialist may be appropriate for further evaluation and testing. Electrophysiology studies (EPS) are utilized to induce arrhythmias in individuals with structural defects and cardiac disease, such as prior MI, conductive disorders, and heart failure (Moya et al., 2009; Saklani et al., 2013). EPS provide a low yield in the structurally normal heart.

Evaluation for structural or functional causes for the TLOC might include an echocardiogram to assess for structural abnormalities and left ventricular function; a cardiac stress test, if ischemia is a concern or if the syncope was exercise induced; and carotid ultrasound to assess for stenosis (Saklani et al., 2013). In the high-risk patient, these studies can be performed in the inpatient setting. For the low-risk patient, if deemed necessary, the evaluation is completed in the outpatient setting. Tilt table testing can be used to determine orthostasis or neurocardiac reflexes as causes for repeated syncopal episodes. Neurologic studies, such as electroencephalogram and brain imaging, should be considered only if there is significant evidence on the initial evaluation that there was a neurologic event or seizure as a cause of the TLOC (Saklani et al., 2013).

RISK STRATIFICATION

By focusing on prognosis at the conclusion of the initial evaluation, a determination can be made concerning the safe disposition of the patient; high-risk features for syncope are listed in Table 23.3. In addition, utilizing clinical decision rules can assist the practitioner in determining the risk of a serious adverse event if there are repeated syncopal episodes among patients experiencing a TLOC. The goal of risk scoring is to differentiate between patients who require inpatient evaluation from those who can be safely evaluated in the outpatient setting (Saklani et al., 2013). The San Francisco Syncope Rule is a prospectively evaluated decision rule with a sensitivity of 98% and specificity of 56% for predicting the likelihood of an adverse event occurring within 30 days (Quinn et al., 2006). In this decision rule, high-risk features for serious sequelae to a syncopal episode are a history of congestive heart

TABLE 23.3 High-Risk Features in Syncope

Male gender
Age >45
Abnormal ECG
History of ventricular arrhythmias
History of heart failure

Sources: Martin et al. (1997); Sheldon, Hersi, Richie, Koshman, and Rose (2010).

failure, hematocrit less than 30%, abnormal ECG, complaint of shortness of breath, and a triage SBP of less than 90 mmHg (Quinn et al., 2006). The mnemonic "CHESS" is utilized to recall the key factors. A positive finding for any of the tool indicators places the patient at high risk. Other clinical decision rules have similar criteria recognizing the significance of the abnormal ECG, structural or functional cardiac disease, and older adult status in predicting adverse outcomes at 1 year post-event (Colivicchi et al., 2003; Martin et al., 1997). Based on scores provided by these tools, the practitioner can determine appropriate management and disposition.

MANAGEMENT

The goal of treatment of patients with TLOC is to reduce occurrences of syncopal episodes, thus limiting future risk for injury and lowering mortality. Identification of the cause of the TLOC is essential to initiating treatment. In the high-risk population experiencing TLOC due to a cardiovascular cause, optimization of cardiac function is the essential strategy. In individuals with ischemic or nonischemic cardiomyopathies with severely depressed left ventricular function or heart failure, insertion of an implantable cardioverter defibrillator (ICD) can reduce the risk for sudden cardiac death (Moya et al., 2009). In individuals with hypertrophic cardiomyopathy, right ventricular cardiomyopathy, Brugada syndrome, long QT syndrome on beta blocker therapy, and ischemic and nonischemic cardiomyopathies without depressed left ventricular function or heart failure, ICD therapy is individualized based on the specific patient's risk analysis (Arnar, 2013; Moya et al., 2009; Olshansky & Sullivan, 2013). If it is determined that an ICD is not indicated, placement of an implantable loop recorder should be considered, thus facilitating identification of symptomatic or asymptomatic dysrhythmias (Arnar, 2013; Moya et al., 2009; Olshansky & Sullivan, 2013). Following ICD implantation in appropriate patients, medication management can be optimized for these individuals.

When cardiac arrhythmia is the precipitating event producing TLOC, electrophysiology evaluation may be indicated for pacemaker therapy, ICD implantation, or ablation (Moya et al., 2009). Situations that may warrant pacing include sinus node disease and conductive disorders—Mobitz Type II heart block or third-degree heart block, and bundle branch blocks—and unexplained syncope or positive EPS (Moya et al., 2009). Individuals with ECG-documented supraventricular tachycardia (SVT) or VT in the absence of structural cardiac disease may benefit from catheter ablation (Moya et al., 2009). Antiarrhythmic agents should be utilized to control syncope related to atrial fibrillation with rapid ventricular response and SVT or VT when catheter ablation cannot be performed or was unsuccessful (Moya et al., 2009).

The final modality to consider in the individual experiencing syncope due to dysrhythmia is the ICD. For individuals with documented VT with structural heart disease, those with prior MI and monomorphic VT induced during EPS, or VT in patients with inherited disorders—such as cardiomyopathies or channelopathies—device therapy with an ICD is indicated to prevent sudden death and repeated TLOC (Moya et al., 2009; Olshansky & Sullivan, 2013). Frequently, the cause of recurrent TLOC is multifactorial. Device therapy to control dysrhythmias may be only one component of the therapy that is necessary to manage the situation. In managing this patient population, reevaluating the patient for orthostatic hypotension and neurally mediated causes for TLOC should be considered. Underlying autonomic neuropathy can still produce orthostasis after a pacemaker or ICD placement. Therefore, it is prudent to reevaluate the patient's medications and co-morbidities to identify any potential of additional causes for the TLOC.

The treatment approach to neurocardiogenic and orthostatic hypotension–induced syncope is similar. The initial intervention is education. Patients must have a clear understanding of the underlying pathophysiology for their presyncopal or syncopal episodes. Individuals who suffer from neurocardiogenic syncope must be aware of and avoid their triggers, such as prolonged standing and painful stimuli. They should also be instructed to drink at least 2 liters of fluid daily (Grub, 2005). For patients with orthostatic hypotension, interventions such as avoiding immobility and gradually arising from a sitting or lying position can help avoid recurrences. For some, increased salt and fluid intake may be important (Fedorowski & Melander, 2013). Among older adults, especially those in nursing homes, avoidance of large meals may help avoid syncope associated with meals (Calkins & Zipes, 2015). For those with more significant autonomic dysfunction, compression stockings may be helpful (Fedorowski & Melander, 2013).

The next step is to scrutinize each patient's medications to identify any medications that can cause hypotension and discontinue if feasible. Some commonly prescribed medications that can cause orthostatic hypotension include diuretics, alpha blockers, beta blockers, vasodilators, clonidine, tricyclic antidepressants, muscle relaxants, and medications prescribed for parkinsonism (Moses, 2012). Because of reduced baroreceptor sensitivity, decreased cerebral blood flow, and other changes that occur with aging, older adults are especially sensitive to these medications (Calkins & Zipes, 2015).

Some patients with orthostatic hypotension may benefit from medications to prevent reductions in BP. The effects of these medications are limited, and often there are significant side effects. Midodrine, a direct alpha-1-adrenergic agonist, increases vascular tone, and fludrocortisone, a mineralocorticoid, may be used when volume expansion is desirable (Fedorowski & Melander, 2013). Midodrine and fludrocortisone can also be used in the treatment of neurocardiogenic syncope. Beta blockers have been used for many years to treat this form of syncope; however, the guidelines from the European Society of Cardiology for the diagnosis and treatment of syncope (Moya et al., 2009) state that beta blockers are not indicated and may be harmful. Regardless of the therapy chosen, follow-up is important to determine the effectiveness of treatment and to make adjustments if required.

For full reference citations to this chapter, please see "Section References" in the back of the book, under the heading "Section V."

Sudden Cardiac Death and Cardiac Arrest

LINDA BRIGGS

Sudden cardiac death (SCD) has several definitions that vary based on the time-span from the initial onset of the problem to the actual death of the patient. What these definitions have in common are the following features: (a) abrupt onset with a loss of consciousness, (b) circulatory collapse, and (c) death of the patient. One of the most stringent definitions stipulates the timeframe from onset of symptoms to death as 1 hour (Myerburg & Castellanos, 2015). The incidence of SCD varies according to how it is defined.

A similar corollary is cardiac arrest (CA), in which there is a loss of consciousness and circulation due to a lack of cardiac activity. If not corrected rapidly, death will occur. *Cardiac arrest* is the term that should be used to stipulate a nonfatal event (Buxton et al., 2006). Despite definitions published by the American College of Cardiology (ACC) and American Health Association (AHA), *sudden cardiac death* and *cardiac arrest* are terms that are often used interchangeably.

Out-of-hospital CA also has a number of definitions. The Resuscitation Outcomes Consortium registry has made estimates of CA occurrence. Based on the 2013 census data, there are approximately 424,000 outside CAs per year in the United States (Go et al., 2013). In-hospital CAs are estimated to be 209,000 per year (Merchant et al., 2011).

ETIOLOGY

Ventricular tachycardia (VT), ventricular fibrillation (VF), or any shockable rhythm has been observed in 23% of out-of-hospital CA instances (Nichol et al., 2008). In a study of hospitalized patients, the first recorded rhythms were pulseless electrical activity (PEA) in 41%, VT in 39%, and asystole in 20%. In this same investigation, 63% of CAs were due to heart disease and 15% to pulmonary causes, such as pulmonary embolism and asthma. Other causes included aortic dissection, exsanguination, alcohol or drugs, metabolic derangements, and sepsis (Wallmuller et al., 2012). Clearly arrhythmias and heart disease are significant mediators of CA, and, by extension, SCD.

Heart disease associated with CA and SCD can either be acquired or congenital. The predominant types of acquired heart disease associated with CA and SCD are coronary heart disease (CHD) and heart failure (HF). Congenital heart diseases connected with CA include congenital long QT syndrome (LQTS), short QT syndrome, and Brugada syndrome. Genetic disorders, such as hypertrophic cardiomyopathy and right ventricular dysplasia, are also associated with increased risk of SCD. Infiltrative diseases, such as sarcoidosis and amyloidosis, are examples of acquired heart disease that are responsible for a small percentage of CAs and SCDs.

Valvular heart disease, such as aortic stenosis or aortic regurgitation, may also cause SCD. However, approximately 80% of all SCD events occur in patients with CHD, with known or unknown coronary disease prior to the SCD event (Myerburg & Castellanos, 2015). Myocardial ischemia and scarring are substrates for arrhythmogenesis (Darby & DiMarco, 2014; Myerburg & Castellanos, 2015).

Myocardial ischemia causes changes in cell membrane function. As a result, potassium leaves the cell, and calcium ions enter, causing a decrease in the resting membrane potential and an increase in automaticity (Myerburg & Castellanos, 2015). A decrease in myocyte resting potential partially inactivates sodium channels, which can lead to slow Na+ influx and slow conduction when the affected cell or myocardial tissue becomes depolarized. Slowed impulse conduction in ischemic myocytes creates a situation where normal, surrounding cells have repolarized and are ready to accept another stimulus when the slowed impulse finally exits the ischemic tissue. This creates a reentry or circuit loop that causes reentry rhythms such as VT. In VF, there are multiple reentry circuits (Hall, 2011a). With the sudden reintroduction of oxygen to ischemic tissues during reperfusion, arrhythmias may develop due to electrical instability caused by the continued entry of calcium into ischemic cells (Myerburg & Castellanos, 2015).

The degree of left ventricular dysfunction in HF is the strongest predictor of SCD. An ejection fraction less than 40% is associated with increased mortality following myocardial infarction (MI) (Multicenter Postinfarction Research Group, 1983). Ventricular ectopy is common among patients with left ventricular dysfunction. In fact, severe dysfunction is associated with more complex ventricular arrhythmias and a higher risk of death (Cleland, Chattopadhyay, Khand, Houghton, & Kaye, 2002). Among patients with chronic HF, ischemic cardiomyopathy is most commonly associated with SCD. Acute HF may also lead to SCD (Myerburg & Castellanos, 2015).

Other forms of cardiomyopathy also confer risk. SCD among young athletes occurs more frequently among men than women. Most often SCD in younger individuals is due to known or previously unrecognized cardiac abnormalities, such as hypertrophic cardiomyopathy or coronary artery anomalies (Myerburg & Castellanos, 2015). Another mode of SCD among young athletes, commotio cordis, is due to blunt chest wall trauma that initiates ventricular arrhythmias (Madias, Maron, Weinstock, Estes, & Link, 2007).

DIAGNOSIS

The diagnosis of CA must be performed quickly and often without benefit of advanced technology. Once emergency measures are initiated, clinicians should consider the potential cause so that reversible conditions can be addressed. For persons of SCD, postmortem investigations may unveil previously unknown CHD or other pathology. Knowledge of the cause of death may be important in determining future risk of SCD among surviving family members.

CLINICAL PRESENTATION

SCD and CA are first evidenced by a sudden loss of consciousness and the cessation of effective respirations and circulation. Depending on the cause of SCD or CA, there may be signs and symptoms that precede the patient's collapse. Patients or their families may indicate that there was a prior syncopal event (Cleland et al., 2002; Myerburg & Castellanos, 2015). Patients with HF may complain of dyspnea and palpitations. Those with pulmonary embolus, aortic dissection, or MI may complain of chest pain. Obtaining a history from the patient, family, or other witnesses may help determine the etiology of the collapse. A history of previous CHD, HF, arrhythmias, syncope, or trauma can help narrow the possible causes of CA. Family histories of sudden death, cardiomyopathy, or arrhythmias are also important clues. While historical information is important, immediate intervention with cardiopulmonary resuscitation (CPR) should not be delayed.

PHYSICAL EXAMINATION

Once unresponsiveness and cessation of effective respirations have been established, a clinician may assess for a carotid pulse. This maneuver should not take longer than 10 seconds. If the patient has monitoring electrodes already in place, the cardiac rhythm should be assessed simultaneously. Defibrillator pads should be placed as soon as the monitor or defibrillator is available. Further assessment is deferred until after 2 minutes of CPR and the first shock is delivered. Once an advanced airway has been placed, auscultation of the lungs should be performed to verify airway placement. Capnography or an exhaled CO_2 detector is recommended as more reliable methods of assessing proper airway positioning (Neumar et al., 2010). Rhythm assessment should occur every 2 minutes to determine if a shockable rhythm exists. If an organized rhythm, such as normal sinus rhythm or sinus bradycardia, returns after defibrillation, a pulse check should be performed to assess for the return of spontaneous circulation (ROSC). If a pulse is noted, a blood pressure should be obtained (Neumar et al., 2010).

In cases where PEA or asystole is the initial rhythm, CPR should be initiated immediately and an IV should be established. During these efforts, a search for a reversible cause for the arrest should be conducted. Details surrounding the patient's initial collapse may provide clues as to the cause (Neumar et al., 2010). For example, the victim of an automobile accident may have a tension pneumothorax or cardiac tamponade. Efforts to correct these problems may improve the likelihood of a successful resuscitation effort.

DIAGNOSTIC TESTING

Most often CA and SCD are related to a combination of an underlying structural abnormality and a triggering event, such as an ischemic insult, electrolyte disturbance, acidosis, or drug-induced prolongation of the QT interval (Myerburg & Castellanos, 2015). Therefore, it is important to perform tests to detect or rule out these issues.

Serum Electrolytes

In addition to a routine electrolyte panel, magnesium and calcium levels should be evaluated. Hypomagnesemia, abnormal potassium levels, and hypocalcemia are associated with ventricular arrhythmias and CA (Myerburg & Castellanos, 2015).

Arterial Blood Gases

Acidosis can exacerbate potential resting membrane problems associated with ischemia (Myerburg & Castellanos, 2015). Correction of acidosis, primarily by increasing ventilation rates, improves the actions of medications and decreases cardiac irritability. Care should be taken to avoid hyperventilation and hypocarbia, which can lead to cerebral vasoconstriction (Peberdy et al., 2010). Hypoxemia should be corrected to improve oxygen delivery to the heart, brain, and other vital organs.

Serum Troponin

While the results may not be immediately available, elevated troponin levels help support a diagnosis of acute MI. Early detection of this problem is key in determining appropriate therapy to limit damage and reduce ongoing cardiac ischemia.

Toxicology Screen

Drugs such as cocaine may cause coronary vasospasm. This, in turn, may create ischemia and cardiac cell membrane instability.

Electrocardiogram

The initial purposes of ECG monitoring are to detect rhythm disturbances and assess the effectiveness of defibrillation. ST-segment elevation noted in monitor leads should be explored further as soon as conditions allow for a full 12-lead ECG. ST elevation in monitoring leads is suspicious for ST-segment elevation myocardial infarction (STEMI) and the patient should be evaluated for emergent transfer to the cardiac catheterization laboratory for coronary angiography and possible percutaneous coronary intervention (PCI) (O'Gara et al., 2013).

Echocardiogram

Once spontaneous circulation has been restored and the patient's condition is stabilized, an echocardiogram may be performed to assess ventricular and valvular function. Presence of ventricular wall motion abnormalities may indicate acute MI, previously existing dysfunction, or myocardial stunning. Valvular abnormalities may indicate other causes of CA. The size of the ventricles and their wall thicknesses may suggest cardiomyopathies predisposing life-threatening arrhythmias.

MANAGEMENT

High-quality CPR and rapid defibrillation are the cornerstones of improving chances for survival and preventing neurologic impairment. Epinephrine and vasopressin can be administered when IV or intraosseous access has been established. Once spontaneous circulation has been restored, post-CA care centers on achieving hemodynamic stability and providing adequate ventilation. The ultimate purpose is to prevent further ischemic injury to the brain and other vital organs. Fluid resuscitation may be appropriate for patients with hypovolemia. Vasopressors and inotropic agents may be required to support an adequate blood pressure if fluid administration is inadequate or inappropriate. Norepinephrine, dopamine, or epinephrine infusion may be used in these circumstances. During the initial resuscitation efforts, if amiodarone was administered to treat ventricular arrhythmias, a maintenance infusion should be initiated if the drug seemed effective (Peberdy et al., 2010).

Airway management outside the hospital may or may not involve the placement of an endotracheal tube (ETT). In the inpatient setting, placement of an ETT usually occurs prior to the ROSC. Once placement has been verified as previously described, ventilations should be delivered at a rate of 8 to 10 breaths per minute (Neumar et al., 2010). Even if spontaneous respirations return with the restoration of circulation, breathing attempts may be inadequate and maintenance of a patent airway may be problematic. Therefore, supporting the patient with mechanical ventilation is usually required. The assistance of an anesthesiologist, intensivist, pulmonologist, and/or respiratory therapist is beneficial for ensuring appropriate ventilator settings for optimal oxygenation. The goal of therapy is to achieve an SpO_2 equal to or greater than 94% and a $PaCO_2$ of 40 to 45 mmHg (Peberdy et al., 2010).

In the best of circumstances, the wishes of the patient concerning CPR are known in advance, communicated effectively, and honored. As medicine and technology improve chances for survival, so too should the methods for determining and following patient wishes. Even when the desires of the patient concerning CPR are known and enacted, additional therapies may require further decision making from the patient, family, and health care team.

Following successful resuscitation, patients surviving CA should be monitored in an intensive care unit for a minimum of 48 to 72 hours (Myerburg & Castellanos, 2015). In this setting, additional testing can be performed to determine possible causes. Patients who demonstrate poor neurologic recovery during the first few days postresuscitation often will not undergo extensive testing to determine future management. Supportive therapies, such as mechanical ventilation and intravenous medications, require careful management by skilled staff. If the likely cause of the arrest was myocardial ischemia, coronary angiography and possible PCI should be considered according to previously discussed guidelines.

Therapeutic hypothermia may be utilized to minimize oxygen demands and improve the chances of neurologic recovery. If a patient is unable to follow commands after circulation has been restored, therapeutic hypothermia should be considered (Peberdy et al., 2010). For individuals with STEMI and CA, this therapy is a Class I recommendation (O'Gara et al., 2013). This specialized support is most successful when provided in centers that have multi-specialty resources and previous hypothermia experience (Peberdy et al., 2010).

Hypothermia can be achieved via a variety of methods. Cooling can be initiated with cold isotonic fluids, lactated Ringer's solution, or normal saline 30 mL/kg at 4°C, but must be maintained by other methods. The most basic hypothermia technique is the application of cooling blankets or ice packs. This method leads to more variability in cooling and is very labor-intensive. Specialized catheter-based and topical hypothermia systems provide more reliable cooling. Patient temperature should be monitored via an esophageal, bladder, or pulmonary artery catheter temperature probe. Hypothermia, with core temperatures of 32°C to 34°C, should be maintained for 12 to 24 hours. After 24 hours, the patient is rewarmed gradually in increments up to 0.25°C per hour. Sedation and muscle relaxants may be necessary to control shivering (Peberdy et al., 2010). Complications of hypothermia include skin breakdown (ice or cooling blankets), arrhythmias, coagulopathies, hyperglycemia, and infection (Peberdy et al., 2010). Interventions to detect and treat any of these problems should be part of protocols for hypothermia patient care.

PREDICTING NEUROLOGIC OUTCOMES

Within the first 24 hours following ROSC there are no physical examination findings or diagnostic studies that can accurately predict poor outcomes for comatose CA patients. In addition, the use of hypothermia renders even the best predictors less reliable. Other factors that may confound neurologic testing results include hypotension, seizures, sedatives, and neuromuscular blockers (Peberdy et al., 2010). In the absence of hypothermia treatment, or confounding factors, lack of pupillary light reactivity and corneal reflexes at equal to or greater than 72 hours of ROSC are highly reliable indicators of poor outcome (Zandbergen et al., 2006). The most reliable diagnostic test for determining prognosis is the somatosensory-evoked potential study, when conducted 3 or more days following ROSC. Absence of bilateral cortical responses following median nerve stimulation is associated with a poor outcome (Wijdicks, Hijdra, Young, Bassetti, & Wiebe, 2006).

LONG-TERM MANAGEMENT OF CA SURVIVORS

One might reason that antiarrhythmic medications would be an important part of long-term therapy for survivors of CA. However, the Cardiac Arrhythmia Suppression Trial (CAST) revealed that the use of Class I antiarrhythmic drugs for arrhythmia suppression in post-MI patients was either ineffective in improving survival or harmful (Echt et al., 1991). A later study, the Antiarrhythmics versus Implantable Defibrillators (AVID) trial, showed that implantable cardioverter defibrillators (ICDs) were superior to antiarrhythmic drugs in reducing mortality in survivors of CA with ejection fractions less than or equal to 40% (Antiarrhythmics versus Implantable Defibrillators [AVID] Investigators, 1997). As a result of these and other studies, ICD implantation has become the main strategy for secondary prevention of SCD.

As mentioned previously, approximately 80% of CA survivors have CHD. Determining the severity of this disease and performing revascularization if indicated is accepted therapy for CA survivors, particularly when the circumstances of the arrest implicate myocardial ischemia as a precipitating factor. Depending on the completeness of revascularization and the degree of left ventricular dysfunction, if ischemia is eliminated, an ICD may not be required. The use of beta blockers in this population may also improve survival (Myerburg & Castellanos, 2015). For patients with STEMI who develop sustained VT or VF more than 48 hours post-MI, an ICD should be implanted before discharge if treatable ischemia, reinfarction, or metabolic disturbances can be ruled out as inciting factors (O'Gara et al., 2013). STEMI patients who do not experience CA but who may be at risk for ventricular arrhythmias due to left ventricular dysfunction, should be reevaluated for possible ICD insertion at least 40 days following discharge.

Implantation of an ICD occurs through a process of shared decision making between patients, their families, and their providers. Whenever possible, patients are provided information regarding the procedure, as well as the risks and benefits of the device. Patients are informed about the sensations and discomfort that might occur with the discharge of the device and the possibility that such experiences can provoke anxiety. Also, they are educated regarding the need for specialized follow-up. Patients' co-morbidities, life expectancy, and desires concerning end-of-life care should all be considered prior to ICD implantation. Patients are also informed that they could request to have the device turned off should they decide that they no longer wish to receive this therapy.

Survivors of CA may suffer anoxic brain injury and damage to other vital organs. They may require extensive physical, occupational, and speech therapy. Kidney damage due to hypoperfusion may require dialysis. Recovery may require days to months of rehabilitation. Smooth transitions in care from hospital to subacute rehabilitation to home or long-term care are critical to the well-being of these patients. Care providers must be aware of ICD implants, if present, and any connected follow-up. Advanced directives should be created and communicated. The support of social and rehabilitative services is essential. An ICD support group can be very helpful to patients and those in close relationships with them.

ICDs AS PRIMARY PREVENTION FOR SCD

The Multicenter Automatic Defibrillator Implantation Trial (MADIT) demonstrated that ICD implantation in patients with a history of MI with an ejection fraction equal to or less than 35%, spontaneous nonsustained VT, and inducible VT via an electrophysiology study experienced a 54% relative risk reduction in mortality (Moss et al., 1996). Other studies, such as MADIT II and the Sudden Cardiac Death in Heart Failure Trial (SCD-HeFT), demonstrated ICD survival benefits for patients with cardiomyopathies and HF (Bardy et al., 2005; Moss et al., 2002). As a result of these trials and other data from registries, ICDs are now recommended preventative therapy for patients at high risk of SCD, especially those with significant left ventricular dysfunction (Tracy et al., 2013).

Acute cardiovascular conditions account for a significant proportion of hospitalizations in the United States. The sudden onset and potential for significant morbidity and mortality requires rapid evaluation for both common and uncommon conditions. Once an assessment is conducted, clinicians must determine appropriate management strategies to match the patient findings with the facilities, specialized equipment, and a comprehensive health care team that is required to improve patient outcomes and quality of life.

For full reference citations to this chapter, please see "Section References" in the back of the book, under the heading "Section V."

Cardiovascular Diagnostics

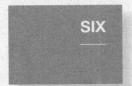

Diagnostic Laboratory Evaluations

BRITTANY C. MOORE, LAUREN WENHOLD,
AND KELLEY M. ANDERSON

Since the ancient Greeks, evaluation of human body fluids has been appreciated as a means to understand health conditions and disease. In the late 1800s, as the etiologies of infectious diseases were discovered and testing was developed to evaluate and detect organisms, diagnostic laboratory evaluations played a larger role in patient care, and the first clinical laboratory opened at Johns Hopkins Hospital in 1896 (Delwiche, 2003). Currently, the clinical laboratory is an integral component of the health care system, with an essential role in the diagnosis, treatment, and monitoring of treatment efficacy for cardiovascular disorders. Diagnostic laboratory evaluation increasingly includes a large number of biochemical tests, which are usually completed on biological specimens obtained from blood, urine, and other bodily fluids. In patients with suspected cardiovascular disease (CVD), the laboratory evaluation not only serves as a diagnostic tool but also allows for risk stratification. This chapter reviews laboratory studies that are the most pertinent to patients at risk for, or with known cardiovascular conditions.

The list of available laboratory tests is extensive, and the accuracy, sensitivity, and specificity of each test vary depending on the level of clinical suspicion. Therefore, the choice of diagnostic laboratory studies for an individual patient is guided by the clinical presentation, comprehensive health history, physical examination, and the findings of other diagnostic studies. In certain conditions, especially lipid metabolism disorders and acute coronary syndromes, the laboratory evaluations are a key element to confirm a diagnosis, guide treatment, and provide prognostic data. As in all testing, risks must be evaluated in concert with the following two considerations: Will the test results impact clinical management? What is the relative importance of knowing the results?

In addition, when considering laboratory testing, determine the relative cost of the laboratory test, including the financial cost of the testing to the patient and the health care system, and the related costs of discomfort and time. In clinical cardiology, decisions about laboratory tests—including risk factors and co-morbidities—must be evaluated in the context of the whole individual.

The clinician must also be cautious in the interpretation of laboratory test results. Results that do not coincide with the clinical presentation may necessitate reevaluation to determine the accuracy of the sample. If samples are insufficient or undergo hemolysis, values may be inaccurate, especially for serum potassium, magnesium, calcium, phosphorus, and creatinine kinase.

Basic laboratory tests are completed routinely in clinical practice, and although there are implications for the findings of these results for many conditions, there are specific considerations regarding cardiovascular disorders of these general studies. The normal reference ranges for these evaluations are presented in Table 25.1.

TABLE 25.1 Normal Reference Ranges for Basic Laboratory Tests

Laboratory Test	Normal	Laboratory Test	Normal
Blood chemistries		Basic lipid panel	
Sodium (Na+)	135–145 mEq/L	Cholesterol	<200 mg/dL
Potassium (K+)	3.3- 4.9 mEq/L	LDL	60–180 mg/dL
Chloride (Cl−)	97–110 mEq/L	HDL	
Magnesium (Mg+)	1.3–2.2 mEq/L	Male	>45 mg/dL
Calcium (Ca+), total	8.9–10.3 mg/dL	Female	>55 mg/dL
Calcium, ionized	4.4–5.3 mg/dL	Triglycerides	
Blood urea nitrogen	8–26 mg/dL	Male	40–160 mg/dL
Creatinine		Female	35–135 mg/dL
Male	0.9–1.4 mg/dL		
Female	0.8–1.3 mg/dL	Thyroid profile	
Glucose	60–90 mg/dL	TSH	0.4–4 mIU/L
		T4 (total)	5–12 mcg/dL
Hemoglobin A1C	<5.7%	T4 (free)	0.8–2.8 ng/dL
		T3	100–200 mcg/dL
Hepatic function			
Alkaline phosphatase (ALP)	30–120 units/L	Coagulation studies	
Alanine aminotransferase (ALT)	4–36 units/L	PT	12–15 s
Aspartate aminotransferase (AST)	0–35 units/L	INR	0–1.3
Lactate dehydrogenase (LDH)	105–333 IU/L	aPTT	35–45 s
Albumin	3.4–5.4 g/dL	Bleeding time	1–9 min
		Activated clotting time	80–160 s
Hematologic studies		D-dimer	<250–600 mcg/L
White blood cell count	4,500–11,000/mm^3		
Hemoglobin		Urinalysis	
Male	13.5–18 g/dL	Bilirubin	negative
Female	12–16 g/dL	Blood	negative
Hematocrit		Clarity	clear or cloudy
Male	40%–50%	Color	yellow
Female	36%–47%	Glucose	<130 mg/day
Red blood cell count		Ketones	negative
Male	4.7–6.1 mil/mm^3	Leukocytes	negative
Female	4.2–5.4 mil/mm^3	Nitrite	negative
Corpuscle indices		Protein	negative—trace
MCV	82–98 fl		(<150 mg/d)
MCH	27–31 pg	Specific gravity	1.005–1.030
MCHC	32–36 g/dL	Urine pH	4.5–8
Platelet count	250,000–500,000/mm^3	Urobilinogen	0.5–1 mg/dL

aPTT, activated partial thromboplastin time; HDL, high-density lipoproteins; INR, international normalized ratio;
LDL, low-density lipoproteins; MCH, mean corpuscular hemoglobin; MCHC, mean corpuscular hemoglobin concentration;
MCV, mean corpuscular volume; PT, prothrombin time; TSH, thyroid-stimulating hormone.

Sources: Pagana and Pagana (2012); Reed (2009).

SERUM CHEMISTRIES

Within the routine biochemistry panel, serum electrolyte levels are important in cardiovascular patients, since their equilibrium regulates the activity of the conduction system and cardiac contractility.

Sodium (Na⁺)

Sodium is the principal cation in the extracellular fluid and is responsible for maintaining osmotic pressure in the blood, regulating acid–base balance, and transmitting nerve impulses. The balance of sodium is associated with the fluid homeostatis and is integral to proper physiologic function. Sodium, a vital element, is not stored in the body and requires an intricate and complex neural and hormonal system to control its balance. Largely regulated by the kidneys and the hypothalamus, sodium levels are continuously monitored and adjusted. Sodium concentration is regulated by aldosterone, atrial natriuretic hormone, and antidiuretic hormone, which cause sodium retention or excretion based on the body's physiologic needs. When kidney perfusion is decreased from reduced cardiac output or low interstitial volume, the renin-angiotensin-aldosterone system is triggered, which prompts vasoconstriction, as well as sodium and water retention. Increased serum sodium levels can be due to loss of a large volume of water without a proportional loss of sodium, as with diarrhea or vomiting. Decreased serum sodium levels are the result of excess fluid volume or natriuresis.

In patients with cardiac disease, including heart failure (HF), hypertension, and cardiac conduction disorders, monitoring serum sodium levels is critically important to assess the overall status of fluid balance, the effect of pharmacologic agents, and dietary and lifestyle modifications. Pharmacologic therapies, including diuretics and angiotensin-modifying medications, have significant implications for sodium and fluid balance. In particular, patients with HF with hyponatremia have higher rates of mortality than those whose sodium levels are considered normal, as evidenced by registry data (Sato et al., 2013). Among 4,837 patients who were hospitalized with HF, this study confirmed that those patients with hyponatremia had significantly higher all-cause death rates, higher cardiac death rates, and longer lengths of hospital stay compared with those patients with normonatremia (Sato et al., 2013).

Potassium (K⁺)

Potassium is primarily an intracellular cation, although there is a small amount of potassium in the extracellular fluid. This extracellular potassium is tightly regulated and essential for cardiac and skeletal muscle contraction. Even minor alterations in serum potassium level can have significant effects on cardiac muscle function. Thus, maintenance of potassium within the normal range is essential, as electrolyte imbalance can result in cardiac conduction abnormalities and arrhythmia. For example, hyperkalemia will result in ECG changes of tall peaked T waves, prolonged PR interval, and widening of the QRS complex. Hypokalemia may be evidenced on the ECG with decreased T-wave amplitude, ST segment depression, and a prominent U wave. Severe hypokalemia may also lead to tachyarrhythmias, including ventricular tachycardia and ventricular fibrillation. Serum potassium can be altered in patients who are prescribed diuretics, as these medications can cause hypokalemia; conversely, patients who are prescribed angiotensin-converting enzyme inhibitors, angiotensin receptor blockers, direct renin inhibitors, and aldosterone inhibitors can experience hyperkalemia, especially if these medications are prescribed in combination. Potassium must be monitored carefully in patients with concomitant renal disease, especially with dialysis, because potassium levels will vary widely, and changes can occur rapidly. Although less common, genetic conditions, including hypokalemic periodic paralysis, will result in unusually low potassium levels.

Chloride (Cl⁻)

Chloride is the principal anion in the extracellular fluid, and in conjunction with sodium, it maintains osmotic pressure in the blood. An increase or decrease in the chloride level is often associated with factors similar to those that influence a loss or gain of sodium. The kidneys selectively excrete chloride to maintain the acid–base balance, and thus chloride excretion can be impaired in patients with renal disorders. An inability to excrete chloride can result in increased serum chloride levels, causing metabolic acidosis. Decreases in serum chloride levels are often related to loss from vomiting, diarrhea, and the use of diuretics. Therefore, it is important to monitor chloride levels when prescribing diuretics, including in patients with hypertension and HF.

Magnesium (Mg⁺⁺)

Magnesium is primarily an intracellular cation and is stored in the bones with very small amounts circulating in the serum. Magnesium is essential for neuromuscular function and enzyme activation. Changes in serum magnesium levels also affect other serum ions, potassium, and calcium, and, therefore, decreases in serum magnesium typically do not occur independent of other electrolyte changes. The kidneys primarily excrete magnesium, and, thus, renal disorders are the most common cause of increased serum magnesium levels. Excess magnesium can result in depressed neuromuscular conduction, which can reduce cardiac conduction. Decreased serum magnesium levels can be the result of impaired absorption, medications, and low intake of dietary magnesium, as seen in alcoholic individuals. Magnesium deficiency can contribute to the induction of cardiac arrhythmias, including atrial fibrillation, ventricular fibrillation, and ventricular tachycardia, so the Advanced Cardiac Life Support algorithm for the treatment of ventricular arrhythmias includes magnesium replacement as a therapy option.

Calcium (Ca⁺⁺)

Calcium, the most abundant mineral in the body, is necessary for bone formation, nerve transmission, coagulation, and cardiac and skeletal muscle contraction. Calcium is primarily located in the teeth and bones with approximately 1% of ionized calcium, also known as free calcium, circulating in the bloodstream unbound to serum albumin and metabolically active. Ionized calcium is essential for cardiac and neuromuscular excitability, although the unbound state is more difficult to measure through a blood analysis, so a total calcium level is usually obtained.

Thiazide diuretics may contribute to hypercalcemia. Abnormal calcium levels are also known to induce cardiac arrhythmias; therefore, it is important to monitor a patient's calcium level prior to beginning many antiarrhythmic therapies. For example, hypocalcemia may cause prolonged ST and QT intervals on the ECG, whereas hypercalcemia can result in a shortened ST segment, shortened QT interval, and widened T wave.

Ionized calcium measures the calcium in the blood not attached to proteins. Total serum calcium levels are more commonly ordered, whereas a separate ionized calcium test may be desired for patients with low albumin levels, because decreased serum albumin can result in decreased total calcium levels. An ionized calcium test should be ordered for patients with hypocalcemia in conjunction with low albumin levels, because this combination of evaluations is a more accurate representation of a patient's calcium level than total serum calcium.

MEASURES OF KIDNEY FUNCTION

Blood Urea Nitrogen

Blood urea nitrogen (BUN) measures the amount of urea nitrogen, a waste product of protein metabolism, in the blood. Urea nitrogen is excreted exclusively by the kidneys, rendering BUN a marker of kidney function. Kidney damage; conditions that decrease renal perfusion, such as HF; and dehydration result in an elevated BUN, referred to as azotemia. BUN levels are often evaluated in conjunction with serum creatinine levels to monitor kidney function, because the BUN level is influenced by an individual's hydration status and protein absorption through the gastrointestinal tract, and therefore may inaccurately represent kidney function.

Renal disease can lead to CVD, and conversely, CVD can result in renal impairment. In the 2009 annual data report of the United States Renal Data System (USRDS), the prevalence of CVD reached 63% in patients with chronic kidney disease (CKD), and approximately 50% of CKD patients died of CVD complications before experiencing end-stage renal disease (Shiba & Shimokawa, 2011). In addition, CKD occurs in up to 70% of individuals with HF (Shiba & Shimokawa, 2011).

Creatinine

Creatinine is a byproduct of skeletal muscle contraction that is excreted entirely by the kidneys. An individual's serum creatinine, therefore, reflects renal excretory function. Serum creatinine is usually evaluated in association with BUN. Individuals with greater muscle mass have higher serum creatinine levels than those with less muscle mass, such as women, elderly people, and amputees. In patients with cardiac disease, serum creatinine should be evaluated prior to procedures that require potentially nephrotoxic contrast agents, including coronary computed tomography, cardiac catheterization, and ventriculograms. In addition, patients prescribed diuretics, angiotensin-converting enzyme inhibitors, and angiotensin receptor blockers require routine monitoring of renal function.

BUN/Creatinine Ratio

When a BUN or creatinine is elevated, a provider may assess the BUN/creatinine ratio in order to determine the etiology of these elevated concentrations. Usually, the BUN/creatinine ratio is between 10:1 and 20:1. An increase in this ratio can be due to decreased renal perfusion in HF, gastrointestinal bleeding, or dehydration. Conversely, the ratio may be decreased in patients with hepatic disease or malnutrition.

Glomerular Filtration Rate, Estimated (eGFR)

The estimated glomerular filtration rate (eGFR) provides an overall value of the filtration rates of the functioning nephrons in the kidney. Although eGFR is difficult to measure directly, serum levels of creatinine along with additional identifying information (such as age, weight, gender, and race) are used to obtain eGFR. The GFR is considered the best clinical indicator of renal function, and an eGFR calculator is available at http://www.nkdep.nih.gov. The Cockcroft and Gault equation is a well-validated and clinically applicable calculation of eGFR:

$$\text{CrCl (mL/min)} = \frac{[(140 - \text{age in years}) \times (\text{weight in kg}) \times (0.85 \text{ if female})]}{72 \times \text{serum creatinine (mg/dL)}}$$

The National Kidney Foundation guidelines also recommend the use of one of the formulas from the Modification of Diet in Renal Disease (MDRD) Study Group for estimation of GFR (Levey et al., 1999). There are four established versions of the formula, which include age, gender, serum creatinine level, and race (defined as African American or non–African American) with the inclusion of serum albumin, serum urea, and urinary urea in some formulas (Jones & Lim, 2003; National Kidney Foundation, 2002). Note that GFR gradually declines with age, even without the presence of known kidney disease. Examples of MDRD formulas are:

$$\text{eGFR (mL/min/1.73 m}^2) = 186 \times \text{serum creatinine (mg/dL)}^{-1.154} \times \text{age}^{-0.203}$$
$$\times [1.210 \text{ if Black}] \times [0.742 \text{ if female}]$$

$$\text{eGFR} = 170 \times \text{serum creatinine}^{-0.999} \times \text{age}^{-0.176} \times \{0.762 \text{ if female}\}$$
$$\times \{1.180 \text{ if Black}\} \times \text{BUN}^{-0.170} \times \text{albumin}^{+0.318}$$

An evaluation of GFR in patients with cardiac disease is essential before prescribing many cardiac medications, especially those that are metabolized or excreted primarily through the kidneys. Individuals with reduced GFR may require dosage adjustments for certain medications—low-molecular-weight heparin and novel anticoagulants, among others. A reduction in GFR may be an indication to withhold certain pharmacologic agents, including some antiarrrhythmics. The GFR estimation assists in determining the safety of patients to undergo certain diagnostic studies—computed tomography and cardiac catheterization, for example—or whether to consider alternative studies that do not require potentially nephrotoxic agents. The GFR levels define the stages of CKD and are described in Table 25.2.

TABLE 25.2 Stages of Chronic Kidney Disease

Stage	Description	GFR (mL/min/1.73 m²)
1	Kidney damage (proteinuria) and normal GFR	≥90
2	Kidney damage and mild decrease in GFR	60–89
3	Moderate decrease in GFR	30–59
4	Severe decrease in GFR	15–29
5	Kidney failure or dialysis	<15

GFR, glomerular filtration rate.

Source: National Kidney Foundation (2014b).

GLUCOSE METABOLISM

Complex carbohydrates, sugars, and starches are metabolized to glucose in the body. Blood glucose is elevated when endogenous epinephrine is released from the adrenal medulla in response to hypoglycemia. Abnormal glucose levels are detectable in the serum and urine as a result of metabolic abnormalities, mainly diabetes mellitus. Glucose levels can be identified in the blood via a finger stick or with a laboratory blood sample. Normal plasma glucose, obtained equal to or greater than 8 hours of fasting, is less than 100 mg/dL. Fasting plasma glucose equal to or greater than 126 mg/dL on two separate occasions, or any random plasma glucose equal to or greater than 200 mg/dL, confirms the diagnosis of diabetes. Hyperglycemia is a common side effect of physiologically stressful conditions, including HF, acute myocardial infarction, cardiac surgery, and infection. Therefore, monitoring glucose in patients with cardiac disease is very important because insulin resistance, glucose intolerance, and every form of diabetes mellitus are related to cardiovascular risk. Glucose control potentially reduces mortality, infection rates, and average length of hospital stay among these populations.

Hemoglobin A1C, Glycated Hemoglobin

Hemoglobin A1C, or glycated hemoglobin, provides information regarding average blood glucose over the past 2 to 3 months. As glucose enters the red blood cells, it glycates or combines with hemoglobin; as more hemoglobin is glycated, there is more glucose present in the bloodstream. By measuring the percentage of glycated hemoglobin in the blood, hemoglobin A1C averages blood glucose readings for the past few months. Table 25.3 provides a comparison of glycated hemoglobin and average glucose levels.

Hemoglobin A1C is utilized for the diagnosis of diabetes mellitus, an A1C of 5.7% to 6.4% is consistent with prediabetes, and A1C equal to or greater than 6.5% confirms the diabetes diagnosis (American Diabetes Association, 2014b). For diabetes management, A1C should be measured at least twice per year, according to the American Diabetes Association. The glycemic recommendation for all nonpregnant adults is less than 7.0%, which is an average blood glucose reading of about 154 mg/dL. Target glycemic control for most adults is listed in Table 25.4, although

TABLE 25.3 Comparison of Glycated Hemoglobin and Average Glucose

Hemoglobin A1C (%)	Average Glucose (mg/dL)
6	126
7	154
8	183
9	212
10	240
11	269
12	298

Source: American Diabetes Association (2014b).

TABLE 25.4 Targets for Glycemic Control in Most Adults

Hemoglobin A1C	<7%
Preprandial (fasting) plasma glucose	70–130 mg/dL
Postprandial (after meal) plasma glucose	<180 mg/dL

Source: American Diabetes Association (2013).

more or less stringent blood glucose control may be appropriate for certain patients. A less stringent glycemic index has been proposed for certain individuals, primarily older adults or those with multiple co-morbidities.

MEASURES OF HEPATIC FUNCTION

Alkaline Phosphatase

Alkaline phosphatase (ALP) is an enzyme in many bodily tissues, with the highest concentrations located in the liver, biliary tract, and bone. In the liver, ALP is located in the Kupffer cells, which line the biliary-collecting system. ALP is significantly elevated in both extrahepatic and intrahepatic obstructive biliary disease and cirrhosis. Bone is the most common source of extrahepatic ALP, with increased levels noted in adolescence due to new bone growth. Other common conditions associated with elevated ALP include hepatic tumors, healing fractures, hyperparathyroidism, Paget's disease, and rheumatoid arthritis. ALP isoenzymes can be used to determine whether elevations are related to bone or liver diseases. Many pharmacologic agents are associated with elevated ALP levels, including lipid-lowering agents such as bile acid resins, nicotinic acid, and 3-hydroxy-3-methylglutaryl-coenzyme (HMG-CoA) reduction inhibitors (statins). ALP, along with other liver enzymes, alanine aminotransferase (ALT) and aspartate aminotransferase (AST), are often measured before initiating and during lipid-lowering therapy.

Alanine Aminotransferase

The enzyme ALT is predominately concentrated in the liver; however, smaller quantities are in other tissues, including the kidneys, heart, and skeletal muscle. The ALT level is a specific and sensitive laboratory test for hepatic disease, as injury or disease to the liver results in the release of ALT into the bloodstream. Possible etiologies of elevated ALT include hepatitis, nonalcoholic fatty liver disease, hepatic necrosis, hepatic ischemia, cirrhosis, cholestasis, hepatic tumor, obstructive jaundice, severe burns, myositis, pancreatitis, myocardial infarction, infectious mononucleosis, and shock. Elevated ALT and other liver enzymes are evident in significant HF due to the hepatic congestion. With hepatocellular disease other than viral hepatitis, the ALT/AST ratio is less than 1.0, and in viral hepatitis, the ALT/AST ratio is greater than 1.0. Pharmacologic agents that may increase ALT levels include acetaminophen, allopurinol, antibiotics, fibrates, codeine, HMG-CoA reduction inhibitors, nicotinic acid, nonsteroidal anti-inflammatory drugs, oral contraceptives, phenytoin, procainamide, propranolol, and salicylates.

Aspartate Aminotransferase

AST is located in the cytoplasm and mitochondria of cells. Levels of AST are measurable in the blood when disease or injury results in cell lysis, releasing AST. This enzyme is highly concentrated in the liver, skeletal muscle, kidneys, red blood cells, and myocardium, with considerably smaller amounts of AST found in the brain, pancreas, and lungs. Although previously applied as a marker to confirm myocardial infarction, the presence of AST in many organs reduces its specificity, limiting its usefulness in cardiac ischemic evaluation. Elevated AST and other liver enzymes are evident in significant HF due to the hepatic congestion. AST is now primarily used in the diagnosis and management of hepatocellular disease.

Lactic Dehydrogenase

Lactic dehydrogenase (LDH) is an enzyme located in body tissues, primarily the heart, liver, kidney, muscles, brain, and blood cells. As a result, LDH is often measured in order to assess for nonspecific tissue damage. An elevated LDH level in the blood may be indicative of myocardial infarction, ischemia, shock or trauma, muscle injury, tissue death, hemolytic anemia, or liver disease.

Albumin

Albumin is the most abundant human protein produced by the liver. This protein functions to maintain blood volume by regulating the osmotic pressure in the vascular system and as a carrier for molecules. Hypoalbuminemia is generally an indicator of hepatic or renal dysfunction. Other causes of hypoalbuminemia are burns, malabsorption, malnutrition, malignancy, protein-losing enteropathy, and genetic variations. Increased serum albumin, or hyperalbuminemia, is generally a sign of dehydration. Albumin monitoring is the most useful in the cardiac patient to evaluate hepatic function, fluid balance, and nutrition and calcium levels and to guide medication management.

HEMATOLOGIC STUDIES

Red Blood Cell Count

The red blood cell count identifies the number of red blood cells circulating in venous blood. Red blood cells are produced in the bone marrow and usually survive in the bloodstream for about 120 days. Hemoglobin molecules are present within each red blood cell, which allows for transport and exchange of oxygen into the tissues. A decrease in red blood cells occurs for many reasons, including hemorrhage, hemolysis, dietary deficiencies, genetic abnormalities, medications, marrow failure, chronic illness, or organ failure. A red blood cell value less than 10% of the expected normal value is consistent with anemia. Increases in the red blood cell count can be related to high altitude, dehydration, polycythemia vera, or congenital heart disease. Evaluation and management of anemia in patients with cardiac disease is essential, as anemia often exacerbates HF, precipitates angina, and generates other ischemic-related symptoms. Extracellular fluid excess or deficit can mislead the accuracy of the red blood cell count, resulting in a potentially false interpretation.

Mean Corpuscular Volume

The mean corpuscular volume (MCV)—obtained as part of the red blood cell indices—is a measure of the average volume, or size, of a single red blood cell. This information is essential for classifying anemia, with an elevated MCV characterized as macrocytic. Anemias associated with macrocytic red blood cells are megaloblastic anemias; some examples include vitamin B_{12} or folic acid–deficiency anemias. A reduced, or microcytic, MCV value is generally associated with iron-deficiency anemia and thalassemia.

Mean Corpuscular Hemoglobin and Concentration.

The mean corpuscular hemoglobin (MCH), a measure of the average mass or weight of hemoglobin within a red blood cell, is evaluated with other red blood cell indices to differentiate hematologic conditions, including anemias. MCH values are categorized as macrocytic cells with more hemoglobin and microcytic cells with less hemoglobin. The average concentration of hemoglobin in a single red blood cell is represented by the mean corpuscular hemoglobin concentration (MCHC). Red blood cells usually have a normal hemoglobin concentration (referred to as normochromic) or a decreased hemoglobin concentration (hypochromic), which results in a lighter color. Although less common, red blood cells are hyperchromic.

Hemoglobin

Each red blood cell contains a hemoglobin molecule that is responsible for transporting oxygen and carbon dioxide, so hemoglobin values reflect the number of serum red blood cells. Decreased hemoglobin values indicate anemia, and elevated values indicate erythrocytosis. Changes in plasma volume are more accurately interpreted by evaluating hemoglobin values rather than the red cell count. According to the Centers for Disease Control and Prevention (CDC) and based on the fifth percentile of the third National Health and Nutrition Examination Survey (NHANES), the hemoglobin values for anemia in individuals equal to or greater than 18 years of age are less than 12.0 g/dL in nonpregnant women and less than 13.5 g/dL in men (CDC, 2014).

Although anemia can contribute to myocardial ischemia, general recommendations favor a conservative transfusion strategy (Carson et al., 2012). In 2012, the American Association of Blood Banks provided clinical practice guidelines based on expert opinion and studies, recommending a restricted, symptom-guided transfusion strategy. In asymptomatic, hemodynamically stable patients without coronary heart disease, consider transfusion for hemoglobin less than 7 g/dL to 8 g/dL. For hospitalized patients with CVD and symptoms of chest pain, orthostasis, or HF, transfusion can be considered for hemoglobin levels less than 8 g/dL, although no specific recommendations are provided for acute coronary syndrome. The recommended maintenance hemoglobin concentration in postoperative patients is equal to or greater than 8 g/dL, unless the patient exhibits symptoms of anemia, in which case transfusion can be considered at higher values.

Hematocrit

The hematocrit is the percentage of total blood volume comprising red blood cells. Both gender and age affect the normal ranges of the hematocrit count. The hematocrit is an indirect measure of red blood cells; thus, fluctuations in the red blood cells are reflected in the hematocrit level. Hematocrit values are generally three times the value of the hemoglobin concentration in percentage points. According to the CDC, and based on the fifth percentile of the third NHANES survey, the hematocrit values for anemia in individuals 18 years old and older are less than 35.7% in nonpregnant women and less than 39.9% in men (CDC, 2014).

White Blood Cell Count

White blood cells, also known as leukocytes, protect a person against foreign substances and maintain tissue integrity by combating infection. There are two components to a white blood cell count—the total number of leukocytes in a specific amount of peripheral venous blood, and the differential count, measuring the percentage of each type of leukocyte present. Five types of leukocytes are listed in order of frequency: neutrophils, eosinophils, basophils, monocytes, and lymphocytes (Table 25.5). An elevation in the total white blood cell count usually indicates infection, inflammation, tissue necrosis, or leukemic aplasia. The elevation can also be related to trauma or stress. In the transient stress states of myocardial infarction and decompensated HF, the total leukocyte count may be elevated. Elevations in specific types of leukocyte can guide the provider to different causes of leukocytosis.

TABLE 25.5 Normal Leukocyte Differential

Leukoctye Type	Percentage	Likely Etiology
Neutrophils	55–70	Bacterial infection
Lymphocytes	20–40	Viral infection
Monocytes	2–8	Chronic infection/fungal infection
Eosinophils	1–4	Allergies
Basophils	0.5–1	Inflammation

Platelet Count

Platelets are small fragments of cells that coalesce at the site of an injury or adhere to an injured vessel to provide a platform on which blood coagulation occurs. This process results in the formation of a fibrin clot, which covers wounds and prevents blood from leaking, and serves as the basis for new tissue formation. Platelets are formed in the bone marrow, and a platelet count is often obtained as part of the complete blood count. Platelet counts higher than normal can lead to unnecessary clotting, potentiating a cerebral vascular accident or myocardial infarction. Many antiplatelet therapies are available to reduce the risk of thromboembolic cardio-vascular events, including aspirin, dipyridamole, and $P2Y_{12}$ adenosine diphosphate receptors, including clopidogrel, prasugrel, and ticagrelor.

Thrombocytopenia poses a serious risk of hemorrhage when platelet counts are less than 50,000 mm^3, which may result in spontaneous bleeding character-ized by petechiae, bleeding from the oral mucosa, or epistaxis. Causes of thrombo-cytopenia include reduced production of platelets, sequestration of platelets, accelerated platelet destruction, consumption of platelets, hemorrhage, heparin-induced thrombocytopenia (HIT), or dilution after administration of massive blood transfusions. Thrombocytopenia may also be induced by many pharmacologic agents, including, but not limited to, acetaminophen, aspirin, chemotherapy agents, chloramphenicol, colchicine, H_2 blocking agents, heparin, hydralazine, indometh-acin, isoniazid, quinolone antibiotics, quinidine, streptomycin, sulfonamides, and thiazide diuretics. Platelet function testing is not recommended routinely, as this testing has not demonstrated improvement in outcomes in the general thrombo-cytopenic population, although it can be considered in certain patients with recur-rent acute coronary syndromes (Anderson et al., 2013).

COAGULATION STUDIES

For cardiovascular conditions, the assessment of coagulation parameters is an important component of the diagnostic evaluation before invasive procedures and during the monitoring of treatment with antithrombotic medications, particularly anticoagulants.

Prothrombin Time

Prothrombin time (PT) assesses the adequacy of the extrinsic and common pathway in the clotting cascade. The PT specifically measures the clotting ability of fibrinogen; prothrombin; and factors V, VII, and X. Any deficiencies in these factors will cause increased PT. The PT may also be increased in HF, vitamin K deficiency, disseminated intravascular coagulation (DIC), and hepatic disease. Some medications, including amiodarone, heparin, warfarin, nonsteroidal anti-inflammatories, and aspirin, are also associated with prolonged PT. Conversely, a decreased PT can be noted in patients with myocardial infarction, pulmonary embolus, thrombophlebitis, and thyroid dysfunction, and in patients who are taking medication such as diuretics, oral contraceptives, and antacids. PT is primarily used for monitoring patients on warfarin therapy. A PT value of 1.5 to 2 times the normal range, measured in seconds, is considered therapeutic with most indications for warfarin therapy. However, a PT greater than 2.5 times the control value significantly increases the risk for bleeding.

International Normalized Ratio

The international normalized ratio (INR) provides standardization of PT results worldwide, independent of reagents or instrument types used to obtain the sample. The individual thromboplastins are calibrated and assigned an International Sensitivity Index. The first sensitivity index was 1, and others are calibrated on this norm. INR is the ratio of a patient's PT to a normal PT value, a control value obtained from the International Reference Preparation, a standard human brain thromboplastin provided by WHO. A normal INR is less than 1.3, with a therapeutic INR for patients on warfarin therapy ranging between 2 and 3.5. Generally, the INR range for deep vein thrombosis (DVT), pulmonary embolism (PE), and atrial fibrillation is between 2 and 3. For patients with mechanical prosthetic heart valves, it is between 2.5 and 3.5, although anticoagulation therapy and INR goals must be individualized, thus accounting for patient and device factors. The blood sample for INR calculation is usually obtained after the last daily warfarin dose—generally, there is an evening dose of warfarin with a morning laboratory evaluation. Dietary practices influence the effect of warfarin and INR levels, and they are considered when adjusting dosages or altering the therapeutic regimen.

Activated Partial Thromboplastin Time

Activated partial thromboplastin time (aPTT) evaluates the intrinsic coagulation pathway and is primarily monitored during unfractionated heparin therapy. The aPTT measures all coagulation factors except factors III, VII, and XIII, and it is obtained by adding test reagents to partial thromboplastin time (PTT) in order to shorten clotting time. When clotting time is reduced, defects in the coagulation system can be identified. The aPTT is prolonged with heparin administration, vitamin K deficiency, clotting factor deficiencies, DIC, and hepatic disease. For patients on heparin therapy, the therapeutic range for aPTT is 1.5 to 2.5 times the patient's baseline value, measured in seconds.

TABLE 25.6 Effect of Warfarin and Aspirin on Coagulation Studies

	PT/ INR	PTT	Bleeding Time	Platelet Count
Warfarin	Prolonged	Normal to prolonged	Normal	Normal
Aspirin	Normal	Normal	Prolonged	Normal

INR, international normalized ratio; PT, prothrombin time; PTT, partial thromboplastin time.

Bleeding Time

The bleeding time test is used infrequently in current clinical practice, and it assesses the ability to achieve hemostasis mainly in postoperative patients. The bleeding time is measured when a small superficial incision is made in the forearm, and the length of time required for the bleeding to stop is recorded. A person's bleeding time will be prolonged if there are deficiencies in platelet quantity or function or if vessel constriction cannot be achieved. Usually, bleeding will stop within 1 to 9 minutes. Table 25.6 describes the effect of warfarin and aspirin on specific coagulation studies.

Activated Clotting Time

Activated clotting time (ACT) is similar to aPTT, and it measures the ability of the intrinsic clotting pathway to initiate clot formation in seconds. The ACT measures the time for whole blood to clot, and it is primarily indicated to monitor the effect of high-dose unfractionated heparin therapy during cardiac surgery, hemodialysis, and cardiac catheterization procedures. The ACT levels are directly and linearly related to heparin concentrations. The test is performed rapidly and often evaluated at the bedside of the patient, in the operating room, or in the procedural area. The ACT informs post-procedure management by evaluating the normalization of the coagulation process, and it informs the dosage of protamine sulfate to reverse the effect of heparin anticoagulation on completion of surgeries or procedures. The ACT can also be used to monitor direct thrombin inhibitors, bivalirudin and argatroban. When monitoring therapy, ACT is more accurate than aPTT in patients with unstable angina, acute myocardial infarction, the presence of lupus anticoagulant, or for high doses of unfractionated heparin.

Heparin Anti-Xa Assay

Heparin antifactor Xa assay measures unfractionated and low-molecular-weight heparin levels during anticoagulation therapy. Heparin increases the anticoagulation time of antithrombin, which also inactivates coagulation factors IIa and Xa. The therapeutic and prophylactic unfractionated heparin ranges are 0.3 to 0.7 units/mL and 0.1 to 0.4 units/mL, respectively, when measured by the anti-Xa assay. This test may be more useful than PTT for monitoring anticoagulation in patients with lupus anticoagulant and other coagulation factor deficiencies that may affect PTT results. Low-molecular-weight heparin inhibits factor Xa more than unfractionated heparin, and it has minimal effect on PTT values. Therapeutic and prophylactic low-molecular-weight heparin levels are 0.5 to 1.2 units/mL and 0.2 to 0.5 units/mL, respectively. Laboratory monitoring using anti-Xa concentrations is suggested for special patient populations such as children, older adults, patients with renal impairment, the obese, and pregnant women (Kearon et al., 2012). Four hours after an injection is the usual time period to obtain a blood sample for anti-Xa, when concentrations peak.

Heparin-Induced Thrombocytopenia (HIT) Assay

Clinical findings must be supplemented with laboratory testing to confirm the diagnosis of HIT. Development of HIT is most common in the postoperative period after cardiac or orthopedic surgery. HIT testing should be considered for patients on heparin therapy who experience a reduction in the platelet count by 50% or a thrombotic event. Two laboratory methods are available to confirm the presence of heparin antibodies: an enzyme-linked serologic immunoassay for antibody detection (ELISA) and a functional test to measure platelet activation. The serologic test for heparin-platelet factor 4 antibodies is most commonly used, because it is widely available, straightforward to interpret, and generally has a rapid turnaround time. Although serologic testing is very sensitive, it lacks specificity, which then results in a high negative but low positive predictive value; therefore, the diagnosis of HIT can largely be excluded if the serologic antibody testing is negative, but if serologic antibody testing is positive, confirmatory functional testing is important to solidify the diagnosis (Arepally & Ortel, 2006). Functional testing is completed with the heparin-induced platelet aggregation assay (HIPA) and the serotonin assay, which is generally used only in the research setting. The sensitivity of HIPA ranges from 39% to 81%, and specificity ranges from 82% to 100% (Chong, Burgess, & Ismail, 1993).

Fibrin Degradation Product/D-Dimer

D-dimer is a fibrin degradation fragment that is produced through the process of fibrinolysis after a thrombus is formed. Usually, D-dimer fragments are undetectable, with levels rising to reflect the amount of fibrin degradation; thus, a positive test indicates the presence of a recent thrombus. Because of the high sensitivity of the test, D-dimer has become valuable in the diagnosis of PE and DVT. For example, when evaluating for DVT, a positive D-dimer test identifies patients who would benefit from further evaluation and consideration for venous ultrasound or chest computed tomography. Alternatively, if the D-dimer test is negative, the patient is unlikely to have a DVT due to the high specificity of the test. In addition to PE and DVT, the D-dimer is elevated in sickle cell anemia and thrombosis associated with malignancy. This evaluation is also a confirmatory test for DIC.

LIPID METABOLISM

The association of lipid metabolism disorders with the development and progression of CVD is well established. Disorders of lipid metabolism and abnormal lipid balance are implicated in a number of pathologic processes that increase risk for, and adverse prognosis of, atherosclerotic cardiovascular disease (ASCVD) of the coronary, peripheral, and cerebral vasculature. Lipid accumulation within the arterial endothelium is a prominent feature of atherosclerosis.

Basic Lipid Panel

Basic tests that measure lipid balance and metabolism are commonly referred to as a "lipid panel" and are completed on a fasting serum sample. Lipids are carried and transported by lipoproteins, globular particles that contain proteins called apoproteins. Apolipoproteins surround the lipid content, creating a water-soluble substance that can be transported throughout the circulatory system. Lipoproteins are classified by density, and common lipoproteins that are measured include cholesterol, high-density lipoprotein (HDL), low-density lipoprotein (LDL), and triglycerides. Table 25.7 provides reference ranges for these measures and non-HDL, which is calculated by subtracting HDL from total cholesterol. Cholesterol,

TABLE 25.7 Lipid Profile Reference Ranges

Total cholesterol (TC)	
Desirable	<200 mg/dL
Borderline high	200–239 mg/dL
High	>240 mg/dL
High-density lipoprotein (HDL)	
Low	<40 mg/dL
High	>60 mg/dL
Low-density lipoprotein (LDL)	
Optimal	<70 or <100 mg/dL
Near or above optimal	100–129 mg/dL
Borderline high	130–159 mg/dL
High	160–189 mg/dL
Very high	>190 mg/dL
Triglyceride	
Optimal	<150 mg/dL
Borderline high	150–199 mg/dL
High	200–499 mg/dL
Very high	>500 mg/dL
Non-HDL cholesterol (TC-HDL)	
Optimal	<130 mg/dL
Borderline high	139–159 mg/dL
High	160–189 mg/dL
Very high	≥190 mg/dL

Source: Stone et al. (2013).

HDL, and triglycerides can be measured directly; however, LDL levels are calculated using the Friedewald formula. The Friedewald equation estimates LDL concentration by subtracting the quantity of other particles and a constant value from the total cholesterol level.

The Friedewald formula is $L \sim C-H-\kappa T$,
where
$L = LDL$
$C = Total\ cholesterol$
$H = HDL$
$\kappa = 0.20$ if the measurement is in mg/dL and 0.45 in mmol/L
$T = Triglycerides$

There are limitations to this calculation methodology, as estimation of LDL requires a 12+ hour fast and LDL values cannot be calculated for triglycerides greater than 400 mg/dL (Friedewald, Levy, & Fredrickson, 1972).

Langsted, Freiberg, and Nordestgaard (2008) evaluated more than 33,000 individuals to compare fasting and nonfasting lipid studies, and they reported that there was minimal change in lipid values in the general population. Lipid values assessed in this study were total cholesterol, HDL, LDL, albumin levels, apolipoprotein A1, and apolipoprotein B (Langsted et al., 2008). However, fasting for 8 or more hours is standard clinical practice due to the potential changes in triglycerides, and the calculated LDL associated with the nonfasting state.

A large number of clinical studies and guidelines exist on the diagnostic role of the lipid panel in terms of risk stratification and as a tool for patient monitoring. Screening and management of individuals with elevated blood lipids through laboratory evaluations is essential in decreasing mortality associated with CVD. The U.S. Preventive Services Task Force (USPSTF) currently recommends obtaining a fasting lipid panel every 5 years for men aged 35 and older and for women aged 45 and older who are at an increased risk for coronary heart disease. However, these recommendations are currently undergoing review and revisions are likely (USPSTF, 2014). The 2013 American College of Cardiology/American Heart Association (ACC/AHA) guidelines for the management of high cholesterol indicate that individuals may benefit from screening for dyslipidemia as early as 21 years of age to decrease the risk of atherosclerotic cardiovascular events (Stone et al., 2013). The Pooled Cohort Risk Assessment Equation, which predicts the 10-year risk for initial ASCVD, factors total cholesterol and HDL into the calculation (Stone et al., 2013). Current guidelines for lipid management suggest early identification and initiation of treatment for patients with an increased risk of ASCVD. Specific groups have been identified in which pharmacologic intervention should be initiated based on risk and LDL levels, with the aim of decreasing atherosclerotic cardiovascular events and conditions (Stone et al., 2013).

Comprehensive Lipid Analysis—Vertical Auto Profile (VAP)

Commonly, a basic lipid panel is obtained, and the basic levels inform the initiation of referral, nonpharmacologic interventions, and pharmacologic therapy. However, because the calculation of LDL level is based on the total cholesterol, HDL, and triglyceride levels in the basic lipid panel, evidence suggests that

TABLE 25.8 Reference Range for the Comprehensive VAP Lipid Analysis

Test	Goal (mg/dL)	Moderate Risk (mg/dL)	High Risk (mg/dL)
VAP total LDL	<130	130–159	>159
LDL-R	<100	100–129	>129
Lp(a) cholesterol	<10.0	10.0–14.9	>14.9
IDL	<20	20–29	>29
Total HDL	>39		<40
VAP HDL2 (female)	>15		<16
VAP HDL2 (male)	>10		<11
VAP HDL3 (female)	>25		<26
VAP HDL3 (male)	>30		<31
VAP total VLDL	<30		>29
VAP VLDL 1+2	<20.0		>19.9
VLDL 3	<10		>9
VAP total cholesterol	<200	200–239	>239
VAP triglycerides	<150	150–199	>199
Non-HDL cholesterol	<160	160–189	>189
Remnant lipoproteins	<30		>29
LDL density (pattern)	A	A/B	B
VAP apolipoprotein A1 (female)	>145		<146
VAP apolipoprotein A1 (male)	>118		<119
VAP apolipoprotein B100	<109	109–126	>126
Apo-B100/A ratio (female)	<0.75	0.75–0.86	>0.86
Apo-B100/A ratio (male)	<0.92	0.92–1.07	>1.07

HDL, high-density lipoproteins; LDL, low-density lipoproteins; VAP, vertical auto profile; VLDL, very low-density lipoproteins.

Source: Cleveland HeartLab (2013).

LDL levels may be underreported in up to 60% of patients (Martin et al., 2013). Patients with established CVD, or who are at risk of developing CVD, benefit from interventions to reduce the risk of atherosclerotic cardiovascular conditions, so a comprehensive lipid analysis may more accurately identify patients with hyperlipidemia.

The comprehensive lipid analysis, VAP, enhances the basic lipid panel and provides a more diverse and accurate presentation of lipid analysis. The test directly measures total cholesterol, LDL, HDL, VLD, Lp(a), and triglycerides. The VAP also provides a qualitative assessment of LDL particle size, HDL subfractions (HDL2 and HDL3), VLDL subfractions (VLDL 1+2, VLDL3, and IDL), and LDL remnants (Table 25.8). A higher percentage of smaller, dense LDL molecules is associated with greater risk for atherosclerosis than a higher percentage of large LDL. The VAP test clarifies risk and enables the clinician to provide a personalized treatment approach based on three categories of residual cardio-metabolic risk: cholesterol, triglycerides, and heredity. The 2013 ACC/AHA guideline on the assessment of cardiovascular risk evaluated Apo-B as a risk marker for CVD (Goff et al., 2013). The guidelines reported that Apo-B has not been evaluated as a screening test for CVD with a randomized controlled trial with clinically important outcome data (Goff et al., 2013). Therefore, there is no recommendation from the guidelines for or against the testing of Apo-B (Goff et al., 2013).

INFLAMMATORY MARKERS

The link between inflammation and CVD has recently been identified and is providing novel insight into the pathophysiology of many conditions affecting patients with CVD. Although the association of inflammation and cardiovascular disorders is strong, the evidence for treating inflammation is less robust, and therapeutic management for inflammatory markers are under continued investigation. However, the following is a review and description of selected inflammatory biomarkers that are important in CVD.

C-Reactive Protein

C-reactive protein (CRP) is a nonspecific, acute-phase reactant protein produced by the liver during acute inflammatory processes. Antigen-immune complexes, bacteria, fungi, or trauma initiate the synthesis of CRP; thus, positive results are helpful in identifying the presence of an inflammatory process, although not the specific cause of disease. Average CRP levels are 1 to 3 mg/dL, with a high result indicated by any value greater than 3 mg/dL. CRP values increase earlier in acute inflammation than most other inflammatory markers such as the erythrocyte sedimentation rate (ESR). CRP levels also return to normal sooner than ESR. A high-sensitivity assay for CRP (hs-CRP) can accurately measure CRP at even lower levels.

Causes of increased CRP levels include increased body mass index, insulin resistance, hypertension, cigarette smoking, and chronic inflammatory or infectious conditions. CRP levels are decreased with physical activity, weight loss, and moderate alcohol consumption. Pharmacologic agents that suppress the inflammatory process may decrease CRP levels, including fibrates, HMG-CoA reductase inhibitors, nicotinic acid, nonsteroidal anti-inflammatory agents, salicylates, corticosteroids, and medications utilized for autoimmune processes. Evidence exists that atherosclerosis is an inflammatory condition. CRP levels may be useful in identifying individuals who are at an increased risk for ASCVD. In 2010, Park et al. implicated high CRP levels in the pathogenesis of atherosclerosis and associated elevated CRP levels with a higher risk for coronary heart disease. Despite this evidence, routine screening of the CRP level as a mechanism to determine risk for CVD is not recommended.

Statin therapy is associated with lower levels of CRP along with a reduction in cholesterol values. In 2008, a trial by Ridker et al. (2008) demonstrated that rosuvastatin significantly reduced the incidence of major cardiovascular events. This study involved 17,802 apparently healthy people with elevated high-sensitivity CRP levels of 2.0 mg/L or higher and with normal LDL cholesterol levels of 130 mg/dL or lower. Participants were randomized to receive rosuvastatin 20 mg daily or placebo. After a median follow-up of 1.9 years, results demonstrated that rosuvastatin reduced high-sensitivity CRP levels by 37% and LDL cholesterol levels by 50%. Moreover, rosuvastatin was found to significantly reduce the incidence of major cardiovascular events, including myocardial infarction, stroke, and death from cardiovascular causes.

The 2013 ACC/AHA guideline on the assessment of cardiovascular risk evaluated hs-CRP as a risk marker for CVD and concluded that hs-CRP has not been evaluated with a randomized controlled trial as a screening test with outcomes of clinically important cardiovascular events (Goff et al., 2013). Therefore, hs-CRP is an optional screening test with a level IIb recommendation if cardiovascular risk is uncertain after risk-based assessment is completed. In addition, the guidelines support revising the risk upward for hs-CRP equal to or greater than 2 mg/L in those individuals with uncertain risks based on the usual assessment criteria (Goff et al., 2013).

Erythrocyte Sedimentation Rate

The ESR test detects inflammation that may be caused by infection, inflammatory disorders, cancers, or autoimmune diseases. This is a nonspecific test for inflammation, however, as it merely indicates the presence of inflammation and does not identify the cause or location of the inflammation. Since ESR can be affected by multiple factors and is a nonspecific marker of inflammation, the results of this test must be considered in conjunction with other pertinent clinical findings to establish any diagnosis of cause. The ESR may be useful for guiding the diagnosis and evaluating risk, since multiple inflammatory disorders, including systemic lupus erythematosus and rheumatoid arthritis, are associated with increased risk of CVD, especially in women (Mosca et al., 2011). In the 2011 Guideline for the Prevention of Cardiovascular Disease in Women from the AHA, systemic autoimmune collagen-vascular disease is listed as a risk factor for CVD in women (Mosca et al., 2011).

OTHER RELATED STUDIES

Homocysteine

Homocysteine is an amino acid that is formed during metabolism of methionine. Essential nutrients, including vitamins B_6, folic acid, B_{12}, and riboflavin, are necessary for this metabolic process to occur. Normal serum homocysteine levels are less than 12 mmol/L, with desirable levels at less than 10 mmol/L. Evidence suggests that elevated homocysteine levels promote atherosclerotic plaque formation by causing endothelial damage, increasing LDL deposition, enhancing thrombus formation, and promoting vascular smooth muscle growth (Park et al., 2010). Thus, elevated levels of homocysteine may be related to increased risk of coronary heart disease, stroke, and peripheral arterial disease. The AHA (2014) suggested that screening of serum homocysteine levels may be useful for individuals with familial predisposition to CVD but who do not demonstrate known risk factors such as elevated blood pressure, obesity, and smoking. However, routine screening of homocysteine levels is not recommended for the general population.

Homocysteine levels can be elevated due to genetic defects in homocysteine metabolism; acquired nutrient deficiencies of folate, vitamin B_6, or vitamin B_{12}, and megoblastic anemias. Children with genetic defects causing hyperhomocysteinemia should be monitored, as they may have accelerated and early-onset atherosclerosis. In addition, assessing homocysteine levels in patients at increased risk for deficiencies in folate and vitamins B_6 and B_{12}, such as older adults, alcoholics, and drug abusers, may uncover these nutritional deficiencies.

Creatine Kinase

Creatine kinase (CK), otherwise known as creatine phosphokinase, is an enzyme that converts creatine to creatinine to allow proper muscle function in the body. A CK test measures the amount of circulating CK in the bloodstream and can be used to detect inflammation, muscle injury, or muscle damage. Elevated CK generally indicates recent muscle damage, although it will not indicate the cause or location of the muscle injury. Clinicians may evaluate CK levels before initiating statin therapy and to monitor changes in patients who experience myalgia, exercise intolerance, or myopathies.

The use of the CK-myocardial band (MB) isoenzyme is less sensitive and specific for myocardial infarction than cardiac troponins; therefore, CK-MB is less widely used as a diagnostic or prognostic test for acute coronary syndromes (Anderson et al., 2013). Due to the short half-life of CK-MB, this test is useful in patients with a recent myocardial infarction for the evaluation of reinfarction, the extension of a previous infarct area, and periprocedural myocardial infarctions. For these situations, a CK-MB is obtained at the onset of clinical suspicion, and it is then repeated 6 to 12 hours later.

Uric Acid

Uric acid is the end product of purine metabolism and is excreted largely by the kidneys and to a smaller degree by the intestinal mucosa. Normal uric acid levels range in men from 4 to 8 mg/dL, and in women from 2.8 to 7.5 mg/dL. Many conditions cause an elevation in serum uric acid levels, but the most common cause is gout. Atherosclerosis, hypertension, and elevated triglycerides can raise uric acid levels. In addition, patients with renal disease may have elevated serum uric acid, as urinary excretion is reduced. Some pharmacologic agents prescribed in the management of cardiac conditions, including thiazide diuretics, elevate serum uric acid levels, predisposing the susceptible patient to develop clinical gout symptoms.

Thyroid Profile

Thyroid function is regulated by the pituitary gland, which releases thyroid-stimulating hormone (TSH) in response to low circulating levels of thyroid hormones, triiodothyronine (T3), and thyroxine (T4). Knowledge of this negative feedback system is essential in the interpretation of the thyroid profile. T3 is less stable than T4 and is present in much smaller quantities, rendering T4 a more reliable indicator of thyroid function. Thyroid hormones are bound to protein carriers called thyroid-binding globulins (TBG). T4 levels can be measured in two different forms: total and free. Total T4 values represent a measurement of the total amount of T4 present in the blood. However, T4 is bound to TBG proteins and an elevation in these proteins, such as in pregnancy and oral contraceptive administration, will result in a falsely elevated T4. In clinical situations that alter protein blood levels, T4 should be measured by obtaining a free T4 level, the metabolically active thyroid hormone that is not bound to proteins. TSH levels are essential as a screening test for thyroid disorders and to differentiate primary from secondary hypothyroidism and hyperthyroidism.

Patients with thyroid dysfunction may present with common cardiac symptoms—including fatigue, dyspnea, and palpitations—that may correlate with brady- or tachyarrhythmias. Obtaining a thyroid profile in patients experiencing the symptoms described earlier assists in confirming or reducing the likelihood of thyroid dysfunction in these individuals.

Amiodarone, a common antiarrhythmic agent used in the management of tachyarrhythmias, is highly concentrated in tissues and can lead to hypothyroidism and, less commonly, hyperthyroidism. The prevalence of amiodarone-induced hypothyroidism ranges from 5% to 22%, whereas that of amiodarone-induced thyrotoxicosis is somewhat lower, affecting 2.0% to 9.6% (Narayana, Woods, & Boos, 2011). Hypothyroidism may develop as early as 2 weeks or as late as 39 months after the initiation of amiodarone treatment (Narayana et al., 2011). Therefore, evaluation of thyroid levels is important prior to initiating amiodarone and for monitoring throughout therapy.

Blood Cultures

Blood cultures are obtained to determine the presence of bacteria in the blood. When patients experience persistent clinical signs of infection or fever of unknown origin, blood cultures should be obtained. Blood cultures should be obtained rapidly if bacteremia is suspected and prior to initiation of treatment, as a delay may alter results. Each institution has specific guidelines to accurately collect samples and prevent contamination. Blood is placed in a culture media with preliminary results usually available within 24 hours; final results are available in approximately 1 week. If obtaining a sample of blood from an IV catheter, it is important to also obtain a peripheral venipuncture sample, as colonization of the IV catheter is probable and can provide false data. The blood culture result, along with antibiotic sensitivity testing, informs the clinician of the likely etiology of infection and the selection of appropriate antibiotic therapy. In cardiology practice, blood cultures are obtained to evaluate patients with known or suspected bacterial endocarditis. A recent international study confirmed that *Staphylococcus aureus* is consistently the most prevalent causative organism associated with the diagnosis of bacterial endocarditis (Murdoch et al., 2009).

CARDIAC BIOMARKERS

As our understanding of the complex pathophysiology of CVDs increases, so has our application of cardiac biomarkers in clinical practice. Cardiac biomarkers have become essential for the diagnosis, management, and prognosis of CVDs, most commonly for the evaluation of suspected acute coronary syndrome and HF.

Troponins

Troponins are a group of proteins located in skeletal and cardiac muscle fibers that assist in muscle contraction. Myofibrillar proteins are found in striated muscles; the thick filament contains myosin and the thin filament contains the proteins actin, tropomyosin, and troponin. The troponin subunits are C, T, and I. Troponin T (cTnT) and I (cTnI) are cardiac-specific markers; troponin T binds troponin and tropomyosin, and unbound troponin T is released in the early stages of myocardial damage. Troponin I inhibits actomyosin ATPase, depending on calcium concentrations. There are multiple assays with different sensitivities for cTnI; therefore, cutoff concentrations are required for interpretation in clinical practice. However, there is a single laboratory test for cTnT that provides standardization in all laboratories (Anderson et al., 2013).

Usually, none or a very small amount of troponin is detectable in blood, rarely exceeding 0.1 ng/mL in healthy individuals (Reed, 2009). The high sensitivity troponin assay is able to quantify smaller amounts of circulating troponin, detecting troponin up to 0.005 ng/mL (Mahajan & Jarolim, 2011). This improved sensitivity, which detects levels in healthy populations, results in somewhat less specificity for acute myocardial damage, necessitating a cutoff or normal value to be established (Mahajan & Jarolim, 2011). An increase of cardiac troponins is a marker of cell necrosis and active thrombogenetic plaque (Anderson et al., 2013). The negative predictive value of troponins is robust, with low or undetectable levels facilitating the exclusion of a diagnosis of myocardial injury. Although an elevated troponin represents myocardial necrosis, additional factors must be considered to determine the etiology of the value, as elevations in troponin can occur due to cardiac and noncardiac conditions (Newby et al., 2012). In addition to myocardial infarction, troponins may be elevated due to strenuous activity, myocarditis, HF, severe infections, cardiomyopathy, bradyarrhythmias, tachyarrhythmia, PE, renal disease, hypotension, pericarditis, valvular heart disease, cardiac trauma, cardiac interventions and surgery, endomyocardial biopsy, ablations, pacing, cardioversion, drug toxicity, and defibrillation (Anderson et al., 2013; Mahajan & Jarolim, 2011). End-stage renal disease is particularly problematic for the interpretation of cardiac troponin values, as 53% of patients with this co-morbidity have increased cTnT, and cTnI is elevated in up to 10% of this population (Anderson et al., 2013). The exact mechanism for this elevation is unknown; however, there is a higher associated morbidity regardless of symptoms or known coronary heart disease with the increased levels of troponin in those with end-stage renal disease.

Troponin levels are the biomarker of choice in the evaluation of chest pain and the diagnosis of acute coronary syndromes (Jneid et al., 2010). The biomarker is considered in conjunction with clinical presentation, pretest likelihood, and a 12-lead ECG. Other less specific markers of myocardial injury—LDH, CK, AST, and myoglobin—are less commonly utilized in current cardiovascular practice, as these values may be affected by noncardiac muscle damage, injections, accidents, medications, and strenuous activity. A series of troponin measurements at baseline and at intervals of 3 to 6 hours is obtained for patients who present with acute coronary syndrome symptoms. A rise and fall of the troponin level represents a dynamic cardiac process, which is often associated with an evolution of

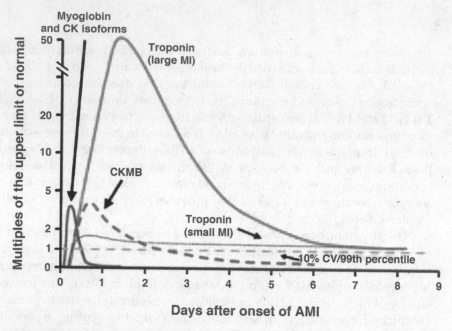

FIGURE 25.1 Timing of release of various biomarkers after acute myocardial infarction.
Reprinted from Anderson et al. (2013, p. e689), with permission from Wolters Kluwer Health.

the myocardial infarction with a 20% change consistent with myocardial damage (Mahajan & Jarolim, 2011; Newby et al., 2012). Typically, the levels increase within 2 to 4 hours after symptom onset, although this rise may be delayed for 8 to 12 hours, and the levels generally peak at 10 to 24 hours. Troponin levels remain elevated for 5 to 14 days (Figure 25.1), limiting their ability to assess early reinfarction; thus, in this setting, CK-MB may be more useful.

Reinfarction is defined as an acute myocardial infarction that occurs within 28 days of the initial myocardial infarction, and troponin values are helpful during the last weeks of this monitoring period. If reinfarction is suspected, troponin values should be obtained immediately with symptoms and a second value should be obtained in 3 to 6 hours. For an initially elevated troponin, a 20% or greater increase in troponin is required to diagnose reinfarction, although if the initial level is normal, the acute myocardial infarction criteria can be applied (Thygesen et al., 2012).

The quantity of troponin measured in the blood provides prognostic information. Increasing troponin levels are associated with more significant infarct size and mortality risk (Anderson et al., 2013), although specific numbers have not been defined (Newby et al., 2012). In addition, an increase in levels that is greater than 50% is associated with increased risk, and a reduction in levels that is greater than 50% is associated with risk reduction (Newby et al., 2012). Serial measurements during the acute phase are generally obtained until the levels begin to decline. In addition to diagnosis and prognostic information, troponin values may identify patients who may benefit from therapeutic antiplatelet medications in the setting of non-ST-elevation myocardial infarction.

The third universal definition of myocardial infarction provides criteria for the interpretation of cardiac troponin values to define acute myocardial infarction (Thygesen et al., 2012). Myocardial infarction can be defined by additional criteria; however, the following are criteria for myocardial infarction that are specifically related to the cardiac troponin value:

- Acute myocardial infarction—cardiac troponin greater than the 99th percentile upper reference limit, with a rise and fall and one of the following—ischemic symptoms, significant ST-T wave changes, new left bundle branch block, development of pathologic Q waves, imaging evidence consistent with loss of myocardial viability or wall motion abnormality, or intracoronary thrombus.
- Percutaneous coronary intervention myocardial infarction—cardiac troponin greater than 5 × 99th percentile with normal baseline values, or a rise greater than 20% for elevated baseline values and one of the following—ischemic symptoms, new ischemic ECG changes, angiographic evidence of procedural complications, or imaging evidence consistent with loss of myocardial viability or wall motion abnormality.
- Stent thrombosis myocardial infarction—cardiac troponin greater than the 99th percentile upper reference limit, with a rise and fall with stent thrombosis and myocardial ischemia.
- Coronary artery bypass graft myocardial infarction—cardiac troponin greater than 10 × 99th percentile with normal baseline values and one of the following—new pathologic Q wave, new left bundle branch block, angiographic evidence of graft or coronary artery occlusion, or imaging evidence consistent with loss of myocardial viability or wall motion abnormality (Thygesen et al., 2012).

Cardiac troponins have a role or potential role in the nonischemic conditions of HF, PE, CKD, sepsis, amyloidosis, cardiac transplant monitoring, blunt cardiac injury, noncardiac surgery, thermal injury, and chemotherapy-associated cardiac toxicity (Newby et al., 2012). In patients who present with acute decompensated heart failure (ADHF), cTnI or cTnT should be measured to evaluate for acute coronary syndrome and to provide prognostic information (Yancy et al., 2013). Elevated troponin values with concomitant HF are associated with a significantly negative prognosis.

Natriuretic Peptides

Cardiomyocytes produce natriuretic peptides in response to changes in cardiac conditions, including myocardial stretch. In response to these triggers, the human BNP gene encodes for pre-proBNP, which is changed to proBNP, then cleaved on secretion into plasma into two main products: BNP, a biologically active C-terminal peptide, and NT-proBNP, a biologically inactive N-terminal peptide. The half-life of BNP is 15 to 20 minutes and that of NT-proBNP is 25 to 70 minutes. In the healthy patient, 15% to 20% of the natriuretic peptides are cleared by the kidneys, with increased levels noted in BNP and NT-proBNP with kidney disease due to decreased clearance. The atria have the highest concentrations of BNP in healthy individuals, although this concentration gradient changes to the ventricles in patients with HF.

Cardiac natriuretic peptides function as part of the neurohormonal system that maintains cardiac homeostasis, promoting natriuresis, diuresis, and vasodilation, and opposing the responses of the renin–angiotensin system. Due to the close correlation of BNP levels to left ventricular pressures, evaluating BNP levels has emerged as a marker for HF diagnosis, prognosis, and treatment. Elevated levels of BNP are a marker of myocardial stress, although the increase in these levels is not cardiac specific. Cardiac causes of elevated natriuretic peptides other than HF include acute coronary syndrome, valvular heart disease, heart muscle disease, myocarditis, cardiac surgery, cardioversion, left ventricular hypertrophy, and cardiac arrhythmia, including atrial fibrillation. Noncardiac causes of elevated BNP include increasing age, anemia, renal failure, pulmonary diseases, sepsis, endocrine disorders, neurologic disease, chronic inflammation, cirrhosis, PE, burns, and toxic substances. Obesity is associated with relatively reduced levels of BNP, with a lower threshold to define HF of 182 pg/mL suggested by some investigators (Daniels et al., 2006).

The BNP has an integral role in providing quantitative information for the diagnosis of HF, particularly in patients who present with dyspnea of uncertain etiology. The 2013 ACCF/AHA guidelines on the management of HF provide an IA recommendation for the measurement of BNP or NT-proBNP for hospitalized and ambulatory patients with dyspnea, especially in the setting of dyspnea with clinical uncertainty, to establish or refute the diagnosis of HF (Yancy et al., 2013). In the emergency department setting, a BNP value less than 100 pg/mL excludes the diagnosis of HF with levels greater than 400 pg/mL, suggestive of an HF diagnosis.

In addition to aiding in the diagnosis of HF, BNP has important implications for HF prognosis. Elevated BNP levels are associated with increased mortality in patients with dyspnea symptoms. For patients hospitalized with HF, a discharge BNP level greater than 250 pg/mL is associated with elevated risk of 6-month rehospitalization or mortality. Higher levels of BNP are associated with HF disease severity. Doust, Pietrzak, Dobson, and Glasziou (2005) performed a systematic review of 19 studies evaluating BNP as a predictor for death and cardiac events. In this review, BNP was a strong predictor of mortality and cardiac events in symptomatic and asymptomatic patients with HF. There was also a demonstrated linear relationship with BNP and risk of death, with each 100 pg/mL increase associated with a 35% greater risk of mortality (Doust et al., 2005).

The use of BNP as a mechanism to guide therapy has revealed some inconsistencies. However, BNP-guided treatment has demonstrated the ability to reduce hospitalization and mortality in some studies of the ambulatory HF population (Lainchbury et al., 2010). When correctly applied, biomarker-guided management appears to improve both the thoroughness of care and the selection of pharmacologic agents (Januzzi & Troughton, 2013). The findings for guideline-directed therapeutic management in the acute heart failure (AHF) setting are less robust (Yancy et al., 2013).

Natriuretic peptides have gained clinical utility for other conditions to predict cardiac events and mortality. Elevated BNP levels are associated with postoperative cardiovascular events, and testing may be indicated as a component of the preoperative evaluation in patients with HF or with increased risk of perioperative cardiovascular risk. The BNP has prognostic importance in the evaluation of early rejection of heart transplants, acute myocardial infarction, stable ischemic heart disease, atrial fibrillation, PE, aortic stenosis, and shock states.

ST2

The ST2 protein is a marker of myocyte stress leading to myocardial fibrosis, with implications for the prognosis and management of HF. The ST2 is a member of the interleukin-1 receptor family that binds to interleukin 33, another marker that is released with increased myocardial stretch. There are two forms of ST2, the circulating, soluble form, and the membrane-bound form. In clinical practice, the soluble form is measured, and it may be notated as sST2. In comparison to BNP, ST2 is less subject to changes associated with age, gender, obesity, and chronic renal disease. However, ST2 is indicated as a complementary biomarker with natriuretic peptides because ST2 is not a diagnostic marker, although it is considered the best predictor of 1-year HF mortality (Rehman, Martinez-Rumayor, Mueller, & Januzzi, 2008). The combination of a high BNP and ST2 provides additive value for risk prediction.

Currently, the main role for ST2 is as a marker of HF prognosis, progression, and risk, and to guide therapeutic management. The 2013 ACCF/AHA HF guidelines provide an IIB recommendation for ST2 for risk stratification in acute and chronic HF for the evaluation of myocardial fibrosis (Yancy et al., 2013). In clinical practice, an ST2 level greater than 35 ng/mL predicts mortality (Januzzi, Mebazaa, & DiSomma, 2015). In the PRIDE study, 593 patients who presented to the emergency department with and without HF underwent evaluation of ST2 levels (Januzzi et al., 2007). The ST2 was predictive of 1-year mortality in those with and without HF, and the combination of ST2 and NT-proBNP was especially predictive of mortality in this time period. In addition, there was a linear relationship in clinical findings with an increased New York Heart Association (NYHA) class associated with increasing ST2 levels (Januzzi et al., 2007).

The ST2 levels have been evaluated in association with left ventricular ejection fraction (LVEF). A study of 447 patients admitted with ADHF assessed LVEF and ST2 levels with preserved LVEF defined as equal to or greater than 50% (Manzano-Fernandez, Mueller, Pascual-Figal, Truong, & Januzzi, 2011). Patients with HF with preserved ejection fraction (HFpEF) had lower ST2 levels compared with those with HF with reduced ejection fraction (HFrEF); however, ST2 concentrations were an independent predictor of 1-year mortality and were associated with symptom severity in both groups independent of LVEF (Manzano-Fernandez et al., 2011).

Changes in ST2 have important clinical implications with persistently high ST2 levels predictive of mortality or HF hospitalization, and reduction of levels associated with reduced risk (Breidthardt et al., 2013). Beta blocker therapy is demonstrating some effect in modulating ST2 levels and in decreasing related cardiovascular events (Gaggin, Motiwala, Bhardwaj, Parks, & Januzzi, 2013).

As ST2 is a relatively new biomarker in clinical practice, in January 2015 a current procedural terminology (CPT) code was assigned for ST2: The code is 83006. An international ST2 consensus panel published a report on ST2 and prognosis for acutely decompensated HF in January 2015, which demonstrates the increasingly compelling clinical implications of this particular cardiac biomarker (Januzzi et al., 2015).

Additional Biomarkers

The evaluation of biomarkers in association with CVD will continue to develop, and many are under investigation in biological and clinical trials. Additional biomarkers that may gain increased clinical importance include markers for oxidative damage—myeloperoxidase, oxidized LDL, midregional proadrenomedullin; inflammation—Fas, adiponectin, interleukins, tumor necrosis factor (TNF)-alpha, osteoprotegerin; hypertrophy and fibrosis—galectin3, matrix metalloproteinases (MMPs), collagen propeptides; apoptosis—GDF-15; neurohormonal activation—renin, angiotensin II, aldosterone; sympathetic nervous system—norepinephrine, chromogranin A; and arginine vasopressin (Sun et al., 2014).

THERAPEUTIC DRUG MONITORING

Certain cardiac medications require therapeutic drug monitoring to determine medication efficacy, prevent organ toxicity, and evaluate adverse effects, such as arrhythmias. Normal therapeutic ranges and toxic serum concentration levels for some commonly prescribed cardiac medications are provided in Table 25.9. Drug serum concentration levels can be affected significantly by intestinal absorption, renal excretion, electrolyte balance, metabolism, and interactions with other medications. Accurate interpretation of serum concentration levels requires identification of the medication administration route and the time of the last dose. Digoxin, a medication generally used in the management of HF and atrial fibrillation, requires therapeutic monitoring, due to its narrow therapeutic range and low threshold for toxicity. Warning signs and symptoms of digoxin toxicity include confusion, visual disturbances, nausea, vomiting, palpitations, and changes in heart rate and rhythm. Potassium competes with digoxin for binding sites, so patients with hypokalemia have an increased risk of digoxin toxicity. Similarly, amiodarone and many other antiarrhythmic medications have narrow therapeutic windows with serious potential for proarrhythmic effects and organ toxicity. Therefore, when caring for cardiac patients who are prescribed these medications, clinicians may monitor drug serum concentration levels regularly and as clinical symptoms arise.

TABLE 25.9 Therapeutic Ranges and Toxic Levels of Commonly Prescribed Cardiac Medications

Medication	Therapeutic Range	Toxic Level
Amiodarone	1.5–2.5 mg/L	>3.5 mg/L
Digoxin		
Atrial fibrillation	0.5–2 ng/mL	>2.5 ng/mL
Heart failure	0.5–0.9 ng/mL	
Diltiazem	40–200 ng/mL	>1 mg/L
Flecainide	0.2–1 mg/L	≥6 mg/L
Lidocaine	1.4–6 mg/L	>12 mg/L
Procainamide	4–8 mg/L	
Propafenone	64–1,044 ng/mL	>1,000 ng/mL
Propranolol	50–100 ng/mL	>7 mg/L
Quinidine	2–5 mg/L	

Source: Reed (2009).

CARDIAC GENETIC TESTING

Genetic Variants With Clopidogrel

Clopidogrel is a prodrug converted to an active form by CPY450 isoenzymes in the liver. Currently, three primary genetic polymorphisms of the CYP2C19 allele impair the conversion of clopidogrel to its active form, decreasing the effectiveness of the medication (Anderson et al., 2013). In 2010, the Food and Drug Administration (FDA) announced a boxed warning regarding the reduction of clopidogrel efficacy in the subgroup of patients with an impaired ability to convert the medication to an active form (Anderson et al., 2013). Routine testing for CYP2C19 genotypes or overall platelet function is not currently recommended, as there have been no prospective studies to demonstrate that testing improves outcomes. Testing is also limited by expense, because it is not routinely covered by insurance. Nevertheless, clinicians should maintain an awareness of this subgroup of patients who may have reduced platelet inhibition with clopidogrel, especially if a patient has recurrent events.

Cardiogenomic Profiles

An increased interest in genetic testing as a mechanism to predict CVD risk led to the 2005 formation of the Evaluation of Genomic Applications in Practice and Prevention (EGAPP), a nonfederal, independent work group supported by the CDC. In 2010, the EGAPP released Cardiogenomic Profiles to Predict Risk of Developing Cardiovascular Disease (EGAPP Work Group, 2010), which evaluated 57 genetic variants in 28 genes for risk of CVD. The report suggests that the independent and combined testing had an overall low benefit, and did not improve outcomes over traditional risk-factor evaluation.

Lipid Storage Disorders

Genetic lipid storage disorders are rare, diverse diseases due to inherited deficiencies of lysosomal hydrolase. These disorders are primarily inherited by an autosomal recessive trait, except Fabry disease, which is transmitted via an X-linked recessive trait. Examples of these disorders include Gaucher disease, Niemann-Pick disease, gangliosidoses, Farber's disease, Fabry disease, metachromatic leukodystrophy, Wolman's disease, and Krabbe disease. Laboratory evaluations include diagnostic assays measuring specific enzymatic activity in peripheral blood leukocytes or cultured fibroblasts.

Inherited Arrhythmogenic Disorders and Cardiomyopathies

In the 1990s, the first causative genes for cardiomyopathy were discovered, followed by those for channelopathies, and since that time our understanding of the genetic basis of arrhythmogenic and structural disorders has increased (Ackerman et al., 2011). In 2011, the Heart Rhythm Society and the European Heart Rhythm Association provided an expert consensus statement on the state of genetic testing for the channelopathies and cardiomyopathies (Ackerman et al., 2011). The key recommendations are that genetic counseling is an integral component of care, and treatment should be guided by a comprehensive evaluation of the patient (Ackerman et al., 2011). In general, genetic testing for these disorders is obtained after evaluation by an electrophysiologist and at centers experienced in genetic evaluation and testing (Ackerman et al., 2011). Specialized laboratories that evaluate these disorders include, but are not limited to, GeneDX (www.genedx.com) and AMBRY Genetics (www.ambrygen.com).

Genetic testing recommendations were provided for the 13 known inherited cardiac conditions for which genetic testing may have diagnostic or prognostic implications. There are no Class I recommendations in the guidelines for atrial fibrillation, although an abbreviated summary of Class I recommendations for other disorders is listed in Table 25.10.

TABLE 25.10 Summary of Class I Recommendations for Genetic Testing of Channelopathies and Cardiomyopathies

Condition	Class I Recommendation	Class I Recommendation for Testing of Family Members in Confirmed Index Cases
Long QT syndrome	Strong clinical index of suspicion Prolonged QT on serial ECG with no known etiology	Yes
Catecholaminergic polymorphic ventricular tachycardia	Strong clinical index of suspicion	Yes
Brugada syndrome		Yes
Cardiac conduction disease		Yes
Short QT syndrome		Yes
Hypertrophic cardiomyopathy	Established clinical diagnosis	Yes
Arrhythmogenic cardiomyopathy/ Arrhythmogenic right ventricular cardiomyopathy		Yes
Dilated cardiomyopathy	Confirmed dilated cardiomyopathy and significant cardiac conduction disease and/or family history of premature sudden death	Yes
Left ventricular non-compaction		Yes
Restrictive cardiomyopathy		Yes
Out-of-hospital cardiac arrest—survivors	Guided by results of evaluation for patient and family	
Postmortem for sudden unexpected death	Tissue sample for testing	Yes

Source: Ackerman et al. (2011).

URINE STUDIES

Urinalysis

Complete urinalysis consists of a gross visual evaluation, dipstick analysis, and microscopic evaluation of the urine sample. To interpret the results accurately, the urine specimen should be collected via the clean-catch technique, capturing the sample midstream in a clean container. On gross evaluation, a normal urine specimen is light yellow in color and clear. The urine dipstick analysis tests for specific gravity, glucose, heme, leukocyte esterase, nitrites, albumin, and hydrogen ions (Table 25.1). Measuring urine specific gravity allows interpretation of urine osmolality. Usually, concentrated urine ranges in specific gravity from 1.005 to 1.030. The microscopic examination provides confirmation and clarification of the dipstick findings, and it identifies structures such as epithelial cells, crystals, and casts that are not visualized by dipstick analysis. A normal urinalysis contains few cells, little or no protein or glucose, no bacteria or fungi, and no casts other than hyaline casts. When caring for patients with cardiac disease who are taking diuretics, the urine specific gravity is monitored in order to ensure that patients are not overly dilute or dehydrated.

Urine Electrolytes

A urine specimen can be evaluated for electrolytes, including calcium, chloride, potassium, and sodium. Normal values are presented in Table 25.11. The specimen can be collected via random urine collection or 24-hour urine collection. Assessment of urine electrolytes is helpful in the diagnostic evaluation of a patient's volume status, hyponatremia, hypokalemia, and metabolic disorders.

TABLE 25.11 Reference Ranges of Urine Electrolytes in 24-Hour Urine Collection

Electrolyte	Normal Range
Calcium	100–300 mg
Chloride	110–250 mEq/L
Potassium	25–125 mEq/L
Sodium	40–220 mEq/L

Source: National Institutes of Health (2014).

Urine Creatinine

Urine creatinine measures the amount of creatinine excreted in the urine over a specified period of time. The clinician can order the urine to be collected over 2, 12, or 24 hours. Urine creatinine provides information for the creatinine clearance test, which is a more direct measure of the GFR. A normal creatinine clearance for men is 95 to 135 mL/min, and that for women is 85 to 125 mL/min. Measurements of 24-hour timed urine collection for creatinine clearance do not enhance the eGFR over the prediction equations, although they may be considered for individuals with extremes of age; extremes of body size due to malnutrition or obesity, skeletal muscle disease, or paraplegia or quadriplegia; vegetarian diet; prior to dosing significantly nephrotoxic medications; and in the setting of rapidly changing kidney function.

Urine Protein

Evaluation of protein in the urine is often performed in individuals with diabetes mellitus or hypertension at the time of diagnosis and then annually. The test is completed with a urine dipstick on a spot urine sample or on a 24-hour urine collection. Normal values for spot-urine albumin and 24-hour urine collection are less than 30 ug/mg (ADA, 2014b) and less than 150 mg of protein, respectively. Urinary albumin equal to or greater than 30 ug/mg is considered increased; persistent proteinuria is an indicator of reduced renal function and requires further evaluation and potentially referral to a nephrologist (ADA, 2014b). Angiotensin-converting enzyme inhibitors delay the progression of renal disease; therefore, patients with hypertension or diabetes mellitus who develop proteinuria are evaluated for angiotensin-converting enzyme inhibitor therapy.

Urine Culture

Confirming or excluding a urinary tract infection requires urine culture analysis. The urine culture identifies the infectious organism and therefore helps the clinician select the appropriate antibiotic. Urine specimens for culture and sensitivity should be obtained midstream via the clean-catch technique or by catheterization. In patients with symptomatology consistent with urinary tract infection, a urine culture may be necessary before any invasive procedures, surgical intervention, or device implantation.

Urine Catecholamines-Pheochromocytoma

Pheochromocytoma is a catecholamine-secreting tumor that arises from chromaffin cells in the adrenal medulla. The tumoral hypersecretion of catecholamines—including dopamine, norepinephrine, and epinephrine—produces symptoms of paroxysmal hypertension, episodic headache, generalized sweating, tachycardia, forceful palpitations, and dyspnea. Patients who present with symptomatic paroxysmal hypertension, tachycardia, or arrhythmia during diagnostic procedures, induction of anesthesia, or ingestion of certain foods or medications may be evaluated for pheochromocytoma. Diagnosis of pheochromocytoma is usually confirmed by 24-hour urine collection measuring the excretion of catecholamines and fractionated metanephrines. In order to verify an adequate urine collection, the 24-hour urine specimen includes a measurement of urinary creatinine. Positive findings consistent with the diagnosis of pheochromocytoma include one or more of the following in a 24-hour urine collection: norepinephrine greater than 170 mcg, epinephrine greater than 35 mcg, dopamine greater than 700 mcg, normetanephrine greater than 900 mcg, or metanephrine greater than 400 mcg.

GENERAL RECOMMENDATIONS

Diagnostic laboratory test selection is an integral component of the diagnosis, treatment, and management of individuals with cardiovascular disorders. Table 25.12 provides general recommendations for the evaluation of selected, common cardiovascular conditions.

TABLE 25.12 General Recommendations for Evaluating Cardiovascular Conditions

Condition	Electrolytes	Glucose	Renal	CBC	Hepatic	Lipids	Thyroid	UA	CK	BNP	Uric Acid
Hypertension	×	×	×	×		×		×			×
Dyslipidemia		×			×	×	×		×		
Coronary heart disease	×	×	×	×	×	×	×				
Heart failure	×	×	×	×	×			×		×	
Atrial fibrillation	×		×	×			×				

BNP, brain natriuretic peptide; CBC, complete blood count; CK, creatine kinase; UA, urinalysis.

Tests may have overlapping and complementary indications in the diagnosis and management of cardiovascular disorders. The practitioner must remember to evaluate the diagnostic laboratory data in the context of the whole patient, along with the clinical presentation, comprehensive health history, and physical examination. Moreover, as with all diagnostic testing and procedures, the risks must be considered with the benefits when deciding whether to obtain the diagnostic study.

For full reference citations to this chapter, please see "Section References" at the back of the book, under the heading "Section VI."

Noninvasive Diagnostic Testing: Electrocardiograph and Ultrasound

BRIAN C. CASE AND MONVADI B. SRICHAI

Diagnostic testing is an essential component of contemporary cardiology practice for evaluating cardiovascular conditions by determining the existence of disorders, characterizing illness, defining severity, and guiding effective treatment modalities. Many older testing strategies remain useful, whereas innovative tests are continually evolving to improve our ability to understand, diagnose, and manage heart disease. Not all individuals will benefit from cardiac evaluations; therefore, before testing, the patient will require individual evaluation to establish the appropriateness of the test, to ensure safety, and to determine the clinical value. Clinical value has increased efficacy when the diagnostic testing results have the potential to influence subsequent treatment planning, including the use of pharmaceuticals, referral for procedures or specialty services, or lifestyle interventions.

Goals of cardiac testing are generally categorized by the ability to (a) identify or exclude various forms of cardiac disease in response to patient symptoms; (b) establish the risk of developing future cardiac disease, including myocardial infarction (MI); and (c) aid in the recommendation for additional medical therapies and procedures. The majority of cardiac diagnostic testing is performed for the evaluation of a cardiac etiology for a patient's presenting symptoms.

Multitudes of testing options are available for the evaluation of cardiovascular disease. Depending on the clinical question, one or more tests may be indicated to provide the required information to inform clinical decisions. Test selection often depends on the type of cardiac disease, a patient's personal health history and preferences, and the availability of testing options based on the facility and clinician expertise. Tests are generally categorized by the type of technology, including electrocardiograph, computed tomography, ultrasound; the information provided, including stress tests, and coronary angiography; or the invasiveness of the test procedure, noninvasive imaging, or invasive testing.

Inherent in testing and evaluation are associated risks based on the specific test and the patient's status. Proper evaluation through health history and physical examination are required prior to initiating most cardiovascular tests. In addition, appropriately trained personnel, suitable facilities, and the availability of emergency equipment and medications are required for many cardiovascular tests.

Another important aspect of diagnostic test selection is the test performance, the ability of the test to accurately detect and exclude disease, sensitivity, and specificity, respectively. The predictive value of any test, however, is dependent on the prevalence of the disorder in the tested population and the probability principles of Bayes' Theorem.

This chapter and Chapter 27 describe common noninvasive cardiovascular diagnostics used in the medical community, including indications, contraindications, risks, and benefits for each test. The diagnostic studies are organized into four broad categories: (1) electrocardiograph tests; (2) ultrasound tests; (3) radiographic tests; and (4) nuclear imaging. Electrocardiograph and ultrasound are discussed in this chapter, with radiographic tests and nuclear imaging detailed in Chapter 27. Invasive diagnostic cardiovascular testing, including coronary angiography, is discussed in a separate chapter. Information is provided on each test procedure, the usual reported results, and considerations for abnormal findings. When selecting an appropriate test, the cardiovascular clinician must consider financial costs, patient preparation and education, duration to complete the test, and interval to obtain results.

ELECTROCARDIOGRAPH TESTS

These noninvasive tests use the electrocardiogram (ECG or EKG) to evaluate the electrical activity generated by the heart at rest or with activity, to evaluate various conditions within the cardiovascular system. These tests include the 12-lead ECG, ambulatory monitors, tilt table test, exercise ECG stress test, and cardiopulmonary exercise test (CPX).

Electrocardiogram

The 12-lead ECG is the most commonly used test for the initial evaluation of the cardiovascular system. The ECG may display abnormal cardiac rhythms and conduction, detect myocardial damage, and indicate widespread cardiac or systemic disease processes. Widely used as a screening tool, the ECG evaluates certain populations who are at risk for developing cardiac disease, individuals with symptoms consistent with cardiovascular disease, and in general evaluations, including preoperative testing (Schlant et al., 1992).

Indications

The ECG is a rapid, simple test indicated for various presenting symptoms and conditions. The ECG may reflect changes associated with primary or secondary myocardial diseases, including coronary heart disease (CHD), hypertension, or cardiomyopathy (Fisch, 1989). The ECG also serves as the gold standard for noninvasive diagnosis of arrhythmias and conduction disturbances, and it may serve as a marker for the presence of heart disease. An ECG is the initial test that is used to evaluate unexplained chest pain, which can be due to an acute MI, myocardial ischemia (angina), or inflammation of the pericardium (pericarditis) (Samson & Scher, 1960). The ECG is also indicated in the evaluation of patients with symptoms that are consistent with cardiac conditions, including shortness of breath, dizziness, syncope, or palpitations, and to screen patients with an increased risk of developing cardiac disease in the future due to hypertension, dyslipidemia, cigarette smoking, diabetes, or a family history of heart disease. Other common indications for ECG include evaluation of metabolic disorders, efficacy and side effects of medications, and management of patients with cardiac implantable electronic devices (CIEDs), defibrillators, and pacemakers.

The American College of Cardiology (ACC) and American Heart Association (AHA) Task Force created a Committee on Electrocardiography in 1992 that developed specific guidelines regarding the indications for ECG in populations of confirmed, suspected, or no known cardiovascular disorders (Table 26.1; Schlant et al., 1992). ECG recommendations are based on initial evaluation, follow-up assessment, response to therapy, or preoperative evaluation.

Contraindications

There are no strict contraindications to ECG testing. However, some patients may have allergies or sensitivities to the adhesive tape used to attach the leads, for which hypoallergenic alternatives are available. Cautious interpretation is also needed in patients who are morbidly obese or in those with chronic obstructive pulmonary disease (COPD), as these conditions may lead to decreased ECG voltage.

TABLE 26.1 Class I Recommendations for Electrocardiography

CV Disorder	Baseline or Initial	Response to Therapy	Follow-Up	Preoperative
Known	All patients with known CV disease or dysfunction	Prescribed therapy with ECG changes associated with therapeutic response, disease progression, or adverse effects	Changes in symptoms, signs, diagnostic findings Implanted devices Interval evaluation of CV disorders—congenital, valvular, conduction, inflammatory, post-revascularization, and co-morbidities	Generally all patients
Suspected or high risk	Suspected CV disease or dysfunction Increased risk for developing CV disease Illicit drug or overdose of pharmaceuticals with CV effects	Prescribed therapies, including cardioactive and other agents that may result in ECG changes	Changes in symptoms, signs, or diagnostic findings indicating cardiac disease or dysfunction Interval evaluation for those at risk for CV disorders	Generally all patients
No apparent	>40 years Before administration of cardiotoxic agents Before stress testing Occupations requiring very high CV performance or associated with public safety	Prescribed therapies with cardiovascular effects	Asymptomatic >40 years	>40 years Evaluation for pretransplantation donor or recipient

CV, cardiovascular; ECG, electrocardiogram.

Adapted from Schlant et al. (1992).

Procedure

The standard 12-lead ECG records tracings of the heart's electrical activity by evaluating the potential differences between prescribed sites on the body surface that vary during the cardiac cycle. The ECG reflects differences in transmembrane voltages in myocardial cells that occur during depolarization and repolarization within each cycle (Hancock et al., 2009; Kligfield et al., 2007; Mason et al., 2007; Rautaharju et al., 2009; Surawicz et al., 2009; Wagner et al., 2009). Pairs of electrodes or a combination of electrodes serve as one of the two electrodes, and the tracings that result are known as leads. The ECG leads are grouped into two electrical planes: The frontal leads (Lead I, II, III, aVR, aVL, aVF) view the heart in a vertical plane, whereas the transverse leads (V1 through V6) view the heart in a horizontal plane. Patients are placed in a supine position with their arms by their sides. The skin is prepared by cleaning and gently abrading, before the application of electrodes to improve the quality of the ECG recording. The electrodes are placed on the limbs and the chest wall in a conventional pattern. At any point in time, the electrical activity of the heart is composed of differently directed forces. These electrical forces are displayed on tracings over a certain period of time, in seconds, onto the ECG printout.

Risks and Benefits

In general, an ECG is a rapid, simple test with minimal to no risks involved. During the test, electricity does not pass through the patient while the electrodes are reading; thus, this test is not harmful. The medical staff should make sure that the patient does not have any integumentary conditions, open wounds, or prior history of an allergy to adhesive tape, which is part of the electrodes. The test itself can be performed in less than 10 minutes.

Results

Important information can be gathered from an ECG tracing. Proper positioning of the electrodes, with good skin contact, is important to minimize artifacts and misinterpretations, as improperly placed leads can yield the appearance of disease when none is present and vice versa (Schijvenaars, Kors, van Herpen, Kornreich, & van Bemmel, 1997). Interpretation involves careful analysis of the waveform components, including morphology and intervals with recognition of specific patterns that may be indicative of a specific disease process, including possible structural abnormalities, myocardial ischemia, MI, conduction disorders, metabolic imbalances, pulmonary disease, pharmacologic therapies, and arrhythmias (Hancock et al., 2009; Kligfield et al., 2007; Mason et al., 2007; Rautaharju et al., 2009; Surawicz et al., 2009; Wagner et al., 2009). Although computer ECG interpretation programs have demonstrated useful adjunctive value, they cannot substitute for interpretations by experienced electrocardiographers and should not be used alone in making clinical decisions (Kadish et al., 2001).

Further Testing

For an ECG that suggests signs of cardiovascular disease, the clinician may recommend further testing to evaluate cardiac function, conduction, or coronary perfusion. In symptomatic individuals with associated ECG findings of ischemia or infarction, invasive testing such as coronary angiography may be indicated. If a patient is exhibiting signs and symptoms suggestive of an arrhythmia, including palpitations, dizziness, or syncope, but demonstrates nondiagnostic findings on a single 12-lead ECG, the patient may be referred for additional testing, including extended ambulatory ECG monitoring. These tests include Holter monitors, event monitors, and loop recorders, which will be discussed later. Further testing is dependent on the clinical presentation and the 12-lead ECG findings, which is typically the first test that all others follow.

Diagnostic Performance

As ECGs are composed of several different waveforms, each influenced differently by a variety of pathologic and physiologic factors, the sensitivity and specificity for diagnosis of specific conditions varies depending on the patient history, clinical scenario, and diagnostic criteria. The ECG demonstrates higher accuracy in the diagnosis of arrhythmias and conduction disturbances compared with the diagnosis of structural or metabolic abnormalities. As there is considerable overlap in the ECG patterns that may be seen with a variety of structural and pathophysiological abnormalities, the ECG often demonstrates high sensitivity but lower specificity in the diagnosis of specific structural and metabolic diseases (Friedberg & Zager, 1961). Skillful ECG interpretation with particular attention to the limitations of the technique enhances its sensitivity, specificity, and overall clinical usefulness.

Ambulatory Electrocardiography Monitors

Ambulatory electrocardiography allows a provider to monitor a patient's heart rhythm for an extended period of time. The three main ambulatory ECG monitoring devices include a Holter monitor, an event monitor, and a loop recorder (Table 26.2). Providers usually recommend one of these monitors if there is clinical suspicion of arrhythmia based on clinical symptoms. Symptoms consistent with arrhythmia include palpitations, shortness of breath, dizziness, syncope, or presyncope. The benefit of ambulatory ECG monitoring is that the duration to evaluate cardiac conduction and rhythm is extended, instead of just a few moments to evaluate with a standard 12-lead ECG. In addition, individuals with known conduction disorders who are treated for cardiac rhythm abnormalities may benefit from ambulatory ECG monitors to evaluate treatment progress. Holter monitors, event monitors, and loop recorders are contrasted in the recording duration and invasiveness of the procedure (Zimetbaum & Josephson, 1999).

TABLE 26.2 Comparison of Different Types of Electrocardiography Monitoring

	What Does This Test Show?	Who Should Get This Test?	Risks	Benefits
12-Lead ECG	Arrhythmias Ischemic heart disease May indicate underlying structural heart disease or metabolic disorders	Patients having signs and symptoms suggestive of arrhythmias or heart disease	Minimal Allergies to adhesive tape	Screening tool evaluation of all cardiac diseases <10 minutes
Holter monitor *External*	Arrhythmias	Patients having signs and symptoms suggestive of arrhythmias not seen on a basic ECG	Extended period of time Avoiding water	Provides continuous monitoring and recording over an extended period of time (24–48 hours)
Event monitor *External*	Arrhythmias	Patients having signs and symptoms suggesting of arrhythmias not seen on a basic ECG	Extended period of time Avoiding water	Provides monitoring over an extended period of time (weeks) and recording of ECG when the patient is symptomatic and/or arrhythmia detection
Loop recorder *External* 3–4 weeks *Internal* up to 36 months	Arrhythmias	Patients having signs and symptoms suggestive of arrhythmias not seen on a basic ECG	Internal—minor surgical procedure for implant and explant with risks of infection, bleeding, and pain	Provides monitoring over an extended period of time (months to years) and recording of ECG when the patient is symptomatic

Indications

Ambulatory ECG monitoring is primarily indicated to assess symptoms that may be related to rhythm disturbances. Specific symptoms may include unexplained syncope, near syncope, episodic dizziness of unknown cause, or unexplained recurrent palpitations. Additional symptoms that may be related to arrhythmia and warrant ambulatory ECG monitoring include episodic shortness of breath, chest pain, fatigue of unknown cause, or neurologic symptoms when transient atrial fibrillation or flutter is suspected. Ambulatory ECG monitoring may also be indicated to assess future risk of cardiac arrhythmia and events in patients with left ventricular systolic dysfunction, CHD, heart failure (HF), and genetic disorders, including hypertrophic obstructive cardiomyopathy. In patients on antiarrhythmic therapy, ambulatory ECG monitoring can assess pharmacologic therapy, detect proarrhythmic response, evaluate rate control in atrial fibrillation, or document recurrent or asymptomatic nonsustained arrhythmias in the outpatient setting. In patients with pacemakers or implanted cardioverter defibrillators (ICD), ambulatory ECG monitoring is effective in evaluating symptomatic patients to assess device function or malfunction and to assist in programming advanced pacer features (Crawford et al., 1999b).

The ACC and AHA Task Force created a Committee on Ambulatory Electrocardiography in 1999 and formed specific guidelines of indications for the use of ambulatory ECG in certain populations (Crawford et al., 1999a). Primary indications for ambulatory electrocardiography monitoring include:

- Symptoms related to rhythm disorders, including unexplained syncope, presyncope, dizziness, or recurrent palpitations
- Evaluation of risk for future cardiac events in asymptomatic patients, including heart rate (HR) variability in patients after MI with left ventricular dysfunction, HF, or idiopathic hypertrophic cardiomyopathy
- Assessment of antiarrhythmic pharmacologic therapy
- Evaluation of device function, including pacemakers and ICDs
- Ischemia monitoring with variant angina, those who cannot exercise, and atypical chest pain presentations (Crawford et al., 1999a)

Contraindications

Ambulatory ECG monitoring is considered a safe procedure in stable outpatients. These monitoring devices should never delay hospitalization or treatment of acute conditions, or be considered in the acute care setting, such as a patient with active chest pain or acute shortness of breath, especially with concerns for acute coronary syndrome. Patients with these findings require urgent evaluation and testing performed in order to rule out potential life-threatening conditions. The ambulatory ECG monitoring devices are not indicated in patients with a clear etiology of symptoms as identified by history, physical examination, or laboratory tests. Although most ambulatory ECG monitors are external and noninvasive, implantable devices may be indicated for prolonged evaluations. Absolute contraindications for receiving an implantable device include patients with active infection or significant bleeding disorder.

Procedure

For Holter monitoring, a patient wears a battery-operated device that is typically connected to three to five electrodes on the chest, which allows continuous recording and storage of ECG signals for the duration of monitoring, usually 24 to 48 hours. Holter monitors can determine average HR and HR range, quantify atrial and ventricular ectopy counts, and detail episodes of supraventricular or ventricular arrhythmia, including the shortest and longest duration, burden, HR, and pattern of initiation and termination of the arrhythmia (DiMarco & Philbrick, 1990).

Event monitors are similar to Holter monitors except that the ECG signal is recorded intermittently. Different types of event monitors perform in slightly different ways. Most are activated by the patient when symptoms occur, although some will record automatically if the monitor detects an abnormal heart rhythm. Since event monitors do not store as much data, the size is smaller than Holter monitors and the duration of use can be several weeks. Some of the smallest event monitors are post-event recorders and are not connected to the chest directly, but rather require the patient to hold the device to the chest or push a button to start the recording when symptoms are experienced. Post-event recorders can only record what happens after symptoms begin, potentially missing an arrhythmia that occurs before and during the onset of symptoms, or if the patient is asymptomatic.

Loop recorders differ from event monitors, as they are programmed to have a retrospective (loop) memory, which continuously records newer data while deleting older ECG data. A patient may activate the device, which results in the storage of a single-lead ECG both before (typically 45–60 sec) and after (typically 15–90 sec) activation. To minimize loss of critical data, immediate transtelephonic data transmission is necessary after a symptomatic episode (Mittal, Movsowitz, & Steinberg, 2011). Loop recorders can be useful in patients with infrequent, short-duration transient symptoms that recur over weeks or months, and thus are unlikely to be diagnosed by conventional 12-lead ECG, Holter, or event monitoring. Loop recorders can be both implantable and external, and the selection is dependent on available devices and frequency of symptoms. External loop recorders are worn similar to Holter monitors, for up to 3 to 4 weeks, and require continual maintenance of the device. Implantable loop recorders involve the invasive placement of a subcutaneous, single-lead, ECG monitoring device usually in the left parasternal region of the chest wall under sterile technique. Although more invasive, implantable loop recorders allow for the longest monitoring capability of up to 36 months before requiring explants under sterile conditions (Brignole et al., 2009).

Risks and Benefits

The benefits of ambulatory ECG monitoring are the ability to improve the likelihood of detecting, and therefore diagnosing, cardiac arrhythmias in patients who have unexplained symptoms and nondiagnostic 12-lead ECGs, to stratify patients at clinically high risk for development of arrhythmia, or to evaluate the efficacy of antiarrhythmic treatment with pharmacotherapeutics or devices. Minimal risks are associated with external-type ambulatory ECG monitoring, outside of the inconvenience of avoiding water around the device. In addition, patients should advise their provider if they are allergic to tape or other adhesives used by the electrodes. With implantable loop recorders, there is a risk of local complications with the implant and explant, including infection, bleeding, scarring, and pain associated with the procedure. In addition, there is the fear or stigma that the patient may have about undergoing a surgical procedure. Prophylactic antibiotics may be administered intravenously or locally to avoid the incidence of infection. In the rare instance of a local-pocket infection, the hardware may be removed. Absolute contraindications from receiving the implantable device include a patient with an active infection or those who suffer from a bleeding disorder, which may preclude implantation. Mild anxiolytics and analgesics can be administered to enhance patient comfort during implantation and explantation. Cost is another disadvantage to receiving an implantable loop recorder. The implantable loop recorder has a high initial cost; however, overall the cost effectiveness may be justified, should the device provide diagnostic or prognostic important information (Farwell, Freemantle, & Sulke, 2004).

Results

Depending on the indication for ambulatory ECG monitoring, the significance of the results will vary. In symptomatic patients, the ultimate goal is to correlate the patient's symptoms with the presence of an arrhythmia, which can inform specific treatment or intervention. The absence of an arrhythmia during a symptomatic event suggests a noncardiac etiology for the patient's symptoms, which often results in further evaluation for noncardiac causes. Asymptomatic arrhythmic events may also be detected, which, depending on the type of rhythm disturbance, may be important for further evaluation, management, and risk stratification.

Further Testing

If symptoms are correlated with arrhythmic events, further invasive evaluation of the electrical system may be indicated by an electrophysiologist or with an electrophysiology study. The patient may be referred for definitive treatment with medications, pacemaker, ablation, or internal cardioverter defibrillator. If symptoms do not appear to be associated with arrhythmias, further considerations and possible additional testing for noncardiac etiologies of the patient's symptoms may be indicated. Figure 26.1 provides a diagnostic algorithm for the evaluation of syncope due to a presumed arrhythmia (Zimetbaum & Josephson, 1999).

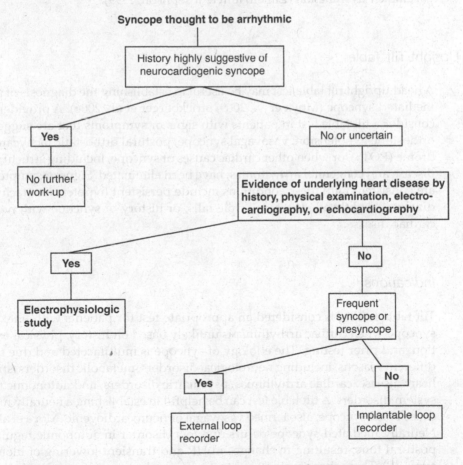

FIGURE 26.1 Suggested diagnostic evaluation algorithm for ambulatory electrocardiographic monitoring for patients presenting with syncope.

Reprinted from Zimetbaum and Josephson (1999), with permission from the American College of Physicians.

Diagnostic Performance

The diagnostic performance of ambulatory ECG monitoring depends on the indication for the test and type of monitoring device. Holter monitors have a diagnostic yield of approximately 35% to 40% for the evaluation of palpitations (Zimetbaum & Josephson, 1999). Event and loop recorders generally have higher success rates with diagnostic yields of 66% to 73% for the evaluation of palpitations. Common rhythms identified by ambulatory ECG monitoring that are associated with palpitations include sinus rhythm, sinus and supraventricular tachycardia, premature atrial and ventricular conductions, atrial fibrillation, and ventricular tachycardia (Zimetbaum & Josephson, 1999). The evaluation of syncope is enhanced with implanted loop recorders, demonstrating diagnostic yields of 50% to 70% (Krahn, Klein, Norris, & Yee, 1995; Solano et al., 2004) compared with external event monitors or loop recorders of approximately 25% to 36% (Zimetbaum & Josephson, 1999). Common arrhythmias identified by ambulatory ECG monitoring that are associated with syncope include sinus bradycardia, sinus pause, second- and third-degree atrioventricular block, supraventricular tachycardia, ventricular tachycardia, and pacemaker dysfunction (Zimetbaum & Josephson, 1999).

Head Upright Tilt Table

A head upright tilt table test may be useful in establishing the diagnosis of neurally mediated syncope (Moya et al., 2009; Strickberger et al., 2006). A provider should consider a tilt table test in patients with signs or symptoms that are suggestive of orthostatic hypotension, vasovagal syncope, postural orthostatic tachycardia syndrome (POTS), or when other cardiac causes of syncope, including structural heart disease and congenital arrhythmias, have been eliminated. Signs or symptoms that are consistent with these conditions include persistent hypotension, tachycardia, dizziness, lightheadedness, multiple falls, or history of syncope with no known cardiac disease.

Indications

Tilt table testing is considered an appropriate test for patients with unexplained syncope when cardiac arrhythmia is unlikely based on history, physical examination, and prior testing. The etiology of syncope is multifaceted and due to many different reasons, including neurological disorders, metabolic disorders, structural heart disease, cardiac arrhythmias, psychiatric disorders, and autonomic nervous system disorders. A tilt table test can be helpful in establishing a neurally mediated cause of the syncope, also termed vasovagal or neurocardiogenic (Moya et al., 2009). Neurally mediated syncope occurs due to a disorder in autonomic regulation in postural tone, resulting in changes in HR and transient lowering of blood pressure (BP). These changes result in a temporary reduction of blood flow to the brain, causing the patient to rapidly lose consciousness, followed by an immediate, spontaneous recovery (Kenny, Ingram, Bayliss, & Sutton, 1986).

POTS is a form of dysautonomia that has orthostatic intolerance as its primary symptom (Grubb, 2008). It is characterized by a sustained HR increase of ≥30 bpm within 10 minutes of standing in the absence of orthostatic hypotension on tilt table testing. POTS is commonly seen in young women and is caused by a heterogeneous group of disorders with similar clinical manifestations. The differential diagnosis for POTS includes other conditions associated with tachycardia, including thyrotoxicosis, inappropriate sinus tachycardia and other tachyarrhythmias, pheochromocytoma, hypoadrenalism, anxiety, dehydration, and side effects from medications. Even though the BP does not decrease, patients with POTS may feel symptoms that are similarly consistent with hypotension, including dizziness, fainting, headache, sweating, shakiness, nausea, and sense of anxiety (Freeman et al., 2011). The usual treatment for POTS is a high fluid intake, compression stockings, careful postural changes, cautious fitness training, and, in some patients, high salt intake and medications, including midodrine or fludrocortisone (Raj, 2006).

Tilt table testing may also be considered when distinguishing neurally mediated syncope from orthostatic hypotension or from epilepsy, especially when abnormal motor movements are associated with the condition. Patients with unexplained falls or frequent syncopal episodes may also benefit from tilt table testing by establishing a cardiac or autonomic nervous system disorder for the syncopal or presyncopal events. The European Society of Cardiology Task Force for the Diagnosis and Management of Syncope provided strict guidelines in 2009 about the methodology, indications (Table 26.3), and diagnostic criteria for the tilt table test (Moya et al., 2009).

TABLE 26.3 Indications for Tilt Table Testing

Class I	First syncopal event with risk of physical injury
	First syncopal event with occupational considerations
	Recurrent syncope without known cardiac disease
	Recurrent syncope with cardiac disease unrelated to syncope
	Importance to demonstrate reflex syncope
Class II	Differentiate syncope due to orthostatic hypotension or reflex syncope
Class III	Differentiate syncope associated with bodily movements of seizures
	Recurrent falls of unknown origin
	Evaluating syncope with psychiatric disorders

Source: Moya et al. (2009).

Contraindications

Tilt table testing is considered a safe procedure with few contraindications. Absolute contraindications include patients with poor baseline mental status; who are unable to stand for long periods; with significant lower extremity or spinal disorders; or who are pregnant. In addition, any patients with recent brain injury, including cerebral vascular accident or aneurysm, or any significant heart disease (critical valvular disease, tachyarrhythmias, HF, shock) should not be considered for this type of testing. Lastly, patients with severe anemia, end-stage renal disease, or electrolyte imbalances are not appropriate candidates to undergo this type of testing, until these metabolic conditions are corrected.

Procedure

During the tilt table test (Figure 26.2), the patient's BP and HR are continuously monitored using a BP cuff and ECG tracing, respectively. The patient is placed in a supine position on the table, and an intravenous access is obtained. Straps are adjusted on the patient to ensure security and safety on the table, without binding or constricting. After approximately 5 minutes in the supine position, the table is tilted as a single unit to raise the patient's body to a head-up position at 60 to 70 degrees for at least 20 minutes. If no event occurs in the initial passive phase, testing will continue based on institutional protocols. Often, the tilt is continued for a further 15 to 20 minutes at the initial angle or the angle may be increased to 90 degrees. A pharmacologic agent, nitroglycerin or isoproterenol, may be administered. During the test, BP, HR, ECG, mental status, and patient symptoms are continuously monitored. The endpoints of a tilt table test are based on the presence of syncope, significant changes in BP, HR, ECG, or symptoms, or the test concludes in the absence of any changes after the protocol is complete. Patients should not eat or drink before the study, to help prevent nausea or vomiting. The patient should also avoid caffeine on the day of the examination to prevent the influence of caffeine on the HR.

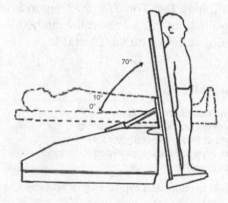

FIGURE 26.2 Example of the tilt table test procedure.

Reprinted with permission from STARS-US—Syncope Trust and Reflex anoxic Seizures®. www.stars-us.org.

Risks and Benefits

A tilt table test is generally safe, and although problems are rare, all patients should be screened for potential complications prior to starting the test. Information gained from tilt table testing can provide confirmation or exclusion of diagnoses and demonstrate patient susceptibility to syncope. Complications include cardiac arrhythmias, hypotension, sinus pause, myocardial ischemia, seizures, transient ischemic attack (TIA), or cerebrovascular accident (CVA). Patients may also experience nonspecific symptoms of fainting, lightheadedness, nausea, or anxiety.

Results

A positive tilt table is based on multiple end points. During the test, if the patient has a syncopal event or is subjectively very lightheaded or dizzy, the test is considered positive for syncope or symptoms, respectively. In addition, if the patient's HR or BP significantly changes after the table is tilted, these changes are also

TABLE 26.4 Diagnostic Criteria for Postural Orthostatic Tachycardia Syndrome (POTS)

1. Sustained heart rate increase of ≥ 30 beats per minute within 10 minutes of standing or tilt in the absence or orthostatic hypotension.
2. Standing heart rate is often ≥ 120 beats per minute.
3. Orthostatic tachycardia may be accompanied by symptoms of cerebral hypoperfusion and autonomic overactivity, relieved by supine position.
4. Criteria not applicable for low resting heart rate.

Source: Freeman et al. (2011).

considered positive findings. Positive tilt table testing is diagnostic for neurally mediated syncope triggered by prolonged standing (Moya et al., 2009), but the test can also be positive in patients with other forms of neurally mediated syncope (Accurso et al., 2001) and in patients with sick sinus syndrome (Brignole et al., 1991). There are specific diagnostic criteria for POTS with tilt table testing that are outlined in Table 26.4.

Further Testing

In general, if the tilt table test is positive, no further evaluation of the patient's syncope needs to be performed, and the patient can be managed accordingly. However, if the test is negative, further testing, diagnostic procedures, specialty care, or referral may be required to determine other causes of syncope. If a cardiac arrhythmia continues to be suspected, referral is generally requested for the subspecialty of electrophysiology.

Diagnostic Performance

The reported sensitivity and specificity of tilt table testing depends on the procedural technique. Sensitivities range from 26% to 80%, and the specificity is approximately 90% for neutrally mediated syncope (Strickberger et al., 2006). Sensitivity is improved with the use of medications such as nitroglycerin, although specificity is reduced (Furukawa, Maggi, Solano, Croci, & Brignole, 2011).

Exercise ECG Stress Testing

Exercise ECG stress testing (EST) is a common diagnostic technique for the investigation and evaluation of patients with known or suspected cardiovascular disease. Although primarily indicated for the evaluation of CHD, additional diagnostic and prognostic findings are derived from EST, which aids in the evaluation and treatment of many cardiovascular disorders.

Indications

EST is recommended as the initial test for the evaluation of patients with known, suspected, or obstructive CHD, and in stable, low- and intermediate-risk patients with symptoms or signs that are suggestive of myocardial ischemia. Prior to

TABLE 26.5 Pretest Probability of Coronary Artery Disease by Age, Gender, and Symptoms

Age (Yrs)	Gender	Typical/Definite Angina Pectoris	Atypical/Probable Angina Pectoris	Nonanginal Chest Pain	Asymptomatic
Younger than 39	Men	Intermediate	Intermediate	Low	Very low
	Women	Intermediate	Very low	Very low	Very low
40–49	Men	High	Intermediate	Intermediate	Low
	Women	Intermediate	Low	Very low	Very low
50–59	Men	High	Intermediate	Intermediate	Low
	Women	Intermediate	Intermediate	Low	Very low
Older than 60	Men	High	Intermediate	Intermediate	Low
	Women	High	Intermediate	Intermediate	Low

High: >90% pretest probability. Intermediate: between 10% and 90% pretest probability. Low: between 5% and 10% pretest probability. Very low: <5% pretest probability.

Reprinted from Patel et al. (2012), with permission from Elsevier.

determining whether a patient qualifies for an EST, providers should determine the pretest likelihood of CHD, based on age, gender, and symptoms. The EST provides the most benefit in patients with intermediate pretest likelihood of CHD. A modified version of the Diamond and Forrester criteria are often used to determine the pretest likelihood of coronary artery disease (Table 26.5) (Gibbons et al., 1997; Patel et al., 2012).

EST is often beneficial in guiding care after MI for activity prescription, evaluating medical therapy, and when considering cardiac rehabilitation (Gibbons et al., 2002). EST may also be considered for assessment of functional capacity and symptomatic responses in patients with chronotropic incompetence, valvular heart disease, and particularly chronic aortic stenosis or aortic insufficiency (Fletcher, Mills, & Taylor, 2006; Nishimura et al., 2014). In patients with rhythm disorders, EST may be useful for evaluating pacemaker activity, diagnosing exercise-induced arrhythmias, and assessing treatment response of exercise-induced arrhythmias. The ACC and AHA Task Force on Practice Guidelines in 1997 provides diagnostic criteria and indications for the use of EST—common indications for EST include the evaluation of:

- Intermediate pretest probability of obstructive CHD
- Symptoms of suspected or known CHD
- Assessment and prognosis of known CHD
- After acute coronary syndromes
- Cardiac and pulmonary conditions with ventilatory gas analysis
- Pre- and post-percutaneous or surgical revascularization
- Cardiac conduction or rhythm abnormalities (Gibbons et al., 1997).

Contraindications

EST requires physical exertion on a treadmill or bicycle; therefore, patients must be physically, mentally, and emotionally capable of performing these activities. If the patient is not able to exercise safely, EST is contraindicated. The 12-lead ECG must also be free from any significant conduction, rhythm, structural, or ST changes that

TABLE 26.6 Contraindications to Exercise Testing

	Contraindications
Absolute	Acute myocardial infarction (within 2 days)
	High-risk unstable angina*
	Uncontrolled cardiac arrhythmias causing symptoms or hemodynamic compromise
	Symptomatic severe aortic stenosis
	Uncontrolled symptomatic heart failure
	Acute pulmonary embolus or pulmonary infarction
	Acute myocarditis or pericarditis
	Acute aortic dissection
Relative[†]	Left main coronary stenosis
	Moderate stenotic valvular heart disease
	Electrolyte abnormalities
	Severe arterial hypertension (systolic blood pressure > 200 mmHg and/or diastolic blood pressure > 110 mmHg)
	Tachyarrhythmia or bradyarrhythmia
	Hypertrophic cardiomyopathy and other forms of outflow tract obstruction
	Mental or physical impairment leading to inability to exercise adequately
	High-degree atrioventricular block

*ACC/AHA Guidelines for the Management of Patients With Unstable Angina/Non-ST-Segment Elevation Myocardial Infarction.

[†]Relative contraindications can be superseded if the benefits of exercise outweigh the risks. Modified from Fletcher et al.

Reprinted with permission from American Heart Association.

will limit the interpretation of the ECG. The ACC and AHA task force practice guidelines outline absolute and relative contraindications for EST (Table 26.6) (Gibbons et al., 1997; Gibbons et al., 2002).

Procedure

A thorough history and physical examination should be performed prior to commencing EST to rule out significant valvular or heart conditions, which may increase the risk for adverse events with the test. The patient should not eat, smoke, or drink beverages containing caffeine or alcohol for 3 to 4 hours before the test. The decision to withhold HR–limiting medications, beta-adrenergic blockers, and calcium channel blockers is determined on an individual basis while considering the necessity of obtaining a target HR to achieve an adequate study. ECG leads are attached to the patient's chest in order to record a 12-lead ECG prior to testing, and continuously during and after exercise for detection of rhythm disturbances, ST-segment changes, and other ECG manifestations of myocardial ischemia. HR, BP, and symptoms are also carefully monitored before, during, and after the test. Exercise can be performed with either treadmill or stationary bicycle ergometer devices using established stress test protocols (Bruce, 1974; Bruce, Blackmon, Jones, & Strait, 1963; Hill & Timmis, 2002). EST is commonly performed as a symptom-limited test, in order to assess functional capacity of patients' exercise until they are fatigued; however, the test may be terminated early for significant angina or arrhythmia, high-risk findings on the ECG (ST-depression > 3 mm), or significant hemodynamic abnormalities (systolic blood pressure [SBP] > 220 mmHg or diastolic blood pressure

[DBP] > 120 mmHg, or BP reduction > 20 mmHg). In the absence of significant findings during the test, the recommendation is that patients exercise to a minimum target HR of 85% of the maximum predicted HR (220 minus age) in order to improve the overall diagnostic test performance.

Risks and Benefits

Information obtained from EST can aid in the diagnosis of a patient's symptoms and guide the management and treatment of cardiovascular disorders. EST is generally a safe procedure, although MI and death have been reported at a rate of up to 1 per 2,500 tests (Stuart & Ellestad, 1980). During the test, patients may experience hemodynamic instability, arrhythmia, or orthopedic injury. In addition, non-limiting or exercise-limiting symptoms of chest discomfort, dyspnea, palpitations, leg discomfort, lightheadedness, or dizziness may occur. Therefore, clinical judgment is required to evaluate which patients may undergo testing safely.

Results

EST interpretation commonly incorporates information on exercise capacity and clinical, hemodynamic, and ECG response. The presence of ischemic chest pain with stress testing is important, particularly if its presence and intensity results in the termination of the test. Abnormalities in exercise capacity, BP response, and HR response are also important diagnostic and prognostic findings in addition to ECG findings of ST depression or elevation. A positive ECG test result, suggestive of ischemia, is associated with the presence of 1 mm or greater horizontal or down-sloping ST-segment depression (Figure 26.3) or elevation measured 0.08 seconds after the end of the QRS complex (Gibbons et al., 1997). An EST result is considered negative for ischemia when there are no significant ECG changes, hemodynamic abnormalities, or symptoms with an adequate study of the HR equal to or greater than 85% of the theoretical maximum age-adjusted HR. An inconclusive ECG test occurs when there are baseline ST-T changes that limit the interpretation of the ECG and contain left bundle branch block pattern, digitalis effect, left ventricular hypertrophy voltage, or other ECG changes or rhythm abnormalities; the patient does not reach 85% of the theoretical maximum age-adjusted HR; or the ECG changes are present without meeting the diagnostic criteria for ischemia.

Further Testing

A patient with a positive EST or with other high-risk features often requires additional testing to evaluate underlying cardiovascular disease, including CHD, structural heart disease, and arrhythmias. Depending on the clinical scenario and severity of test results, patients may be referred for additional testing, including stress testing with imaging, advanced imaging techniques, or coronary angiography. A positive test will also likely affect the management and pharmaceutical therapy for that patient. Similarly, in a patient with an inconclusive ECG stress test,

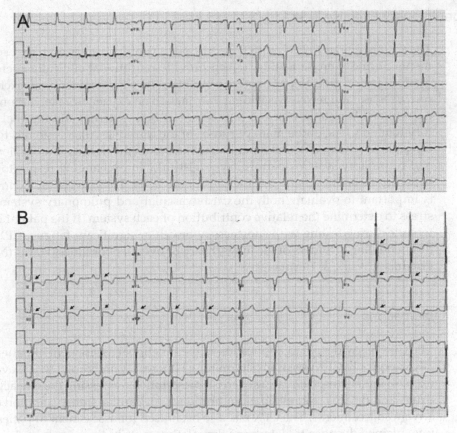

FIGURE 26.3 Pre- (A) and post- (B) stress ECG demonstrating 1–2 mm ST (arrows) at peak stress.

additional testing will likely be required depending on the clinical scenario. In a patient with a negative stress test, depending on the clinical findings, no further workup may be required. However, in high-risk patients with multiple underlying CHD risk factors, a negative stress test does not necessarily exclude the presence of CHD, and further workup may be necessary.

Diagnostic Performance

EST has reported a sensitivity of 69% (range 45%–92%) and a specificity of 70% (17%–92%) for the diagnosis of CHD (Gibbons et al., 1997). A more recent meta-analysis focusing on prospective studies found similar performance between exercise modalities. Treadmill ECG testing had a positive likelihood ratio of 3.57 for the diagnosis of CHD and a negative likelihood ratio of 0.38; whereas with bicycle ECG stress testing, the positive likelihood ratio was 2.94 and the negative likelihood ratio was 0.4 (Banerjee, Newman, Van den Bruel, & Heneghan, 2012). However, test performance is variable depending on the institutional criteria to determine a positive test, the presence of ECG abnormalities on baseline ECG, and the influence of certain pharmacologic therapies, such as digoxin. The sensitivity and specificity of EST is lower in women compared with men (Banerjee et al., 2012).

Cardiopulmonary Exercise Test

The CPX is similar to EST, with the addition of ventilatory gas exchange measurements during exercise testing, which provides additional clinically useful information. In addition to parameters with EST, the CPX analyzes gas exchange at rest, exercise, and recovery, yielding information on oxygen uptake, carbon dioxide output, and ventilation for the assessment of both external and internal respiratory function. One of the main purposes of the cardiovascular system is to supply O_2 while removing CO_2 and other metabolites from the tissues. The cardiovascular and respiratory systems perform synergistically in exchanging respiratory gases between the environment and the cells of the body. Thus, in certain conditions, it is important to evaluate both the cardiovascular and pulmonary systems under stress to determine the relative contribution of each system. If the patient is symptomatic during testing with shortness of breath or significant fatigue, CPX aids in differentiating disorders of the lungs, heart, or overall poor fitness status (Neuberg, Friedman, Weiss, & Herman, 1988).

Indications

The CPX has widespread application in the functional assessment of patients with HF. Specifically, CPX assists in determining HF severity and prognosis by evaluating exercise limitations, facilitating exercise prescriptions, assessing the efficacy of new drugs and devices, and evaluating candidacy for cardiac transplantation or other advanced treatments. The CPX has also been used for assessment of patients with unexplained dyspnea to determine the relative contributions from cardiovascular

TABLE 26.7 Indications for Cardiopulmonary Stress Testing

Evaluation of exercise tolerance	Determination of functional impairment or capacity (peak VO_2) Determination of exercise-limiting factors and pathophysiologic mechanisms
Evaluation of undiagnosed exercise intolerance	Assessing contribution of cardiac and pulmonary etiology in coexisting disease Symptoms disproportionate to resting pulmonary and cardiac tests Unexplained dyspnea when initial cardiopulmonary testing is nondiagnostic
Evaluation of patients with cardiovascular disease	Functional evaluation and prognosis in patients with heart failure Selection for cardiac transplantation Exercise prescription and monitoring response to exercise training for cardiac rehabilitation
Evaluation of patients with respiratory disease	Functional impairment assessment Chronic obstructive pulmonary disease Interstitial lung disease Pulmonary vascular disease Cystic fibrosis Exercise-induced bronchospasm
Specific clinical applications	Preoperative evaluation Exercise evaluation and prescription for pulmonary rehabilitation Exercise evaluation and prescription for cardiac rehabilitation Evaluation for impairment—disability Evaluation for lung, heart–lung transplantation

Source: Piepoli et al. (2006).

(chronic HF) and pulmonary (obstructive airways disease) causes for a patient's symptoms in those with multiple co-morbidities. The CPX is also indicated for derivation of an exercise prescription or disability assessment. Table 26.7 provides general indications for CPX (Piepoli et al., 2006).

Contraindications

Contraindications to CPX are similar to EST, and neither are recommended in situations with patients experiencing acute symptoms. In acute circumstances, more direct, invasive procedures must be provided in the acute settings to evaluate and treat the condition. Absolute contraindications include acute or recent MI, unstable angina, uncontrolled cardiac arrhythmias, symptomatic severe aortic stenosis, symptomatic HF, acute pulmonary embolus or infarction, pneumothorax, acute myocarditis or pericarditis, and acute aortic dissection. Other relative contraindications include known significant left main stenosis, moderate stenotic valvular heart disease, electrolyte abnormalities, severe arterial hypertension, tachyarrhythmias or bradyarrhythmias, hypertrophic cardiomyopathy, mental or physical impairments leading to inadequate exercise ability, and high-degree atrioventricular block. There are relative and absolute contraindications for CPX as listed in Table 26.8 (Piepoli et al., 2006).

TABLE 26.8 Contraindications to Cardiopulmonary Stress Testing

Absolute	Acute myocardial infarction (3–5 days)
	Unstable angina
	Uncontrolled arrhythmia causing symptoms or hemodynamic compromise
	Syncope
	Active endocarditis
	Acute myocarditis or pericarditis
	Symptomatic severe aortic stenosis
	Uncontrolled heart failure
	Acute pulmonary embolus or pulmonary infarction
	Thrombosis of lower extremities
	Suspected dissecting aneurysm
	Uncontrolled asthma
	Pulmonary edema
	Room air desaturation at rest < 85%
	Respiratory failure
	Acute noncardiopulmonary disorder that may affect exercise performance or aggravated by exercise
	Mental impairment leading to inability to cooperate
Relative	Left main coronary stenosis or its equivalent
	Moderate stenotic valvular heart disease
	Severe untreated arterial hypertension at rest (> 200 mmHg systolic, > 120 mmHg diastolic)
	Tachyarrhythmia or bradyarrhythmia
	High-degree atrioventricular block
	Hypertrophic cardiomyopathy
	Significant pulmonary hypertension
	Advanced or complicated pregnancy
	Electrolyte abnormalities
	Orthopedic impairment that compromises exercise performance

Source: Piepoli et al. (2006).

Procedure

The procedure for CPX is very similar to that for EST. Before the procedure, patients must refrain from eating, drinking, ingesting caffeine, or smoking anything for a minimum of 4 hours. The procedure is performed in a similar manner to EST, with continuous ECG monitoring of HR, rhythm and ECG changes, and measurement of BP periodically throughout the test. In addition, the patient will be asked to breathe through a mouthpiece or facemask at rest, during exercise, and during recovery, which allows for the calculation of airflow, volumes, and both oxygen and carbon dioxide concentrations usually breath by breath. Recommended exercise test protocols with CPX have more modest increases in work rate per stage than EST (Balady et al., 2010), and they can be performed with either treadmill exercise or bicycle ergometry with a goal to yield a symptom-limited exercise duration of 8 to 12 minutes. The CPX is performed as a symptom-limited test in order to assess functional capacity, although it may be terminated early if a patient experiences significant angina, symptoms, arrhythmia, high-risk findings on the ECG, or significant hemodynamic abnormalities (Koike et al., 2002).

Risks and Benefits

Complications with CPX include the potential for death, MI, arrhythmia, hemodynamic instability, and orthopedic injury. Information obtained from CPX is particularly useful in the diagnosis and management of patients with known HF. In addition, CPX is useful in the evaluation of patients with unexplained dyspnea; aids the diagnosis of cardiac, pulmonary, or mixed disorders; and guides management and treatment.

Results

As CPX includes EST, similar information provided by an EST is also available with CPX, depending on the laboratory. Additional parameters that can be obtained with CPX include maximal aerobic capacity (VO_2 max or peak VO_2), ventilatory threshold, peak respiratory exchange ratio, minute ventilation-carbon dioxide output relationship, exercise breathing reserve, post-exercise FEV_1, $PaCO_2$, PaO_2, or O_2 saturation, and dead space to tidal volume ratios (Arena & Sietsema, 2011). Further analysis of these parameters provides data to determine whether there are abnormalities of oxygen delivery, oxygen utilization, gas exchange efficiency, or breathing mechanics.

Further Testing

The CPX provides a number of parameters that are useful in the evaluation of patients with unexplained dyspnea, HF, or pulmonary disorders that are associated with limited exercise tolerance. Further testing may be needed depending on the primary indication of the test and the associated findings. The CPX that is performed for unexplained dyspnea that reveals a significant pulmonary component to the patient's symptoms may indicate the need for further management, such as pulmonary imaging and disease-specific therapy. For CPX demonstrating significantly limited exercise capacity that is primarily due to HF, patients may be referred for cardiac transplantation or other advanced therapeutic cardiovascular options.

Diagnostic Performance

There have been no randomized trials addressing the diagnostic and prognostic applications of CPX. However, maximal aerobic capacity (peak VO_2) has demonstrated prognostic importance in patients with HF in many studies (Cahalin et al., 2013; Cohn et al., 1993; Likoff, Chandler, & Kay, 1987; Mancini et al., 1991; Szlachcic, Massie, Kramer, Topic, & Tubau, 1985).

ULTRASOUND TESTS

Ultrasound technology provides noninvasive dynamic imaging of the cardiovascular system. Cardiovascular studies that rely on ultrasound as part of their performance include carotid artery duplex ultrasound, transthoracic echocardiogram, transesophageal echocardiogram, and stress echocardiography, with exercise and dobutamine.

Carotid Ultrasound (Carotid Artery Duplex Ultrasound)

Carotid ultrasound is a painless and harmless test that uses high-frequency sound waves to create pictures of the bilateral carotid arteries, the main arteries that supply blood to the brain. Carotid ultrasound evaluates the carotid arteries for atherosclerotic, cardiovascular, and cerebrovascular disease, by assessing abnormal thickening of the vessel walls, plaque, and blood flow to the brain.

Indications

The goal of carotid ultrasound is to distinguish normal from diseased vessels, classify disease states, and assess cerebral collateral circulation. Indications for carotid ultrasound include evaluation of cervical bruits, amaurosis fugax, hemispheric stroke, focal cerebral or ocular TIAs, drop attacks or syncope, vasculitis, pulsatile masses in the neck, or neck trauma. For patients with known carotid disease, carotid ultrasound is indicated for follow-up after carotid revascularization and for surveillance with moderate to severe stenosis, defined as occlusions equal to or greater than 50% to 69%. The 2012 Appropriate Use Criteria for peripheral vascular ultrasound provides detailed guidelines for the clinical application of carotid ultrasound and duplex imaging endorsed by multiple cardiovascular societies; general indications are listed next (Mohler et al., 2012). General indications for carotid ultrasound include:

- Findings consistent with cerebrovascular disease
- Atherosclerotic risk factors or co-morbidities
- Surveillance of known carotid artery stenosis 50% to 69%
- Evaluation after carotid artery intervention

Carotid ultrasound has also been used to evaluate intimal media thickness (IMT) as a screening test for cardiovascular disease, specifically CHD. Patients with increased carotid IMT have an increased risk of cardiovascular disease (O'Leary et al., 1999). The 2010 ACCF/AHA guideline for assessment of cardiovascular risk in asymptomatic adults recommends measurement of carotid IMT in asymptomatic adults at intermediate risk of cardiovascular disease based on clinical risk factors (Greenland et al., 2010). However, in the new 2013 AHA guidelines, carotid IMT is not recommended for routine measurement in clinical practice for risk assessment for a first atherosclerotic cardiovascular event (Goff et al., 2014).

Contraindications

There are no specific contraindications to carotid ultrasound. However, the examination may be of limited diagnostic value in patients with poor or limited acoustic windows such as markedly obese patients due to a thick neck, or in patients with recent neck surgery who have limitations in positioning the ultrasound probe.

Procedure

In general, no preparation is necessary prior to the test. Patients are placed in the supine position, and an ultrasound probe with gel is placed on the patient's neck to assess the vascular anatomy and blood flow through each of the carotid arteries, right and left. In general, the test duration is about 15 to 30 minutes.

Risks and Benefits

There are no specific risks related to carotid duplex ultrasound. Patients who have had recent cervical surgery or are unable to lie flat or to be still may not tolerate the procedure. In general, carotid ultrasound is a rapid, painless, and harmless test for evaluation of cerebrovascular and cardiovascular disease.

Results

Carotid artery ultrasound includes information on the common carotid artery, internal carotid artery, external carotid artery, and the carotid artery bifurcation, bilaterally. Two-dimensional anatomic imaging of the arterial walls enables assessment of intimal medial thickening and atherosclerotic plaque (Figure 26.4). Spectral waveforms of pulse Doppler images in combination with anatomic imaging allow

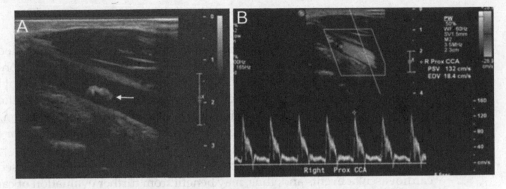

FIGURE 26.4 Carotid ultrasound images of the proximal right internal carotid artery.
(A) Demonstrates plaque (arrow) with only mildly elevated velocities on Doppler imaging
(B) Suggestive of mild stenosis (<50%). See color insert.

for grading of stenosis severity. Stenosis severity is categorized as normal, low grade less than 50%, moderate grade 50% to 69%, severe greater than 70%, subtotal occlusion, and total occlusion, based on parameters including peak systolic velocities, end-diastolic velocity, and the extent of spectral broadening (Gerhard-Herman et al., 2006; Grant et al., 2003). A normal ultrasound indicates blood flow within the carotid arteries is adequate and there are no significant blockages or critical narrowing. Conversely, an abnormal result suggests that the carotid arteries may be narrowed or completely blocked—by either atherosclerosis or rarely, emboli. A positive carotid artery duplex suggests critical narrowing (>70%) or occlusion of the artery, which increases the risk of a cerebrovascular event.

Carotid IMT is the measured distance between the luminal–intimal interface and the media–adventitial interface (Figure 26.5) (Pignoli, Tremoli, Poli, Oreste, & Paoletti, 1986; Wikstrand & Wendelhag, 1994). This measurement should be obtained from the distal 2 cm of the common carotid artery, proximal to the bifurcation, preferably in a region free of plaque (Touboul et al., 2004), and it should be reported as an absolute mean and maximum measurement with percentile ranking based on comparison with normal IMT measurements adjusted for age and sex (Stein et al., 2008). The presence or absence of carotid plaque is also commonly reported. The presence of carotid plaque is associated with similar or slightly higher risk as those with increased carotid IMT measurement (Stein et al., 2008).

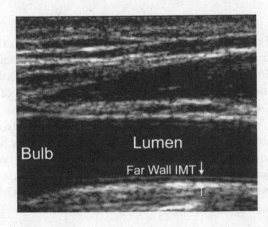

FIGURE 26.5 Carotid IMT measurement.
IMT, intimal media thickness.

Further Testing

As a positive carotid ultrasound suggests a critically narrowed or occluded carotid artery, additional studies are often performed to confirm the findings. Noninvasive magnetic resonance angiography, computed tomography angiography of the neck and brain, or invasive cerebral angiography may be required to detail the carotid arteries for determination of location and degree of stenoses. In addition, referral to a vascular or cardiovascular specialist may be required to evaluate for invasive or surgical management of carotid artery stenoses.

Patients with significantly increased carotid IMT are at an increased risk of cardiovascular events and, thus, may benefit from further evaluation of cardiovascular disease or aggressive risk factor management.

Diagnostic Performance

Carotid artery duplex has a reported sensitivity of 99% and specificity of 84% for distinguishing between normal and diseased internal carotid arteries (Gerhard-Herman et al., 2006; Langlois, Roederer, Chan, Phillips, et al., 1983; Langlois, Roederer, Chan, & Strandness, 1983). The accuracy for detecting 50% to 99% stenosis is 93% (Gerhard-Herman et al., 2006). Both carotid plaques and carotid IMT have demonstrated high diagnostic accuracy for the prediction of future CHD events (Inaba, Chen, & Bergmann, 2012).

Transthoracic Echocardiogram

Transthoracic echocardiography (TTE), cardiac ultrasound, is one of the most commonly used noninvasive diagnostic tools in cardiology. The TTE provides accurate information about cardiac structure and function, and it is indicated for the diagnosis of a multitude of cardiovascular disorders, surveillance of known abnormalities, and guidance of management decisions. The term *transthoracic* indicates that the ultrasound probe is placed on different areas of the chest and upper abdomen to acquire images.

Indications

TTE provides a multitude of information about the heart, which aids in the diagnosis and management of numerous cardiac conditions, including the comprehensive assessment for underlying myocardial, valvular, pericardial, congenital, and vascular disease. TTE is frequently indicated for the general evaluation of cardiac structure and function in patients presenting with signs or symptoms that are suggestive of cardiac disease, such as shortness of breath, palpitations, stroke, syncope, or murmurs. In the acute setting, TTE may be indicated to evaluate hemodynamic or respiratory compromise and to guide therapy in the setting of myocardial ischemia or infarction, endocarditis, pulmonary embolism, or cardiac trauma. Finally, an echocardiogram is indicated for suspected cardiac masses or tumors, as identified on other imaging modalities (CT) or findings on physical examination. The 2011

Appropriate Use Criteria for echocardiography provides detailed guidelines for the clinical application of echocardiography endorsed by multiple cardiovascular societies (Douglas et al., 2011). General indications for transthoracic echocardiogram include:

- Suspected cardiovascular diseases
- Cardiac conditions
  - Arrhythmia
  - Hypertension
  - Heart failure
  - Cardiomyopathies
  - Congenital heart disease
  - Acute hypotension or hemodynamic instability
  - Myocardial ischemia or infarction
  - Post-acute coronary syndrome
  - Cardiac trauma
  - Valvular heart disease
    - Native valve disease
    - Prosthetic valves
    - Signs or symptoms of valvular disease
    - Endocarditis
  - Structural heart disease
  - Cardiac transplantation
  - Cardiac devices
    - Implanted devices
    - Ventricular assist device
- Pulmonary conditions
  - Pulmonary hypertension
  - Respiratory failure
  - Pulmonary embolism
- Evaluations of presyncope or syncope
- Evaluation of aortic disease

Contraindications

There are no specific contraindications for transthoracic echocardiography. However, the examination may be of limited diagnostic value in patients with poor or limited acoustic windows, such as markedly obese patients due to a thick chest wall, severely underweight patients due to overcrowded ribs, or patients with recent chest or abdominal surgery with limited areas for positioning the ultrasound probe.

Procedure

No preparation is required prior to the TTE. Patients lie on their left side or in the supine position, and an ultrasound probe is placed in various locations on the patient's chest and upper abdomen in order to record dynamic images of the heart and adjacent blood vessels. Usually, a small amount of ultrasound gel is placed on the patient's chest wall to increase the magnitude of the ultrasound waves to improve the image quality. Electrodes are placed on the chest to record an ECG tracing in conjunction with the images. Depending on the study indication and quality of the images, an intravenous injection of agitated saline micro-bubbles or echocardiographic contrast agents, protein or lipid-based microspheres, may be administered during the procedure. Standard echocardiography protocols for the performance and interpretation of TTE are available (Mulvagh et al., 2008; Picard et al., 2011). In general, the test duration is 30 to 45 minutes, although focused studies can be performed in 5 to 10 minutes.

Risks and Benefits

Minimal risks are associated with TTE imaging, and there are no radiation exposures or harmful effects with ultrasound. Patients may experience transient discomfort with positioning or pressure from the ultrasound probe on the chest and upper abdomen during the procedure. The benefits of the procedure are that TTE provides a rapid, portable, and noninvasive imaging method for obtaining structural and functional information about the heart and surrounding structures. In cases requiring an injection of agitated saline micro-bubbles, there is a risk (0.062%) of TIAs and CVAs from paradoxical embolization, although proper technique minimizes this risk (Bommer, Shah, Allen, Meltzer, & Kisslo, 1984; Romero et al., 2009). In patients requiring use of echocardiographic contrast agents, protein, or lipid-based microspheres, there is a risk of back pain, headache, urticaria, and, rarely, anaphylactic reactions, estimated at 1 per 10,000 (Dolan et al., 2009; Main et al., 2008). Current contraindications to the use of echocardiographic contrast agents are right to left or bidirectional cardiac shunts, hypersensitivity to perflutren, intra-arterial injection, and hypersensitivity to blood or albumin.

Results

TTE uses a combination of two-dimensional Doppler and color-flow Doppler imaging for the evaluation of the heart (Figure 26.6). In select cases, three-dimensional anatomic and color Doppler images can be obtained. The most common information provided with TTE is an evaluation of left ventricular size and function, including an estimation of left ventricular ejection fraction. This information is extremely useful in diagnosing a cardiac etiology for a patient's symptoms, to guide treatment, and for risk stratification of many cardiovascular disorders. In a completed TTE study, additional information includes right ventricular size and function, atrial sizes, valvular structure and function, pericardial abnormalities (constriction, tamponade physiology, and effusion), great vessel anatomy, and estimation of intracardiac pressures in individual cardiac chambers. Color and spectral Doppler provide functional findings of hemodynamic parameters, in addition to blood flow data of two-dimensional and three-dimensional anatomic imaging. Depending on the indication, information on the presence or absence and characterization of cardiac masses such as tumors, thrombi, or vegetations can also be obtained (Cheitlin et al., 1997).

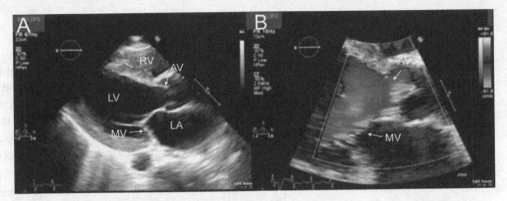

FIGURE 26.6 Transthoracic echocardiography images in 2D (A) and color doppler (B), showing the aortic valve (AV), mitral valve (MV), left ventricle (LV), left atrium (LA), and right ventricle (RV). See color insert.

Further Testing

The TTE is often the initial imaging test in a patient with known or suspected cardiac structural or functional abnormalities. Patients with significant structural abnormalities may need further testing to delineate the findings, which may include additional imaging studies with higher resolution (TEE), improved tissue characterization (cardiac MRI), or for confirmation of hemodynamic significance of valvular lesions or elevated intracardiac pressures (right heart or left heart catheterization). Depending on the presence and severity of cardiac disease, a follow-up evaluation with serial TTE assesses stability or worsening of disorders and guides treatment or referral for therapeutic interventions (Richards, 1985).

Diagnostic Performance

Several aspects of cardiac disease may be discerned on TTE imaging. The diagnostic performance of TTE is dependent on the specific parameter being measured. As such, appropriate use guidelines have been developed to aid in determining whether TTE is an appropriate test depending on the specific indication and performance characteristics of the test (Douglas et al., 2011; Picard et al., 2011). In general, TTE is indicated for the initial evaluation of cardiac structure and function when there is a high suspicion for a cardiac condition. These include patients with frequent premature ventricular contractions, sustained atrial or ventricular arrhythmias, HF, suspected pulmonary hypertension, acute hypotension or hemodynamic instability with suspected cardiac etiology, acute respiratory failure of uncertain etiology, and suspected cardiac injury. TTE is also beneficial in the evaluation and management of patients with MI or ischemia; suspected valvular disease, including prosthetic valves; suspected infective endocarditis; cardiac mass; pericardial conditions; ascending aortic disease; suspected hypertensive heart disease; known cardiomyopathy; and congenital heart disease.

Transesophageal Echocardiogram

Transesophageal echocardiography (TEE) is similar to TTE, except images of the heart are obtained with the ultrasound probe positioned within the esophagus or stomach, rather than on the external chest wall. A TEE is a more invasive study, and it is usually performed when TTE does not provide sufficient information to answer an important diagnostic question. With the ultrasound probe positioned in the esophagus, which is usually located directly posterior to the heart, this study prevents the air-filled lung tissues and associated acoustic shadowing that may occur with TTE. For this reason, a TEE is excellent in producing images of the posterior structures such as the atria, the atrial appendages, the interatrial septum, and the aorta.

Indications

A TEE is generally performed when a TTE has not adequately answered a clinical diagnostic question. Common indications for TEE include the evaluation of a predisposing cardioembolic condition, suspected endocarditis, or prior to cardioversion in a patient with atrial arrhythmias (Douglas et al., 2011; O'Brien et al., 1998). Other indications for TEE include the evaluation of the aorta in acute aortic dissection; acute hemodynamic compromise; adult congenital heart disease such as atrial septal defect or ventricular septal defect; mitral and aortic valves prior to interventional procedures such as valvuloplasty and transcatheter aortic-valve implantation; and perioperative status (Douglas et al., 2011). The 2011 Appropriate Use Criteria for Echocardiography provides guidelines on the use of TEE as endorsed by multiple societies; Table 26.9 highlights these recommendations (Douglas et al., 2011).

Contraindications

As TEE requires pharmacologic sedation and insertion of the probe into the esophagus, evaluation of the cardiovascular, respiratory, neurologic, upper gastrointestinal, oropharynx, and musculoskeletal condition of the neck is required prior to the test. There are absolute contraindications to performing a TEE, although relative contraindications are more frequently encountered in clinical practice. Table 26.10 provides information on specific contraindications for TEE (Douglas et al., 2011).

Procedure

The TEE is commonly performed with topical anesthetic spray and moderate sedation; thus, the patient's BP, HR, respiratory status, and oxygen saturation should be monitored before, during, and after the procedure. The TEE is a highly involved procedure and should only be performed by a team of providers, including physicians who have been adequately trained in TEE. Patients are required to fast for a minimum of 4 hours prior to the procedure to prevent aspiration of gastric contents. A detailed history and examination is performed to evaluate indications, contraindications, and risks of the test. Once the patient is placed in the correct position and sedated, the ultrasound probe is placed in the posterior pharynx and guided to the

TABLE 26.9 Highlights From the 2011 Appropriate Use Guidelines for Transesophageal Echocardiography

	Appropriate	Uncertain	Inappropriate
General evaluation	High likelihood of a nondiagnostic TTE due to patient characteristics or inadequate visualization of structures Reevaluation of prior TEE finding for interval change, when a change in management is anticipated (for example, thrombus evaluation after anticoagulation, vegetation evaluation after antibiotics) Guide percutaneous noncoronary cardiac interventions (for example, closure device placement, radiofrequency ablation, and percutaneous valve procedures) Suspect acute aortic pathology (for example, dissection or transection)		Use of TEE when a diagnostic TTE is likely diagnostic and can guide management Survey of prior TEE finding for interval change, when no change in management is anticipated Assessment of pulmonary veins in an asymptomatic patient status post–pulmonary vein isolation
Valvular disease	Evaluate valvular structure and function to assess suitability or planning of an intervention Diagnose infective endocarditis with a moderate or high pretest probability		Diagnose infective endocarditis with a low pretest probability
Embolic event	Evaluate for cardiovascular source of embolus with no identified noncardiac source	Evaluate cardiovascular source of embolus with a previously identified noncardiac source	Evaluate for cardiovascular source of embolus with a known cardiac source; no change in management is anticipated
Atrial fibrillation or atrial flutter	Evaluate to facilitate clinical decision making (for example, anticoagulation, cardioversion, and/or radiofrequency ablation		Evaluate when a decision has been made to anticoagulate and not to perform cardioversion; no change of management is anticipated

TEE, transesophageal echocardiography.

Source: Douglas et al. (2011).

mid-esophagus to the level of the heart. Guidelines for the safe performance of a comprehensive TEE examination detail recommendations for procedure performance (Hahn et al., 2013; Reeves, 2013).

Risks and Benefits

Potential major complications with TEE include death, esophageal perforation, serious arrhythmia, HF, and laryngospasm; however, these are very rare. Minor complications are usually related to the conscious sedation or trauma in the oropharynx or esophagus. Minor complications include transient hypoxia, hypotension, hypertension, angina, bronchospasm, atrioventricular block, supraventricular tachycardia, and non-sustained ventricular arrhythmia, all of which are usually rare. Sore throat and mild dysphagia are common after the procedure, although they are rarely experienced for more than 24 hours (Daniel et al., 1991).

TABLE 26.10 Contraindications to Performance of TEE

Absolute	Uncooperative patient
	Severe respiratory depression
	Unstable cardiorespiratory status
	Esophageal obstruction (stricture or mass)
	Previous esophagectomy or esophagogastrectomy
	Tracheoesophageal fistula
	Perforated viscus
	Active upper gastrointenstinal bleeding
Relative	Esophageal diverticulum
	Esophageal varices
	Previous esophageal surgery
	History of dysphagia
	Recent upper gastrointestinal bleed
	Severe cervical arthritis with restricted mobility
	Atlantoaxial joint disease with restricted mobility
	Severe coagulopathy

TEE, transesophageal echocardiography.

Reprinted from Burwash and Chan (2012), with permission from Elsevier.

Benefits must be weighed against the risks of the procedure. The TEE is a more invasive procedure; however, it provides higher resolution images compared with TTE, particularly of the posterior cardiac structures and the aorta. Interference or acoustic shadowing from prosthetic material in the chest wall is also less of a concern when a TEE is performed. Consultation with the cardiovascular specialist is often acquired before the scheduling of a TEE.

Results

The TEE uses a combination of two-dimensional, Doppler, and color-flow Doppler imaging for evaluation of the heart (Figure 26.7). In select cases, three-dimensional anatomic and color Doppler images can be obtained. Results are dependent on the indication for the study, and most common indications include evaluation for cardiac source of embolism, intracardiac vegetations, significance of valvular disease, acute aortic disease (dissection), and intracardiac thrombus evaluation prior to

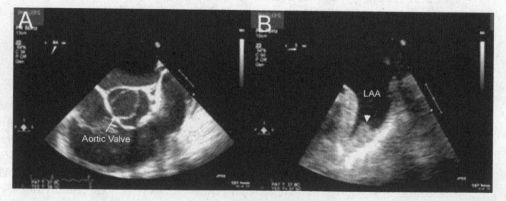

FIGURE 26.7 Transesophageal echocardiography 2D images demonstrating a bicuspid aortic valve (A) and thrombus (arrowhead) in the left atrial appendage (LAA) (B).

cardioversion of an arrhythmia, usually atrial fibrillation. The TEE can also provide much of the same information obtained with the TTE and can serve as confirmation on the presence and significance of cardiac disease.

Further Testing

As described earlier with TTE, if a TEE reveals significant structural abnormalities, the patient may undergo additional evaluations or specific treatments for the disorder. Follow-up echocardiograms may be indicated for surveillance of the progress of therapies or of the identified disease. On occasion, a TEE may be nondiagnostic or unobtainable, and further testing such as cardiac MRI or CT may be required.

Diagnostic Performance

Diagnostic performance of TTE is dependent on the specific parameter being measured. As such, appropriate use guidelines have been developed to aid in selecting the appropriate test, dependent on the specific indication and performance characteristics of the test in question (Douglas et al., 2011; Picard et al., 2011). In general, TEE is often indicated when there is a high likelihood of a nondiagnostic TTE due to patient characteristics or inadequate visualization of relevant structures. Common indications include evaluation of cardiac source of embolism; vegetations; further evaluation of valvular structure and function, particularly with prosthestic valves; evaluation of atrial thrombi to direct management of atrial arrhythmias; and evaluation of the thoracic aorta.

Stress Echocardiogram

Stress echocardiogram uses ultrasound technology to assess stress-induced changes in cardiac or pulmonary vascular function, as defined by wall thickening, wall motion, ventricular volumes, and hemodynamic pressures to infer the presence of myocardial ischemia, viability, valvular function, and pulmonary hypertension. The echocardiogram technology can be used with physical exercise or pharmacologic agents to induce a stress response. Stress echocardiogram is beneficial in patients with baseline ECG changes, such as repolarization changes, which limit the interpretation of ischemic changes on a basic ECG stress test without imaging. In addition, stress echocardiogram allows for localization of ischemic and viable tissue. Finally, stress echocardiogram may guide the management and characterization of valvular heart disease, primary myocardial disease, pulmonary vascular disease, and some obstructive lesions under stress-induced conditions.

Indications

The most common indication for stress echocardiography is the detection of CHD in patients with ischemic symptoms such as chest pain, palpitations, or shortness of breath. Other indications include functional assessment for significance of known coronary stenoses, evaluation after a nondiagnostic or non-interpretable exercise ECG stress test, risk assessment prior to vascular or other high-risk non-cardiac surgery, evaluation of HF, myocardial viability, arrhythmias, syncope, and hemodynamic assessment in known valvular heart disease or pulmonary vascular disease. The 2011 Appropriate Use Criteria for Echocardiography provides guidelines on the use of stress echocardiography as endorsed by multiple societies (Douglas et al., 2011). General indications for stress echocardiogram include:

- Evaluation of symptoms consistent with CHD
- Evaluation of known CHD
  - After acute coronary syndrome
  - Post-revascularization
  - Prior to cardiac rehabilitation
- Evaluation of asymptomatic individuals with likelihood of coronary heart disease
  - Ventricular arrhythmias
  - Syncope
  - Heart failure
  - Cardiomyopathy
  - Elevated troponin
- Abnormal cardiac testing
  - Coronary calcium score
  - Coronary angiography
  - Cardiac stress studies
- Valvular heart disease
- Pulmonary hypertension
- Preoperative evaluation

Contraindications

Contraindications to exercise stress echocardiogram are similar to those detailed for exercise stress testing (Table 26.6). For patients undergoing pharmacologic stress echocardiogram, specific contraindications depend on the stressor agent. Table 26.11 details contraindications for dobutamine (Henzlova, Cerqueira,

TABLE 26.11 Contraindications for Dobutamine

Stress Agent	Test Type	Contraindications
Dobutamine	Stress echocardiogram	MI < 1 week
		Unstable angina
		Significant aortic stenosis or obstructive cardiomyopathy
	Nuclear MPI	Severe aortic stenosis
	MRI	Atrial tachyarrhythmias with uncontrolled ventricular response
		History of ventricular tachycardia
		Uncontrolled hypertension
		Aortic aneurysm or dissection
		Obstruction of the left ventricular outflow tract

MI, myocardial infarction; MPI, myocardial perfusion image; MRI, magnetic resonance imaging.

Mahmarian, & Yao, 2006). Dobutamine is the typical pharmacologic agent for stress echocardiogram. Adenosine, regadenoson, and dipyridamole are primarily utilized for radiographic and nuclear stress tests; these agents have similar contraindications, with known hypersensitivity as a contraindication for all of them.

Procedure

Stress echocardiography with physical exercise is performed in a similar manner to an ECG EST, in which the patient's BP, HR, ECG, and symptoms are monitored while a patient is exercising on a treadmill or stationary bicycle. During an exercise stress echocardiogram, a baseline echocardiogram is performed prior to exercise at rest. Immediately after maximal tolerated exercise, the patient is quickly placed in the left lateral decubitus position, a repeat echocardiogram is performed in similar views as the resting echocardiogram, and the images are compared. On both resting and post-stress image acquisitions, at least four views of the heart, parasternal long axis, parasternal short axis, and apical four-chamber and apical two-chamber views, are acquired to allow evaluation of each left ventricular wall segment.

Although exercise-induced physiologic stress is preferred, patients who are unable to exercise on a treadmill or bicycle due to orthopedic, rheumatologic, cardiac, or pulmonary co-morbidities are administered a pharmacological agent, commonly dobutamine, to induce a cardiac stress response. Dobutamine is an adrenergic agonist that acts on beta1-adrenergic receptors to increase cardiac contractility and HR, and on beta2-adrenergic receptors to cause peripheral vasodilatation. Dobutamine temporarily increases myocardial oxygen consumption, thereby probably provoking ischemia. The onset of action for dobutamine is 1 to 2 minutes, and the plasma half-life is approximately 2 minutes (Hays, Mahmarian, Cochran, & Verani, 1993). As with exercise stress echocardiography, a baseline echocardiogram is performed first. Next, a graded infusion of dobutamine is given, typically at a starting dose of 5 or 10 µg/kg per minute and increased every 3 to 5 minutes by 5 to 10 µg/kg per minute to a maximal dose of 40 µg/kg per minute, with continuous echocardiographic imaging performed at each stage. The goal of dobutamine infusion is to achieve an HR of 85% of the maximal predicted HR (MPHR) based on the patient's age. Each echocardiography laboratory may specify a local protocol of minimal and maximal doses and stages. If the HR target is not achieved with standard dobutamine infusion alone, up to 2 mg atropine is given in divided doses. Increased dobutamine (50 µg/kg per minute); additional pharmacologic agents; and gentle hand, arm, or leg exercises are often used to augment chronotropic response. End points of the protocol include achievement of target HR, detection of moderate wall motion abnormalities in at least two coronary artery territories, symptomatic or sustained arrhythmias, hypotension or severe hypertension (SBP > 220–240 mmHg or DBP > 120 mmHg), or the patient's inability to tolerate the examination. The administration of beta-adrenergic blocking agents in recovery can be used for reversal of stress-induced wall motion abnormalities or to unmask subendocardial wall motion abnormalities that may be difficult to distinguish from hyperdynamic contraction of mid- and epicardial layers (Karagiannis et al., 2006; Mathias et al., 2003).

Risks and Benefits

The stress echocardiogram test is rapid, noninvasive, and inexpensive. The possible risks associated with an exercise stress echocardiogram are similar to those with exercise ECG stress testing, and include, but are not limited to, chest pain, elevated BP, arrhythmia, dizziness, nausea, or in rare cases MI.

The incidence of life-threatening complications of dobutamine stress echocardiography is less than 0.01% (Geleijnse et al., 2009). Ventricular arrhythmias are more common in patients with high-grade ischemic disease and in those with left ventricular dysfunction, and they occur more frequently with higher doses of dobutamine.

Results

Stress echocardiography with exercise provides all the same information obtained with exercise ECG stress tests (exercise capacity, clinical, hemodynamic, and ECG response to exercise), with the addition of echocardiographic information, including global and regional left ventricular function at rest and stress, along with the significance of the findings. For stress echocardiography with a pharmacologic stressor agent, information on clinical, hemodynamic, and ECG response to stress in addition to echocardiographic information is obtained. Regional wall motion is graded using either the 16-segment (Figure 26.8) (Smart et al., 1997) or 17-segment model (Cerqueira et al., 2002) of the left ventricle (Pellikka, Nagueh, Elhendy, Kuehl, &

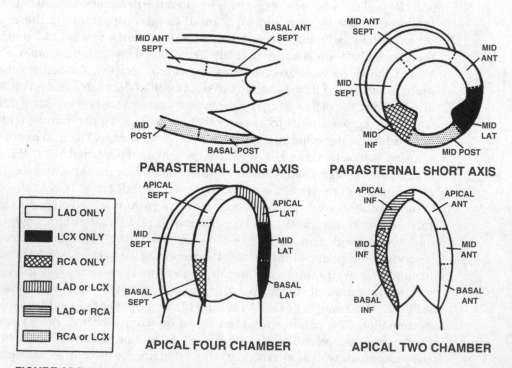

FIGURE 26.8 16-segment model of the left ventricle.

Reprinted from Smart et al. (1997), with permission from Wolters Kluwer Health.

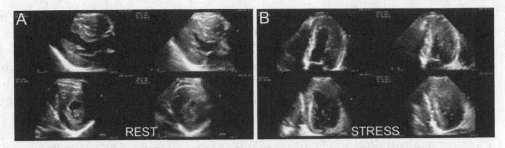

FIGURE 26.9 Stress echocardiogram: End-systolic images in rest (A) and exercise (B) stress echocardiogram. Normal augmentation of wall motion is noted during exercise stress.

Sawada, 2007), and post-stress images are compared with rest images (Figure 26.9). A normal or negative test is consistent with no significant clinical, hemodynamic, or ECG changes; normal augmentation of left ventricular function with stress; and normal global and regional wall motion at rest and after stress. A positive ischemic response is demonstrated by worsening of regional wall motion on stress images compared with rest images occurring in at least one segment, although specificity increases when an ischemic response is noted in two or more contiguous segments. Additional cardiovascular parameters such as viability, arrhythmias, degree of valvular stenosis or regurgitation, and estimation of right ventricular systolic pressure or diastology can also be measured depending on the test indication and study protocol.

Further Testing

Patients with a positive stress echocardiogram test have a high likelihood of obstructive CHD. Depending on the test indication and the extent and degree of ischemia, a patient may be referred for additional cardiovascular testing with invasive coronary angiography or treated with pharmaceutical and lifestyle interventions. In rare cases, a test may be equivocal, demonstrating some abnormal findings, ECG changes, or clinical symptoms, with normal echocardiographic imaging findings. Alternatively, a test may be considered of limited diagnostic value if the patient is unable to achieve 85% of the MPHR response with stress. These patients may require further evaluation with alternative noninvasive imaging tests such as nuclear myocardial perfusion imaging, coronary CT angiography, cardiac MRI, or invasive coronary angiography. It is important to note that a negative stress echocardiography test does not exclude subclinical CHD, because the test is designed to diagnose obstructive CHD.

Diagnostic Performance

Echocardiographic measures of inducible wall-motion abnormalities and global or regional left ventricular function are predictive of long-term outcomes (Shaw, Vasey, Sawada, Rimmerman, & Marwick, 2005). Stress echocardiography with exercise has a reported sensitivity of 85% and specificity of 77% for detection of obstructive CHD (Fleischmann, Hunink, Kuntz, & Douglas, 1998). Various studies report sensitivities ranging from 61% to 96% and specificities ranging from 70% to 100% for dobutamine stress echocardiography (Marwick, 2007). Certain factors or conditions may interfere with the accuracy of stress echocardiography results, including the presence of preexisting wall-motion abnormalities, which reduces the specificity of the test. Smoking or ingesting caffeine within 3 hours before the procedure, COPD, and beta-adrenergic blocking medications may limit the interpretation of results or the ability to obtain an adequate study (Mertes et al., 1993).

For full reference citations to this chapter, please see "Section References" at the back of the book, under the heading "Section VI."

Noninvasive Diagnostic Testing: Radiographic and Nuclear Imaging

BRIAN C. CASE AND MONVADI B. SRICHAI

RADIOGRAPHIC TESTS

Radiographic tests vary greatly in the types of tests performed and the quality of images produced; however, all of these studies use x-ray machines or other specialized equipment with computerized technology to obtain images of the cardiovascular system. These tests can be grouped by technology type and include chest x-ray, computed tomography (CT), and magnetic resonance imaging (MRI).

Chest Radiographs

Chest radiographs (x-rays) use various quantities of radiation to produce images of the lungs, heart, blood vessels, small portions of the gastrointestinal tract, and bony structures in the chest area. Even though there has been tremendous advancement in cardiac imaging over the past 20 years, the chest x-ray continues to be frequently obtained in the diagnosis and management of cardiac disease.

Indications

Beneficial diagnostic information is revealed in a chest x-ray that assists the clinician in evaluating a patient with presumed or known cardiac disease. Specific cardiovascular indications include the evaluation of dyspnea, chest pain, cough, and heart failure; the monitoring of patients with implanted cardiac devices; preoperative assessment in patients with cardiac symptoms; and the evaluation after cardiac surgery or other interventional procedures.

Contraindications

Given the low risk associated with chest x-rays, there are no specific contraindications. A chest x-ray neither details the structures within the heart nor provides information on the electrical activity of the heart. Thus, alternative tests should be considered when evaluating patients for possible valvular heart disease, arrhythmias, or ischemia.

Procedure

A standard chest x-ray includes an erect posterior–anterior and left lateral projection made during full inspiration to include both of the lung apices and the costophrenic sulci. A technologist positions the patient next to the x-ray film; then, an x-ray machine emits a small beam of x-rays that passes through the chest, producing an image on the film. By changing the position of the patient, the standard examination may be modified to highlight other areas, depending on the specific indication.

Risks and Benefits

A chest x-ray is a noninvasive, painless test that is used to evaluate the heart, lungs, and structures of the chest. The quantity of radiation exposure is very small and not considered dangerous for most individuals. Table 27.1 provides radiation exposure doses for a chest x-ray and other cardiac diagnostic studies (Einstein et al., 2007; http://www.healthcommunities.com/heart-tests/cardiac-imaging-tests-radiation-exposure_jhmwp.shtml). However, considerations in pregnancy and for the safety of the developing fetus should be evaluated in all women of childbearing age. In addition, sequential and frequent x-rays over an extended period of time are potentially harmful to all individuals.

TABLE 27.1 Typical Radiation Exposure for Cardiac Diagnostic Tests

Diagnostic Medical Test	Radiation Exposure (mSv)
Echocardiogram	0
Magnetic resonance imaging (MRI)	0
Chest x-ray	0.02
Calcium score CT scan	2 (1–1.5 mSv with new technology)
Stress PET MPI	2.5–3
Coronary angiography	5
MUGA (multi-gated acquisition scan)	6–7
Nuclear medicine stress test with Tc-99m	11
Coronary CT angiography	12 (5–10 mSv with new technology)
PET viability	15
Nuclear medicine stress test with thallium-201	22

CT, computed tomography; MPI, myocardial perfusion imaging; PET, positron emission tomography.

Average background radiation patients receive from natural sources is 2.5–3 mSv per year.

Source: Health Communities (2014).

Results

Information on the heart size, shape, and silhouette margins, particularly heart borders, can be used to infer underlying cardiac disease from the chest x-ray (Figure 27.1). The left heart border consists of the subclavian artery and vein, aortic arch, pulmonary artery, left atrium, and left ventricular contours. The right heart border contains the superior vena cava, ascending aorta and right atrium, and inferior vena cava contours. Lastly, an x-ray enables assessment of the parenchymal pulmonary vascularity.

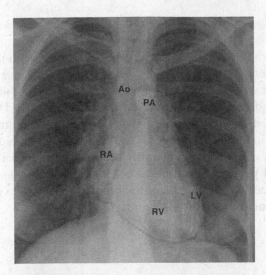

FIGURE 27.1 Chest x-ray showing approximate location of heart structures. See color insert.

Ao, ascending aorta; LV, left ventricle; PA, pulmonary artery; RA, right atrium; RV, right ventricle.

Reprinted from Kirk (2014), with permission. www.transplantkids.org.uk

Another important feature to be examined on the plain chest film is the cardiac position. The cardiac position is described by the primary location of the cardiac silhouette. In a normal x-ray, one expects the cardiac apex and most of the ventricle to be shifted to the left of the image. Dextrocardia refers to the presence of a heart in the right chest, due to an abnormality of embryologic cardiac rotation, whereas dextroposition describes a heart in the right chest; however, this is caused by noncardiac abnormalities that affect a normally formed heart.

Many cardiac abnormalities are associated with an enlarged cardiac silhouette or a heart contour of the left ventricular portion of the left heart border, which appears larger in curvature than expected. Although both cases are sensitive indicators of cardiac abnormalities, these are nonspecific findings and require further diagnostic evaluation. Finally, the presence of pulmonary edema on a chest x-ray can be highly indicative of congenital heart disease or heart failure with congestion. Pulmonary edema has the characteristic, homogeneous-appearing infiltrates and vascular changes in the bilateral lung fields.

Further Testing

If the chest x-ray reveals the presence of an enlarged heart, altered heart borders, or changes in cardiac position, these findings will likely result in further diagnostic testing. An echocardiogram or more detailed radiographic studies can be performed to obtain detailed studies of the heart and surrounding structures. The presence of pulmonary edema or signs of cardiomegaly may also lead to more invasive testing, such as cardiac catheterization, to evaluate the pressures within the heart.

Diagnostic Performance

Information about cardiac structure and function can be discerned from a chest x-ray, and the diagnostic performance of the chest x-ray for the evaluation of cardiovascular disease depends on the specific parameter measured. In general, though, chest x-rays are commonly performed as a screening tool, although they are usually not the sole test used for diagnosis of cardiac disease.

Cardiac CT

CT, commonly referred to as a CT scan, uses multiple x-ray images with the aid of a computer to create cross-sectional images of the body. Cardiac CT refers to the use of CT technology with or without intravenous contrast to visualize heart anatomy, coronary circulation, and great-vessel structure. Commonly utilized CT scans of the heart include the non-contrast calcium-score CT scan and cardiac CT angiography (CTA), which includes coronary CTA. Non-contrast calcium-score CT scans, as the name implies, identify and quantify coronary artery calcifications, which have proved to be of prognostic value for coronary heart disease (CHD) (Agatston et al., 1990). Cardiac CTA produces contrast-enhanced scans to visualize the coronary arteries and structures in the heart and great vessels.

Indications

Non-contrast calcium-score CT scans are generally performed to evaluate CHD presence and severity to determine risk for cardiovascular events. This test is particularly valuable for reclassifying patients initially classified as intermediate risk by clinical evaluation into either a high- or low-risk category (Greenland, LaBree, Azen, Doherty, & Detrano, 2004).

Cardiac CTA with contrast provides unique two- and three-dimensional images for understanding complex coronary anatomy. This test is commonly performed for the diagnosis of CHD, coronary artery anomalies, and complex CHD assessment, including bypass-graft evaluation. Noncoronary indications include the pre-procedural evaluation of the left atrium and pulmonary veins prior to pulmonary vein isolation, detailed assessment of aortic valve and great-vessel anatomy prior to transcatheter aortic valve replacement, assessment of cardiac structure and function in complex congenital heart disease, or other clinical scenarios where alternative imaging modalities are limited or nondiagnostic.

Cardiac CTA can be used in the evaluation of patients experiencing chest pain. The CTA is indicated for patients with intermediate risk profiles for CHD with suspicious cardiac symptoms of anginal chest pain or shortness of breath. The CTA may also be useful in patients who experience atypical symptoms, including chest pain unrelated to physical exertion, with low to intermediate risk profiles for CHD or after unclear or inconclusive stress-test results.

The 2010 Appropriate Use Criteria for Cardiac CT are endorsed by multiple societies (Taylor et al., 2010). In these guidelines, non-contrast calcium-score CT scans may be appropriate in individuals with a family history of premature CHD or in asymptomatic individuals with no known CHD, based on CHD clinical risk estimates (Taylor et al., 2010). General indications for contrast cardiac CTA are listed in Table 27.2 (Taylor et al., 2010).

TABLE 27.2 Potential Indications for Contrast Cardiac CT Angiography

Coronary Heart Disease	Cardiac Structure and Function
Symptomatic patients	Cardiac chambers
Asymptomatic patients, based on clinical risk estimates	Coronary arterial or venous anatomy
Asymptomatic patients after heart transplantation	Thoracic vessels
New onset heart failure	Left ventricular function
Preoperative evaluation	Right ventricular function
Arrhythmias	Pericardial anatomy
Elevated troponins	Myocardial viability
Post-revascularization	Valvular heart disease
Uncertain, unclear, or equivocal prior cardiac testing	Congenital heart disease
	Cardiac masses

CT, computed tomography.

Source: Taylor et al. (2010).

Contraindications

Given the low risk associated with non-contrast calcium-score CT scan, there are no specific contraindications. Cardiac CTA is often associated with higher radiation exposure and additional risks related to the use of intravenous iodinated contrast administered during the study. Contraindications to cardiac CTA (Hoffmann, Ferencik, Cury, & Pena, 2006) are listed in Table 27.3.

TABLE 27.3 Absolute and Relative Contraindications for Coronary CTA

Contraindication	Description
Absolute	Hypersensitivity to iodinated contrast agent
Relative	History of allergies or allergic reactions to other medications
	Renal insufficiency (serum creatinine level of >1.5 mg/dL)
	Congestive heart failure
	History of thromboembolic disorders
	Multiple myeloma
	Hyperthyroidism
	Pheochromocytoma
	Atrial fibrillation
	Inability to perform breath hold for 15 seconds

CTA, computed tomography angiography.

Reprinted from Hoffmann et al. (2006), with permission from the Society of Nuclear Medicine and Molecular Imaging.

Procedure

Cardiac CT studies are performed in a similar manner to CT scans of other parts of the body; in addition, ECG gating, or synchronization, is commonly added to image acquisition to correspond with the cardiac cycle. Medications, including beta adrenergic blockers, calcium channel blockers, and nitroglycerin, are commonly administered before or during cardiac CT scan to improve image quality.

Patients are in a supine position on the CT scanner table with ECG electrodes placed on the chest to monitor heart rate and rhythm, and to allow timing of the image acquisition with the cardiac cycle. No further preparation is needed for non-contrast calcium-score CT scans, and the patient is scanned according to a standard protocol.

Patients undergoing cardiac CTA require a large gauge intravenous access for administration of iodinated contrast dye timed with image acquisition. Depending on the CT scanner characteristics, local protocols, and study indication, patients may be administered oral or intravenous medications, including beta-adrenergic blockers or calcium channel blockers, prior to scanning in order to slow the heart rate (ideally < 65 bpm) and sublingual nitroglycerin in order to dilate the coronary vessels to improve visualization. The CT scan duration is usually 10 to 15 minutes once the preparation is complete.

Risks and Benefits

A non-contrast calcium-score CT scan is a rapid, noninvasive test that is used for the assessment of CHD and that carries a risk of exposure to radiation. The small amount of radiation exposure is equal to the amount of radiation that most people are naturally exposed to in a single year (Table 27.1). However, considerations for the benefits must be weighed against the risks with any diagnostic test that involves radiation exposure, as continuous exposure over time is potentially harmful. A patient's pregnancy status should always be considered in all women of childbearing age before this study is performed.

Contrast cardiac CTA is usually associated with higher amounts of radiation exposure compared with a calcium-score CT scan (Table 27.1). Additional CTA risks are associated with the intravenous administration of iodinated contrast. The risks specific to intravenous iodinated contrast are outlined in Table 27.4.

Mild idiosyncratic reactions to contrast agents are usually self-limited, but moderate or severe reactions usually require treatment. Risk factors for idiosyncratic contrast reactions include a previous reaction to contrast; a strong history of allergic tendencies or multiple allergies; and active asthma, which increases the frequency of bronchospasm after contrast administration. Severe or life-threatening reactions can occur without any specific risk factor and with any type of contrast agent. Premedication with corticosteroids, antihistamines, and histamine H_2 antagonists before the contrast administration can decrease the frequency of contrast reactions up to 10 times (Bui, Horner, Herts, & Einstein, 2007). Many premedication regimens exist, although no particular one has demonstrated superiority over another. In general, a corticosteroid should be administered at least 6 hours before contrast administration (Bui et al., 2007). A common protocol includes the administration of 50 mg of oral prednisone at 13 hours, 7 hours, and 1 hour before scanning, with 50 mg of oral diphenhydramine, with or without a histamine antagonist, 1 hour before scanning.

Non-idiosyncratic reactions reflect the physiologic effects of contrast media and direct organ toxicity. Contrast-induced nephropathy has been estimated to occur in 2% to 7% (Bui et al., 2007) of all patients undergoing contrast CT scans, reflected in rising serum creatinine within the first 24 hours, peaking by 3 to 7 days, and returning to the baseline in 1 to 2 weeks. In rare cases, temporary or permanent dialysis

TABLE 27.4 Iodinated Contrast Reactions

Idiosyncratic (allergic) reactions	Mild	Mild urticaria Rhinorrhea Dizziness
	Moderate	Symptomatic or diffuse urticaria Mild bronchospasm Facial edema Mild laryngeal edema
	Severe	Hypotension Arrhythmias Moderate or severe bronchospasm Moderate or severe laryngeal edema Pulmonary edema Respiratory arrest
Non-idiosyncratic reactions	Mild	Warmth sensation Metallic taste in mouth Bradycardia Vasovagal reactions Neuropathy
	Organ toxicity	Nephropathy
	Metformin	Lactic acidosis

Source: Bui et al. (2007).

may be required. There are many risk factors for contrast-induced nephropathy, including diabetes mellitus with nephropathy, dehydration, concomitant nephrotoxic medications, high dosages of contrast, age older than 70 years, cardiovascular disease, and preexisting renal insufficiency, defined as a serum creatinine greater than or equal to 1.5 mg/dL. Pre- and postprocedural hydration, use of N-acetylcysteine, delaying 72 hours or longer between multiple contrast studies, and the use of iso-osmolar contrast agents are recommended for patients with a high risk for contrast-induced nephropathy. Patients on metformin should hold their dose for at least 48 hours after the contrast study to prevent the development of lactic acidosis. There is also the theoretical risk of teratogenicity in pregnant patients as iodinated contrast agents cross the human placenta. However, breastfeeding is considered safe, as less than 1% of the contrast dose is excreted into breast milk, and of the amount ingested, only about 1% is absorbed from the infant's gastrointestinal tract (Bui et al., 2007; Media, 2013).

Results

Information on cardiac anatomy and pathology can be obtained from cardiac CT studies. Non-contrast calcium-score CT scans allow for detection and quantification of coronary artery calcium (Figure 27.2), which correlates with total coronary artery atherosclerotic plaque burden. The coronary calcium score is commonly reported using the Agatston calcium score, which is based on a quantification of the total calcium in the coronary arteries for the entire heart (Agatston et al., 1990). A calcium volumetric score, a lesion-specific calcium score, or an absolute calcium mass score have also been used to show prognostic significance (Callister et al.,

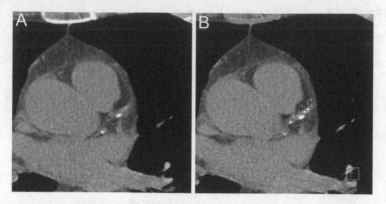

FIGURE 27.2 Non-contrast cardiac CT scan performed for calcium scoring (A). Postprocessing software identifies coronary artery calcification lesions for scoring (B). See color insert.

1998; Hong, Bae, & Pilgram, 2003). All these scoring systems characterize the total amount of calcium found within the coronary arteries. An Agatston score of 0 suggests no coronary artery calcification and is associated with a very low risk of cardiovascular events. Agatston scores are often graded as minimal (1–10), mild (11–100), moderate (101–400), and severe (>400) with higher grades correlating with a higher burden of atherosclerotic disease and a higher risk of events (Shaw, Raggi, Schisterman, Berman, & Callister, 2003).

Cardiac CTA allows further delineation of coronary atherosclerosis, with direct visualization of calcified and noncalcified plaques, and the associated degree of luminal stenosis (Figure 27.3). The location and patency of bypass grafts and intracoronary stents can often be evaluated. Depending on the indication for the study and the protocol used, chamber sizes, global and regional ventricular function, and cardiac valve structure and function can be visualized in two- and three-dimensional formats. Additional information on great-vessel anatomy, including evaluation for aortic aneurysm or dissection, and pulmonary embolism can be obtained, using certain study protocols (triple rule-out protocol).

Further Testing

Patients with a positive cardiac CT scan may require further testing, depending on the indication for the study. Calcium-score CT scans are commonly performed in asymptomatic patients, and based on the findings, further studies or recommendations regarding risk factor modification may be indicated.

Cardiac CTA studies are commonly performed for the evaluation of coronary artery disease in symptomatic and asymptomatic individuals. Evidence of significant coronary artery stenosis or blockage may lead to further studies and interventions. Stress testing with imaging may be indicated in cases with intermediate coronary artery lesions. Alternatively, patients may be referred for invasive coronary angiography with possible percutaneous intervention if there is evidence of severe coronary artery disease.

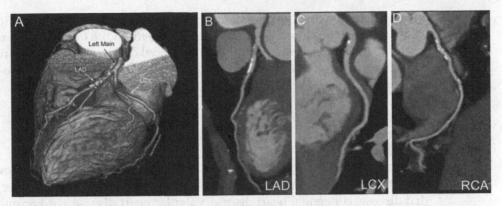

FIGURE 27.3 Coronary CT (computed tomography) Angiography demonstrating 3D view of the heart (A) and curved reformats (B–D) of the left anterior descending (LAD), left circumflex artery (LCX), and right coronary artery (RCA).

Diagnostic Performance

Cardiac CT scans are performed for a variety of indications, and the diagnostic performance is dependent on the specific indication. Non-contrast calcium-score CT scans are highly correlated with the risk of future cardiovascular events (Stein Yaekoub, Matta, & Sostman, 2008). However, these studies demonstrate a modest predictive value for the determination of obstructive CHD. Coronary CTA demonstrates high diagnostic accuracy compared with other noninvasive imaging studies used for the detection of significant CHD. On a per-patient basis, coronary CTA demonstrates a sensitivity of 98% (93%–99%) and a specificity of 82% (63%–93%) for the diagnosis of CHD (Nielsen et al., 2014). The advantage of coronary CTA lies in its ability to exclude significant coronary artery disease with reported negative predictive values of 96% to 100% (Stein et al., 2008). Cardiac CTA for the evaluation of left ventricular size and function has been shown to have good correlation with other noninvasive imaging modalities, including cardiovascular MRI and echocardiography (Van der Vleuten et al., 2009; Tadamura et al., 2005). There have been no specific comparisons on the use of cardiac CTA with other modalities for evaluation of valvular heart disease, although cardiac CTA has become important for accurate valve sizing in patients undergoing transcatheter aortic valve implantation (Kempfert et al., 2012).

Cardiovascular MRI

Cardiovascular MRI is an evolving technology combining magnets, radio waves, and a computer to create detailed, cross-sectional images of the cardiovascular system based on the activity of the hydrogen atom. Cardiovascular MRI plays a significant role as a diagnostic modality in all facets of cardiovascular conditions. Cardiovascular MRI is well suited for the morphologic and physiologic evaluation of a range of acquired and congenital disease processes, pericardium, and great arteries and veins of the thorax. This test is commonly used to distinguish soft tissues as normal or abnormal, accurately assess cardiovascular flow and function, and evaluate the anatomic relationship between intra- and extra-cardiovascular structures. Furthermore, MRI's potential is evident in the fields of atherosclerosis imaging, molecular imaging, and interventional cardiovascular medicine (Kim et al., 2007). An advantage of this technology, unlike an x-ray or a CT scan, is that MRI images are created without the use of radiation.

Indications

Common indications for a cardiovascular MRI examination include the evaluation of aortic disease, ischemic heart disease, nonischemic cardiomyopathies, pericardial disease, congenital heart disease, valvular heart disease, cardiac masses, and pulmonary veins. In particular, cardiac MRI is one of the best diagnostic imaging tests for tissue characterization and distinguishing different forms of cardiomyopathies by differentiating myocardial tissue states, including normal, ischemic, inflammatory, necrotic, fibrotic, hypertrophic, and iron laden. The 2006 Appropriate Use Criteria for Cardiovascular MRI are endorsed by multiple societies (Hendel et al., 2006). General indications for cardiovascular MRI are detailed in Table 27.5.

TABLE 27.5 Potential Indications for Cardiovascular MRI

Cardiac MRI	Coronary MR Angiogram	Stress Cardiac MRI
Left ventricular function	Chest pain syndromes	Acute chest pain
Cardiomyopathies	Intracardiac structures	Chest pain syndromes
Valvular heart disease	Coronary anomalies	Uncertain, unclear, or equivoca
Arrhythmias	Post-revascularization	prior cardiac testing
Preoperative evaluation		
Congenital heart disease		
Syncope		
Cardiac masses		
Pericardial disease		
Aortic disorders		
Pulmonary vein evaluation		
Location of myocardial scar		
Myocardial necrosis or viability		

MRI, magnetic resonance imaging.
Source: Hendel et al. (2006).

Contraindications

A safety evaluation will be completed prior to MRI scanning to screen for potential contraindications (Table 27.6). Patients with absolute contraindications either should not undergo MRI scanning or should do so only with special MRI safety precautions, as in the case of implanted cardiac devices (Jung, Zvereva, Hajredini, & Jackle, 2011; Kodali, Baher, & Shah, 2013; Shinbane, Colletti, & Shellock, 2011). Relative contraindications may pose hazards and should be investigated prior to the MRI examination. Orthopedic implants are usually well anchored and thus do not pose a risk of movement, although there is potential for heating of the implant and degradation of image quality, which should be considered prior to scanning. Special considerations are necessary for patients with possible ferromagnetic devices or

TABLE 27.6 Contraindications to Cardiac MRI

MRI scanning	Absolute contraindications	Electronically, magnetically, and mechanically activated implants
		Ferromagnetic or electronically operated active devices
		Cardiac pacemakers
		Metallic splinters in the eye
		Ferromagnetic hemostatic clips in the brain
	Relative contraindications	Cochlear implants
		Other pacemakers, e.g., for the carotid sinus
		Insulin pumps and nerve stimulators
		Lead wires or similar wires
		Prosthetic heart valves in high fields, if dehiscence suspected
		Hemostatic clips (body)
		Non-ferromagnetic staples
	Special considerations	Pregnancy
		Claustrophobia
		Tattoos
		Bullet fragments
Gadolinium contrast	Absolute contraindications	Previous or preexisting nephrogenic systemic fibrosis
	Relative contraindications	Previous anaphylactic/anaphylactoid reaction to gadolinium containing contrast agent
		Pregnancy (risk–benefit analysis)
		Severe renal insufficiency (eGFR < 30 mL/min/1.73 m^2)
		Unstable renal impairment
		Hepatorenal syndrome
		Breastfeeding

MRI, magnetic resonance imaging.
Source: Hendel et al. (2006).

implants, pregnant women, or those who have claustrophobia (Table 27.7) (Shellock, 2014). A comprehensive list of implants and devices that have been evaluated for MRI safety can be found at www.mrisafety.com. For patients receiving gadolinium contrast, specific contraindications exist as listed in Table 27.6, and for patients undergoing pharmacologic stress testing with MRI, patients should be screened for potential contraindications to the stressor agent (Table 27.8).

Procedure

Cardiovascular MRI examinations are performed in a similar fashion as MRI scans that are performed in other parts of the body, with the addition of ECG gating, or synchronization, of the image acquisition with the cardiac cycle. In addition, for stress cardiac MRI studies, pharmacologic stressor agents (Table 27.8) are utilized.

Patients are supine on the MRI scanner table with ECG electrodes placed on the chest in order to monitor the patient's heart rate and rhythm, and this allows for timing of the image acquisition with the cardiac cycle. Earplugs or headphones are usually provided for the patient, because of the loudness of the radio waves during MRI scanning. No further preparation is needed for non-contrast MRI scans, and the patient is scanned according to a standard protocol. Intravenous administration of a gadolinium-based contrast agent is needed for most cardiovascular MRI protocols.

TABLE 27.7 Specific Devices and Special Issues With MRI

Cerebral aneurysm clips	Certain cerebral aneurysm clips have the potential for displacement when exposed to a magnetic field. Aneurysm clips classified as "nonferromagnetic" or "weakly ferromagnetic" are considered safe.
Cardiac pace-makers and ICDs	Cardiac pacemakers/defibrillators have several potential problems when exposed to a magnetic field, including (1) movement, (2) malfunction, (3) heating induced in the leads, and (4) current induced in the leads. In addition, artifact from the leads may significantly degrade image quality of the cardiovascular structures. Consultation with an electrophysiology team is vital. The FDA has approved an MRI-safe pacing system (Revo MRI by Medtronic, Inc) that allows for patients to undergo MRI of certain body regions (e.g., brain and knees) outside the chest. At present, this system is not FDA approved for MRI scans in the chest region.
Cardiovascular catheters	Catheters with conductive metallic components (e.g., pulmonary artery catheters with temperature probes) have the potential for excessive heating. Thus, patients with these devices should not undergo MRI scanning with the catheter in place.
Cochlear implants and hearing aids	Most implants either utilize a strong magnet or are electronically activated. When exposed to a magnetic field, there is the potential of injury or damage to the function of these implants. External hearing aids should be removed before the MRI procedure is conducted.
Intravascular coils, stents, and filters	These implants typically become securely incorporated into the vessel wall within 6–8 weeks after placement. Thus, most are considered safe. However, specific information on the type of device should be obtained before MRI scanning. Most intracoronary stents have been shown to be safe during MRI, even when performed on the day of implantation, although many stent manufacturers recommend waiting for 6–8 weeks.
ECG electrodes	MRI-safe ECG electrodes are recommended for use during MRI scanning to ensure patient safety and proper ECG recording.
Foley catheters	Foley catheters with temperature sensors have the potential for excessive heating. These catheters are generally safe if properly positioned and disconnected from the temperature monitor during MRI scanning.
Heart valve prostheses	All types of heart valve prostheses have been shown to be safe during MRI. Although certain prostheses exhibit relatively minor magnetic field interactions, these forces are minimal compared to the force exerted by the beating heart. The prosthetic material may cause artifacts in the MRI images.
Metallic foreign bodies	All patients with a history of injury with metallic foreign bodies such as shrapnel or bullets should be thoroughly screened and evaluated since serious injury could result from movement, dislodgement, or excessive heating of the foreign body, particularly if located in or adjacent to sensitive body sites such as vital neural, vascular, or soft tissue structures. Plain film radiography is commonly used to screen for the presence of metallic foreign bodies in the body.
Metallic cardiac closure devices	The MRI is considered safe for non-ferromagnetic devices immediately after implantation. Weakly ferromagnetic devices are safe approximately 6–8 weeks after placement.
Retained epicardial pacing wires	Retained epicardial pacing wires after cardiac surgery are safe for MRI scanning. Retained intracardiac, transvenous pacing wires, however, are considered a contraindication due to their potential for significant heating of the wire.
Tattoos, perma-nent cosmetics, and eye makeup	Permanent cosmetics and tattoos may be associated with minor, short-term skin reactions and artifacts in the image with MRI scanning, related to use of a ferromagnetic pigment. Decorative tattoos have been associated with first-and second-degree skin burns.
Pregnant patients	MRI environment-related risks are difficult to assess for pregnant patients, and to date, there has been no indication that MRI during pregnancy is associated with deleterious effects. Current standard-of-care policy is that MRI may be used in pregnant women if other nonioniz-ing forms of diagnostic imaging are inadequate or if the examination provides important information that would otherwise require exposure to ionizing radiation (e.g., CT, fluoroscopy).
Claustrophobia, anxiety, and emotional distress	Patient distress can lead to adverse outcomes during MRI scanning, including unintentional exacerbation of patient distress, compromise in the quality and diagnostic aspects of the imaging study, and delayed, prematurely terminated, or cancelled studies.

CT, computed tomography; FDA, Food and Drug Administration; ICD, implanted cardioverter defibrillators; MRI, magnetic resonance imaging.

Source: Shellock (2014).

TABLE 27.8 Test Type and Contraindications for Various Pharmacologic Stressor Agents

Stress Agent	Test Type	Contraindications	Type of Contraindication
Adenosine (Adenocard®) Dipyridamole (Persantine)	Nuclear MPI MRI CTP	Absolute contraindications	Active bronchospasm Active treatment for reactive airway disease Second- or third-degree heart block without a pacemaker Sick sinus syndrome Systolic blood pressure <90 mmHg Recent use of dipyridamole-containing medications <12-hour use of methylxanthines, caffeine, aminophylline, theophylline
		Relative contraindications	Remote history of reactive airway disease, ≥1 year Acute coronary syndrome Profound sinus bradycardia (heart rate <40 bpm)
Regadenoson (Lexiscan®)	Nuclear MPI MRI CTP	Absolute contraindications	Second- or third-degree heart block unless pacemaker in place Sinus node dysfunction unless pacemaker in place Systolic blood pressure <90 mmHg Myocardial ischemia <12-hour use of methylxanthines, caffeine, aminophylline, theophylline
		Relative contraindications	Profound sinus bradycardia (heart rate <40 bpm) Reactive airway disease Seizure disorder

CTP, computed tomography perfusion; MPI, myocardial perfusion image; MRI, magnetic resonance imaging.

Risks and Benefits

Unlike other imaging tests, MRI does not use ionizing radiation, and thus does not carry the risk of potential malignancy; however, there are a number of other potential risks with MRI scanning. The strong, static magnetic fields produced by the MRI scanners may result in ferromagnetic interactions in which an object or a device with certain properties is attracted to the center of the magnet and may be moved, rotated, dislodged (metallic splinters, vascular clips, or cochlear implants), or accelerated (helium or oxygen cylinders, wheelchairs, etc.) toward the magnet when placed within the magnetic field, possibly causing severe injuries and damage. The strong magnetic field may also affect an implanted device's performance, including cardiac pacemakers. Pulsed, gradient magnetic fields used when acquiring images have the ability to induce electrical currents in implanted devices and may directly cause neuromuscular stimulation. Pulsed radiofrequency fields, which are used when acquiring images, may cause local heating and can also generate electrical currents in wires and leads that may induce arrhythmias (Dill, 2008).

Patients with renal insufficiency who require intravenous gadolinium-based contrast for the examination have a risk of nephrogenic systemic fibrosis, a debilitating disease characterized by fibrosis of the skin and internal organs, similar to but distinct from scleroderma or scleromyxedema (Cowper, 2008). Symptoms usually develop up to 4 weeks after exposure, with no specific treatment available, although extracorporeal photopheresis appears to provide the best therapy for this chronic, progressive condition (Elmholdt, Buus, Ramsing, & Olesen, 2011; Kafi et al., 2004; Kintossou et al., 2007; Schmook et al., 2005). Other potential risks include anaphylactic reaction (1 in 10,000) and transient headache, nausea, and dizziness. Available data suggest that it is safe for mothers who are breastfeeding to continue nursing after receiving gadolinium contrast (Hylton, 2000; Media, 2013). No harmful effects of MRI during pregnancy have been reported; however, more research on the safety of MRI during pregnancy is needed.

Patients undergoing cardiac MRI with pharmacologic stress have the same risks as other imaging stress studies using pharmacologic agents. These risks include development of chest pain, blood pressure changes, arrhythmias, myocardial infarction, and death, particularly with higher doses. Finally, patients should be evaluated for claustrophobia or fear of small spaces, because the test is performed in a confined space with an approximate duration of an hour, depending on the indication for the MRI. As with any test, risks of the test must be weighed against the potential benefits of the information gained from the examination. In particular, cardiovascular MRI has the potential to provide a wealth of information unavailable with other imaging tests, without the use of ionizing radiation.

Results

Cardiovascular MRI uses a number of different MRI acquisition techniques for evaluation of the cardiovascular system. Tissue-characterization information such as identification of fat or edema can be obtained using T1- and T2-weighted imaging sequences. Bright blood cine imaging and myocardial tagging sequences facilitate qualitative and quantitative evaluation of myocardial function. In addition, assessment for pericardial tethering can be performed to assess for signs of constrictive pericarditis. Dynamic first-pass perfusion imaging at rest and stress are used for stress-perfusion cardiovascular MRI studies. Late gadolinium enhancement imaging has been utilized for assessment of myocardial fibrosis and scarring (Figure 27.4). Phase-contrast velocity mapping provides information on blood velocity and flow, and it is used for quantification of cardiac output, shunts,

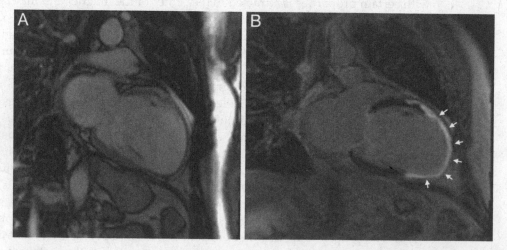

FIGURE 27.4 Cardiac MRI (magnetic resonance imaging) cine image in end-systole (A) and late gadolinium enhancement image (B) showing dilated left ventricle with nonviable, transmural scar (arrows) involving a large portion of the left ventricular myocardium.

and valvular dysfunction. Magnetic resonance angiography (MRA) refers to three-dimensional MRI acquisition, commonly after the injection of gadolinium contrast, for evaluation of the vasculature, including great vessels and coronary arteries. Depending on the study indication, one or more of the types of image acquisition techniques described earlier may be utilized in a single examination.

Further Testing

Cardiovascular MRI is often performed in patients with suspected cardiac structural or functional abnormalities, supplementing prior imaging studies such as echocardiography. Depending on the presence and severity of cardiac disease, patients may be referred for further invasive evaluation, including coronary angiography, therapeutic interventions of percutaneous intervention or cardiovascular surgery, or medical therapy with continued follow-up. Patients with inconclusive results on cardiovascular MRI may need additional noninvasive tests, possibly TEE or cardiac CT, for further clarification of underlying cardiac disease.

Diagnostic Performance

Diagnostic performance of cardiovascular MRI is dependent on the specific parameter being measured. Stress-perfusion MRI has a reported sensitivity of 89% to 91% and a specificity of 76% to 85% for detection of CHD (de Jong, Genders, van Geuns, Moelker, & Hunink, 2012; Desai & Jha, 2013; Jaarsma et al., 2012; Nandalur, Dwamena, Choudhri, Nandalur, & Carlos, 2007). Dobutamine stress MRI has a reported sensitivity of 83% and a specificity of 86% (Nandalur et al., 2007). The diagnostic accuracy of cardiovascular MRI for viability assessment is dependent on the technique, with the highest sensitivity reported with late gadolinium enhancement imaging and the highest specificity (91%) reported with low-dose dobutamine stress for assessment of improvement in wall-motion abnormalities (Allman, 2013; Romero, Xue, Gonzalez, & Garcia, 2012). Appropriate-use guidelines have been developed to aid in choosing the appropriate test, depending on the specific indication and performance characteristics of the test in question (Hendel et al., 2006).

NUCLEAR IMAGING

Nuclear imaging modalities use techniques with intravenous radioactive tracers to provide images and information about cardiac function and the presence of disease. Cardiovascular imaging studies utilizing nuclear imaging include multi-gated acquisition (MUGA) scans, stress tests with single-photon emission computed tomography (SPECT) imaging, and positron emission tomography (PET) scans.

Multi-Gated Acquisition Scan

A MUGA scan is a type of nuclear imaging test utilizing radioactive tracer, a radionuclide, and a special camera to view the heart throughout the cardiac cycle. This test is primarily indicated to determine global and regional measures of ventricular function at rest, during exercise stress, or during pharmacologic intervention. A MUGA scan can be performed as first-pass radionuclide angiography or equilibrium radionuclide angiocardiography.

Indications

There are few indications for a MUGA study. The most common indications are for the assessment of left ventricular function, including ventricular volumes and ejection fraction, that are unreliable with other imaging studies or for baseline and serial assessment in patients starting chemotherapy, especially with cardiotoxic agents, including doxorubicin (Hendel et al., 2009).

Contraindications

Given the low risk associated with the radiotracers used in MUGA scans, there are no specific contraindications.

Procedure

No special preparation is required for a resting MUGA scan, although a fasting state is generally preferred. For a stress MUGA scan, the patient should be fasting for at least 3 to 4 hours prior to the study and should be hemodynamically and clinically stable. Exercise stress is generally preferred, but pharmacologic stress with a positive inotropic agent may be performed in patients who are unable to exercise. The patient's red blood cell pool is labeled with a radioactive tracer, technetium-99m-pertechnetate (Tc-99m). Labeling can be performed using the in vivo method, in which stannous chloride is injected initially to "prime" the blood cells, followed by an injection of the Tc-99m for labeling. With the in vitro method, some of the patient's blood is drawn, and stannous chloride is injected into the drawn blood followed by Tc-99m. Then, the blood is re-injected into the patient. The in vivo method is less time consuming, less expensive, and more convenient for patients, although the in vitro method provides more efficient labeling of the red blood cells. After the red blood cells are tagged, a gamma-ray camera captures images of the heart throughout the cardiac cycle as the blood circulates. Imaging is performed either immediately as first pass or after equilibrium, approximately 20 to 30 minutes after injection, usually in three standard views of the heart: anterior, left anterior oblique, and septal. The duration of the scan is approximately 20 minutes. The images can be reviewed and analyzed to provide quantitative measurement of ventricular volumes and ejection fraction.

Risks and Benefits

The radioactive tracer utilized for the MUGA scan is safe for most people and excreted by the kidneys within 24 hours, with no known long-term harmful effects. As with any test that involves radiation exposure (Table 27.1), consideration of the benefit must be weighed against the risk as continuous exposure over an extended period of time is potentially harmful. A patient's pregnancy status should always be considered prior to this study. This test provides a detailed and accurate assessment of cardiac ejection fraction, which is very beneficial, especially in patient populations that receive cardiotoxic medications.

Results

Information on left and right ventricular volumes, filling, emptying, wall motion, and ejection fraction can be evaluated both qualitatively and quantitatively (Figure 27.5). Rest and stress imaging parameters can be compared with each other to assess for underlying ischemia, which may manifest as a reduction in ejection fraction or new wall motion abnormalities.

Further Testing

In current practice, MUGA scans are commonly used for baseline and serial assessment of left ventricular function in a patient receiving medication associated with cardiotoxicity. A significant change in ventricular function may indicate cardiotoxicity and the need to withhold the offending medication, at least temporarily,

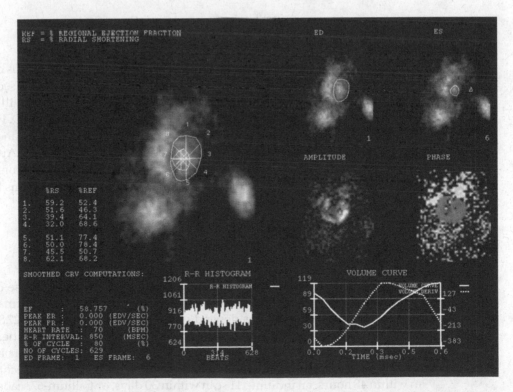

FIGURE 27.5 MUGA (multi-gated acquisition) scan demonstrating calculation of left ventricular volume and ejection fraction.

to prevent further deterioration in ventricular function and allow for potential recovery of ventricular function. In the setting of abnormal stress MUGA, further evaluation of ischemia, such as coronary angiography, may be indicated.

Diagnostic Performance

The MUGA scans for ejection fraction measurements demonstrate diagnostic performance similar to echocardiography (Canclini, Terzi, et al., 2001), although considered less accurate compared with cardiac MRI. Average relative errors in ejection fraction range from 7% to 22% (Debatin et al., 1992). There are very limited data on the diagnostic performance of MUGA for detection of significant CHD.

Single Photon Emission Computed Tomography, Myocardial Perfusion Imaging

SPECT scans are the most common type of nuclear stress test used to diagnose CHD. The SPECT myocardial perfusion imaging (MPI) study uses radionuclide tracers to detail blood flow to the myocardium under rest and stress conditions, with stress induced with exercise or pharmacologically. The SPECT MPI can confirm the diagnosis and estimate the severity of CHD. In addition, this examination provides prognostic data to determine subsequent risk of cardiovascular events.

Indications

The SPECT MPI studies are generally indicated to establish the diagnosis of CHD. In general, they are useful for patients in whom CHD is suspected, based on the symptoms and risk factors, without a confirmed diagnosis. In addition, this imaging modality can provide information on the progression of known CHD. Finally, a SPECT MPI is able to measure the size and shape of the patient's heart and, therefore, able to calculate the left ventricular ejection fraction. The 2009 Appropriate Use Criteria for cardiac radionuclide imaging provides guidelines on the use of SPECT MPI as endorsed by multiple societies, with general indications listed in Table 27.9 (Hendel et al., 2009).

Contraindications

Contraindications to exercise nuclear stress testing are similar to those detailed for exercise stress testing (Table 26.6). For patients undergoing pharmacologic stress, specific contraindications depend on the stressor agent (Table 27.8) (Henzlova et al., 2006). The SPECT imaging is contraindicated when the patient has a prior allergic reaction to the tracer or has recently completed a nuclear imaging including iodine-131 therapy within 12 weeks, nuclear imaging using technetium-99m within 48 hours, an indium-111 scan within 30 days, or gallium-67 scans within 30 days.

TABLE 27.9 Potential Indications for SPECT and PET MPI

Symptomatic patients, based on pretest probability and clinical findings
Asymptomatic patients, based on clinical risk estimates
Risk assessment after acute coronary syndrome
New onset heart failure with reduced LVEF
Preoperative evaluation
New onset atrial fibrillation
Ventricular arrhythmias
Syncope
Elevated troponins
Post-revascularization
Uncertain, unclear, abnormal, or equivocal prior to cardiac testing
Assessment of myocardial scar or viability
Left ventricular function
Cardiac rehabilitation

LVEF, left ventricular ejection fraction; MPI, myocardial perfusion imaging; PET, positron
emission tomography; SPECT, single-photon emission computed tomography.

Source: Hendel et al. (2009).

Procedure

A stress SPECT MPI is performed in a similar manner to an exercise stress ECG and
stress echocardiography, in which the patient's blood pressure, heart rate, ECG, and
symptoms are monitored while a patient is exercising on a treadmill or stationary
bicycle or receiving a pharmacologic stressor agent, most commonly a vasodilator
agent, adenosine or regadenoson, although dobutamine can be used. The minimum
goal for exercise is to obtain 85% of the maximum predicted heart rate, although
patients are requested to exert themselves until they are fatigued, unless there is
an indication to stop sooner due to the development of moderate to severe chest
pain, severe shortness of breath, abnormally high or low blood pressure, abnormal
heart rhythm, severe dizziness, or other significant symptoms. The vasodilators
produce maximal coronary hyperemia, creating flow heterogeneity by causing a
greater increase in blood flow in normal coronary arteries than in arteries with
flow-limiting stenosis. Dobutamine temporarily increases myocardial oxygen consumption and heart rate, thereby probably provoking ischemia. Pharmacologic stress
with a vasodilator agent or dobutamine is performed according to test protocol,
depending on the agent (Henzlova et al., 2006). A myocardial perfusion radiotracer,
thallium-201 or technitium-99m labeled compounds (sestamibi or tetrofosmin), is
injected intravenously at rest and during peak stress. The patient is positioned
supine while a gamma camera rotates around the patient and creates images of the
heart muscle. Depending on the radiotracer and protocol, resting images of the heart
may be acquired either before or after stress. For vasodilator stress, adenosine and
regadenoson, patients should avoid caffeine for more than 12 hours, theophylline
for more than 48 hours, and fast for at least 6 hours.

Risks and Benefits

These cardiac nuclear stress tests are generally safe, and complications are rare. Possible risks associated with an exercise SPECT MPI stress test are similar to those

with exercise ECG stress testing, and include, but are not limited to, the following: chest pain, blood pressure changes, arrhythmias, dizziness, nausea, or, rarely, a myocardial infarction or death. Pharmacologic stress SPECT MPI study medications carry risks that are related to the stressor agent (Table 27.8) and may include hypotension, heart block, and, rarely, life-threatening arrhythmia and myocardial infarction. The SPECT MPI stress scans are associated with radiation exposure (Table 27.1). Consideration of the benefit must be weighed against the risk with any test that involves radiation exposure, as continuous exposure over an extended period of time is potentially harmful. Before the study is conducted, a patient's pregnancy status should always be considered in the case of childbearing women.

Results

A normal SPECT MPI stress test indicates normal blood flow during rest and stress, and the patient is unlikely to have significant CHD. An abnormal study that is suggestive of myocardial ischemia will demonstrate normal blood flow during rest, but not during stress (Figure 27.6). The location, degree, and extent of these perfusion abnormalities carry important implications, both for treatment and for prognosis (Brown, 1996; Hachamovitch et al., 2011; Heller & Brown, 1994; Iskander & Iskandrian, 1998). The study may also show decreased regional blood flow during both rest and stress, which is suggestive of prior myocardial infarction. Viability testing is often needed to determine whether infarct regions represent a scarred or hibernating myocardium.

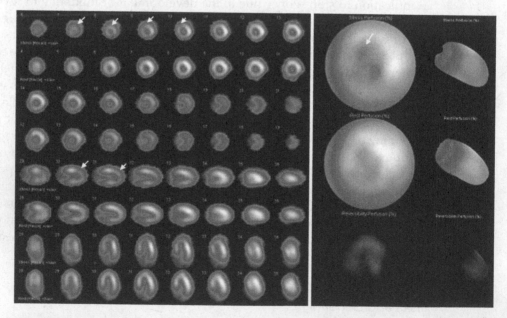

FIGURE 27.6 SPECT MPI study showing reversible perfusion defect involving the mid- and apical anterior walls (arrows) suggestive of ischemia in the LAD territory. See color insert.

Further Testing

A normal SPECT MPI stress test generally implies that further testing to diagnose CHD is not warranted. If the results demonstrate evidence of myocardial ischemia, considerations for further evaluation, including coronary angiography with possible coronary revascularization, may be indicated, depending on the initial indication for the SPECT MPI, the severity of the patient's symptoms, and the extent of the abnormalities.

Diagnostic Performance

Cardiac stress SPECT MPI scans demonstrate an 88% sensitivity and a 76% specificity for detection of significant CHD (Parker et al., 2012). There is no significant difference in diagnostic performance for SPECT MPI with exercise compared with pharmacologic stress (Parker et al., 2012). In general, stress SPECT scans are clinically the most suitable for the evaluation of patients at intermediate risk for CHD. In addition, abnormalities on stress SPECT MPI studies have been identified as independent predictors of cardiovascular events (Brown, 1995). Normal findings are associated with good prognosis and a yearly mortality rate less than 1% (Metz et al., 2007).

Cardiac Positron Emission Tomography

A cardiac PET scan is an imaging test using specific positron-emitting radionuclide tracers to evaluate the heart. The PET myocardial perfusion imaging (MPI), similar to SPECT MPI, measures blood flow to the heart muscle under rest and stress. The PET viability imaging in patients with cardiomyopathy assesses whether the myocardium is scarred or viable. The radiotracers used in PET imaging emit two high-energy photons in opposite directions, 180 degrees from each other, that are simultaneously detected, coincidence detection, by a PET scanner. The radiotracers and scanners used in PET imaging lead to improved image quality compared with SPECT imaging (Beanlands & Youssef, 2010; Yoshinaga et al., 2006), which may result in an improvement in diagnostic accuracy and overall cost effectiveness (Merhige et al., 2007); however, PET imaging is not as accessible as SPECT imaging (Cerqueira, 2010).

Indications

Cardiac PET studies are generally indicated to identify, diagnose, and assess severity of CHD and to identify myocardial viability in patients with left ventricular dysfunction to estimate benefit for revascularization. The 2009 Appropriate Use Criteria for cardiac radionuclide imaging provides guidelines on the use of myocardial perfusion imaging with PET or SPECT as endorsed by multiple societies and general guidelines (Hendel et al., 2009). Specific indications and contraindications for PET myocardial perfusion and metabolic imaging are noted in Table 27.10.

TABLE 27.10 Specific Indications and Contraindications for PET Perfusion and Metabolic Imaging

	Perfusion Imaging	Metabolic Imaging
Indications	Diagnosis of patients with suspected or known CHD	Assessment of myocardial viability
	Risk stratification of patients with suspected or known CHD	Evaluation for cardiac sarcoidosis
	Detection of CHD and assessment of resting perfusion in patients undergoing PET myocardial viability/metabolic imaging	
Contraindications	Standard contraindications to exercise or pharmacologic stress	
	Inability to lie flat or lie still for the duration of the acquisition	
	Claustrophobia	

CHD, coronary heart disease; PET, positron emission tomography.

Source: Hendel et al. (2009).

Contraindications

Contraindications to PET MPI exercise stress testing are similar to those detailed for exercise stress testing (Table 26.6) and pharmacologic stress agents (Table 27.8) (Henzlova et al., 2006). In addition, the inability to lie flat or to be still for the duration of the examination and claustrophobia are other potential contraindications (Table 27.10).

Procedure

Patient preparation for PET MPI studies is similar to that for pharmacologic stress SPECT MPI. For vasodilator stress, adenosine and regadenoson, patients should avoid caffeine for more than 12 hours, theophylline for more than 48 hours, and fast for at least 6 hours. The ECG monitors heart rate, cardiac rhythm, and ST-T segments, as well as allows for ECG gating, synchronization of the images with the cardiac cycle. A PET perfusion tracer is injected into the bloodstream at rest and during peak hyperemia for pharmacologic stress. Exercise PET MPI is potentially feasible, but challenging due to the short half-life of the PET perfusion tracers, potential high radiation dose to personnel, coordination with use of the cyclotron for production of the tracers, and patient motion. Commonly used PET perfusion tracers include rubidium-82, N-13 ammonia, and O-15 water or carbon dioxide.

For myocardial viability studies, F-18 fluorodeoxyglucose (FDG) is the PET tracer. Patients should fast for 6 or more hours before the study, and metabolic preparation is essential to stimulate myocardial F-18 FDG uptake. Different approaches of preparation have been used, but the hyperinsulinemic euglycemic clamp appears to provide the best imaging quality, although it is time consuming. The most common preparation is the use of 25 to 100 g of oral glucose, followed by supplemental IV insulin as needed to promote maximum uptake of F-18 FDG. The actual study duration is about 30 minutes (Amanullah et al., 2000). Rest–stress PET MPI and viability PET protocols may be combined to provide information on both myocardial ischemia and viability.

Risks and Benefits

Cardiac PET is generally considered a safe study for most people. The PET radio-tracer is usually removed from the patient's body within 24 hours. Possible risks associated with a PET MPI stress test are dependent on the stressor agent used (Table 27.8) and are similar to risks with pharmacologic stress SPECT MPI, including but not limited to chest pain, dyspnea, hypotension, heart block, and, rarely, life-threatening arrhythmia and myocardial infarction. The amount of radiation exposure in a PET study is small (Table 27.1). As with all studies, consideration of the benefit must be weighed against the risk with any test that involves radiation exposure, as continuous exposure over an extended period of time is potentially harmful. A patient's pregnancy status should always be considered prior to this study being performed in all women of childbearing age.

Results

The PET MPI provides similar information to SPECT MPI with the possibility of quantifying blood flow. A normal PET MPI stress test demonstrates normal blood flow during rest and stress; therefore, the patient is unlikely to have significant CHD. An abnormal study that is suggestive of myocardial ischemia may demonstrate normal blood flow during rest, although not during stress (Figure 27.7). Gated PET provides assessment of left ventricular volumes as well as global and regional ventricular function. F-18 FDG viability imaging provides information on the perfusion–metabolism pattern, with mismatched patterns, decreased blood flow with normal metabolism, suggestive of underlying myocardial viability. This indicates that there is decreased coronary blood flow to a particular area of tissue, usually due to coronary artery disease, although the myocardial cells remain functional. This viability study is generally performed to determine the usefulness of revascularization.

Further Testing

If a patient suffers from CHD or had a known myocardial infarction, a PET scan demonstrating viable myocardium may result in further testing or interventions. The patient may benefit from a coronary angiogram and possible percutaneous intervention in order to improve vascularization of the viable tissue. Based on the distribution of the damaged coronary arteries, although still viable tissue, a cardiac interventionalist may recommend referral for coronary artery bypass grafting referral.

Diagnostic Performance

The PET MPI demonstrates high diagnostic accuracy for detection of CHD with a sensitivity of 93% and a specificity of 81% (Parker et al., 2012). Evidence from nonrandomized studies of 8,000 patients with moderate to severe ischemic left

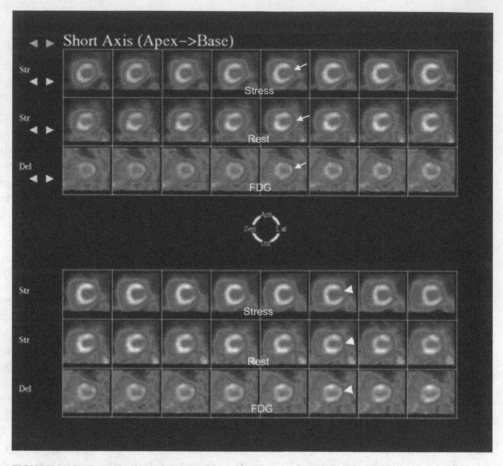

FIGURE 27.7 Rest and stress PET MPI with metabolic FDG imaging showing ischemia (arrowheads) and viability (arrow) in the lateral wall. See color insert.

FDG, fluorodeoxyglucose; MPI, myocardial perfusion imaging; PET, positron emission tomography.

ventricular dysfunction suggests that PET viability imaging with F-18 FDG can identify segments that will recover contractile function after revascularization (Parker et al., 2012). Prognostic literature indicates that the best survival occurs in patients who undergo revascularization with evidence of viable myocardium on PET FDG imaging (Parker et al., 2012).

CLINICAL DECISION MAKING

Diagnostic test selection is an integral component of the care of individuals with cardiovascular disorders. Tests may have overlapping and complementary indications. The lists and tables given next assist the clinician in understanding the testing options and in comparing the various tests for specific indications to facilitate appropriate test selection. Clinical considerations should also include cost and referral to cardiovascular specialists for test selection as needed. When considering testing and interpretation of results, it is vital that clinicians treat the patient, rather than the results or the test.

Noninvasive stress tests, by exercise or pharmacologic methods:
Exercise
    Exercise Tolerance Test (ETT)
    Exercise Stress Echocardiogram (ESE)
    Exercise Single-Photon Emission Computed Tomography (SPECT),
        Myocardial Perfusion Imaging (MPI)
Pharmacologic
    Adenosine Single-Photon Emission Computed Tomography (SPECT),
        Myocardial Perfusion Imaging (MPI)
    Adenosine Positron Emission Computed Tomography (PET), Myocardial
        Perfusion Imaging (MPI)
    Adenosine Cardiac Magnetic Resonance Imaging (MRI)
    Adenosine Cardiac Computed Tomography Perfusion (CTP)
    Regadenoson Single-Photon Emission Computed Tomography (SPECT),
        Myocardial Perfusion Imaging (MPI)
    Regadenoson Positron Emission Computed Tomography (PET), Myocardial
        Perfusion Imaging (MPI)
    Regadenoson Cardiac Magnetic Resonance Imaging (MRI)
    Regadenoson Cardiac Computed Tomography Perfusion (CTP)
    Dipyridamole Single-Photon Emission Computed Tomography (SPECT),
        Myocardial Perfusion Imaging (MPI)
    Dipyridamole Positron Emission Computed Tomography (PET), Myocardial
        Perfusion Imaging (MPI)
    Dipyridamole Cardiac Magnetic Resonance Imaging (MRI)
    Dipyridamole Cardiac Computed Tomography Perfusion (CTP)
    Dobutamine Stress Echocardiogram (DSE)
    Dobutamine Single-Photon Emission Computed Tomography (SPECT),
        Myocardial Perfusion Imaging (MPI)
    Dobutamine Positron Emission Computed Tomography (PET), Myocardial
        Perfusion Imaging (MPI)
    Dobutamine Cardiac Magnetic Resonance Imaging (MRI)

Noninvasive stress tests with imaging, by imaging type:
Echocardiogram
    Exercise
    Dobutamine

Single-Photon Emission Computed Tomography (SPECT), Myocardial Perfusion
Imaging (MPI)
    Exercise
    Adenosine
    Regadenoson
    Dipyridamole
    Dobutamine

TABLE 27.11 Noninvasive Stress Test Administration

Test Type	Administration	Usual Duration	Common Transient Effects	Before Test Evaluation	Patient Instructions
Exercise	Bruce protocol	Seven stages, 3 min/stage 21-min total exercise	Fatigue Dyspnea Palpitations Chest pain Leg discomfort	Physical condition—walk/jog on treadmill or ride stationary bicycle ECG Medications	No food or fluids 4 hr Walking or running shoes Exercise clothing Medication Instructions
Adenosine (Adenocard, Adenoscan®)	140 mcg/kg/min IV	6-min infusion	Flushing Chest pain Bronchospasms Dizziness Nausea Symptomatic hypotension Conduction disturbances	Conduction abnormalities Bradycardia Chronic airway disease Weight limit of camera Claustrophobia Hypotension Medications Able to be supine for 20–30 min	No caffeine or methylxanthines for 48 hr No phosphodiesterase inhibitors No food or fluids 4–8 hr Medication instructions Nitrates, beta blockers, calcium channel blockers, insulin, pulmonary inhalers
Regadenoson (Lexiscan®)	0.4 mg IV	10-sec infusion	Headache Chest discomfort Nausea Flushing	Tachycardia Hypotension Methylxanthines Weight limit of camera Claustrophobia Medications Able to be supine for 20–30 min	No caffeine for 48 hr No phosphodiesterase inhibitors No food or fluids 4–8 hr Medication instructions Nitrates, beta blockers, calcium channel blockers, insulin, pulmonary inhalers
Dobutamine	10–40 to 50 mcg/kg/min IV, begin at 5–10 mcg/kg/min, then increase 10 mcg/kg/min every 3 min	Four to five stages, 3 min/stage, 12–15-min total infusion	Headache Chest pain Palpitations Nausea Tremor Hypertension or hypotension Atrial or ventricular arrhythmias	Blood pressure Glaucoma Cardiac medications	No food or fluids 4–8 hr Medication instructions Nitrates, beta blockers, calcium channel blockers, insulin, pulmonary inhalers

Reprinted from Anderson, Murphy, and Balaji (2014), with permission from John Wiley and Sons.

Positron Emission Computed Tomography (PET), Myocardial Perfusion Imaging (MPI)
>   Adenosine
>   Regadenoson
>   Dipyridamole
>   Dobutamine

Cardiac Magnetic Resonance Imaging (MRI)
>   Adenosine
>   Regadenoson
>   Dipyridamole
>   Dobutamine

Cardiac Computed Tomography Perfusion (CTP)
>   Adenosine
>   Regadenoson
>   Dipyridamole

TABLE 27.12 Dipyridamole Stress Test Administration and Considerations

Stressor Agent	Administration	Usual Duration	Common Transient Effects	Before Test Evaluation
Dipyridamole (Persantine®)	0.142 mg/kg/min (0.56 mg/kg total) IV	4-min infusion	Flushing Chest pain Bronchospasms Headache Dizziness Hypotension Conduction disturbances	Conduction abnormalities Bradycardia Chronic airway disease Weight limit of camera Claustrophobia Hypotension Medications Able to be supine 20–30 min

Tables 27.11 and 27.12 describe common methods of noninvasive stress tests and general considerations for evaluation before the tests and administration of the tests.

Table 27.13 describes the relative efficacy of common cardiac diagnostic tests for specific cardiac conditions.

TABLE 27.13 Relative Efficacy of Cardiac Diagnostic Tests

	Echocardiogram	SPECT Nuclear MPI	Cardiac CT	Cardiac MRI
Acute coronary syndrome	+	++	++	++
Valvular heart disease	+++	+	++	+++
Ischemic evaluation	+	++	++	++
Differentiating cardiomyopathies	++	+	++	Most useful test +++
Ejection fraction	+++	+++	+++	+++

CT, computed tomography; MPI, myocardial perfusion imaging; MRI, magnetic resonance imaging; SPECT, single-photon emission computed tomography.

Invasive Testing

Invasive cardiovascular procedures include cardiac angiogram, intravascular ultrasound, cardiac venogram, peripheral angiography, and electrophysiology study. These are the most invasive tests with catheters placed into the vasculature, and they will be discussed in greater detail in other chapters. This chapter and Chapter 26 were designed in a format to help practitioners choose the best and most effective noninvasive diagnostic test to evaluate a patient's symptoms to guide evaluation and management strategies. When selecting an imaging modality or diagnostic test, consider the type of information required for diagnosis and management, risk and benefits of the test, and prognostic implications of any findings. Prior to choosing an imaging modality or diagnostic test, the examiner also needs to consider the pretest probability of the particular test and anticipate how certain results will change the clinical management. Through evidence-based medicine and guidelines outlined by professional health organizations, health care practitioners can become more confident in their choice of diagnostic testing strategies to best manage their patients.

For full reference citations to this chapter, please see "Section References" in the back of the book, under the heading "Section VI."

Cardiovascular Therapeutics and Interventions

SEVEN

Integration of Therapeutic Lifestyle Interventions

PATRICIA MATTICOLA AND RACHEL BARISH

A growing number of effective treatment modalities are now available for patients with cardiovascular disease (CVD), from aspirin to sophisticated invasive procedures, as highlighted in other chapters. However, the beneficial effect of a pharmacologic treatment or a surgical procedure is unlikely to result in a sustained survival benefit or improved quality of life if not accompanied by appropriate lifestyle changes. Indeed, neither taking a statin while eating fast food regularly nor being on antihypertensive medications while consuming excess salt in the diet is likely to obtain the desired health outcome. Even the best pharmacologic treatment and the most sophisticated invasive procedures to prevent and treat CVD will be unsuccessful if not integrated with lifestyle modifications. The integration of lifestyle modifications within a treatment plan has become important not only in CVD but also in other chronic conditions such as diabetes and obesity. This chapter addresses the specific evidence-based therapeutic lifestyle interventions for integration into primary care and specialty cardiovascular practices to improve patient-care outcomes, including a review of the role of diet and nutrition, weight management, physical activity, stress reduction, cardiac rehabilitation, sexual activity, smoking cessation, and substance abuse as they relate to CVD.

CVD is prevalent in our society, and CVD incidence and prevalence have increased worldwide over the past three decades (Gaziano & Gaziano, 2012); since 2000, CVD has become the leading cause of death worldwide. The high prevalence of CVD and the associated morbidity and mortality are directly related to specific risk factors and lifestyle habits. The evaluation for risk factors and the integration of therapeutic lifestyle interventions are key components to the prevention and management of CVD.

Studies such as the landmark Framingham study first identified the role of lipid management, physical activity, and smoking prevention or cessation for CVD risk reduction (Kannel, Dawber, Kagan, Revotskie, & Stokes, 1961; Ridker & Libby, 2008). Repeated, large-scale studies have identified these and other modifiable risk factors, which are responsible for the overwhelming majority of CVD (Hill, Fleming, & Kris-Etherton, 2009; Lim et al., 2012; Rees, Dyakova, Ward, et al., 2013; Ridker & Libby, 2008). In addition to lipid abnormalities, tobacco, and sedentary lifestyle, the World Health Organization (WHO) has added high blood pressure (BP) and overweight/obesity to a list of well-researched risk factors for the development of CVD (Lim et al., 2012). In order to determine the burden of risk factors for CVD, a research group organized by the WHO (Lim et al., 2012) analyzed both deaths and disability-adjusted life years (DALYs) to quantify mortality and morbidity from 67 different identified risk factors. The findings of this research substantiates that over the past decade, non-communicable diseases related to lifestyle have replaced communicable diseases as the leading causes of morbidity and mortality throughout the world (Gaziano & Gaziano, 2012; Lim et al., 2012). Elevated BP and high blood cholesterol were found to be the most significant contributors to CVD, followed by physical inactivity, overweight/obesity, and tobacco use (Gaziano & Gaziano, 2012; Lim et al., 2012).

Although diabetes mellitus (DM) is known to be a significant contributor to the development of CVD, it was classified as a separate disease, rather than a risk factor, and its impact on CVD was not quantified in the WHO research (Lim et al., 2012). The Action for Health in Diabetes, or Look AHEAD trial, aimed at quantifying the major cardiovascular event reduction in more than 5,000 overweight patients with DM in an intensive lifestyle-intervention group, with a control group receiving diabetes support and education (Wing et al., 2013). The study group received intensive on-site counseling, meal replacement products, and numerous strategies to engage in at least 175 minutes of vigorous physical activity per week. The trial was stopped early, after 9.6 years, as the study group failed to achieve a decrease in major CVD events during that time period. Although major CVD event reduction was not achieved, patients in the high-intensity intervention group obtained and sustained a 6% weight loss, lowered their glycated hemoglobin, were less likely to be treated with insulin, and had greater overall improvement in cardiovascular fitness than the control group (Wing et al., 2013). Previously, the INTERHEART study (Yusuf et al., 2004) analyzed data from patients in 262 centers in 52 countries experiencing their first myocardial infarction (MI), and it found that 90% of MIs were attributable to smoking, dyslipidemia, abdominal obesity, DM, hypertension, stress, poor diet, physical inactivity, and excess alcohol consumption.

The majority of Americans have one or more CVD risk factors; therefore, lifestyle modifications are identified as essential tools in CVD prevention and management (Eckel et al., 2013; Hsu et al., 2013; Pearson et al., 2013; Rees, Dyakova, Ward, Thorogood, & Brunner, 2013). These lifestyle modifications, which must be tailored to the individual patient's goals, include eating a healthy and nourishing diet, engaging in regular physical activity, avoiding cigarette smoking, achieving and maintaining a normal body size, managing stress appropriately, avoiding heavy alcohol intake, and abstaining from illicit drug use. With the increased awareness in the United States and elsewhere of the effects of poor diet and a sedentary lifestyle, dietary health and increased physical activity are ongoing health issues for the overall population (Pearson et al., 2013).

Within the American population, certain ethnicities experience worse CVD outcomes than others. Although overall mortality related to CVD has decreased, mortality remains disproportionately high in Black men and women (Go et al., 2014), with the CVD mortality rate for Black men 1.6 times that for Whites (Yancy, 2012). Black and Hispanic patients are more likely than their White and Asian counterparts to have CVD risk factors, including obesity, hypertension, and DM (Go et al., 2014). Black Americans have one of the highest rates of hypertension in the world, and many have genetic factors resulting in reduced effectiveness of certain pharmaceuticals in population (James et al., 2013; Yancy, 2012). Other populations, such as Asian Americans, have a lower overall risk of CVD (Hill et al., 2009; Rees, Dyakova, et al., 2013), with ongoing research focusing on both the genetic and behavioral bases for this reduced risk.

Racial and ethnic minorities are often underrepresented in CVD research with studies on risk reduction enrolling relatively small percentages of non-White participants, such as Latinos and African Americans (Bell, Lutsey, Windham, &

Folsom, 2013). Well-proven strategies among Caucasians have often been extended to non-White patients without the benefit of evidence to substantiate their usefulness in these populations. In addition, poorer health outcomes are documented among low-income populations, of which non-Whites are disproportionately represented (Kumar et al., 2013). Clinicians should, therefore, be aware that there may be additional challenges in adhering to dietary interventions among patients of certain ethnicities or diverse socioeconomic status, for access to healthy foods may be limited by virtue of where a patient resides or his or her ability to afford fresh fruits and vegetables (Dong et al., 2012).

Patients who are able to maintain a healthy body mass index (BMI), report a healthy diet, and engage in regular physical activity should still be reassessed for their CVD risk at regular intervals (Bell, Hayen, et al., 2013). Patients with low baseline risk and a low-to-intermediate risk as determined by the Framingham equation are recommended to continue to have their risk reevaluated at least every 2 years (Bell, Hayen, et al., 2013). Any significant alteration in clinical status, such as weight gain, change in smoking status, or self-reported change in level of physical activity, should also prompt clinicians to recalculate a patient's CVD risk, using the Framingham equation or an equivalent predictor of CVD risk (Bell, Hayen, et al., 2013).

In 2013, the American Heart Association (AHA)/American College of Cardiology (ACC) released the Pooled Risk Equation to provide a method to evaluate a 10-year risk for the development of atherosclerotic CVD in non–Hispanic African Americans and non–Hispanic White Americans, 40 to 79 years of age (Goff et al., 2013b). Unlike the Framingham Risk Score, the new equation represents a more diverse ethnic population and evaluates the development of a broader scope of atherosclerotic diseases, rather than coronary heart disease (CHD) alone. Atherosclerotic CVDs are defined as first nonfatal MI, CHD death, and nonfatal and fatal cerebral vascular accident. Components of the Pooled Risk Equation include age, gender, ethnicity, total cholesterol, high-density lipoprotein (HDL) cholesterol, systolic blood pressure (SBP), treatment for hypertension, diabetes, and smoking status. Risk-factor evaluation is recommended in all adults at 20 to 79 years of age who are free from atherosclerotic disease, and reevaluation is recommended every 4 to 6 years, with formal 10-year risk evaluation beginning at the age of 40 years (Goff et al., 2013b).

Regardless of risk stratification, all adults require healthy lifestyle behaviors (Eckel et al., 2013). Depending on a patient's history and current health status, lifestyle modifications are individualized to include a range of appropriate interventions. Primary prevention strategies for patients with relatively low risk of CVD include dietary modification, weight loss, and exercise, creating the benefit of risk reduction without the harms of potential side effects and other problems related to long-term medication usage (Rees, Dyakova, et al., 2013). Lifestyle modifications are generally as effective as medication and have been found to be more cost effective (Go et al., 2014). Secondary prevention strategies include weight loss programs for patients with morbid obesity and exercise rehabilitation programs for patients after MI. Although some patients may appear reluctant to make changes to their diet and exercise routines, these changes are as integral as prescribed medications in ensuring optimal BP and lipid levels (Gaziano & Gaziano, 2012).

When directing patients to make lifestyle changes, both clinicians and patients have an array of available recommendations and interventions to be considered. The cardiovascular clinician collaborates with individual patients to address current positive lifestyle choices and to determine the priority for improvements, as indicated. There are tools and theoretical frameworks to assess a person's readiness for lifestyle changes (Prochaska & Norcross, 2001), but initially, any patient needing to lose weight, increase physical activity, or quit smoking should simply be asked whether he or she is ready to make the change (Hochman, Feinstein, & Stauter, 2013) and should be provided with information on the benefits of lifestyle modification. A well-regarded framework that is used to guide patients through the process of changing health behaviors is the Transtheoretical Model developed by Prochaska, utilized in health care settings for behaviors, including diet modification, treatment for alcoholism and drug addiction, and smoking cessation (Prochaska & Norcross, 2001). The Transtheoretical Model consists of five stages, from the initial stages of precontemplation (not yet ready to make a change) and contemplation (considering a change), through preparation, action, and the final stage of maintenance after successful incorporation of the change (Prochaska & Norcross, 2001).

A motivated patient may make significant lifestyle changes, although others may respond to modifications in an incremental manner. Therefore, clinicians may consider repeat visits to follow up on complex lifestyle changes of smoking cessation, increasing exercise, or dietary modifications, or they may consider referral to other specialty providers. Table 28.1 provides a list of health professionals who may be a part of the team that promotes therapeutic lifestyle changes.

NUTRITIONAL INTERVENTIONS

With increased focus on the role of diet, current research offers definitive recommendations on conveying information to patients regarding specific dietary modifications, which can be adopted to reduce the risk of CVD. A meta-analysis conducted by Rees, Dyakova, et al. (2013) demonstrated that counseling on specific dietary interventions is beneficial in high-risk as well as in low-risk patients (Pearson et al., 2013). These conclusions were based on research findings of numerous prior studies of varying quality and duration. For example, a study by Buller et al. (1999) employed peer education to increase the daily intake of fruits and vegetables among low-income workers. The study was limited by the use of self-report in its methodology, although findings described that peer education provided statistically significant benefit in the daily intake of fruits and vegetables.

Health care providers evaluate patients to properly identify individual nutritional practices and to determine whether medical nutritional interventions are indicated. For clinicians who are unable to provide appropriate dietary counseling during the course of an office visit, presenting patients with information regarding improved diet can be accomplished by providing prepared written materials, or can be offered in a group setting, with equal benefit (Taylor, Ashton, Moxham, Hooper, & Ebrahim, 2011). Large-scale studies showed modest benefits with any of these interventions, so providers may select the method that works best within their area of practice, or the method to which they believe their patient would be the most receptive (Rees, Dyakova, et al., 2013).

The benefits of dietary counseling include reduced BP; decreased self-reported saturated fat consumption; decreased total cholesterol; and increased self-reported intake of fruits, vegetables, and fiber (Rees, Dyakova, et al., 2013). Ammerman et al. (2003) performed an randomized controlled trial (RCT) of more than 500 patients

TABLE 28.1 Health Professionals to Promote Therapeutic Lifestyle Interventions

Provider	Professional Qualifications	Service Offered	Potential Barriers
Registered dietician (RD) Registered dietician nutritionist (RDN)	Baccalaureate degree or higher An expert in food and nutrition Professional certification; licensure required in 46 states	Individualized or general meal planning Knowledge of appropriate diets for specific disease processes (diabetes, renal disease) Meal plans targeted for weight loss and ideal weight maintenance	Not always covered by insurance plans Not widely available in underserved communities
Personal trainer	High school diploma Professional certification	Individualized exercise programs Exercise plans targeted for weight loss	Not covered by insurance plans; cost may be prohibitive
Cognitive behavioral therapist (CBT)	Master's degree or doctorate in psychology or social work (PhD, PsyD, LCSW); professional certification and licensure as a therapist; postgraduate work as a CBT Certification awarded by the National Association of Cognitive-Behavioral Therapists	Talk therapy focused on one or more specific behavioral modifications	Not universally covered by insurance plans Not widely available in underserved areas
Certified tobacco treatment specialist	Associate's degree and health licensure (respiratory therapist, RN) or bachelor's degree or higher in any field Completion of an accredited course in tobacco treatment and maintenance of certification through continuing education	Reactive counseling for patients attempting to quit Referral to local support groups May be accessed in person or via telephone	May require telephone access
Certified diabetes educator	Health professional (clinical psychologist, registered nurse, occupational therapist, optometrist, pharmacist, physical therapist, physician (MD or DO), podiatrist, dietician or dietician nutritionist, physician assistant, exercise specialist, exercise physiologist, health educator, or a health professional with a master's degree or higher in social work who is trained and certified in diabetes education)	Individualized education and plans for management of DM Health care professional with specialized knowledge and expertise in diabetes care	May not be covered by insurance May not be widely available in underserved areas
Board certified advanced diabetes management certification (BC-ADM)	Registered nurse, registered dietician, registered pharmacist, physician assistant, physician (MD or DO)		

DM, diabetes mellitus; DO, doctor of osteopathy; MD, medical doctor.

Sources: Gulliksson et al. (2011); Jensen et al. (2013); Stead et al. (2013).

living in a rural area to examine the effects of dietary counseling on dietary changes and blood cholesterol levels. The participants who received face-to-face diet recommendations combined with reinforcement phone calls and newsletters had a statistically significant improvement in self-reported dietary intake, defined as a decrease in consumption of oils, high-fat dairy, and meats. Beckmann et al. (1995) studied the effect of dietary advice delivered by a nutritionist on BP, urinary sodium excretion, and circulating catecholamines in patients with moderate hypertension. The study authors reported that patients who were provided specific advice on reducing dietary sodium intake and losing weight at regular intervals over a 12-month period had improved BP measurements, as well as reduced levels of urinary sodium excretion, decreased body weight, and a decrease in blood levels of norepinephrine (Beckmann et al., 1995).

Challenges are inherent in conducting research on dietary interventions—specifically, it is difficult to enroll patients in long-term RCTs with complete control of food intake and accurate measurements to verify dietary adherence. To address these concerns, more recent studies have employed specific biomarkers, which improve accuracy of adherence to a healthier diet. These biomarkers include periodic measurements of micronutrients such as cholesterol, blood glucose, and urine sodium, as well as indicators of plant intake, such as beta-carotene (Rees, Dyakova, et al., 2013). Obtaining these measurements will be impractical for most clinicians due to associated costs and other logistical constraints, so in general practice, it is not possible to verify patient adherence to a recommended diet. However, it is essential for providers to evaluate dietary habits via noninvasive treatments such as weight measurement, BP checks, and use of a food diary or diet recall.

One population-specific diet widely studied for CVD prevention is the Mediterranean diet. Over the past several decades, the Mediterranean diet has been recognized due to the association of lower risk of CVD mortality among people living in southern Europe who consume a similar dietary pattern (Rees, Hartley, Flowers, et al., 2013). Numerous studies have substantiated the benefits of this dietary pattern, including a decrease in many of the co-morbidities associated with CVD, such as DM and metabolic syndrome (Rees, Hartley, Flowers, et al., 2013). One of the most recent RCTs studying the effect of the Mediterranean diet on CVD is the Spanish Prevención con Dieta Mediterránea, or PREDIMED, study (Estruch et al., 2013). In the PREDIMED trial, a group of 7,447 patients with confirmed CVD risk factors, but no documented CVD, were randomized into three groups: standard diet with advice to reduce dietary fat intake; Mediterranean diet supplemented with olive oil; and Mediterranean diet supplemented with nuts, primarily walnuts, almonds, and hazelnuts (Estruch et al., 2013). Dietary adherence was measured by patient self-report, and by measurement of a total of 16 specific biomarkers, including urinary hydroxytyrosol levels to determine adherence to olive oil intake and plasma alpha-lineolic acid to determine adherence to nut intake. After a period of 4.8 years, the trial ended, with findings of a statistically significant reduction in major cardiovascular events in the Mediterranean diet groups. This research has substantiated smaller studies that linked a reduction in endothelial dysfunction and inflammatory markers (Vincent-Baudry et al., 2005) with lower incidence of stroke in patients adhering to a Mediterranean diet (Samieri et al., 2011).

Ongoing research seeks to determine the specific micronutrients and enzymes that explain the cardioprotective features of this diet, but for the cardiology clinician, there are several key features to emphasize with patients. The "Mediterranean diet" is, in itself, a misleading term, since it does not refer to a weight-loss plan or a diet that should be followed for a brief period, but rather an eating pattern that is centered around fresh fruits and vegetables, whole-grain breads and cereals, healthy fats (primarily nuts and olive oil), and fish. Dairy products, red meat, and concentrated sweets are consumed sparingly. In addition, low to moderate amounts of red wine are consumed regularly with meals (Rees, Hartley, Flowers, et al., 2013). A high intake of fruits, vegetables, whole grains, and fish has been documented in other populations known to have lower risk of CVD, such as those living in Japan and the Pacific Rim (Kris-Etherton, Harris, & Appel, 2002).

Other diets specifically targeted at reducing CVD risk are listed in Table 28.2 and include the Dietary Approaches to Stop Hypertension (DASH), the American Diabetes Association (ADA) diet, and the AHA diet (Eckel et al., 2013; Hill et al., 2009). As with the Mediterranean diet, the DASH diet emphasizes the adoption of dietary strategies as consistent patterns of eating, even beyond the achievement of a particular weight or BP measurement. Although the DASH diet was initially developed to improve the BP of patients with known hypertension, it is established as an eating pattern for primary prevention of CVD (Go et al., 2014).

For some patients, the idea of undertaking an entirely new pattern of eating may seem overwhelming. In this situation, providers may choose to focus on certain elements of the Mediterranean, DASH, ADA, or AHA diets. Some research report benefits related to smaller interventions, such as increasing the daily intake of fruits and vegetables, increasing fiber intake, and decreasing total fat intake, with specific attention to decreasing saturated fats (Eckel et al., 2013; Hill et al., 2009; Rees, Hartley, Flowers, et al., 2013). Patients may consider making one small change at a time until eventually developing an eating pattern that more closely resembles those described earlier.

Specific foods in the Mediterranean diet are beneficial for CVD prevention in conjunction with an overall healthy diet and are recommended as small steps toward CVD risk reduction. Nuts, particularly walnuts and almonds, are associated with a decrease in all-cause and CVD mortality, as well as a reduced risk of major CV events (Bao et al., 2013). For those who are able to drink alcohol, moderate

TABLE 28.2 Common Dietary Recommendations

Dietary Approaches to Stop Hypertension (DASH)	American Diabetes Association (ADA) Diet	American Heart Association (AHA) Diet
Determination of daily caloric needs based on age, gender, and activity level	1,600–2,800 kCal/day based on gender and activity level	Dietary pattern that emphasizes:
Daily caloric intake ranges from 1,200 to 1,800 kCal/day based on the earlier criteria	Healthy carbohydrates—fruits, vegetables, whole grains, legumes, low-fat dairy products	Fruits Vegetables Whole grains Low-fat dairy products
Food intake consisting mainly of whole grains, fruits, and vegetables	Fiber-rich foods—vegetables, fruits, nuts, legumes, whole-wheat flour, bran	Poultry, fish, and nuts
Limited intake of low-fat dairy, lean meats, and nuts	Heart-healthy fish	Limiting: Red meat, high sugar foods, and high sugar beverages
Sweets and added sugars limited to three or fewer servings per week for most people	Good fats—avocados, almonds, pecans, walnuts, olives, canola oil, olive oil	
	Limiting: Saturated fats, trans fats, sodium, cholesterol	

consumption of one serving per day for women or two drinks per day for men has demonstrated cardioprotective effects (King, Mainous, & Geesey, 2008). Caffeine intake, in the form of coffee or green or black tea, has also demonstrated a modestly beneficial effect on the risk of CVD, including cardiovascular mortality and the prevention of heart failure (HF; Hartley et al., 2013; Lopez-Garcia, van Dam, Li, Rodriguez-Artalejo, & Hu, 2008; Mostofsky, Rice, Levitan, & Mittleman, 2012).

Dietary Modifications

Sodium

One of the most commonly recommended dietary modifications with respect to decreasing CVD risk is reducing salt intake, with recommendations provided by various organizations, including the U.S. Department of Agriculture, the WHO, and the Institute of Medicine (Table 28.3). Sodium reduction has been identified as a desired outcome at a population-wide level, based on the supposition that decreased salt intake will benefit healthy patients as well as those with known CVD risk factors such as hypertension (Go et al., 2014; Pearson et al., 2013; Rees, Dyakova, Flowers, et al., 2013; Taylor et al., 2011). On average, American adults consume 3,400 mg of sodium daily, generally attributable to processed foods, including canned and prepackaged foods, and food ordered in restaurants (Bibbins-Domingo, 2014; Eckel et al., 2013; Pearson et al., 2013). African Americans have been identified as being more sodium sensitive and should therefore receive specific advice regarding restricted salt intake (Kaplan, 2012). All patients should be advised to limit their sodium intake, and for certain patient populations, including patients with hypertension and HF, specific recommendations for sodium intake are often required. A starting point is to recommend reducing the addition of table salt and to select only prepackaged foods labeled as "low-sodium" (Eckel et al., 2013).

TABLE 28.3 General Dietary Recommendations for Sodium Intake by Organizations

Organization	Sodium Recommendation
U.S. Dept of Agriculture Dietary Guidelines for Americans, 7th edition 2010	< 2,300 mg/d for > 2 year olds < 1,500 mg/d for high-risk subgroups 　Hypertension 　DM 　Chronic kidney disease 　Older than 50 years 　African American
WHO	Recommends a reduction in sodium intake to reduce blood pressure and risk of CVD, stroke, and CHD Adults < 2 g/day sodium (5 g/day salt)
Institute of Medicine (IOM) Report 2014	1,500 mg/day minimum for essential nutrition 2,300 mg/day as upper limit

CHD, coronary heart disease; CVD, cardiovascular disease; DM; diabetes mellitus; WHO, World Health Organization.

Findings from the Institute of Medicine Report (Bibbins-Domingo, 2014) indicate that CVD is associated with higher sodium intake. Although reduced sodium intake is associated with decreased BP readings, controversy exists because the duration of this effect is not well established due to a lack of studies that included follow-up periods of greater than 12 months (DiNicolantonio et al., 2013; Taylor et al., 2011). However, a recent meta-analysis (Taylor et al., 2011) revealed that there was no mortality benefit of following a low-salt diet among normotensive or hypertensive patients. In addition, there are reports of higher mortality rate among advanced HF patients following a severely restricted sodium diet. Nevertheless, guideline recommendations on sodium reduction in patients with HF exist from professional organizations, as increased sodium intake is associated with HF exacerbations and clinical symptoms (Table 28.4). Evidence for these recommendations is generally based on expert opinion; therefore, dietary sodium recommendations must be individualized based on pharmacologic management, usual sodium intake, renal function, clinical status, and HF stage.

TABLE 28.4 Guideline Recommendations for Dietary Sodium in Patients With Heart Failure

Organization	Recommendation
ACCF/AHA 2013 Guideline for the management of HF 7.3.1.3	Stage A and B < 1,500 mg/day Stage C and D < 3,000 mg/day
HFSA 2010 comprehensive HF practice guidelines recommendation 6.2	2,000–3,000 mg/day < 2,000 mg/day for moderate to severe HF

ACCF, American College of Cardiology Foundation; AHA, American Heart Association; HF, heart failure.

Refined Sugar

After decades of intense focus on the role of salt and saturated fat in CVD, research is emerging that demonstrates that sugar intake contributes significantly to the development of CVD (Thornley, Tayler, & Sikaris, 2012). It has been established that diabetics and other patient populations with impaired glucose regulation, such as those with the metabolic syndrome, have an increased risk of developing CVD (Go et al., 2014; Thornley et al., 2012). However, the relationship between high sugar intake and CVD morbidity and mortality has not been well established (Thornley et al., 2012). Providers can certainly advise patients that a high intake of refined sugars, such as soft drinks and other sweetened beverages, is linked to conditions that are known to increase CVD risk, including type 2 DM and obesity (Thornley et al., 2012). Recently, drafted guidelines released by the WHO have called for a daily refined sugar intake of no more than 25 grams for adults, which equates to about six teaspoons, or less than is contained in one can of sugar-sweetened soda (WHO, 2014). In addition, there is little role for the use of refined carbohydrates and simple sugars in cardioprotective diets, such as the Mediterranean diet, which incorporates primarily whole grains with a very limited intake of foods with high concentrations of sugar (Hill et al., 2009).

Omega-3 and Omega-6 Fatty Acids

As most clinicians are aware, many patients take nutritional or herbal supplements in addition to prescribed medications for perceived or actual health benefits, and patients should be asked at each visit about over-the-counter supplements in addition to prescribed medications (Hill et al., 2009). Some nutritional supplements, such as omega-3 fatty acids, demonstrate a reduction of CVD risk (Hill et al., 2009; Hooper et al., 2006). Providers should be well versed in the role that supplements play in cardiovascular health, since they are a frequent topic of news reports in popular media and are likely to gain attention from patients accordingly. In addition, as more research emerges on the role of specific biochemicals, which contribute to the development of atherosclerosis, more specific enzymes and micronutrients may be associated with beneficial effects on CVD prevention and treatment (Ros & Hu, 2013).

The role of omega-3 and omega-6 fatty acids in CVD prevention was initially noted through population-specific research, which established lower incidence of CVD in groups, such as Eskimos, with a very high intake of oily fish (Hooper et al., 2006; Ros & Hu, 2013). Recently, research has also identified plant sources of omega-3s, such as flaxseed and linseed. Based on the purported benefits of omega-3s, substantial research has been conducted with mixed results. Several large-scale studies have demonstrated a decrease in CVD morbidity with increased intake of omega-3s from a number of sources, including both food (Table 28.5) and supplements (Hill et al., 2009; Kris-Etherton et al., 2002), whereas others have failed to demonstrate a decrease in CV events or mortality related to CVD (Hooper et al., 2006). Research in this area, including RCTs, is ongoing, with significant studies attributing a cardioprotective effect to omega-3s (Eckel et al., 2013; Hill et al., 2009).

TABLE 28.5 Food Sources of Omega-3 Fatty Acids

Fish	Nuts and Seeds	Oils	Vegetables
Salmon	Walnuts	Canola	Spinach
Halibut	Flaxseed	Olive	Kale
Albacore tuna	Soybeans	Flaxseed	Brussels sprouts
Herring	Chia	Fish	Watercress
Mackerel			
Sardines			
Trout			

There is an established link between omega-3 fatty acid consumption and reduced levels of total blood cholesterol and triglycerides (Krauss, 2012; Kris-Etherton et al., 2002). Omega-3s have demonstrated, in both animal and human models, to have antiplatelet and anti-inflammatory effects, which would explain the finding that high intake is correlated with decreased incidence of coronary artery disease (CAD) and sudden cardiac death (Krauss, 2012). Most researchers suggest that patients with and without known CVD should obtain most of their omega-3 intake through foods, primarily fish, and should only consume high doses of supplements such as fish oil under the guidance of their health care provider (Kris-Etherton et al., 2002).

Vitamin Supplementation

Apart from omega-3 fatty acids, there is conflicting research that demonstrates a reduced CVD risk related to the ingestion of specific vitamins and minerals (Rees, Hartley, Day, et al., 2013). The cardioprotective benefit of many specific vitamins and supplements is at least partially theoretical, based on the relationship between arteriosclerosis and an increase in circulating levels of C-reactive protein (CRP) and homocysteine (Marti-Carvajal, Sola, Lathyris, Karakitsiou, & Simancas-Racines, 2013). Therefore, antioxidant supplements, which reduce the blood homocysteine level, have been theorized to decrease the risk of CVD (Hill et al., 2009; Marti-Carvajal et al., 2013). B-complex vitamins, including vitamins B_6 and B_{12}, have been studied extensively to determine their role in CVD prevention, as determined by the rate of fatal and nonfatal MI as well as stroke (Hill et al., 2009; Marti-Carvajal et al., 2013). Based on a recent meta-analysis, there was no significant relationship between intake of B-complex vitamins and CVD morbidity and mortality reduction (Marti-Carvajal et al., 2013). Similarly, large-scale studies that have evaluated selenium, vitamin E, or antioxidant supplements have failed to demonstrate an effect on CV events, including nonfatal MIs and death (Hill et al., 2009; Myung et al., 2013; Qaseem et al., 2012; Rees, Hartley, Day, et al., 2013). At this time, there is no recommendation for patients to use any specific supplement for CVD risk reduction; instead, patients should attempt to eat a healthy diet, as previously described, with the knowledge that this is the best route to reduce CVD risk.

Studies in the past decade suggest that vitamin D (25-hydroxyvitamin D) deficiency is associated with higher rates of CVD and mortality, even when controlling for traditional CVD risk factors (Deo et al., 2011; Hsia et al., 2007). The exact mechanism for this relationship is poorly understood, although experimental models indicate decreased levels of vitamin D are associated with activation of the renin-angiotensin-aldosterone system and subsequent vasoconstriction. Similarly, a relationship between high levels of vitamin D and lower BP and triglycerides has been reported (Williams, Fraser, & Lawlor, 2011). One study (Deo et al., 2011) reported a statistically significant relationship between vitamin D deficiency in patients with hypoparathyroidism and increased risk of sudden cardiac death. However, in this study, patients with vitamin D deficiency alone were not found to be at increased risk of SCD. In addition, a large-scale RCT by Hsia et al. (2007) found no benefit from vitamin D supplementation on the development of CVD in generally healthy women.

WEIGHT MANAGEMENT AND WEIGHT LOSS

The AHA estimates that in 2014, 68% of all adults were obese or overweight (Go et al., 2014). Dietary changes are integrally related to weight management and weight loss to decrease or moderate risk for CVD. In addition, clinicians should be prepared to measure and address a patient's height and weight at every visit, with a minimum of once per year, because increased BMI leads to increased risk for CVD, as well as for developing CVD risk factors such as type 2 DM (Eckel et al., 2013; Jensen et al., 2013; Qaseem et al., 2012). General classifications for BMI are less than 18.5 kg/m^2, 18.5 to 24.9 kg/m^2, 25.0 to 29.9 kg/m^2, and greater than 30 kg/m^2

for underweight, normal weight, overweight, and obese patients, respectively. A patient's waist circumference should also be measured annually, since waist circumference greater than 88 cm in women or greater than 102 cm in men has been linked to increased risk for CVD (Jensen et al., 2013). Increased waist circumference is a criterion for the diagnosis of metabolic syndrome, which has been linked to increased CVD risk (Eckel et al., 2013; Taylor et al., 2011). Patients who have a BMI greater than 25 kg/m², or who are found to have increased waist circumference, should receive specific advice from their providers to lose weight, achieve a lower BMI, and reduce their waist circumference.

Clinicians can inform patients that there are numerous benefits associated with weight loss in terms of CVD risk reduction and related co-morbidities. Although the exact relationship between overweight or obesity and CVD has not been physiologically defined, there is an identified relationship between overweight and increased BP dating back to the Framingham study (Kannel et al., 1961). For hypertensive patients, the relationship between weight loss and BP reduction has been well established, although the exact amount of BP reduction achieved has varied among studies (Harsha & Bray, 2008). A meta-analysis of 25 randomized controlled trials by Neter, Stam, Kok, Grobbee, and Geleijnse (2003) calculated a decrease of 1 mmHg per 1 kg of body weight lost, for approximately 5 kg of weight reduction. There was a greater reduction in BP with losses of weight greater than 5 kg (Neter et al., 2003). Similarly, patients with type 2 DM experience a significant benefit from weight loss, with some cases of DM resolving after significant weight reduction (Sjostrom, Peltonen, Wedel, & Sjostrom, 2000).

Although the relationship between weight loss and DM is well established, there is more controversy regarding the connection between weight loss and hypertension, with some studies failing to show a significant benefit over time (Harsha & Bray, 2008). In a long-term study, overweight subjects were followed for an 8-year period after bariatric surgery (Sjostrom et al., 2000). There was a statistically significant impact on DM throughout follow-up, with some patients being effectively cured of DM through weight loss of 27 kg or more, but the impact on BP measurements did not persist beyond the initial 1-year period of dramatic weight reduction (Sjostrom et al., 2000).

Weight-Loss Strategies

For patients who are overweight or obese, clinicians must undertake a frank discussion about the risks associated with increased BMI, which include increased incidence of type 2 diabetes and all-cause mortality, in addition to increased CVD risk. The overall focus should be to encourage a weight loss of 1 to 2 pounds per week until the desired weight is achieved (Eckel et al., 2013; Jensen et al., 2013). Counseling regarding weight loss can be coordinated with discussions of dietary modifications and physical activity, and patients should be advised that even modest amounts of weight loss produce meaningful health benefits in terms of risk reduction (Jensen et al., 2013).

Patients may select from a wide range of healthier eating patterns, with a focus on long-term changes that will allow for slow, sustained weight reduction and then maintenance (Jensen et al., 2013). Table 28.6 includes a list of diets that result in sustained patterns of weight loss or maintenance of a healthy weight when

TABLE 28.6 Dietary Patterns for Weight Loss

Higher protein—25% of total calories protein

Higher protein Zone™-type diet—five meals/day, each with 30% of total calories protein

Lacto-ovo-vegetarian-style diet

Low-calorie diet

Low-carbohydrate (initially <20 g/day carbohydrate) diet

Low-glycemic-load diet

Lower fat (≤30% fat), high dairy (four servings/day) diets with or without increased fiber

Macronutrient-targeted diets (protein, fat, carbohydrate)

Mediterranean-style diet

Moderate protein (12% of total calories protein, 58% of total calories carbohydrate, 30% of total calories fat)

The AHA-style Step 1 diet (1,500–1,800 kcal/day, <30% of total calories from fat, <10% of total calories from saturated fat)

AHA, American Heart Association.

Adapted from Jensen et al. (2013).

combined with a recommended calorie deficit. Overweight and obese patients should be referred for nutrition and exercise counseling with health professionals, as previously described, to help navigate the complex process of making appropriate lifestyle changes. Follow-up, either in person or by electronic means, including telephone calls, is essential to assess progress and maintain motivation (Jensen et al., 2013). Any patient wishing to attempt a very restricted calorie diet consisting of less than 800 calories per day should be carefully followed and supervised medically to monitor vital signs and electrolytes, but an intensely calorie-restricted diet is not advised for the majority of patients (Jensen et al., 2013). Low-quality evidence suggests that meal replacement, in the form of bars or liquids, can result in weight loss for obese and overweight women. Further evidence is required to determine the extent of this benefit beyond a period of 6 months (Ashley et al., 2001; Jensen et al., 2013). However, the most effective weight-loss therapy provides a comprehensive approach of nutrition, physical activity, and behavioral strategies by a trained weight-loss interventionist, with equal to or more than 14 sessions in a 6-month period (Jensen et al., 2013).

Pharmacologic Treatments for Weight Loss

In spite of the obesity epidemic, primary-care providers and cardiology specialists do not routinely prescribe medications for weight loss. Although weight-loss medications are not a mainstay of treatment for obesity, they may be considered for short- or long-term use in appropriate patients (Jensen et al., 2013; Ryan & Bray, 2013). Pharmacologic weight-loss therapy should generally be used in patients with a BMI greater than 30, and administered with careful follow-up by the prescriber (Ryan & Bray, 2013) and concomitant use of lifestyle interventions as discussed throughout this chapter. Locaserin, a schedule IV medication, and phentermine-topiramate are approved for a BMI equal to or greater than 30 or a BMI equal to or greater than 27 with a related health condition, including hypertension, diabetes, or dyslipidemia. Table 28.7 addresses current medications, which can be prescribed for weight loss,

TABLE 28.7 Pharmacologic Therapies for Weight Loss

Medication	Adverse Effects	Contraindications

Orlistat
  Prescription 120 mg, Xenical
  Over the counter 60 mg, Alli®
	Stomach pain
	Flatus
	Diarrhea
	Stool leakage
	Severe liver injury (rare)
		Liver disease
		Eating disorders
		Renal calculi
		Pancreatitis
		Gallbladder disease
		Pregnancy category X

Lorcaserin (Belviq®) 10 mg twice a day	Headaches Dizziness Nausea Fatigue Constipation Dry mouth Hypoglycemia with diabetes	Concomitant use of SSRI, SSNRI, tricyclic antidepressents, bupropion, triptans, lithium, tramadol, antipsychotics, or MAOI Medications that cause valvular heart disease Pregnancy
8 mg Naltrexone and 90 mg Bupropion (Contrave) U.S. Approval 9/2014 Extended release tablets Week 1—1 tablet a.m. Week 2—1 tablet a.m. and p.m. Week 3—2 tablets a.m. and 1 tablet p.m. Week 4 onward—2 tablets a.m. and p.m.	Nausea Constipation Headache Vomiting Dizziness Insomnia Dry mouth Diarrhea	Suicidal thoughts and behaviors Uncontrolled hypertension

Phentermine-topiramate (Qsymia®)
  Begin 3.75 mg/23 mg daily for
  14 days, then 7.5 mg/46 mg,
  and then consider discontinuing
  or escalating
	Dizziness
	Paraesthesia
	Insomnia
	Constipation
	Dry mouth
	Dysgeusia
		Pregnancy or planned pregnancy
		Glaucoma
		Hyperthyroidism
		Within 14 days of MAOI
		Known hypersensitivity
		Suicidal thoughts or behaviors

MAOI, monoamine oxidase inhibitor; SSNRI, serotonin-norepinephrine reuptake inhibitor; SSRI, selective serotonin reuptake inhibitor.

as well as their general contraindications. The most effective medication, phentermine-topiramate, has produced a mean weight loss of 10% of total body mass in patients observed in clinical trials (Ryan & Bray, 2013). Lorcaserin and orlistat have achieved a more modest weight loss of 5% and 4% of body mass, respectively (Ryan & Bray, 2013).

Bariatric Surgery

For patients with a BMI greater than 40, or a BMI greater than 35 with obesity-related co-morbidities such as CAD and DM, bariatric surgery may be considered when attempted lifestyle interventions, including diet and exercise, have failed to produce sustained weight loss (Jensen et al., 2013; Pories, 2008). Referral to a bariatric specialty practice for further consultation is warranted (Pories, 2008), as there are several types of bariatric surgery, which are listed in Table 28.8. When referring, consider preoperative risk evaluation for abdominal surgery, or whether cardiac testing is warranted before proceeding. Bariatric surgery is contraindicated in patients with severe untreated emotional or substance abuse disorders, and the surgery is relatively contraindicated in patients older than 70 years or younger than 18 years and in patients lacking adequate social or emotional support (Pories, 2008).

TABLE 28.8 Types of Bariatric Surgery

Commonly in current practice
■ Gastric bypass
■ Adjustable gastric band
■ Biliopancreatic bypass with duodenal switch

Rare
■ Intestinal bypass
■ Vertical banded gastroplasty
■ Minigastric loop bypass

SMOKING CESSATION AND SUBSTANCE ABUSE

Any discussion of lifestyle modification to decrease CVD risk must address alcohol, tobacco, and illicit drugs, all of which are known to play a significant role in specific types of CVD morbidity and mortality (van Sluijs, van Poppel, & van Mechelen, 2004; World Health Organization, 2013). In particular, tobacco is the most common preventable cause of death among all causes, as well as a major contributor to CVD mortality (WHO, 2013). Smoking has been implicated as a major risk factor in numerous cardiovascular morbidities, including CHD, cerebral vascular disease, abdominal aortic aneurysm, and peripheral vascular disease. Large-scale, population-based efforts have focused on the prevention of smoking in young people and smoking cessation in adults, and although the exact benefits of these mass media interventions are unclear, smoking rates in the United States have declined over the past several decades (Bala, Strzeszynski, Topor-Madry, & Cahill, 2013). However, providers should continue to evaluate smoking at every visit, and encourage patients who smoke to stop. This single intervention of providing a suggestion to quit and assessing readiness in every patient who smokes has demonstrated benefits (Okuyemi, Nollen, & Ahluwalia, 2006). An initial assessment of the patient's interest in quitting can be made at the first visit, and follow-up discussions, including encouragement, counseling, and advice, can be delivered during subsequent encounters (Okuyemi et al., 2006; van Sluijs et al., 2004). Clinicians may also consider providing contact information for outside programs that provide telephone support and counseling for patients who are attempting to stop smoking (Stead et al., 2013). For patients who prefer a pharmacologic aid, or for patients who have tried to discontinue smoking unsuccessfully, several possible interventions are discussed in Table 28.9 (Cahill, Stead, & Lancaster, 2012; Okuyemi et al., 2006; MainHealth Center for Tobacco Independence, 2011; van Sluijs et al., 2004).

Moderate alcohol intake, defined as no more than two drinks a day for men and one drink a day for women, confers a cardioprotective effect, whereas excessive alcohol consumption can have cardiotoxic effects (Bonow, Mann, Zipes, & Libby, 2012). Excessive alcohol has direct, harmful effects on the myocardium, and it contributes to co-morbidities such as hypertension, arrhythmias, and cardiomyopathy (Bonow et al., 2012). Patients who regularly consume alcohol are at significantly increased risk for developing left ventricular dysfunction, even if they are considered social drinkers rather than alcoholics (Bonow et al., 2012). Heavy alcohol intake is associated with increased risk of other cardiovascular disorders, including

TABLE 26.9 Tobacco Treatment Medication Dosing Chart

Product	Nicotine Patch	Nicotine Gum	Nicotine Lozenge	Nicotine Nasal Spray	Nicotine Inhaler	Bupropion SR	Varenicline
Brand name/generic available	Nicoderm CQ® habitrol generic	Nicorette® generic	Nicorette® generic Mini form also available	Nicotrol NS®	Nicotrol® inhaler	Zyban® Wellbutrin SR® generic	Chantix®
Product strength	21 mg, 14 mg, 7 mg	2 mg, 4 mg	2 mg, 4 mg	10 mg/mL (10 mL bottle ~ 200 applications)	10 mg/cartridge	150 mg SR	0.5 mg, 1 mg
Standard dosing— (adjustments in dose and/or duration may be needed for optimal benefit and/or reducing risk of side effects)	1 patch / 24 hours 11+ cigarettes per day, use 21 mg for 6 weeks, 14 mg for 2 weeks, 7 mg for 2 weeks 6–10 cigarettes per day, use 14 mg for 6 weeks, 7 mg for 2 weeks	Use one piece every 1–2 hours 25+ cigarettes/ day or if first cigarette within 30 minutes of walking—start with 4 mg Maximum 20 per day Taper over past few weeks	Use one lozenge every 1–2 hours 20+ cigarettes/day or if first cigarette within 30 minutes of waking—start with 4 mg Maximum 24 lozenges/day Taper over past few weeks	1 spray each nostril/hour Do not exceed 5 doses/hour or 40 doses/day	6–16 cartridges/ day Use for 6 months, taper over past 3 months	150 mg daily for 7 days, then twice daily Start 7 days before target quit date	Begin 1 week before quit date Starter pack includes dose titration from 0.5 mg to 1 mg twice daily
Common side effects	Mild skin reactions: rotate site, apply 1% cortisone cream Sleep disturbance (vivid dreams, insomnia not from withdrawal): may remove at night	Mouth soreness, hiccup, jaw ache, indigestion	Nausea, hiccups, heartburn, headache, coughing	Nose, throat, or eye irritation; runny nose Higher dependence potential compared with other NRT	Mouth or throat irritation, cough, taste change	Insomnia, dry mouth, gastrointestinal symptoms	Nausea, vomiting, gas, constipation, appetite change, headache, sleep disturbance, unusual dreams, drowsiness
Less common, rare, or serious side effects may include, but are not limited to	Signs of excessive nicotine include rapid heart rate, chest pain, dizziness, stomachache, diarrhea, nausea, vomiting, drooling, cold sweat, weakness, headache, confusion, shaking, seizure.					*Behavioral:* include suicidality, agitation, violence, depressed or manic mood, confusion, hallucinations, impulsivity, anxiety *Medical:* seizures, hypertension, tremor	*Behavioral:* include suicidality, agitation, violence, depressed mood, confusion, hallucinations, impulsivity *Cardiovascular:* possible serious events such as MI

	Patch	Gum	Lozenge	Nasal spray	Inhaler	Bupropion	Varenicline
Brief instructions	Apply 1 patch to healthy, clean, dry, hairless skin such as upper arm, upper back, shoulders, lower back, or hip. Replace daily after waking. Rotate skin site. Wash hands after handling. Avoid moisturizers under patch	Chew gum until a peppery taste and slight tingle occurs, and park between cheek and gum. Repeat when taste fades, then park in another area of mouth. Avoid eating and drinking for 15 minutes before and after use	Allow lozenge to dissolve slowly without chewing or swallowing. Occasionally move lozenge from one side of mouth to the other. Avoid eating and drinking for 15 minutes before and after use	Blow nose if not clear and tilt head back. Insert bottle tip as far as comfortable, angling toward wall of nostril; do not sniff while spraying; wait 2–3 minutes before blowing nose	Inhale using short breaths or puffs to get vapor in mouth and throat but not lungs. Protect cartridges from excessive heat and light. Less effective if temperature <60°F	Take with food	Swallow with water. Avoid taking at bedtime. Do not make up a missed dose by doubling up the next dose. Avoid using nicotine replacement therapy (NRT) with Chantix. May need dose reduction: renal disease, elderly, weight less than 100 pounds
Cost (average)	$1.36 per day *generic / 1 patch per day	$7.14 per day *generic / 24 per day	$11.74 per day *generic / 20 per day	$15.00 per day / 40 doses per day	$19.36 per day / 16 cartridges per day	$1.24 per day *generic / 2 tablets per day	$2.78 per day / 2 tablets per day
Relative contraindications—partial list	Severe eczema or other skin disorder. Adhesive allergy	Dental disease, TMJ disease, dentures or other dental appliances, toothless	Oral thrush, oral lesions	Rhinitis, nasal polyps, sinusitis, asthma, or other severe reactive airway disease	Asthma or other severe reactive airway disease. COPD, allergy to menthol	Seizure history or risk for seizures (e.g. bulimia, head injury, alcohol detox); some mental health conditions; uncontrolled hypertension	Suicidal, some serious mental health conditions (may be difficult to determine illness from adverse medication effect), recent cardiac event

Unstable CVD and some acute post-op conditions—consult with physician.

Monitor or consider alternatives if: peptic ulcer disease, endocrine disorders, severe kidney or liver disease, malignant hypertension.

Special populations: Must consider risks/benefits/alternatives to medication. *Pregnant/lactating women:* limited safety testing, no medicines are FDA approved for tobacco treatment. *Youth:* no evidence for efficacy; probably safe; no FDA-approved medication. *Cardiovascular disease:* NRT considered safe for most, but caution if recent MI or stroke, arrhythmia, unstable angina; 2011 CVD warnings with varenicline; bupropion may increase BP; consult with physician. *Psychiatric disorders:* all are generally safe, but potential for psychiatric destabilization with nicotine withdrawal, changes in psych med metabolism, and/or some of these medications, consider psychiatric consultation.

Allergic reactions: Possible for any of these medications. Symptoms include: difficulty in breathing or swallowing; swelling of face, mouth, tongue; lips; hives; blistering rash. Immediate medical assistance recommended. Past hypersensitivity or allergic reactions to the medication or any of its components is a contraindication for use.

Rx duration: Treatment is recommended for 3 months for most medications, but a longer time is appropriate for many people. Consultation with a health care provider is recommended for a longer duration.

(continued)

TABLE 28.9 Tobacco Treatment Medication Dosing Chart (*continued*)

	Medication Dosing Guidelines for the Treatment of Smokeless Tobacco and Cigars
Smokeless tobacco	If using 1 can/week, suggest starting dose of 21-mg patch/day *OR* 4 mg gum *OR* 4 mg lozenge. If using < 1 can/week, suggest starting dose of 14-mg patch/day *OR* 2 mg gum *OR* 2 mg lozenge. Consider bupropion at same dose for cigarette use.
Cigar/Stogie	If using small cigars, consider dosing similar to that of smoking cigarettes. If using 2 or more medium-sized cigars/day suggest starting with 21-mg patch *OR* 4 mg gum *OR* 4 mg lozenge. If using 1 or more large, stogie-sized cigars/day, suggest starting with 21-mg patch *OR* 4 mg gum *OR* 4 mg lozenge. Consider bupropion at the same dose for cigarette use.

The PHS Clinical Practice Guideline 2008 update does not recommend use of tobacco treatment medications for smokeless tobacco use due to lack of sufficient evidence of its efficacy. The variety of products and individual differences in use patterns make it difficult to have precise dose guidelines. We recommend that tobacco treatment specialists discuss this with their clients and help clients monitor and adjust dose and frequency of NRT based on symptoms, increasing dose if withdrawal symptoms are high and decreasing it if there are symptoms of nicotine excess.

This chart is strictly for the convenience of consumers and providers. Information is simplified and may not reflect the most recent safety updates. Consumers are advised to consult a physician, nurse, or tobacco treatment specialist for more information regarding individual circumstances. Providers are advised to consult MedlinePlus® or the manufacturer for more product information. Prices are approximations based on those found at www.drugstore.com in September 2011. By comparison, the average price of cigarettes in Maine as of 02/09 is $6–$7/pack.

- **STORE ALL MEDICATIONS OUT OF THE REACH OF PETS AND CHILDREN.**

Dispose of used medications properly.   *Updated 10/11*

FDA, Food and Drug Administration.

Reprinted with permission from MainHealth Center For Tobacco Independence.

cardiac arrhythmias of atrial fibrillation and flutter, as well as infective endocarditis (Mukamal, Tolstrup, Friberg, Jensen, & Gronbaek, 2005; Murdoch et al., 2009). Therefore, providers should encourage patients who are unable to adhere to the recommendations for moderate consumption to abstain from alcohol intake.

All patients presenting for cardiovascular evaluation should be evaluated for illicit drug use. Though cocaine use is much less common than alcohol or tobacco, it is the most frequent substance utilized by patients presenting to the emergency department, and it is known to have direct effects on the coronary arteries and the myocardium. Even occasional cocaine use can have serious effects on the heart, including increased risk of cerebral vascular accident, MI, life-threatening arrhythmias, aortic dissection, and sudden cardiac death (Bonow et al., 2012; Hsue, Salinas, Bolger, Benowitz, & Waters, 2002). Extended cocaine use can result in hypertension, angina, and myocarditis or endocarditis (Bonow et al., 2012). In addition, there are potential serious effects on the cardiac structure due to intravenous (IV) drug use, a route for any number of substances, including heroin, methamphetamine, and cocaine. Due to the potential introduction of pathogens into the bloodstream, IV drug use is a common etiology of tricuspid valve endocarditis, with *Staphylococcus aureus* being a common infectious organism (Murdoch et al., 2009).

PHYSICAL ACTIVITY

More than 60 years ago, a study revealed that the incidence of CHD was lower in British bus conductors climbing up and down stairs of double-deck buses and in postal carriers delivering mail on foot than peer bus drivers or postal workers who spent most of the day sitting (Morris et al., 1953). This was the first scientific demonstration of the important role of physical activity in the prevention of CVD. Since then, several studies documented the deleterious effects of physical inactivity on CVD (Hamilton, Healy, Dunstan, Zderic, & Owen, 2008). In 1992, the AHA included physical inactivity as a major risk factor for development of CAD, adding to established risk factors (Fletcher et al., 1996). In addition, physical inactivity has been recognized as having a negative impact on other chronic conditions, including type 2 DM, obesity, osteoporosis, depression, and cancer (Lee et al., 2012).

Among numerous strategies used to prevent CVD, regular physical activity reduces mortality risk. Several studies indicate that the higher the level of cardiorespiratory fitness, the less likely an individual will suffer premature cardiovascular death (Lee, 2010). As an example, it has been estimated that reducing sitting to less than 3 hours/day and television watching to less than 2 hours/day results in a gain-of-life expectancy of 2 years and 1.4 years, respectively (Katzmarzyk & Lee, 2012). As a result, all major cardiovascular professional societies have included physical activity among the strongest (Class I) recommendations for the prevention of CVD (Franklin et al., 2011).

Cardiovascular exercise refers to activities that cause a sustained increase in heart rate and breathing with an increase in the circulation of blood and oxygen throughout the body to the muscles. The mechanism by which exercise produces beneficial effects on the cardiovascular system includes modifications in the myocardium, skeletal muscle, and vascular system. For example, in patients with hypertension who perform regular aerobic exercise, arterial stiffness is lower when compared with their sedentary peers (Tanaka et al., 2000). At a molecular level, it has been demonstrated that the production of nitric oxide, a potent vasodilator, by the endothelium is increased during physical exercise (Hambrecht et al., 2003), resulting in lower peripheral resistance and increased tissue perfusion. Exercise also induces the mobilization of endothelial progenitor cells from the bone marrow, thereby enhancing the process of neovascularization and endothelial repair after a cardiovascular event (Conti & Macchi, 2013; Lenk, Uhlemann, Schuler, & Adams, 2011). On a broader scale, exercise is one of the physiologic mechanisms in CVD prevention that exerts antiatherogenic, anti-inflammatory, antithrombotic, and anti-ischemic effects, in addition to inducing autonomic functional changes and reducing age-related disability (Fletcher et al., 2001).

Indeed, a sedentary lifestyle is a major modifiable risk factor for the prevention of CVD. A recent analysis estimated that by eliminating physical inactivity, 6% of CHD worldwide may be prevented and life expectancy could be increased by 0.68 years (Lee et al., 2012). There are numerous reasons that people are less active these days as compared with a few decades ago: more widespread use of technology and mass transportation, and the rising incidence of sedentary jobs in developed nations. The average work week is now longer, with Americans working 47 hours per week (164 more hours a year than 20 years ago), and sedentary jobs have increased by 83% since 1950, with physically active jobs constituting about 25% of the workforce, which is 50% less than 1950. Simultaneously, the increased availability of food, including fast food and other forms of prepared foods, has resulted in a higher incidence of obesity.

In May 2013, the CDC reported that only one in five Americans is meeting the overall physical-activity recommendations. Not only is inactivity common, but it is also expensive. Amid rising overall health care costs, inactivity-related diseases affect employers directly through health plan–related costs and indirectly due to higher rates of absence, injury, and disability. Based on data from medical expenditures and productivity loss, it has been calculated that in 2003 the impact of physical inactivity for all U.S. adults reached approximately $251 billion (Chenoweth & Leutzinger, 2006).

Physical activity has been defined as "any bodily movements produced by skeletal muscles that result in energy expenditure" (Caspersen, Powell, & Christenson, 1985). Energy expenditure is commonly quantified in terms of kilocalories or metabolic equivalents (METs). One MET represents the resting energy expenditure during quiet sitting and is commonly defined as $3.5 \text{ mLO}_2 \cdot \text{kg}^{-1} \cdot \text{min}^{-1}$ or $\approx 250 \text{ mL/min}$ of oxygen consumed, which represents the average value for a standard 70-kg person. The METs can be converted to kilocalories (1 MET = 1 kcal $\cdot$ $\text{kg}^{-1} \cdot \text{h}^{-1}$). These values represent approximations, because factors of gender, age, and body composition affect measures of resting energy expenditure, and, thus, actual MET values may vary (Katch, McArdle, & Katch, 2011). Clinicians should assist patients in setting reasonable and achievable goals for physical activity based on factors such as age and co-morbidities; not everyone has to be a marathon runner to meet physical activity guidelines. For those who are starting an exercise program from a sedentary lifestyle, a practical tip would be 10,000 steps per day, which is equivalent to 5 miles. In fact, walking is a safe low-impact exercise that usually keeps the heart rate within 40% to 70% of the maximum predicted value (Fletcher et al., 2013).

TABLE 28.10. Energy Expenditure for 1 Hour of Activity, Based on Body Weight

Physical Activity	100 lbs (kcal)	150 lbs (kcal)	200 lbs (kcal)
Walking, 2 miles per hr	160	240	312
Bicycling, 6 miles per hr	160	240	312
Swimming, 25 yards per min	185	275	358
Walking, 3 miles per hr	210	320	416
Tennis, singles	265	400	535
Walking, 4.5 miles per hr	295	440	572
Jogging, 7 miles per hr	610	920	1,230
Running, 10 miles per hr	850	1,280	1,664

Source: American Heart Association (2015).

Table 28.10 provides estimates, in increasing order, of the approximate calories spent per hour by a 100-, 150-, and 200-pound person for particular activities. As a rough estimate, it has been determined that an expenditure of 3,500 kilocalories (kcal) corresponds to a weight loss of 1 pound.

Resistance training is a form of physical activity made of movements against resistance of low to moderate intensity, using weights or bands. This allows for increased strength and improved muscle mass, which increases activity and raises the basal metabolic rate; among the older adult, it decreases fall risk and improves performance of activities of daily living (Fletcher et al., 1996).

Guidelines for Physical Activity

From a practical perspective, the AHA suggests one of the following recommendations for physical activity in adults:

- At least 30 minutes of moderate-intensity aerobic activity at least 5 days per week for a total of 150 minutes, and/or
- At least 25 minutes of vigorous aerobic activity at least 3 days per week for a total of 75 minutes. For additional health benefits, a moderate- to high-intensity muscle-strengthening activity at least 2 days per week is also recommended when feasible (Smith et al., 2011).

When the recommendations for physical exercise given earlier are adhered to, they are effective. A study of more than 250,000 adults between the ages of 50 and 70 years found that in those achieving levels of moderate activity according to recommendations, the mortality risk was 27% lower compared with inactive people (Leitzmann et al., 2007).

Given the inherent risks associated with a sedentary lifestyle, physical-activity assessment should be considered a vital health measurement that is tracked regularly by medical providers. There are subjective and objective means to assess the level of physical activity in an individual person. Easy subjective methods are self-report via physical activity questionnaires and physical activity diaries or logs. Objective methods include pedometers, heart rate monitoring, indirect calorimetry, the doubly labeled water method, direct observation, accelerometers, and motion sensors (Strath et al., 2013). Fortunately, the current explosion of electronic devices in our society has made high-tech and convenient modalities available to monitor physical activity.

Pre-Exercise Screening and Clearance

There are multiple considerations before beginning an exercise program. In general, contraindications to physical exercise include unstable ischemic symptoms, severe valvular heart disease, decompensated HF, and potentially life-threatening arrhythmias that exercise may worsen. Healthy adults do not generally require formal medical screening before starting a low- to moderate-intensity exercise program. However, if a person is experiencing chest pain, palpitations, dyspnea, lightheadedness, or joint pain with exercise, he or she should seek evaluation. Likewise, medical screening is advisable before engaging in vigorous exercise programs, especially in the elderly or for patients known to be at high risk for CHD based on risk factors. For example, patients with known CVD should generally undergo a baseline exercise stress test before the start of cardiac rehabilitation or exercise. Patients who do not have a stress test after acute coronary syndrome or surgery and are not referred to cardiac rehabilitation should initiate a low-intensity program, such as walking, under the direction of a health care provider, with attention to any cardiac symptoms.

As a general rule, different types of physical activity for specific conditions are individualized based on age, body weight, and medical co-morbidities. The tolerability of physical exercise, as well as the prognosis in patients with heart disease, generally worsens with the extent of the disease, reduced left ventricular function, inducible ischemia, valvular disorders, and the presence of arrhythmia. In addition, in people older than 75 years, it is important to start exercise at low levels and to increase in small increments with intermittent rest periods. In patients with balance disorders, bicycle ergometer is usually a good choice of physical exercise. The description of an individually tailored and safe exercise program for CVD prevention is out of the scope of this chapter and should be discussed in consultation with a health care provider; however, Table 28.11 provides physical activity considerations for different cardiac conditions.

For patients who have undergone coronary artery bypass graft (CABG), an examination is required before initiating exercise to rule out wound infections and instability of the sternum; upper-extremity resistance training exercise is also generally delayed for 4 to 6 weeks post-CABG. Similarly, a delay in resuming physical exercise after MI or percutaneous coronary intervention should be considered to guarantee safe recovery of myocardial function. Patients who have a cardiac transplant usually enter a medically supervised exercise program after discharge. Although the denervated donor heart has altered physiologic responses to exercise, endurance capacity is improved with exercise. In patients with peripheral vascular disease, intermittent bouts of walking exercise can be performed until mild to moderate claudication symptoms develop, followed by rest until pain has completely subsided. Then, activity may be resumed to a similar level for 50 minutes daily.

TABLE 28.11 Physical Activity Considerations in Select Cardiovascular Conditions

Condition	Considerations
Atrial fibrillation	Regularly scheduled moderate exercise as long as rate is controlled
Heart failure	If compensated
Implantable cardioverter defibrillator (ICD)	Evaluate device's cutoff rate before beginning exercise
Myocardial infarction	Exercise training can be initiated 1 week after acute coronary syndrome, if clinically stable
Permanent pacemaker (PPM)	Evaluate type of PPM, setting, and sensor to detect activity in rate responsive pacemakers
Percutaneous coronary intervention (PCI)	1–2 weeks of recovery time before start of exercise
Valvular disease	Evaluate degree of abnormality, generally contraindicated in severe aortic stenosis

Source: Fletcher et al. (2013).

Benefits of Physical Activity

There are numerous documented benefits on cardiovascular health from regular physical activity, including an improvement of mental and physical wellness, prolonging health, reducing risk factors, and strengthening the immune system (Fletcher et al., 2001). In addition, regular physical activity can relieve tension, anxiety, depression, and anger. Not only do patients experience a "feeling good" sensation immediately after physical activity but, in general, most people also note an improvement in overall well-being over time, as physical activity becomes a part of a daily or weekly routine. Exercise increases the flow of oxygen to the brain, which directly affects mental acuity and memory. It also enhances the immune system and decreases the risk of developing chronic diseases such as cancer. Becoming more active can lower the BP by as much as 5 to 7 mmHg (Fagard & Cornelissen, 2007; Pescatello, 2004), the same reduction in BP obtained with some antihypertensive medications, and reduce levels of low-density lipoprotein (LDL) and non-HDL cholesterol (Eckel et al., 2013). On the contrary, without regular physical activity, the body slowly loses its strength, stamina, and ability to function well, impacting overall survival. In July 2013, the AHA stated that for each hour of regular exercise, about 2 hours of additional life expectancy are gained, even when beginning in middle age. Moderate exercise, such as brisk walking for as little as 30 minutes a day, has the proven health benefits listed earlier. Other benefits of general health include weight control, prevention of bone loss, and improvement in the quality of sleep (American Heart Association [AHA], 2013).

Challenges to Following Physical Activity Recommendations

One of the major challenges related to maintaining exercise programs is consistent adherence. Adherence is a major determinant for obtaining the beneficial effects of regular physical activity, and multiple reasons contribute to reduced adherence. In the elderly, the reasons for reduced adherence include sickness, pain, or associated co-morbidities. In the younger population, lack of education, economics, and time limitations are reported as significant (Leijon, Faskunger, Bendtsen, Festin, & Nilsen, 2011). Changing sedentary habits in adults and the elderly is often a difficult and unrewarding task. The strategic impact goals from the AHA will target a 20% improvement in cardiovascular health. "Ideal cardiovascular health" is defined as the absence of disease and the presence of seven key health factors, including BP control, adequate physical activity, normal cholesterol levels, healthy diet, normal weight, normal glucose levels and the absence of smoking (Go et al., 2013). It is speculated that a legitimate approach commences with increasing physical activity in school children, postulating that an early adoption of an active lifestyle may continue through adulthood. Other measures that could improve implementation are a reward-based system for employees who participate in regular exercise programs, funding for gym membership fees, as well as tax deductions for sports equipment.

The literature on controlling hypertension, diabetes, hyperlipidemia, and obesity encourages the reduction of risks for cardiovascular events regardless of whether it is geared at primary or secondary prevention. Exercise is a way to improve all of these risk factors. This highlights the underlying principles that medications, surgery, and invasive treatments obtain limited results if not accompanied by lifestyle modifications, including consistent physical activity.

Initiating an Exercise Program

Simple, practical habits, such as taking 10,000 steps daily and maintaining an exercise diary, help maintain a regular schedule of physical activity. Physical activity at home may be more convenient and comfortable than going to an outside facility. Activity also provides a good example for family members, including children. At home, exercise can be combined with other activities, such as watching television. Buying exercise equipment for the home is a one-time expense that benefits other family members and allows patients to have short bouts of activity several times a day. Other practical tips that combine exercise with ordinary daily activities include doing housework, gardening, walking or biking to the corner store instead of driving, and parking farther away at the shopping mall and walking the extra distance. The AHA supports the implementation of a comprehensive set of wellness initiatives at workplaces. Such programs can be an important means of addressing the nation's rising obesity rates, sedentary behavior, and increasing prevalence of chronic disease.

COMPLEMENTARY THERAPIES

Stress Management

Stress can be defined as any physical, chemical, or emotional factor that generates bodily or mental tension and may be a factor in disease causation. Under physiologic circumstances, stress is part of a normal physical reaction to events that are threatening or upsetting to balance. Stress can be physical or emotional, and there is an established connection between stress and CVD. Physical stress due to surgery, trauma, or intense physical exertion is a well-known trigger of cardiovascular events. Psychological stress in the absence of physical stress or illness has also been associated with cardiovascular effects. For example, during an earthquake, individuals living in the affected city and surrounding county who did not undergo direct physical trauma or increased physical exertions suffered a two- to five-times higher number of cardiac deaths compared with the usual rate (Kloner, Leor, Poole, & Perritt, 1997). The consequences of both physical and psychological stress are often determined by the intensity and duration of the stressor.

Though not included in the list of traditional risk factors for CVD, numerous mental and psychological states are increasingly recognized as important risk factors for increased cardiac morbidity. These include psychological stress; major depressive disorder; posttraumatic stress disorder; personality types with trends toward hostility, pessimism, and social isolation; and chronic anxiety (Barefoot & Schroll, 1996). This highlights the relevance of the mind–body connection in maintaining overall health. This connection was first described a century ago, observing the physiologic changes occurring in animals and humans exposed to stress experiencing a "fight or flight response" (Cannon, 1914). The stress response, modulated by the sympathetic nervous system, was better characterized years later in humans and includes increased heart rate, increased BP, increased respiratory rate, and metabolic shifts that liberate energy (Selye, 1956). Similarly, a relaxation response is associated with decreased oxygen consumption, decreased respiratory rate, decreased BP, and overall improved well-being (Dusek & Benson, 2009; Wallace, Benson, & Wilson, 1971).

The pathophysiologic mechanisms that link stress to CVD have been analyzed extensively (Bairey Merz et al., 2002). These mechanisms involve the hypothalamic–pituitary–adrenocortical and sympatho–adrenomedullary axes (Steptoe & Kivimaki, 2012; Figure 28.1) and provide compelling biologic plausibility of the positive effects of stress reduction using relaxation techniques that modify indices of autonomic activation (Brotman, Gloden, & Wittstein, 2007). Indeed, although there is still limited documented clinical efficacy of behavioral and psychological stress-reduction techniques in the prevention of cardiovascular events, stress-reduction strategies have an important role in the overall plan for the maintenance of cardiovascular health. Some of these strategies will be discussed later.

Due to growing evidence for stress as a major risk factor that contributes to CVD, multiple alternative therapies can be considered, some of which have demonstrated research to have specific benefits for preventing or treating CVD.

Yoga

Yoga is a practice centered on meditation, breathing, and postures. Although its purpose is to unite mind, body, and spirit, there are documented physical benefits of yoga, including better muscle flexibility, lower BP (Hagins, Rundle, Consedine, & Khalsa, 2014; Hagins, States, Selfe, & Innes, 2013), and fewer arrhythmic episodes (Dhanunjaya et al., 2013). Mechanisms attributed to the cardiovascular benefits of yoga are a decrease in activation of the sympathetic nervous system, an alteration in neuroendocrine status, and an alteration in inflammatory responses (Innes & Vincent, 2007).

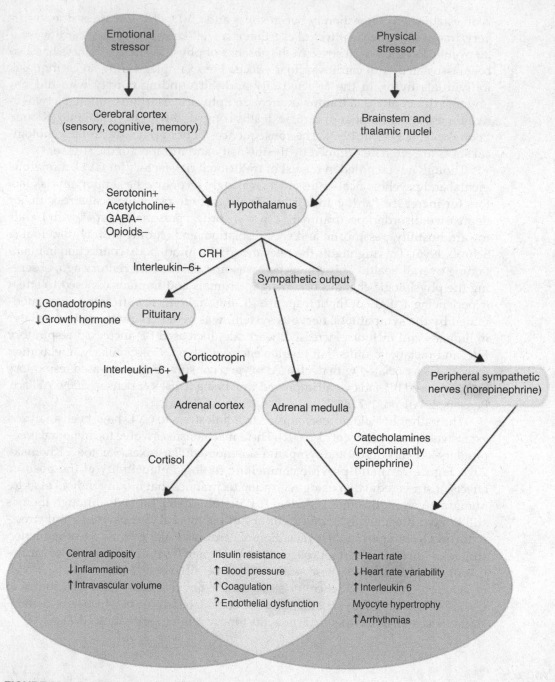

FIGURE 28.1 Cardiovascular effects of the stress response.

CRH, corticotropin-releasing hormone; GABA, γ-aminobutyric acid.

Reprinted from Brotman et al. (2007), with permission from Elsevier.

Massage Therapy

Massage is the manipulation of tissues (rubbing and kneading of muscles and joints) of the body with the hands in order to relieve tension or pain and can be effective for stress relief (AMTA, 2006). In many small studies, subjects in the massage group have shown significant changes in emotional states and stress levels (Field, 1996; Field, Hernandez-Reif, Diego, Schanberg, & Kuhn, 2005). In addition, a significant decrease in heart rate, SBP and diastolic blood pressure (DBP), and cortisol levels has been measured after receiving massage (Delaney, Leong, Watkins, & Brodie, 2002). Application of these effects on larger subject populations with CVD has not been studied.

Tai Chi and Qi Gong

Tai chi originated in China, and was developed by Taoist monks to honor and cultivate a person's innate healing ability and connections with others and the world. It involves gentle exercises of slow and graceful movements by following a set pattern; to improve balance, strength, and calmness; and to facilitate the flow of chi, or life-force energy, in order to restore internal balance and harmony. Tai chi is considered a low- to moderate-level physical exercise that teaches participants to be mindful of their capacity to perceive greater self-control and empowerment. Tai chi is believed to benefit cardiorespiratory function, the immune system, mental control, flexibility, and balance control; it also improves muscle strength and reduces the risk of falls in the elderly (Li, Hong, & Chan, 2001). Tai chi may improve symptoms, quality of life, and mood, but it does not appear to increase exercise capacity in HF (Yeh et al., 2011). Randomized trials are needed to substantiate the effects of tai chi on stress reduction.

Qi gong is another traditional Chinese exercise that uses meditation, breathing, and physical movement to promote body energy, or qi. Studies describe the effectiveness of the practice of qi gong in reducing levels of stress and anxiety (Wang et al., 2014). Self-practiced qi gong has been shown to reduce BP (Guo, Zhou, Nishimura, Teramukai, & Fukushima, 2008). More robust, randomized, and controlled trials are needed to prove the relevance of these studies.

Acupuncture

Acupuncture, which originated in China, is a practice of inserting fine needles through the skin at specific points to cure disease or relieve pain. Acupuncture is not indicated for the purposes of improving symptoms or reducing cardiovascular risk in patients with stable ischemic heart disease (Qaseem et al., 2012).

Thermal Stimulation

Hyperthermia involves increasing the core body temperature through sauna and other methods. Hyperthermia induced by sauna-level heat causes thermal stimulation, which may markedly increase endorphin level (Vescovi et al., 1992). Increasing core body temperature reduces BP and has significant benefits in patients with HF, including improvement in hemodynamics, endothelial function, and exercise tolerance (Kihara et al., 2002). Contraindications to thermal stimulation are unstable angina, recent MI, decompensated HF, severe aortic stenosis, hypotension, and concomitant alcohol use; relative contraindications include pregnancy, pulmonary hypertension, and use of certain antiepileptic medications (Hanuksela & Ellahham, 2001). Larger studies are needed to establish the clinical relevance of these findings.

Hypnosis

Hypnosis is the induction of a deeply relaxed and focused state through therapeutically provided suggestions, resulting in alterations of perception or behavior. Hypnosis has demonstrated effectiveness in the treatment of insomnia, smoking cessation, weight reduction (through adherence to diet modifications), and stress reduction (Wark, 2008). Improvement of these factors can positively affect a patient's cardiac-risk profile.

Meditation

Meditation is the act or process of spending time in quiet thought, allowing the mind to rest in an effort to obtain a higher realization. Transcendental meditation, promulgated by an international organization founded by the Indian guru Maharishi Mahesh Yogi, is a form of meditation that involves detaching oneself from anxiety and promoting harmony and self-realization by meditation, repetition of a mantra, and other yogic practices. The potential effects of meditation are decreases in anxiety, anger, worry, and depression. Transcendental meditation is reported to reduce mortality in patients with mild hypertension (Warburton et al., 2005). Research in this field suggests that cardiovascular benefits arise from normalization of neuroendocrine and autonomic nervous systems (Greeson, 2009).

Mindfulness-based stress reduction (MBSR) is a structured group program that employs mindfulness meditation (constantly focusing attention on thoughts that enter the minds and observing them without judgment) to alleviate the suffering associated with physical, psychosomatic, and psychiatric disorders. The program is based on a systematic procedure to develop enhanced awareness of a moment-to-moment experience of perceptible mental processes (Grossman, Niemann, Schmidt, & Walach, 2004). An MBSR program was reported to be effective in reducing anxiety and depressive symptoms, perceived stress, BP, and BMI in patients with CHD (Parswani, Sharma, & Iyengar, 2013).

Spirituality/Faith-Based Interventions

Many patients report engaging in some form of religious or spiritual practice, and some may feel that this has a beneficial effect on their health. Faith-based interventions have been documented to contribute to reducing SBP in African American women (Duru, Sarkisian, Leng, & Mangione, 2010).

Biofeedback

Biofeedback, a method of learning to control one's bodily functions by monitoring one's own brain waves, BP, and degree of muscle tension, has also been studied in patients with CVD and shown to provide some benefit in controlling hypertension (Lin et al., 2012).

Cognitive Behavioral Therapy

According to the British Association of Behavioral and Cognitive Psychotherapies, cognitive behavioral therapy (CBT) includes a range of therapies based on concepts and principles derived from psychological models of human emotion and behavior. There are different treatment approaches for emotional disorders that may have, as a secondary effect, modification of risk factors for CVD. The CBT intervention programs decrease the risk of recurrent CVD and recurrent acute MI. This may have implications for secondary preventive programs in patients with CHD (Gulliksson et al., 2011).

CARDIAC REHABILITATION

Cardiac rehabilitation is a behavior-modification program that consists of programmed regular exercise, dietary modification, smoking cessation, and education to control modifiable risk factors. Cardiac rehabilitation allows patients to regain their autonomy after developing cardiovascular problems that limit their regular physical activities. It decreases cardiovascular events; reduces modifiable risk factors by decreasing body weight, waist circumference, glucose levels, LDL cholesterol, and CRP levels; increases compliance with preventive medications; boosts exercise capacity; improves function in daily life and overall quality of life; and lends itself to lifelong healthy behaviors (Roca-Rodriguez et al., 2014). The demonstrated evidence-based benefits of cardiac rehabilitation as outlined by the American Association of Cardiovascular and Pulmonary Rehabilitation (AACPVR) in 2007 include: 20% to 30% reduction in all-cause mortality rates and reduced mortality risk at 5 years, improved adherence with preventive medications, reduced hospitalizations and use of medical resources, increased exercise performance, and improved health-related quality of life (Ries et al., 2007).

Class I indications for cardiac rehabilitation include CHD after MI or acute coronary syndrome, coronary angioplasty with or without stents, HF, chronic stable angina, coronary bypass surgery, peripheral artery disease, and CVD prevention in women (Ries et al., 2007). Cardiac rehabilitation programs are also indicated for patients with a left ventricular assist device, a heart or heart/lung transplant, or who have undergone a surgical valve repair. In February 2014, the Centers for Medicare and Medicaid Services (CMS) approved coverage for cardiac rehabilitation services to beneficiaries with stable, chronic HF, defined as patients with a left ventricular ejection fraction of 35% or less and those of the New York Heart Association (NYHA) experiencing Class II to IV symptoms and who have received optimal HF therapy for at least 6 weeks.

Expanding applications for cardiac rehabilitation are DM, HF with preserved ejection fraction, congenital heart disease, and pulmonary artery hypertension. Contraindications to cardiac rehabilitation include unstable angina, ventricular arrhythmias, decompensated HF, pulmonary arterial hypertension, intracavity thrombus, recent thrombophlebitis with or without pulmonary embolism, severe obstructive cardiomyopathy, severe aortic stenosis, uncontrolled inflammatory or infectious pathologies, and any musculoskeletal condition that prevents physical exercise (Warner, 2012).

As with programs of physical exercise, a close relationship between compliance to a cardiac rehabilitation program and outcomes has been observed: Patients who attended 36 sessions versus those who attended one session showed a 47% lower risk of death and a 31% lower risk of MI (Hammill, Curtis, & Whelihan, 2010). Unfortunately, despite the overwhelming improvement in mortality, cardiac rehabilitation remains underutilized, with only 14% to 35% of eligible MI survivors and approximately 31% of patients after CABG participating in programs. In addition, participation in cardiac rehabilitation tends to be lower in women, minorities, socioeconomically disadvantaged patients, and the elderly (Suaya, Shepard, Normand, Prottas, & Stason, 2007).

Timely referral to outpatient cardiac rehabilitation is essential to promote its appropriate use and to prevent deconditioning in this patient population. A medical order is required prior to starting a cardiac rehabilitation program, and the order is often provided to the patient prior to discharge from an acute-care facility. Patients usually wait for 6 weeks and until medically approved, after cardiac surgery, to begin an exercise program. In the interim, evaluation of patients prior to exercise initiation should include a symptom-limited exercise test while on medical therapy. This allows the provider to establish the patient's baseline exercise capacity. Exercise testing is a tool for assessment of any ischemic symptoms or arrhythmias that would require intervention prior to start of a formal exercise program. Patients not undergoing formal exercise testing after MI can safely exercise 20 beats per minute above their resting heart rate value or at a certain percentage above their resting heart rate (20%–30%), with incremental increases over the time span of the cardiac rehabilitation program (Bonow, Mann, Zipes, & Libby, 2012).

Cardiac rehabilitation programs are usually organized into three phases:

Phase 1 is the in-hospital program after an acute cardiac event or intervention: This helps with early mobilization and self-care, and it progresses to walking and stair climbing to include activities similar to the home environment.

Phase 2 consists of a physician-supervised exercise program after discharge in the outpatient setting, with heart rate and BP monitoring; it may include stress management, nutritional counseling, and smoking cessation. Usually, three sessions a week for a total of 36 sessions over a 3- to 4-month period, with gradual increases of activity level.

Phase 3 is the long-term maintenance program at home, a local gym, or at the cardiac rehabilitation center without monitoring.

A cardiac rehabilitation staff includes an on-site supervising physician/medical director, registered nurses, and other individuals with exercise-physiology training, all of whom must be trained in administering advanced cardiac life support (ACLS). Patients usually exercise under physician supervision for 12 weeks, typically involving three visits per week. Sessions generally consist of a 10- to 15-minute warm-up and stretching period, followed by 30 to 50 minutes of continuous aerobic exercise at an intensity of 50% to 80% of heart rate reserve calculated from the entry exercise treadmill test. Sessions end with a 15- to 20-minute cooldown period (Balady et al., 2000). Although there are risks associated with cardiac rehabilitation programs, estimated as one cardiac arrest for every 115,000 patient hours of cardiac rehabilitation and one death for every 750,000 patient hours of participation (Fletcher et al., 2013), nonetheless, on a large scale these risks are far outweighed by the numerous benefits in CV recovery and health. In the United States, private health insurance, Medicare, or Medicaid usually provide coverage for exercise training three times weekly for the duration of 12 or more weeks.

SEXUAL FUNCTION

Sexual activity, as an essential part of human function and quality of life, has potential implications in cardiovascular health and, simultaneously, is affected by CVD. Among the many benefits of maintaining sexual activity are lowered BP, increased physical activity, partner intimacy, lowered risk of heart attack in men, improved bladder control in women, stress reduction, and increased self-esteem, among other benefits. Studies have also documented the benefit of sexual activity on longevity in men and women (Palmore, 1982). CVD may contribute to sexual dysfunction in both men and women. A common complaint in the clinic setting for men is erectile dysfunction (ED). Erectile dysfunction, a pathologic alteration in the endothelium of penile vasculature or erectile tissue or impairment of neurovascular processes, increases in prevalence with aging and can result from either physiologic or psychological factors. Rates of erectile dysfunction among men with CVD are observed twice as frequently than in the general population (Steinke et al., 2013). Hypertension, diabetes, hyperlipidemia, depression, smoking, sedentary lifestyle, and obesity are recognized contributing factors of ED (Bacon et al., 2006). Sexual dysfunction is observed in women with CVD with similar rates.

Interestingly, ED has been identified as a sentinel marker for subsequent CVD (Thompson et al., 2005). Men with ED were found at risk for developing cardiac events over the next 10 years, thus identifying ED as a risk factor comparable to smoking or premature family history of CAD (Bohm et al., 2010). Studies have suggested that incidence of ED can be reduced through increased levels of physical activity. In 2007, a meta-analysis on erectile dysfunction and exercise estimated a 40% to 60% reduction in ED risk with moderate to higher levels of exercise (Cheng, Ng, Ko, & Chen, 2007). On the other hand, sexual activity can trigger MI, arrhythmia, or sudden death in a small minority of patients (Dahabreh & Paulus, 2011). Possible mechanisms for fatal cardiac events are the increase in heart rate and BP associated with sexual activity. As a result, some patients abstain from sexual activity after a coronary event for fear of reoccurrence of angina, MI, or sudden death. The use of phosphodiesterase inhibitors for ED is generally considered safe in the setting of CVD but is contraindicated with concomitant use of nitrates. It is important to emphasize to patients that medications prescribed for CVD should not be discontinued because of concerns about potential impact on sexual function.

According to the AHA, sexual activity is reasonable for male and female patients who can exercise more than 3 to 5 METs without angina, excessive dyspnea, ischemic ST-segment changes, cyanosis, hypotension, or arrhythmia. Patients with unstable, decompensated, and/or severe symptomatic CVD or patients with CVD who experience cardiovascular symptoms precipitated by sexual activity should defer sexual activity until their condition is stabilized and optimally managed. Women with CVD should be counseled regarding the safety and advisability of contraceptive methods and pregnancy when appropriate (Glenn et al., 2012).

Lifestyle factor modifications in conjunction with alternative therapies and traditional medicine are components of cardiovascular care. The integration of therapeutic lifestyle interventions have proved beneficial in improving quality of life and survival benefit in the setting of both primary and secondary prevention of CVD and serves as the cornerstone of all therapies.

For full reference citations to this chapter, please see "Section References" in the back of the book, under the heading "Section VII."

Pharmacotherapeutics of Hypertension and Hypertensive Emergencies

DEV CHATTERJI AND CONNIE H. YOON

PHARMACOTHERAPEUTICS OF CHRONIC HYPERTENSION

Hypertension is the most common chronic cardiovascular (CV) disease in the United States. Defined as elevated arterial blood pressure (BP), hypertension can contribute to the development of diseases of the heart, kidneys, brain, and many other systems. Although a healthy lifestyle is an integral component of the management of hypertension, proper pharmacologic management can significantly reduce morbidity and mortality associated with this condition. The Eighth Joint National Committee on the Detection, Evaluation, and Treatment of High Blood Pressure (JNC-8) and the American Society of Hypertension (ASH), in collaboration with the International Society of Hypertension (ISH), provide guidance to prescribers on the management of hypertension (James et al., 2013; Weber et al., 2013).

Pathophysiology

Adequate knowledge of the determinants of BP and the regulation of BP homeostasis is important to understand the pharmacologic basis of antihypertensive agents. In most patients, hypertension has no identifiable cause—this is classified as essential or primary hypertension, most likely a genetic condition. Secondary hypertension occurs when an underlying condition or medication is responsible for causing an elevation in BP.

Numerous mechanisms contribute to the pathogenesis of hypertension. The primary determinants of BP are cardiac output and total peripheral resistance. BP is maintained with intricate regulation, primarily by the autonomic nervous system and the kidneys. The autonomic nerves mediate the baroreceptor reflex to maintain BP at a preset level. If baroreceptors sense a decrease in BP, impulses are transmitted along sympathetic nerves to stimulate the heart and blood vessels to increase cardiac output and cause vasoconstriction in order to increase BP to the original preset level. If baroreceptors identify an increase in BP, the opposite response occurs. The kidneys play an important role in controlling blood volume and, therefore, BP. When the kidneys detect a decrease in BP, the body responds by retaining sodium and water. This results in an increase in blood volume, which subsequently augments cardiac output, thereby elevating BP. In addition, the renin-angiotensin-aldosterone system (RAAS) contributes to BP control via angiotensin II–mediated vasoconstriction and aldosterone-mediated water retention.

BP is controlled by the same mechanisms in both hypertensive patients and patients with normal BP. The pathologic difference in hypertensive patients is that the baroreceptors and renal blood volume control systems appear to "reset" the BP to a new, higher "normal" level. When this occurs, the control mechanisms described earlier respond to a "drop" in BP when, in fact, there is no true drop. All antihypertensive medications specifically target these various mechanisms of BP regulation.

Pharmacologic Therapy

There are approximately 10 different classes of medications for the treatment and management of hypertension. These are:

- Diuretics
- Angiotensin-converting enzyme inhibitors (ACEI)
- Angiotensin II receptor blockers (ARBs)
- Direct renin inhibitors
- Calcium channel blockers (CCBs)
- Beta-adrenergic receptor blockers (beta blockers)
- Alpha-1 receptor blockers
- Centrally acting alpha-2 agonists
- Peripheral adrenergic antagonists
- Direct acting vasodilators

Diuretics for Hypertension

Diuretics are agents that increase urine output. They have two major clinical applications—treatment of hypertension and reducing excess extracellular fluid volume associated with heart failure, cirrhosis, or kidney disease. There are four categories of diuretics with indications for the treatment of CV conditions: thiazide, loop, aldosterone antagonists, and potassium-sparing diuretics (Table 29.1). Among these, thiazide diuretics are the preferred agents for the treatment of hypertension. In general, diuretics exhibit their hypotensive actions by inhibiting sodium reabsorption at different segments of the renal tubular system. This results in decreased blood volume, leading to decreased cardiac filling (preload). The net result is a reduced cardiac output, which results in a lower BP. The degree of diuresis and natriuresis attributable to the diuretic is directly related to the amount of sodium reuptake that is blocked. Therefore, diuretics that exhibit their actions earlier in the nephron (Figure 29.1), where a greater degree of sodium reabsorption takes place, produce a greater degree of diuresis (Ernst & Moser, 2009).

Thiazide Diuretics

Thiazide diuretics are the preferred diuretic for most patients with hypertension. The ALLHAT (Antihypertensive and Lipid-Lowering Treatment to Prevent Heart Attack Trial) study provides strong evidence justifying their use in hypertension management (ALLHAT, 2002). These agents inhibit sodium reabsorption by antagonizing the $Na^+ Cl^-$ cotransporter in the distal convoluted tubule, where

TABLE 29.1 Diuretic Agents for Hypertension

Class	Agents (Brand Name)	Dosage* (mg/day)	Dosing Frequency	Clinical Pearls/Monitoring	Significant Drug Interactions
Thiazide	Chlorthalidone	12.5–100	Once daily	■ Usually once daily dosing	■ NSAIDs
	Hydrochlorothiazide (Microzide®)	12.5–50	1 to 2 divided doses	■ Avoid evening use to reduce nocturia ■ Side effects generally more prevalent in higher doses ■ Ineffective if CrCl <30 mL/min	■ Lithium
	Indapamide (Lozol®)	1.25–2.5	Once daily	■ Periodically monitor	
	Metolazone (Zaroxolyn®)	2.5–5	Once daily	• Electrolytes • Uric acid • Glucose • Lipid levels	
Loop	Furosemide (Lasix®)	40–80	2 divided doses	■ Most potent diuretics	■ NSAIDs
	Bumetanide (Bumex®)	0.5–10	1 to 2 divided doses for edema/heart failure	■ Monitor electrolytes ■ All agents with the exception of ethacrynic acid contain a sulfa moiety. Do not use in patients with a true sulfa allergy.	■ Aminoglycosides (increases risk of ototoxicity)
	Torsemide (Demadex®)	10–200	Once daily for edema/heart failure		
	Ethacrynic acid (Edecrin®)	50–400	1 to 2 divided doses for edema/heart failure		
Potassium sparing	Amiloride	5–20	Once daily	■ Onset of action is faster than aldosterone antagonists	■ NSAIDs
	Triamterene (Dyrenium®)	50–300	1 to 2 divided doses for edema	■ Weak diuretics ■ Often in combination with other diuretics ■ May cause hyperkalemia ■ Avoid in patients if CrCl <30 mL/min	■ ACEI ■ ARBs ■ Direct renin inhibitors
Aldosterone antagonists	Eplerenone (Inspra®)	50–100	1 to 2 divided doses	■ Diuretic effects of these agents are delayed and it takes about 1–2 days to see effects from these agents	■ NSAIDs
	Spironolactone (Aldactone®)	25–50	1 to 2 divided doses	■ Weak diuretics, often used in combination with other diuretics ■ May cause hyperkalemia ■ Avoid in patients if CrCl <30 mL/min	■ ACEI ■ ARBs ■ Direct renin inhibitors

ACEI, angiotensin-converting enzyme inhibitors; ARBs, angiotensin II receptor blockers; CrCl, creatinine clearance; NSAIDs, nonsteroidal anti-inflammatory drugs.

*Unless indicated, dosing recommendations listed are for the treatment of hypertension only. Doses may vary for heart failure and other indications. Only oral doses are listed; intravenous formulations may be available for certain agents.

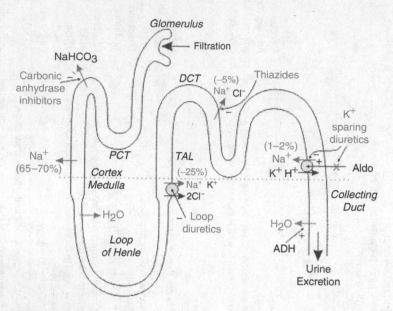

FIGURE 29.1 Diuretic sites of action.
Reprinted with permission from www.cvpharmacology.com.

approximately 5% to 10% of sodium is reabsorbed. With long-term use, thiazide diuretics also decrease total peripheral resistance, which is understood to be due to a reduction in sodium content of arteriolar smooth muscle cells. Among the thiazide diuretics, previous guidelines recommended hydrochlorothiazide as the thiazide of choice in hypertensive patients. New guidelines do not specify which thiazide should be selected, although chlorthalidone and indapamide have more compelling evidence for improving CV outcomes. Thiazide diuretics are very effective BP agents, but most agents in this class are ineffective when creatinine clearance (CrCl) is less than 30 mL/min. Adverse effects of these agents include hypokalemia, hypomagnesemia, hypercalcemia, hyperuricemia, hyperglycemia, and hypercholesterolemia. Thiazide diuretics are contraindicated in patients with severe hypersensitivity to sulfonamides because these agents are sulfonamide derivatives (Brater, 2000).

Loop Diuretics

Despite the greater diuretic and natriuretic effects of loop diuretics, they are usually less effective than thiazide diuretics in the management of hypertension. In general, loop diuretics are utilized in hypertension only in patients with chronic kidney disease (CKD) when estimated CrCl is less than 30 mL/min. Loop diuretics inhibit sodium reabsorption in the ascending loop of Henle, where approximately 20% to 25% of sodium is reabsorbed. Similar to thiazide diuretics, loop diuretics can cause hypokalemia and hypomagnesemia, but effects on serum lipids and glucose are not clinically significant. Loop diuretics can cause a dose-related ototoxicity, which is usually, but not always, reversible. Loop diuretics should be used with extreme caution in patients with a sulfonamide hypersensitivity, because the majority of the agents in this class are sulfonamide derivatives. Ethacrynic acid is a therapeutic option in patients with a "sulfa allergy," as this agent is not a sulfonamide derivative (Brater, 2000).

Potassium-Sparing Diuretics and Aldosterone Antagonists

Potassium-sparing diuretics are very weak diuretics. Their role in hypertension is primarily to counteract the potassium-wasting properties of the other diuretic agents. Potassium-sparing diuretics directly inhibit sodium channels on the aldosterone-sensitive Na^+/K^+-ATPase pump. Aldosterone antagonists, technically potassium-sparing agents, antagonize aldosterone in the distal segment of the nephron. Aldosterone acts to promote sodium uptake and retention, in exchange for potassium secretion, so blocking the actions of aldosterone produces the opposite effect. Notable adverse reactions with these agents include hyperkalemia and gynecomastia, which is more prevalent with spironolactone (Brater, 2000).

Angiotensin-Converting Enzyme Inhibitors

The RAAS is essential in the regulation of BP. The ACEI suppress RAAS activation by blocking angiotensin-converting enzyme (ACE), which converts angiotensin I to angiotensin II (Figure 29.2). This leads to less angiotensin II–mediated vasoconstriction and a reduction in the release of aldosterone. ACEI also prevent the breakdown of the peptide bradykinin, which results in vasodilation of blood vessels.

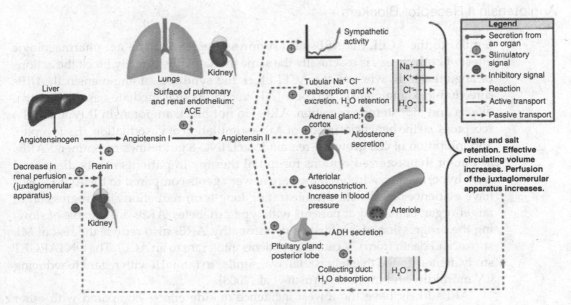

FIGURE 29.2 The renin-angiotensin-aldosterone system (RAAS).

ACE, angiotensin-converting enzyme; ADH, antidiuretic hormone; H_2O, water.

Source: Rad (2006).

JNC-8 guidelines recommend ACEI as one of the initial pharmacologic options in the treatment of hypertension (Table 29.2). In addition, ACEI have evidence-based compelling indications for patients with hypertension and coexisting conditions, including type 2 diabetes mellitus, heart failure, stroke prevention, and chronic renal insufficiency. The Heart Outcomes Prevention Evaluation (HOPE) study was one of the first to demonstrate the efficacy of ACEI in reducing rates of death, MI, and stroke in a broad range of high-risk CV patients. The study results also demonstrated that ACEI were beneficial in patients with renal insufficiency, reducing progression of proteinuria and development of new microalbuminuria (Yusuf et al., 2000). Furthermore, data from the PROGRESS trial demonstrated combination therapy with a thiazide diuretic and ACEI reduced the risk of secondary stroke (PROGRESS, 2001). Thereafter, a number of landmark trials justify the role of ACEI as primary agents used as monotherapy or in combination therapy for treatment of hypertension (Rosendorff et al., 2007).

ACEI are generally well tolerated, with a few notable adverse effects. Up to 20% of patients can experience a persistent dry cough, pharmacologically explained by the inhibition of bradykinin breakdown. ARBs do not have this effect, so patients may be switched to an ARB if they experience a dry cough from an ACEI. ACEI decrease the production of aldosterone, which may result in hyperkalemia. A rare and serious adverse effect of ACEI is angioedema. Angioedema is likely due to inhibition of bradykinin breakdown, but a clear mechanism for this effect remains unknown. Symptoms of angioedema include lip and tongue swelling, as well as difficulty breathing. If a patient experiences ACEI–induced angioedema or has a history of angioedema, these agents are contraindicated. Other contraindications to the use of ACEI are bilateral renal artery stenosis and pregnancy.

Angiotensin II Receptor Blockers

Similar to the ACEI, the ARBs also suppress the RAAS. The net pharmacologic effect of both classes is essentially the same in that ARBs directly block the actions of angiotensin II, whereas the ACEI block the synthesis of angiotensin II. ARBs directly block angiotensin II type 1 (AT_1) receptors that mediate vasoconstrictive effects and aldosterone secretion. ARBs do not block angiotensin II type 2 (AT_2) receptors, so the beneficial effects of AT_2—stimulation of vasodilation, tissue repair, and inhibition of cell growth—remain intact. JNC-8 guidelines recommend ARBs as one of the preferred options for initial therapy in patients newly diagnosed with hypertension. Although they are newer agents compared to the ACEI, ARBs have evidence-based data demonstrating long-term reductions in progression of target-organ damage. For patients with type 2 diabetes, ARBs are capable of slowing the progression of established nephropathy. ARBs also reduce the risk of MI, stroke, and death from CV causes in patients intolerant to an ACEI. The ONTARGET study demonstrated that telmisartan was similar to ramipril with regard to reducing CV morbidity and mortality (Yusuf et al., 2008).

ARBs likely have the lowest incidence of side effects compared with other hypertensive agents. Adverse effects with ARBs are similar to ACEI due to similar effects on the RAAS; however, because ARBs do not affect bradykinin, dry cough is not an adverse effect. ARBs are also contraindicated in pregnancy.

TABLE 29.2 Antihypertensive Agents That Act on the RAAS

Class	Agents (Brand Name)	Dosage (mg/day)	Dosing Frequency	Clinical Pearls/Monitoring	Significant Drug Interactions
Angiotensin-converting enzyme inhibitors (ACEI)	Benazepril (Lotensin®)	10–40	Once daily	■ African Americans do not respond as well to these agents; concurrent use of a thiazide diuretic may improve efficacy ■ Use caution in patients with acute renal failure (efferent arteriole vasodilation) ■ Monitor serum creatinine, electrolytes ■ Rare side effect of angioedema ■ Contraindicated with bilateral renal artery stenosis ■ Pregnancy category X	■ NSAIDs ■ Lithium ■ K⁺ sparing diuretics
	Captopril	25–150	BID to TID		
	Enalapril (Vasotec®)	5–40	Once daily		
	Fosinopril (Monopril®)	10–40	Once daily		
	Lisinopril (Zestril®, Prinivil®)	10–40	Once daily		
	Moexipril (Univasc®)	7.5–30	Once daily		
	Perindopril (Aceon®)	4–16	Once daily		
	Quinapril (Accupril®)	10–80	Once daily		
	Ramipril (Altace®)	2.5–10	Once daily		
	Trandolapril (Mavik®)	1–4	Once daily		
Angiotensin II receptor blockers (ARBs)	Candesartan (Atacand®)	8–32	Once daily	■ Can be substituted for an ACE inhibitor in patients developing dry cough ■ Use caution in patients with acute renal failure (efferent arteriole vasodilation) ■ Monitor serum creatinine, electrolytes ■ Pregnancy category X	■ NSAIDs ■ Lithium ■ K⁺ sparing diuretics
	Eprosartan (Teveten®)	600–800	Once daily		
	Irbesartan (Avapro®)	150–300	Once daily		
	Losartan (Cozaar®)	50–100	Once daily		
	Olmesartan (Benicar®)	20–40	Once daily		
	Telmisartan (Micardis®)	20–80	Once daily		
	Valsartan (Diovan®)	80–320	Once daily		
Direct renin inhibitor	Aliskiren (Tekturna®)	150–300	Once daily	■ Monitor serum creatinine, electrolytes ■ May cause hyperkalemia ■ Pregnancy category X	■ NSAIDs ■ K⁺ sparing diuretics ■ Lithium

BID, twice daily; NSAID, nonsteroidal anti-inflammatory drug; RAAS, renin-angiotensin-aldosterone system; TID, three times daily.

Direct Renin Inhibitors

Direct renin inhibitors are the newest class of agents that suppress the RAAS. Currently, only one direct renin inhibitor, aliskiren (Tekturna®), is available. Aliskiren binds tightly with renin to inhibit the conversion of angiotensinogen to angiotensin I, the rate-limiting step in the production of angiotensin II. Aliskiren is approved as monotherapy or in combination for the management of hypertension. In clinical trials, it reduced BP to a similar extent as ACEI or ARBs (Oh et al., 2007). However, aliskiren's therapeutic ability is limited by lack of long-term outcomes data for CV event reduction. Clinicians generally consider this agent for add-on therapy to achieve additive BP–lowering effects and proteinuria reduction. Adverse effects of these agents are similar to ACEI and ARBs, and pregnancy is a contraindication to the use of direct renin inhibitors.

Calcium Channel Blockers

In addition to thiazide diuretics, ACEI, and ARBs, CCBs are first-line antihypertensive agents. Calcium has an important role in the function of vascular smooth muscle and cardiac cells, as contraction of these cells requires an increase in intracellular calcium. CCBs prevent calcium ions from entering the voltage-sensitive channels in the cell membranes. There are two primary subclasses of CCBs, the dihydropyridines and nondihydropyridines (Table 29.3). The dihydropyridines cause peripheral vasodilation, primarily by preventing contraction of smooth muscle in the vasculature. The nondihydropyridines act on the arterioles to cause peripheral vasodilation and affect the heart by decreasing heart rate and slowing atrioventricular (AV) nodal conduction. Both subclasses undergo hepatic metabolism and are prone to extensive first-pass metabolic effects.

Dihydropyridine CCBs have been extensively studied in patients with hypertension and are as effective at lowering CV events as other first-line agents. In the ALLHAT study, there was no difference in the primary outcome between chlorthalidone and amlodipine. Further, a subgroup analysis of ALLHAT directly compared lisinopril with amlodipine and found no difference in the primary outcome of fatal coronary heart disease or nonfatal MI (ALLHAT, 2002). The VALUE study revealed no difference between valsartan and amlodipine in the primary outcome of first CV event in high-risk patients (Julius et al., 2004).

The dihydropyridines are selective for calcium channels in the vasculature and therefore are associated with adverse effects of flushing, dizziness, peripheral edema, and other vasodilation-related symptoms. The short-acting dihydropyridine, nifedipine, can cause reflex sympathetic discharges in response to the vasodilating properties and should be avoided in the treatment of hypertension. Agents with a longer half-life, including amlodipine or sustained release forms of the other agents, are preferred in treatment of hypertension.

The *nondihydropyridine* CCBs have similar antihypertensive effects as the dihydropyridine CCBs; in addition, by blocking calcium channels in the heart they also decrease heart rate and slow AV nodal conduction. Therefore, they are often used to treat cardiac arrhythmias, especially atrial fibrillation. Adverse effects with nondihydropyridines include cardiac-conduction abnormalities, such as bradycardia and AV nodal block. These agents also inhibit multiple cytochrome P450 (CYP450)

TABLE 29.3 Calcium Channel Blockers for Hypertension

Class	Agents (Brand Name)	Dosage (mg/day)	Dosing Frequency	Clinical Pearls/Monitoring	Significant Drug Interactions
Dihydropyridines (DHP)	Amlodipine (Norvasc®)	2.5–10	Once daily	Avoid short-acting dihydropyridines (i.e., nifedipine IR); can cause severe hypotension, acute MI, syncope, stroke and other serious adverse events	CYP450-mediated drug interactions
	Felodipine (Plendil®)	5–20	Once daily		
	Isradipine (DynaCirc®)	5–10	Twice daily		
	Nicardipine (Cardene®)	60–120	Twice daily		
	Nifedipine (Procardia XL®)	30–90	Once daily		
	Nisoldipine (Sular®)	10–40	Once daily		
Nondihydropyridines (non-DHP)	Diltiazem (Cardizem):			Avoid non-DHP in patients with LV dysfunction due to negative inotropic effects; may worsen outcomes	CYP450-mediated drug interactions: digoxin, simvastatin, tacrolimus
	Cardizem SR®	180–360	Twice daily		
	Cardizem CD®	120–480	Once daily		
	Verapamil (Calan®)	180–480	Once or twice daily		

CYP450, cytochrome P450; IR, immediate release; LV, left ventricular; MI, myocardia infarction.

enzymes and are prone to drug–drug interactions with agents that are substrates for CYP450 enzymes. Verapamil is frequently associated with constipation, and patients should be advised to increase dietary fiber and utilize over-the-counter stool softeners if this occurs.

Beta-Adrenergic Receptor Blockers

Beta-adrenergic receptor blockers (beta blockers) antagonize beta receptors of the sympathetic nervous system and inhibit sympathetic effects of those receptors. A change from previous guidelines, the JNC-8 guidelines do not recommend beta-adrenergic receptor blockers for the initial treatment of hypertension (James et al., 2013). However, beta blockers are appropriate first-line agents in the treatment of hypertension associated with specific compelling indications, such as coronary heart disease or after MI (Weber et al., 2013). Clinical trial data suggest that beta blockers do not exhibit as extensive CV event reduction as ACEI, ARBs, CCBs, or thiazide diuretics. In the Losartan Intervention for Endpoint reduction (LIFE) in hypertension trial, for example, losartan was statistically better than atenolol at lowering the combined rate of death, stroke, and MI (24% and 28%, respectively) in patients with isolated systolic hypertension and left ventricular hypertrophy (Dahlöf et al., 2002).

Beta-1 and beta-2 receptors are distributed throughout the body, concentrating differently in certain organs and tissues. Beta-1 receptors are primarily located in the heart and kidney, and beta-2 receptors are located in the lungs, liver, and pancreas. A blockade of beta-1 receptors in the kidney reduces the release of renin, causing less angiotensin II–mediated vasoconstriction. A blockade of beta-1 receptors in the heart decreases cardiac contractility and heart rate. A blockade of beta-2 receptors causes bronchoconstriction and vasoconstriction.

There are important pharmacokinetic and pharmacodynamic considerations within the beta-adrenergic receptor blocker class of medications. One property that distinguishes beta blockers is their cardioselectivity. Cardioselective beta-receptor blockers have a greater affinity for beta-1 receptors and therefore have a clinically significant advantage for the treatment of hypertension (Table 29.4). Cardioselective agents are also safer than nonselective agents in patients with coexisting asthma, chronic obstructive pulmonary disease (COPD), and peripheral arterial disease. Some beta blockers have a property known an intrinsic sympathomimetic activity (ISA), and act as partial agonists upon binding to the beta-receptor; therefore, their effect on heart rate and cardiac output is less than that of full antagonists. The partial agonists may be beneficial in patients who are prone to bradycardia or certain patients with heart failure. However, agents with ISA do not reduce CV events as effectively as other beta blockers do and are very rarely prescribed for the management of hypertension.

Most adverse effects associated with the beta blockers are directly related to the antagonizing effects on the beta receptors. Adverse effects of beta-1 blockade include bradycardia, AV nodal conduction abnormalities, fatigue, and reduced myocardial contractility. Adverse effects of beta-2 blockade include bronchoconstriction and decreased peripheral blood flow. Additional systemic effects that can occur include alterations in serum cholesterol and the blunting of symptoms of

TABLE 29.4 Beta-Adrenergic Receptor Blockers for Hypertension

Class	Agents (Brand Name)	Dosage (mg/day)	Dosing Frequency	Clinical Pearls/Monitoring
Cardio-selective beta-receptor blockers	Atenolol (Tenormin®)	25–100	Once daily	Atenolol is the least lipophilic
	Betaxolol (Kerlone®)	5–20	Once daily	Agents of choice post-MI and CHD
	Bisoprolol (Zebeta®)	2.5–10	Once daily	Bisoprolol and metoprolol succinate agents of choice in HF
	Metoprolol tartrate (Lopressor®)	100–400	Twice daily	May adversely affect serum cholesterol values
	Metoprolol succinate (Toprol XL®)	50–200	Once daily	Cardioselectivity decreases as doses increase
				Abrupt discontinuation may cause rebound hypertension
Non-selective beta-receptor blockers	Nadolol (Corgard®)	40–120	Once daily	Propranolol is the most lipophilic
	Propranolol (Inderal®)	160–480	Twice daily	Use with caution in patients with asthma, COPD, and PAD
	Timolol (Blocadren®)	10–40	Once daily	May blunt symptoms of hypoglycemia in those with DM
				May adversely affect serum cholesterol values
				Non-selective BB may have clinical benefit in patients with migraines, thyrotoxicosis, and essential tremor
Agents with ISA	Acebutolol (Sectral®)	200–800	Twice daily	Do not use in patients post-MI or with CHD
	Penbutolol (Levatol®)	10–40	Once daily	May blunt symptoms of hypoglycemia in DM
	Pindolol	10–60	Twice daily	
Mixed alpha and beta blockers	Carvedilol (Coreg®)	12.5–50	Twice daily	Evaluate for orthostatic hypotension due to added alpha blockade
	Labetalol (Trandate®)	200–800	Twice daily	Carvedilol is an agent of choice in HF

BB, beta blocker; CHD, coronary heart disease; COPD, chronic obstructive pulmonary disease; DM, diabetes mellitus; HF, heart failure; ISA, intrinsic sympathomimetic activity; MI, myocardial infarction; PAD, peripheral arterial disease.

hypoglycemia in patients with diabetes mellitus. Rebound hypertension and tachycardia can occur with abrupt withdrawal of beta blocker therapy, and tapering is advised, if possible.

Alpha-1 Receptor Blockers

Alpha-1 selective blockers antagonize alpha-1 receptors in the vasculature, resulting in arterial and venous vasodilation. These adjunctive agents are not first-line antihypertensive medications (Table 29.5). They are primarily used to augment the lowering of BP to obtain therapeutic BP goals or if contraindications exist to the traditional agents of ACEI, ARBs, diuretics, CCBs, and beta blockers. Alpha-1 blockers have a special niche in therapy by providing symptomatic benefits in men with hypertension and concurrent benign prostatic hyperplasia (BPH). The primary adverse effect with alpha-1 antagonists is orthostatic hypotension and patients should be educated on orthostasis symptoms. The first dose of these medications or dose increase can be administered in the presence of a health care provider to evaluate symptoms or at night prior to sleep to reduce the concern for first-dose hypotension. Other adverse effects include nasal congestion and central nervous system effects of dizziness and headache.

Centrally Acting Alpha-2 Agonists

Centrally acting alpha-2 agonists are also adjunctive medications in the management of hypertension, to be considered after first-line agents (ALLHAT, 2002) (Table 29.5). Centrally acting alpha-2 agonists lower BP by stimulating alpha-2 receptors within the brain stem. Activation of alpha-2 receptors in the brain stem is associated with autonomic regulation, and these agents decrease the release of norepinephrine from sympathetic nerves, thereby reducing activation of peripheral adrenergic receptors. The net effect is decreased heart rate and a decrease in cardiac output by suppression of sympathetic signals to the heart. In the periphery, these agents cause vasodilation by suppression of sympathetic signals to the blood vessels. The most common adverse effects with centrally acting alpha-2 agonists are sedation and dry mouth. Other adverse effects include the retention of sodium and water and potential rebound hypertension with abrupt withdrawal. These agents should generally be avoided in the elderly due to a high incidence of anticholinergic effects of sedation, dry mouth, constipation, urinary retention, and blurred vision. Methyldopa is a drug of choice for the management of hypertension in pregnancy.

Peripheral Adrenergic Antagonists

Reserpine is the only available peripheral adrenergic antagonist. Reserpine depletes norepinephrine from postganglionic sympathetic nerve terminals and reduces sympathetic stimulation of the heart and blood vessels. In addition, reserpine depletes

TABLE 29.5 Adjunctive Antihypertensive Agents

Class	Agents (Brand Name)	Dosage (mg/day)	Dosing Frequency	Clinical Pearls/Monitoring	Significant Drug Interactions
Alpha-1 antagonists	Doxazosin (Cardura®)	1–8	Once daily	▪ Give first dose at bedtime or under supervision	
	Prazosin (Minipress®)	2–20	Two or three times daily	▪ Evaluate for orthostatic hypotension	
	Terazosin (Hytrin®)	1–20	Once or twice daily	▪ Drugs of choice for men with concomitant BPH	
Centrally acting alpha-2 agonists	Clonidine (Catapres®)	0.1–0.8	Twice daily	▪ For withdrawing agents—if on concurrent beta blocker therapy, discontinue beta blocker first and then gradually withdraw clonidine	Beta blockers: AV nodal blocking effect of beta blockers may be enhanced; beta blockers may enhance rebound hypertensive effects when abruptly withdrawing alpha-2 agonists
	Clonidine patch (Catapres-TTS®)	0.1–0.3	Once weekly		
	Methyldopa	250–1,000	Twice daily	▪ Methyldopa is the drug of choice for chronic management of hypertension in pregnancy	
Peripheral adrenergic antagonist	Reserpine	0.05–0.25	Once daily	▪ Use with a diuretic to diminish fluid retention ▪ Avoid with a history of depressive illness	
Direct acting vasodilator	Hydralazine (Apresoline®)	20–100	Two or three times daily	▪ Be aware of reflex sympathetic response ▪ Administer with beta blocker and diuretic to reduce tachycardia and fluid retention	
	Minoxidil	10–40	Once or twice daily		

AV, atrioventricular; BPH, benign prostatic hypertrophy.

serotonin and other catecholamines from the brain, which may cause depression. Other than the implications as a cause of mental depression, reserpine is well tolerated. Other notable adverse effects are due to the inhibition of sympathetic activity, which enhances parasympathetic activity, including nasal stuffiness, increased gastric acid secretion, diarrhea, and bradycardia.

Direct-Acting Vasodilators

Direct-acting vasodilators are adjunctive medications in the management of hypertension (Table 29.5). Direct-acting vasodilators cause dilation of the arterioles, leading to a marked decrease in peripheral-vascular resistance. Rapid reduction in arterial pressure causes a reflex sympathetic response with tachycardia, renin release, and fluid retention. Therefore, patients receiving either of the agents in this class, hydralazine or minoxidil, for the treatment of hypertension should receive concurrent therapy with a beta blocker and diuretic. Hydralazine is the more commonly prescribed agent in this class and is especially useful in resistant hypertension in patients with renal failure. A unique side effect of hydralazine is a dose-dependent lupus-like syndrome. Other adverse effects include headache, dizziness, and fatigue. Minoxidil® produces more intense vasodilation than hydralazine, resulting in an exaggerated compensatory response. Minoxidil® is, therefore, reserved for patients with severe hypertension resistant to hydralazine and other primary treatment options. A high percentage of patients prescribed minoxidil for a longer period of time develop hypertrichosis, excessive growth of hair. Topical minoxidil, marketed as Rogaine, is used to promote hair growth in balding men and women.

Pharmacotherapy of Hypertension Management

The overall goal of treating hypertension is to reduce associated morbidity and mortality from CV events. The choice of initial drug therapy depends on the degree of BP elevation, presence of compelling indications, scientific evidence for efficacy and safety, individual patient factors, and cost. Per the most recent JNC-8 guidelines, a thiazide diuretic, ACEI, ARB, or CCB is recommended as primary antihypertensive options for all non-Black patients, including those with diabetes. Initial therapy recommended for African Americans, including those with diabetes, is a thiazide diuretic or CCB. These agents are recommended based on evidence from landmark placebo-controlled clinical trials, including ALLHAT, that demonstrated CV risk-reduction benefits with these classes of agents.

Most patients require combination therapy to achieve goal BP values. In some cases, especially patients diagnosed with Stage 2 hypertension, initial therapy with a combination of two drugs is recommended. The ACCOMPLISH trial evaluated the efficacy and safety of initial combination therapy by comparing an ACEI–thiazide diuretic combination with an ACEI–CCB combination (Jamerson et al., 2008). This study demonstrated that initial two-drug combination therapy is an effective, evidence-based strategy to manage hypertension. Consideration of which combinations of agents are optimal is somewhat patient specific. The ASH has recommended three categories of combination therapy—preferred, acceptable, and less effective (Weber et al., 2013).

The preferred categories for combination therapy include:

ACEI/CCB
ARB/CCB
ACEI/diuretic
ARB/diuretic

The acceptable categories for combination therapy include:

Beta blocker/diuretic
CCB/Beta blocker
CCB/diuretic
Direct renin inhibitor/diuretic
Thiazide diuretic/potassium-sparing diuretic

The less-effective categories for combination therapy include:

ACEI/beta blocker
ARB/beta blocker
CCB (nondihydropyridine)/beta blocker
Alpha-2 agonist/beta blocker

Certain combinations are not effective for long-term treatment of hypertension. For example, in the ONTARGET trial, ramipril, telmisartan, and the combination of both agents were assessed, demonstrating that the use of an ACEI and an ARB together results in no additional reduction in the incidence of CV events. Combination therapy with this regimen was also associated with more adverse events (Yusuf et al., 2008). Similar findings were discovered when an ARB was combined with the direct renin inhibitor, aliskiren.

Unlike prior recommendations, the new JNC-8 guidelines do not promote the choice of an agent based on compelling indications. The ASH guidelines, however, do maintain recommendations for patients with compelling indications. For patients with concomitant CKD, diabetes mellitus, or a history of stroke, the antihypertensive regimen should include an ACEI or ARB. For patients with CAD, the antihypertensive regimen should include a beta blocker plus an ACEI or ARB. For patients with heart failure with left ventricular dysfunction, regimens should include an ACEI or ARB, beta blocker, a diuretic, and an aldosterone antagonist (Weber et al., 2013).

PHARMACOTHERAPEUTICS OF HYPERTENSIVE EMERGENCIES

The JNC defines a hypertensive crisis as a systolic blood pressure (SBP) greater than 180 mmHg or diastolic blood pressure (DBP) greater than 120 mmHg (Chobanian et al., 2003). A hypertensive crisis is further divided into two categories, hypertensive urgency and hypertensive emergency. The differentiating factor between the two categories is the presence of target end-organ damage, which necessitates the need for immediate BP reduction. Patients presenting with hypertensive urgency may complain only of shortness of breath, headache, or appear asymptomatic and do not require immediate and aggressive BP reductions. Hypertensive emergency, however, is associated with the presence of end-organ damage, including but not limited to acute ischemic stroke (AIS), hemorrhagic stroke, aortic dissection, myocardial ischemia, MI, acute pulmonary edema, acute decompensated heart failure, hypertensive encephalopathy, acute kidney injury, or preeclampsia/eclampsia in pregnant women (Marik & Varon, 2007). Whereas end-organ damage often manifests with DBP greater than or equal to 120 mmHg, such severe elevations in BP may not always accompany hypertensive emergency (Ramos & Varon, 2014; Rodriguez, Kumar, & DeCaro, 2010). In pregnant women, preeclampsia is defined as BP greater than or equal to 140/90 mmHg associated with proteinuria after 20 weeks of gestation. This section will discuss the management of BP in the setting of hypertensive emergency for selected end-organ events. Table 29.6 provides specific details regarding pharmacologic options for the management of hypertensive emergencies.

Acute Ischemic Stroke

For patients with AIS, target BP goals are as follows: SBP less than 185 mmHg or DBP less than 110 mmHg (Rhoney & Peacock, 2009a). There is an increased risk of mortality when SBP is less than 155 mmHg or greater than 220 mmHg and DBP less than 70 mmHg or greater than 105 mmHg. Intravenous (IV) antihypertensive therapy should be initiated for SBP greater than 220 mmHg and DBP greater than 120 mmHg, targeting BP reduction by 15% within the first 24 hours (Jaunch et al., 2013). For patients eligible for reperfusion therapy with a thrombolytic agent, initiate antihypertensive therapy for SBP greater than 185 mmHg and DBP greater than 110 mmHg. Preferred agents in the setting of AIS are nicardipine and labetalol (Marik & Varon, 2007).

Hemorrhagic Stroke/Intracerebral Hemorrhage

For patients with intracerebral hemorrhage (ICH), the immediate goal is to prevent the expansion of the hematoma. Currently no evidence suggests decreasing BP will affect the expansion of the hematoma (Marik & Varon, 2007). Decreasing BP can lead to decreased cerebral perfusion and worsen ischemia. Antihypertensive agents should be initiated only if SBP greater than 180 mmHg or mean arterial pressure (MAP) greater than 130 mmHg. For patients with ICH, nicardipine or labetalol is the preferred agent (Rhoney & Peacock, 2009a). Aggressive reduction with continuous infusion of these agents should be administered for SBP greater than 200 mmHg or MAP greater than 150 mmHg.

Aortic Dissection

According to the Stanford Classification System, there are two types of aortic dissections: Type A, which affects the ascending aorta and/or the aortic arch, and Type B, which affects the descending aorta or the aortic arch distal to the left subclavian artery. Type A dissections require emergent surgical intervention. First-line therapy for Type B dissections is aggressive BP control with medications, as there is limited evidence for differences in mortality between surgical interventions and medical

TABLE 29.6 Intravenous Pharmacologic Agents for the Treatment of Hypertensive Emergencies

Class	Agent	Dose	Mechanism of Action	Pharmacokinetics	Clinical Considerations
Calcium channel blockers	Nicardipine	Initial: 5 mg/hr IV infusion Increase by 2.5 mg/hr q5 min Max: 15 mg/hr	■ Dihydropyridine calcium channel blocker ■ Inhibits Ca^{2+} influx into cardiac and vascular smooth muscle, causing muscle relaxation ■ Coronary and peripheral vasodilator ■ Minimal negative inotropic or chronotropic effects	Onset: 5–15 min Duration: 4–6 hr Elimination $t_{1/2}$: 2–4 hr	■ Once at goal BP, wean by 3 mg/hr as tolerated ■ Beneficial effects on cardiac ischemia, improving blood distribution and flow to ischemic areas ■ Predictable and consistent BP effects ■ Use with caution in decompensated HF, angina, and increased ICP ■ May cause reflex tachycardia, headache, and flushing ■ Indication: AIS, ICH, aortic dissection, ACS, preeclampsia, eclampsia, AKI, hepatic encephalopathy
	Clevidipine	Initial: 1–2 mg/hr IV infusion Increase by doubling dose every 90 sec to goal BP Once at goal BP, increase by less than double every 5–10 min PRN Max: 32 mg/hr Max DOT: 72 hr	■ Third-generation dihydro-pyridine calcium channel blocker ■ MOA similar to nicardipine ■ Dilates arterioles, reduces afterload, does not affect cardiac-filling pressures or cause reflex tachycardia	Onset: 2–4 min Duration: 5–15 min Metabolism: plasma esterases $t_{1/2}$: 1 min	■ Can be used in patients with either hepatic or renal insufficiency ■ TPN patients—adjust for calories due to lipid component in formulation ■ Monitor TGs with prolonged administration ■ CI: allergies to soy or eggs ■ Indication: ACS, AKI

(continued)

TABLE 29.6 Intravenous Pharmacologic Agents for the Treatment of Hypertensive Emergencies *(continued)*

Class	Agent	Dose	Mechanism of Action	Pharmacokinetics	Clinical Considerations
Vasodilators	Nitroprusside	Initial: 0.25–0.5 mcg/kg/min IV infusion Increase by 0.5 mcg/kg/min Max: 10 mcg/kg/min	▪ Direct vasodilator ▪ Nitroso-group in molecule (NO) causes arteriolar and venous smooth muscle relaxation (intravenous form only) ▪ Decrease in preload and afterload	Onset: 30–60 sec Duration: 1–10 min $t_{1/2}$ of nitroprusside: 2 min $t_{1/2}$ of thiocyanate: 3–4 days (renally excreted)	▪ Vasodilatory and BP effect not as predictable ▪ Risk of coronary steal syndrome—shunting of blood away from ischemic areas of the heart by reduction of diastolic perfusion pressure ▪ Pulmonary shunting can occur—reversal of vasoconstriction of pulmonary vessels in patients with acute/chronic hypoxemia ▪ May increase cerebral blood volume and ICP ▪ Risk of rebound hypertension and tachycardia ▪ Safe in patients with AS and LV systolic dysfunction ▪ Cyanide toxicity due to thiocyanate accumulation—can monitor via lactate levels, evaluate lactic acidosis ▪ Use with caution in renal or hepatic disease ▪ Caution with use >72 hr ▪ CI: Do not use within 24 hr of sildenafil or vardenafil use or 48 hr of tadalafil use due to profound hypotension ▪ Indication: aortic dissection, APE, HF
	Nitroglycerin	Initial: 5 mcg/min IV infusion Increase by 5 mcg/min every 3–5 min Inadequate response by 20 mcg/min, can increase by 10 mcg/min every 3–5 min Max: 200 mcg/min	▪ Venodilator ▪ Converted into NO, causing smooth muscle relaxation of venous system, decrease in preload and cardiac output ▪ Arteriolar dilation occurs at high doses	Onset: 2–5 min Duration: 5–10 min $t_{1/2}$: 1–4 min	▪ Not for patients with compromised cerebral and renal perfusion ▪ Indication: ACS, APE, HF

	Drug	Dosing	Mechanism	Pharmacokinetics	Notes
	Hydralazine	Initial: 10 mg IV bolus (slow infusion) Repeat every 4–6 hr PRN Max initial bolus: 20–40 mg/dose	▪ Peripheral vasodilator ▪ Relaxation of arteriolar smooth muscle causes arterial vasodilation and reduction in arterial vascular resistance, thus decreases afterload ▪ Has no effect on venous smooth muscle	Onset: 10–20 min Duration: 1–4 hr $t_{1/2}$: 2–8 hr	▪ Generally not preferred as first line due to unpredictable response and prolonged duration of action ▪ Risk of reflex tachycardia, headache, flushing ▪ Caution in patients with angina, increased ICP and aortic dissection
Adrenergic-receptor antagonists	Esmolol	Initial: 0.5–1.0 mg/kg LD IVP over 1 min + infusion: 50 mcg/kg/min Can repeat bolus and increase infusion by 50 mcg/kg/min Max: 300 mcg/kg/min	▪ beta-1 antagonist (cardioselective) ▪ Negative inotrope and chronotrope, reduction myocardial oxygen consumption	Onset: 1 min Duration: 10–20 min $t_{1/2}$: 9 min Metabolism: plasma esterases	▪ Can be used in patients with either hepatic or renal insufficiency ▪ CI: decompensated HF, bradycardia, heart block, asthma ▪ Indication: aortic dissection, ACS
	Labetalol	Initial: 20 mg bolus Repeat 20–80 mg bolus every 10 min if needed or infusion at 2 mg/min Max: 300 mg/24 hr	▪ Alpha and non-selective beta blocker ▪ alpha-1 antagonism = direct vasodilation → ↓SVR (afterload); prevents reflex vasoconstriction ▪ beta-1 antagonism = ↓ HR ▪ beta-2 antagonism = vasodilation and inhibit neuronal uptake of NE ▪ Reduces systemic vascular resistance ▪ Maintains cardiac output and cerebral and renal blood flow ▪ IV form binds to 1 alpha-receptor for every 7 beta-receptors ▪ PO form binds to 1 alpha receptor for every 3 beta receptors	Onset: 2–5 min Duration: 8–18 hr Elimination $t_{1/2}$: 5.5 hr	▪ Long $t_{1/2}$, difficult to titrate ▪ Use with caution in asthma and severe COPD ▪ CI: decompensated HF, AV block, bradycardia, asthma ▪ Does NOT increase ICP/minimal effects on cerebral blood flow ▪ Indication: AIS, ICH, preeclampsia, eclampsia, ACS, hypertensive encephalopathy

(continued)

TABLE 29.6 Intravenous Pharmacologic Agents for the Treatment of Hypertensive Emergencies (continued)

Class	Agent	Dose	Mechanism of Action	Pharmacokinetics	Clinical Considerations
	Phentolamine	Initial: 5–15 mg IV bolus Max: 15 mg	alpha-1 and alpha-2 receptor antagonist	Onset: 1–2 min Duration: 10–30 min	▪ Use with caution in CAD patients; precipitates angina/MI ▪ Manage compensatory tachycardia with beta blocker (i.e. esmolol) ▪ Indication: Sympathetic crisis—HTN emergencies due to excess catecholamines (i.e., pheochromocytoma, food or DDIs with MAOIs, amphetamine overdose, cocaine toxicity, clonidine withdrawal)
Dopamine agonist	Fenoldopam	Initial: 0.1–0.3 mcg/kg/min Increase 0.05–0.1 mcg/kg/min every 15 min Max: 1.6 mcg/kg/min	▪ Peripheral dopamine 1 agonist causes relaxation of vascular smooth muscle ▪ Vasodilation of peripheral arteries; decreases total peripheral resistance ▪ Stimulates dopamine receptors on renal tubular cells, preserves renal blood flow and increases urinary flow rate	Onset: <5 min Duration: 30 min $t_{1/2}$: 9.8 min Metabolism: hepatic via conjugation not via CYP450	▪ Increase IOP, questionable increase in ICP; avoid in glaucoma patients ▪ CI: sulfite allergy ▪ Renal protective effect not proven ▪ Tolerance can develop after 48 hr of infusion ▪ Indication: AKI, hypertensive encephalopathy
Angiotensin-converting enzyme inhibitor	Enalaprilat	Initial: 1.25 mg IVP over 5 min every 4–6 hr CrCl ≤30 mL/min: initial dose = 0.625 mg Increase by 1.25 mg every 6 hr Max: 5 mg every 6 hr	▪ Blocks conversion of AngI to AngII → vasodilation (AngII = potent vasoconstrictor) ▪ Decreases peripheral resistance without affecting cardiac output and HR	Onset: 15–30 min Duration 12–24 hr	▪ Longer DOA, concerns for hypotension ▪ CI: pregnancy ▪ Avoid in acute MI, renal artery stenosis or renal failure ▪ Most effective in patients with higher renin levels

↓, decrease; ACS, acute coronary syndromes; AIS, acute ischemic stroke; AKI, acute kidney injury; Ang, angiotensin; APE, acute pulmonary edema; AS, aortic stenosis; AV, atrioventricular; BP, blood pressure; CAD, coronary artery disease; CI, contraindications; cont., continuous; COPD, chronic obstructive pulmonary disease; CrCl, creatinine clearance; CYP450, cytochrome P450; DDI, drug-drug interaction; DOA, duration of action; DOT, duration of therapy; HF, heart failure; hr, hour(s); HR, heart rate; HTN, hypertension; ICH, intracerebral hemorrhage; ICP, intracranial pressure; IOP, intraocular pressure; IV, intravenous; IVP, intravenous push; LD, loading dose; LV, left ventricular; MAOI, monoamine oxidase inhibitor; min, minute(s); MI, myocardial infarction; MOA, mechanism of action; NE, norepinephrine; NO, nitric oxide; PO, oral; PRN, as needed; sec, second(s); SVR, systemic vascular resistance; $t_{1/2}$, half-life; TG, triglycerides; TPN, total parental nutrition.

management (Marik & Varon, 2007). Type B dissections require immediate treatment with an IV beta blocker, esmolol or labetalol. Beta blockers are preferred as they decrease aortic wall stress. Beta blockers must be administered before any vasodilators, as vasodilators can exacerbate the dissection due to the associated reflex tachycardia (Marik & Varon, 2007). The patient's SBP goal is less than or equal to 120 mmHg, and the agent of choice for Type B aortic dissection is esmolol. Nicardipine or nitroprusside may be added if additional agents are required to achieve the BP goal.

Preeclampsia and Eclampsia

Preeclampsia is a medical emergency characterized by elevated BP and significant proteinuria in pregnant women. Preeclampsia can progress to eclampsia, which includes the occurrence of seizures. Antihypertensive therapy should be initiated for SBP greater than 155 to 160 mmHg, as SBP greater than 160 mmHg increases the risk of cerebrovascular accidents (Marik & Varon, 2007). The target SBP is 140 to 160 mmHg and DBP 90 to 105 mmHg. Labetalol and nicardipine are considered the agents of choice. Nicardipine is generally well tolerated and provides a relatively predictable response (Marik & Varon, 2007; Rhoney & Peacock, 2009b). Hydralazine was considered first line; however, the American College of Chest Physicians no longer recommends its use due to a delayed onset of action and the side effects of headache, nausea, and vomiting, which mimic deteriorating preeclampsia (Marik & Varon, 2007). ACEI should never be used in any stage of pregnancy as teratogenic effects may occur. Nitroprusside should also be avoided in pregnant patients. Additional therapeutic interventions for preeclampsia are warranted but not discussed, as they are not specific to hypertension management.

For full reference citations to this chapter, please see "Section References" in the back of the book, under the heading "Section VII."

Pharmacotherapeutics of Hyperlipidemia

DEV CHATTERJI AND JONATHAN RICHARD E. PUHL

Hyperlipidemia is one of the most common pharmacologically treated diseases in the United States and worldwide. Epidemiologic studies confirm that abnormalities of plasma lipoproteins result in the predisposition to coronary disease, and there is a graded relationship between cholesterol levels and coronary risk (Menotti et al., 2006). The etiology of hyperlipidemia is multifactorial and is related to genetics, dietary consumption, and lifestyle habits.

PATHOPHYSIOLOGY

Cholesterol is an important component of cell membranes and for the synthesis of essential hormones. The source of cholesterol can be exogenous—from dietary sources—or endogenous—synthesized by cells in the liver. The majority of our cholesterol originates from endogenous synthesis rather than dietary sources. A critical step in hepatic cholesterol synthesis is catalyzed by an enzyme *3-hydroxy-3-methylglutaryl coenzyme A reductase*, HMG-CoA reductase. As will be discussed next, drugs that inhibit this enzyme are our most effective and widely prescribed lipid-lowering agents. In its most basic state, cholesterol is minimally water-soluble. To travel through the bloodstream, cholesterol is bound to proteins and grouped into lipoproteins for transport through the body. Lipoproteins are available in six different forms; however, from a pharmacotherapeutic standpoint, three of them are of primary importance in the development of coronary atherosclerosis:

- Very-low-density lipoproteins (VLDLs)
- Low-density lipoproteins (LDLs)
- High-density lipoproteins (HDLs)

The lipoproteins are identified to correspond to their density. The various classes of lipoproteins differ in density due to the relative percent composition of lipid and protein. The differences in density also provide the basis for the physical isolation and subsequent measurement of plasma lipoproteins by laboratories, the lipid panel. VLDLs primarily contain triglycerides (TG) and their main physiologic role is to deliver TG from the liver to adipose tissue and muscle, to allow TG to be used as fuel. LDLs contain mainly cholesterol; their main physiologic role is to deliver cholesterol to non-hepatic tissues. Cells absorb cholesterol through engulfment of LDLs from the bloodstream, binding to LDL receptors on the cell surface. When cellular demand for cholesterol increases, cells synthesize more LDL receptors to enhance their capacity for LDL engulfment. Accordingly, when cells are unable to make more LDL receptors or the plasma levels of LDL are too high, cholesterol absorption is hindered, resulting in elevated LDL cholesterol in the plasma. LDLs are the primary lipid type associated with the development of coronary atherosclerosis. The probability of developing coronary heart disease (CHD) is directly related to LDL levels in the blood; therefore, lowering LDL levels is a major target of hyperlipidemia drug therapy. HDLs also contain cholesterol as their primary core lipid, although in contrast to LDLs, HDLs carry cholesterol from peripheral tissues back to the liver—this promotes cholesterol removal. Therefore, high HDL levels actively protect against CHD (Kannel, 1995).

Pharmacologic agents for the treatment of hyperlipidemia include several classes of drugs: HMG-CoA reductase inhibitors (statins), fibric acid derivatives, bile acid sequestrants, nicotinic acid, and a cholesterol absorption inhibitor, ezetimibe. The major benefit of pharmacologic therapy for hyperlipidemia is primary prevention of CHD. In 2013, the American Heart Association (AHA) along with the National Heart, Lung, and Blood Institute released an update to the guidelines for the management of elevated blood cholesterol (Stone et al., 2013). The subsequent sections will review the various pharmacological treatment options for hyperlipidemia and recommendations from expert groups regarding lipid management for both primary and secondary prevention.

HMG-CoA REDUCTASE INHIBITORS (STATINS)

Of the pharmacologic therapies for lipid management, statins are the first-line agents as they exhibit substantial potential for reduction in LDL. Several randomized trials support the use of statins to reduce the risk of CHD, total mortality, myocardial infarctions, stroke, and peripheral vascular disease (Stone et al., 2013). Currently available statins include: atorvastatin, fluvastatin, lovastatin, pitavastatin, pravastatin, rosuvastatin, and simvastatin. Statins have varying potencies (Table 30.1), with atorvastatin (Lipitor) and rosuvastatin (Crestor) the most potent statins approved in the United States.

Statins inhibit the enzyme 3-hydroxy-3-methylglutaryl coenzyme A reductase (HMG-CoA), which catalyzes the conversion of HMG-CoA to mevalonate. The mevalonate pathway is the rate-limiting step in the ultimate synthesis of cholesterol; therefore, by inhibiting this step, statins cause upregulation of hepatic LDL receptors and reduction in LDL cholesterol concentrations. Statins reduce LDL 20% to 60%, raise HDL cholesterol 5% to 15%, and reduce TG 7% to 30%; Table 30.2 provides the approximate change to lipid levels by individual statin.

In general, statins have similar side effect profiles, with the most common side effect being myalgias. The muscle cramps associated with the use of statins occur frequently enough to be problematic in clinical practice. Sometimes initiating statin therapy with lower doses and slowly titrating up can mediate this side effect. Also, switching to another agent may improve myalgias, necessitating the trial of more than one agent before characterizing a patient as statin-intolerant. Rhabdomyolysis, a severe breakdown of muscle tissue, is another potential side effect, although very rare, occurring in 0.1% to 0.5% of patients. Prior to initiating statin therapy, evaluate liver function tests (LFTs) and baseline creatinine kinase; during therapy, these laboratory studies should be monitored periodically, especially if a patient is exhibiting adverse effects. Concurrent use of fibric acid derivatives, fibrates, with statins is also not recommended due to increased risk of myopathy and rhabdomyolysis.

TABLE 30.1 High-, Moderate-, and Low-Intensity Statin Therapy (Used in the RCTs Reviewed by the Expert Panel)*

High-Intensity Statin Therapy+	Moderate-Intensity Statin Therapy++	Low-Intensity Statin Therapy+++
Daily dose lowers LDL-C, on average, by approximately ≥50%	Daily dose lowers LDL-C, on average, by approximately 30% to <50%	Daily dose lowers LDL-C, on average, by <30%
Atorvastatin (40)–80 mg	**Atorvastatin 10 (20) mg**	*Simvastatin 10 mg*
Rosuvastatin 20 (40) mg	**Rosuvastatin (5) 10 mg**	**Pravastatin 10–20 mg**
	Simvastatin 20–40 mg	**Lovastatin 20 mg**
	Pravastatin 40 (80) mg	*Fluvastatin 20–40 mg*
	Lovastatin 40 mg	*Pitavastatin 1 mg*
	Fluvastatin XL 80 mg	
	Fluvastatin 40 mg BID	
	Pitavastatin 2–4 mg	

RCTs, randomized controlled trials.

*Individual responses to statin therapy varied in randomized, controlled trials and vary in clinical practice. A less-than-average response may have a biological basis. Statins and dosages in bold reduced major cardiovascular events in randomized, controlled trials. Statins and doses in italics were approved by the U.S. Food and Drug Administration (FDA) but were not tested in randomized, controlled trials.

+Daily dose decreases low-density lipoprotein cholesterol (LDL-C) levels by an average of >=50%

++Daily dose decreases LDL-C levels by an average of 30% to <50%.

+++Daily dose decreases LDL-C levels by average of <30%

Boldface type indicates specific statins and doses that were evaluated in RCTs.

Reprinted from Stone et al. (2013), with permission from Wolters Kluwer.

TABLE 30.2 Approximate Change in Lipid Levels by Statins

Statin	Reduction In Total Cholesterol (%)	Reduction in LDL (%)	Elevation in HDL (%)	Reduction in TGs (%)
Atorvastatin	25–45	26–60	5–13	17–53
Fluvastatin	16–27	22–36	3–11	12–25
Lovastatin	16–34	21–42	2–10	6–27
Pitavastatin	16–37	26–48	7–18	13–22
Pravastatin	16–25	22–34	2–12	15–24
Rosuvastatin	33–46	45–63	8–14	10–35
Simvastatin	19–36	26–47	8–16	12–34

HDL, high-density lipoprotein; LDL, low-density lipoprotein; TGs, triglycerides.

Drug interactions with statins are also an important consideration, and it is always important to check potential drug interactions prior to prescribing these agents. Of the available statins, atorvastatin, lovastatin, and simvastatin are substrates for CYP3A4. Therefore, it is advisable to avoid, if possible, strong CYP3A4 inhibitors, including grapefruit juice, HIV protease inhibitors, amiodarone, verapamil, itraconazole, and ketoconazole, for patients on those specific statin medications. If concurrent therapy is required, it is preferable to administer pravastatin or rosuvastatin, as these agents have minimal to no effect on CYP3A4.

The 2013 American College of Cardiology and the AHA (ACC/AHA) cholesterol guidelines recommend pharmacologic therapy of hyperlipidemia based on their primary evaluation tool, the atherosclerotic cardiovascular disease (ASCVD) pooled-risk equation. The guidelines focus on the identification of four groups who may benefit from the use of statins for both primary and secondary prevention of cardiovascular events due to ASCVD. There is identification of both high- and moderate-intensity statin therapy dosing, and the management of statin-associated adverse effects. The four groups that will benefit from ASCVD risk reduction with statin therapy are the following:

- Patients with clinical ASCVD
- Primary elevations of LDL equal to or greater than 190 mg/dL
- Age 40 to 75 years with diabetes with LDL 70–189 mg/dL
- Age 40 to 75 years without clinical ASCVD or diabetes with LDL 70–189 mg/ dL with an estimated 10-year ASCVD risk of equal to or greater than 7.5%, based on the pooled-risk equation

If the patient qualifies for one of the statin benefit groups, the intensity of therapy is determined. The statin intensity levels are low, moderate, and high. High-intensity statin therapy is recommended in patients with known ASCVD or similar risk. The two most potent regimens for intensive statin therapy are rosu-vastatin 40 mg and atorvastatin 80 mg (Nicholls et al., 2011). The PROVE IT-TIMI 22 trial demonstrated that high-intensity lipid- lowering therapy with atorvastatin 80 mg/day had reduction in cardiovascular clinical events compared with moderate-intensity lipid-lowering therapy with pravastatin 40 mg/day (Cannon et al., 2004).

While statins are beneficial in the primary and secondary prevention of CHD, these agents are also understood to have secondary beneficial effects beyond cholesterol lowering. There is data suggesting cholesterol-independent or "pleiotropic" effects of statins. The ASTEROID trial, for example, demonstrated that statins improve endothelial function, modulate inflammatory responses, maintain plaque stability, and contribute to the prevention of thrombus formation (ASTEROID Investigators, 2006).

NICOTINIC ACID

Nicotinic acid (vitamin B3, niacin) is a water-soluble inhibitor of metabolism of free fatty acids from the adipose tissue, causing a reduction in triglyceride synthesis and VLDL. The reduction of VLDL is directly correlated to a reduction in LDL synthesis. One of the major advantages of nicotinic acid is the ability to increase HDL. Nicotinic acid acts directly to inhibit the metabolism of Apo-A1, a primary structural component of HDL that is responsible for removing excess cholesterol esters from the plasma. With the use of nicotinic acid, there is an approximate reduction in LDL by 10% to 20%, increase in HDL by 20% to 35%, and reduction in TG by approximately 30% to 70%. The available nicotinic acid products are the following:

- Nicotinic acid immediate release (Niacor®)
- Nicotinic acid extended release (Niaspan®)

The primary adverse effect of nicotinic acid is dose-dependent facial flushing. Flushing is caused by a dilation of subcutaneous blood vessels presenting as redness, warmth, and itching. To reduce flushing as a side effect of nicotinic acid, use extended-release formulations, titrate the dose slowly, administer aspirin prior to niacin, avoid hot fluids prior to administration, and administer with food. Other common adverse effects associated with nicotinic acid include gastrointestinal upset, flatulence, nausea, diarrhea, and activation of peptic ulcer disease. The clinical use of niacin is limited by poor tolerability (Guyton & Bays, 2007).

BILE ACID SEQUESTRANTS

Bile acid sequestrants are a class of medications that act within the gut to provide lipid-lowering effects. These agents promote the excretion of bile acids by binding to them and preventing their reabsorption, resulting in increased liver uptake of cholesterol from the plasma. Reductions in LDL vary, but range from 10% to 35%. A negative effect of bile acid sequestrants is a potential for an increase in serum TG levels.

Primarily, the adverse effects of bile acid sequestrants are gastrointestinal, including severe constipation, flatulence, nausea, and vomiting. Most patients benefit from a stool softener in combination with a bile acid sequestrant to avoid these side effects. There have been reports of reduced folate levels with long-term use of bile acid sequestrants, so folate levels should be monitored closely. Drug interactions are also common, mainly due to decreased absorption of the medication caused by altered gastrointestinal emptying and gastric absorption. Separating other medications from the administration of bile acid sequestrants is important.

Available bile acid sequestrant agents include the following:

- Colestipol (Colestid®)
- Cholestyramine (Questran®)
- Colesevelam (Welchol®)

FIBRATES

The fibrates act by activating the peroxisome-proliferator–activated receptor alpha (PPAR-a). This nuclear receptor subtype is primarily located in the liver, heart, kidney, and muscle, where fatty acids are metabolized. Fibrates increase HDL production, increase lipolysis of TGs, and increase LDL particle size. Fibrates have demonstrated an approximate reduction in TG by 20% to 50%, a 5% to 20% reduction in LDL, and a 10% to 35% increase in HDL. Adverse drug events are relatively minimal; the most common are dyspepsia, myalgia, gallstones, and elevations of creatinine kinase. There is a risk of rhabdomyolysis, and fibrates are typically not prescribed with statins concurrently due to the additive potential for rhabdomyolysis and general muscle aches. Fibrates are contraindicated in patients with gallbladder disease and severe renal or hepatic impairment. Fibrates have not demonstrated lower cardiovascular mortality and therefore are not considered first-line agents to treat hyperlipidemia. Their primary clinical use is for the treatment of hypertriglyceridemia. Available fibrate agents include the following:

- Gemfibrozil (Lopid®)
- Fenofibrate (TriCor®)
- Fenofibric acid (Trilipix®)

CHOLESTEROL ABSORPTION INHIBITOR

Ezetimibe (Zetia®) acts by inhibiting a cholesterol transporter located within the brush-border of the small intestine, leading to reduced absorption of cholesterol in the intestine. With monotherapy, there are relatively small reductions in LDL (12%–20%), and minimal changes in HDL and TG. The primary clinical role of ezetimibe is in conjunction with statins for additive effect on LDL reduction. However, recent data have questioned the role of ezetimibe. The SEAS trial compared the effect of simvastatin and ezetimibe in patients with aortic valve stenosis, and there was no statistically significant difference in progression of stenosis or cardiovascular events with the combination (Rossebo et al., 2008). The SEAS trial also found an increased risk of cancer and cancer death in the active treatment arm. Statins do not appear to increase the risk of cancer, which raised the possibility that ezetimibe treatment could cause cancer. Because of this concern, an interim analysis of two other trials of simvastatin and ezetimibe (IMPROVE-IT and SHARP) was performed. This analysis found no increased risk of incident cancer but a trend toward an increase in cancer deaths (Peto et al., 2008). Another large surrogate endpoint trial attempting to demonstrate clinical benefits with the addition of ezetimibe was the ENHANCE trial (ENHANCE Investigators, 2008). ENHANCE was a double-blind, randomized, 24-month trial comparing the effects of daily therapy with 80 mg of simvastatin either with placebo or with 10 mg of ezetimibe in 720 patients with familial hypercholesterolemia. Although there was an additive reduction in LDL, there was no statistically significant difference in the primary outcome of change in carotid intima-media thickness from baseline.

Since enhanced cardiovascular benefit remains undetermined, the role of ezetimibe as a lipid-lowering agent is somewhat suboptimal. Additive reductions in LDL can often be achieved simply by maximizing the dose of statins, which have a number of potential health benefits in addition to lipid lowering. One potential role in therapy for ezetimibe is for patients who cannot tolerate high-dose statin therapy (due to increased myopathy) but fail to meet cholesterol goals with low- or moderate-intensity statin therapy.

FISH OIL

Fish oil may be associated with a decreased risk of CHD and CHD-related death. Fish oil contains eicosapentaenoic acid (EPA) and docosahexaenoic acid (DHA), both of which are long-chain omega-3 polyunsaturated fatty acids (Harper & Jacobson, 2001). Fish oils can reduce levels of TG through inhibition of the synthesis of VLDL-TG and apolipoprotein B. Although available as a dietary supplement over the counter, a commercial preparation of omega-3 acid ethyl esters (Lovaza) is approved by the U.S. Food and Drug Administration (FDA) for prescription use. Lovaza contains a combination of EPA and DHA, and, in patients with hypertriglyceridemia, can reduce TG levels between 20% and 50%. The recommended dose is 4 g/day. The principal adverse effects of this product are gastrointestinal, including diarrhea, nausea, and abdominal pain.

For full reference citations to this chapter, please see "Section References" in the back of the book, under the heading "Section VII."

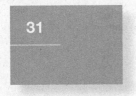

Antithrombotic Therapy and Pharmacotherapeutics of Thrombotic Disease States

CONNIE H. YOON AND DEV CHATTERJI

PHARMACOTHERAPEUTICS OF THROMBOEMBOLIC DISEASE STATES

Antithrombotic therapy, which includes anticoagulant, antiplatelet, and thrombolytic agents, is indicated for the treatment or prophylaxis of thromboembolic disease states. These agents may be used for the treatment of venous thromboembolisms (VTE), myocardial infarction, peripheral arterial disease, acute ischemic or cardioembolic stroke, and heparin-induced thrombocytopenia (HIT). Additionally, various antithrombotics have been studied for the prevention of cardioembolic stroke—due to either atrial fibrillation (AF) or heart valve replacement—and for the secondary prevention of ischemic stroke. The choice of therapy can be complex and difficult, often determined by the required duration of therapy and individual patient factors. This section discusses the relevant pathophysiology and mechanism of the antithrombotic drug classes, as well as the individual agents studied for each thromboembolic disease state.

HEMOSTASIS

Hemostasis is a complex process involving numerous enzymes and cofactors. Formation of thrombi depends on the activation of the coagulation cascade either through the intrinsic, contact-activation pathway or through the extrinsic, tissue-factor pathway (Figure 31.1). The intrinsic pathway is initiated when factor XII comes into contact with a charged or damaged surface. Activation of factor XII triggers a sequential reaction of factor XI, IX, and X. Factor Xa, the activated form of factor X, marks the start of the common pathway, where the intrinsic and extrinsic pathways converge (Gailani & Renne, 2007).

The extrinsic pathway becomes activated when some form of vessel injury activates factor VII in the plasma and releases the tissue factor (TF) from the endothelial cell membranes (Mackman, Tilley, & Key, 2007). Activated factor VII (VIIa) and TF form a complex, which subsequently leads to the activation of factor X. Platelets rapidly adhere to the site of vessel-wall injury as the coagulation cascade magnifies, starting the initial thrombus formation.

As stated before, the common pathway of the coagulation cascade begins with the activation of factor X. Factor Xa activates prothrombin (factor II) into thrombin (factor IIa), utilizing factor Va as a cofactor. Thrombin then converts fibrinogen

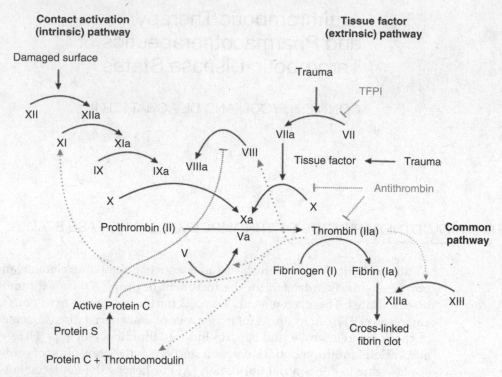

FIGURE 31.1 The coagulation cascade.

TFPI, tissue factor pathway inhibitor.

Source: Wikimedia Commons (2007).

(factor I) into fibrin (factor Ia). Fibrin consumes factor XIIIa as a cofactor for the final stage in the development of a clot. Fibrin deposits cross-link to the activated platelets to stabilize the thrombus (Mackman et al., 2007).

PHARMACOLOGY OF THE ANTITHROMBOTIC AGENTS

Anticoagulants

Anticoagulant agents primarily target the various factors in the coagulation pathway either through indirect or through direct inhibition of factor Xa or IIa. The final common mechanism of this class of antithrombotics is to prevent the cleavage of fibrinogen to fibrin.

Unfractionated Heparin

Unfractionated heparin (UFH) inhibits the formation of fibrin by inhibiting factor Xa and factor IIa (thrombin) through the activation of antithrombin. UFH is a mixture of long polysaccharide chains of varying lengths. The active binding site, a pentasaccharide sequence, can be found in random locations along the entire length of the chain. This pentasaccharide sequence binds to antithrombin, which induces a conformational change in antithrombin, allowing for greater affinity to bind both factor Xa and IIa. In order to inactivate factor IIa, UFH must bind to both antithrombin and factor IIa (Hirsh, Anand, Halperin, & Fuster, 2001). Thus, only the UFH molecules of sufficient chain lengths are able to inactivate thrombin (Figure 31.2). However, inactivation of factor Xa relies only on the pentasaccharide sequence to activate antithrombin; therefore, shorter sequences of UFH can inhibit factor Xa. UFH inactivates factor Xa and IIa in a 1:1 ratio. A major limitation of UFH and other heparin derivatives is the lack of activity against clot-bound thrombin and factor Xa.

UFH is normally administered as a continuous infusion for treatment, and subcutaneously for prophylaxis. Infusion rates for treatment are titrated according to lab monitoring of anti-Xa levels to determine the quantity of heparin in the body or either activated partial thromboplastin time (aPTT) or activated clotting time

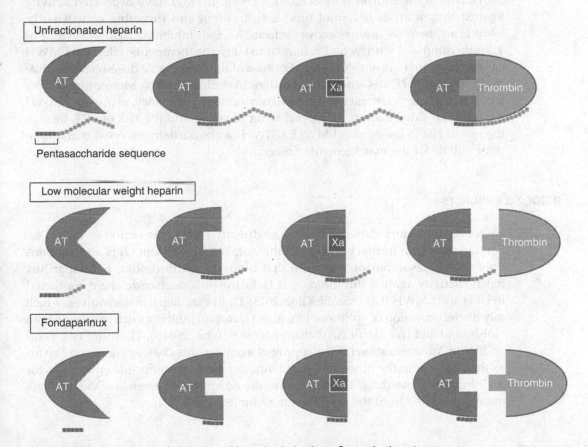

FIGURE 31.2 Mechanism of heparin and heparin derivatives. See color insert.

AT, antithrombin; Xa, factor Xa; UFH, unfractionated heparin, LMWH, low molecular weight heparin.

UFH: The pentasaccharide sequence binds to antithrombin, inducing a conformational change to increase its affinity for factor Xa or IIa. Inactivation of factor IIa requires UFH chains of sufficient length to bind to both antithrombin and thrombin.

LMWH: Similar to UFH, the pentasaccharide sequence activates antithrombin, which binds and inactivates factor Xa. Due to the shorter chain length, its activity against thrombin is limited.

Indirect factor Xa inhibitor/Fondaparinux: Only the pentasaccharide sequence is present; thus, only factor Xa can be inactivated through the antithrombin-dependent mechanism utilized by UFH and LMWH.

(ACT) to monitor therapeutic targets. As UFH can also bind to plasma proteins, resulting in an unpredictable dose-response relationship, lab monitoring is always performed using one of the three parameters.

The predominant adverse effect of heparin is bleeding, which can be treated with protamine sulfate to reverse the effects of UFH. A major but rare adverse event is HIT, with or without associated thrombosis. HIT is a serious, acute condition with associated morbidity of limb loss and mortality, the management of which will be discussed later in this section.

Low Molecular Weight Heparin

Low molecular weight heparins (LMWHs) are derived from UFH, but the pentasaccharide sequence fragments are about a third of the length of UFH (Hirsh et al., 2001). Due to the shorter polysaccharide chain, LWMH have decreased activity against thrombin, as it cannot bind antithrombin and thrombin concurrently. LMWH are therefore more selective for factor Xa, thus inhibiting factor Xa in a 2:1 or 4:1 ratio compared with factor IIa. Similar to UFH, the therapeutic effects of LMWH can be monitored via anti-Xa levels. Because of the predictable dose-response relationship of LMWH, this is not routinely done in clinical practice. Monitoring anti-Xa levels is generally recommended in renal impairment, pregnancy, or obesity. LMWH have similar side effects to UFH, including bleeding and the risk of HIT, though the risk of HIT is lower with LMWH. LMWH can be partially reversed with protamine sulfate for the management of bleeding.

Factor Xa Inhibitors

Factor Xa inhibitors either indirectly or directly inhibit the action of factor Xa. Fondaparinux, an indirect factor Xa inhibitor, is derived from UFH and contains only the pentasaccharide sequence that binds to antithrombin. Fondaparinux has no activity against thrombin, as it lacks the polysaccharide chain contained in UFH and LMWH (GlaxoSmithKline, 2013). Unlike the heparin derivatives, which rely on the activation of antithrombin, direct factor Xa inhibitors can inactivate both clot-bound and free factor Xa (Bristol-Myers Squibb, 2014b). There are two Food and Drug Administration (FDA)-approved agents in this class, apixaban and rivaroxaban. Similar to the other anticoagulants, the most common side effect of factor Xa inhibitors is bleeding. There are currently no approved agents for the management of bleeding from the direct factor Xa inhibitors.

Direct Thrombin Inhibitors

Direct thrombin inhibitors (DTI) directly inhibit the action of clot-bound or free factor IIa, thus acting independently of antithrombin. Hirudin was the first anticoagulant used in humans. It was initially isolated from the salivary glands of medical leeches for its anticoagulant properties (Greinacher & Warkentin, 2008) but is no longer used today. The first recombinant hirudin used clinically was lepirudin, a bivalent DTI, binding to two sites on thrombin. The bivalent DTIs bind to both the active-site pocket of thrombin and the fibrinogen-binding exosite. Lepirudin was discontinued in 2012 due to its high immunogenicity potential. The only bivalent DTI available today is bivalirudin, which is administered as a continuous infusion.

In contrast to bivalent DTIs, univalent DTIs, such as argatroban and dabigatran, bind only to the active site of thrombin. Argatroban is also administered as a continuous infusion, while dabigatran is the first approved oral DTI. The most common adverse event for all three of these agents is bleeding. There are currently no available medications approved for the reversal of these agents.

Vitamin K Antagonists

Warfarin is a coumarin derivative that binds to the C1 subunit of vitamin K epoxide reductase enzyme complex (VKORC1), thus preventing the synthesis of vitamin K–dependent clotting factors, factors II, VII, IX, X, as well as the anticoagulants protein C and protein S (Bristol-Myers Squibb, 2014a; Hirsh, Fuster, Ansell, & Halperin, 2003). While peak plasma concentrations occur around 4 hours after oral administration, the anticoagulation effect begins within 24 hours. The peak antithrombotic effect, however, requires 72 to 96 hours, as warfarin requires the reduction of factor II and X in order to exhibit its full anticoagulant effect. Thus, the duration of action of a single dose of warfarin ranges from 2 to 5 days, based on the half-lives of the targeted clotting factors (factor II: 60 hours; factor VII: 4 to 6 hours; factor IX: 24 hours; factor X: 48 to 72 hours; protein C: 8 hours; protein S: 30 hours).

Warfarin is a racemic mixture of two active isomers, the S-enantiomer and the R-enantiomer. The S-enantiomer generates two to five times the anticoagulant effects of the R-enantiomer. The S-enantiomer is primarily metabolized by the cytochrome P450 (CYP) 2C9 enzyme. Specific genetic variants of CYP2C9 and the VKORC1 gene contribute significantly to the variability in warfarin dose requirements. The anticoagulant effect of warfarin is also influenced by drug–drug interactions and drug–food interactions. Drugs can affect the absorption, metabolism, or clearance of warfarin, or result in a decrease in the synthesis of vitamin K. Table 31.1 identifies drug interactions with warfarin that occur with a high probability (Ageno et al., 2012). This list is not all-inclusive, and each drug interaction may impact patients to varying degrees. Drugs that inhibit the clearance of the S-enantiomer

TABLE 31.1 Major Drug Interactions With Warfarin

Drug	Effect on INR	Mechanism of Interaction
Amiodarone	Increase	Inhibits clearance of R- and S-enantiomers
Carbamazepine	Decrease	Increases metabolism of warfarin
Cholestyramine	Decrease	Decreases absorption of warfarin
Ciprofloxacin	Increase	Precise mechanism unknown
Fluconazole	Increase	Inhibits metabolism of R- and S-enantiomers
Metronidazole	Increase	Inhibits clearance S-enantiomer
Nafcillin	Decrease	Increases metabolism of warfarin
Omeprazole	Increase	Inhibits clearance R-enantiomer
Sulfamethoxazole/Trimethoprim	Increase	Inhibits clearance S-enantiomer
Voriconazole	Increase	Inhibits metabolism of R- and S-enantiomers

INR, international normalized ratio.

have a greater impact on potentiating the anticoagulant effects of warfarin compared with the R-enantiomer. Foods also contain variable concentrations of vitamin K, which can impact the effectiveness of warfarin. Patients are often instructed to maintain a consistent serving of vitamin K in their weekly diet to allow for a more consistent anticoagulant effect from warfarin.

Warfarin dosing varies for each patient due to the previously discussed genetic predispositions and interactions with drugs and food. Initial doses are primarily prescribed by adjusting for the patient's age, with elderly patients receiving lower doses of warfarin. The standard coagulation parameter utilized to monitor the anticoagulant effect of warfarin is the international normalized ratio (INR) (Hirsh et al., 2003). INR is a calculated value that allows for the standardization of prothrombin time across various laboratories. INR target ranges vary depending on the indicating disease states. Table 31.2 identifies the most common indications and their goal INR (January et al., 2014; Kearon et al., 2012; Nishimura et al., 2014).

TABLE 31.2 Common Indications for Warfarin and INR Goals

Indication	Goal INR (Target Range)
Atrial fibrillation	2.5 (2.0–3.0)
Mechanical heart valve*	3.0 (2.5–3.5)
DVT/PE	2.5 (2.0–3.0)

*Specific INR goals depend on the type and location of valve as well as patient risk factors.

DVT, deep vein thrombosis; INR, international normalized ratio; PE, pulmonary embolism.

Warfarin tablets are color-coded based on the specific strength of each tablet (Table 31.3), and the color is the same regardless of the manufacturer. This added feature is helpful in situations where patients may not be aware of the strength of their tablet but can easily identify its color.

TABLE 31.3 Warfarin Tablet Color and Corresponding Strength

Tablet Strength (mg)	Tablet Color
1	Pink
2	Lavender (light purple)
2.5	Green
3	Tan
4	Blue
5	Peach (light orange)
6	Teal (blue-green)
7.5	Yellow
10	White

Reprinted with permission from University of Utah Health Care Thrombosis Service (2007).

Antiplatelet Agents

Inhibition of platelet aggregation is a component of the management of various thromboembolic disease conditions, including ischemic stroke, ischemic heart disease, and various cardioembolic disease states. Pharmacologic options for therapy differ primarily by mechanism of action and degree of platelet inhibition. All agents in this class work to decrease platelet activation and aggregation.

Aspirin

Acetylsalicyclic acid or aspirin is a nonsteroidal anti-inflammatory drug that irreversibly inhibits cyclooxygenase (COX)-1 and COX-2 (Bjorkman, 1998). Inhibiting COX-1 completely inactivates this enzyme, thus impacting the synthesis of thromboxane, prostacyclin, and prostaglandins. Thromboxane, prostacyclin, and prostaglandins are responsible for protecting the stomach mucosa, activating platelet aggregation, and maintaining renal blood flow. COX-2 inhibition leads to a reduction in the synthesis of the prostaglandins that contributes to the inflammatory process. Aspirin is 170 times more potent in inactivating COX-1 than COX-2. This relative potency is likely the reason for its primary role in cardiovascular protection but also explains the gastrointestinal (GI) toxicities of aspirin (Awtry & Loscalzo, 2000). Relatively low doses of aspirin, less than 100 mg, halt the production of thromboxane, thus inhibiting platelet activation and aggregation. Higher doses do not appear to be more efficacious in this regard and often increase the side effects, including GI bleeding.

Platelet inhibition occurs within an hour of ingesting aspirin. While the half-life of this agent is only 20 minutes, the effects on platelets continue for the lifetime of the platelet, approximately 7 to 10 days (Awtry & Loscalzo, 2000). This is due to the inability of platelets to generate new COX.

P2Y₁₂ ADP Receptor Inhibitors

The $P2Y_{12}$ adenosine diphosphate (ADP) receptors can be found on platelet membranes. Activation of these receptors is required for platelet aggregation. While clopidogrel is the most extensively studied ADP inhibitor, three other agents exist in this class: ticlopidine, prasugrel, and ticagrelor. Ticlopidine will not be discussed, as it is rarely used due to its black box warning of severe hematologic toxicity of neutropenia, agranulocytosis, thrombotic thrombocytopenia purpura (TTP), and aplastic anemia, the requirement for extensive monitoring, and the existence of newer ADP-inhibiting agents. Prasugrel and ticagrelor are approved for use only in the setting of acute coronary syndromes and will be discussed in the ischemic heart disease section.

Clopidogrel is a second-generation thienopyridine. Before prescribing clopidogrel, one must take into consideration two major factors, CYP polymorphisms and drug interactions. Clopidogrel is a prodrug that undergoes hepatic metabolism through the CYP2C19 enzyme. Patients with a CYP2C19*2 allele have a reduction in enzyme function leading to decreased activity of clopidogrel and an increased rate of cardiovascular events and in-stent thrombosis. While testing for genetic polymorphisms is available, routine testing is not recommended at this time (Anderson et al., 2013a; Jneid et al., 2010). Also, as clopidogrel is metabolized with the CYP2C19 enzyme, drugs that inhibit CYP2C19 can inhibit the activity of clopidogrel, leading to an increased risk of cardiovascular events. The most predominant drug class that interacts with clopidogrel is the proton pump inhibitors. Omeprazole demonstrates the most significant interaction and should never be concomitantly administered with clopidogrel (Anderson et al., 2013a). For patients who require proton pump inhibition, pantoprazole is preferred, as it does not inhibit CYP2C19 as extensively as other agents in this class. The two major side effects associated with clopidogrel are bleeding and TTP, which rarely occurs.

Dipyridamole

Dipyridamole is a pyrimidopyrimidine derivative that has both antiplatelet and vasodilator properties. Dipyridamole elicits its antiplatelet effects by inhibiting the uptake of adenosine into platelets, resulting in increased concentrations of adenosine and ultimately an increase in cyclic-3'5',-adenosine monophosphate (cAMP) levels, thereby reducing platelet function (Boehringer Ingelheim Pharmaceuticals, Inc., 2012). Additionally, dipyridamole inhibits phosphodiesterase, subsequently increasing the production of nitric oxide and resulting in vasodilation.

Fibrinolytics

The formation of a clot and the ultimate breakdown of the clot are a naturally occurring homeostatic mechanism within the body. The breakdown of the clot is mediated primarily by plasmin, a naturally occurring fibrinolytic. Plasmin circulates in its inactive form, plasminogen, which is produced by the liver. The conversion of plasminogen to its active form, plasmin, occurs naturally by tissue plasminogen activator (tPA), and can also be mediated by medications. Fibrinolytic agents are used in scenarios with the potential for complications of thrombosis, ST-segment elevation myocardial infarctions (STEMI), acute ischemic strokes, or massive pulmonary emboli. Alteplase, reteplase, and tenecteplase are all versions of naturally occurring tPA. Only alteplase is approved for the treatment of pulmonary embolism (PE) and ischemic stroke. Reteplase and tenecteplase are reviewed in the subsequent section on ischemic heart disease, as these agents are approved only for the treatment of STEMI.

PHARMACOTHERAPY OF THROMBOEMBOLIC DISEASE STATES

This section specifically reviews common thromboembolic disease states, which utilize the previously discussed antithrombotic agents for treatment and prophylaxis.

Venous Thromboembolism

PE and deep vein thrombosis (DVT) represent the spectrum of one disease, collectively referred to as VTE. VTE is an important cause of morbidity and mortality, particularly in hospitalized patients, and represents a national health problem in our society. VTE is responsible for approximately 15% of all in-hospital deaths, and the U.S. Surgeon General has estimated that VTE accounts for more than 100,000 deaths annually (Turpie, Chin, & Lip, 2002). In February 2012, the American College of Chest Physicians (ACCP) released the ninth edition of its antithrombotic and thrombolytic therapy evidence-based clinical practice guidelines. These are the most well-recognized guidelines for the prevention and treatment of VTE and assist in providing clinical recommendations on medication treatment and duration of therapy (Kearon et al., 2012).

VTE Prophylaxis

VTE is a common preventable cause of morbidity and mortality in hospitalized medical and surgical patients. Despite evidence and cost-effectiveness of VTE prophylactic measures, adherence to widely accepted guidelines for VTE prophylaxis remains suboptimal. The International Medical Prevention Registry on Venous Thromboembolism (IMPROVE) suggests that only 60% of hospitalized medical patients who meet criteria for VTE prophylaxis actually receive therapy (IMPROVE Investigators, 2007). For this reason, the Agency for Healthcare Research and Quality (AHRQ) has identified VTE prophylaxis as a main strategy for improvement in patient safety.

The pharmacologic options with established roles in VTE prophylaxis include low-dose UFH, LMWH, and selective factor Xa inhibitors. The optimal agent and dose to use for VTE prophylaxis is based on the patient's level of risk for thrombosis versus potential complications of bleeding (Table 31.4).

Low-dose UFH, LMWH, and fondaparinux are all evidence-based options recommended by ACCP for VTE prophylaxis. The Prophylaxis in Medical Patients with Enoxaparin (MEDENOX) and the Prevention of Venous Thromboembolism in Acutely Ill Medical Patients (PREVENT) trials provided initial evidence to establish the role of the LMWH, enoxaparin, and dalteparin in VTE prophylaxis in

TABLE 31.4 Risk Stratification for VTE Prophylaxis

Risk Level	Patient Characteristics	Pharmacological Options for Prophylaxis
Low	Minor surgery Fully ambulatory	None generally recommended
Moderate	Most surgical patients Acutely ill medical patients with limited mobility	Low-dose UFH LMWH Fondaparinux
High	Major orthopedic surgical patients Major trauma Medical patients with high thromboembolic risk	LMWH Fondaparinux Warfarin

LMWH, low molecular weight heparin; UFH, unfractionated heparin; VTE, venous thromboembolism.

TABLE 31.5 Subcutaneous Dosing of UFH, LMWH, and Fondaparinux for VTE Prophylaxis

Agent	VTE Prophylaxis Dose	Clinical Pearls
Unfractionated heparin	General surgery and acute medical illness: 5,000 units SQ TID	Can be used in patients with renal impairment including patients on hemodialysis
Dalteparin	Surgery and acute medical illness: 5,000 units SQ daily	
Enoxaparin	General surgery and acute medical illness: ■ 40 mg SQ daily ■ CrCl < 30 mL/min: 30 mg SQ daily Hip/knee surgery ■ 30 mg SQ BID ■ CrCl < 30 mL/min: 30 mg SQ daily	Advantages: less frequent dosing, lower incidence of HIT Contraindicated in patients on hemodialysis
Fondaparinux	Surgery and acute medical illness: 2.5 mg SQ daily	Contraindicated in renal impairment, CrCl < 30 mL/min

BID, twice daily; CrCl, creatinine clearance; HIT, heparin-induced thrombocytopenia; SQ, subcutaneously; TID, three times daily; VTE, venous thromboembolism.

acutely ill medical patients (Leizorovicz et al., 2004; Samama et al., 1999). The Arixtra for Thromboembolism Prevention in a Medical Indications Study (ARTEMIS) established a role for fondaparinux (ARTEMIS Investigators, 2006). Table 31.5 lists dosing information for these agents.

Treatment of VTE

Since DVT and PE are manifestations of the same disease process, they are treated similarly. The goals of treatment are to prevent further clot extension, prevent recurrence of thrombosis, and prevent development of late complications. Anticoagulants are the mainstay in therapy for VTE, but there are substantial concerns with use of these high-risk drugs. The optimal use of antithrombotic drugs requires in-depth knowledge of their pharmacodynamic and pharmacokinetic properties. Treatment options for initial anticoagulation include the following:

■ UFH
■ LMWH
■ Fondaparinux
■ Vitamin K antagonists: warfarin
■ Oral factor Xa inhibitors: apixaban and rivaroxaban
■ Oral direct thrombin inhibitors: dabigatran

Unfractionated Heparin

Acute treatment of VTE with parenteral UFH followed by warfarin has been a treatment modality for patients with VTE for decades. The antithrombotic response to standard doses of UFH varies widely among patients, necessitating the monitoring of the anticoagulant effect using a suitable coagulation study—measured by the aPTT or heparin anti-Xa assay. While heparin dosing and monitoring protocols are institution specific, the general therapeutic level of heparin for VTE measured by the aPTT is 1.5 to 2.5 times the mean control value of the normal aPTT range. This corresponds to a heparin level of 0.3 to 0.7 units/mL when measured by the anti-Xa assay. It is critical to achieve a therapeutic level of heparin within the first 24 hours of initiating therapy to prevent recurrent VTE.

UFH can be safely and effectively used in patients with renal insufficiency, including patients on hemodialysis. Heparin compounds can also be safely used in pregnancy. Because UFH does not cross the placenta, it is not associated with teratogenicity or fetal-bleeding complications. UFH is also not excreted in breast milk and is considered safe to use by women who are breastfeeding.

Low Molecular Weight Heparin

The LMWHs have a number of advantages over UFH. The LMWHs have favorable pharmacokinetics and pharmacodynamics compared with UFH. They have greater bioavailability and simplified dosing. Three LMWHs have been used clinically for VTE in the United States: dalteparin, enoxaparin, and tinzaparin (Table 31.6). Their pharmacokinetic properties allow for body-weight adjusted subcutaneous dosing once or twice daily without laboratory monitoring.

In special patient populations such as children, patients with kidney failure, obese patients, and pregnant women, laboratory monitoring using anti-Xa concentrations has been suggested (Kearon et al., 2012). The usual time to obtain a blood sample for anti-Xa is after concentrations are expected to peak, around 4 hours after an injection. A target range of 0.6 to 1.0 IU/mL is suggested for twice-daily dosing, and a target of 1 to 2 IU is recommended for once-daily administration.

Fondaparinux (Arixtra)

Fondaparinux was approved by the FDA for the acute treatment of DVT and PE in 2004, and it remains a safe and effective alternative to UFH and LMWH for the treatment of VTE. Two major clinical trials demonstrated the safety and efficacy

TABLE 31.6 Dosing of LMWHs in Treatment of VTE

Agent	VTE Treatment Dose	Clinical Pearls
Enoxaparin	1 mg/kg SQ every 12 hr 1.5 mg/kg every 24 hr Renal impairment (CrCl <30 mL/min): 1 mg/kg every 24 hr	Contraindicated in HD
Dalteparin*	200 units/kg SQ every 24 hr	No specific dose adjustment recommended in renal impairment
Tinzaparin	175 units/kg SQ every 24 hr	No specific dose adjustment recommended in renal impairment

CrCl, creatinine clearance; HD, hemodialysis; SQ, subcutaneously; VTE, venous thromboembolism.

*Off-label use in the United States in non-cancer patients.

of fondaparinux. In the MATISSE-DVT trial, a fixed-dose regimen of fondaparinux (7.5 mg every 24 hours) given by subcutaneous (SQ) injection was compared with the standard weight-adjusted dosing of enoxaparin (1 mg/kg every 12 hours) for the acute treatment of DVT followed by 3 months of warfarin therapy (Büller et al., 2004). In the MATISSE-PE trial, fondaparinux (7.5 mg SQ every 24 hours) was compared with UFH administered by IV infusion (Büller et al., 2003). In both trials, the dose of fondaparinux was increased to 10 mg SQ every 24 hours for patients who weighed more than 100 kg and reduced to 5 mg SQ every 24 hours for those who weighed less than 50 kg. Renal function must be carefully monitored for patients on fondaparinux, as the drug is contraindicated if creatinine clearance is less than 30 mL/min.

Warfarin

Warfarin is not a suitable option for the acute treatment of VTE because it does not produce a rapid antithrombotic effect. However, warfarin is highly effective for the long-term management of VTE and should be started concurrently with rapid-acting injectable anticoagulant therapy—UFH, LMWH, or fondaparinux—on the first treatment day. The recommended target INR for VTE is 2.5 (goal between 2 and 3). The injectable anticoagulant should overlap with warfarin until an INR greater than 2 has been achieved for 24 hours. A starting dose of 5 mg/day is recommended for the first 2 days for most patients, with subsequent dosing based on the INR. A reduced starting dose of less than 5 mg/day, for example, 2.5 mg, is recommended in patients who are older than 65 years, are debilitated, have poor nutritional status or liver disease, or who are taking drugs known to elevate the INR. Higher warfarin doses, for example, 10 mg, may be appropriate for young, otherwise healthy patients.

Direct Factor Xa and Direct Thrombin Inhibitors

Two novel groups of oral anticoagulants include the oral factor Xa inhibitors—apixaban or rivaroxaban—and the oral DTI dabigatran. These are fixed-dose oral anticoagulants that, compared with warfarin, do not require routine laboratory monitoring or frequent dose adjustments. In addition, these oral options are rapid acting and can be used in both the acute and long-term treatment of VTE. The major disadvantages of these agents are the lack of long-term efficacy studies and the nonavailability of antidote for bleeding events. Dosing recommendations for the treatment of VTE are listed in Table 31.7.

APIXABAN
Apixaban is a factor Xa inhibitor that was FDA approved in August 2014 for treatment of VTE. Data regarding the safety and efficacy for the treatment of acute VTE and prevention of recurrent VTE are demonstrated in the AMPLIFY and AMPLIFY-EXT trials. AMPLIFY was a prospective randomized double-blind trial that compared apixaban (10 mg twice daily for 7 days followed by 5 mg twice daily for 6 months) with conventional anticoagulation (enoxaparin followed by warfarin) for the treatment of acute VTE (DVT and/or PE). There was no difference in the rates

TABLE 31.7 Factor Xa Inhibitors and Direct Thrombin Inhibitors in the Treatment of VTE

Agent	Class	VTE Dosing
Apixaban (*Eliquis®*)	FXa inhibitor	Initial: 10 mg BID for 7 days Maintenance: 5 mg BID Prevention of recurrence: 2.5 mg BID
Rivaroxaban (*Xarelto®*)	FXa inhibitor	Initial: 15 mg BID for 21 days Maintenance & prevention of recurrence: 20 mg daily
Dabigatran (*Pradaxa®*)	DTI	Initial: 5 to 10 days injectable anticoagulant Maintenance & prevention of recurrence: 150 mg BID

BID, twice daily; DTI, direct thrombin inhibitor; FXa, factor Xa; VTE, venous thromboembolism.

of recurrent symptomatic VTE or VTE-related death between the groups, and fewer bleeding events were reported in the apixaban group (AMPLIFY Investigators, 2013). In AMPLIFY-EXT, two doses of apixaban, a prophylactic dose of 2.5 mg twice daily or a therapeutic dose of 5 mg twice daily, were compared with placebo in patients with VTE who had already completed 6 to 12 months of conventional anticoagulation. Compared with placebo, treatment with apixaban for 12 months at 2.5 mg and 5 mg resulted in lower rates of symptomatic VTE or VTE-related death (AMPLIFY-EXT Investigators, 2013).

RIVAROXABAN

Rivaroxaban is a factor Xa inhibitor that is FDA approved for the treatment of VTE. The EINSTEIN-DVT and EINSTEIN-PE were randomized open-label, controlled noninferiority trials in patients with acute DVT or PE; the trials demonstrated that oral rivaroxaban alone is noninferior to traditional therapy for a treatment period of 3, 6, or 12 months with similar rates of recurrent VTE and clinically relevant bleeding. Traditional therapy was defined as initial warfarin with a target INR 2 to 3 overlapping with enoxaparin. The dosing of rivaroxaban used in the study was 15 mg for 3 weeks followed by 20 mg once daily (EINSTEIN Investigators, 2010; EINSTEIN-PE Investigators, 2012).

DABIGATRAN

Dabigatran is the first and only oral DTI approved for the treatment of VTE. One of the major trials demonstrating safety and efficacy of dabigatran for the treatment and prevention of VTE is known as the RE-COVER study. In this randomized, double-blind trial, patients with acute VTE were treated for 6 months with either dabigatran (150 mg by mouth twice per day) or warfarin, each after 7 days of initial parenteral anticoagulation. Dabigatran had a similar incidence of recurrent VTE, VTE-related deaths, and major bleeding compared with warfarin (RE-COVER Study Group, 2009).

Thrombolysis

A majority of cases of VTE are treated with anticoagulant therapy alone. The routine use of thrombolytic therapy is not indicated and should be considered only for life-threatening VTE, for example, acute massive PE. For patients with DVT, thrombolytic therapy should be considered only for patients who present with shock, hemodynamic instability, right ventricular dysfunction, or massive DVT with limb gangrene. Similarly, for patients with acute PE, thrombolytic therapy is indicated only in patients with hemodynamic instability or right ventricular dysfunction. Furthermore, the diagnosis of acute DVT or PE must be confirmed via objective diagnostic tools prior to initiation of a thrombolytic.

When thrombolysis is indicated for the treatment of VTE, alteplase is the preferred agent in the United States. The FDA-approved dose for acute massive or submassive PE is a fixed dosage of 100 mg infused over 2 hours. Bleeding is the major adverse reaction, and factors that increase the risk of bleeding must be evaluated before therapy is initiated. These include recent surgery, trauma, intracranial bleeding, recent stroke, or other active bleeding (Konstantinides, Heusel, Heinrick, & Kasper, 2002).

Treatment of VTE in Special Populations

Certain patient populations with acute VTE require special consideration. The use of anticoagulants in pregnant women is quite common. UFH and LMWH are preferred agents to use during pregnancy, with LMWH being the preferred agent to use for long-term anticoagulation. Warfarin is absolutely contraindicated in pregnancy. The novel oral agents, including factor Xa and DTI, have not been adequately studied in pregnant women and therefore cannot be recommended at this point. If a pregnant patient with a history of HIT requires anticoagulation, the ACCP guidelines recommend fondaparinux as an alternative to heparin since the preferred agent, danaparoid, is unavailable in the United States (Bates et al., 2012).

For patients with malignancy and VTE, LMWH is the preferred anticoagulant for long-term use. In this case, oral therapy with warfarin is not contraindicated; however, warfarin therapy in these patients can be complicated by factors such as drug interactions with chemotherapeutic agents, patient's inconsistent dietary intake, and the need to interrupt therapy for invasive procedures. Therefore, maintaining a stable INR in this patient population is very difficult. This was further demonstrated in the CLOT trial where continuous treatment with a LMWH was compared with conventional therapy of LMWH followed by warfarin in cancer patients with an acute VTE. The probability of recurrent VTE was reduced by nearly 50% in the long-term LMWH treatment group (CLOT investigators, 2003). Clinical trials with the newer oral anticoagulants in the treatment of VTE either excluded or had very few patients with malignancy. Therefore, until data from adequately powered trials in patients with active cancer are available, their safety and efficacy as VTE therapy in cancer patients cannot be proven.

Duration of Therapy

The ACCP guidelines recommend at least 3 months of anticoagulation therapy for VTE associated with an identifiable risk factor, for example, after surgery (Kearon et al., 2012). For patients with unprovoked VTE, at least 3 months of treatment is recommended, after which risk and benefits of indefinite treatment should be considered. Indefinite anticoagulation is recommended for most patients after a second unprovoked VTE. In patients with VTE associated with cancer, a minimum of 3 months of treatment with LMWH monotherapy is recommended, followed by continued treatment with LMWH or a change to warfarin for long-term treatment or until the cancer resolves (Kearon et al., 2012).

Cardioembolic Stroke Secondary to AF

AF can account for 10% to 12% of ischemic stroke cases annually (Meschia et al., 2014). In patients with AF, their annual risk of stroke can be estimated using the CHA2DS2VASc scoring tool. The letters within this scoring tool form an acronym for the various risk factors, which can contribute toward a patient's risk for a cardioembolic stroke secondary to AF. Table 31.8 lists the risk factors used in this scoring system and the points assigned to each risk factor (January et al., 2014). The total score correlates to an individual's annual stroke risk (Table 31.9). Preventative antithrombotic therapy is determined based upon the patient's CHA2DS2VASc score. In low-risk patients—defined as a CHA2DS2VASc score of 0—primary prevention is not indicated; however, aspirin may be implemented by a prescriber who prefers therapy over no therapy. In patients with moderate risk—defined as a CHA2DS2VASc score of 1—prescribers can opt to initiate anticoagulation therapy or antiplatelet therapy with aspirin, or choose not to initiate therapy. The

TABLE 31.8 CHA2DS2VASc Scoring System

Risk Factor	Point(s) Awarded
Congestive heart failure	1
Hypertension	1
Age 65–74	1
Age ≥ 75	2
Diabetes mellitus	1
Female sex	1
Vascular disease (other than cerebrovascular)	1
History of stroke or transient ischemic attack	2

TABLE 31.9 Annual Stroke Risk and Recommended Antithrombotic Class

CHA2DS2VASc Score	Annual Stroke Risk (%)	Risk Level and Recommended Antithrombotic Therapy
0	0	Low risk: no therapy
1	1.3	Moderate risk: anticoagulation, antiplatelet, or no therapy
2	2.2	High risk: anticoagulation
3	3.2	
4	4.0	
5	6.7	
6	9.8	
7	9.6	
8	6.7	
9	15.2	

primary drug class recommended for stroke prophylaxis in patients with high risk of stroke is anticoagulants. For primary prevention, warfarin is recommended as first line, followed by rivaroxaban, apixaban, and dabigatran.

All patients who have had a history of previous stroke or transient ischemic attack (TIA) are automatically considered high risk. In these patients, first-line therapies are warfarin and apixaban, followed by dabigatran for secondary prevention of stroke or TIA. The American Stroke Association (Kernan et al., 2014) recommends rivaroxaban as second-line therapy, while the American College of Cardiology (January et al., 2014) makes no distinction among the available oral anticoagulants. For patients requiring triple therapy—aspirin, clopidogrel, and warfarin— the American Stroke Association guidelines for secondary prevention recommend using a lower INR target (2.0–2.5) for warfarin, compared with the usual INR target range (2.0–3.0), given the high risk of bleeding with combined therapies (Kernan et al., 2014). The American College of Cardiology (January et al., 2014) recommends using only clopidogrel (no aspirin) with anticoagulation following coronary revascularization for high-risk patients. This regimen was associated with less bleeding and no differences in thrombotic rates. For patients immediately post stroke or TIA, initiation of any anticoagulation should be deferred until 14 days after the initial onset of stroke symptoms (Kernan et al., 2014).

The most studied anticoagulant for the primary and secondary prevention of stroke due to AF is warfarin. Numerous clinical trials have proven the superiority of warfarin compared with placebo in preventing a first stroke. Additionally, warfarin was compared with high-dose aspirin (300 mg) and placebo in the European Atrial Fibrillation Trial (EAFT) for the secondary prevention of stroke (EAFT Study Group, 1993). Anticoagulation with warfarin was effective in reducing the annual risk of stroke in this trial.

Prior to the development of the newer, target-specific oral anticoagulant agents, the other oral antithrombotic agents available were aspirin and clopidogrel. For patients who were unable to tolerate warfarin, the efficacy of combining aspirin and clopidogrel was compared with aspirin monotherapy. In the Atrial Fibrillation Clopidogrel Trial with Irbesartan for Prevention of Vascular Events (ACTIVE Investigators, 2006; ACTIVE Investigators, 2009), dual antiplatelet therapy was superior to aspirin monotherapy in reducing the rate of stroke. However, there was a significantly higher incidence of major bleeding in those receiving a combination of clopidogrel and aspirin. The net benefit of dual antiplatelet therapy was underwhelming compared to monotherapy with aspirin.

Dual antiplatelet therapy was then compared with warfarin in the ACTIVE W trial (ACTIVE Investigators, 2006). Warfarin was superior to the combination of clopidogrel and aspirin for the primary prevention of stroke and was associated with a significantly lower rate of bleeds. This study was terminated early due to the distinct superiority of warfarin over antiplatelet therapy. Anticoagulation is therefore considered first line over antiplatelet therapy for patients with moderate to high risk of stroke.

The efficacy of dabigatran, an oral DTI, was evaluated in the Randomized Evaluation of Long-Term Anticoagulant Therapy (RE-LY) trial (Connolly et al., 2009). Dabigatran was compared with warfarin for the primary prevention of cardioembolic stroke in patients with nonvalvular AF. For the primary outcome of stroke or systemic embolism, dabigatran was superior to warfarin with no major differences in bleeding. However, while dabigatran was associated with lower rates of intracranial hemorrhage, there were significantly higher rates of GI bleeding and a trend toward an increased risk of myocardial infarctions. The risk of GI bleeds was greater in subjects 75 years or older.

Two oral factor Xa inhibitors were also studied for the primary and secondary prevention of stroke. Rivaroxaban was compared with warfarin in the Rivaroxaban Once Daily Oral Direct Factor Xa Inhibition Compared with Vitamin K Antagonism for Prevention of Stroke and Embolism Trial in Atrial Fibrillation (ROCKET AF trial; Patel et al., 2011). In patients with nonvalvular AF with a high risk for stroke, rivaroxaban given once daily was noninferior to dose-adjusted warfarin. While major bleeding rates were similar between the two, rivaroxaban had significantly lower rates of intracranial hemorrhage (ICH) but a greater risk of GI bleeding. However, the overall results must be considered carefully, as subjects in the warfarin group were only within the therapeutic INR range 55% of the time, which is lower than other comparable trials. Given this limitation, rivaroxaban is recommended only as second line for the *secondary* prevention of stroke (Kernan et al., 2014), but it can be considered a first-line agent for the primary prevention of stroke (Meschia et al., 2014).

Apixaban was evaluated in the Apixaban Versus Acetylsalicyclic Acid to Prevent Strokes (AVERROES) study (Connolly, Eikelboom, et al., 2011). Patients with nonvalvular AF and moderate to high stroke risk who were unable to tolerate warfarin therapy were included in this trial. Compared with aspirin, apixaban had a significantly lower risk of stroke or systemic embolism. There were also no differences in the rates of bleeding between the two groups. Given the favorable outcomes of apixaban, the trial was stopped prematurely. Apixaban was also compared with warfarin in the Apixaban for Reduction in Stroke and Other Thromboembolic Events in AF (ARISTOLE) trial (Granger et al., 2011). In individuals with one or more stroke risk factors, apixaban was superior to warfarin for the prevention of ischemic or hemorrhagic stroke or systemic embolism. Similar to the previous trials, rates of ICH were lower with apixaban than warfarin. However, rates of GI bleeding remained the same.

All patients with AF should be evaluated for the need for antithrombotic therapy regardless of their prior stroke history. The selection of that agent is dependent on their risk score and various patient-specific factors. Table 31.10 discusses the various antiplatelet and anticoagulant agents approved for the primary and secondary prevention of cardioembolic stroke for patients with nonvalvular AF. This table also describes the various dosing regimens and clinical considerations for selecting each agent.

Addendum

The FDA approved edoxaban (Savaysa), an oral factor Xa inhibitor, in January 2015. Edoxaban is approved for the prevention of stroke secondary to nonvalvular AF and for the treatment of VTE. Edoxaban was compared to warfarin in two major phase 3 trials (ENGAGE AF-TIMI48 and Hokusai VTE), which subsequently led to the approval of this agent (Daiichi Sankyo Co., LTD, 2015). In both trials, edoxaban was found to be noninferior to warfarin. Edoxaban has not been compared directly with other oral anticoagulant agents.

TABLE 31.10 Agents Utilized for the Primary and Secondary Prevention of Cardiogenic Stroke

Drug (Brand Name)	Therapeutic Class	Dosage	Role in Therapy	Pharmacokinetics	Side Effects	Additional Information
Aspirin	COX inhibitor	■ 75–325 mg daily (doses <100 mg preferred)	Primary prevention in moderate risk	$t_{1/2}$: 20 min Peak: 1–2 hr	GI ulcers, abdominal pain, dyspepsia, gastritis	■ Antiplatelet effects last for lifetime of platelet (~7–10 days) ■ Reverse effects by transfusing platelets
Clopidogrel (Plavix)	ADP receptor inhibitor; thienopyridine	■ 75 mg daily	Primary prevention if unable to tolerate aspirin	$t_{1/2}$: 6 hr Peak: 0.75 hr	Bleeding, rash, TTP	■ Antiplatelet effects last for lifetime of platelet (~7–10 days)
Rivaroxaban (Xarelto)	Factor Xa inhibitor	■ 20 mg daily with evening meal ■ CrCl 15–50 mL/min: 15 mg daily ■ CrCl <15 mL/min or HD: avoid	Primary prevention: 1st line Secondary prevention: 2nd line	$t_{1/2}$: 5–9 hr Peak: 2–4 hr	Hemorrhage	■ No reversal agent currently available ■ Coagulation monitoring not required ■ May have elevated INR
Apixaban (Eliquis)	Factor Xa inhibitor	■ 5 mg BID ■ SCr ≥1.5 and age ≥80 or weight ≤60 kg: 2.5 mg BID ■ HD: 5 mg BID ■ HD and age ≥80 or weight ≤60 kg: 2.5 mg BID	Primary and secondary prevention: 1st line	$t_{1/2}$: 12 hr Peak: 3–4 hr	Hemorrhage	

Drug	Class	Dosing	Indication	Pharmacokinetics	Adverse effects	Monitoring
Dabigatran (Pradaxa)	Direct thrombin inhibitor	150 mg BID; CrCl 15–30 mL/min: 75 mg BID; CrCl 15–30 mL/min + P-gp inhibitor: avoid; CrCl <15 mL/min: avoid	Primary and secondary prevention: 1st line	$t_{1/2}$: 12–17 hr; Peak: 1 hr	Hemorrhage, gastritis, dyspepsia	
Warfarin (Coumadin, Jantoven)	Vitamin K antagonist	Initial dose: 5 mg daily (elderly ≤5 mg), then dose adjusted for target INR range of 2.0–3.0	Primary and secondary prevention: 1st line (preferred over all other oral anticoagulants)	$t_{1/2}$: 20–60 hr; Peak: 4 hr; DOA: 2–5 days	Hemorrhage; skin necrosis; calciphylaxis	■ INR increases will not be seen until 4–5 days of therapy ■ Do not dose adjust until 4 doses have been administered; check INR daily when initiating therapy ■ Once therapeutic INR has been maintained for 2 consecutive days, may check INR weekly ■ If the regimen is stable, with INR within goal, may decrease monitoring intervals to every 4 weeks ■ Any changes in medications and diet may impact the anticoagulant effect of warfarin ■ A consistent diet of foods containing vitamin K is preferred ■ Anticoagulant effects can be reversed with vitamin K (phytonadione)

ADP, adenosine diphosphate; BID, twice daily; COX, cyclooxygenase; CrCl, creatinine clearance; DOA, duration of action; GI, gastrointestinal; HD, hemodialysis; hr, hour(s); INR, international normalized ratio; P-gp, P-glycoprotein; SCr, serum creatinine; t½, half-life; min, minute(s); TTP, thrombotic thrombocytopenic purpura.

Edoxaban is available in the following strengths: 15 mg, 30 mg, 60 mg. For the treatment of DVT and PE, the recommended dose is 60 mg once daily after 5 to 10 days of parenteral anticoagulation. For patients with renal insufficiency (CrCl less than 15 mL/min) or those weighing less than 60 kg, the recommended dose is 30 mg once daily. The recommendation for nonvalvular AF is 60 mg once daily for patients with a CrCl between 50 mL/min and 95 mL/min. A reduced dose of 30 mg should be prescribed for patients with a CrCl of 15 to 50 mL/min. Unlike the other oral factor Xa inhibitors, edoxaban is *not* recommended for patients with a CrCl greater than 95 mL/min for the treatment of nonvalvular AF due to a decrease in efficacy.

Ischemic Stroke

The primary class of medications for the primary and secondary prevention of noncardioembolic stroke is the antiplatelet agents. Aspirin, clopidogrel, and the combination of dipyridamole plus aspirin have been extensively studied for stroke prophylaxis and can decrease the risk of recurrent stroke, myocardial infarction, and cardiac death by 22% (Kernan et al., 2014). At this time, the American Stroke Association recommends the use of antiplatelet agents as first line over the anticoagulants (Table 31.11).

The American Stroke Association does *not* recommend use of antiplatelet agents, specifically aspirin, for the primary prevention of stroke (Meschia et al., 2014). However, aspirin for primary prevention can be considered in patients with a 10-year cardiovascular risk greater than 10%, in women, or in patients with diabetes mellitus. In these patient populations, the benefits of aspirin outweigh the adverse effects. Aspirin is recommended at 81 mg daily or 100 mg every other day. For secondary prevention, aspirin 50 to 325 mg/day as monotherapy is preferred (Kernan et al., 2014). When compared with placebo, aspirin prophylaxis reduces the risk of recurrent stroke, either ischemic or hemorrhagic (Johnson et al., 1999).

The combination of aspirin plus dipyridamole, twice daily, can also be considered in lieu of aspirin monotherapy for secondary prevention. The efficacy and safety of dipyridamole in combination with aspirin was studied in the ESPS 2 (European Stroke Prevention Study 2) for the secondary prevention of stroke or TIA (Diener et al., 1996). Dipyridamole in combination with aspirin resulted in a decreased

TABLE 31.11 Antiplatelet Agents Utilized for the Prevention of Ischemic Stroke

Drug	Dose	Available Formulations	Pharmacokinetics	Common Adverse Events
Aspirin	75–325 mg daily (doses < 100 mg preferred)	Tablet: 81 mg, 325 mg Chewable tablets: 81 mg	$t_{1/2}$: 20 min peak: 1–2 hr	Gastrointestinal ulcer, abdominal pain, dyspepsia, gastritis
Clopidogrel (Plavix)	75 mg daily	Tablet: 75 mg, 300 mg	$t_{1/2}$: 6 hr peak: 0.75 hr	Hemorrhage, rash, thrombotic thrombocytopenic purpura
Dipyridamole/ Aspirin (Aggrenox)	200 mg/25 mg twice daily	Capsule: dipyridamole 200 mg/aspirin 25 mg	Dipyridamole: $t_{1/2}$: 10–12 hr peak: 2–2.5 hr	Headache, dyspepsia, nausea, diarrhea, abdominal pain

$t_{1/2}$, half life.

risk of recurrent stroke compared with aspirin alone, dipyridamole alone, and placebo. The ESPS 2 trial resulted in the FDA approval of dipyridamole plus aspirin for the secondary prevention of stroke or TIA.

Clopidogrel monotherapy is a potential option for secondary prophylaxis, but it is recommended for only those patients who are unable to tolerate aspirin. Clopidogrel was compared with aspirin in the Clopidogrel Versus Aspirin in Patients at Risk of Ischemic Events (CAPRIE) trial (CAPRIE Steering Committee, 1996). Clopidogrel had a lower incidence of the primary outcome of stroke, MI, or vascular death. However, in a subgroup analysis of patients with a previous history of stroke, no difference was found between clopidogrel and aspirin. Clopidogrel was also compared with aspirin plus dipyridamole in the Prevention Regimen for Effectively Avoiding Second Strokes (PRoFESS) trial (Sacco et al., 2008). There were no differences between the two groups in the rate of the primary outcome of recurrent stroke. The combination of aspirin and clopidogrel was also evaluated in the Management of Atherothrombosis With Clopidogrel in High-Risk Patients With Recent Transient Ischemic Attacks or Ischemic Stroke (MATCH) trial (Diener et al., 2004). The combination of clopidogrel 75 mg plus aspirin 75 mg daily was compared with clopidogrel 75 mg monotherapy in patients with an ischemic stroke occurring 3 months prior to enrollment. No difference was found between the two groups for recurrent stroke, MI, vascular death, or rehospitalization for an ischemic event. However, there was a significant increase in the rate of major hemorrhage in the group that received the combination of clopidogrel and aspirin.

Contrary to the results of the MATCH trial, the Clopidogrel in High-Risk Patients with Acute Non-Disabling Cerebrovascular Events (CHANCE) trial (Wang et al., 2013) demonstrated a lower rate of ischemic or hemorrhagic stroke with combination therapy. In this study, patients were randomized within 24 hours of a minor ischemic stroke or TIA to two treatment arms. All subjects received 75 mg to 300 mg of aspirin on day 1. Those in the combination group received 75 mg of aspirin daily on days 2 to 21 and 300 mg of clopidogrel on day 1, then 75 mg of clopidogrel daily on days 2 to 90. Subjects in the aspirin only arm received 75 mg of aspirin daily on days 2 to 90. The design of the CHANCE trial in comparison with the MATCH trial suggests timing of these agents plays a key role. Administering aspirin and clopidogrel within 24 hours of an acute minor stroke event may be beneficial in preventing recurrent stroke in the first 90 days. Beyond the 90-day time period, prophylactic strategies should involve either aspirin monotherapy or aspirin plus dipyridamole combination therapy only (Kernan et al., 2014). Combination therapy with aspirin and clopidogrel should not be initiated days to years after a minor stroke or TIA, as this is associated with an increased risk of hemorrhage and no additional benefit.

For patients already on prophylaxis who present with a new or recurrent stroke, there is currently no data that suggests additional benefit by increasing the aspirin dose or switching to a different antiplatelet agent or combination agent.

Acute Ischemic Stroke

Intravenous (IV) fibrinolytic therapy is now considered the standard for the emergent treatment of acute ischemic stroke (Jaunch et al., 2013). Alteplase is the only FDA-approved fibrinolytic agent for ischemic stroke. Treatment with alteplase is associated with neurological improvement within 24 hours and complete or nearly complete recovery in 3 months. Because of the mechanism of alteplase, there is a considerable risk of bleeding upon administration. Therefore, it is imperative to evaluate the risks versus the benefits of administering a thrombolytic. Several studies have evaluated the efficacy and safety of IV fibrinolytics. These studies were pivotal in identifying a time period during which the benefits of administering fibrinolytics outweighed the risk of bleeding. The ideal time period for alteplase (tPA) administration is within 3 hours of symptom onset. Depending on the individual patient's criteria, he or she may be eligible for fibrinolytic therapy within 3 to 4.5 hours of symptom onset. Tables 31.12 and 31.13 list the inclusion and exclusion criteria for treatment with IV tPA as recommended by the American Stroke Association (Jaunch et al., 2013). All patients should be ruled out for intracranial bleeding with a non-contrast head CT or MRI prior to administration of alteplase. The recommended dose is 0.9 mg/kg of alteplase, with a maximum total dose of 90 mg. Ten percent of the dose should be administered as an IV bolus over 1 minute, then the remaining dose should be infused over 60 minutes. All patients must be admitted to the intensive care unit for close monitoring. Neurological assessments should be conducted every 15 minutes during and for 2 hours after tPA infusion. Then the frequency of assessments can decrease to every 30 minutes for 6 hours and then every hour for 24 hours after tPA. Patients should also be monitored for headaches and acute hypertension and a repeat CT or MRI should be conducted 24 hours after tPA but before starting any antiplatelet or anticoagulant therapy. All patients should be started on aspirin within 24 to 48 hours after stroke but not within 24 hours of IV tPA administration. The recommended initial dose of aspirin is 325 mg. Aspirin dose should then be modified and the regimen followed as outlined in the CHANCE trial (Wang et al., 2013).

Heparin-Induced Thrombocytopenia

HIT is a rare but serious complication associated with exposure to heparin. It is a prothrombotic state associated with the development of heparin/platelet factor 4 (PF4) antibodies. HIT antibodies activate platelets and can cause severe clinical consequences, ranging from uncomplicated thrombocytopenia to catastrophic venous or arterial thrombosis. Patients experiencing HIT-associated thrombosis may develop manifestations such as skin necrosis, gangrene of limbs, PE, DVT, or stroke.

Diagnosis and Evaluation

Patients who develop HIT usually present with thrombocytopenia, a platelet count less than 150,000 mm^3, or a 50% reduction in platelet count after more than or equal to 4 days of heparin treatment. The diagnosis of HIT takes into consideration clinical characteristics as well as laboratory evidence. HIT should be suspected in patients with a large reduction in platelet count, for example, 50%; when the thrombocytopenia occurs within 5 to 14 days of heparin exposure; if there is associated thrombosis; and finally, if no other obvious causes of thrombocytopenia are present. These clinical findings must then be supplemented with laboratory testing to confirm the diagnosis of HIT. Two laboratory methods are available to

TABLE 31.12 Inclusion and Exclusion Criteria of Patients With Ischemic Stroke Who Could Be Treated With IV rtPA Within 3 Hours From Symptom Onset

Inclusion criteria
  Diagnosis of ischemic stroke causing measurable neurological deficit
  Onset of symptoms <3 hr before beginning treatment
  Age ≥18

Exclusion criteria
  Significant head trauma or prior stroke in previous 3 months
  Symptoms suggest subarachnoid hemorrhage
  Arterial puncture at noncompressible site in previous 7 days
  History of previous intracranial hemorrhage
  Intracranial neoplasm, arteriovenous malformation, or aneurysm
  Recent intracranial or intraspinal surgery
  Elevated blood pressure (systolic >185 mmHg or diastolic >110 mmHg)
  Active internal bleeding
  Acute bleeding diathesis, including but not limited to
    Platelet count <100,000/mm³
    Heparin received within 48 hr, resulting in abnormally elevated aPTT greater than the upper
      limit of normal
    Current use of anticoagulant with INR >1.7 or PT >15 seconds
    Current use of direct thrombin inhibitors or direct factor Xa inhibitors with elevated sensitive
      laboratory tests (such as aPTT, INR, platelet count, and ECT; TT; or appropriate factor Xa
      activity assays)
  Blood glucose concentration <50 mg/dL (2.7 mmol/L)
  CT demonstrates multilobar infarction (hypodensity >1/3 cerebral hemisphere)

Relative exclusion criteria
  Recent experience suggests that under some circumstances—with careful consideration and
    weighting of risk to benefit—patients may receive fibrinolytic therapy despite one or more
    relative contraindications. Consider risk to benefit of IV rtPA administration carefully if any of
    these relative contraindications are present:
  Only minor or rapidly improving stroke symptoms (clearing spontaneously)
  Pregnancy
  Seizure at onset with postictal residual neurological impairments
  Major surgery or serious trauma within previous 14 days
  Recent gastrointestinal or urinary tract hemorrhage (within previous 21 days)
  Recent acute myocardial infarction (within previous 3 months)

aPTT, activated partial thromboplastin time; CT, computed tomography; ECT, ecarin clotting time; FDA, Food and Drug Administration; INR, international normalized ratio; IV, intravenous; PT, partial thromboplastin time; rtPA, recombinant tissue plasminogen activator; TT, thrombin time.

The checklist includes some FDA-approved indications and contraindications for administration of IV rtPA for acute ischemic stroke. Recent guideline revisions have modified the original FDA-approved indications. A physician with expertise in acute stroke care may modify this list.

Onset time is defined as either the witnessed onset of symptoms or the time last known normal if symptom onset was not witnessed.

In patients without recent use of oral anticoagulants or heparin, treatment with IV rtPA can be initiated before availability of coagulation test results but should be discontinued if INR is greater than 1.7 or PT is abnormally elevated by local laboratory standards.

In patients without history of thrombocytopenia, treatment with IV rtPA can be initiated before availability of platelet count but should be discontinued if platelet count is less than 100,000/mm³.

Reprinted from Jaunch et al. (2013, 44, pp. 870–947, Table 10, p. 898), with permission from Wolters Kluwer Health.

TABLE 31.13 Additional Inclusion and Exclusion Characteristics of Patients With Acute Ischemic Stroke Who Could Be Treated With IV rtPA Within 3 to 4.5 Hours From Symptom Onset

Inclusion criteria
    Diagnosis of ischemic stroke causing measurable neurological deficit
    Onset of symptoms within 3 to 4.5 hr before beginning treatment

Relative exclusion criteria
    Age > 80
    Severe stroke (NIHSS > 25)
    Taking an oral anticoagulant regardless of INR
    History of both diabetes and prior ischemic stroke

INR, international normalized ratio; IV, intravenous; NIHSS, National Institutes of Health Stroke Scale; rtPA, recombinant tissue plasminogen activator.

Reprinted from Jaunch et al. (2013), with permission from Wolters Kluwer Health.

confirm the presence of heparin antibodies—a serologic assay for antibody detection (ELISA) and a functional test to measure platelet activation (serotonin release assay or heparin-induced platelet aggregation assay). The method most commonly used is the serologic test for heparin/PF4 antibodies, because it is widely available, straightforward to interpret, and generally has a more rapid turnaround time. Although serologic testing is very sensitive, it lacks specificity, which then results in a high negative but low positive predictive value. The diagnosis of HIT can largely be excluded if the serologic antibody testing is negative, but if serologic antibody testing is positive, confirmatory functional testing is important to solidify the diagnosis (Arepally & Ortel, 2006).

Treatment

The goal of therapy in patients with HIT is to reduce the risk of thrombosis associated with this condition. Once the diagnosis of HIT is confirmed or strongly suspected, all heparin products should be immediately discontinued and therapy with a non-heparin anticoagulant initiated. At minimum, non-heparin anticoagulation should continue until the diagnosis of HIT is either confirmed or excluded.

The non-heparin anticoagulants available for use in the initial treatment phase of HIT include the parental DTI—argatroban and bivalirudin—and the selective anti-Xa inhibitor fondaparinux (Table 31.14). Argatroban and bivalrudin are generally considered first-line options for the initial treatment of HIT. Fondaparinux does not interact with PF4 and can therefore have a role in the treatment of HIT. Fondaparinux has the advantage of subcutaneous dosing, but efficacy data in the initial treatment of HIT are lacking, leading to a weaker recommendation for treatment of HIT (Warkentin, Greinacher, Koster, & Lincoff, 2008).

Warfarin should not be used in the initial treatment phase of HIT before platelet-count recovery because it can exacerbate hypercoagulability by depleting antithrombotic protein C, leading to increased risk of skin necrosis and venous limb gangrene. However, once initial anticoagulation has been started, warfarin can be used for continued oral anticoagulation in the subsequent phases of HIT treatment. According to the ACCP guidelines, warfarin should not be initiated until the patient has been stable on anticoagulation with a non-heparin anticoagulant and the platelet count has increased to at least 150,000 mm^3. The starting dose should

TABLE 31.14 Medications for the Treatment of Heparin-Induced Thrombocytopenia

Agent	Dosage	Dose Adjustments	Pharmacokinetics	Monitoring	Side Effects	Clinical Pearls
Argatroban DTI	≤2 mcg/kg/min continuous infusion	Hepatic impairment: 0.5 mcg/kg/min	$t_{1/2}$: 39–51 min Peak: 1–3 hr Metabolism: hepatic Elimination: 20% renal	aPTT: at baseline; 2 hr after start and post dose adjustments Goal: 1.5–3 times baseline aPTT	Chest pain, hypotension, hematuria	Can falsely elevate INR First-line agent for HIT Also preferred in renal insufficiency
Bivalirudin DTI	0.15–0.2 mg/kg/hr continuous infusion	CrCl 30–60 mL/min: 0.08–0.1 mg/kg/hr CrCl <30 mL/min: 0.04–0.05 mg/kg/hr HD: 0.07 mg/kg/hr	$t_{1/2}$: 25 min Peak: immediate Metabolism: proteolytic cleavage Elimination: 20% renal; 80% enzymatic	Goal aPTT: 1.5–2.5 times baseline aPTT	Hypotension, minor hemorrhage, nausea, pain	Can cause moderate elevations in INR Primarily utilized in the setting of PCI with or without HIT May be preferable in hepatic impairment; avoids metabolism via CYP3A4 (unlike argatroban)
Fondaparinux Xa inhibitor	<50 kg: 5.0 mg 50–100 kg: 7.5 mg >100 kg: 10 mg doses administered SQ once daily	CrCl <30 mL/min: contraindicated	$t_{1/2}$: 17–20 hr Peak: 2–3 hr Elimination: renal	None recommended	Anemia, thrombocytopenia, increases in AST/ALT	No effect on INR Possible alternative to DTIs Not preferred for peri-procedural use due to long half-life

ALT, alanine transaminase; aPTT, activated partial thromboplastin time; AST, aspartate aminotransferase; CrCl, creatinine clearance; CYP, cytochrome; DTI, direct thrombin inhibitor; HD, hemodialysis; HIT, heparin-induced thrombocytopenia; hr, hour; INR, international normalized ratio; PCI, percutaneous coronary intervention; SQ, subcutaneously; $t_{1/2}$, half-life.

not exceed 5 mg, and the non-heparin anticoagulant should be continued for at least 5 days and until the INR has reached the intended goal (2.0–3.0; Linkins et al., 2012).

It is important to note that argatroban can falsely elevate the INR, making INR interpretation during the transition period difficult. The appropriate INR target during the transition to warfarin for patients concurrently on argatroban is based on clinician- and institution-specific protocols. The use of fondaparinux during this transition period may alleviate some of the challenges, as fondaparinux does not interfere with the INR, and its subcutaneous dosing option can facilitate hospital discharge.

The duration of treatment with warfarin or other non-heparin anticoagulants in the setting of HIT has yet to be clearly defined. Experts have recommended treatment for a minimum of 2 to 3 months and for 6 months if a thrombotic event occurred (Alving, 2003).

For full reference citations to this chapter, please see "Section References" in the back of the book, under the heading "Section VII."

Pharmacotherapeutics of Ischemic Heart Disease

CONNIE H. YOON

Ischemic heart disease (IHD) involves a spectrum of diagnoses including chronic stable angina, unstable angina (UA), non-ST-segment elevation myocardial infarction (NSTEMI), and ST-segment elevation myocardial infarction (STEMI). Chronic stable angina is related to the progression of obstructive coronary heart disease (CHD); however, UA, NSTEMI, and STEMI involve plaque rupture and manifest as an acute coronary syndrome (ACS). This section discusses the pharmacologic therapies involved in the management of chronic stable angina, UA, NSTEMI, and STEMI. The mechanism of action and specific details related to antiplatelet and antithrombotic agents are further described in the section on antithrombotic therapy.

CHRONIC STABLE ANGINA

Interventions related to chronic stable angina are primarily directed at a healthy lifestyle; the management of the chronic conditions of hypertension, hyperlipidemia, and diabetes mellitus; and pharmacologic therapies. As the management of hypertension and hyperlipidemia was already discussed in the previous sections, they will not be discussed specifically for the management of chronic stable angina. The medication classes utilized in the management of chronic stable angina are aspirin, clopidogrel, short-acting nitrates, beta blockers, calcium channel blocker (CCB), long-acting nitrates, and ranolazine.

All patients with chronic stable angina should receive 75 to 162 mg of aspirin daily to prevent plaque rupture and progression of coronary disease (Fihn et al., 2012). There is no added benefit of high-dose aspirin (325 mg) compared with low-dose aspirin (75–100 mg) for secondary prevention, with high-dose aspirin associated with increased bleeding complications. Clopidogrel 75 mg daily may be substituted in patients with contraindications to aspirin. In the CAPRIE (Clopidogrel versus Aspirin in Patients at Risk of Ischemic Events) trial, daily aspirin 325 mg was compared with clopidogrel 75 mg for secondary prevention in patients with previous myocardial infarction (MI), stroke, or established peripheral artery disease (CAPRIE Steering Committee, 1996). Clopidogrel was found to be superior in the prevention of recurrent MI and death; however, as the difference between the two groups was marginal, clopidogrel continues to serve as an alternative to aspirin. The CHARISMA (Clopidogrel for High Atherothrombotic Risk and Ischemic Stabilization Management, and Avoidance) trial evaluated the use of aspirin (75–162 mg) to dual antiplatelet therapy (DAPT) with aspirin (75–162 mg) and clopidogrel (75 mg daily; Bhatt et al., 2006). This study specifically evaluated primary prevention in patients either with established cardiovascular disease or at high risk for cardiovascular disease. This trial revealed no difference in MI, stroke, or cardiovascular death, but did show an increased risk of bleeding with DAPT. The results of the CHARISMA trial supported the use of low-dose aspirin monotherapy for the primary prevention of cardiovascular events.

Patients with angina symptoms, which occur from either an increase in myocardial oxygen demand or a decrease in supply, should be prescribed a short-acting nitrate—various formulations are described in Table 32.1. Sublingual nitroglycerin (0.3 mg or 0.4 mg) is indicated for the immediate relief of acute angina pain. The tablet is placed under the tongue and allowed to dissolve. If after 5 minutes, the patient does not experience relief or if symptoms worsen, the patient is then instructed to call for emergent medical attention and take a second dose. If symptoms improve but continue to persist despite a maximum of three doses (one dose administered every 5 minutes), the patient should also seek immediate medical care (Anderson et al., 2013a). Nitrates cause vascular smooth muscle relaxation, increasing coronary and collateral blood flow. Nitrates also reduce preload, which decreases cardiac wall tension and myocardial oxygen demand. Therefore, nitrates are contraindicated in severe aortic stenosis, right ventricular infarction, and hypertrophic obstructive cardiomyopathy, as these patients depend heavily on preload for forward flow of blood. In addition, nitrates are contraindicated with hypotension and bradycardia. Do not use any nitrates within 24 hours of sildenafil or vardenafil use, or within 48 hours of tadalafil use.

TABLE 32.1 Short-Acting Nitrates*

Agent	Dose	Patient Instructions	Onset/Duration of Action	Other Considerations
Sublingual nitroglycerin tablets	0.3 mg to 0.6 mg tablet	Place one tablet under the tongue and allow to dissolve May repeat in 5 min Maximum of 3 tablets in 15 min	Onset: 1–3 min DOT: 25 min	■ Store tablets in original manufacturer container to maintain drug potency ■ Store in a cool place, not in the refrigerator ■ Protect from sunlight ■ Open bottle expires 6–12 months after opening
Nitroglycerin spray	0.4 mg/spray	Spray once onto or under tongue Do not swallow or inhale Do not shake Repeat every 5 min as needed, maximum of 1.2 mg per 15 min	Onset: 1–3 min DOT: 30–40 min	
Nitroglycerin 2% ointment	0.5–2.0 inches	Apply ointment on chest, rotating application sites Cover area with plastic cover Wash hands	Onset: 30 min DOT: 4–6 hr	■ Must include a 10- to 12-hr nitrate-free interval to prevent the development of tolerance ■ Ointment may discolor clothing

DOT, duration of therapy.

*Do not use any nitrates within 24 hours of sildenafil or vardenafil use or 48 hours of tadalafil use.

Patients with chronic angina may be prescribed a beta blocker to control anginal symptoms. These agents reduce myocardial oxygen demand by decreasing heart rate, contractility, and afterload. Increasing the duration of diastole allows for improved coronary perfusion and oxygen supply. A beta blocker should be a component of therapy in patients with prior MI or heart failure with reduced ejection fraction (HFrEF), based on the validated mortality benefit. For patients with contraindications to beta blockers or who continue to have persistent angina symptoms on beta blockers, a CCB or a long-acting nitrate may be substituted or added as a second agent (Anderson et al., 2013a).

CCBs decrease coronary vascular resistance, which augments blood flow and oxygen supply. The dihydropyridine CCBs—such as diltiazem and verapamil—have significant negative inotropic effects, slowing down cardiac conduction and therefore decreasing myocardial oxygen demand. These agents are contraindicated in patients with sick-sinus syndrome or severe heart block, and in post-MI patients with left ventricular ejection fraction (LVEF) less than 40% due to an increase in cardiac events (MDPIT Research Group, 1988). Nondihydropyridine CCBs cause coronary muscle relaxation and vasodilation, thus increasing oxygen delivery. Currently the American Heart Association (AHA) guidelines recommend beta blockers as first line for chronic angina management, due to a meta-analysis that compared the efficacy and safety of beta blockers, CCBs, and long-acting nitrates for stable angina (Anderson et al., 2013a; Heidenreich et al., 1999). Though no difference in efficacy was found between beta blockers and CCBs, there were less adverse events and drug interactions with beta blockers.

Ranolazine is an additional adjunctive therapy for persistent angina despite therapy with a beta blocker, CCB, or nitrate. Ranolazine is an antianginal agent thought to inhibit sodium influx during repolarization—specifically in ischemic cardiac myocytes—to decrease myocardial oxygen consumption and cause myocardial relaxation. Unlike other agents utilized for chronic angina, ranolazine has no impact on blood pressure (BP); therefore, it is a favorable agent for angina in the setting of borderline to low BP. Ranolazine is typically initiated at 500 mg twice daily with a maximum dose of 1,000 mg twice daily. For patients on diltiazem, verapamil, or other cytochrome 3A4 inhibitors, the maximum recommended dose is 500 mg of ranolazine twice daily. Dose adjustments for renal or hepatic insufficiency are not required. Ranolazine can increase digoxin serum concentrations by 1.5-fold; thus, a lower dosage of digoxin (0.125 mg daily or every other day) is recommended. Ranolazine has also been found to increase QTc by approximately 6 msec, and caution should be exercised if used in combination with other QT prolonging agents.

A recent meta-analysis compared the clinical efficacy—defined as a reduction in weekly angina rate and frequency of short-acting nitrate use—of add-on agents for patients with stable angina (Belsey, Savelieva, Mugelli, & Camm, 2015). This review evaluated the addition of beta blockers, CCBs, long-acting nitrates, or ranolazine to currently existing beta blocker or CCB monotherapy. The weekly rate of angina symptoms was reduced when a CCB was added to existing beta blocker therapy; a long-acting nitrate was added to either existing beta blocker or CCB therapy; or ranolazine was added to beta blocker or CCB therapy. No differences in angina rates were seen when a beta blocker was added to existing CCB therapy. A reduction in nitrate use was seen when ranolazine was added to beta blocker or CCB therapy or beta blocker was added to existing CCB treatment and vice versa. This meta-analysis supports the use of add-on therapy for patients with persistent angina despite beta blocker or CCB therapy. If anginal symptoms persist despite medical therapy, the evaluation for revascularization therapy is recommended.

ACUTE CORONARY SYNDROMES: UA, NSTEMI, AND STEMI

The management of ACS varies upon whether the patient presents with UA, NSTEMI, or STEMI. The recommendations for the management of UA or NSTEMI are grouped together and involve medication management and/or percutaneous coronary intervention (PCI). The management of STEMI focuses primarily on PCI, though medications are available for immediate treatment for non-PCI institutions.

Unstable Angina/Non-ST-Segment Elevation Myocardial Infarctions

For patients presenting with UA or NSTEMI, the initial management strategy involves medications for symptom relief and mortality reduction with the immediate goals of restoring myocardial blood flow and salvaging myocardium. The majority of these medications have been studied in clinical trials to reduce mortality. The medication classes utilized in the management of UA/NSTEMI include the following:

- Antiplatelet therapy
- Anticoagulation
- High-dose statin therapy
- Beta adrenergic receptor blockers
- Angiotensin-converting enzyme inhibitors or angiotensin II receptor blockers

Antithrombotic therapy for UA/NSTEMI includes antiplatelet therapy and anticoagulation, depending on the planned management strategy. Figure 32.1 provides a general algorithm for antithrombotic approaches in the management of UA/NSTEMI.

DUAL ANTIPLATELET THERAPY

For all patients presenting with UA/NSTEMI, DAPT is the cornerstone of management. Everyone must receive a high dose of aspirin, usually 162 mg to 325 mg, chewed and swallowed immediately, unless there is a severe contraindication to aspirin therapy (Amsterdam et al., 2014b). Aspirin prevents platelet aggregation and thrombus formation while exerting anti-inflammatory properties. Clinical

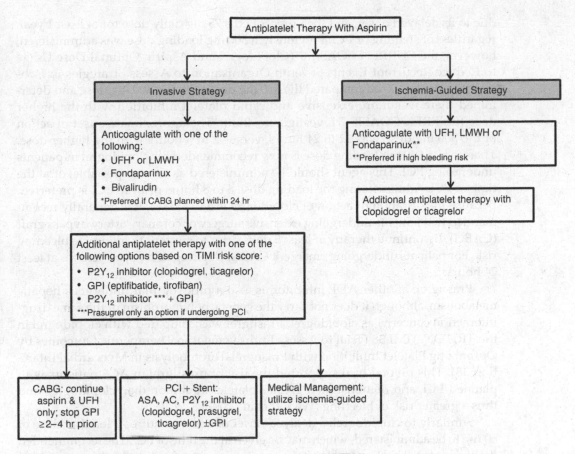

FIGURE 32.1 General algorithm for the management of UA/NSTEMI.

AC, anticoagulant; ASA, aspirin; CABG, coronary artery bypass graft; GPI, glycoprotein IIb/IIIa inhibitor; LMWH, low molecular weight heparin; NSTEMI, non-ST-segment elevation myocardial infarction; PCI, percutaneous coronary intervention; TIMI, thrombolysis in myocardial infarct; UA, unstable angina; UFH, unfractionated heparin.

Adapted from Amsterdam et al. (2014b).

trials demonstrate that aspirin reduces mortality in patients with UA/NSTEMI. After the first administration of high-dose aspirin, all patients should receive 81 to 325 mg of aspirin once daily, indefinitely. Clopidogrel may be substituted for those unable to take aspirin. A loading dose should be followed by a daily maintenance dose of 75 mg.

The use of $P2Y_{12}$ adenosine diphosphate (ADP) receptor antagonist, clopidogrel, prasugrel, and ticagrelor in combination with aspirin is the standard of care. Results from the CURE (Clopidogrel in Unstable Angina to Prevent Recurrent Events) trial, which compared DAPT—clopidogrel and aspirin—to monotherapy with aspirin, showed a significant reduction in mortality, nonfatal MI, and strokes in the dual-agent group (CURE Trial Investigators, 2001). This trial solidified the role of ADP inhibitors for the management of UA/STEMI. Patients who are administered clopidogrel for UA/NSTEMI are initially loaded with 600 mg due to its delayed onset, and then prescribed a 75 mg daily dose for at least 1 year, regardless of stenting or PCI. Previously, a 300 mg loading dose was administered; however, the CURRENT-OASIS 7 (Clopidogrel and Aspirin Optimal Dose Usage to Reduce Recurrent Events-Seventh Organization to Assess Strategies in Ischemic Syndromes) trial compared the 600 mg dose with the 300 mg dose and determined there was more extensive and rapid platelet inhibition with the higher dose (CURRENT-OASIS 7 Investigators, 2010). The approximate onset of action of the 300 mg dose was 12 to 24 hours, versus 2 to 6 hours with the higher dose. Therefore, a 600 mg loading dose is now recommended for clopidogrel in patients undergoing PCI. This agent should be administered as soon as possible, or at the time of PCI. Administering the loading dose 6 to 8 hours prior to PCI is preferred. Because the duration of action of clopidogrel is 5 to 8 days, it is generally recommended that patients undergoing extensive surgery or coronary artery bypass graft (CABG) discontinue therapy at least 5 days prior to surgery to minimize bleeding risk. For patients undergoing emergent CABG, clopidogrel must be held for at least 24 hours.

Prasugrel, another ADP inhibitor, is also a prodrug that undergoes hepatic metabolism, although it does not carry the genetic polymorphism or the same drug-interaction concerns as clopidogrel. Prasugrel was compared with clopidogrel in the TRITON-TIMI 38 (Trial to Assess Improvement in Therapeutic Outcomes by Optimizing Platelet Inhibition with Prasugrel-Thrombolysis in Myocardial Infarction 38). This pivotal trial supported the use of prasugrel in ACS patients with planned PCI, and demonstrated greater platelet inhibition than clopidogrel, and thus a greater risk of bleeding (Wiviott et al., 2007).

Similarly to clopidogrel, a delayed onset of action requires a loading dose of 60 mg to be administered, which may be given at the time of PCI. The recommended daily maintenance dose is 10 mg. In specific subsets of patients—those weighing less than 60 kg or those older than 75 years of age—prasugrel is generally contraindicated, because there is no net benefit with its use. Prasugrel is absolutely contraindicated in patients with a history of stroke or transient ischemic attack (TIA), due to an overall net harm found in this group. Currently prasugrel has been approved at a reduced daily maintenance dose of 5 mg for patients weighing less than 60 kg. While this dose has been studied in pharmacokinetic trials to exhibit similar platelet inhibition to the 10 mg dose in patients weighing more than 60 kg, it has not been studied in clinical trials. Thus, mortality data are unknown with the 5 mg dose. A greater benefit from prasugrel was found in patients with STEMI, making its use more preferable; however, the TRITON–TIMI 38 study was not powered to evaluate the subset alone.

After the Food and Drug Administration (FDA) approval of prasugrel, the TRIOLOGY ACS (Targeted Platelet Inhibition to Assess Improvement in Therapeutic Outcomes by Optimizing Platelet Inhibition with Prasugrel) and ACCOAST (A Comparison of Prasugrel at the Time of Percutaneous Coronary Intervention or as Pretreatment at the Time of Diagnosis in Patients with Non-ST-Elevation Myocardial Infarction) trials were published. In the TRIOLOGY ACS trial, subjects 10 days post-ACS were enrolled to evaluate the efficacy of prasugrel compared to clopidogrel (Roe et al., 2012). Unlike the TRITON TIMI 38 trial, subjects specifically did not undergo PCI and were strictly medically managed. In this superiority trial, prasugrel failed to demonstrate superiority of the primary endpoint of death due to stroke, MI, or other cardiovascular causes. The ACCOAST trial evaluated the efficacy of pretreatment with prasugrel for ACS patients undergoing PCI (Montalescot et al., 2013). Patients were randomized to receive either a 60 mg loading dose at the time of PCI or a 30 mg pretreatment loading dose prior to angiography and an additional 30 mg loading dose at the time of PCI. Pretreatment with prasugrel was not superior to dosing at the time of PCI and was associated with an increased rate of bleeds. Based on these two trials, the American Heart Association (AHA)/American College of Cardiology (ACC) guidelines do *not* recommend the use of prasugrel outside of the setting of PCI (Amsterdam etal., 2014b).

Because prasugrel has a longer duration of action than clopidogrel, at 5 to 10 days, prasugrel must be held for at least 7 days prior to surgery or CABG. Similar to clopidogrel, prasugrel also has two major side effects—bleeding and TTP.

The newest ADP inhibitor is ticagrelor. Unlike clopidogrel and prasugrel, ticagrelor is not a prodrug and does not need to be metabolized into its active form. It is however, hepatically eliminated through the CYP3A4 enzyme, and thus concurrent use with strong CYP3A4 inhibitors is cautioned due to an increased risk of bleeding from higher ticagrelor concentrations. Ticagrelor was compared with clopidogrel in the PLATO (Study of Platelet Inhibition and Patient Outcomes) trial (Wallentin et al., 2009). Ticagrelor had a greater mortality reduction compared with clopidogrel; however, there was an increased risk of intracranial hemorrhages (ICH) with ticagrelor. The increased risk of bleeding may be due to the enhanced platelet inhibition compared with clopidogrel. The results of the PLATO trial led to the approval of ticagrelor for the management of ACS, although unlike prasugrel, ticagrelor does not need to be used in patients undergoing PCI. Ticagrelor is loaded with a 180 mg dose, and a maintenance dose of 90 mg twice daily that must be started 12 hours after the loading dose. Prescribers must be diligent in utilizing low-dose aspirin (doses less than 100 mg daily) concurrently with ticagrelor, as the subset of patients who received high-dose aspirin with ticagrelor experienced a decreased efficacy of ticagrelor. Patients should still receive the initial high dose of aspirin at the onset of UA/NSTEMI symptoms. Ticagrelor has a duration of action of 3 to 5 days; however, it must still be held for 5 days prior to extensive surgery or CABG. For patients undergoing emergent CABG, ticagrelor must be held for at least 24 hours. Ticagrelor is contraindicated in patients with a history of ICH and severe hepatic disease. Unlike the other agents in this class, ticagrelor has a unique set of side effects, including dyspnea, ventricular pauses, elevated creatinine, and elevated uric acid levels.

ANTICOAGULATION

Anticoagulation therapy with unfractionated heparin (UFH), enoxaparin, fondaparinux, or bivalirudin aids in reducing thrombus formation. The selection of anticoagulation therapy is dependent on several factors, including patient symptoms; the extent of the infarction; medications administered, including fibrinolytics; and the appropriateness of an invasive versus ischemia-guided approach. Several studies have compared UFH to low molecular weight heparin (LMWH), specifically enoxaparin. Patients treated with enoxaparin had a decreased incidence of death and nonfatal MI. Unlike UFH, enoxaparin can be administered subcutaneously without the need for a continuous infusion and requires no monitoring. Additionally, enoxaparin is less likely to activate platelets and has a lower incidence of heparin-induced thrombocytopenia (HIT). In the majority of the studies that compared UFH to enoxaparin, there was no difference in major bleeding rates between the two treatment agents. UFH should be administered for at least 48 hours or until PCI is performed (Amsterdam et al., 2014). Enoxaparin should be administered for the duration of the hospitalization or until PCI is performed.

Anticoagulation with fondaparinux, a subcutaneously administered factor Xa inhibitor, in patients with ACS was evaluated in the OASIS-5 (Fifth Organization to Assess Strategies in Acute Ischemic Syndromes) trial. Fondaparinux was noninferior to enoxaparin in preventing ischemic events and also had a decreased risk of major bleeds (OASIS-5 Investigators, 2006). Fondaparinux is therefore recommended in place of enoxaparin or UFH in patients with higher bleeding risk. However, in patients treated with fondaparinux and undergoing PCI, an additional anticoagulant with anti-factor IIa activity—for example, 60 to 80 IU/kg IV UFH—is required to prevent catheter thrombosis (Amsterdam et al., 2014b).

For patients undergoing CABG, UFH may be continued, but enoxaparin should be discontinued 12 to 24 hours prior to surgery and fondaparinux 24 hours prior to surgery. Once enoxaparin and fondaparinux are discontinued, all anticoagulation should be switched to UFH.

Direct thrombin inhibitors (DTIs) are anticoagulation agents primarily administered in patients undergoing initial invasive strategy with PCI. Bivalirudin is the predominant drug in this class. DTIs bind directly to circulating and clot-bound thrombin to prevent thrombin-mediated conversion of fibrinogen to fibrin. DTIs also prevent thrombin-mediated platelet activation and aggregation. The effects of these agents can be monitored via activated clotting time (ACT). Patients undergoing PCI with a high risk of bleeding may be administered bivalirudin for anticoagulation in place of heparin. Patients with a history of HIT should be administered bivalirudin with or without a glycoprotein (GP) IIb/IIIa inhibitor in place of heparin for anticoagulation. Bivalirudin can also be administered in conjunction with heparin for additional anticoagulation during PCI. Argatroban, another DTI, is also an option for patients undergoing PCI with HIT or suspected HIT. Argatroban is recommended in patients with renal insufficiency as it is primarily hepatically metabolized (Amsterdam et al., 2014b).

GP IIB/IIIA INHIBITORS

GP IIb/IIIa inhibitors are generally indicated in ACS when an initial invasive management strategy is selected; in patients with high-risk elements—including elevated troponins and significant ST-segment depression, and in patients with diabetes. These agents are given in addition to aspirin and ADP inhibitors as part of triple-antiplatelet therapy to prevent cardiac ischemic complications. GP IIb/IIIa inhibitors work in the final platelet aggregation pathway and prevent fibrinogen binding and platelet aggregation. GP IIb/IIIa is a complex found on the surface of platelets, which serves as a receptor for fibrinogen and von Willebrand factor, thereby causing platelet aggregation (Armstrong & Peter, 2012). GP IIb/IIIa inhibitors bind to GP IIb/IIIa receptors to prevent this effect (Merck & Co., Inc., 2014b). Of the three agents in this class (tirofiban, eptifibatide, and abciximab), only abciximab binds irreversibly to the GP IIb/IIIa receptor and continued inhibition of platelets may persist for up to 10 days post-infusion (Eli Lilly and Company, 2013). Abciximab should only be administered in patients undergoing PCI within 24 hours. While reversing the effects of abciximab requires platelet transfusions, tirofiban and eptifibatide's effects are reversed with drug elimination. GP IIb/IIIa inhibitors have been extensively studied to determine the optimal timing for initiation, although there is no known difference in outcomes whether these agents are administered early in ACS or late. GP IIb/IIIa inhibitors are not recommended in patients at high risk of bleeding, with normal baseline troponin levels, without a history of diabetes, or more than or equal to 75 years. Table 32.2 details pharmacologic management considerations of patients who present with ACS.

TABLE 32.2 Pharmacologic Treatment Options for ACS

Immediate therapy for all patients	**ANTIPLATELET AGENT:** All patients must receive aspirin, unless serious contraindication
	Aspirin 162–325 mg chew and swallow at onset of ACS, then 81–325 mg (81 mg preferred) once daily indefinitely
	
	P2Y₁₂ INHIBITOR/ANTIPLATELET AGENT: Administer one of the following:
	Clopidogrel
	■ 300–600 mg load
	  • 300 mg for initial ischemia-guided strategy
	  • 600 mg recommended for PCI and administered at least 6–8 hr prior to PCI
	  • >75 years old, do not administer loading dose
	■ Maintenance dose: 75 mg daily
	■ Onset: 2–6 hr
	■ Reduced effectiveness with impaired metabolism to convert to active form
	■ DDI: Proton pump inhibitors (with the exception of pantoprazole)
	
	Prasugrel *ONLY USE THIS AGENT IF UNDERGOING PCI*
	■ 60 mg load no later than 1 hr post-PCI
	■ Maintenance dose: 10 mg (5 mg for <60 kg)
	■ Onset: <30 min
	■ CI: weight <60 kg; age ≥75 years; history of stroke/TIA; active, pathologic bleeding
	
	Ticagrelor
	■ 180 mg load given as soon as possible or at time of PCI
	■ Maintenance dose: 90 mg twice daily
	■ Onset: 30 min
	■ BBW: ASA >100 mg a day reduces effectiveness, only the first/loading dose should be >100 mg
	■ CI: ICH; severe hepatic impairment; active bleeding

(continued)

TABLE 32.2 Pharmacologic Treatment Options for ACS (*continued*)

ANTICOAGULATION therapy with one of the following:

Unfractionated Heparin (UFH)
- Initial bolus 60 IU/kg IV (max 4000 IU), then 12 IU/kg/hr infusion (max of 1,000 IU/hr)
- Adjust to goal aPTT of 1.5–2.5x control (or Anti-Xa levels between 0.3 and 0.7)
- Check aPTT 6 hr post-infusion
- Continue for at least 48 hr or until PCI is performed
- STEMI:
  - With GPI: use bolus dosing of 50–70 IU/kg IV; goal ACT 200–250s
  - Without GPI: 70–100 IU/kg IV bolus, goal ACT 250–300s

Enoxaparin
- 1 mg/kg subcutaneously every 12 hr
- CrCl < 30 mL/min: 1 mg/kg every 24 hr
- Additional 0.3 mg/kg IV dose should be given if < 2 doses of enoxaparin given at time of PCI or last dose was 8–12 hr prior to PCI
- Enoxaparin should be continued for duration of hospitalization or until PCI is performed
- STEMI with fibrinolytic therapy:
  - ≤ 75 years: 30 mg IV bolus, then 1 mg/kg subcutaneous every 12 hr (max of 100 mg/dose for first two doses)
  - > 75 years: 0.75 mg/kg subcutaneous every 12 hr (max of 75 mg/dose for first two doses); no bolus
  - CrCl < 30 mL/min: 1 mg/kg every 24 hr regardless of age

Fondaparinux
- 2.5 mg subcutaneously once daily for duration of hospitalization or until PCI is performed
- Must give additional anticoagulant with anti-factor IIa activity (80 IU/kg UFH; 60 IU/kg if GPI used) at time of PCI due to risk of catheter thrombosis
- Contraindicated with creatinine clearance < 30 mL/min
- STEMI with fibrinolytic therapy:
  - 2.5 mg IV initial dose then 2.5 mg subcutaneously once daily beginning the following day
  - Not recommended as sole anticoagulant

STATIN THERAPY: Administer high-intensity statin within 24 hr

Atorvastatin
- 80 mg daily
- Draw lipid panel at presentation as lipid levels may be falsely decreased post-ACS (obtain preferably within 24 hr)

BETA ADRENERGIC BLOCKER:
- Administer oral BB agent within 24 hr (give maximum possible dose or goal HR 50–60 bpm)
- **Metoprolol, propranolol,** and **atenolol** studied in acute settings
- CI: Prinzmetal/variant angina-coronary vasospasms, active asthma or reactive airway disease, ADHF, cardiogenic shock, symptomatic bradycardia or second- or third-degree heart block
- Relative CI: Use of non-selective BB in patients with recent cocaine use (unopposed beta-blocking causes alpha activation from cocaine effects, leading to vasoconstriction and ↑BP)
- Other considerations:
  - HF/LVEF < 40%: use bisoprolol, carvedilol ER or IR; metoprolol ER (these agents are studied in HF and demonstrate decreased mortality)
  - COPD/asthma: Beta-1 selective agents preferred (metoprolol, atenolol)

ACEI/ARB:
- Indicated only for patients with LVEF < 40% or pulmonary congestion
- Administer within 24 hr

NonDHP CCBs
- No role in MI; consider only if BBs are contraindicated

(continued)

TABLE 32.2 Pharmacologic Treatment Options for ACS (*continued*)

Agents utilized for symptom relief only—no mortality benefit associated with use	**SHORT-ACTING NITRATES:** ■ May administer one of the following or can start with oral and transition to IV if necessary ■ CI: sildenafil or vardenafil use within 24 hr (48 hr of tadalafil use), SBP <90 mmHg, severe bradycardia; do not administer in right ventricular infarction because compromises preload: these patients need fluids **Sublingual Nitroglycerin Tablet** ■ 0.3–0.6 mg ■ Venous vasodilation only; decreases preload **Nitroglycerin spray** 0.4 mg per spray **Nitroglycerin paste** 0.2–0.8 mg per hr, every 12 hr **Intravenous Nitroglycerin** ■ Initial infusion rate=5 mcg/min then ↑q3–5 min by 5 mcg/min ■ Medication should be provided only in GLASS BOTTLE with non-PVC tubing (PVC leeches into IV solution, tubing absorbs medication) ■ Unlike sublingual tablets, IV produces both venous and arteriolar vasodilation **ANALGESIA:** May administer other analgesics; however, morphine is generally preferred **Morphine sulfate** 2–4 mg IV, ↑in increments of 2–8 mg IV every 5–10 min as needed ■ May mask ongoing angina symptoms
Initial invasive management strategy, optional for ischemia-guided strategy	**GLYCOPROTEIN IIb/IIIa INHIBITORS:** Use as adjunct to heparin in PCI to prevent cardiac ischemic complications **Eptifibatide** ■ 180 mcg/kg IV bolus, then 10 min later 2nd bolus of 180 mcg/kg (2nd bolus if undergoing PCI) ■ Start continuous infusion of 2 mcg/kg/min after first bolus, continue until discharge or 18–24 hr post-PCI (max 15 mg/hr), whichever is shorter ■ CrCl <50 mL/min: adjust to 1 mcg/kg/min (calculate CrCl using actual body weight, max 7 mg/hr) ■ Bolus dose is not affected by CrCl (failure to reduce dose in renal dysfunction leads to ↑↑bleeding risk) ■ CI: hemodialysis due to massive bleed; stroke within 30 days ■ Max infusion time: 96 hr **Abciximab** *USE THIS AGENT ONLY IF UNDERGOING PCI WITHIN 24 HR* ■ 0.25 mg/kg IV bolus given 10–60 min prior to PCI, then continuous infusion 0.125 mcg/kg/min (max of 10 mcg/min) × 12–18 hr ■ Conclude infusion 1 hr after PCI ■ This is a monoclonal antibody; thus, readministration not recommended due to development of human anti-chimeric antibodies increasing risk of anaphylaxis **Tirofiban** ■ 25 mcg/kg IV bolus, then continuous infusion 0.15 mcg/kg/min for up to 18 hr ■ CrCl <30 mL/min: reduce rate by 50%

(*continued*)

TABLE 32.2 Pharmacologic Treatment Options for ACS (*continued*)

DIRECT THROMBIN INHIBITORS: Use in patients undergoing PCI with HIT or suspected HIT, as an **alternative** to heparin

Bivalirudin
- ACT goal 200–250 sec
- PCI with HIT/suspected HIT or STEMI:
  - 0.75 mg/kg IV bolus (can give 0.3 mg/kg additional bolus if ACT not at goal 5 min post-initial bolus)
  - Then infusion of 1.75 mg/kg/hr for duration of PCI
  - CrCl < 30 mL/min: reduce continuous infusion rate to 1 mg/kg/hr
  - Can continue up to 4 hr post-PCI; if additional infusion needed, can give for up to 20 hr at rate of 0.2 mg/kg/hr
- UA/NSTEMI with early invasive strategy:
  - 0.1 mg/kg IV bolus
  - Then 0.25 mg/kg/hr infusion.
  - Once PCI deemed necessary, may give additional bolus of 0.5 mg/kg and increase infusion rate to 1.75 mg/kg/hr
  - Discontinue post-PCI or up to 4 hr post-PCI

Argatroban
- aPTT goal 1.5 to 3x baseline (but ≤ 100 s)
- PCI with HIT/suspected HIT: 2 mcg/kg/min continuous IV

Antiplatelet dose and duration of therapy for patients after ACS with or without stent placement	AGENT AND DOSE	NO STENT/ NO PCI	BARE METAL STENT	DRUG-ELUTING STENTS			
				Cypher (Sirolimus)	Taxus (Paclitaxel)	Xience (Everolimus)	Medtronic (Zotarolim-us)
	Aspirin 81–325 mg daily	Indefinitely	Indefinitely	Indefinitely			
	Plavix 75 mg daily, prasugrel 10 mg daily, or ticagrelor 90 mg twice daily	12 months; do not use prasugrel	PCI due to ACS: 12 months Elective PCI: 1 month at minimum; ideally 1 year	PCI due to ACS: at least 12 months Elective PCI: 12 months at minimum STEMI patients: prasugrel preferred if prior stroke or TIA			

↑, increase(d); ACS, acute coronary syndrome; ACT, activated clotting time; ADHF, acute decompensated heart failure; ADP, adenosine diphosphate; aPTT, activated partial thromboplastin time; BB, beta blocker; BP, blood pressure; CABG, coronary artery bypass graft; cath, catheterization; CBC, complete blood count; CI, contraindication/contraindicated; COPD, chronic obstructive pulmonary disease; CrCl, creatinine clearance; DES, drug-eluting stent; ER, extended release; HF, heart failure; HIT, heparin-induced thrombocytopenia; HR, heart rate; ICH, intracranial hemorrhage; hr, hour(s); IR, immediate release; LVEF, left ventricular ejection fraction; MI, myocardial infarction; PCI, percutaneous coronary intervention; PVC, polyvinyl chloride; q, every; RV, right ventricular; SBP, systolic blood pressure; SL, sublingual; TIA, transient ischemic attack.

HIGH-DOSE STATIN THERAPY

High-dose statin therapy has demonstrated decreased mortality and a reduction in recurrent ischemic events in two pivotal trials, MIRACL (Myocardial Ischemia Reduction with Aggressive Cholesterol Lowering) and PROVE-IT (Pravastatin or Atorvastatin Evaluation and Infection Therapy–Thrombolysis in Myocardial Infarction 22). MIRACL evaluated atorvastatin 80 mg to placebo (Schwartz et al., 2001) and

PROVE-IT (Cannon et al., 2004) evaluated atorvastatin 80 mg to pravastatin 40 mg. In both trials, atorvastatin 80 mg demonstrated a reduction in morbidity and mortality in patients presenting with ACS. There is some debate among clinicians regarding the choice of statin therapy and dose, as the mechanism of benefit from these studies remains unclear. While high-dose statins certainly play a large role in significantly decreasing low-density-lipoprotein levels, statins have been proposed to be pleiotropic, including an antiinflammatory effect. Thus, it is unclear whether the benefit is derived specifically from atorvastatin versus a class effect, from the high-dose impacting LDL levels, or from the pleiotropic property. While some clinicians routinely prescribe only atorvastatin 80 mg to all patients with ACS, others may select different statin agents or lower doses. Selecting an agent requires clinical considerations and an understanding of specific patient- and agent-related variables.

BETA ADRENERGIC RECEPTOR BLOCKERS

The use of oral beta adrenergic receptor blocker therapy is recommended within 24 hours of ACS symptoms. Beta blockers are proven to limit infarct size, recurrent ischemia, ventricular tachycardia, ventricular fibrillation, and other arrhythmias associated with ACS, thereby decreasing mortality rates. Mechanistically, beta blockers decrease myocardial oxygen demand by reducing heart rate, contractility, and cardiac workload. Several studies have evaluated the utility of beta blockers in acute MI, one being the MIAMI (Metoprolol in Acute Myocardial Infarct) trial (MIAMI trial research group, 1985), which specifically evaluated metoprolol. Beta blockers are indicated in all ACS patients, unless there are significant contraindications.

ANGIOTENSIN-CONVERTING ENZYME INHIBITORS AND ANGIOTENSIN II RECEPTOR BLOCKERS

Angiotensin-converting enzyme inhibitors (ACEI) and angiotensin II receptor blockers (ARBs) decrease afterload and preload by dilating coronaries via increased nitric oxide production. They also have a neurohormonal effect, which decreases remodeling of the heart. ACEI/ARBs have been shown to reduce mortality in the ISIS-4 (Fourth International Study of Infarct Survival; ISIS-4 collaborative group, 1995) and GISSI-3 (Gruppo Italiano per lo Studio della Sopravvivenza nell'infarto Micardico; GISSI-3 study group, 1994) trials and are specifically indicated in patients post-MI with an LVEF less than 40% or with pulmonary congestion.

PROTEASE-ACTIVATED RECEPTOR-1

Vorapaxar is the first agent in a new class called protease-activated receptor-1 (PAR-1) antagonists (Merck & Co., Inc., 2014a). This agent was FDA approved in May 2014 and acting as an antiplatelet agent through inhibition of thrombin-induced and thrombin receptor agonist peptide (TRAP)-induced platelet aggregation. Vorapaxar competes with thrombin to block PAR-1 and PAR-4 receptors on platelets. Unlike the ADP inhibitors and aspirin, vorapaxar does not exert its antiplatelet aggregation activity via ADP or thromboxane. The recommended dose of vorapaxar is 2.08 mg once daily in conjunction with aspirin with or without clopidogrel in patients with a history of MI or peripheral arterial disease (PAD). This agent is 100% bioavailable, and peak effects can be seen 1 to 2 hours after ingestion. Vorapaxar is hepatically metabolized and eliminated primarily through the feces. Administration of vorapaxar has no impact on PT, ACT, or activated partial thromboplastin time (aPTT).

Vorapaxar was studied in two major phase 3 trials, the TRACER (Thrombin Receptor Antagonist for Clinical Event Reduction in Acute Coronary Syndrome) trial (Tricoci et al., 2012) and the TRA 2P-TIMI 50 (Thrombin Receptor Antagonist in Secondary Prevention of Atherothrombotic Ischemic Events-Thrombolysis in Myocardial Infarction 50) trial (Morrow et al., 2012). The TRACER trial evaluated subjects with non-ST segment elevation ACS, but no differences in cardiovascular mortality, MI, or stroke were seen when vorapaxar was given in addition to standard therapy. Increased bleeding rates were found in the vorapaxar group. Given these results, vorapaxar should not be administered to patients for the management of ACS.

The TRA 2P-TIMI 50 trial evaluated the use of vorapaxar in conjunction with standard therapy (aspirin, ADP inhibitor, or dipyridamole) in patients with a recent MI or ischemic stroke (within 2 weeks to 12 months) or with symptomatic PAD. Patients in the vorapaxar group had a significant reduction in the rates of cardiovascular death and ischemic events but had a higher risk of bleeding, specifically ICH. An increased bleeding risk was found in the subgroup with a history of stroke, TIA, or ICH. Vorapaxar is therefore contraindicated in those patients and is only approved in patients with established MI or PAD when given in conjunction with aspirin and/or clopidogrel. Because of its newly approved status, the clinical role of vorapaxar for patients with MI has not been firmly established.

ST-SEGMENT ELEVATION MYOCARDIAL INFARCTIONS

The primary treatment for patients with STEMI is reperfusion therapy, preferentially with PCI. If the patient arrives to a non-PCI capable hospital and transport to a PCI-capable hospital is anticipated to be more than 120 minutes from the initial medical contact, fibrinolytic therapy is recommended for reperfusion (O'Gara et al., 2013b). If the patient has a contraindication to fibrinolytic therapy, the patient should be transported to a PCI-capable hospital regardless of the time delay. Table 32.3 lists the contraindications for fibrinolytic therapy.

For patients who are evaluated to be appropriate candidates for fibrinolytic therapy, the agent must be administered within 30 minutes of arrival to the hospital and within 12 hours of symptom onset. Clinical trials demonstrate time-related reductions in morbidity and mortality, and administration as close to symptom onset as possible provides the greatest benefit. For patients within 12 to 24 hours of symptom onset, fibrinolytic therapy should be administered if there is ECG evidence of ongoing ischemia or hemodynamic instability. The overall benefit of administering fibrinolytic therapy beyond 12 hours of symptom onset is not well established and is only considered in ongoing STEMI or hemodynamic instability. Table 32.4 details various fibrinolytic agents used for STEMI management.

TABLE 32.3 Contraindications and Cautions for Fibrinolytic Therapy in STEMI

Absolute contraindications
- Any prior ICH
- Known structural cerebral vascular lesion (e.g., arteriovenous malformation)
- Known malignant intracranial neoplasm (primary or metastatic)
- Ischemic stroke within 3 mo
  - EXCEPT acute ischemic stroke within 4.5 hr
- Suspected aortic dissection
- Active bleeding or bleeding diathesis (excluding menses)
- Significant closed-head or facial trauma within 3 mo
- Intracranial or intraspinal surgery within 2 mo
- Severe uncontrolled hypertension (unresponsive to emergency therapy)
- For streptokinase, prior treatment within the previous 6 mo

Relative contraindications
- History of chronic, severe, poorly controlled hypertension
- Significant hypertension on presentation (SBP > 180 mmHg or DBP > 110 mmHg)
- History of prior ischemic stroke > 3 mo
- Dementia
- Known intracranial pathology not covered in absolute contraindications
- Traumatic or prolonged (> 10 min) CPR
- Major surgery (< 3 wk)
- Recent (within 2 to 4 wk) internal bleeding
- Noncompressible vascular punctures
- Pregnancy
- Active peptic ulcer
- Oral anticoagulant therapy

CPR, cardiopulmonary resuscitation; DBP, diastolic blood pressure; ICH, intracranial hemorrhage; SBP, systolic blood pressure; STEMI, ST-elevation myocardial infarction.

*Viewed as advisory for clinical decision making and may not be all-inclusive or definitive.

Reprinted from O'Gara et al. (2013b), with permission from Elsevier.

TABLE 32.4 Fibrinolytic Agents

Agent	Dose	Mechanism of Action	Other Considerations
Alteplase (tPA)	Bolus 15 mg IV over 1–2 min, then infuse 0.75 mg/kg (not to exceed 50 mg) over next 30 min, followed by 0.5 mg/kg over next 60 min (not to exceed 35 mg). Total dose not to exceed 100 mg.	Binds to fibrin in clot and converts plasminogen to plasmin	▪ Available as 50 mg or 100 mg reconstituted solutions ▪ DOA: fibrinolysis continues up to 1 hr post-infusion ▪ Relatively fibrin selective
Reteplase (rPA)	10 units IV over 2 min, then a second dose 30 min later of 10 units over 2 min; withhold second dose if serious bleeding or anaphylaxis occurs.		▪ Available as full kit or half-kit (half-kit only provides a single dose, while full kit provides both doses) ▪ Produced using recombinant DNA technology using *E. coli* ▪ Thrombolysis occurs in 30–90 min ▪ Lacks relative fibrin specificity
Tenecteplase (TNK-tPA)	Administer as IV bolus over 5 sec < 60 kg: 30 mg ≥ 60 to < 70 kg: 35 mg ≥ 70 to < 80 kg: 40 mg ≥ 80 to < 90 kg: 45 mg ≥ 90 kg: 50 mg (max dose of 50 mg)		▪ Available as 50 mg IV kit ▪ More fibrin specific than alteplase and reteplase ▪ Similar structure to alteplase, varies by 3-point mutations ▪ Terminal $t_{1/2}$: 90–130 min ▪ Highly selective for fibrin

DNA, deoxyribonucleic acid; DOA, duration of action; hr, hour(s); IV, intravenous; min, minute(s); rPA, reteplase plasminogen activator; sec, second(s); $t_{1/2}$, half-life; TNK-tPA, tenecteplase tissue-type plasminogen activator; tPA, tissue-type plasminogen activator.

Similar to UA/NSTEMI, adjunctive antiplatelet and anticoagulant therapies are indicated in addition to the administration of a fibrinolytic agent (Table 32.2). While the agents are the same, specific medications may have different dosing recommendations for STEMI compared to UA/NSTEMI.

With all anticoagulants, antiplatelets, and fibrinolytic agents, the patient should be monitored closely for bleeding. For anticoagulation with heparin derivatives, the patient should also be monitored for HIT. All patients should be transferred to a PCI-capable hospital after the administration of fibrinolytic therapy.

CABG POST-ANGIOGRAPHY

In patients undergoing CABG surgery, specific antithrombotic agents must be held prior to surgery given the high risk for bleeding. The specific recommendations on holding or continuing these agents can be found in Table 32.5.

TABLE 32.5 Pharmacologic Considerations of Anticoagulants and Antithrombotics Prior to CABG

Pharmacologic Agent	Action
Prasugrel	Hold for 7 days prior
Clopidogrel	Hold for 5 days (24 hr if urgent)
Ticagrelor	Hold for 5 days (24 hr if urgent)
Fondaparinux	Hold for 24 hr prior and transition to UFH
Enoxaparin	Hold for 12–24 hr prior and transition to UFH
Glycoprotein IIb/IIIa inhibitors: Abciximab, Eptifibatide, Tirofiban	Discontinue 4 hr prior
Bivalirudin	Hold for 3 hr prior and transition to UFH
Unfractionated heparin (UFH)	Continue
Aspirin	Continue

CABG, coronary artery bypass graft.

For full reference citations to this chapter, please see "Section References" in the back of the book, under the heading "Section VII."

Pharmacotherapeutics of Heart Failure and Acute Decompensated Heart Failure

DEV CHATTERJI

Heart failure (HF), which affects more than 5.8 million individuals in the United States, is an epidemic and the only cardiovascular condition with an increasing incidence (Go et al., 2014). HF results when the heart fails to provide sufficient blood to meet the metabolic requirements of the body. In response to the decline in cardiac function and significantly decreased cardiac output, the body activates a number of compensatory mechanisms (Figure 33.1). These mechanisms include an increase in sympathetic tone or activation of the sympathetic nervous system and the renin angiotensin aldosterone system (RAAS), which results in vasoconstriction, sodium and water retention, and cardiac remodeling. Although these responses attempt to compensate for reduced cardiac output, it begins a vicious cycle that promotes further cardiac deterioration and damage. HF characterized by reduced left ventricular systolic ejection fraction (HFrEF) has the most evidence to support the use of pharmacologic agents to mediate these processes (Yancy et al., 2013).

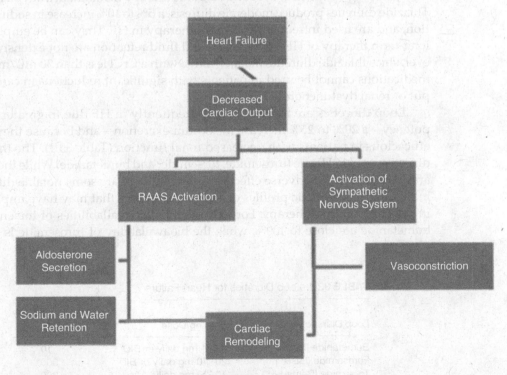

FIGURE 33.1 Compensatory mechanisms in heart failure.

RAAS, renin angiotensin aldosterone system.

PHARMACOLOGIC THERAPY: CHRONIC HF

The goal of pharmacologic therapy in HF is to block the compensatory mechanisms caused by decreased cardiac output, enhance cardiac function, prevent further cardiac damage, and improve symptoms. The agents used in the treatment and management of chronic HF include the following:

- Diuretics
- Agents that inhibit the RAAS
    - Angiotensin-converting enzyme inhibitors (ACEIs)
    - Angiotensin II receptor blockers (ARBs)
    - Aldosterone antagonists
- Beta adrenergic receptor blockers (beta blockers)
- Nitrates and other vasodilators
- Cardiac glycosides

Diuretics for HF

Diuretics are utilized in patients with HF who have clinical evidence of fluid overload. The primary goal of diuretic therapy is to reduce symptoms associated with sodium and water retention. Diuretics have no proven effect on delaying disease progression or improving mortality and therefore should never be used as monotherapy for HF. Diuretic agents may be utilized intermittently for symptom improvement, although patients may require chronic therapy to maintain a euvolemic state. Thiazide diuretics produce moderate diuresis, a 5% to 10% increase in sodium excretion, and are used infrequently as monotherapy in HF. They can be employed for long-term therapy of HF when edema and fluid retention are not extensive. However, since thiazide diuretics are ineffective with a CrCl less than 30 mL/min, these medications cannot be used in patients with significant reductions in cardiac output or renal dysfunction.

Loop diuretics are indicated more frequently in HF due to greater diuretic potency—a 20% to 25% increase in sodium excretion—and because they remain efficacious in patients with decreased renal function (Table 33.1). The three loop diuretics used in HF are furosemide, torsemide, and bumetanide. While their mechanism of action and adverse effects are similar, there are some notable differences in the pharmacokinetic profiles of the loop diuretics that may have implications in selecting optimal therapy. For example, the bioavailabilities of torsemide and bumetanide are close to 100%, while the bioavailability of furosemide is approxi-

TABLE 33.1 Loop Diuretics for Heart Failure

Loop Diuretic	Starting Dose	Maximum Daily Dose (mg)
Bumetanide (Bumex®)	0.5–1 mg daily or BID	10
Furosemide (Lasix®)	20–40 mg daily or BID	600
Torsemide (Demadex®)	10–20 mg daily	200

BID, twice daily.

mately 50%. There are also differences in the half-lives among the agents. Although pharmacokinetic considerations can help clinicians optimize use of the diuretics, many patients can develop diuretic resistance with chronic use of loop diuretics. In patients with diuretic resistance or severe fluid overload, the addition of a thiazide diuretic to loop diuretics may provide synergy. By blocking distal tubule sodium reabsorption, thiazide-type diuretics can antagonize the renal adaptation to chronic loop diuretic therapy and potentially improve diuretic resistance due to rebound sodium retention. Of the thiazide or thiazide-like diuretics, metolazone has been evaluated for this purpose most frequently in clinical trials. However, there is no evidence that any specific agent is superior to the other. Dosing recommendations for thiazide diuretics in combination with loop diuretics include oral metolazone, 2.5 to 10 mg once daily or 2.5 to 5 mg twice daily, or hydrochlorothiazide 25 to 100 mg once or twice daily (Jentzer, DeWald, & Hernandez, 2010).

ACEIs for HF

As discussed, the RAAS plays an important role both in cardiac remodeling and in the hemodynamic changes that occur in response to reduced cardiac output. ACEIs block production of angiotensin II, decrease release of aldosterone, and suppress degradation of bradykinins. As a result, ACEIs improve hemodynamics and favorably alter cardiac remodeling. Accordingly, ACEIs are cornerstones of HF therapy, and common dosing is listed in Table 33.2. The benefits of ACEIs have been studied in numerous trials and positive outcomes include decreased mortality, decreased hospitalizations, symptom improvement, and improved clinical status. One of the first studies that evaluated the influence of ACEIs on the prognosis of HF was the Cooperative North Scandinavian Enalapril Survival Study (CONSENSUS). The study reported dramatic reduction in mortality with ACEI therapy and set the stage for further research confirming the pivotal role of these agents in HF management (CONSENSUS Trial Study Group, 1987). Current American Heart Association (AHA) guidelines indicate that HF patients with reduced ejection fraction should receive therapy with an ACEI unless there is a medical contraindication (Yancy et al., 2013).

TABLE 33.2 ACEIs for Heart Failure

ACEI	Initial Dose	Target Dose
Captopril	6.25 mg TID	50 mg TID
Enalapril (Vasotec®)	2.5 mg BID	10–20 mg BID
Fosinopril (Monopril®)	5–10 mg daily	40 mg daily
Lisinopril (Zestril®, Prinivil®)	2.5–5 mg daily	20–40 mg daily
Quinapril (Accupril®)	5 mg BID	20 mg BID
Ramipril (Altace®)	1.25–2.5 mg daily	10 mg daily
Trandolapril (Mavik®)	1 mg daily	4 mg daily

ACEI, angiotensin-converting enzyme inhibitor; BID, twice daily; TID, three times daily.

ARBs for HF

The effects of ARBs are similar to those of ACEIs. Clinical trials demonstrate that ARBs improve left ventricular ejection fraction (LVEF), reduce HF symptoms, decrease hospitalizations, and decrease mortality. ARBs, however, do not increase the levels of kinins, so their effects on cardiac remodeling are potentially less favorable than ACEIs. The primary niche for ARBs in HF is for those patients unable to tolerate ACEI due to an ACEI–induced cough. The primary clinical trials supporting the use of ARBs in HF studied either candesartan or valsartan (Table 33.3). The Candesartan in HF: Assessment of Reduction in Mortality and Morbidity (CHARM) trials are examples of key trials evaluating the use or ARBs in patients with HF. CHARM was designed as three studies: CHARM, CHARM-Added, and CHARM-Alternative. All of the CHARM trials found significant reductions in hospitalizations or cardiovascular deaths for HF patients on candesartan. AHA guidelines, therefore, call for an ARB for patients who cannot tolerate ACEI (Granger et al., 2003; McMurray et al., 2003; Pfeffer et al., 2003; Yancy et al., 2013).

TABLE 33.3 Angiotensin Receptor Blockers (ARBs) for Heart Failure

ARB	Initial Dose	Target Dose
Candesartan (Atacand®)	4–8 mg daily	32 mg daily
Valsartan (Diovan®)	20–40 mg BID	160 mg BID

BID, twice daily.

Aldosterone Antagonists

Current guidelines promote the addition of an aldosterone antagonist, spironolactone or eplerenone, for patients with New York Heart Association (NYHA) Class II to IV HF and an LVEF less than 30% (Table 33.4). These agents improve symptoms, decrease hospitalizations, and decrease mortality for patients with HF. The role of aldosterone in HF is multifaceted. Aldosterone is a mineralocorticoid that promotes renal retention of sodium in exchange for excretion of potassium. In addition, other pathophysiologic effects of HF that aldosterone mediates are cardiac remodeling, myocardial fibrosis, and activation of the sympathetic nervous system. Aldosterone antagonists block the effects of aldosterone in the kidneys, heart, and vasculature, resulting in decreased potassium loss, decreased sodium retention, reduced fibrosis on the myocardium, and decreased fluid retention. These agents are not recommended for patients with hyperkalemia or decreased renal function.

TABLE 33.4 Aldosterone Antagonists for Heart Failure

Agent (Brand)	Initial Dose	Target Dose
Eplerenone (Inspra®)	25 mg daily	50 mg daily
Spironolactone (Aldactone®)	12.5–25 mg daily	25 mg daily to BID

BID, twice daily.

Three major trials have demonstrated prolonged survival in HF patients with the use of aldosterone antagonists. The benefits of adding spironolactone to an ACEI was examined in the Randomized Aldactone Evaluation Study (RALES) (Pitt et al., 1999). Patients treated with spironolactone in addition to other standard HF therapies had a 30% reduction in the primary endpoint of overall mortality. The EPHESUS trial assessed the impact of eplerenone on mortality in patients after an acute myocardial infarction (AMI) with an LVEF less than 40% and clinical signs of HF. Eplerenone demonstrated significant reductions in all-cause mortality at 30 days in addition to conventional therapy (Pitt et al., 2003). Lastly, the EMPHASIS-HF trial evaluated the effects of eplerenone in patients with chronic systolic HF and mild symptoms. The trial was stopped prematurely because of a significant benefit with eplerenone (Zannad et al., 2011).

Beta Adrenergic Receptor Blockers for HF

There is sufficient evidence from a number of trials demonstrating that beta blockers decrease mortality in patients with HF and left ventricular dysfunction in combination with an ACEI. Primarily, three beta blockers have been studied extensively in the management of HF and have demonstrated reduced mortality compared with placebo: carvedilol, metoprolol succinate, and bisoprolol. When added to conventional therapy, beta blockers can improve LVEF, increase exercise tolerance, slow the progression of HF, reduce hospitalizations, and, most importantly, reduce mortality. An overview of landmark trials that led to the recommendation of these particular agents is reviewed in Table 33.5.

TABLE 33.5 Landmark Trials With Beta Blockers in Heart Failure

Study	Inclusion Criteria	Treatment	Results
MERIT-HF	■ NYHA Class II–IV for ≥3 months before randomization ■ LVEF < 40% within 3 months prior to study	Initial dose: Metoprolol succinate 12.5 mg daily Target dose: Metoprolol succinate 200 mg once daily	Significant reduction in: ■ All-cause mortality ■ All-cause mortality or all-cause hospitalization
U.S. Carvedilol study	■ NYHA Class II–III ■ HF for at least 3 months ■ LVEF < 35% for at least 2 months	Initial dose: Carvedilol 6.25 mg twice daily Target Dose: Carvedilol 25 mg twice daily	Significant improvement in: ■ Survival Significant reduction in: ■ Hospitalizations
COPERNICUS	■ NYHA Class IV w/HF symptoms at rest or w/ minimal exertion ■ LVEF < 25%	Initial dose: Carvedilol 3.125 mg twice daily Target Dose: Carvedilol 25 mg twice daily	Significant reduction in: ■ Survival
CIBIS II	■ NYHA Class III or IV ■ LVEF < 35%	Initial dose: Bisoprolol 1.25 mg once daily Target dose: Bisoprolol 10 mg once daily	Significant reduction in: ■ All-cause mortality

HF, heart failure; LVEF, left ventricular ejection fraction; NYHA, New York Heart Association.

• AHA guidelines recommend that one of the beta blockers proven to reduce mortality should be used in all stable patients with left ventricular dysfunction (HFrEF) unless there is a medical contraindication (CIBIS-II, 1999; MERIT-HF, 1999; Packer et al., 1996; Packer et al., 2002). Target doses listed in Table 33.6 are associated with reductions in mortality, so proper titration to target doses is necessary. Since beta blockade decreases cardiac contractility, begin administration at a low dose and gradually increase to recommended target doses.

TABLE 33.6 Beta Adrenergic Blockers for Heart Failure

Agent (Brand)	Initial Dose	Target Dose
Bisoprolol (Zebeta®)	1.25 mg daily	10 mg daily
Carvedilol *immediate release* (Coreg®)	3.125 mg BID	25 mg BID 50 mg BID in patients > 85 kg
Carvedilol *extended release* (Coreg CR®)	10 mg daily	80 mg daily
Metoprolol succinate (Toprol XL®)	12.5–25 mg daily	200 mg daily

BID, twice daily.

Nitrates and Hydralazine

Nitrates and hydralazine are usually combined when used for the treatment of HF and may provide both symptomatic and mortality benefit in this patient population. Nitrates cause direct, selective vasodilation—primarily of veins—by enhancing nitric oxide (NO) production in vascular endothelium and arterial smooth muscle. This process effectively reduces preload. Hydralazine is a direct-acting vasodilator with selective dilation of the arterioles to reduce systemic vascular resistance and increase stroke volume and cardiac output. Hydralazine also has antioxidant properties and appears to prevent nitrate tolerance. The combination of hydralazine and nitrates may hinder HF progression due to the vasodilatory effects as well as the hemodynamic benefits. The combination of hydralazine and isosorbide dinitrate, available as a fixed-dose combination marketed as BiDil® (Table 33.7), has been evaluated in clinical trials and found to decrease mortality and hospitalizations in patients with HF. Subsequent analysis suggests that this combination was particularly effective in African Americans and is recommended in African American patients with NYHA Class II to IV HF who are symptomatic with standard therapy, including an ACEI and beta blocker (Taylor et al., 2004). This combina-

TABLE 33.7 Vasodilators for Heart Failure

Agent (Brand)	Initial Dose	Target Dose
Hydralazine	25–50 mg three to four times/day	300 mg daily in divided doses
Isosorbide dinitrate (Isordil®)	20–30 mg three to four times/day	120 mg daily in divided doses
Isosorbide dinitrate/hydralazine (BiDil®) [fixed-dose combination]	20/37.5 mg three times/day (1 tablet three times/day)	40/75 mg three times/day (2 tablets three times/day)

tion is also a reasonable alternative in patients unable to take ACEI or ARBs due to contraindications or disease-state implications. Adverse effects with these agents are headache, dizziness, tachycardia, postural hypotension, and gastrointestinal (GI) effects. Nitrates should be administered with caution in association with cyclic guanine monophosphate (cGMP)-dependent phosphodiesterase inhibitors due to hypotension.

Cardiac Glycosides: Digoxin

Digoxin is the only available cardiac glycoside in the United States. Digoxin has a number of effects on the mechanical and electrical properties of the heart. In patients with HF, digoxin increases myocardial contractility and has indirect effects on neurohormonal systems, including the RAAS. Digoxin exerts a positive inotropic action on the heart by increasing the force of ventricular contraction and cardiac output, by inhibiting an enzyme known as Na^+-K^+ adenosine triphosphate. This action indirectly results in calcium buildup inside the myocardial cell, resulting in enhanced cardiac contraction. The systemic effects of digoxin in HF patients are unlikely related to the positive ionotropic actions, but rather, are related to the neurohormonal effects of decreasing sympathetic outflow and decreasing renal reabsorption of sodium. The benefits of digoxin in HF include symptom improvement, improved exercise tolerance, and decreased hospitalizations; however, as demonstrated in the Digitalis Investigation Group (DIG) trial, digoxin has *no effect on mortality* (Digitalis Investigation Group, 1997). Digoxin's electrical effects on cardiac conduction are discussed in the antiarrhythmic Chapter 34.

There are numerous adverse effects and important monitoring considerations with digoxin. Digoxin has a narrow therapeutic index, in which serum concentrations higher than therapeutic levels greatly increase the risk of toxicity. The starting dose of digoxin is 0.125 mg daily, achieving the desired concentrations in the majority of patients. The DIG trial recommended target serum concentrations of digoxin in HF between 0.5 and 0.8 ng/mL, obtained at least 6 hours after the dose is administered. This target serum level minimizes the risk of cardiac arrhythmias, one of the principal adverse effects of concern. Other noncardiac adverse effects involve the GI system and the central nervous system. Anorexia, nausea, and vomiting are the most commonly reported GI symptoms. Visual disturbances of blurred vision, yellow vision, and appearance of halos around dark objects are also relatively common with digoxin. Digoxin is subject to a number of drug–drug interactions and increased digoxin concentrations occur with amiodarone, dronedarone, clarithromycin, azole antifungals, verapamil, and medications that cause hypokalemia, such as diuretics. Therapeutic responses to digoxin can be decreased with drugs that cause hyperkalemia, including ACEI, ARBs, and aldosterone antagonists. The AHA guidelines suggest initiating digoxin in patients with LVEF less than 40% who continue to have HF symptoms despite appropriate therapy with an ACEI, beta blocker, aldosterone antagonist, and a diuretic if needed (Yancy et al., 2013).

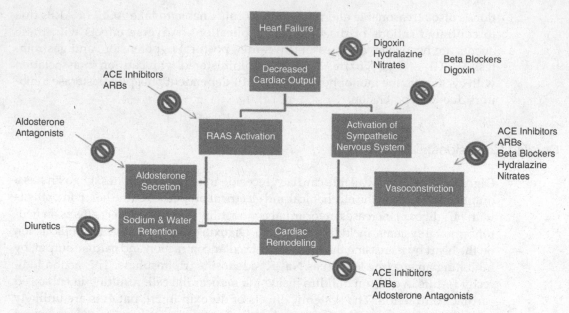

FIGURE 33.2 Summary of sites of action for agents used in the management of heart failure.
ACE, angiotensin-converting enzyme; ARB, angiotensin II receptor blocker; RAAS, renin angiotensin aldosterone system.

PHARMACOTHERAPY OF HF MANAGEMENT

Pharmacotherapy for HF management can be complex, and agents may have multiple sites of action; Figure 33.2 provides a summary.

HF is often accompanied by concomitant conditions and polypharmacy can be problematic. Clinicians must be mindful of optimizing therapy to provide the safest, most effective pharmacotherapy. A number of medications commonly used in clinical practice have the potential to exacerbate HF symptoms. Table 33.8 summarizes major medications or classes of medications to avoid or to prescribe with caution in patients with HF, and provides recommendations to optimize therapy.

ACUTE DECOMPENSATED HEART FAILURE

Acute decompensated heart failure (ADHF) is a sudden worsening of symptoms in patients with existing HF, or due to a precipitating acute coronary syndrome. The overall goals of therapy in the patient with decompensated HF are to relieve congestive symptoms, optimize volume status, and improve symptoms of low cardiac output. The mainstays of therapy ADHF include diuretic and vasodilator therapy.

Diuretics for ADHF

Patients with ADHF are usually volume overloaded and ACC/AHA guidelines recommend diuretic therapy in all patients with significant fluid overload (Yancy et al., 2013). Loop diuretics, including furosemide, bumetanide, and torsemide, are

TABLE 33.8 Medications to Avoid or Use With Caution in Heart Failure

Agent or Drug Class	Reason to Avoid or Use Caution	Recommendations
Corticosteroids	▪ Can cause sodium and fluid retention	▪ Use the lowest dose for the shortest duration ▪ Select corticosteroid with less mineralocorticoid activity
NSAIDs	▪ Can blunt diuretic response; sodium and water retention; increased systemic vascular resistance; renal compromise	▪ Avoid in patients with left ventricular dysfunction if possible
Class I and Class III antiarrhythmics	▪ Negative inotropic activity ▪ Proarrhythmic effects	▪ Avoid use of all Class I and III agents ▪ Except for amiodarone and dofetilide
Calcium channel blockers	▪ Negative ionotropic activity ▪ Neurohormonal activation	▪ Avoid use of calcium channel blockers, especially diltiazem and verapamil ▪ Amlodipine and felodipine can be used safely in patients with HF
Thiazolidinediones	▪ Fluid retention	▪ Avoid use
Metformin	▪ Increased risk of lactic acidosis	▪ Generally avoid use ▪ However, patients with well-controlled HF symptoms, without pulmonary edema and with good renal function, should not be denied the benefits of metformin for diabetes treatment
Carbamazepine	▪ Negative inotropic and chronotropic effects; suppression of sinus nodal automaticity and atrioventricular conduction	▪ Avoid use if possible
Pregabalin	▪ Lower extremity edema ▪ Inhibition of calcium channels	▪ Use caution

HF, heart failure; NSAIDs, nonsteroidal anti-inflammatory drugs.
Source: Amabile and Spencer (2004).

used commonly in the management of ADHF (Yancy et al., 2013), and furosemide is the most widely studied and utilized of these medications. Loop diuretic dosing is generally individualized and titrated based on patient symptoms and response to diuresis. Intravenous (IV) diuretic administration is recommended in ADHF due to more consistent and rapid drug bioavailability. Initial IV furosemide dosing generally begins at 40 mg IV bolus or continuous infusion of furosemide 0.1 mg/kg/hr (max 0.4 mg/kg/hr). Data have not validated a significant difference in efficacy or safety endpoints for bolus versus continuous infusion dosing (Felker et al., 2011). HF is the most common clinical scenario where diuretic resistance is observed, resulting in some patients responding poorly to large doses of loop diuretics. The mechanisms responsible for diuretic resistance in these patients may have a pharmacologic basis. It is hypothesized that the decreased response in HF patients can be explained by the high concentrations of sodium reaching the distal tubule as a result of blocked sodium reabsorption in the loop of Henle by the loop diuretic. As a result, the distal tubule undergoes hypertrophy, which enhances its ability to reabsorb sodium, potentially leading to refractory therapy and subsequent edema. Several pharmacologic strategies may be employed to overcome diuretic resistance. First, higher doses of loop diuretics may be administered, with IV furosemide having a ceiling effect at 160 to 200 mg. A second approach is to administer a continuous infusion of a loop diuretic, although this strategy has produced conflicting results in clinical trials. Lastly, a second diuretic with a different mechanism may be used to potentiate the effects of the loop diuretic; reasonable choices include oral hydrochlorothiazide (HCTZ) 12.5 to 25 mg daily, oral metolazone 2.5 to 5 mg daily, or, in severe refractory cases, IV chlorthalidone 250 to 500 mg daily (Cleland, Coletta, & Witte, 2006).

Vasodilator Therapy for ADHF

In patients with severely symptomatic fluid overload, who are not experiencing concomitant hypotension, vasodilators such as IV nitroglycerin, nitroprusside, or nesiritide can be beneficial in combination with diuretic therapy (Table 33.9).

TABLE 33.9 Vasodilator Therapy for Acute Decompensated Heart Failure

	Sodium Nitroprusside (Nipride®)	Nesiritide (Natrecor®)	Nitroglycerin (Nitronal®)
Mechanism of action	Nitric oxide induced stimulation of GC to convert GTP to cGMP	Recombinant B-type natriuretic peptide that binds to natriuretic peptide receptor A to stimulate GC and production of cGMP	Combines with sulfhydryl groups in the vascular endothelium to create S-nitrosothiol compounds that mimic nitric oxide's stimulation of GC and production of cGMP
Pharmacokinetics	Half-life: 10 minutes	Half-life: 20 minutes	Half-life: 1–4 minutes
Dosing	0.3–0.5 mcg/kg/min IV, then titrate (max: 3 mcg/kg/min)	2 mcg/kg IV bolus, then 0.01 mcg/kg/min IV	5 mcg/minute IV, then titrate (max: 200 mcg/min)
Adverse effects	Hypotension, cyanide toxicity	Hypotension, tachycardia	Hypotension, reflex tachycardia, headache
Clinical pearls	Arterial and venous vasodilator	Has hemodynamic, natriuretic, and neurohormonal effects	Primarily a venous vasodilator

cGMP, cyclic guanine monophosphate; GC, guanylate cyclase; GTP, guanosine triphosphate; IV, intravenous.

Inotropic Therapy for ADHF

Inotropic therapy is used in select patients to manage hypoperfusion as a result of severe left ventricular systolic dysfunction, low cardiac output, or inadequate response to vasodilator and diuretic therapy (Table 33.10). IV inotropes are not recommended unless elevations of left heart filling pressures are confirmed or cardiac index is severely impaired based on direct measurement or clear clinical signs.

TABLE 33.10 Inotropic Therapy for Acute Decompensated Heart Failure

	Dobutamine (Dobutrex®)	Milrinone (Primacor®)
Mechanism of action	Beta-1 agonist: stimulates AC to convert ATP into cAMP to increase cardiac output	PDE inhibitor: inhibits cAMP breakdown in the heart to increase cardiac output and in vascular smooth muscle to decrease total peripheral resistance
Pharmacokinetics	Half-life: 2 minutes	▪ Half-life: 2.5 hr ▪ Prolonged clearance in renal impairment
Dosing	2.5–5 mcg/kg/min IV infusion, then titrate (max: 20 mcg/kg/min)	Optional 50 mcg/kg IV bolus; then 0.375 mcg/kg/min infusion, titrate (max: 0.75 mcg/kg/min)
Adverse effects	Proarrhythmia, tachycardia, hypokalemia, myocardial ischemia	Hypotension, proarrhythmia, tachycardia
Clinical pearls	▪ Exhibits positive inotropic, chronotropic effects ▪ Possible increased mortality with long-term use	▪ Positive inotropic effects ▪ No chronotropic effects ▪ Avoid bolus dose to minimize hypotension ▪ Possible increased mortality with long-term use

AC, adenylate cyclase; ATP, adenosine triphosphate; cAMP, cyclic adenosine monophosphate; IV, intravenous; max, maximum; PDE, phosphodiesterase.

For full reference citations to this chapter, please see "Section References" in the back of the book, under the heading "Section VII."

34

Pharmacotherapeutics of Cardiac Arrhythmias

CONNIE H. YOON

A commonly utilized classification of antiarrhythmic medications is the Vaughan Williams classification. Based on this classification scheme, drugs are divided into four major classes (Class, I, II, III, and IV) with a fifth miscellaneous category. Medications are grouped into each category based on ion fluctuations during the slow- and fast-action potentials. For many antiarrhythmic medications it is necessary to evaluate the ECG, serum electrolytes, liver function, and kidney function prior to administering and to periodically monitor these parameters based on the medication selected. Antiarrhythmic medications are indicated for the management of supraventricular tachycardia, atrial fibrillation, atrial flutter, ventricular tachycardia, and ventricular fibrillation (Anderson et al., 2013b).

CLASS I

Vaughan Williams Class I agents are sodium channel blockers. These agents block the influx of sodium into cardiac cells of the atrial and ventricular myocardium as well as the His-Purkinje system (fast potential), thereby delaying depolarization of the cell. Class I medications are further divided into three subclasses, IA, IB, and IC.

Class IA agents block the influx of sodium and also block the efflux of potassium, thus also delaying repolarization. This effect can increase the QT interval, potentially precipitating torsades de pointes (TdP), a polymorphic ventricular tachycardia with prolonged QT. Because of this mechanism, Class I antiarrhythmic medications are proarrhythmic, meaning they can induce arrhythmias, though their main indication is to prevent or disrupt arrhythmias.

Class IB agents display selective delay in depolarization, specifically targeting ischemic tissue. They also reduce the duration of the action potential, thus decreasing the refractory period. Of note, phenytoin, an anticonvulsant agent, also contains antiarrhythmic properties similar to Class IB agents and was studied as an antiarrhythmic but is not currently used in this capacity.

Class IC agents produce significant delays in depolarization compared with Class IA and IB agents, slowing electrical conduction and increasing the refractory period. In general, Class I antiarrhythmic medications, specifically Class IC agents, are rarely prescribed due to the results of the CAST (Cardiac Arrthymia Suppression Trial). The CAST trial evaluated two Class IC antiarrhythmic agents versus placebo in patients who were within 6 days to 2 years of a myocardial infarction (MI; Echt et al., 1991). There was an increased risk of cardiac death in the antiarrhythmic groups, with the majority of deaths due to arrhythmias, and the remaining deaths secondary to acute MI with shock or heart failure (HF).

CLASS II

Medications in Vaughan Williams Class II are beta blockers. Beta blockers inhibit the influx of calcium, which decreases cardiac contractility and automaticity of the sinoatrial (SA) node. These actions slow the conduction velocity through the atrioventricular (AV) node, which causes a delayed repolarization and increased refractory period.

CLASS III

Vaughan Williams Class III agents are potassium channel blockers. Drugs in this class primarily prevent the efflux of potassium during the fast potential, delaying repolarization, thereby prolonging the action potential and thus the refractory period. Some agents in this class also possess beta-blocking properties, although their primary mechanism categorizes them as a Class III antiarrhythmic. Ibutilide increases the action potential, similar to the other Class III agents, but its proposed mechanism is not based on an interaction with potassium channels.

CLASS IV

Class IV agents are the nondihydropyridine calcium channel blockers. The antiarrhythmic mechanism of calcium channel blockers is blocking the influx of calcium, having a similar effect as the Class II agents, beta blockers.

CLASS V

The final class, sometimes referred to as Class V, consists of antiarrhythmic agents that do not fall into the above four categories. Digoxin and adenosine are the primary agents in this class. Digoxin produces an antiarrhythmic effect by inhibiting the sodium/potassium ATPase pump, which blocks the influx of sodium in exchange for potassium and also prevents the influx of calcium. Both digoxin and adenosine work primarily to decrease AV nodal conduction and automaticity of the SA node.

Additional details related to specific medications can be found in Table 34.1. Details regarding adenosine can also be found under the cardiac emergencies section in Chapter 35 as part of the advanced cardiac life support algorithm. Anticoagulation therapy for atrial fibrillation is reviewed in Chapter 31.

For full reference citations to this chapter, please see "Section References" in the back of the book, under the heading "Section VII."

TABLE 34.1 Antiarrhythmic Medications

Class	Class Mechanism	Drugs	Indication and Dose	Dose and Formulations Available	Pharmacokinetics	Clinical Considerations
IA	Sodium channel blockers	Disopyramide	VT conversion: 300 mg IR (≥50 kg) or 200 mg IR (<50 kg) PO q6h VT maintenance: >50 kg: 150 mg IR q6h or 300 mg CR PO q12h <50 kg: 100 mg IR q6h or 200 mg CR PO q12h	IR and CR Caps: 100 mg, 150 mg	Onset: 0.5–3.5 hr DOA: 1.5–8.5 hr for IR t½: 4–10 hr	■ Must be renally dose adjusted for CrCl <40 mL/min ■ t½ prolonged in renal or hepatic insufficiency ■ Correct electrolyte imbalances prior to use ■ SE: hypotension, TdP, anticholinergic effects, proarrhythmic ■ Caution in MG due to anticholinergic effects ■ Caution in HF can precipitate an exacerbation ■ CI: 2nd or 3rd degree heart block without pacer, congenital long QT syndrome, SSS ■ DDI: do not use within 48 hr of verapamil, may precipitate HF
		Procainamide	VT conversion: 20–50 mg/min IV until total of 17 mg/kg given or QRS widens by >50% or arrhythmia ceases VT maintenance: 1–4 mg/min IV infusion	Inj: 100 mg/mL, 500 mg/mL	t½: 2.5–4.7 hr NAPA t½: 6–8 hr	■ Must be renally dosed for CrCl <50 mL/min; active metabolite NAPA can accumulate producing class II antiarrhythmic effects ■ Correct electrolyte imbalances prior to use ■ SE: drug-induced lupus-like syndrome, TdP, agranulocytosis ■ CI: HF, may precipitate exacerbation ■ Caution: MG, may exacerbate condition
		Quinidine	AF maintenance: 200–300 mg IR PO q6h ER: Quinidine sulfate: 300 mg PO q8–12h; Quinidine gluconate: 324 mg PO q8–12h	IR Tabs: 200 mg, 300 mg, XR Tabs: 300 mg (sulfate), 324 mg (gluconate) Inj: 80 mg/mL	Peaks: 2 hr for sulfate; 3–6 hr for gluconate t½: 6–8 hr	■ Renally dose adjust for CrCl <10 mL/min ■ Correct electrolyte imbalances prior to use ■ In AF patients, must control AV conduction prior to use as drug can ↑ventricular response rates ■ SE: hepatotoxicity, proarrhythmic, TdP, N/V, diarrhea ■ CI: MG, 2nd or 3rd degree heart block, long QT, thrombocytopenia, TTP ■ Caution: G6PD deficit, HF, SSS ■ May increase mortality in non–life-threatening ventricular arrhythmias

(continued)

TABLE 34.1 Antiarrhythmic Medications (continued)

Class	Class Mechanism	Drugs	Indication and Dose	Dose and Formulations Available	Pharmacokinetics	Clinical Considerations
IB		Lidocaine	VF/pulseless VT conversion: 1–1.5 mg/kg IV/IO bolus, repeat q5–10 min with 0.5–0.75 mg/kg bolus as needed (max total of 3 mg/kg); or 2–3.75 mg/kg LD only via ET diluted in 5–10 mL NS or SWFI VT maintenance: 1–4 mg/min IV infusion (can bolus 0.5 mg/kg if arrhythmia reappears during maintenance) Must dose reduce in HF, shock, or hepatic disease: 10 mcg/kg/min with max of 20 mcg/kg/min or 1.5 mg/min	Inj: 4 mg/mL (0.4%), 5 mg/mL (0.5%), 8 mg/mL (0.8%), 10 mg/mL (1%), 15 mg/mL (1.5%), 20 mg/mL (2%) Premix: 1,000 mg/250 mL (0.4%) in D_5W, 2,000 mg/250 mg (0.8%) in D_5W Prefilled syringe: 100 mg/5 mL (2%)	Onset: 45–90 sec DOA: 10–20 min $t_{1/2}$: biphasic; initial 7–30 min, terminal 1.5–2 hr	■ Increase risk of lidocaine toxicity with prolonged use or higher doses ■ Dose must be adjusted for hepatic disease due to increased risk of lidocaine toxicity ■ SE: N/V, proarrhythmic ■ Lidocaine toxicity typically appears as CNS effects (confusion, dizziness, drowsiness, tinnitus, perioral numbness/tingling, visual disturbances, seizures) ■ CI: WPW, Adam Stokes syndrome, heart block without pacer ■ DDI: Amiodarone can increase lidocaine levels
		Mexiletine	VT maintenance: 200–300 mg PO q8h (max of 1,200 mg/day)	Caps: 150 mg, 200 mg, 250 mg	Peak: 2–3 hr $t_{1/2}$: 10–14 hr (↑ in hepatic disease or HF)	■ When converting from other antiarrhythmic, take 1st dose 6–12 hr after DC of other agent (or 3–6 hr after DC of procainamide) ■ SE: lightheadedness, dizziness, ataxia, hypotension, N/V, hepatotoxicity, QT prolongation ■ CI: 2nd or 3rd degree heart block without pacer, cardiogenic shock ■ Caution: may exacerbate HF, correct K^+ and Mg^{2+} abnormalities prior to use
IC		Flecainide	VT conversion: 100 mg PO q 12 hr, can titrate by 50–100 mg/day every 4 days (max 400 mg/day) PSVT: 50 mg PO q 12 hr, can titrate by 50 mg BID every 4 days (max 300 mg/day) Paroxysmal AF: 200 mg PO once (<70 kg) or 300 mg PO once (≥70 kg); do not repeat dose within 24 hr ["Pill in Pocket" dose]	Tabs: 50 mg, 100 mg, 150 mg	Onset: rapid Peak: 1.5–3 hr $t_{1/2}$: 7–22 hr (prolonged in HF or renal dysfunction)	■ Patient must be on an AV nodal blocker prior to initiating ■ SE: prolonged QT, dizziness, visual disturbance, dyspnea ■ CI: 2nd or 3rd degree heart block, RBBB, cardiogenic shock, CAD/MI ■ Caution: may exacerbate HF, correct electrolyte imbalances prior to use, SSS ■ DDI: Digoxin concentrations may ↑ by 24%

	Drug	Dosing	Formulations	Pharmacokinetics	Notes
	Propafenone	AF conversion: 600 mg IR PO once Paroxysmal AF, PSVT, VT: 150 mg IR PO q 8 hr, can ↑q3–4 days to 225 mg q8h (max 300 mg q8h) Secondary AF prevention: 225 mg ER PO q 12 hr, can ↑q5 days to 325 mg q 12 hr (max of 425 mg q 12 hr)	Tabs: IR: 150 mg, 225 mg, 300 mg SR: 225 mg, 325 mg, 425 mg	Onset for AF conversion dose: 2–6 hr Peak: 3.5 hr (IR), 3–8 hr (ER) $t_{1/2}$: 2–32 hr	■ Must give with AV nodal blocker prior to initiating ■ SE: agranulocytosis, drug-induced lupus-like syndrome, QT prolongation ■ CI: HF (mortality risk, precipitates exacerbation), CAD/MI, SA or AV conduction disorder, cardiogenic shock, severe hypotension, electrolyte abnormalities, severe COPD or bronchospastic disorder, sinus bradycardia, Brugada syndrome ■ Caution: MG (condition may be exacerbated) ■ DDI: Digoxin concentrations can ↑by 30%–100% due to decreased renal elimination, warfarin concentrations ↑
Ⅱ	Beta blockers				
	Acebutolol	Ventricular arrhythmia maintenance: 200 mg PO BID, can increase 600–1,200 mg/day; max of 1,200 mg/day	Caps: 200 mg, 400 mg	Onset: 1–2 hr Peak: 2–4 hr DOA: 12–24 hr $t_{1/2}$: 3–4 hr (parent), 8–13 hr (metabolite)	■ Renally adjust dose for CrCl <50 mL/min ■ Possess intrinsic sympathetic activity (ISA) in addition to its beta blocking properties ■ SE: Hypotension, severe bradycardia, fatigue, headache, dizziness ■ CI: Cardiogenic shock, severe bradycardia, 2nd or 3rd degree heart block without pacer ■ Caution: SSS, bronchospastic disease, HF (this agent's ISA activity may increase mortality), hyperthyroidism (abrupt DC can precipitate thyroid storm), pheochromocytoma without adequate alpha-1 blocker ■ DDI: CCB and digoxin–use of either agent with acebutolol can cause heart block or bradycardia
	Esmolol	AF rate control: 0.5 mg/kg LD IVP over 1 min + cont. infusion: 50 mcg/kg/min. Can repeat bolus & ↑ infusion by 50 mcg/kg/min q 4 min (max dose of 300 mcg/kg/min SVT: 0.5 mg/kg LD IVP over 1 min + cont. infusion: 50 mcg/kg/min, can ↑q 4 min by 50 mcg/kg/min (max 200 mcg/kg/min)	Inj: 100 mg/10 mL Premixed IV solution: 2,500 mg/250 mL, 2,000 mg/100 mL	Onset: 1 min DOA: 10–20 min $t_{1/2}$: 9 min	■ Abrupt DC can cause tachycardia, exacerbating angina or precipitate a MI ■ SE: Hypotension, severe bradycardia, injection site reaction, ↑K⁺ ■ CI: ADHF, SSS, 2nd or 3rd degree heart block without pacer, cardiogenic shock, pulmonary HTN ■ Caution: bronchospastic disease, hyperthyroidism (abrupt DC can precipitate thyroid storm), pheochromocytoma without adequate alpha-1 blocker ■ DDI: CCB can cause heart block or bradycardia

(continued)

TABLE 34.1 Antiarrhythmic Medications (continued)

Class	Class Mechanism	Drugs	Indication and Dose	Dose and Formulations Available	Pharmacokinetics	Clinical Considerations
		Metoprolol	AF rate control, SVT: 2.5–5 mg IVP q2–5 min (max of 15 mg in 10–15 min period) Maintenance: 25–100 mg PO BID	Tabs: IR: 25 mg, 50 mg, 100 mg; ER: 25 mg, 50 mg, 100 mg, 200 mg Inj: 1 mg/mL	Onset: 20 min (IV) DOA: 5–8 hr (IV) $t_{\frac{1}{2}}$: 3–4 hr (IV)	▪ Oral to IV conversion is a 2.5:1 ratio ▪ SE, CI, and cautions similar to esmolol
		Propranolol	Tachyarrhythmias: 1–3 mg/dose slow IVP q 2–5 min, total of 5 mg Maintenance: 10–30 mg PO (IR formulation) q 6–8 hr	Tabs: IR: 10 mg, 20 mg, 40 mg, 60 mg, 80 mg Caps: ER: 60 mg, 80 mg, 120 mg, 160 mg PO solution: 20 mg/5mL, 40 mg/5 mL Inj: 1 mg/mL	Onset: 1–2 hr (PO) Peak: 1–4 hr (PO, IR formulation) $t_{\frac{1}{2}}$: 3–6 hr (PO, IR)	▪ SE, CI, and cautions similar to esmolol
III	Potassium channel blockers	Amiodarone	AF conversion: 5–7 mg/kg IV over 30–60 min then 1.2–1.8 gm daily until 10 gm load; 1.2–1.8 gm/day PO in divided doses until 10 gm total load AF maintenance: 200–400 mg/day PO VF/pulseless VT conversion: 300 mg IVP, can repeat in 3–5 min with 150 mg bolus (max daily dose: 2.2 gm) VF/VT maintenance: 1 mg/min×6 hr then 0.5 mg/min×18 hr	Tabs: 100 mg, 200 mg, 400 mg Inj: 50 mg/mL, 150 mg/100 mL, 360 mg/200 mL Prefilled syringe: 150 mg/3 mL (must be diluted prior to use)	Onset: 2 days–3 weeks (PO) Peak: 1 week–5 months (IV & PO) DOA: 7–50 days after DC (IV & PO) $t_{\frac{1}{2}}$: 40–55 days	▪ Possesses beta-blocking properties ▪ SE: pulmonary fibrosis, blue/gray skin discoloration, hyper- or hypo-thyroidism, N/V, constipation, vision changes from corneal deposits, neurotoxicity, heart block, hypotension, hepatitis, proarrhythmic ▪ CI: 2nd or 3rd degree heart block, cardiogenic shock, bradycardia ▪ Caution: hepatic impairment, thyroid disease, electrolyte abnormalities ▪ DDI: numerous, including phenytoin, lidocaine, simvastatin, warfarin, digoxin. Must check for DDIs before initating ▪ Obtain baseline pulmonary, liver and thyroid function tests prior to initiation

Drug	Dosing	Formulation	PK	Notes
Dofetilide	AF conversion and maintenance: 500 mcg PO BID Check QTc 2–3 hr post-1st dose, if QTc >15% baseline or >500 msec, 50% dose reduction If post-2nd dose QTc >500 msec, must DC drug	Caps: 0.125 mg, 0.25 mg, 0.5 mg	Peak: 2–3 hr $t_{1/2}$: 10 hr	■ Renally adjust dose for CrCl <60 mL/min ■ Patients and providers must be enrolled in T.I.P.S, the dofetilide REMS program ■ SE: headache, dizziness, VT, TdP (especially during initial 3 days of therapy, HF patients, or in recent MI) ■ CI: QTc >440 msec, long QT syndrome, CrCl <20 mL/min ■ Caution: SSS, 2nd or 3rd degree heart block, electrolyte abnormalities must be corrected, hepatic, and renal impairment ■ DDI: verapamil, hydrochlorthiazide, and numerous other agents, check DDIs prior to use ■ Agent initiated in hospital setting with continuous EKG monitoring
Dronedarone	AF maintenance: 400 mg PO BID	Tabs: 400 mg	Peak: 3–6 hr. $t_{1/2}$: 13–19 hr	■ Analog of amiodarone without iodine groups ■ Less effective in preventing recurrent AF than amiodarone in persistent AF patients (DIONYSOS trial) but better tolerated than amiodarone (ATHENA trial) ■ SE: hepatotoxicity, ↑SCr (in 5–7 days after initiation), rash, N/V, diarrhea ■ CI: permanent AF (↑mortality found in PALLAS trial), HF or LVEF <35% (↑mortality and new or worsened symptoms in ANDROMEDA trial), 2nd or 3rd degree heart block, HR <50 bpm, QTc ≥500 msec or PR >280 msec, sever hepatic impairment ■ Caution: hepatic insufficiency, QT prolongation ■ DDI: multiple agents, including drugs that prolong QT
Ibutilide	AF conversion: 0.01 mg/kg over 10 min (<60 kg), 1 mg over 10 min ≥60 kg	Inj: 1 mg/10 mL	Onset: 90 min $t_{1/2}$: 2–12 hr	■ Do not use in chronic AF, does not maintain NSR ■ SE: nonsustained and sustained VT, SVT, hypotension, BBB, TdP, bradycardia, fatal proarrhythmic events ■ CI: QTc >440 msec

(continued)

TABLE 34.1 Antiarrhythmic Medications (continued)

Class	Class Mechanism	Drugs	Indication and Dose	Dose and Formulations Available	Pharmacokinetics	Clinical Considerations
		Sotalol	AF/VT maintenance: 80 mg PO BID, increase q3 days if no QTc prolongation to 120 mg BID and then to 160 mg BID for AF; in VT can increase to 240–320 mg/day in q3day increments Stable monomorphic VT (ACLS protocol): 1.5 mg/kg IV over 5 min	Inj: 150 mg/10 mL Tabs: 80 mg, 120 mg, 160 mg, 240 mg	Onset: 5–10 min (IV), 1–2 hr (PO) Peak: 2.5–4 hr (PO) $t_{1/2}$: 12 hr	■ Possesses beta-blocking properties ■ SE: bradycardia, chest pain, palpitations, fatigue, dizziness, lightheadedness ■ CI: QTc >450 msec, K^+ <4 mEq/L, CrCl <40 mL/min, SSS, bronchospastic disease, cardiogenic shock, uncontrolled HF, 2nd or 3rd degree heart block, long QT syndrome, sinus bradycardia ■ Agent initiated in hospital setting with continuous EKG monitoring
IV	Calcium channel blockers	Diltiazem	AF rate control, PSVT: 0.25 mg/kg IV bolus over 2 min, can repeat in 15 min at 0.35 mg/kg over 2 min Maintenance rate: 5–15 mg/hr IV cont. infusion; or 120 mg–480 mg PO TDD IV drip to PO conversion: PO TDD (mg daily) = (infusion rate (in mg/hr) × 3 + 3) × 10 (i.e. 5 mg/hr rate = 180 mg PO TDD)	Inj: 5 mg/mL Tabs: IR 30 mg, 60 mg, 90 mg, 120 mg Caps: 12-hr ER: 60 mg, 90 mg, 120 mg Caps: 24-hr CD, XR, XT, LA: 120 mg, 180 mg, 240 mg, 300 mg, 360 mg, 420 mg	Onset: 3 min (IV) 30–60 min (PO, IR formulation) DOA 1–10 hr (IV, range includes bolus and after cont infusion is DC) $t_{1/2}$: 3.4–5 hr (IV & PO)	■ SE: bradycardia, edema, headache, hypotension ■ CI: LVEF <40% (increased cardiac death), SSS, SBP <90 mmHg or cardiogenic shock, WPW, VT, 2nd or 3rd degree heart block ■ DDI: Concurrent use of beta blockers and CCBs increase risk of bradycardia; both drug classes block the AV node
		Verapamil	SVT: 2.5–5 mg IV over 2 min, can repeat in 15–30 min with 5–10 mg (0.15 mg/kg), max total dose of 20–30 mg AF rate control, PSVT prophylaxis: 240 mg–480 mg PO divided in 3–4 doses	Inj 2.5 mg/mL Tabs: IR: 40 mg, 80 mg, 120 mg; ER: 120 mg, 180 mg, 240 mg Caps: ER: 100 mg, 120 mg, 180 mg, 200 mg, 240 mg, 300 mg, 360 mg	Onset: 1–5 min (IV) DOA: 10–20 min (IV) $t_{1/2}$: 3–7 hr	■ SE: severe constipation, headache, gingival hyperplasia, peripheral edema, pulmonary edema, bradycardia, dizziness, fatigue, dyspepsia ■ CI: same as for diltiazem

Class	Drug	Dosing	Formulation	Kinetics	Notes
Other	Na⁺-K⁺ ATPase inhibitor; cardiac glycoside	Digoxin	AF rate control: 0.25 mg IV LD q 2 hr up to 1.5 mg/24 hr period AF maintenance of 0.125–0.375 mg IV/PO once daily SVT: 0.5–1 mg IV; give 1/2 TDD as initial load, then 1/4 TDD q 6 hr SVT maintenance: 0.125–0.5 mg PO daily or 0.1–0.4 mg IV daily	Tabs/caps: 125 mcg, 250 mcg Inj: 0.25 mg/mL	Onset: 5–60 min (IV) Peak 1–6 hr (IV) $t_{1/2}$: 36–48 hr	▪ Renally adjust for CrCl ≤50 mL/min ▪ ↓K⁺ increases risk of digoxin toxicity as there is less K⁺ to compete with digoxin for binding-site ▪ Works on resting heart as digoxin is drawn into skeletal muscles during exercise ▪ SE: proarrhythmic, heart block, visual disturbances, N/V, hallucinations, confusion, dizziness ▪ CI: VF, acute MI, 2nd or 3rd degree heart block ▪ Caution: WPW, K⁺ and Ca²⁺, HF (mortality when trough >0.9 ng/mL) ▪ Digoxin trough goal 0.5–2 ng/mL for AF (rate control typically requires higher doses for AF than in HF), if patient has concurrent HF, target trough of 0.5–0.9 ng/mL
	Transient AV nodal blocker	Adenosine	PSVT: 1st dose: 6 mg IVP over 1–3 sec 2nd dose: Give 1–2 min after 1st dose if rhythm ongoing; 12 mg IVP 3rd dose: May repeat 1–2 min after 2nd dose; 12 mg IVP Follow all doses by 20 mL saline flush	Inj: 2 mg/mL, 6 mg/2mL	Onset: rapid DOA: extremely brief $t_{1/2}$: <10 sec	▪ Dose reduce initial dose only to 3 mg if concurrently on carbamazepine or dipyridamole ▪ SE: flushing, chest pain/tightness, bradycardia, brief asystole ▪ CI: 2nd or 3rd degree heart block ▪ Safe for use in pregnancy

↑, increase; ↓, decrease; ACLS, adult cardiac life support; ADHF, acute decompensated heart failure; AF, atrial fibrillation; AV, atrioventricular; BBB, bundle branch block; BID, twice daily; Ca²⁺, serum calcium; CAD, coronary artery disease; Caps, capsules; CCB, calcium channel blocker; CD, XT, LA, long acting; CI, contraindicated; CNS, central nervous system; COPD, chronic obstructive pulmonary disease; CR, controlled release; CrCl, creatinine clearance; DC, discontinue or discontinuation; DDI, drug–drug interaction; DOA, duration of action; ER, extended release; ET, endotracheal route; HF, heart failure; HTN, hypertension; inj, injection; IO, intraosseous; IR, immediate release; IV, intravenous; IVP, intravenous push; K⁺, serum potassium; LD, loading dose; LVEF, left ventricular ejection fraction; MG, myasthenia gravis; Mg²⁺, serum magnesium; MI, myocardial infarction; NAPA, N-acetylprocainamide; N/V, nausea/vomiting; NS, normal saline; NSR, normal sinus rhythm; PO, by mouth or orally; PSVT, paroxysmal supraventricular tachycardia; q, every; QTc, corrected QT; RBBB, right bundle branch block; REMS, risk evaluation and mitigation strategy; SA, sinoatrial; SCr, serum creatinine; SE, side effect; SR, sustained release; SSS, sick sinus syndrome; SVT, supraventricular tachycardia; SWFI, sterile water for injection; Tabs, tablets; TDD, total daily dose; TdP, torsades de pointes; T.I.P.S., Tikosyn In Pharmacy System; $t_{1/2}$, half-life; TTP, thrombocytopenia purpura; G6PD, glucose-6-phosphate dehydrogenase; VF, ventricular fibrillation; VT, ventricular tachycardia; WPW, Wolff-Parkinson-White; XR, extended release.

Sources: DIONYSOS study (Le Heuzey et al., 2010); ATHENA trial (Hohnloser et al., 2009); PALLAS trial (Connolly et al., 2011); ANDROMEDA study (Kober et al., 2008); Campbell and Williams (1998); Yancy et al. (2013).

Pharmacotherapeutics of Cardiac Emergencies

CONNIE H. YOON

CARDIAC ARREST AND ADVANCED CARDIAC LIFE SUPPORT

Cardiac arrest is a significant public health concern with an estimated annual incidence of over 400,000 in 2014 (Go et al., 2014). Sympathomimetic agents are the most widely studied agents for the treatment of cardiac arrest. Epinephrine and vasopressin, along with antiarrhythmic drugs discussed earlier in Section VII, are the primary medications used in the management of cardiac arrest. This chapter highlights select pharmacologic treatment algorithms and recommendations from the 2010 American Heart Association Guidelines for Advanced Cardiac Life Support (ACLS; Neumar et al., 2010). Interventions related to medication management of cardiac emergencies are the focus of this section. Note that the dosing recommendations for vasopressors and inotropes in the setting of ACLS may vary from doses used for shock states.

Epinephrine, an alpha and beta receptor agonist, has been the vasopressor of choice for the management of cardiac arrest. Administration of epinephrine causes vasoconstriction of the peripheral vasculature while also increasing cardiac contractility. When compared with placebo, epinephrine improved the likelihood of achieving return of spontaneous circulation (ROSC) during out-of-hospital cardiac arrest (Jacobs, Finn, Jelinek, Oxer, & Thompson, 2011). However, there was no difference in survival to hospital discharge between placebo and epinephrine. Epinephrine was also compared with norepinephrine in the setting of out-of-hospital cardiac arrest, but norepinephrine was not associated with improved outcomes (Callaham, Madsen, Barton, Saunders, & Pointer, 1992). Similarly, a lack of efficacy was found with phenylephrine in animal models when compared with epinephrine for cerebral blood flow (Brown, Werman, Davis, Katz, & Hamlin, 1987).

Vasopressin, an endogenous antidiuretic hormone, also causes peripheral vasoconstriction but dilates cerebral blood vessels. Its role in cardiac arrest was evaluated in several studies. Vasopressin administered concurrently with epinephrine resulted in no improvement in survival to hospital admission or ROSC (Callaway et al., 2006; Gueugniaud et al., 2008). However, when vasopressin is administered after epinephrine, rates and ROSC were significantly higher in patients with asystole but not in patients with ventricular fibrillation (VF) or pulseless electrical activity (PEA) (Wenzel et al., 2004).

VF/PULSELESS VENTRICULAR TACHYCARDIA (VT)

For VF or VT, initiate cardiopulmonary resuscitation (CPR) and direct current cardioversion (DCC) as appropriate. After 2 minutes of CPR and the delivery of at least one shock, a vasopressor such as epinephrine or vasopressin may be administered in an effort to increase blood flow to the heart (Table 35.1). Epinephrine should be administered every 3 to 5 minutes. Vasopressin may be administered one time in place of the first or second dose of epinephrine. Epinephrine and vasopressin are the only two vasopressors for ACLS, as there are no survival benefits with norepinephrine and phenylephrine compared with epinephrine. Amiodarone is the antiarrhythmic drug of choice in refractory VF and pulseless VT. Amiodarone may be administered if the patient is unresponsive to the initial interventions described above. Amiodarone has been clinically proven to increase rates of ROSC compared with placebo or lidocaine, which is considered a second-line agent. Finally, magnesium sulfate, 1 to 2 grams, may be administered in patients with prolonged QT interval and torsades de pointes (TdP). The reversible causes of rhythm abnormalities should be identified and addressed.

ASYSTOLE OR PULSELESS ELECTRICAL ACTIVITY

For asystole or PEA, initiate CPR for 2 minutes, as asystole and PEA are nonshockable rhythms and DCC is not indicated. A vasopressor, such as epinephrine or vasopressin, should be administered in an effort to increase blood flow to the heart and brain (Table 35.1). Epinephrine should be administered every 3 to 5 minutes if the patient continues in asystole or PEA. Vasopressin may be administered one time in place of the first or second dose of epinephrine. Reversible causes of the abnormal rhythm should be identified and treatment to address the underlying etiology instituted.

SYMPTOMATIC BRADYCARDIA

For symptomatic bradycardia, identify the underlying cause of symptomatic bradycardia. If patient is unstable, as indicated by hypotension, altered mental status, ischemic chest discomfort, acute heart failure (HF), or signs of shock, administer atropine. Atropine (Table 35.1) is considered the drug of choice for symptomatic and unstable bradycardia. Atropine is clinically proven to improve signs and symptoms associated with symptomatic bradycardia; however, due to its short duration of action, it is only considered a temporary intervention. Transcutaneous pacing or administration of dopamine or epinephrine infusion should be initiated if atropine does not provide the desired heart-rate effect.

TABLE 35.1 Select Advanced Cardiac Life Support (ACLS) Medications

Agent	Dosing for ACLS	Considerations	Available Formulations
Adenosine	■ 1st dose: 6 mg rapid IVP, over 1–3 sec; followed by 20 mL saline flush; dose reduce to 3 mg if on carbamazepine or dipyridamole ■ 2nd dose: Administer 1–2 mins after first dose if rhythm continues; 12 mg IVP followed by rapid 20 mL saline flush ■ 3rd dose: may repeat 12 mg in 1–2 mins after second dose	■ Indications: stable, narrow complex PSVT; regular wide complex tachycardia (i.e., SVT with aberrancy) ■ AE: flushing, chest pain/tightness, bradycardia, brief asystole ■ CI: second- or third-degree heart block ■ Safe for use in pregnancy	■ IV vial (preservative and PF): 3 mg/mL, 6 mg/2 mL, 12 mg/4 mL
Atropine	■ 0.5 mg IV every 3–5 mins ■ Max total dose of 3 mg or 0.4 mg/kg	■ Indication: Acute symptomatic bradycardia ■ Doses <0.5 mg may paradoxically slow HR ■ Use with caution in setting of ACS or myocardial ischemia; may worsen ischemia or infarct ■ Caution with glaucoma ■ May be ineffective in heart transplant patients	■ IV vial: 0.4 mg/mL, 0.8 mg/mL, 1 mg/mL ■ Prefilled syringe: 1 mg/10 mL
Epinephrine	■ 1 mg IV/IO every 3–5 mins followed by 20 mL flush ■ 2–2.5 mg diluted in 10 mL NS via ET route	■ Indications: VF or pulseless VT; asystole or PEA ■ 1 mg is equivalent to 10 mL of 1:10,000 solution ■ Increases BP, HR, and myocardial O₂ demand; may cause myocardial ischemia or angina	■ IV vial: 1 mg/mL, 1 mg/10 mL ■ Prefilled syringe: 1 mg/10 mL
Magnesium sulfate	■ 1–2 gm diluted in 10 mL D₅W IV/IO, infuse over 5–20 mins	■ Indications TdP (polymorphic VT with prolonged QT interval); ventricular arrhythmias secondary to hypomagnesemia ■ Rapid administration associated with hypotension ■ Use with caution in patients with renal failure	■ IV vial: 1 gm/2 mL, 5 gm/10 mL, 10 gm/20 mL, 25 gm/50 mL ■ IV bags: 1 gm/100 mL, 2 gm/50 mL, 4 gm/50 mL, 4 gm/100 mL, 10 gm/500 mL, 20 gm/500 mL, 40 gm/1,000 mL
Vasopressin	■ 40 units IV/IO once	■ Indications: VF or pulseless VT ■ Alternative to 1st or 2nd dose of epinephrine ■ May cause myocardial ischemia or angina due to potent vasoconstrictive properties	■ IV vial: 20 units/mL

ACS, acute coronary syndromes; AE: adverse events; BP, blood pressure; CI, contraindication; D₅W, 5% dextrose; ET, endotracheal route; HR, heart rate; IO, intraosseous; IV, intravenous; IVP, intravenous push; NS, normal saline; O₂, oxygen; PEA, pulseless electrical activity; PF, preservative free; PSVT, paroxysmal supraventricular tachycardia; SVT, supraventricular tachycardia; TdP, torsades de pointes; VF, ventricular fibrillation; VT, ventricular tachycardia.

SYMPTOMATIC TACHYCARDIA

For symptomatic tachycardia, evaluate the patient to ascertain the underlying rhythm and to identify the underlying cause of the tachycardia. If the patient is unstable, administer synchronized cardioversion. In stable patients, determine whether the QRS complex is wide (> 120 milliseconds) or narrow. A wide-QRS-complex tachycardia may indicate VT, VF, supraventricular tachycardia (SVT) with aberrancy, preexcited tachycardias (i.e., Wolff–Parkinson–White syndrome) or ventricular-paced rhythms. A narrow-complex SVT may be caused by the following rhythms: sinus tachycardia, atrial fibrillation (AF), atrial flutter, AV nodal reentry, accessory pathway-mediated tachycardia, atrial tachycardia, multifocal atrial tachycardia, or junctional tachycardia.

A regular wide-complex tachycardia is most likely to be VT or SVT with aberrancy. Adenosine may be administered in this setting. If the rhythm is SVT with aberrancy, adenosine will either slow down or convert the patient into sinus rhythm. If the patient does not respond to the first dose of adenosine, a second and third bolus may be administered. Adenosine will have minimal impact on VT. For patients with monomorphic VT, administer DCC or an intravenous (IV) antiarrhythmic agent, such as amiodarone, procainamide, or sotalol. Refer to Chapter 34 for additional details regarding antiarrhythmic agents. Lidocaine may be considered; however, it is less successful in terminating VT compared with the other three agents.

Polymorphic or irregular VT should be managed as outlined for the management of VF. These patients require rapid defibrillation. TdP is a polymorphic VT associated with a long QT interval. Magnesium is an appropriate agent for the treatment of TdP. The arrhythmia may also be managed with pacing and/or beta blocker therapy. A polymorphic VT without QT prolongation is commonly due to myocardial ischemia, and the administration of amiodarone or beta blockers are appropriate pharmacologic agents in this setting.

An irregular wide-complex or irregular narrow-complex tachycardia is often AF. Hemodynamically unstable patients should receive DCC in an effort to convert to normal sinus rhythm. In patients who are stable, therapeutic interventions focus on controlling the rapid heart rate with either IV beta blockers or nondihydropyridine calcium channel blockers. Digoxin or amiodarone are preferred in patients with HF. Special consideration of medication selection is indicated for patients with AF greater than 48 hours, as the risk of thrombosis increases with prolonged AF. Amiodarone may convert AF to a normal sinus rhythm, which places the patient at risk for cardioembolic clots. Additional medications for the management of AF are listed in the antiarrhythmia section.

The most common narrow-complex tachycardia is sinus tachycardia. Often, no drug therapy is required and treatment should be targeted toward the underlying cause. Reentry SVTs typically have an abrupt onset and offset, also known as paroxysmal supraventricular tachycardia (PSVT). PSVT may be terminated using vagal maneuvers or adenosine. If the rhythm does not convert despite both interventions, a second dose of adenosine should be administered. Amiodarone may be helpful in terminating PSVT, although this agent has a longer onset of action compared with adenosine. Recurrent PSVT may be managed with adenosine or other AV nodal blocking agents, including nondihydropyridine calcium channel blockers or beta blockers, which have longer durations of action allowing for continued

TABLE 35.2 Inotropes and Vasopressors

Agent	Target Receptors and Mechanism of Action	Hemodynamic Effects	Infusion Rate	Pharmacokinetics	Monitoring	Adverse Effects	Considerations
INOTROPES							
Dobutamine	Strong beta1 agonist: ↑contractility and HR Mild beta 2 agonist: causes muscle relaxation and peripheral vasodilation Minimal alpha-1 effects	■ ↓SVR (afterload) ■ ↓preload & afterload ■ ↑CI & CO (increases tissue perfusion due to vasodilatory effects) ■ ↔ MAP	2.5–20 mcg/kg/min [2–10 mcg/kg/min = targets beta 1] [10–20 mcg/kg/min = also targets beta 2]	Onset: 1–10 min Peak: 10–20 mins $t_{1/2}$: 2 mins (hepatic elimination)	CI HR	■ Tachycardia ■ Tachyarrhythmias ■ ↓K+ ■ Myocardial ischemia	■ First line in shock when CI or CO is low ■ May be add-on therapy to vasopressors ■ Indicated in cardiogenic shock/myocardial dysfunction or ADHF ■ Counteracts effects of beta blockers ■ Tolerance develops due to down regulation of beta receptors ■ Easier to titrate than milrinone ■ Positive inotropic and chronotropic effects
Milrinone	PDE3-inhibitor: ↑intracellular cAMP, activating cardiac calcium channels and ↑myocardial contractility; also relaxes vascular smooth muscle	■ ↑CO via ↓SVR and ↓PVR ■ ↑SV & CI ■ ↓right atrial, pulmonary venous and pulmonary arterial pressure secondary to venodilation	50 mcg/kg LD over 10 minutes, then maintenance infusion of rate of 0.375–0.75 mcg/kg/min	Onset: 5–15 min $t_{1/2}$: 2.5 hr 80% renally eliminated; $t_{1/2}$ may be longer in renal failure	BP HR Fluids Electrolytes Renal function	■ Hypotension due to vasodilation ■ Arrhythmias ■ Vasodilation effects may lead to reflex tachycardia (rare)	■ Indicated in cardiogenic shock of ADHF due to poor CO and no response to dobutamine or epinephrine ■ Drug of choice in right-sided HF; RV dysfunction due to pulmonary vascular resistance (i.e., PAH, LVAD patients whose right heart starts to fail) ■ Can use in HF patients concurrently on beta blockers ■ Harder to titrate than dobutamine ■ Less dysrhythmias than dobutamine ■ Must use lower doses in renal failure ■ Slow onset and long half-life ■ Synergistic effect on ventricular perfusion ■ Positive inotrope only, does not have chronotropic effects
Isoproterenol	Targets beta receptors only. No effects on alpha receptors beta 1: ↑contractility & HR → ↑CI beta 2: ↓PVR	■ ↑HR & contractility ■ ↑CI ■ ↓DBP	2–10 mcg/min	Onset: immediate DOA: 10–15 mins $t_{1/2}$: 2.5–5 mins Renal elimination	BP HR Electrolytes RR	■ Hyper- or hypo-tension ■ Tachyarrhythmias ■ ↓K+ ■ Pulmonary edema	■ Indicated for bradycardia or heart block ■ Dose-dependent vasodilation may occur from unopposed beta 2 agonism

(continued)

TABLE 35.2 Inotropes and Vasopressors (continued)

Agent	Target Receptors and Mechanism of Action	Hemodynamic Effects	Infusion Rate	Pharmacokinetics	Monitoring	Adverse Effects	Considerations
VASOPRESSORS							
Norepinephrine	alpha 1 effects > alpha 2 > beta 1 Primarily alpha agonism: vasoconstricts arterioles → ↑SVR & BP Some beta 1: ↑SV and contractility	■ ↑↑SVR & BP ■ ↔CO	0.01–3 mcg/kg/min For infusion rates >30 mcg/min, add a second vasopressor	Onset: immediate DOA: 1–2 mins Elimination: renal	■ MAP ■ SVR ■ Signs of organ damage (↓UOP, cold extremities) ■ Serum lactate	■ Tissue necrosis due to severe peripheral vaso-constriction ■ Worsening ventricular function from ↑afterload ■ Metabolic acidosis ■ Tachyarrhythmias ■ Renal ischemia due to ↓hepato-splanchnic perfusion ■ Extravasation	■ First line in septic or cardiogenic shock; indicated for low BP and SVR ■ Powerful vasoconstrictor w/inotropic effects ■ Administer via central line due to extravasation risk (can treat with diluted phentolamine 5–10 mg IV) ■ Preferred over dopamine due to increased side effects and dysrhythmias with dopamine ■ NE potency is greater than dopamine
Epinephrine	Potent beta 1: inotrope & chronotrope effects → ↑CO Moderate beta 2 & alpha 1, effects dose dependent Doses <2 mcg/kg/min beta 2 agonism > alpha 1 → mild peripheral vasodilation, ↑CO, ↓SVR, effects on MAP variable Doses >2 mcg/kg/min: alpha 1 agonism > beta 2 → ↑SVR and BP	■ ↑CO ■ ↓SVR ■ ↑MAP, HR	0.1–5 mcg/kg/min Rates <0.05 mcg/kg/min has inotropic effects only, not in dose range for vasopressor effects	Onset: rapid Elimination: renal	■ MAP ■ HR ■ Glucose ■ Signs of organ damage (↓UOP, SCr) ■ Lactate	■ Dysrhythmias ■ Myocardial ischemia due to an ↑ in myocardial O₂ demand ■ Splanchnic vasoconstriction leading to gut ischemia ■ Metabolic ketoacidosis ■ Lactic acidosis ■ Hyperglycemia ■ Digital necrosis ■ Extravasation	■ Second line for cardiogenic shock; use when refractory to other vasopressors ■ Also indicated for anaphylactic shock ■ Administer via central line due to extravasation risk (can treat with diluted phentolamine 5–10 mg IV) ■ Promotes peripheral vascular resistance ■ Preferred in HF patients

Drug	Mechanism	Hemodynamic Effects	Dose	Pharmacokinetics	Monitoring	Adverse Effects	Clinical Pearls
Vasopressin	Antidiuretic hormone; Targets V2 receptors in renal tubules to ↑free water reabsorption → ↑BP Targets V1a receptors in vascular tissue causing arterial vasoconstriction → ↑SVR Proposed vasoconstriction of efferent arterioles of nephrons → ↑GFR	■ ↑SVR ■ ↑SBP ■ ↑MAP ■ ↔HR,CI	0.03–0.04 units/min Max rate: 0.06 units/min	Onset: rapid $t_{1/2}$ = 10–20 mins Elimination: renal	■ BP ■ HR ■ Input/output volumes	■ MI ■ Negative changes in CI ■ Ischemia (ischemic skin lesions due to ↓tissue perfusion) ■ Hyponatremia from ↑ADH & water reabsorption	■ Indicated for refractory vasodilatory hypotension (i.e., septic shock) as add-on therapy to adrenergic agents. Thought to reduce catecholamine agent dose due to relative vasopressin deficiency in septic shock ■ No titration required, use a high dose and wean off ■ Once adrenergic agent has been discontinued, must slowly taper off by 0.01 units/min every 30 min to prevent hypotension with withdrawal of vasopressin ■ Useful in acidotic states due to vasoconstrictive actions which are not dependent on adrenergic receptors ■ Infusion rates >0.04 units/min associated with coronary vasoconstriction and peripheral necrosis ■ Vasopressin adjunct therapy does not decrease mortality when compared to NE
Phenylephrine	Pure alpha 1 agonist: peripheral vasoconstriction, ↑afterload	■ ↑MAF ■ ↑SVR ■ May ↓HR	100–500 mcg/dose bolus every 10–15 min or IV infusion of 0.5–8 mcg/kg/min	Onset: immediate DOA: 15–20 mins $t_{1/2}$: 5 mins	■ MAP ■ SVR ■ Signs of end-organ damage (↓UOP, cold extremities)	■ Reflex bradycardia due to rapid ↑ in SBP and DBP ■ Severe peripheral & visceral vasoconstriction ■ Pallor ■ Tissue necrosis ■ Extravasation	■ Generally not recommended in septic shock, but may be used in patients with arrhythmias from NE use, high CO and low BP, salvage therapy if failed inotrope & vasopressor combination ■ ↓Renal perfusion ■ Caution in patients with narrow angle glaucoma ■ Administer via central line due to extravasation risk (can treat with phentolamine)

(continued)

TABLE 35.2 Inotropes and Vasopressors (continued)

Agent	Target Receptors and Mechanism of Action	Hemodynamic Effects	Infusion Rate	Pharmacokinetics	Monitoring	Adverse Effects	Considerations
Dopamine	Precursor to NE and epinephrine → dose dependent stimulation of adrenergic receptors Induce NE release → alpha stimulation → vasoconstriction Dopamine itself is an indirect vasopressor	Dopamine (D) receptor agonism: vasodilation at splanchnic, renal, & coronary vascular beds beta 1 agonism: ↑inotropy & HR alpha 1 & beta 1 agonism: ↑HR, ↑BP, vasoconstriction and afterload; ↑MAP, HR & CO	Rate <5 mcg/kg/min targets D-receptor Rate of 5–10 mcg/kg/min targets beta1 Rate >10 mcg/kg/min targets alpha 1 & beta 1 Titrate by 1–4 mcg/kg/min every 10–30 min; max of 50 mcg/kg/min	Onset: 5 mins DOA: <10 mins $t_{\frac{1}{2}}$: 2 min	▪ MAP ▪ HR ▪ CI ▪ UOP	▪ May impair hepatosplanchnic metabolism ▪ Tachyarrhythmias ▪ ↑venous & arterial pressure → ↑preload & afterload → ischemia ▪ Hypoxemia/ARDS ▪ Extravasation	▪ Indicated for septic and cardiogenic shock when low CO states when SVR is low and BP is marginal ▪ Use only as alternative to NE in patients at low risk for bradycardia or tachyarrhythmias ▪ If infusion rate is >20–30 mcg/kg/min, consider using NE or epinephrine (direct acting vasopressors) ▪ May improve renal perfusion when used with fenoldopam ▪ Should not be used for renal protection; renal dose has not been shown to have benefit ▪ Improvement of cardiac function and effects on renal blood flow ↓ at higher doses ▪ Prolonged infusions can ↓endogenous NE stores and ↓vasopressor response

↑, increase; ↓, decrease; →, leading to; ↔, neutral effect; ADH, antidiuretic hormone; ADHF, acute decompensated heart failure; ARDS, acute respiratory distress syndrome; BP, blood pressure; cAMP, cyclic adenosine monophosphate; CI, cardiac index; CO, cardiac output; DBP, diastolic blood pressure; DOA, duration of action; GFR, glomerular filtration rate; HF, heart failure; HR, heart rate; IV, intravenous; K⁺, serum potassium; LD, loading dose; LVAD, left ventricular assist device; MAP, mean arterial pressure; MI, myocardial infarction; NE, norepinephrine; O₂, oxygen; PAH, pulmonary arterial hypertension; PDE3, phosphodiesterase 3; PVR, peripheral vascular resistance; RR, respiratory rate; RV, right ventricle; SBP, systolic blood pressure; SCr, serum creatinine; SV, stroke volume; SVR, systemic vascular resistance; t₁/₂, half-life; UOP, urine output.

termination of PSVT. Use caution in patients with Wolff–Parkinson–White (WPW) syndrome when using an AV nodal blocking agent. A defibrillator should be made available during administration of adenosine in patients with WPW, as there is an increased risk of converting the rhythm into AF with rapid ventricular rate upon blocking the AV node.

SYMPTOMATIC HYPOTENSION AND SHOCK

Hypotension and shock can cause decreased tissue perfusion, leading to organ damage. Early goal-directed therapy, which includes immediate resuscitation strategies to maintain a mean arterial blood pressure (MAP) equal to or greater than 65 mmHg, has been associated with good clinical outcomes (Dellinger et al., 2013). Vasopressor and inotropic agents are indicated in the setting of life-threatening hypotension in order to maintain adequate blood flow to vital organs. Generally norepinephrine is recommended as the first-line vasopressor for shock. Epinephrine may be considered as an add-on or a substitute for norepinephrine. Despite the proposed renal-protective properties of vasopressin (Bragadottir, Redfors, Nygren, Sellgren, & Ricksten, 2009), this agent has not been shown to decrease mortality compared with norepinephrine (Russell et al., 2008). Vasopressin is therefore used only as adjunctive therapy to norepinephrine to increase MAP. Several studies have compared the efficacy and safety of dopamine with norepinephrine. Norepinephrine is the preferred agent as it is more potent than dopamine and associated with fewer cardiac arrhythmias (De Backer et al., 2010). Inotropic agents may be utilized in place of or in addition to a vasopressor for specific patient conditions. Table 35.2 summarizes medications that may be used in patients who are hemodynamically unstable, due to bradycardia, hypotension, reduced cardiac output, and various shock states. Clinical considerations are also listed for selecting between the various inotropes and vasopressors.

For full reference citations to this chapter, please see "Section References" in the back of the book, under the heading "Section VII."

Diagnostic and Therapeutic Catheterization Procedures

VENKATESH K. RAMAN

As a young surgical trainee outside of Berlin in the 1920s, Werner Forssmann was preoccupied with a picture from an old French medical journal. The manuscript reported a technique in animals—specifically in horses—for direct cardiovascular evaluation through the insertion of a catheter tip via the jugular vein into the right ventricle, with the external end positioned near a toy drum. The researchers described the sound and feel of each impulse. The medical community continued to regard the heart with wonder but respected its mystique, while Forssmann and a select few others pondered methods for better understanding this essential organ (Fenster, 2003). By the end of the decade, Forssmann began working in earnest toward a more direct assessment of the right heart. Knowing the peripheral veins of the upper arm provided a relatively direct route to the heart, he was determined to proceed. After being forbidden by his superiors, Forssmann enlisted the help of a surgical nurse, inserted the catheter via his cubital vein, pushed it in nearly two feet, and then had an x-ray taken demonstrating the catheter tip in the right ventricle, heralding the advent of heart catheterization. It would take more than a decade before systematic work by others, including Dickinson Richards and Andre Cournand, demonstrated the importance of this technique in the diagnosis and management of cardiovascular disease. For this, Dr. Forssmann was a corecipient of the Nobel Prize for Medicine and Physiology in 1956 (Fenster, 2003).

The subsequent development of selective coronary angiography in the 1960s, along with the pioneering work of radiologist Dr. Charles Dotter in sequential dilatation of lower-extremity arteries, established the foundation for the next phase in therapeutic catheterization procedures. At the American Heart Association (AHA) meeting in 1977, Dr. Andreas Gruentzig presented a well-received poster on the results of coronary angioplasty with a balloon catheter in dogs (Cohen, 2014). Shortly thereafter, he performed the first human coronary angioplasty intraoperatively. Percutaneous coronary interventions (PCIs), encompassing a myriad of techniques to relieve obstructive atherosclerotic stenosis, grew exponentially. Since that time, the field of interventional cardiology has broadened to include structural heart disease, most recently the transcatheter delivery and implantation of prosthetic aortic valves (Moscucci, 2013).

Interventional procedures and techniques are invasive diagnostic studies that require expert decision making to ensure that the decision to proceed is guided by appropriate patient selection and assessment. In addition, these diagnostic studies require consideration of health care costs and safety, especially with the use of conscious sedation. Specialized equipment and a trained interventional team are required, as well as surgical capabilities for potential complications during certain procedures.

RIGHT HEART CATHETERIZATION AND HEMODYNAMIC STUDIES

Right heart catheterization is performed to obtain hemodynamic measurements—either alone or in conjunction with left heart catheterization and/or coronary angiography—during evaluation of valvular heart disease, cardiomyopathy, pulmonary hypertension, pericardial disease, shock states, and other conditions. When this is performed under fluoroscopic guidance in the catheterization laboratory, percutaneous access is often obtained in the common femoral, the internal jugular, or the subclavian veins. The femoral approach is favored when the catheter is to be removed upon completion of the study or if the catheter will remain for a few days in a patient who is immobilized or intubated. The jugular or subclavian veins are preferable if the system remains in place for a number of days and in a conscious patient who can subsequently sit or ambulate. Depending upon whether thermodilution cardiac output measures are desired, a series of balloon-tipped flow-directed or nonflow-directed catheters, varying in size from 5 French to 8 French, may be used.

In a typical right heart study, pressure measurements are obtained in the right atrium, right ventricle, main pulmonary artery, and pulmonary capillary wedge (PCW) position. Both absolute measures and the shape of the pressure curve provide useful information in pathophysiologic assessment. For example, elevated pulmonary artery pressures with normal PCW values confirm precapillary pulmonary hypertension and prompt consideration for vasodilator testing. When evaluating refractory right-sided volume overload, the characteristic "square root" sign in the diastolic phase of a right ventricular pressure tracing may suggest pericardial constriction and lead to additional diagnostic maneuvers.

Cardiac output may be assessed by oximetric analysis of concomitant samples from the pulmonary artery (mixed venous blood) and the systemic circulation (arterial blood). Alternatively, a pulmonary artery catheter with embedded distal thermistor can provide similar estimates using the indicator dilution method with room-temperature saline. A combination of pressure and cardiac output measurements provides a complete hemodynamic assessment; Table 36.1 provides the normal hemodynamic measurements. Understanding these hemodynamic values can readily elucidate volume status and differentiate among the various categories of shock, including cardiogenic, hypovolemic, distributive, and obstructive. Table 36.2 outlines the hemodynamic profiles for different states of shock.

TABLE 36.1 Normal Hemodynamic Values

Right atrium (RA)	0–8 mmHg
Right ventricle (RV)	Systolic 15–30 mmHg Diastolic 0–8 mmHg
Pulmonary artery (PA)	Systolic 15–30 mmHg Diastolic 3–12 mmHg Mean 8–20 mmHg
Pulmonary capillary wedge pressure (PCWP)	Mean 6–12 mmHg
Cardiac output (CO)	4–8 L/min
Systemic vascular resistance (SVR)	770–1,550 dynes $\times$ sec $\times$ cm^{-5}
Pulmonary vascular resistance (PVR)	20–120 dynes $\times$ sec $\times$ cm^{-5}

TABLE 36.2 Hemodynamic Profiles in Shock

Type of Shock	PCWP	CO	SVR
Cardiogenic	↑	↓	↑
Hypovolemic	↓	↓	↑
Distributive	↓ or =	↓, =, or ↑	↓
Obstructive (tamponade, PE)	↓, =, or ↑	↓	↑

CO, cardiac output; PCWP, pulmonary capillary wedge pressure; PE, pulmonary embolism; SVR, systemic vascular resistance.

Simultaneous right heart and left heart catheterization facilitates evaluation of certain valvular, pericardial, and myocardial abnormalities. Using this technique to superimpose PCW position and left ventricular pressure tracings allows for measures of the transvalvular pressure gradients and estimates the valve area in mitral stenosis.

There are few absolute contraindications to right heart catheterization besides the lack of informed consent in a nonemergent setting. These absolutes include the presence of a mechanical tricuspid or pulmonic valve prosthesis (very uncommon) and a significant thrombus or tumor in right-sided chambers. Relative contraindications are severe coagulopathy (INR [international normalized ratio] > 2–3), thrombocytopenia (platelets < 20,000 mm³), and newly implanted pacemaker or implantable cardioverter-defibrillator leads. Preexisting left bundle-branch block should prompt preparation for temporary pacing, as the pulmonary artery (PA) catheter may cause temporary stunning of the right bundle during passage from right ventricle to pulmonary artery, leading to complete heart block. Complications from right heart catheterization are relatively infrequent, but may include access-site injury; arrhythmia, including ventricular tachycardia and heart block; and perforation or rupture of the right-sided chambers or pulmonary artery.

LEFT HEART CATHETERIZATION AND CORONARY ANGIOGRAPHY

With more than 1 million diagnostic catheterization procedures performed annually in the United States (Riley, Don, Powell, Maynard, & Dean, 2011), the vast majority include coronary angiography to delineate the coronary vessels and assess for evidence of significant luminal narrowing. Arterial access is obtained percutaneously via the common femoral artery or, increasingly, via the radial artery. Preformed catheters of sizes 6 French (~2 mm outer diameter) or smaller are used to selectively engage the right and left coronary arteries while pressure is continuously monitored. Aqueous, iodine-based contrast dye is injected manually or by power injector to transiently replace blood and opacify the lumen during image acquisition. Due to the use of projection imaging, the complex three-dimensional course of the arterial tree, and the possibility of eccentric narrowing or stenosis, angiograms must be acquired from multiple views to adequately map the major epicardial coronary vessels and branches.

In order to be evaluated with invasive cardiovascular testing, the pretest probability of coronary heart disease (CHD) or other cardiac abnormalities must be significant. However, upon evaluation through these modalities some individuals may not have evident disease. In this circumstance, the information from the testing continues to be useful for excluding disease, prognostication, and follow-up. For those with apparent coronary disease, coronary angiography demonstrates the location, number, length, and severity of atherosclerotic lesions. The purpose is twofold: (1) to stratify the risk of cardiovascular events and (2) to guide recommendations for management, whether medical, percutaneous, or surgical. Use of simple categories based upon the anatomic extent of significant disease, defined as diameter stenosis greater than 70% compared with adjacent reference vessel, in 1-vessel, 2-vessel, 3-vessel, or left main disease, provides important prognostic information (Alderman et al., 1990). Although this categorization is not complicated, it is relevant despite well-known limitations of coronary angiography. By necessity, the stated degree of stenosis is somewhat subjective and associated with substantial interobserver variability (Leape et al., 2000). As noted earlier, coronary angiography is an anatomic test that by itself does not provide physiologic information about coronary flow and ischemia. Adjunctive studies, including intravascular ultrasound (IVUS) and fractional flow reserve (FFR), can be incorporated during catheterization to further evaluate lesion severity and will be discussed in the section on PCI.

Before the widespread availability of noninvasive imaging methods, assessment of left ventricular systolic function by contrast ventriculography was a standard component of catheterization studies. This method continues to have an important role in describing global and regional wall motion, particularly in the setting of acute coronary syndromes. Ventriculography is usually performed with a side-hole, pigtail catheter and power injector. Overall ejection fraction can be estimated visually or quantitated using standard postprocessing techniques.

As with right heart catheterization, there are few, if any, absolute contraindications to coronary angiography and left heart catheterization. Relative contraindications are similar with more conservative thresholds warranted by arterial, rather than venous, access. These include severe coagulopathy (INR > 1.8 is commonly used), thrombocytopenia (platelets < 50,000 mm^3), severe anemia (hematocrit < 21%) and/or active bleeding, severe metabolic derangements (particularly hypokalemia and hyperkalemia), radiocontrast allergy, renal insufficiency, and the patient's inability to lie flat or keep relatively still.

The incidence of complications during diagnostic catheterization has continued to decline over time. The 2012 American College of Cardiology Foundation (ACCF) Consensus Document on Cardiac Catheterization Laboratory Standards usefully categorizes potential complications into coronary, vascular, and systemic nonvascular types (Bashore et al., 2012). Major complications, including death, stroke, myocardial infarction, and emergency coronary artery bypass graft (CABG), occur in less than 0.1% of diagnostic procedures. Other adverse events include vascular access site complications leading to hematoma, retroperitoneal bleeding, pseudoaneurysm formation, and arteriovenous fistula. Contrast nephropathy is another recognized consequence of iodinated radiocontrast use and occurs more frequently in patients with certain clinical risk factors described earlier.

Indications for Left Heart Cardiac Catheterization

The ACCF collaborated with the Society for Cardiovascular Angiography and Interventions, the AHA, and many other specialty and subspecialty organizations to write an appropriate use criteria (AUC) document that offers guidance on the indications for and the optimal role of diagnostic cardiac catheterization and coronary angiography (Patel et al., 2012). The 2012 document includes 166 indications developed by a writing group to encompass common clinical scenarios that represent the majority of clinically relevant situations. Most of these indications focus on coronary angiography for coronary artery disease (CAD), while the remaining indications involve hemodynamic assessment for valvular heart disease, cardiomyopathy, and pulmonary hypertension. An independent technical panel scored these indications on a scale of 1 to 9. Median scores between 7 to 9 represent appropriate use of diagnostic catheterization, indicating it is a generally acceptable and reasonable approach; scores of 4 to 6 represent uncertain use, meaning that it *may* be acceptable and *may* be a reasonable approach; scores 1 to 3 represent probable inappropriate use of diagnostic catheterization, meaning it is *not* generally acceptable or is *not* a reasonable approach. The statement goes to great lengths to acknowledge the ambiguity often present in clinical medicine as well as the necessity for clinical judgment to determine the appropriateness of these procedures for individual patients. As such, the AUC document is intended to serve as a guideline for evaluation and policy making at the institution and systemwide levels (Patel et al., 2012).

The AUC document reports 75 indications scored as appropriate, 49 rated uncertain, and 42 indications labeled inappropriate. A significant emphasis is placed upon the following patient-specific parameters: symptom status, noninvasive imaging results, pretest probability of CHD, and global CHD risk. Pretest probability can be calculated using published algorithms (Gibbons et al., 1997; Morise, Haddad, & Beckner, 1997) and global 10-year risk can be estimated with standard methods, such as those described in recent ACC/AHA guidelines (Goff et al., 2013b). In general, patients with suspected or definite acute coronary syndromes are considered appropriate for coronary angiography. While few studies have focused on the diagnostic angiogram, there is considerable literature supporting the value of angiography to guide risk stratification and management in this setting (Anderson et al., 2011; O'Gara et al., 2013a, 2013c). Patients with high-risk findings on noninvasive stress testing, regardless of symptoms, are considered appropriate for coronary angiography. In addition, those patients with symptoms and either intermediate-risk noninvasive testing or discordant/equivocal testing, for example, negative treadmill ECG with typical exertional symptoms, are candidates for angiography as well. Angiography in patients without known CHD and no prior noninvasive testing is considered appropriate only in those with a high pretest probability for CHD.

On the other end of the AUC spectrum, coronary angiography is considered inappropriate in asymptomatic patients without high pretest probability or high global risk, and in symptomatic patients with low pretest probability. Angiography is also rated inappropriate in asymptomatic patients post revascularization, as well as in those with stable CHD and low-risk noninvasive testing but no change in symptoms (Patel et al., 2012).

In those patients studied for primary non-CHD indications, coronary angiography is rated appropriate prior to planned valve surgery and for evaluation of unexplained global or regional left ventricular dysfunction. Discordant clinical and noninvasive findings warrant hemodynamic assessment by catheterization in valvular heart disease, heart failure, and pericardial disease, for example, to differentiate constrictive versus restrictive cardiomyopathy. Catheterization is rated inappropriate for evaluation of mild or moderate valvular disease in asymptomatic patients and in symptomatic patients for whom noninvasive findings are concordant with the clinical impression (Patel et al., 2012).

PERCUTANEOUS CORONARY INTERVENTION

Andreas Gruentzig furthered the concept of nonsurgical dilation of obstructive arterial stenoses from the periphery to the coronary circulation in 1977, first intraoperatively and subsequently through a percutaneous approach. The technique was initially confined to a carefully selected patient population with short, proximal noncalcified lesions that could be safely approached with the rudimentary equipment available. Despite a significant need for emergency CABG due to abrupt vessel closure in 5% to 10% of patients, the procedure evolved and thrived due to the foresight of Gruentzig and his contemporaries, who established a comprehensive registry for tracking and reporting (King, 1996). In the ensuing 35 years, interventional cardiology has experienced a series of transformative developments, including the current era of transcatheter valve replacement.

As with diagnostic catheterization, arterial access is typically obtained via the femoral or radial route with 5- to 8-French sheaths. When possible, particularly for a known or elective PCI, the patient is administered 162 to 325 mg chewable aspirin preprocedure, if not prescribed aspirin chronically. An antiplatelet thienopyridine, such as clopidogrel, prasugrel, or ticagrelor, is also administered prior to or immediately following intervention. Therapeutic anticoagulation is achieved during the procedure, typically with unfractionated heparin or bivalirudin, a direct thrombin inhibitor. In order to accommodate interventional devices, the guiding catheters used to selectively engage coronary ostia are additionally reinforced; however, they are thinner-walled than their diagnostic counterparts of the same French size. A 0.014" guidewire is passed across the obstructive lesion(s) to be treated, serving as a rail over which balloons, stents, and other devices are delivered. The coronary balloon dilatation, or percutaneous transluminal coronary angioplasty (PTCA), catheter was first used to effect a "controlled" dissection and relieve obstructive stenoses in patients with stable CAD syndromes. The success of this technique was limited in the acute setting by abrupt vessel closure, and in the 3- to 6-month intermediate period by exuberant smooth muscle cell migration and proliferation, leading to obstructive neointimal hyperplasia and/or restenosis, in more than one-quarter of patients (Fischman et al., 1994).

Intracoronary stents were first introduced in the mid-1980s for rescue in the setting of post-PTCA flow-limiting dissection and abrupt vessel closure, markedly reducing the incidence of emergency CABG to less than 1%. Widespread use was constrained by the occurrence of stent thrombosis despite intensive anticoagulation regimens, including dextran, heparin, and warfarin. After the introduction of dual antiplatelet therapy (DAPT) with aspirin and a thienopyridine, initially ticlopidine, the rates of subacute thrombosis fell below 1% (Leon et al., 1998). The pivotal BENESTENT and STRESS studies confirmed an important reduction in restenosis and the need for repeat revascularization (George et al., 1998; Macaya et al., 1996). Improvements in stent design and materials led to superior profile and deliverability, allowing the treatment of increasingly complex lesion subsets. Despite these advances, significant residual restenosis rates in up to one third of cases remained an important limitation of this approach.

A large quantity of preclinical work identified medial smooth muscle proliferation as a key element of the vascular injury response to PCI that resulted in restenosis. An equally large number of preclinical studies used local and systemic administration of a variety of agents to mitigate this pathologic event. Eventually, two agents targeting the cell division and growth phases, sirolimus and paclitaxel, were applied to stent surfaces in proprietary polymers to control elution kinetics. These first-generation drug-eluting stents (DES) were profoundly effective in reducing restenosis rates to the single digits compared with bare-metal stents (BMS). The pivotal RAVEL trial, with sirolimus-coated stents, modest in size with almost 240 patients, revealed a remarkable 0% angiographic restenosis rate at 6 months versus BMS (Morice et al., 2002). A series of trials in increasingly challenging lesion and clinical subsets proved the efficacy of this platform for "real-world" cases. Exuberant clinical use of first-generation DES was quickly tempered by a signal for increased risk of stent thrombosis extending far beyond the 1-month timeframe of vulnerability for BMS (Pfisterer et al., 2006). Subsequent trial and registry data with second- and third-generation DES suggest an improved safety profile similar to BMS (Kirtane et al., 2013). Tables 36.3 and 36.4 list commercially available BMS and DES.

TABLE 36.3 Commercially Available and Commonly Used Bare-Metal Stents (BMS)

Company Name	Coronary Stent	Stent Type	Stent Size Range (mm)	Stent Length Range (mm)
Abbott Vascular	Multi-link (8 series, Vision series, Zeta)	Cobalt chromium or 316L stainless steel	2.0–4.5	8–38
Boston Scientific	VeriFLEX	316L stainless steel	2.75–4.5	8–32
Medtronic	Integrity, driver series	Cobalt alloy	2.25–4.0	8–30

The choice of device during PCI is operator- and patient-specific, relying upon a number of clinical and anatomic factors. PTCA, or balloon angioplasty, without coronary stenting is relatively infrequent and comprises fewer than 10% of all PCI procedures in contemporary registries. PTCA alone may be used to address lesions

TABLE 36.4 Commercially Available and Commonly Used Drug-Eluting Stents (DES)

Company Name	Coronary Stent	Stent Type and Drug Coating	Stent Size Range (mm)	Stent Length Range (mm)
Abbott Vascular	XIENCE Xpedition	Cobalt chromium, everolimus coating	2.25–4.0	8–38
Boston Scientific	Promus PREMIER	Platinum chromium, everolimus coating	2.25–4.0	8–38
Boston Scientific	TAXUS ION	Platinum chromium, paclitaxel coating	2.25–4.0	8–38
Medtronic	Resolute	Cobalt alloy, zotarolimus coating	2.25–4.0	8–38

or segments of disease (1) where stents cannot be delivered due to severe tortuosity or calcification, (2) when there is expected to be an extremely high risk of short-term bleeding on DAPT, or (3) if noncardiac surgery and/or interruption of DAPT study will be necessary within 4 to 6 weeks. BMS are used in a substantial minority of PCI cases, often in the setting of ST-segment elevation myocardial infarction (STEMI) or other urgent acute coronary syndrome (ACS) presentations where there is not adequate time to discuss and gauge the probability of adherence to extended courses of DAPT. BMS is also a reasonable consideration in situations where PCI is beneficial but (1) the intermediate-term bleeding risk with DAPT is considered unacceptable (e.g., patients also requiring anticoagulation for DVT/PE or atrial fibrillation) or (2) a nonemergency but necessary surgery is planned within 2 to 3 months. DES are used during the majority of PCI procedures due to the lower rates of restenosis, particularly for small vessels, for longer lesions, and in patients with diabetes or chronic kidney disease. The current guidelines recommend 12 months of uninterrupted DAPT, which may pose a challenge for some patients as outlined earlier.

Contemporary data from the ACCF's CathPCI Registry indicates a PCI in-hospital mortality rate ranging from less than 1% for elective procedures up to nearly 5% for patients with STEMI (Peterson et al., 2010). This analysis also revealed a low incidence of PCI-related stroke at 0.22%. The need for emergency CABG due to coronary injury during PCI has steadily fallen over the past decades and is now reported at less than 0.5% (Kutcher et al., 2009). As with diagnostic procedures, noncoronary vascular complications typically occur at the site of arterial access and include hematoma, retroperitoneal bleeding, pseudoaneurysm, and arteriovenous fistula. Rates of access-site complications are higher with PCI than with diagnostic studies due to the use of larger sheaths as well as intensive antiplatelet and anticoagulation therapy, reported in the range of 2% to 6%.

PCI for STEMI

For patients with transmural STEMI, restoring flow in the infarct artery is the cornerstone of care. From the available strategies to achieve this goal, primary PCI (PPCI) performed in a timely fashion is the preferred mode for reperfusion by multiple trials and meta-analyses (Andersen et al., 2003; Keeley, Boura, & Grines, 2003). There is a clear time dependence for reperfusion and outcomes, with an increase in mortality with each 30-minute delay (McNamara et al., 2006). As such, the ACC-sponsored D2B (Door-to-Balloon) Alliance has promoted a strategy of implementing regional care systems, identifying all components of care that affect reperfusion times, sharing best practices, and achieving a D2B reperfusion time of less than 90 minutes in a substantial percentage of patients. PPCI has a Class I indication in the treatment of STEMI by the 2013 ACCF/AHA Guidelines (O'Gara et al., 2013a) when performed in a timely fashion and within 12 hours of symptom onset. This window for PPCI is extended in those with severe heart failure or those in cardiogenic shock, the latter group gaining significant mortality benefit as shown in the Should We Emergently Revascularize Occluded Coronaries for Cardiogenic Shock (SHOCK) trial (Hochman et al., 1999). PPCI remains a Class IIa indication for patients with STEMI who present with ongoing evidence of ischemia between 12 and 24 hours after onset of symptoms.

PCI for Non-ST-Elevation Acute Coronary Syndromes (NSTEACS)

Unstable angina (UA) and non-ST-elevation myocardial infarction (NSTEMI) are closely related conditions along the spectrum of acute coronary syndromes, and are often considered together for purposes of diagnosis and management. Patients presenting with NSTEACS comprise a broad spectrum of risk for cardiovascular death, reinfarction, and refractory ischemia, as demonstrated by stratification algorithms like the Thrombolysis in Myocardial Infarction (TIMI) Risk Score (Antman et al., 2000). Immediate goals at the time of presentation are to triage patients and focus aggressive management strategies on those at highest risk. Early cardiac catheterization with appropriate revascularization by PCI or surgery is supported as a Class I indication in those at high risk, as identified by clinical and testing criteria (Table 36.5) to include positive cardiac biomarkers, troponin I or T, and dynamic ECG changes (Anderson et al., 2013b). A meta-analysis of NSTEMI trials concludes that an early invasive strategy confers long-term morbidity and mortality benefits compared with a conservative or selective invasive approach to management (Bavry, Kumbhani, Rassi, Bhatt, & Askari, 2006).

TABLE 36.5 High-Risk Features Favoring Early Invasive Strategy in NSTEACS

Refractory angina
Elevated cardiac biomarkers (TnT or TnI)
Dynamic ST-segment depression
Heart failure or new/worsening mitral regurgitation
Hemodynamic compromise
Left ventricular systolic dysfunction (EF < 40%)
PCI within 6 months or prior CABG
Refractory ventricular arrhythmia

CABG, coronary artery bypass graft; EF, ejection fraction; NSTEACS, non-ST-elevation acute coronary syndromes; PCI, percutaneous coronary intervention; TnI, troponin I; TnT, troponin T.

Adapted from Anderson et al. (2013b).

PCI for Stable Ischemic Heart Disease (SIHD)

While PCI reduces cardiovascular events across the acute coronary syndromes, demonstrating a similar effect in stable CAD has proven elusive. The 2011 ACCF/AHA/SCAI PCI Guideline has reformatted revascularization recommendations to focus on (1) improved survival and (2) improved symptoms (Levine et al., 2011). Notably, PCI is not given a Class I indication for any SIHD scenario to improve survival compared with medical therapy. The Guideline does provide a Class IIa recommendation for PCI in unprotected left main disease in high-risk surgical patients as long as the coronary anatomy is not predictive of procedural complications. PCI may be considered for symptomatic improvement and is a Class I recommendation when angina remains unacceptable despite guideline-directed medical therapy (GDMT), including the administration of at least two antianginal medications.

Of contemporary studies comparing PCI with medical therapy, the COURAGE trial has substantially impacted current practice. In this trial, almost 2,300 patients having angina or abnormal stress tests following angiographic demonstration of severe CAD were randomized to an initial strategy of optimal medical therapy (OMT) or to PCI plus OMT. At a median of 4.6 years, there was no statistical difference in the occurrence of a composite endpoint of all-cause mortality and nonfatal myocardial infarction between the PCI group and the OMT group, 19.01% and 18.5%, respectively (Boden et al., 2007). PCI was associated with more rapid improvement in angina, but the difference was eliminated by the end of the follow-up period. Notably, one third of patients in the OMT group crossed over to PCI within the first year of the trial.

There have been a number of studies comparing operative revascularization by CABG with PCI from balloon angioplasty, BMS, and DES. The SYNTAX trial randomized 1,800 patients with left main or three-vessel CAD to CABG or PCI with the paclitaxel-eluting stent, after an interventional cardiologist and cardiac surgeon determined that both modalities would yield equivalent anatomical revascularization (Serruys et al., 2009). A noninferiority comparison was made at 12 months for a composite endpoint of death, stroke, myocardial infarction, or repeat revascularization. The trial did not confirm this primary endpoint, leading the authors to conclude that CABG remains the standard for revascularization of severe CAD. A prospectively defined SYNTAX score was used to define the aggregate severity of CAD by grading the angiographic findings based on lesion location, morphology, and severity, with the coronary tree divided into 16 segments. Post hoc analyses led to the following categories: low score equal to or less than 22, intermediate 23 to 32, and high score equal to or greater than 33. In the low SYNTAX score group, 12-month outcomes were similar for both PCI and CABG. Patients in the intermediate and high SYNTAX score groups, however, experienced major adverse cardiac event (MACE) rates, almost double in those undergoing PCI compared with CABG.

ADJUNCTIVE DIAGNOSTIC DEVICES

As noted in the section on coronary angiography, both visual and quantitative estimates are prone to the limitations of projection imaging and may lead to over- or underestimation of stenosis severity. IVUS and FFR assessments provide additional information to guide care. IVUS allows high-resolution axial imaging from within the coronary artery to identify lesion characteristics, specifically calcification, lumen diameter, and cross-sectional area. Anatomic thresholds for flow-limiting stenosis using lumen diameters and areas have been empirically determined from correlation with physiologic studies like SPECT myocardial perfusion and FFR (Nishioka et al., 1999). Nevertheless, clinical trials comparing IVUS-guided PCI to standard techniques have not consistently demonstrated any reduction in either restenosis or in composite major cardiovascular event rates, including target vessel revascularization and myocardial infarction (De Jaegere et al., 1998).

FFR assessment uses a guidewire or catheter with distal pressure transducer to generate a ratio of the maximal blood flow beyond a stenosis to the normal maximal blood flow at the tip of the guiding catheter. Values less than 0.75 to 0.80 correlate with ischemia on stress SPECT perfusion testing with accuracy of more than 90% (Pijls et al., 1996). Investigators in the DEFER study demonstrated superior outcomes with medical therapy for stenoses judged significant by angiography but without evidence of flow limitation by FFR values above 0.75 (Pijls et al., 2007). When used to guide PCI in multivessel disease in the FAME and FAME 2 trials, FFR reduced the need for revascularization and reduced cardiovascular event rates (De Bruyne et al., 2012; Tonino et al., 2009).

PREPROCEDURAL CONSIDERATIONS

Preparation of the patient for cardiac catheterization requires meticulous attention to detail that ensures patient safety and optimal outcomes, with procedural risks mitigated by proper patient selection and preprocedural evaluation. An expert consensus statement published by the Society for Cardiovascular Angiography and Interventions serves as a resource for recommended "best practices" (Naidu et al., 2012). All patients must have a history and physical examination documented in the chart, dated within 30 days for outpatient studies, and updated within 24 hours of the procedure. The history should include recent cardiovascular symptoms and status; medications; co-morbidities; allergies; indications; and a review of systems that focuses on any cardiac, pulmonary, gastrointestinal, renal, and hematologic issues (Table 36.6). Bleeding diatheses and potential difficulty maintaining DAPT following PCI, for example, planned necessary surgery, should be documented. Prior reactions to iodinated contrast should be detailed, and consideration given to pretreatment with steroids and/or histamine antagonists based upon the severity and suspected type of reaction. When feasible, three or four doses of oral prednisone or equivalent can be prescribed beginning the day before the procedure at 6- to 8-hour intervals. In an emergency or without prior notice, intravenous methylprednisolone, hydrocortisone, or an equivalent can be administered as soon as possible prior to contrast administration. Allergy to shellfish or seafood is no longer considered a predictor of adverse reaction to iodinated contrast, as a history of significant atopy is a better predictor of a reaction. An assessment of the risk of contrast nephropathy should be included if the patient has acute or chronic renal dysfunction, particularly in the setting of diabetes, heart failure, periprocedural

TABLE 36.6 Sample of Items for Preprocedure Checklist

H&P documented within 30 days (outpatient)/24 hr (inpatient)?
History of prior PCI? CABG?
Stable angina vs ACS?
Noninvasive testing? Reports and risk category available?
Significant anemia (Hct < 30)? Significant thrombocytopenia (Plt < 50K)?
Major surgery within past month or planned over the next year?
Clinically evident bleeding? History GI or intracranial bleeding?
History of medication noncompliance?
Contrast allergy? Pretreated?
Oral or intravenous anticoagulation? Last dose? PT/INR or PTT checked?
CBC and basic metabolic panel within 30 days (outpatient) or 24 hr (inpatient)?
ECG within 24 hr?
ASA and Mallampati class documented?

ACS, acute coronary syndrome; ASA, American Society of Anesthesiologists; CABG, coronary artery bypass graft; CBC, complete blood count; ECG, electrocardiogram; GI, gastrointestinal; H&P, history and physical; Hct, hematocrit; INR, international normalized ratio; PCI, percutaneous coronary intervention; Plt, platelet count; PT, prothrombin time; PTT, partial thromboplastin time.

Adapted from Naidu et al. (2012).

diuretic use, or hypotension. Published risk calculators (Mehran et al., 2004) incorporate clinical and procedural factors including age, gender, diabetes, contrast volume, and preexisting renal excretory dysfunction to provide useful estimates. Consideration of mitigating strategies for contrast-induced acute kidney injury includes intravenous hydration, sodium bicarbonate, and n-acetylcysteine. Hafiz et al. (2012) evaluated the incidence of contrast-induced kidney injury by comparing intravenous normal saline to sodium bicarbonate with and without oral n-acetylcysteine in 320 patients with baseline renal insufficiency. The findings suggest that there was no difference in the development of contrast-induced kidney injury between the groups (Hafiz et al., 2012). N-acetylcysteine is a Class III, no-benefit recommendation according to the ACCF/AHA guidelines for percutaneous interventions (Levine et al., 2011). Diabetics should have oral hypoglycemics and insulin regimens reviewed and modified as appropriate.

A focused but thorough examination of the cardiovascular system is essential to provide a baseline and to facilitate identification of periprocedural changes. Documentation of peripheral lower extremity pulses and of the presence of femoral arterial bruits should be included. Prior to planned radial artery access, many operators perform a modified Allen's or Barbeau test to assess continuity of the palmar arch (Patel, Shah, & Pancholy, 2013); however, the utility of this practice has been called into question and has long been abandoned by the highest volume centers abroad (Valgimigli et al., 2014). Evidence should be noted for left ventricular systolic dysfunction and heart failure symptoms, including elevated jugular venous pressure, pulmonary crackles, and peripheral edema. Systolic murmurs consistent with valvular stenosis should be identified along with ancillary criteria that refine estimates of severity such as any decrease in amplitude or delay in peripheral pulses. Because most cardiac catheterization procedures are performed with the use of moderate sedation, a careful assessment of the patient's oropharynx, neck, and lungs is mandatory to identify cases that may benefit from anesthesia consultation and support. Those with a history of stroke and residual deficits should have a baseline screening neurologic exam.

While ancillary testing should be individually tailored, all patients should have a baseline ECG, particularly those with recurring or persistent cardiovascular symptoms. Beta human chorionic gonadotropin (HCG) levels should be checked within 2 weeks of the procedure in women of childbearing age. A complete blood count and basic metabolic panel with serum creatinine should be obtained within 30 days for elective procedures. Testing is usually convenient for hospitalized patients and becomes particularly important with suspected or active bleeding and with fluctuating renal function. Unrecognized anemia should be noted and should raise the threshold for proceeding with nonurgent studies. Prothrombin time (PT)/INR should be measured for patients on chronic warfarin anticoagulation therapy, and an INR greater than 1.8 is a reasonable threshold to consider deferral of the procedure in the absence of an emergent or high-risk presentation (STEMI), or if there is an underlying, uncorrectable coagulopathy, for example, with advanced hepatic dysfunction (Naidu et al., 2012).

POSTPROCEDURAL CONSIDERATIONS

Access site care is a critical component of safety and the patient experience post catheterization or PCI. The most technically challenging procedure may go unappreciated by patient and primary teams if there is a significant vascular complication requiring transfusion or surgical repair. Careful evaluation of the patient and inspection of the access site can identify hematoma, pseudoaneurysm, arteriovenous fistula, retroperitoneal bleeding, and compartment syndrome, with radial or brachial access. Distal pulses should be assessed with special care if the patient complains of pain or paresthesias suggesting arterial occlusion, which may warrant emergency operative or endovascular management. Pseudoaneurysms should be confirmed by Doppler. Those smaller than 2 cm often thrombose spontaneously, while larger pseudoaneurysms may require ultrasound therapy or surgery. AV fistulas rarely require treatment but can be successfully compressed, excluded by endograft, or surgically ligated when necessary. Retroperitoneal bleeding, heralded by abdominal and/or back pain and hypotension, is best managed by supportive care with fluids, blood transfusion, and analgesia. Surgical evacuation is necessary only for large hematomas with ongoing bleeding, local compression, or significant nerve irritation. For femoral artery hemostasis, vascular hemostasis devices using compression (e.g., FemoStop™), collagen plug (e.g., Angio-Seal™), and suture closure (e.g., Perclose) have been evaluated and found to reduce time to ambulation compared with manual pressure, but not to decrease vascular complications (Levine et al., 2011).

Aspirin after PCI should be continued indefinitely at a daily dose of 81 to 325 mg, although the lower dose may be preferred due to a lower risk of bleeding. In patients undergoing PCI for stable CAD, clopidogrel is used as a periprocedural load, then 75 mg daily and continued for at least 1 month, and ideally up to 12 months with BMS and at least 12 months with DES. When patients have PCI for ACS indications, then additional antiplatelet options include either prasugrel 10 mg daily or ticagrelor 90 mg twice daily in lieu of clopidogrel for at least 12 months. Importantly, prasugrel is contraindicated in patients with a history of prior stroke or transient ischemic attack. Ticagrelor should be used with concomitant aspirin dosed at or less than 100 mg daily, as higher doses of aspirin may limit the effectiveness of ticagrelor. Proton pump inhibitor (PPI) use is a Class I recommendation in patients with a history of prior GI bleeding, for example, peptic ulcer disease, on DAPT following PCI (Levine et al., 2011). Other subpopulations for whom concomitant PPI therapy is reasonable include those on warfarin, steroids, or nonsteroidal antiinflammatory drugs (NSAIDs), as well as patients with *H. pylori* infection. As clopidogrel is a prodrug and metabolized with the CYP2C19 enzyme, drugs that inhibit CYP2C19 can inhibit the activity of clopidogrel, resulting in an increased risk of cardiovascular events. The most predominant drug class that interacts with clopidogrel is the PPI, with omeprazole and esomeprazole demonstrating the most significant in vitro interactions. Despite the paucity of evidence for reduced in vivo efficacy or an increase in clinical events, the Food and Drug Administration (FDA) has issued a warning to avoid the use of these two agents with clopidogrel (Anderson et al., 2013b; Jneid et al., 2012). For patients who require proton pump inhibition, pantoprazole may be preferred, as it does not inhibit CYP2C19 as extensively as other agents in this class (Jneid et al., 2012).

ADDITIONAL THERAPEUTIC INTERVENTIONS

Catheter-based cardiovascular therapies have evolved beyond the coronary arteries to address structural heart disease, including valvular stenotic and regurgitant lesions as well as congenital abnormalities such as atrial septal defect (ASD), often treated during adulthood.

Valvular Heart Disease

No procedure has garnered as much attention and enthusiasm as transcatheter aortic valve replacement (TAVR). With FDA's 2011 approval of the first device for patients with severe aortic stenosis and considered to have risks prohibitive for surgery, TAVR numbers are growing rapidly. The pivotal PARTNER I trial demonstrated a remarkable 2-year reduction in mortality with TAVR compared with medical therapy in this inoperable cohort (43% vs 68%; Makkar, 2012). Since then, additional devices have been approved for commercial use, with many more in clinical trials. Procedure indications have been expanded to allow TAVR as an alternative to surgery in patients at high surgical risk. Balloon valvuloplasty remains an available tool for short-term symptomatic relief in patients who are not candidates for replacement or who can benefit from "bridging" before definitive therapy, for example, in patients requiring time-sensitive noncardiac surgery.

Unlike the stenotic aortic valve, mitral valve stenosis, typically a long-term consequence of rheumatic heart disease, often can be treated with a durable response by balloon valvuloplasty. Sonographic characteristics such as degree of calcification, fibrosis of the subvalvular apparatus, and degree of concomitant insufficiency can guide selection of appropriate cases for valvuloplasty. Mitral regurgitation (MR), while much more common, is considerably more challenging to treat. A novel transcatheter implementation of a surgical edge-to-edge repair technique, devised by Dr. Ottavio Alfieri, offers a nonoperative alternative to patients with symptomatic MR who are at high surgical risk. This device, the MitraClip® system, was shown in the pivotal EVEREST II study to have similar clinical outcomes to surgery in reducing symptoms and improving left ventricular indices (Feldman, 2011).

Atrial Septal Defect

The *secundum* ASD may be considered for percutaneous closure in the setting of paradoxical embolism, significantly elevated pulmonary artery pressures, or right-sided chamber enlargement. The two commercially available devices are made of nitinol, a self-expanding alloy with shape memory, and have a "clamshell" morphology with discs on either side of the interatrial septum joined in the middle across the defect. *Sinus venosus* and *primum* ASDs are not amenable to a catheter-based procedure and must be addressed surgically, if necessary.

Alcohol Septal Ablation

Alcohol septal ablation, first described in the mid-1990s, was developed to effect a circumscribed, controlled infarction in the basal-septal myocardium that contributes to the dynamic outflow obstruction with systolic anterior mitral leaflet excursion. Conventional coronary tools are used to access the first or second septal perforator of the left anterior descending artery. With fluoroscopic or sonographic contrast guidance, the perforator supplying the target myocardium is identified. A slow delivery of pure ethanol, with proximal balloon occlusion, infarcts the desired territory while protecting the left anterior descending (LAD) artery from reflux. It is considered an appropriate alternative to surgical myomectomy in patients with medically refractory symptoms who are not surgical candidates or who are at high risk (Gersh et al., 2011).

SPECIAL POPULATIONS

Although women comprise approximately 30% of the STEMI presentations and older adults are ever growing in number, registry data clearly indicate that both populations suffer from lower rates of reperfusion therapy in eligible patients (O'Gara et al., 2013a). Approximately one third of patients with STEMI do not experience typical, severe chest pain or pressure, and this occurs more frequently in women and the older adult, contributing to delays in seeking care or in diagnosis by providers. Women appear to be at higher risk for periprocedural bleeding with antithrombotic therapy, even after adjustment for baseline clinical characteristics. Analysis of NSTE-ACS data reveals similar findings. The incidence of, and absolute risk from, NSTE-ACS are highest in older adults, who benefit as much or more than younger patients from GDMT and early invasive strategies (Amsterdam et al., 2014). Women with high-risk features also benefit from GDMT and an early invasive approach; however, in the absence of elevated cardiac biomarkers, troponin I or T, a conservative or ischemia-guided strategy is associated with better outcomes. In both women and the older adult, particular evaluation is required for body weight, renal function, and bleeding risk. In the older adult, co-morbidities, functional status, and life expectancy also must be evaluated. SIHD—the most common initial manifestation of advanced CAD in women—typically presents at a later age than in men and is more often associated with nonobstructive disease in those that undergo coronary angiography. In the older adult, diffuse and severe multivessel disease is more likely. Co-morbidities and polypharmacy must be considered in devising a management strategy. Revascularization outcomes tend to be less favorable in both groups, but remain important in the presence of high-risk anatomy, for example, three-vessel or left main coronary disease, or with limiting symptoms on appropriate antianginal therapy.

For full reference citations to this chapter, please see "Section References" in the back of the book, under the heading "Section VII."

Appendix: Tables of Cardiovascular Guidelines

TABLE A.1 Cardiovascular Conditions

	Guideline/Year	Source
Acute coronary syndrome	2012 ACCF/AHA Focused Update of the Guidelines for the Management of Patients With Unstable Angina/Non–ST-Elevation Myocardial Infarction (Updating the 2007 Guideline and Replacing the 2011 Focused Update) **2012**	A Report of the American College of Cardiology/American Heart Association Task Force on Practice Guidelines
	2014 AHA/ACC Guideline for the Management of Patients With Non-ST-Elevation Acute Coronary Syndrome **2014**	A Report of the American College of Cardiology/American Heart Association Task Force on Practice Guidelines Developed in Collaboration With the Society of Thoracic Surgeons Endorsed by the American Association for Clinical Chemistry
	2013 ACCF/AHA Guideline for the Management of ST-Elevation Myocardial Infarction **2013**	A Report of the American College of Cardiology/American Heart Association Task Force on Practice Guidelines
Arrhythmia	2014 AHA/ACC/HRS Guideline for the Management of Patients With Atrial Fibrillation **2014**	A Report of the American College of Cardiology Foundation/American Heart Association Task Force on Practice Guidelines and the Heart Rhythm Society
	Treatment of Atrial Fibrillation **2013**	(Prepared by the Duke Evidence-Based Practice Center Under Contract No. 290-2007-10066-I) AHRQ Publication
	Recommendations for Stroke Prevention and Rate/Rhythm Control **2012**	Update of the Canadian Cardiovascular Society Atrial Fibrillation Guidelines
	Oral Antithrombotic Agents for the Prevention of Stroke in Nonvalvular Atrial Fibrillation **2012**	A Science Advisory for Healthcare Professionals From the American Heart Association/American Stroke Association
	Expert Consensus Statement on Catheter and Surgical Ablation of Atrial Fibrillation: Recommendations for Patient Selection, Procedural Techniques, Patient Management and Follow-Up, Definitions, Endpoints, and Research Trial Design **2012**	A Report of the Heart Rhythm Society (HRS) Task Force on Catheter and Surgical Ablation of Atrial Fibrillation. Developed in Partnership With the European Heart Rhythm Association (EHRA), a Registered Branch of the European Society of Cardiology (ESC) and the European Cardiac Arrhythmia Society (ECAS); and in Collaboration With the American College of Cardiology (ACC), American Heart Association (AHA), the Asia Pacific Heart Rhythm Society (APHRS), and the Society of Thoracic Surgeons (STS)

(continued)

TABLE A.1 Cardiovascular Conditions (*continued*)

	Guideline/Year	Source
	ACC/AHA/ESC Guidelines for the Management of Patients With Supraventricular Arrhythmias **2003**	A Report of the American College of Cardiology/American Heart Association Task Force and the European Society of Cardiology Committee for Practice Guidelines (Writing Committee to Develop Guidelines for the Management of Patients With Supraventricular Arrhythmias)
	ACC/AHA/ESC 2006 Guidelines for Management of Patients With Ventricular Arrhythmias and the Prevention of Sudden Cardiac Death **2006**	A Report of the American College of Cardiology/American Heart Association Task Force and the European Society of Cardiology Committee for Practice Guidelines (Writing Committee to Develop Guidelines for Management of Patients With Ventricular Arrhythmias and the Prevention of Sudden Cardiac Death)
	ACCF/AHA/HRS Focused Update Incorporated Into the ACCF/AHA/HRS 2008 Guidelines for Device-Based Therapy of Cardiac Rhythm Abnormalities **2012**	A Report of the American College of Cardiology Foundation/American Heart Association Task Force on Practice Guidelines and the Heart Rhythm Society
Cardio-myopathy	2011 ACCF/AHA Guideline for the Diagnosis and Treatment of Hypertrophic Cardiomyopathy **2011**	Report of the American College of Cardiology/American Heart Association Task Force on Practice Guidelines
Coronary heart disease/ischemic heart disease	Performance Measures for Adults With Coronary Artery Disease and Hypertension **2011**	A Report of the American College of Cardiology Foundation/American Heart Association Task Force on Performance Measures and the American Medical Association–Physician Consortium for Performance Improvement
	2014 ACC/AHA/AATS/PCNA/SCAI/STS Focused Update of the Guideline for the Diagnosis and Management of Patients With Stable Ischemic Heart Disease **2014**	A Report of the American College of Cardiology/American Heart Association Task Force on Practice Guidelines, and the American Association for Thoracic Surgery, Preventive Cardiovascular Nurses Association, Society for Cardiovascular Angiography and Interventions, and Society of Thoracic Surgeons
	2012 ACCF/AHA/ACP/AATS/PCNA/SCAI/ STS Guideline for the Diagnosis and Management of Patients With Stable Ischemic Heart Disease **2012**	A Report of the American College of Cardiology Foundation/American Heart Association Task Force on Practice Guidelines, and the American College of Physicians, American Association for Thoracic Surgery, Preventive Cardiovascular Nurses Association, Society for Cardiovascular Angiography and Interventions, and Society of Thoracic Surgeons
	ACCF/ACG/AHA 2010 Expert Consensus Document on the Concomitant Use of Proton Pump Inhibitors and Thienopyridines: A Focused Update of the ACCF/ACG/AHA 2008 Expert Consensus Document Reducing the Gastrointestinal Risks of Antiplatelet Therapy and NSAID Use **2010**	A Report of the American College of Cardiology Foundation Task Force on Expert Consensus Documents

(*continued*)

TABLE A.1 Cardiovascular Conditions (*continued*)

	Guideline/Year	Source
	2013 Multimodality Appropriate Use Criteria for the Detection and Risk Assessment of Stable Ischemic Heart Disease **2013**	A Report of the American College of Cardiology Foundation Appropriate Use Criteria Task Force, American Heart Association, American Society of Echocardiography, American Society of Nuclear Cardiology, Heart Failure Society of America, Heart Rhythm Society, Society for Cardiovascular Angiography and Interventions, Society of Cardiovascular Computed Tomography, Society for Cardiovascular Magnetic Resonance, and Society of Thoracic Surgeons
Endocarditis	Infective Endocarditis: Diagnosis, Antimicrobial Therapy, and Management of Complications: A Statement for Health Care Professionals From the Committee on Rheumatic Fever, Endocarditis, and Kawasaki Disease **2005**	Council on Cardiovascular Disease in the Young, and the Councils on Clinical Cardiology, Stroke, and Cardiovascular Surgery and Anesthesia, American Heart Association: Endorsed by the Infectious Diseases Society of America
Heart failure	2013 ACCF/AHA Guideline for the Management of Heart Failure **2013**	A Report of the American College of Cardiology Foundation/American Heart Association Task Force on Practice Guidelines
	The 2010 Heart Failure Society of America Comprehensive Heart Failure Practice Guidelines **2010**	Heart Failure Society of America
	2013 ACCF/ACR/ASE/ASNC/SCCT/SCMR Appropriate Utilization of Cardiovascular Imaging in Heart Failure **2013**	A Joint Report of the American College of Radiology Appropriateness Criteria® Committee and the American College of Cardiology Foundation Appropriate Use Criteria Task Force
	ACCF/AHA/AMA-PCPI 2011 Performance Measures for Adults With Heart Failure **2012**	A Report of the American College of Cardiology Foundation/American Heart Association Task Force on Performance Measures and the American Medical Association–Physician Consortium for Performance Improvement
Hypertension	Evidence-Based Guideline for the Management of High Blood Pressure in Adults **2014**	Report From the Panel Members Appointed to the Eighth Joint National Committee (JNC-8)
	Clinical Practice Guidelines for the Management of Hypertension in the Community **2013**	A Statement by the American Society of Hypertension and the International Society of Hypertension
	ACCF/AHA 2011 Expert Consensus Document on Hypertension in the Elderly **2011**	A Report of the American College of Cardiology Foundation Task Force on Clinical Expert Consensus Documents Develop in Collaboration With the American Academy of Neurology, American Geriatrics Society, American Society of Preventive Cardiology, American Society of Hypertension, American Society of Nephrology, Association of Black Cardiologists, and European Society of Hypertension

(*continued*)

TABLE A.1 Cardiovascular Conditions (*continued*)

	Guideline/Year	Source
	An Effective Approach to High Blood Pressure Control **2014**	A Science Advisory From the American Heart Association, the American College of Cardiology, and the Centers for Disease Control and Prevention
	The Seventh Report of the Joint National Committee on Prevention, Detection, Evaluation, and Treatment of High Blood Pressure: The JNC-7 Report **2003**	Joint National Committee on Prevention, Detection, Evaluation, and Treatment of High Blood Pressure
	Blood Pressure and Treatment of Persons With Hypertension as it Relates to Cognitive Outcomes Including Executive Function **2012**	American Society of Hypertension Writing Group
Lipid metabolism disorder	The ACC/AHA Guideline on the Treatment of Blood Cholesterol to Reduce Atherosclerotic Cardiovascular Risk in Adults **2013**	American College of Cardiology/American Heart Association
Peripheral vascular disease	ACCF/AHA Focused Update of the Guideline for the Management of Patients With Peripheral Artery Disease (Updating the 2005 Guideline) **2011**	A Report of the American College of Cardiology Foundation/American Heart Association Task Force on Practice Guidelines
	Appropriate Use Criteria for Peripheral Vascular Ultrasound and Physiological Testing Part I: Arterial Ultrasound and Physiological Testing **2012**	A Report of the American College of Cardiology Foundation Appropriate Use Criteria Task Force, American College of Radiology, American Institute of Ultrasound in Medicine, American Society of Echocardiography, American Society of Nephrology, Intersocietal Commission for the Accreditation of Vascular Laboratories, Society for Cardiovascular Angiography and Interventions, Society of Cardiovascular Computed Tomography, Society for Interventional Radiology, Society for Vascular Medicine, and Society for Vascular Surgery
	2013 Appropriate Use Criteria for Peripheral Vascular Ultrasound and Physiological Testing Part II: Testing for Venous Disease and Evaluation of Hemodialysis Access **2013**	A Report of the American College of Cardiology Foundation Appropriate Use Criteria Task Force
Stroke	AHA/ASA Guidelines for the Early Management of Patients With Acute Ischemic Stroke **2013**	A Guideline for Healthcare Professionals From the American Heart Association and the American Stroke Association

(*continued*)

TABLE A.1 Cardiovascular Conditions (*continued*)

	Guideline/Year	Source
	AHA/ASA Guidelines for the Prevention of Stroke in Patients With Stroke and Transient Ischemic Attack 2014	A Guideline for Healthcare Professionals From the American Heart Association and the American Stroke Association
Syncope	AHA/ACCF Scientific Statement on the Evaluation of Syncope 2006	From the American Heart Association Councils on Clinical Cardiology, Cardiovascular Nursing, Cardiovascular Disease in the Young, and Stroke, and the Quality of Care and Outcomes Research Interdisciplinary Working Group; and the American College of Cardiology Foundation in Collaboration With the Heart Rhythm Society
	Guideline for the Diagnosis and Management of Syncope 2009	The Task Force for the Diagnosis and Management of Syncope of the European Society of Cardiology (ESC), Developed in Collaboration With European Heart Rhythm Association (EHRA), Heart Failure Association (HFA), and Heart Rhythm Society (HRS)
Valvular heart disease	2014 AHA/ACC Guideline for the Management of Patients With Valvular Heart Disease 2014	A Report of the American College of Cardiology/ American Heart Association Task Force on Practice Guidelines

TABLE A.2 Diagnostic Testing

	Guideline/Year	Source
12-Lead ECG	Assessment of the 12-Lead Electrocardiogram as a Screening Test for Detection of Cardiovascular Disease in Healthy General Populations of Young People (12–25 Years of Age) **2014**	A Scientific Statement From the American Heart Association and the American College of Cardiology
	ACC/AHA Clinical Competence Statement on Electrocardiography and Ambulatory Electrocardiography **2001**	A Report of the ACC/AHA/ACP-ASIM Task Force on Clinical Competence (ACC/AHA Committee to Develop a Clinical Competence Statement on Electrocardiography and Ambulatory Electrocardiography, Endorsed by the International Society for Holter and Noninvasive Electrocardiology)
	ACC/AHA Guidelines for Ambulatory Electrocardiography **1999**	A Report of the American College of Cardiology/ American Heart Association Task Force on Practice Guidelines (Committee to Revise the Guidelines for Ambulatory Electrocardiography)
	AHA/ACCF/HRS Recommendation for the Standardization and Interpretation of the Electrocardiogram **2007–2009**	Scientific Statements From the American Heart Association Electrocardiography and Arrhythmias Committee, Council on Clinical Cardiology, the American College of Cardiology Foundation, and the Heart Rhythm Society, Endorsed by the International Society for Computerized Electrocardiology
Advanced imaging (cardiac CT and MRI)	ACCF/ACR/AHA/NASCI/SAIP/ SCAI/SCCT 2010 Expert Consensus Document on Coronary Computed Tomographic Angiography **2010**	A Report of the American College of Cardiology Foundation Task Force on Expert Consensus Documents
	Safety of Magnetic Resonance Imaging in Patients With Cardiovascular Devices **2007**	An American Heart Association Scientific Statement From the Committee on Diagnostic and Interventional Cardiac Catheterization, Council on Clinical Cardiology, and the Council on Cardiovascular Radiology and Intervention
	ACCF/SCCT/ACR/AHA/ASE/ ASNC/NASCI/SCAI/SCMR 2010 Appropriate Use Criteria for Cardiac Computed Tomography **2010**	A Report of the American College of Cardiology Foundation Appropriate Use Criteria Task Force, the Society of Cardiovascular Computed Tomography, the American College of Radiology, the American Heart Association, the American Society of Echocardiography, the American Society of Nuclear Cardiology, the North American Society for Cardiovascular Imaging, the Society for Cardiovascular Angiography and Interventions, and the Society for Cardiovascular Magnetic Resonance
	ACCF/ACR/AHA/NASCI/SCMR 2010 Expert Consensus Document on Cardiovascular Magnetic Resonance **2010**	A Report of the American College of Cardiology Foundation Task Force on Expert Consensus Documents

(continued)

TABLE A.2 Diagnostic Testing (*continued*)

	Guideline/Year	Source
	Appropriateness Criteria for Cardiac Computed Tomography and Cardiac Magnetic Resonance Imaging **2006**	A Report of the American College of Cardiology Foundation Quality Strategic Directions Committee Appropriateness Criteria Working Group, American College of Radiology, Society of Cardiovascular Computed Tomography, Society for Cardiovascular Magnetic Resonance, American Society of Nuclear Cardiology, North American Society for Cardiac Imaging, Society for Cardiovascular Angiography and Interventions, and Society of Interventional Radiology
	Appropriate Utilization of Cardiovascular Imaging in Heart Failure **2013**	A Joint Report of the American College of Radiology Appropriateness Criteria Committee and the American College of Cardiology Foundation Appropriate Use Criteria Task Force
	2013 Appropriate Utilization of Cardiovascular Imaging **2013**	A Methodology for the Development of Joint Criteria for the Appropriate Utilization of Cardiovascular Imaging by the American College of Cardiology Foundation and American College of Radiology
Cardiac catheterization	ACCF/SCAI/AATS/AHA/ASE/ASNC/HFSA/HRS/SCCM/SCCT/SCMR/STS 2012 Appropriate Use Criteria for Diagnostic Catheterization **2012**	A Report of the American College of Cardiology Foundation Appropriate Use Criteria Task Force, Society for Cardiovascular Angiography and Interventions, American Association for Thoracic Surgery, American Heart Association, American Society of Echocardiography, American Society of Nuclear Cardiology, Heart Failure Society of America, Heart Rhythm Society, Society of Critical Care Medicine, Society of Cardiovascular Computed Tomography, Society for Cardiovascular Magnetic Resonance, and Society of Thoracic Surgeons
Cardiopulmonary exercise testing	Clinician's Guide to Cardiopulmonary Exercise Testing in Adults **2010**	Scientific Statement From the American Heart Association
Cardiovascular risk assessment	Assessment of Cardiovascular Risk in Asymptomatic Adults **2010**	A Report of the American College of Cardiology Foundation/American Heart Association Task Force on Practice Guidelines Developed in Collaboration With the American Society of Echocardiography, American Society of Nuclear Cardiology, Society of Atherosclerosis Imaging and Prevention, Society for Cardiovascular Angiography and Interventions, Society of Cardiovascular Computed Tomography, and Society for Cardiovascular Magnetic Resonance
	2013 Guideline on the Assessment of Cardiovascular Risk **2013**	A Report of the American College of Cardiology/American Heart Association Task Force on Practice Guidelines
	Lifestyle Management to Reduce Cardiovascular Risk **2013**	A Report of the American College of Cardiology/American Heart Association Task Force on Practice Guidelines

(*continued*)

TABLE A.2 Diagnostic Testing (*continued*)

	Guideline/Year	Source
	AHA/ACCF Secondary Prevention and Risk Reduction Therapy for Patients With Coronary and Other Atherosclerotic Vascular Disease: 2011 Update **2011**	A Guideline From the American Heart Association and American College of Cardiology Foundation
Cardiovascular technology	2013 ACCF Appropriate Use Criteria Methodology Update **2013**	A Report of the American College of Cardiology Foundation Appropriate Use Criteria Task Force
Carotid intima-media thickness	Consensus Statement From the American Society of Echocardiography Carotid Intima-Media Thickness Task Force **2008**	American Society of Echocardiography, Endorsed by the Society for Vascular Medicine
Echocardiogram	American College of Cardiology/ American Heart Association Clinical Competence Statement on Echocardiography **2003**	A Report of the American College of Cardiology/ American Heart Association/American College of Physicians—American Society of Internal Medicine Task Force on Clinical Competence
	Guidelines for Performing a Comprehensive Transesophageal Echocardiographic Examination **2013**	Recommendations From the American Society of Echocardiography and the Society of Cardiovascular Anesthesiologists
	2011 Appropriate Use Criteria for Echocardiography **2011**	A Report of the American College of Cardiology Foundation Appropriate Use Criteria Task Force, American Society of Echocardiography, American Heart Association, American Society of Nuclear Cardiology, Heart Failure Society of America, Heart Rhythm Society, Society for Cardiovascular Angiography and Interventions, Society of Critical Care Medicine, Society of Cardiovascular Computed Tomography, and Society for Cardiovascular Magnetic Resonance *Endorsed by the American College of Chest Physicians*
	ACCF/ASE/ACEP/AHA/ASNC/ SCAI/SCCT/SCMR 2008 Appropriateness Criteria for Stress Echocardiography **2008**	A Report of the American College of Cardiology Foundation Appropriateness Criteria Task Force, American Society of Echocardiography, American College of Emergency Physicians, American Heart Association, American Society of Nuclear Cardiology, Society for Cardiovascular Angiography and Interventions, Society of Cardiovascular Computed Tomography, and Society for Cardiovascular Magnetic Resonance
Electrocardio-graphy	ACC/AHA Guidelines for Ambulatory Electrocardiography **1999**	A Report of the American College of Cardiology/ American Heart Association Task Force on Practice Guidelines (Committee to Revise the Guidelines for Ambulatory Electrocardiography. Developed in Collaboration With the North American Society for Pacing and Electrophysiology)

(*continued*)

TABLE A.2 Diagnostic Testing (*continued*)

	Guideline/Year	Source
	ACC/AHA Clinical Competence Statement on Electrocardiography and Ambulatory Electrocardiography **2001**	A Report of the ACC/AHA/ACP-ASIM Task Force on Clinical Competence (ACC/AHA Committee to Develop a Clinical Competence Statement on Electrocardiograph and Ambulatory Electrocardiography)
	Recommendation for the Standardization and Interpretation of the Electrocardiogram **2007**	A Scientific Statement From the American Heart Association Electrocardiography and Arrhythmias Committee, Council on Clinical Cardiology; the American College of Cardiology Foundation; and the Heart Rhythm Society
	Guidelines for Electrocardiography **1992**	A Report of the American College of Cardiology/ American Heart Association Task Force on Assessment of Diagnostic and Therapeutic Cardiovascular Procedures (Committee on Electrocardiography)
Electrophysiology studies	American College of Cardiology/ American Heart Association Clinical Competence Statement on Invasive Electrophysiology Studies, Catheter Ablation, and Cardioversion **2000**	A Report of the American College of Cardiology/ American Heart Association/American College of Physicians-American Society of Internal Medicine Task Force on Clinical Competence
	HRS/EHRA Expert Consensus Statement on the State of Genetic Testing for the Channelopathies and Cardiomyopathies **2011**	Partnership Between the Heart Rhythm Society (HRS) and the European Heart Rhythm Association (EHRA)
Exercise stress testing	Clinician's Guide to Cardiopulmonary Exercise Testing in Adults A Scientific Statement From the American Heart Association **2010**	On Behalf of the American Heart Association Exercise, Cardiac Rehabilitation, and Prevention Committee of the Council on Clinical Cardiology; Council on Epidemiology and Prevention; Council on Peripheral Vascular Disease; and Interdisciplinary Council on Quality of Care and Outcomes Research
	ACC/AHA Guideline Update for Exercise Testing **2002**	A Report of the American College of Cardiology/ American Heart Association Task Force on Practice Guidelines (Committee on Exercise Testing)
Implantable loop recorder	ACC/AHA Guidelines for Ambulatory Electrocardiography: Executive Summary and Recommendations **1999**	A Report of the American College of Cardiology/ American Heart Association Task Force on Practice Guidelines (Committee to Revise the Guidelines for Ambulatory Electrocardiography) Developed in Collaboration With the North American Society for Pacing and Electrophysiology

(*continued*)

TABLE A.2 Diagnostic Testing (*continued*)

	Guideline/Year	Source
Nuclear stress imaging	Appropriate Use Criteria for Cardiac Radionuclide Imaging **2009**	A Report of the American College of Cardiology Foundation Appropriate Use Criteria Task Force, the American Society of Nuclear Cardiology, the American College of Radiology, the American Heart Association, the American Society of Echocardiography, the Society of Cardiovascular Computed Tomography, the Society for Cardiovascular Magnetic Resonance, and the Society of Nuclear Medicine Endorsed by the American College of Emergency Physicians
Peripheral vascular ultrasound	ACCF/ACR/AIUM/ASE/ASN/ICAVL/SCAI/SCCT/SIR/SVM/SVS/SVU 2012 Appropriate Use Criteria for Peripheral Vascular Ultrasound and Physiological Testing **2012**	A Report of the American College of Cardiology Foundation Appropriate Use Criteria Task Force, American College of Radiology, American Institute of Ultrasound in Medicine, American Society of Echocardiography, American Society of Nephrology, Intersocietal Commission for the Accreditation of Vascular Laboratories, Society for Cardiovascular Angiography and Interventions, Society of Cardiovascular Computed Tomography, Society for Interventional Radiology, Society for Vascular Medicine, Society for Vascular Surgery, and Society for Vascular Ultrasound

TABLE A.3 Therapeutic Interventions

	Guideline/Year	Source
Advanced cardiac life support	2010 American Heart Association Guidelines for Cardiopulmonary Resuscitation and Emergency Cardiovascular Care Science, Part 8: Adult Advanced Cardiovascular Life Support 2010	2010 American Heart Association Guidelines for Cardiopulmonary Resuscitation and Emergency Cardiovascular Care
Cardiovascular implantable electronic devices	2012 ACCF/AHA/HRS Focused Update of the 2008 Guidelines for Device-Based Therapy of Cardiac Rhythm Abnormalities 2012	A Report of the American College of Cardiology Foundation/American Heart Association Task Force on Practice Guidelines and the Heart Rhythm Society
	HRS/ACC/AHA Expert Consensus Statement on the Use of Implantable Cardioverter-Defibrillator Therapy in Patients Who Are Not Included or Not Well Represented in Clinical Trials 2014	Heart Rhythm Society, American College of Cardiology, American Heart Association Expert Consensus Statement
	Appropriate Use Criteria for Implantable Cardioverter-Defibrillators and Cardiac Resynchronization Therapy 2013	A Report of the American College of Cardiology Foundation Appropriate Use Criteria Task Force, Heart Rhythm Society, American Heart Association, American Society of Echocardiography, Heart Failure Society of America, Society for Cardiovascular Angiography and Interventions, Society of Cardiovascular Computed Tomography, and Society for Cardiovascular Magnetic Resonance
	Update on Cardiovascular Implantable Electronic Device Infections and Their Management 2010	A Scientific Statement From the American Heart Association
Lifestyle interventions	2013 AHA/ACC/TOS Guideline for the Management of Overweight and Obesity in Adults 2014	A Report of the American College of Cardiology/American Heart Association Task Force on Practice Guidelines and the Obesity Society
	2013 AHA/ACC Guideline on Lifestyle Management to Reduce Cardiovascular Risk 2013	A Report of the American College of Cardiology/American Heart Association Task Force on Practice Guidelines
	Implementing American Heart Association Pediatric and Adult Nutrition Guidelines 2009	A Scientific Statement From the American Heart Association Nutrition Committee of the Council on Nutrition, Physical Activity and Metabolism, Council on Cardiovascular Disease in the Young, Council on Arteriosclerosis, Thrombosis and Vascular Biology, Council on Cardiovascular Nursing, Council on Epidemiology and Prevention, and Council for High Blood Pressure Research

(continued)

TABLE A.3 Therapeutic Interventions (*continued*)

	Guideline/Year	Source
	Interventions to Promote Physical Activity and Dietary Lifestyle Changes for Cardiovascular Risk Factor Reduction in Adults **2010**	A Scientific Statement From the American Heart Association
	Tobacco Control Interventions in the Emergency Department **2006**	A Joint Statement of Emergency Medicine Organizations
Coronary revascularization	2011 ACC/AHA/SCAI 2005 Guideline for Percutaneous Coronary Intervention **2011**	A Report of the American College of Cardiology Foundation/American Heart Association Task Force on Practice Guidelines and the Society for Cardiovascular Angiography and Intervention
	SCAI/ACC/AHA 2014 Update on Percutaneous Coronary Intervention Without On-Site Surgical Backup **2014**	SCAI/ACC/AHA Expert Consensus Document
	Appropriate Use Criteria for Coronary Revascularization Focused Update **2012**	A Report of the American College of Cardiology Foundation Appropriate Use Criteria Task Force, Society for Cardiovascular Angiography and Interventions, Society of Thoracic Surgeons, American Association for Thoracic Surgery, American Heart Association, American Society of Nuclear Cardiology, and the Society of Cardiovascular Computed Tomography

TABLE A.4 Pharmacological Therapy

	Guideline/Year	Source
Angiotensin-converting enzyme inhibitors	Angiotensin-Converting Enzyme Inhibitor-Induced Cough: ACCP Evidence-Based Clinical Practice Guidelines 2006	ACCPA Evidence-Based Clinical Practice Guidelines
Antiarrhythmics	ACC/AHA/ESC Guidelines for the Management of Patients With Atrial Fibrillation: Executive Summary 2001	A Report of the American College of Cardiology/American Heart Association Task Force on Practice Guidelines and the European Society of Cardiology Committee for Practice Guidelines and Policy Conferences (Committee to Develop Guidelines for the Management of Patients With Atrial Fibrillation)
Anticoagulants and antithrombotics	Guide to Anticoagulant Therapy: Heparin 2001	A Statement for Health care Professionals From the American Heart Association
	Antithrombotic Therapy 2012	Antithrombotic Therapy and Prevention of Thrombosis, 9th ed: American College of Chest Physicians Evidence-Based Clinical Practice Guidelines
Antiplatelets	ACCF/ACG/AHA 2008 Expert Consensus Document on Reducing the Gastrointestinal Risks of Antiplatelet Therapy and NSAID Use 2008	A Report of the American College of Cardiology Foundation Task Force on Clinical Expert Consensus Documents
Fibrinolytics/thrombolytics	Clinical Policy: Indications for Reperfusion Therapy in Emergency Department Patients With Suspected Acute Myocardial Infarction 2006	American College of Emergency Physicians Clinical Policies Subcommittee (Writing Committee) on Reperfusion Therapy in Emergency Department Patients With Suspected Acute Myocardial Infarction
	2013 ACCF/AHA Guideline for the Management of ST-Elevation Myocardial Infarction 2013	A Report of the American College of Cardiology Foundation/American Heart Association Task Force on Practice Guidelines

TABLE A.5 Additional Topics

	Guideline/Year	Source
Cardiovascular risk assessment	Assessment of Cardiovascular Risk in Asymptomatic Adults 2010	A Report of the American College of Cardiology Foundation/American Heart Association Task Force on Practice Guidelines Developed in Collaboration With the American Society of Echocardiography, American Society of Nuclear Cardiology, Society of Atherosclerosis Imaging and Prevention, Society for Cardiovascular Angiography and Interventions, Society of Cardiovascular Computed Tomography, and Society for Cardiovascular Magnetic Resonance
	2013 Guideline on the Assessment of Cardiovascular Risk 2013	A Report of the American College of Cardiology/American Heart Association Task Force on Practice Guidelines
	Lifestyle Management to Reduce Cardiovascular Risk 2013	A Report of the American College of Cardiology/American Heart Association Task Force on Practice Guidelines
	AHA/ACCF Secondary Prevention and Risk Reduction Therapy for Patients With Coronary and Other Atherosclerotic Vascular Disease: 2011 Update 2011	A Guideline From the American Heart Association and American College of Cardiology Foundation
Preoperative and perioperative cardiovascular evaluation	2014 ACC/AHA Guideline on Perioperative Cardiovascular Evaluation and Management of Patients Undergoing Noncardiac Surgery 2014	A Report of the American College of Cardiology/American Heart Association Task Force on Practice Guidelines
	ACR Appropriateness Criteria® Routine Admission and Preoperative Chest Radiography 2011	American College of Radiology (ACR)
	Guidelines for Performing a Comprehensive Transesophageal Echocardiographic Examination 2013	Recommendations From the American Society of Echocardiography and the Society of Cardiovascular Anesthesiologists
	Practice Guidelines for Perioperative Transesophageal Echocardiography 2010	An Updated Report by the American Society of Anesthesiologists and the Society of Cardiovascular Anesthesiologists Task Force on Transesophageal Echocardiography
	The Heart Rhythm Society (HRS)/American Society of Anesthesiologists (ASA) Expert Consensus Statement on the Perioperative Management of Patients With Implantable Defibrillators, Pacemakers and Arrhythmia Monitors: Facilities and Patient Management 2011	American Society of Anesthesiologists (ASA), and in Collaboration With the American Heart Association (AHA), and the Society of Thoracic Surgeons (STS)
Women and cardiovascular disease	Effectiveness-Based Guidelines for the Prevention of Cardiovascular Disease in Women—2011 Update 2011	A Guideline From the American Heart Association

Section References

SECTION I

Agency of Healthcare Research and Quality (AHRQ). (2014). About TeamSTEPPS. Retrieved from http://teamstepps.ahrq.gov/

American Heart Association. (2012). *Lifestyle changes for heart failure.* Retrieved from http://www.heart.org/HEARTORG/Conditions/HeartFailure/PreventionTreatmentofHeart Failure/Lifestyle-Changes-for-Heart-Failure_UCM_306341_Article.jsp

American Heart Association. (2014). *Alcohol and heart health.* Retrieved from http://www .heart.org/HEARTORG/GettingHealthy/NutritionCenter/HealthyEating/Alcohol-and-Heart-Health_UCM_305173_Article.jsp

American Society of Anesthesiologists. (2014). ASA physical status classification system. Retrieved from http://www.asahq.org/For-Members/Clinical-Information/ASA-Phy sical-Status-Classification-System.aspx. Accessed June 16, 2014. Permission obtained from the ASA June 17, 2014.

American Society of Anesthesiologists Task Force. (2005). Practice advisory for the perioperative management of patients with cardiac rhythm management devices: Pacemakers and implantable cardioverter-defibrillators. *Anesthesiology, 103*(1), 186–189.

Archer, C., Levy, A. R., & McGregor, M. (1993). Value of routine preoperative chest x-rays: A meta-analysis. *Canadian Journal of Anaesthesia, 40,* 1022–1027.

Barash, P. G., Cullen, B. F., Stoelting, R. K., Cahalan, M. K., Stock, M. C., & Ortega, R. (2013). *Clinical anesthesia* (7th ed.). Philadelphia, PA: Wolters Kluwer.

Barbeau, G. R., Arsenault, F., Dugas, L., Simard, S., & Lariviere, M. M. (2004). Evaluation of the ulnopalmar arterial arches with pulse oximetry and plethysmography: Comparison with the Allen's test in 1010 patients. *American Heart Journal, 147*(3), 489–493.

Barnes, P. M., Bloom B., & Nahin, R. L. (2008). Complementary and alternative medicine use among adults and children: United States, 2007. *National Health Statistics Reports, 12,* 1–24.

Baumann, M. H., & Sahn, S. A. (1992). Hamman's sign revisited. Pneumothorax or pneumo-mediastinum? *Chest, 102*(4), 1281–1282.

Beutler, E., & Waalen, J. (2006). The definition of anemia: What is the lower limit of normal of the blood hemoglobin concentration? *Blood, 107*(5), 1747–1750.

Biancaniello, T. (2005). Innocent murmurs. *Circulation, 111,* e20–e22.

Bickley, L. S., & Szilagyi, P. G. (2008). *Bates' guide to physical examination and history taking* (10th ed.). Philadelphia, PA: Lippincott Williams & Wilkins.

Boersma, E., Kertai, M. D., Schouten, O., Bax, J. J., Noordzij, P., Steyerberg, E. W., . . . Poldermans, D. (2005). Perioperative cardiovascular mortality in noncardiac surgery: Validation of the Lee cardiac risk index. *The American Journal of Medicine, 118,* 1134–1141.

Bonnema, R. A., McNamara, M. C., & Spencer, A. L. (2010). Contraception choices in women with underlying medical conditions. *American Family Physician, 82*(6), 621–628.

Bonow, R. O., Mann, D. L., Zipes, D. P., & Libby, P. (2012). *Braunwald's heart disease: A textbook of cardiovascular medicine* (9th ed.). Philadelphia, PA: Saunders Elsevier.

Bosner, S., Beckera, A., Hania, M. A., Kellera, H., Sonnichsen, A. C., Konstantinos, K., . . . Donner-Banzhoff, N. (2010). Chest wall syndrome in primary care patients with chest pain: Presentation, associated features and diagnosis. *Family Practice, 27,* 363–369.

Botto, F., Alonso-Coello, P., Chan, M. T., Villar, J. C., Xavier, D., Srinathan, S., . . . Wildes, T. (2014). Myocardial injury after noncardiac surgery: A large, international, prospective cohort study establishing diagnostic criteria, characteristics, predictors, and 30-day outcomes. *Anesthesiology, 120*(3), 564–578.

Brinds, R., Rodgers, G. P., & Hanberg, E. M. (2011). President's page: Team-based care: A solution for our health care delivery challenges. *Journal of American College of Cardiology, 57*(9), 1123–1125.

Burger, W., Chemnitius, J. M., Kneissl, G. D., & Rucker, G. (2005). Low-dose aspirin for secondary cardiovascular prevention: Cardiovascular risks after its perioperative withdrawal versus bleeding risks with its continuation: Review and meta-analysis. *Journal of Internal Medicine, 257,* 399–414.

Carson, J. L., Grossman, B. J., Kleinman, S., Tinmouth, A. T., Marques, M. B., Fung, M. K., . . . Djulbegovic, B. (2012). Red blood cell transfusion: A clinical practice guideline from the AABB. *Annals of Internal Medicine, 157,* 49–58.

Centers for Disease Control and Prevention (CDC). (2010). *Occupational heart disease.* Retrieved from http://www.cdc.gov/niosh/topics/heartdisease

Centers for Disease Control and Prevention (CDC). (2012). Community Preventive Services Task Force. Cardiovascular disease prevention: Team-based care to improve blood pressure control. Task Force findings and rationale statement. April 2012. Retrieved from http://www.thecommunityguide.org/cvd/RRteambasedcare.html

Centers for Medicare & Medicaid Services (CMS). (2010). *Evaluation and management services guide.* Retrieved from http://www.cms.gov/Outreach-and-Education/Medicare-Learning-Network-MLN/MLNProducts/downloads/eval_mgmt_serv_guide-ICN006764.pdf

Chizner, M. A. (2002). The diagnosis of heart disease by clinical assessment alone. *Disease-a-Month, 48*(1), 7–98.

Cole, S. A., & Bird, J. (2014). *The medical interview* (3rd ed.). Philadelphia, PA: Elsevier Saunders.

Dahlin, C. (Ed.). (2013). *Clinical practice guidelines for quality palliative care* (3rd ed.). Pittsburgh, PA: National Consensus Project for Quality Palliative Care, http://www.nationalconsensusproject.org

Dardiotis, E., Giamouzis, G., Mastrogiannis, D., Vogiatzi, C., Skoularigis, J., Triposkiadis, F., & Hadjigeorgiou, G. M. (2012). Cognitive impairment in heart failure. *Cardiology Research and Practice,* 1–9. doi:10.1155/2012/595821

Deakin, C. D., & Low, J. L. (2000). Accuracy of the advanced trauma life support guidelines for predicting systolic blood pressure using carotid, femoral, and radial pulses: Observational study. *The British Medical Journal, 321*(7262), 673–674.

Department of Health and Human Services, Centers for Medicare & Medicaid Services. (2010). CMS—billing and coding—Evaluation and Management Services Guide.

Devereaux, P. J., Chan, M. T., Alonso-Coello, P., Walsh, M., Berwanger, O., Villar, J. C., . . . Yusuf, S. (2012). Association between postoperative troponin levels and 30-day mortality among patients undergoing noncardiac surgery. *Journal of the American Medical Association, 307,* 2295–2304.

Devereaux, P. J., Xavier, D., Pogue, J., Guyatt, G., Sigmani, A., Garutti, I., . . . Yusuf, S. (2011). Characteristics and short-term prognosis of perioperative myocardial infarction in patients undergoing non-cardiac surgery: A cohort study. *Annals of Internal Medicine, 154,* 523–528.

Devereaux, P. J., Yang, H., Yusuf, S., Guyatt, G., Kate, L., Villar, J. C., & Choi, P. (2008). Effects of extended-release metoprolol succinate in patients undergoing non-cardiac surgery (poise trial): A randomized controlled trial. *The Lancet, 371,* 1839–1846. doi:10.1016/S0140-6736(08)60601-7

Donati, A., Ruzzi, M., Adrario, K., Pelaia, F., Coluzzi, F., Gabbanelli, V., & Pietropaoli, P. (2004). A new and feasible model for predicting operative risk. *The British Journal of Anaesthesia, 93*(3), 393–399.

Ewing, J. A. (1984). Detecting alcoholism. The CAGE questionnaire. *Journal of the American Medical Association, 252*(14), 1905–1907.

Feely, M. A., Collins, S., Daniels, P. R., Kebede, E. B., Jatoi, A., & Mauck, K. F. (2013). Preoperative testing before noncardiac surgery: Guidelines and recommendations. *American Family Physician, 87*, 414–418.

Fisher, S. P., Bader, A., & Sweitzer, B. (2010). Preoperative evaluation. In R. D. Miller (Ed.), *Miller's anesthesia* (pp. 1001–1066). Philadelphia, PA: Churchill Livingstone Elsevier.

Fleisher et al. (2007). ACC/AHA 2007 guidelines on perioperative cardiovascular evaluation and care for noncardiac surgery.

Fleisher, L. A., Fleischmann, K. E., Auerbach, A. D., Barnason, S. A., Beckman, J. A., Bozkurt, B., . . . Wijeysundera, D. N. (2014). ACC/AHA guideline on perioperative cardiovascular evaluation and management of patients undergoing noncardiac surgery. *Journal of the American College of Cardiology, 130*. doi:10. 1016/j.jacc.2014.07.944

Fleischmann, K. E., Beckman, J. A., Buller, C. E., Calkins, H., Fleisher, L. A., Freeman, W. K., . . . Valentine, R. J. (2009). 2009 ACCF/AHA focused update on perioperative beta blockade. *Journal of the American College of Cardiology, 54*(22), 2017. doi:10.1016/j.jacc.2009.07.004

Flu, W. J., Van Kuijk, J. P., Hoeks, S., Bax, J. J., & Poldermans, D. (2010). Preoperative evaluation of patients with possible coronary artery disease. *Current Cardiology Reports, 12*, 286–294.

Freeman, R., Wieling, W., Axelrod, F. B., Benditt, D. G., Benarroch, E., Biaggioni, I., . . . van Dijk, J. G. (2011). Consensus statement on the definition of orthostatic hypotension, neutrally mediated syncope and the postural tachycardia syndrome. *Clinical Autonomic Research, 21*, 69–72.

Freeman, W. K., & Gibbons, R. J. (2009). Perioperative cardiovascular assessment of patients undergoing noncardiac surgery. *Mayo Clinic Proceedings, 84*(1), 79–80.

Frisch, A., Chandra, P., Smiley, D., Peng, L., Rizzo, M., Gatcliffe, C., . . . Umpierrez, G. E. (2010). Prevalence and clinical outcome of hyperglycemia in the perioperative period in noncardiac surgery. *Diabetes Care, 33*(8), 1783–1788.

Garrow, J. S., & Webster, J. (1985). Quetelet's index (W/H2) as a measure of fatness. *International Journal of Obesity, 9*, 147–153.

Gibbons, R. J., Balady, G. J., Beasley, J. W., Bricker, J. T., Durvernoy, W. F., Froelicher, V. F., . . . Yanowitz, F. G. (1997). ACC/AHA guidelines for exercise testing: Executive Summary. A report of the American College of Cardiology/American Heart Association Task Force on Practice Guidelines (Committee on Exercise Testing). *Circulation, 96*(1), 345–354.

Giles, T. G., Martinez, E. C., & Burch, G. C. (1974). Gallavardin phenomenon in aortic stenosis: A possible mechanism. *Archives of Internal Medicine, 134*(4), 747–749. doi:10.1001/archinte.1974.00320220149021

Goldman, L. (2013). The revised cardiac risk index delivers what it promised. *Annals of Internal Medicine, 152*(1), 57–58.

Goldman, L., Caldera, D. L., Nussbaum, S. R., Southwick, F. S., Krogstad, D., Murray, B., . . . Slater, E. E. (1977). Multifactorial index of cardiac risk in noncardiac surgical procedures. *The New England Journal of Medicine, 297*, 845–850.

Gorelick, P. B., Scuteri, A., Black, S. E., DeCarli, C., Greenberg, S. M., Iadecola, C., . . . Seshadri, S. (2011). Vascular contributions to cognitive impairment and dementia: A statement for health care professionals from the American Heart Association/American Stroke Association. *Stroke, 42*, 2672–2713.

Grocott, M. P., Mythen, M. G., & Gan, T. J. (2005). Perioperative fluid management and clinical outcomes in adults. *Anesthesia and Analgesia, 100*(4), 1093–1106.

Gupta, P. K., Gupta, H., Sundaram, A., Kaushik, M., Fang, X., Miller, W. J., . . . Mooss, A. N. (2011). Development and validation of a risk calculator for prediction of cardiac risk after surgery. *Circulation, 124*, 381–387. Retrieved from http://www.qxmd.com/calculate-online/cardiology/gupta-perioperative-cardiac-risk

Gurudevan, S. V., Nelson, M. D., Rader, F., Tang, X., Lewis, J., Johannes, J., . . . Victor, R. G. (2013). Cocaine-induced vasoconstriction in the human coronary microcirculation: New evidence from myocardial contrast echocardiography. *Circulation, 128*, 598–604.

Hata, T. M., & Hata, J. S. (2013). Preanesthetic evaluation and preparation. In P. G. Barash, B. F. Cullen, R. K. Stoelting, M. K. Cahalan, M. C. Stock, & R. Ortega (Eds.), *Clinical anesthesia* (pp. 589–590, 897). Philadelphia, PA: Wolters Kluwer.

Health Resources and Services Administration (HRSA). (2012). U.S. Department of Health and Human Services, Bureau of Health Professions, Coordinating Center for Interprofessional Education and Collaborative Practice. Funding Opportunity Announcement, HRSA-12-184.

Helfrich, C. D., Dolan, E. D., Simonetti, J., Joos, S., Wakefield, B. J., Stark, R., & Fihn, S. D. (2014). Elements of team-based care in a patient-centered medical home are associated with lower burnout among VA primary care employees. *Journal of General Internal Medicine.* Retrieved from http://www.ncbi.nlm.nih.gov/pubmed/24715396

Hill, E. (2011). E/M coding and the documentation guidelines: Putting it all together. *Family Practice Management, 18*(5), 33–38.

Hlatky, M. A., Boineau, R. E., Higginbotham, M. B., Lee, K. L., Mark, D. B., Califf, R. M., . . . Pryor, D. B. (1989). A brief self-administered questionnaire to determine functional capacity (the Duke Activity Status Index). *The American Journal of Cardiology, 64*, 651–654.

Holler, T. (2008). *Cardiology essentials.* Sudbury, MA: Jones and Bartlett.

Hung, Y., Lin, S., Hung, S., Huang, W., & Wang, P. (2012). Preventing radiocontrast-induced nephropathy in chronic kidney disease patients undergoing coronary angiography. *World Journal of Cardiology, 4*(5), 157–172.

Institute of Healthcare Improvement (IHI). (2014). The IHI triple aim initiative. Retrieved from http://www.ihi.org/Engage/Initiatives/TripleAim/Pages/default.aspx

Institute of Medicine (IOM). (1999). *To err is human: Building a safer health system.* Retrieved from http://www.nap.edu/catalog/9728/to-err-is-human-building-a-safer-health-system

Institute of Medicine (IOM). (2001). *Crossing the quality chasm: A new health system for the 21st century.* Retrieved from http://www.iom.edu/Reports/2001/Crossing-the-Quality-Chasm-A-New-Health-System-for-the-21st-Century.aspx

Institute of Medicine (IOM). (2010). *The future of nursing: Leading change, advancing health.* Retrieved from http://books.nap.edu/openbook.php?record_id=12956&page=R1

Institute of Medicine (IOM). (2012). *Best care at lower cost: Path to continuous learning health care in America.* Retrieved from http://www.nap.edu/catalog/13444/best-care-at-lower-cost-the-path-to-continuously-learning

Jaarsma, T. (2005). Interprofessional team approach to patients with heart failure. *Heart, 91*(6), 832–838.

James, P. A., Oparil, S., Carter, B. L., Cushman, W. C., Dennison-Himmelfarb, C., Handler, J., . . . Ortiz, E. (2014). 2014 Evidence-based guideline for the management of high blood pressure in adults. *Journal of the American Medical Association, 311*(5), 507–520.

Jaroszewski, D., Notrica, D., McMahon, L., Steidley, D. E., & Deschamps, C. (2010). Current management of pectus excavatum: A review and update of therapy and treatment options. *Journal of the American Board of Family Medicine, 23*(2), 230–239.

Johansson, T., Fritsch, G., Flamm, M., Hansbauer, B., Bachofner, N., Mann, E., & Sönnichsen, A. C. (2013). Effectiveness of non-cardiac preoperative testing in non-cardiac elective surgery: A systematic review. *British Journal of Anaesthesia, 110*, 926–939.

Joy, B. F., Elliot, E., Hardy, C., Sullivan, C., Backer, C. L., & Kane, J. M. (2011). Standardized multidisciplinary protocol improves handover of cardiac surgery patients to the intensive care unit. *Pediatric Critical Care Medicine, 12*(3), 204–208.

Kertai, M. D., Boersma, E., Bax, J. J., Heijenbrok-Kal, M. H., Hunink, M. G., L'talien, G. J., . . . Roelandt, J. R. (2003). A meta-analysis comparing the prognostic accuracy of six diagnostic tests for predicting perioperative cardiac risk in patients undergoing major vascular surgery. *Heart, 89*(11), 1327–1334.

Khandaker, M. H., Espinosa, R. E., Nishimura, R. A., Sinak, L. J., Hayes, S. N., Melduni, R. M., . . . Oh, J. K. (2010). Pericardial disease: Diagnosis and management. *Mayo Clinical Proceedings, 85*(6), 572–593.

Lee, T. H., Marcantonio, E. R., Mangione, C. M., Thomas, E. J., Polanczyk, C. A., Cook, E. F., . . . Goldman, L. (1999). Derivation and prospective validation of a simple index for prediction of cardiac risk of major noncardiac surgery. *Circulation, 100,* 1043–1049.

Levine, B. S. (2010). History taking and physical examination. In S. A. Woods, E. S. S. Froclicher, S. U. Motzer, & E. J. Bridges (Eds.), *Cardiac nursing* (6th ed., pp. 211–244). Philadelphia, PA: Wolters Kluwer Health.

Levine, G. N., Steinke, E. E., Bakaeen, F. G., Bozkurt, B., Cheitlin, M. D., Conti, J. B., . . . Stewart, W. J.; on behalf of the American Heart Association Council on Clinical Cardiology, Council on Cardiovascular Nursing, Council on Cardiovascular Surgery and Anesthesia, and Council on Quality of Care and Outcomes Research. (2012). Sexual activity and cardiovascular disease: A scientific statement from the American Heart Association. *Circulation, 125,* 1058–1072.

Levinson, D. C., Meehan, J. P., Schwartz, L. H., & Griffith, G. C. (1956). Graphic registration of cardiac thrills in acquired and congenital heart disease. *Circulation, 14,* 784–789.

Lindenauer, P. K., Pekow, P., Wang, K., Gutierrez, B., & Benjamin, E. M. (2004). Lipid-lowering therapy and in-hospital mortality following major noncardiac surgery. *JAMA, 291,* 2092–2099.

Lobo, D. N., Macafee, D. A., & Allison, S. P. (2006). How perioperative fluid balance influences postoperative outcomes. *Best Practice & Research Clinical Anesthesiology, 20*(3), 439–455.

Lotrionte, M., Biondi-Zoccai, G., Abbate, A., Lansetta, G., D'Ascenzo, F., Malavasi, V., . . . Palazzoni, G. (2013). Review and meta-analysis of incidence and clinical predictors of anthracycline cardiotoxicity. *The American Journal of Cardiology, 112,* 1980–1984.

Lyznicki, J. M., Nielsen, N. H., & Schneider, J. F. (2000). Cardiovascular screening of student athletes. *The American Family Physician, 62*(4), 765–774.

Mangano, D. T. (1990). Perioperative cardiac morbidity. *Anesthesiology, 72,* 153–184.

Marley, R. A., Calabrese, T., & Thompson, K. J. (2014). Preoperative evaluation and preparation of the patient. In J. J. Nagelhout & K. Plaus (Eds.), *Nurse anesthesia* (5th ed., pp. 332–352). St. Louis, MO: Saunders Elsevier.

Mason, J. M., Freemantle, N., Gibson, J. M., & New, J. P. (2005). Specialist nurse-led clinics to improve control of hypertension and hyperlipidemia in diabetes: Economic analysis of the SPLINT trial. *Diabetes Care, 28*(1), 40–46.

McAlister, F. A., Stewart, S., Ferrua, S., & McMurray, J. J. J. V. (2004). Multidisciplinary strategies for the management of heart failure patients at high risk for admission. *Journal of the American College of Cardiology, 44,* 810–819.

Mei, Z., Grummer-Strawn, L. M., Pietrobelli, A., Goulding, A., Goran, M. I., & Dietz, W. H. (2002). Validity of body mass index compared with other body-composition screening indexes for the assessment of body fatness in children and adolescents. *The American Journal of Clinical Nutrition, 7597*–7985.

Mills, E., Eyawo, O., Lockhart, I., Kelly, S., Wu, P., & Ebbert, J. O. (2011). Smoking cessation reduces postoperative complications: A systematic review and meta-analysis. *The American Journal of Medicine, 124*(2), 144–154.

Moore, K. J. (2010). Documenting history in compliance with Medicare's guidelines. *Family Practice Management, 17*(2), 22–27.

Mosca, L., Benjamin, E. J., Berra, K., Bezanson, J. L., Dolor, R. J., Lloyd-Jones, D. M., . . . Wenger, N. K. (2011). Effectiveness-based guidelines for the prevention of cardiovascular disease in women—2011 update: A guideline from the American Heart Association. *Circulation, 123,* 1243–1262.

National Center for Interprofessional Practice and Education (NCIPE). (2013). Vision and goals. Retrieved from https://nexusipe.org/funding

National Institute for Occupational Safety and Health. (2013). *Cancer, reproductive, and cardio-vascular disease*. Retrieved from http://www.cdc.gov/niosh/programs/crcd/default.html

Nishimura, R. A., Otto, C. M., Bonow, R. O., Carabello, B. A., Erwin, J. P., Guyton, R. A., . . . Thomas, J. D. (2014). 2014 AHA/ACC guideline for the management of patients with valvular heart disease. *Journal of the American College of Cardiology, 129*(23), 2440–2449. doi:10.1016/j.jacc.2014.02.536

Pacala, J. T. (2012). Promoting quality of life in chronically ill and older people. In P. D. Sloane, L. M. Slatt, M. H. Ebell, M. A. Smith, D. Power, & A. J. Viera (Eds.), *Essentials of family medicine* (pp. 77–86). Philadelphia, PA: Lippincott Williams & Wilkins.

Pandey, A. K., Pandey, S., Blaha, M. J., Agatston, A., Feldman, T., Ozner, M., . . . Nasir, K. (2013). Family history of coronary heart disease and markers of subclinical cardiovascular disease: Where do we stand? *Atherosclerosis, 288*(2), 285–294.

Pape, G. A., Hunt, J. S., Butler, K. L., Stemienczuk, J., LeBlanc B. H., & Gillander, W., . . . Bonin, K. (2011). Team based care approach to cholesterol management in diabetes mellitus: Two-year cluster randomized controlled trial. *Archives Internal Medicine, JAMA Internal Medicine, 171*(16), 1480–1486.

Pickering, T. G., Hall, J. E., Appel, L. J., Falkner, B. E., Graves, J., Hill, M. N. . . . Roccella, E. J. (2005). Recommendations for blood pressure measurement in humans and experimental animals part 1: Blood pressure measurement in humans: A statement for professionals from the subcommittee of professional and public education of the American Heart Association Council on High Blood Pressure Research. *Hypertension, 45*, 142–161.

Poldermans, D., Bax, J. J., Boersma, E., Hert, S. D., Eeckhout, E., Fowkes, G., . . . Tubaro, M. (2009). Guidelines for pre-operative cardiac risk assessment and perioperative cardiac management in non-cardiac surgery. *European Heart Journal, 30*, 2769–2812.

Proulx, A. M., & Zryd, T. W. (2009). Costochondritis: Diagnosis and treatment. *American Family Physician, 80*(6), 617–620.

Puchalski, C., & Romer, A. L. (2000). Taking a spiritual history allows clinicians to understand patients more fully. *Journal of Palliative Medicine, 3*(1), 129–137.

Qaseem, A., Snow, V., Fitterman, N., Hornbake, R., Lawrence, V. A., Smetana, G. W., . . . Owens, D. K. (2006). Risk assessment for and strategies to reduce perioperative pulmonary complications for patients undergoing noncardiothoracic surgery: A guideline from the American College of Physicians. *Annals of Internal Medicine, 114*, 575–580.

Rivin, A. U. (1966). The neck venous hum in adults. *Western Journal of Medicine, California Medicine, 105*(2), 102–103.

Roger, V. L., Go, A. S., Lloyd-Jones, D. M., Benjamin, E. J., Berry, J. D., Borden, W. B., . . . Turner, M. B. (2012). Heart disease and stroke statistics—2012 update: A report from the American Heart Association. *Circulation, 125*, e2–e220.

Roussel, M. G., Gorham, N., Wilson, L., & Mangi, A. A. (2013). Improving recovery time following heart transplantation: The role of the multidisciplinary health care team. *Journal of Multidisciplinary Healthcare, 6*, 293–302.

Rozanski, A., Blumenthal, J. A., Davidson, K. W., Saab, P. G., & Kubzansky, L. (2005). The epidemiology, pathophysiology, and management of psychosocial risk factors in cardiac practice. *Journal of the American College of Cardiology, 45*(5), 637–651.

Sarkar, M., Mahesh, D. M., & Madabhavi, I. (2012). Digital clubbing. *Lung India, 29*(4), 354–362.

Schabelman, E., & Witting, M. (2010). The relationship of radiocontrast, iodine, and seafood allergies: A medical myth exposed. *Journal of Emergency Medicine, 39*(5), 701–707.

Scheie, H. G. (1953). Evaluation of ophthalmoscopic changes of hypertension and arteriolar sclerosis. *AMA Archives of Ophthalmology, 49*(2), 117–138. doi:10.1001/archopht.1953.00920020122001

Schlant, R. C., Adolph, R. J., DiMarco, J. P., Dreifus, L. S., Dunn, M. I., Fisch, C., . . . Murray, J. A. (1992). Guidelines for electrocardiography. *Journal of American College Cardiology, 19*, 473–481.

Seidel, H. M., Ball, J. W., Dains, J. E., Flynn, J. A., Solomon, B. S., & Stewart, R. W. (2011). *Mosby's guide to physical examination* (7th ed.). St. Louis, MO: Mosby Elsevier.

Sharma, U., & Klocke, D. (2014). Attitudes of nursing staff toward interprofessional in-patient-centered rounding. *Journal Interprofessional Care, 28,* 475–477.

Shevchenko, Y. L., & Tsitlik, J. E. (1996). 90th anniversary of the development by Nikolai S. Korotkoff of the ausculatory method of measuring blood pressure. *Circulation, 94,* 116–118.

Shrader, A., & Grigg, C. (2014). Multiple interprofessional education activities delivered longitudinally within a required clinical assessment course. *The American Journal of Pharmaceutical Education, 78,* 1–6.

Silow-Carroll, S., Edward, J. N., & Lashbrook, A. (2011). Reducing hospital readmissions: Lessons from top performing hospitals. The Commonwealth Fund. Retrieved November 4, 2014, from http://www.commonwealthfund.org/~/media/Files/Publications/Case%20Study/2011/Apr/1473_SilowCarroll_readmissions_synthesis_web_version.pdf

Sloane, P. D., Slatt, L. M., Ebell, M. H., Smith, M. A., Power, D., & Viera, A. J. (2012). *Essentials of family medicine* (6th ed.). Philadelphia, PA: Lippincott Williams & Wilkins.

Stevens, R. D., Burri, H., & Tramer, M. R. (2003). Pharmacologic myocardial protection in patients undergoing noncardiac surgery: A quantitative systematic review. *Anesthesia and Analgesia, 97,* 623–633.

Swartz, M. H. (2014). *Textbook of physical diagnosis* (7th ed.). Philadelphia, PA: Elsevier Saunders.

Tachjian, A., Maria, V., & Jahangir, A. (2010). Use of herbal products and potential interactions in patients with cardiovascular disease. *Journal of the American College of Cardiology, 55*(6), 515–525.

UCSF, University of California, San Francisco, School of Nursing. (2014). Science of Caring. Training nurse practitioners and physicians for the next generation of primary care. Retrieved from http://scienceofcaring.ucsf.edu/future-nursing/training-nurse-practitioners-and-physicians-next-generation-primary-care

United States Bureau of the Census. (2008). *Population projections of the United States, by age, sex, race, and Hispanic origin: July 1, 2000–2050.* Washington, DC: Bureau of the Census.

U.S. Preventive Services Task Force. (2013). Screening for intimate partner violence and abuse of elderly and vulnerable adults: Recommendation statement. *Annals of Internal Medicine, 158*(6), 478–486.

Vinik, A. I., Maser, R. E., Mitchell, B. D., & Freeman, R. (2003). Diabetic autonomic neuropathy. *Diabetes Care, 26*(5), 1553–1556.

Wahr, J. A., Parks, R., Boisvert, D., Comunale, M., Fabian, J., Ramsay, J., & Mangano, D. T. (1999). Preoperative serum potassium levels and perioperative outcomes in cardiac surgery patients. *Journal of the American Medical Association, 281*(23), 2203–2210.

Walsh, J., McDonald, K., Shojania, K., Sundaram, V., Nayak, S., Lewis, R., . . . Goldstein, M. K. (2006). Quality improvement strategies for hypertension management: A systematic review. *Medical Care, 44*(7), 646–657.

Wang, S., Xu, L., Jona, J. B., Wang, Y. S., Wang, Y. X., You, Q. S., . . . Zhou, J. Q. (2012). Five year incidence of retinal microvascular abnormalities and associations with arterial hypertension: The Beijing eye study 2001/2006. *Ophthalmology, 119*(12), 2592–2599. doi:10.1016/j.ophtha.2012.06.031

Weber, M. A., Schiffrin, E. L., White, W. B., Mann, S., Lindholm, L. H., Kenerson, J. G., . . . Harrap, S. B. (2013). Clinical practice guidelines for the management of hypertension in the community. *Journal of Clinical Hypertension, 16*(1), 14–26.

Whinney, C. (2009). Perioperative medication management: General principles and practical applications. *Cleveland Clinic Journal of Medicine, 76*(4), 126–128. doi:10.3949/ccjm.76.s4.20

Wijeysundera, D. N., Naik, J. S., & Beattie, W. S. (2003). Alpha-2 adrenergic agonists to prevent perioperative cardiovascular complications: A meta-analysis. *The American Journal of Medicine, 114,* 742–752.

Wikimedia Commons. (2011). Jugular Venous Pressure Waveform. Retrieved from http://upload.wikimedia.org/wikipedia/commons/4/48/Jugular_Venous_Pulse.png By Ecgtocardiology (Own work) [CC BY-SA 3. 0 (http://creativecommons.org/licenses/by-sa/3.0)], via Wikimedia Commons

Wikimedia Commons. (2013). Cardiac cycle vs heart sounds. Anatomy & physiology. Open-Stax College. Retrieved from http://upload.wikimedia.org/wikipedia/commons/f/f3/2029_Cardiac_Cycle_vs_Heart_Sounds.jpg

Willard-Grace, R., Hessler, D., Rogers, E., Dube, K., Bodenheimer, T., & Grumback, K. (2014). Team structure and culture are associated with lower burnout in primary care. *Journal of the American Board of Family Medicine, 27*(2), 229–238.

Wolkove, N., & Baltzan, M. (2009). Amiodarone pulmonary toxicity. *Canadian Respiratory Journal, 16*(2), 43–48.

Wood, D. M., Mould, M. G., Ong, S. B. Y., & Baker, E. H. (2005). "Pack year" smoking histories: What about patients who use loose tobacco? *Tobacco Control, 14*, 141–142.

Woods, S. L., Froelicher, E. S., Motzer, S. A., & Bridges, E. J. (2010). *Cardiac nursing*. Philadelphia, PA: Lippincott Williams & Wilkins.

World Health Organization (WHO). (2010). Framework for action on interprofessional education and collaborative practice. Retrieved from http://www.who.int/hrh/resources/framework_action/en/

World Heart Federation. (2012). *Rheumatic heart disease*. Retrieved from http://www.world-heart-federation.org/fileadmin/user_upload/documents/Fact_sheets/2012/RHD.pdf

Wu, W., Schifftner, T. L., Henderson, W. G., Eaton, C. B., Poses, R. M., Uttley, G., . . . Friedmann, P. D. (2007). Preoperative hematocrit levels and postoperative outcomes in older patients undergoing noncardiac surgery. *Journal of the American Medical Association, 297*(22), 2481–2488.

Yusuf, S. W., Sami, S., & Daher, I. N. (2011). Radiation-induced heart disease: A clinical update. *Cardiology Research and Practice, 2011*, 1–9.

SECTION II

AIM_HIGH Investigators. (2011). Niacin in patients with low HDL cholesterol on intensive statin therapy. *The New England Journal of Medicine, 365*, 2255–2267.

ALLHAT Officers & Coordinators for the ALLHAT Collaborative Research Group. (2002). Major outcomes in high-risk hypertensive patients randomized to angiotensin-converting enzyme inhibitor or calcium channel blocker vs diuretic: The Antihypertensive and Lipid-Lowering Treatment to Prevent Heart Attack (ALLHAT). *Journal of the American Medical Association, 288*(23), 2981–2997.

Amabile, C. M., & Spencer, A. P. (2004). Keeping your patient with heart failure safe: A review of potentially dangerous medications. *Archives of Internal Medicine, 164*(7), 709–720.

American Diabetes Association. (2012). Standards of medical care in diabetes-2012. *Diabetes Care, 35*(1), s11–s64.

American Diabetes Association (ADA). (2014). Standards of medical care in diabetes—2014. *Diabetes Care, 37*, s14–s80.

Anderson, J. W., Hanna, T. J., Peng, X., & Kryscio, R. J. (2000). Whole grain foods and heart disease risk. *Journal of the American College of Nutrition, 19*(Suppl. 3), 291S–299S.

Antithrombotic Trialists' Collaboration. (2002). Collaborative meta-analysis of randomized trials of antiplatelet therapy for prevention of death, myocardial infarction, and stroke in high risk patients. *The British Medical Journal, 324*, 71–86. doi:10/1136/bmj.324.7329.71

Appel, L. J., Champagne, C. M., Harsha, D. W., Cooper, L. S., Obarzaanek, E., Elmer, P. J., . . . Young, D. R. (2003). Effects of comprehensive lifestyle modification on blood pressure control. *Journal of the American Medical Association, 289*(16), 2083–2093.

Arzt, M., Young, T., Finn, L., Skatrud, J. B., Ryan, C. M., Newton, G. E., . . . Bradley, T. D. (2006). Sleepiness and sleep in patients with both systolic heart failure and obstructive sleep apnea. *Archives of Internal Medicine, 166,* 1716–1722.

Baumgartner, H., Hung, J., Bermego, J., Chambers, J. B., Evangelista, A., Griffin, B. P., . . . Quinoses, M. (2009). Echocardiographic assessment of valve stenosis: EAE/ASE recommendations for clinical practice. *Journal of the American Society of Echocardiography, 22,* 1–23.

Ben Farhat, M., Ayari, M., Maatouk, F., Betbout, F., Gamra, H., Jarra, M., . . . Addad, F. (1998). Percutaneous balloon versus surgical closed and open mitral commissurotomy: Seven-year follow-up results of a randomized trial. *Circulation, 97,* 245–250.

Bhatt, D. L., Fox, K. A. A., Hacke, W., Berger, P. B., Black, H. R., Boden, W. E., . . . Topol, E. J. (2006). Clopidogrel and aspirin versus aspirin alone for the prevention of atherothrombotic events. *The New England Journal of Medicine, 354,* 1706–1717.

Bickley, L. S. (2013). Bates' guide to physical exam and history taking (11th ed.). Philadelphia, PA: Lippincott, Wilson & Wilkins.

Blake, G. J., & Ridker, P. M. (2000). Are statins anti-inflammatory? *Current Controlled Trials in Cardiovascular Medicine, 1*(3), 161–165.

Bonow, R. O., Carabello, B. A., Chatterjee, K., de Leon, A. C., Faxon, D. P., Freed, M. D., . . . Shanewise, J. S. (2008). Focused update incorporated into the ACC/AHA 2006 guidelines for the management of patients with valvular heart disease. *Journal of the American College of Cardiology, 52,* e1–e142.

Bonow, R. O., Carabello, B. A., Chatterjee, K., de Leon, A. C., Faxon, D. P., Gasch, W. H., . . . Shanewise, J. S. (2006). ACC/AHA 2006 guidelines for the management of patients with valvular heart disease: A report of the American College of Cardiology/American Heart Association Task Force on Practice Guidelines. *Circulation, 114,* e84–e231.

Bradley, T. D., Logan, A. G., Kimoff, R. J., Senes, F., Morrison, D., Ferguson, K., . . . Floras, J. S. (2005). Continuous positive airway pressure for central sleep apnea and heart failure. *The New England Journal of Medicine, 353,* 2025–2033.

Bristow, M. R., Saxon, L. A., Boehmer, J., Krueger, S., Kass, D. A., . . . Feldman, A. M. (2004). Cardiac resynchronization therapy with or without an implantable defibrillator in advanced chronic heart failure. *The New England Journal of Medicine, 350,* 2140–2150.

Brownlee, M., Aiello, L. P., Cooper, M. E., Vinik, A. I., Nesto, R. W., & Boulton, A. J. (2011). Complications of diabetes mellitus. In S. Melmed, K. S. Polonsky, P. R. Larsen, & H. M. Kronenberg (Eds.), *Williams textbook of endocrinology* (12th ed., pp. 1462–1551). Philadelphia, PA: Elsevier.

Bruckert, E., & Rosenbaum, B. (2011). Lowering LDL-cholesterol through diet: Potential role in the statin era. *Current Opinion in Lipidology, 22*(1), 43–48.

Bursi, F., Weston, S. A., Redfield, M. M., Jacobsen, S. J., Pakhomov, S., . . . Roger, V. L. (2006). Systolic and diastolic heart failure in the community. *Journal of the American Medical Association, 296,* 2209–2216.

Butalia, S., Leung, A. A., Ghali, W. A., & Rabi, D. M. (2011). Aspirin effect on the incidence of major adverse cardiovascular events in patients with diabetes mellitus: A systematic review and meta-analysis. *Cardiovascular Diabetology, 10,* 25.

Campbell, S. C., Moffatt, R. J., & Stamford, B. A. (2008). Smoking and smoking cessation—The relationship between cardiovascular disease and lipoprotein metabolism: A review. *Atherosclerosis, 201*(2), 225–235.

Campeasu, L. (1976). Grading of angina pectoris. *Circulation, 54,* 522–523.

CAPRIE Steering Committee. (1996). A randomized, blinded, trial of clopidogrel versus aspirin in patients at risk of ischaemic events (CAPRIE). *The Lancet, 348*(9038), 1329–1339.

Carabello, B. A., & Paulus, W. K. (2009). Aortic stenosis. *The Lancet, 373*(9680), 2026.

Carapetis, J. R., Steer, A. C., Mulholland, E. K., & Weber, M. (2005). The global burden of group A streptococcal diseases. *The Lancet Infectious Diseases, 5,* 685–694.

Caulfield, M. P., Li, S., Lee, G., Blanche, P. J., Salameh, W. A., Benner, W. H., . . . Krauss, R. M. (2008). Direct determination of lipoprotein particle size and concentrations by ion mobility analysis. *Clinical Chemistry, 54*(8), 1307–1316.

Centers for Disease Control and Prevention (CDC). (2011). National Diabetes Fact Sheet: National estimates and general information on diabetes and prediabetes in the United States, 2011. Atlanta, GA: U.S. Department of Health and Human Services, Centers for Disease Control and Prevention.

Centers for Disease Control and Prevention (CDC). (2013). Number (in Millions) of Civilian, Non-institutionalized Adults with Diagnosed Diabetes, United States, 1980–2011. *Diabetes Public Health Resource*. Retrieved from http://www.cdc.gov/diabetes/statistics/prev/national/figadults.htm

Centers for Medicare & Medicaid Services (CMS). (2013). Decision memo for cardiac rehabilitation (CR) program-chronic heart failure. Retrieved from http://www.cms.gov/medicare-coverage-database/details/nca-decision-memo.aspx?NCAId=270 on May 30, 2014

Cholesterol Treatment Trialists' Collaboration. (2010). Efficacy and safety of more intensive lowering of LDL cholesterol: A meta-analysis of data from 170,000 participants in 26 randomised trials. *The Lancet, 376*(9753). doi:10.1016/S0140-6736(10)61350-5

CIBIS-II Investigators and Committees. (1999). The cardiac insufficiency bisoprolol study II (CIBIS-II): A randomized trial. *The Lancet, 353*, 9–11.

Cleland, J. G. F., Daubert, J. C., Erdmann, E., Freemantle, N., Gras, D., Kappenberger, L., . . . Tavazzi, L. (2005). Cardiac resynchronization-heart failure (CARE-HF) study investigators: The effect of cardiac resynchronization on morbidity and mortality in heart failure. *The New England Journal of Medicine, 352*, 1539–1549J.

Clopidogrel in Unstable Angina to Prevent Recurrent Events Trial Investigators. (2001). Effects of clopidogrel in addition to aspirin in patients with acute coronary syndromes without ST-segment elevation. *The New England Journal of Medicine, 345*, 494–502. doi:10.1056/NEJMoa010746

Constantino, M. I., Molyneaux, L., Limacher-Gisler, F., Al-Saeed, A., Luo, C., Wu, T., . . . Wong, J. (2013). Long term complications and morality in young onset diabetes: Type 2 diabetes is more hazardous and lethal than type 1 diabetes. *Diabetes Care, 36*(12), 3863–3869.

Corrado, D., Thiene, G., Cocco, P., & Frescura, C. (1992). Non-atherosclerotic coronary artery disease and sudden death in the young. *The British Heart Journal, 68*(6), 601–607.

Cuchel, M., Meagher, E. A., du Toit Theron, H., Blom, D. J., Marais, A. D., Hegele, R. A., . . . Rader, D. J. (2013). Efficacy and safety of a microsomal triglyceride transfer protein inhibitor in patients with homozygous familial hypercholesterolaemia: A single-arm, open-label, phase 3 study. *The Lancet, 381*(9860), 40–46.

Cui, J., Hopper, J. L., & Harrap, S. B. (2002). Genes and family environment explain correlations between blood pressure and body mass index. *Hypertension, 40*, 7–12.

Dailey, G. (2011). Early and intensive therapy for management of hyperglycemia and cardiovascular risk factors in patients with type 2 diabetes. *Clinical Therapeutics, 33*(6), 665–678.

Davidson, M. H., Ballantyne, C. M., Jacobson, T. A., Bittner, V. A., Braun, L. T., Brown, A. S., . . . Ziajka, P. E. (2011). Clinical utility of inflammatory markers and advanced lipoprotein testing: Advice from an expert panel of lipid specialist. *Journal of Clinical Lipidology, 5*, 338–367.

Davies, S. W. (2001). Clinical presentation and diagnosis of coronary artery disease: Stable angina. *The British Medical Bulletin, 59*(1), 17–27.

Deng, M. C., Edwards, L. B., Hertz, M. I., Rowe, A. W., Keck, B. M., Kormos, R., . . . Kirklin, J. (2005). Mechanical circulatory support device database of the International Society for Heart and Lung Transplantation: Third annual report. *Journal of Heart and Lung Transplant, 24*, 1182–1187.

Diaz, A., Bourassa, M. G., Guertin, M. C., & Tardif, J. C. (2005). Long term prognostic value of resting heart rate in patients with suspected or proven coronary artery disease. *European Heart Journal, 26*, 967–974.

Domanski, M. J. (2000). Beta-blocker evaluation of survival trial (BEST) (abstract). *Journal of the American College of Cardiology, 35*, 202A.

Dormandy, J. A., Charbonnel, B., Eckland, D. J., Erdmann, E., Massi-Benedetti, M., Moules, I. K., . . . Taton, J., the PROactive investigators. (2005). Secondary prevention of macro-vascular events in patients with type 2 diabetes in the PROactive Study (PROspective pioglitAzone Clinical Trial In macroVascular Events): A randomised controlled trial. *The Lancet, 366*(9493), 1279–1289.

Duckworth, W., Abraira, C., Moritz, T., Reda, D., Emanuele, N., Reaven, P. D., . . . Huang, G. D., the VADT Investigators. (2009). Glucose control and vascular complications in veterans with type 2 diabetes. *The New England Journal of Medicine, 360*(2), 129–139.

Eckel, R. H., Jakicic, J. M., Ard, J. D., de Jesus, J. M., Houston Miller, N., Hubbard, V. S., . . . American College of Cardiology/American Heart Association Task Force on Practice Guidelines. (2013). 2013 AHA/ACC guideline on lifestyle management to reduce car-diovascular risk: A report of the American College of Cardiology/American Heart Association Task Force on Practice Guidelines. *Journal of the American College of Cardiol-ogy, 63*(25 Pt B), 2960–2984.

Egan, B. M., Li, J., Qanugo, S., & Wolfman, T. (2014). Blood pressure and cholesterol control in hypertensive hypercholesterolemic patients: National health and nutrition examina-tion surveys 1988–2010. *Circulation, 128*(1), 29–41.

Eichhorn, E. J., & Bristow, M. R. (2001). The carvedilol prospective randomized cumulative survival (COPERNICUS) trial. *Current Control Trials in Cardiovascular Medicine, 2*(1), 20–23.

Elkayam, U., Amin, J., Mehra, A., Vasquez, J., Weber, L., & Rahimtoola, S. H. (1990). A pro-spective, randomized, double-blind, crossover study to compare the efficacy and safety of chronic nifedipine therapy with that of isosorbide dinitrate and their combination in treatment of chronic congestive heart failure. *Circulation, 82*(6), 1954–1956.

Evangelista, A., Tornos, P., Sambola, A., Permanyer-Miralda, G., & Soler-Soler, J. (2005). Long-term vasodilatory therapy in patients with severe aortic regurgitation. *The New England Journal of Medicine, 353*(13), 1342–1349.

Evangelista, L. S., Doering, L. V., & Dracup, K. (2000). Usefulness of a history of tobacco and alcohol use in predicting multiple heart failure readmissions among veterans. *The American Journal of Cardiology, 86*(12), 1339–1342.

Feldman, T. (2014). 2014 Hot topic: Rollout of the mitraclip. Retrieved from http://www.cardiosource.org/Science-And-Quality/Hot-Topics/2014/03/Rollout-of-the-MitraClip.aspx?w_nav=Search&WT.oss=mitraclip&WT.oss_r=109&

Feldman, T., Wasserman, H. S., Herrmann, H. C., Gray, W., Block, P. C., . . . Foster, E. (2005). Percutaneous mitral valve repair using the edge-to-edge technique: Six-month results of the EVEREST phase I clinical trial. *Journal of the American College of Cardiology, 46*, 2134–2140.

Festa, A., Hanley, A. J., Tracy, R. P., D'Agostino, R., Jr., & Haffner, S. M. (2003). Inflammation in the prediabetic state is related to increased insulin resistance rather than decreased insulin secretion. *Circulation, 108*(15), 1822–1830.

Fihn, S. D., Blankenship, J. C., Alexander, K. P., Bittle, J. A., Byrne, J. G., Fletcher, B. J., . . . Smith, P. K. (2014). 2014 ACC/AHA/AATS/PCNA/SCAI/STS focused update of the guideline for the diagnosis and management of patients with stable ischemic heart disease. *Journal of the American College of Cardiology*. doi:10.1016/j.jacc.2014.07.017

Fihn, S. D., Gardin, J. M., Abrams, J., Berra, K., Blankenship, J. C., Dallas, A. P., . . . Williams, S. V. (2012). 2012 ACCF/AHA/ACP/AATS/PCNA/SCAI/STS guideline for the diag-nosis and management of patients with stable ischemic heart disease. *Journal of the American College of Cardiology, 60*(24), e44–e164.

Fonarow, G. C., Albert, N. M., Curtis, A. B., Stough, W. G., Gheorghiade, M., Heywood, J. T., . . . Yancy, C. W. (2010). Improving evidence-based care for heart failure in outpatient cardi-ology practices: Primary results of the registry to improve the use of evidence-based heart failure therapies in the outpatient setting (IMPROVE HF). *Circulation, 122*, 585–596.

Fonarow, G. C., Stevenson, L., Walden, J. A., Livingston, N. A., Steimle, A. E., Hamilton, M. A., . . . Woo, M. A. (1997). Impact of a comprehensive heart failure management program on hospital readmissions and functional status of patients with advanced heart failure. *Journal of the American College of Cardiology, 30*(3), 725–732.

Food & Drug Administration. (2012). FDA drug safety communication: Important safety label changes to cholesterol-lowering statin drugs. Retrieved from www.fda.gov

Foreman, R. D., Linderoth, B., Ardell, J. L., Barron, K. W., Chandler, M. J., Hull, S. S., . . . Armour, J. A. (2000). Modulation of intrinsic cardiac neurons by spinal cord stimulation: Implications for its therapeutic use in angina pectoris. *Cardiovascular Research, 47*(2), 367–375.

Fox, C. S., Coady, S., Sorlie, P. D., D'Agostino, R. B., Pencina, M. J., Ramachandran, S. V., . . . Savage, P. J. (2007). Increasing cardiovascular disease burden due to diabetes mellitus: The Framingham heart study. *Circulation, 115,* 1544–1550.

Franceschini, N., & Le, T. H. (2014). Genetics of hypertension: Discoveries from the bench to human populations. *The American Journal of Physiology, 306*(1), f1–f11.

Freed, L. A., Levy, D., Levine, R. A., Larson, M. G., Evans, J. C., Fuller, D. L., . . . Benjamin, E. J. (1999). Prevalence and clinical outcomes of mitral valve prolapse. *The New England Journal of Medicine, 341,* 1–7.

Gaudet, D., Kereiakes, D. J., McKenney, J. M., Roth, E. M., Hanotin, C., Gipe, D., . . . Stein, E. A. (2014). Effect of alirocumab, a monoclonal proprotein convertase sustilisen/kexin 9 antibody, on lipoprotein(a) concentrations (a pooled analysis of 150 mg every two weeks dosing from Phase 2 trial). *The American Journal of Cardiology, 114*(5), 711–715.

Gerstein, H. C., Miller, M. E., Byington, R. P., Goff, D. C., Jr., Bigger, J. T., Buse, J. B., . . . Action to Control Cardiovascular Risk in Diabetes Study Group. (2008). Effects of intensive glucose lowering in type 2 diabetes. *The New England Journal of Medicine, 358*(24), 2545–2559.

Go, A. S., Mozaffarian, D., Roger, V. L., Benjamin, E. J., Berry, J. D., Blaha, M. J., . . . American Heart Association Statistics Committee and Stroke Statistics Subcommittee. (2014). Heart disease and stroke statistics–2014 update: A report from the American Heart Association. *Circulation, 129*(3), e28–e292.

Go, A. S., Mozaffarian, D., Roger, V. L., Benjamin, E. J., Berry, J. D., Borden, W. B., . . . Turner, M. B. (2013). Heart disease and stroke statistics—2013 update: A report from the American Heart Association. *Circulation, 127,* e6–e245.

Goff, D. C., Lloyd-Jones, D. M., Bennett, G., Coady, S., D'Agostino, R. B., Gibbons, R., . . . Wilson, P. W. F. (2013). 2013 ACC/AHA guideline on the assessment of cardiovascular risk. *Circulation, 129*(Suppl. 2), s49–s73.

Grines, C. L., Bonow, R. O., Casey, D. E., Gardner, T. J., Lockhart, P. B., Moliterno, D. J., . . . Whitlow, P. (2007). Prevention of premature discontinuation of dual antiplatelet therapy in patients with coronary artery stents. *Circulation, 115*(6), 813.

Gylling, H., Plat, J., Turley, H. N., Ellegard, L., Jessup, W., . . . the European Atherosclerosis Society Consensus Panel on Phytosterols. (2014). Plant sterols and plant stanols in the management of dyslipidaemia and prevention of cardiovascular disease. *Atherosclerosis, 232*(2), 236–260.

Haffner, S. M., Lehto, S., Ronnemaa, T., Pyorala, K., & Laakso, M. (1998). Mortality from coronary heart disease in subjects with type 2 diabetes and in nondiabetic subjects with and without prior myocardial infarction. *The New England Journal of Medicine, 339,* 229–234.

Hallikainen, M., Sinonen, P., & Gylling, H. (2014). Cholesterol metabolism and serum non-cholesterol sterols: Summary of 13 plant stanol ester interventions. *Lipids in Health and Disease, 13,* 72–79.

Hannan, E. L., Wu, C., Bennet, E. V., Carlson, R. E., Culliford, A. T., Gold, J. P., . . . Jones, R. H. (2006). Risk stratification of in-hospital mortality for coronary artery bypass graft surgery. *Journal of the American College of Cardiology, 47,* 661–668.

Hansson, G. K. (2005). Inflammation, atherosclerosis, and coronary artery disease. *The New England Journal of Medicine, 352*(16), 1685–1695.

Hauptman, P. J. (2008). Medication adherence in heart failure. *Heart Failure Review, 13,* 99–106.

Hayek, E., Gring, C. N., & Griffin, B. P. (2005). Mitral valve prolapse. *The Lancet, 365,* 507–518.

He, F. J., Li, J., & Macgregor, G. A. (2013). Effects of longer-term modest salt reduction on blood pressure. *Cochrane Database of Systematic Reviews.* doi:10.1002/14651858 .CD004937.pub2

Heart Protection Study Collaborative Group. (2002). MRC/BHF Heart Protection Study of cholesterol lowering with simvastatin in 20,536 high-risk individuals: A randomised placebo-controlled trial. *The Lancet, 360*(9326), 7–22.

Heidenreich, P. A., McDonald, K. M., Hastie, T., Fadel, B., Hagen, V., Lee, B. K., & Hlatky, M. A. (1999). Meta-analysis of trials comparing beta blockers, calcium antagonists, and nitrates for stable angina. *Journal of the American Medical Association, 281*(20), 1927–1936.

Heidenreich, P. A., Trogdon, J. G., Khavjou, O. A., Butler, J., Dracup, K., Ezekowitz, M. D., . . . American Heart Association Advocacy Coordinating Committee, Stroke Council, Council on Cardiovascular Radiology and Intervention, Council on Clinical Cardiology, Council on Epidemiology and Prevention, Council on Arteriosclerosis, Thrombosis and Vascular Biology, Council on Cardiopulmonary, Critical Care, Perioperative and Resuscitation, Council on Cardiovascular Nursing, Council on the Kidney in Cardiovascular Disease, Council on Cardiovascular Surgery and Anesthesia, and Interdisciplinary Council on Quality of Care and Outcomes Research. (2011). Forecasting the future of cardiovascular disease in the United States: A policy statement from the American Heart Association. *Circulation, 123*(8), 933–944.

Hemmingsen, B., Christensen, L. L., Wetterslev, J., Vaag, A., Gluud, C., Lund, S. S., & Almdal, T. (2012). Comparison of metformin and insulin versus insulin alone for type 2 diabetes: Systematic review of randomised clinical trials with meta-analyses and trial sequential analyses. *The British Medical Journal, 344,* 1–19.

Henderson, B., Csordas, A., Backovic, A., Kind, M., Bernhard, D., & Wick, G. (2008). Cigarette smoke is an endothelial stressor and leads to cell cycle arrest. *Atherosclerosis, 201*(2), 298–305.

Henkin, Y., Shai, I., Zuk, R., Brickner, D., Zuilli, I., Neumann, L., & Shany, S. (2000). Dietary treatment of hypercholesterolemia: Do dietitians do it better? A randomized, controlled trial. *The American Journal of Medicine, 109*(7), 549–555.

Hjalmarson, A., Goldstein, S., Fagerberg, B., Wedel, H., Waagstein, F., . . . Deedwania, P. (2000). Effects of controlled-release metoprolol on total mortality, hospitalizations, and well-being in patients with heart failure: The metoprolol CR/XL randomized intervention trial in congestive heart failure (MERIT-HF). *Journal of the American Medical Association, 8*(283), 1295–1302.

Home, P. D., Pocock, S. J., Beck-Nielsen, H., Curtis, P. S., Gomis, R., Hanefeld, M., . . . the RECORD Study Team. (2009). Rosiglitazone evaluated for cardiovascular outcomes in oral agent combination therapy for type 2 diabetes (RECORD): A multicentre, randomised, open-label trial. *The Lancet, 373*(9681), 2125–2135.

HPS2-THRIVE Collaborative Group. (2014). Effects of extended-release niacin with laropiprant in high risk patients. *The New England Journal of Medicine, 371*(3), 203–212.

Huynh, Q. L., Reid, C. M., Chowdhury, E. K., Hug, M. M., Billah, B., Wing, L. M., . . . Nelson, M. R. (2014). Prediction of cardiovascular and all-cause mortality at 10 years in the hypertensive aged population. *The American Journal of Hypertension.* doi:10.1093/ajh/hpu213

IDEAL Study Group. (2005). High-dose atorvastatin vs usual-dose simvastatin for secondary prevention after myocardial infarction, the IDEAL study: A randomized controlled trial. *Journal of the American Medical Association, 294*(19), 2437–2445.

Institute of Medicine. (2013). *Sodium intake in populations: Assessment of evidence.* Washington, DC: The National Academies Press.

Isaacs, A. J., Critchley, J. A., Tai, S. S., Buckingham, K., Westley, D., Harridge, S. D., . . . Gottlieb, J. M. (2007). Exercise Evaluation Randomised Trial (EXERT): A randomised trial comparing GP referral for leisure centre-based exercise, community-based walking and advice only. *Health Technology Assessment, 11*(10), 1–165, iii–iv.

Jaarsma, T., Stromberg, A., Martensson, J., & Dracup, K. (2003). Development and testing of the European heart failure self-care behavior scale. *The European Journal of Heart Failure, 5,* 363–370.

Jaeger, B. R., Richter, Y., Nagel, D., Heigl, F., Vogt, A., Roeseler, E., . . . Seidel, D. (2009). Longitudinal cohort study on the effectiveness of lipid apheresis treatment to reduce high lipoprotein(a) levels and prevent major adverse coronary events. *Nature Clinical Practice. Cardiovascular Medicine, 6*(3), 229–239.

James, P. A., Oparil, S., Carter, B. L., Cushman, W. C., Dennison-Himmelfarb, C., & Handler, J. (2014). 2014 Evidence-based guideline for the management of high blood pressure in adults report from the panel members appointed to the Eighth Joint National Committee (JNC 8). *Journal of the American Medical Association, 311*(5), 507–520.

Jamil, H., Dickson, J. K., Jr., Chu, C. H., Lago, M. W., Rinehart, J. K., Biller, S. A., . . . Wetterau, J. R. (1995). Microsomal triglyceride transfer protein: Specificity of lipid binding and transport. *Journal of Biological Chemistry, 270*(12), 6549–6554.

Jerling, M., & Abdallah, H. (2005). Effects of renal impairment on multiple-dose pharmacokinetics of extended-release ranolazine. *Clinical Pharmacology and Therapeutics, 78*(3), 288–297.

Joint National Committee. (2003). *The seventh report of the Joint National Committee on prevention, detection, evaluation and treatment of high blood pressure.* National Institutes of Health, National Heart, Lung, and Blood Institute. Washington, DC: Author.

Jouven, X., Empana, J. P., Schwartz, P. J., Desnos, M., Courbon, D., & Ducimetiere, P. (2005). Heart-rate profile during exercise as a predictor of sudden death. *The New England Journal of Medicine, 352*(19), 1951–1958.

Kaneko, Y., Floras, J. S., Usui, K., Plante, J., Tkacova, R., Kubo, T., . . . Bradley, T. D. (2003). Cardiovascular effects of continuous positive airway pressure in patients with heart failure and obstructive sleep apnea. *The New England Journal of Medicine, 348,* 1233–1241.

Kastelein, J. J., Sager, P. T., de Groot, E., & Veltri, E. (2005). Comparison of ezetimibe plus simvastatin versus simvastatin monotherapy on atherosclerosis progression in familial hypercholesterolemia. Design and rationale of the Ezetimibe and Simvastatin in Hypercholesterolemia Enhances Atherosclerosis Regression (ENHANCE) trial. *American Heart Journal, 149*(2), 234–239.

Kernis, S. J., Harjai, K. J., Stone, G. W., Grines, L. L., Boura, J. A., O'Neill, W. W., & Grines, C. L. (2004). Does beta-blocker therapy improve clinical outcomes of acute myocardial infarction after successful primary angioplasty? *Journal of the American College of Cardiology, 43*(10), 1773–1779.

Klingbeil, A. U., Schneider, M., Martus, P., Messerli, F. H., & Schmieder, R. E. (2003). A meta-analysis of the effects of treatment on left ventricular mass in essential hypertension. *The American Journal of Medicine, 115*(1), 41–46.

Kochanek, K. D., Xu, J. Q., Murphy, S. L., Minino, A. M., & Kung, H. C. (2011). Deaths: Final data for 2009. *National Vital Statistics Report, 60*(3). Retrieved from http://www.cdc.gov

Komajda, M., Carson, P. E., Hetzel, S., McKelvie, R., McMurray, J., Ptaszynska, A., . . . Massie, B. M. (2011). Factors associated with outcome in heart failure with preserved ejection fraction findings from the irbesartan in heart failure with preserved ejection fraction study (I-PRESERVE). *Circulation, 4,* 27–35. doi:10.1161/CIRCHEARTFAILURE.109.932996

Kontos, M. C., Diercks, D. B., & Kirk, J. D. (2010). Emergency department and office based evaluation of patients with chest pain. *Mayo Clinic Proceedings, 85*(2), 284–299.

Krumholz, H. M., Amatruda, J., Smith, G. L., Mattera, J. A., Roumanis, S. A., Radford, M. J., . . . Vaccarino, V. (2002). Randomized trial of an education and support intervention to prevent readmission of patients with heart failure. *Journal of the American College of Cardiology, 39*(1), 83–89.

Kühnast, S., van der Hoorn, J. W., Pieterman, E. J., van den Hoek, A. M., Sasiela, W. J., Gusarova, V., . . . Princen, H. M. (2014). Alirocumab inhibits atherosclerosis, improves the plaque morphology, and enhances the effects of a statin. *Journal of Lipid Research*, 55(10), 2103–2112.

Kumbhani, D. (2011). Prospective randomized On-X anticoagulation clinical trial: Reduced anticoagulation for a mechanical heart valve. Retrieved from http://www.cardiosource .org/Science-And-Quality/Clinical-Trials/P/PROACT.aspx?w_nav=Search&WT.oss= valve%20anticoagulation&WT.oss_r=1247&

Kwak, S. M., Myung, S. K., Lee, Y. J., & Seo, H. G., the Korean Meta-Analysis Study Group. (2012). Efficacy of omega-3 fatty acid supplements (eicosapentaenoic acid and docosahexaenoic acid) in the secondary prevention of cardiovascular disease: A meta-analysis of randomized, double-blind, placebo-controlled trials. *Archives of Internal Medicine*, 172(9), 686–694.

Lane, R. E., Cowie, M. R., & Chow, A. W. C. (2005). Prediction and prevention of sudden cardiac death in heart failure. *Heart*, 91, 674–680.

Latini, R., Masson, S., Anand, I., Salio, M., Hester, A., Judd, D., . . . Cohn, J. N. (2004). The comparative prognostic value of plasma neurohormones at baseline in patients with heart failure enrolled in Val-HeFT. *European Heart Journal*, 25, 292–299.

Leon, M. B., Smith, C. R., Mack, M., Miller, C., Moses, J. W., Svensson, L. G., . . . Pocock, S. (2010). Transcatheter aortic-valve implantation for aortic stenosis in patients who cannot undergo surgery. *The New England Journal of Medicine*, 363(17), 1597–1607.

Levy, W. C., Mozaffarian, D., Linker, D. T., Sutradhar, S. C., Anker, S. D., Cropp, A. B., . . . Packer, M. (2006). Heart failure: The Seattle Heart Failure Model. *Circulation*, 113, 1424–1433. doi:10.1161/CIRCULATIONAHA.105.584102

Lieberman, E. B., Bashore, T. M., Hermiller, J. B., Willson, J. S., Pieper, K. S., Keeler, G. P., . . . Davidson, C. J. (1995). Balloon aortic valvuloplasty in adults: Failure of procedure to improve long-term survival. *Journal of the American College of Cardiology*, 26(6), 1522–1528.

Lietz, K., Long, J. W., Kfoury, A. G., Slaughter, M. S., Silver, M. A., Milano, C. A., . . . Miller, L. W. (2007). Outcomes of left ventricular assist device implantation as destination therapy in the Post-REMATCH era. *Circulation*, 116, 497–505.

Lilja, J. J., Kivistö, K. T., & Neuvonen, P. J. (2000). Duration of effect of grapefruit juice on the pharmacokinetics of the CYP 3A4 substrate simvastatin. *Clinical Pharmacology and Therapeutics*, 68(4), 384–390.

Lim, S., Kar, S., Fail, P., Whisenant, B., Gray, W., Bajwa, T., . . . Feldman, T. (2013). The EVEREST II high surgical risk cohort: Effectiveness of transcatheter reduction of significant mitral regurgitation in high surgical risk patients (abstr). *Journal of the American College of Cardiology*, 61, e1958.

Lindenfeld, J., Albert, N. M., Boehmer, J. P., Collins, S. P., Ezekowitz, J. A., Givertz, M. M., . . . Walsh, M. N. (2010). Executive summary: HFSA 2010 comprehensive heart failure practice guideline. *Journal of Cardiac Failure*, 16(6), 475–539.

Long, E. F., Swain, G. W., & Mangi, A. A. (2014). Comparative survival and cost effectiveness of advanced therapies for end-stage heart failure. *Circulation: Heart Failure*. doi:10.1161/ circheartfailure.113.000807

Mackey, R. H., Greenland, P., Goff, D. C., Lloyd-Jones, D., Sibley, C. T., & Mora, S. (2012). High-density lipoprotein cholesterol and particle concentrations, carotid atherosclerosis and coronary events: The multi-ethnic study of atherosclerosis. *Journal of the American College of Cardiology*, 60(6), 508–516.

MADIT Executive Committee. (1991). Multicenter Automatic Defibrillator Implantation Trial (MADIT): Design and clinical protocol. *Pacing and Clinical Electrophysiology*, 14, 920–927.

Mancia, G., Fagard, R., Narkiewicz, K., Redon, J., Zanchetti, A., Bohm, M., . . . Wood, D. A. (2013). 2013 ESH/ESC guidelines for the management of arterial hypertension: The

Task Force for the Management of Arterial Hypertension of the European Society of Hypertension and the European Society of Cardiology. *European Heart Journal, 34*(28), 2159–2219.

Mann, D. L., McMurray, J. J., Packer, M., Swedberg, K., Borer, J. S., Colucci, W. S., . . . Fleming, T. (2004). Targeted anticytokine therapy in patients with chronic heart failure: Results of the Randomized Etanercept Worldwide Evaluation (RENEWAL). *Circulation, 109*(13), 1594–1602.

Mann, D. L., Zipes, D. P., Libby, P., & Bonow, R. O. (2015). *Braunwald's heart disease: A textbook of cardiovascular medicine* (100th ed.). Philadelphia, PA: Elsevier.

Mansfield, D. R., Gollogly, N. C., Kaye, D. M., Richardson, M., Bergin, P., & Naughton, M. T. (2004). Controlled trial of continuous positive airway pressure in obstructive sleep apnea and heart failure. *The American Journal of Respiratory Critical Care Medicine, 169*, 361–366.

Mant, J., Doust, J., Roalfe, A., Barton, P., Cowie, M. R., Glasziou, P., . . . Hobbs, F. D. (2009). Systematic review and individual patient data meta-analysis of diagnosis of heart failure, with modelling of implications of different diagnostic strategies in primary care. *Health Technology Assessment, 13*(32). doi:10.3310/hta13320

Marks, A. R., Choong, C. Y., Sanfilippo, A. J., Ferre, M., & Weyman, A. E. (1985). Identification of high-risk and low-risk subgroups of patients with mitral-valve prolapse. *The New England Journal of Medicine, 320*, 1031–1036.

McAlister, F. A., Stewart, S., Ferrua, S., & McMurray, J. (2004). Multidisciplinary strategies for the management of heart failure patients at high risk for admission. *Journal of the American College of Cardiology, 44*(4), 810–819.

McKee, P. A., Casteilli, W. P., McNamara, P. M., & Kannel., W. B. (1971). The natural history of congestive heart failure: The Framingham study. *The New England Journal of Medicine, 285*(26), 1441–1446.

McVeigh, G. E., Gibson, W., & Hamilton, P. K. (2013). Cardiovascular risk in young type 1 diabetes population with a low 10-year, but high lifetime risk of cardiovascular disease. *Diabetes, Obesity, & Metabolism, 15*(3), 198–203.

Mendis, S., Puska, P., & Norrving, B. (Eds.). (2011). *Global atlas on cardiovascular disease prevention and control*. Geneva, Switzerland: World Health Organization.

Mestroni, L., Maisch, B., McKenna, W. J., Schwartz, K., Charron, P., Rocco, C., . . . Komajda, M. (1999). Guidelines for the study of familial dilated cardiomyopathies. *European Heart Journal, 20*, 93–102.

Metlay, J. P., Hennessy, S., Localio, A. R., Han, X., Yang, W., Cohen, A., . . . Strom, B. L. (2008). Patient reported receipt of medication instructions for warfarin is associated with reduced risk of serious bleeding events. *Journal of General Internal Medicine, 23*(10), 1589.

Michalsen, A., Konig, G., & Thimme, W. (1998). Preventable causative factors leading to hospital admission with decompensated heart failure. *Heart, 80*, 437–441.

Monmeneu, M. J. V., Marin, O. F., Reyes, G. F., Torrent, J. A., Martinez, G. M., . . . deBurgos de Rico, G. E. (2002). Beta-blockade and exercise capacity in patients with mitral stenosis in sinus rhythm. *Journal of Heart Valve Disease, 11*, 199–203.

Moran, A., Katz, R., Smith, N. L., Fried, L. F., Sarnak, M. J., Seliger, S. L., . . . Shlipak, M. G. (2008). Cystatin c concentration as a predictor of systolic and diastolic heart failure. *Journal of Cardiac Failure, 14*(1), 19–26.

Morrow, D. A., Scirica, B. M., Karwatowska-Prokopczuk, E., Murphy, S. A., Budaj, A., Barshavsky, S., . . . Braunwald, E. (2007). Effects of ranolazine on recurrent cardiovascular events in patients with non-ST-elevation acute coronary syndromes: The MERLIN-TIMI 36 randomized trial. *Journal of the American Medical Association, 297*(16), 1775–1783.

Moss, A. J., Hall, W. J., Cannom, D. S., Daubert, J. P., Higgins, S. L., Klein, H., . . . Heo, M. (1996). Improved survival with an implanted defibrillator in patients with coronary disease at high risk for ventricular arrhythmia. Multicenter automatic defibrillator implantation trial investigators. *The New England Journal of Medicine, 335*, 1933–1940.

Mozaffarian, D., Nye, R., & Levy, W. C. (2003). Anemia predicts mortality in severe heart failure: The Prospective Randomized Amlodipine Survival Evaluation (PRAISE). *Journal of the American College of Cardiology, 41*, 1933–1939.

Muntner, P., Levitan, E. B., Brown, T. M., Sharma, P., Zhao, H., Bittner, V., . . . Rosenson, R. S. (2013). Trends in the prevalence, awareness, treatment and control of high low density lipoprotein-cholesterol among United States adults from 1999–2000 through 2009–2010. *The American Journal of Cardiology, 112*(5), 664–670.

Musunuru, K., Orho-Melander, M., Caulfield, M. P., Li, S., Salameh, W. A., Reitz, R. E., . . . Krauss, R. M. (2009). Ion mobility analysis of lipoprotein subfractions identifies three independent axes of cardiovascular risk. *Arteriosclerosis, Thrombosis, and Vascular Biology, 29*(11), 1975–1980.

National Cholesterol Education Program (NCEP). (2002). Adult Treatment Panel III: Detection, evaluation, and treatment of high blood cholesterol in adults. *National Institutes of Health: National Heart, Lungs, and Blood Institute.* Retrieved from www.nhlbi.nih.gov

Nauck, M., Frid, A., Hermansen, K., Shah, N. S., Tankova, T., Mitha, I. H., . . . Matthews, D. R.; the LEAD-2 Study Group. (2009). Efficacy and safety comparison of Liraglutide, Glimepiride, and Placebo, all in combination with metformin, in type 2 diabetes: The LEAD (Liraglutide Effect and Action in Diabetes)-2 study. *Diabetes Care, 32*(1), 84–90.

Nauck, M., Warnick, G. R., & Rifai, N. (2002). Methods for measurement of LDL-cholesterol: A critical assessment of direct measurement by homogeneous assays versus calculation. *Clinical Chemistry, 48*(2), 236–254.

Nishimura, R. A., Carabello, B. A., Faxon, D. P., Freed, M. D., Lytle, B. W., O'Gara, P. T., . . . Shah, P. M. (2008). ACC/AHA 2008 guideline update on valvular heart disease: Focused update on infective endocarditis. *Journal of the American College of Cardiology, 52*(8), 676–685.

Nishimura, R. A., McGoon, M. D., Shub, C., Miller, F. A., Ilstrup, D. M., & Tajik, A. J. (1985). Echocardiographically documented mitral valve prolapse. Long-term follow up of 237 patients. *The New England Journal of Medicine, 313*, 1305–1309.

Nishimura, R. A., Otto, C. M., Bonow, R. O., Carabello, B. A., Erwin, J. P., Guyton, R. A., . . . Thomas, J. D. (2014). 2014 AHA/ACC guideline for the management of patients with valvular heart disease. *Journal of the American College of Cardiology, 129*(23), 2440–2449. doi:10.1016/j.jacc.2014.02.536

Nkomo, V. T., Gardin, J. M., Skelton, T. N., Gottdiener, J. S., Scott, C. G., & Enriquez-Sarano, M. (2006). Burden of valvular heart disease. *The Lancet, 368*(9540), 1005–1011.

Nohria, A., Mielniczuk, L. M., & Stevenson, L. W. (2005). Evaluation and monitoring of patients with acute heart failure syndromes. *The American Journal of Cardiology, 96*(6A), 32g–40g.

Nohria, A., Tsang, S. W., Fang, J. C., Lewis, E. F., Jarcho, J. A., Mudge, G. H., & Stevenson, L. W. (2003). Clinical assessment identifies hemodynamic profiles that predict outcomes in patients admitted with heart failure. *Journal of the American College of Cardiology, 41*(10), 1797–1804.

O'Connor, C. M., Whellan, D. J., Lee, K. L., Keteyian, S. J., Lawton, S., Cooper, M. D., . . . Pina, I. L. (2009). Efficacy and safety of exercise training in patients with chronic heart failure: HF-ACTION randomized controlled trial. *Journal of the American Medical Association, 30*, 1439–1450.

Ogawa, H., Nakayama, M., Morimoto, T., Uemura, S., Kanauchi, M., Doi, N., . . . Japanese Primary Prevention of Atherosclerosis With Aspirin for Diabetes (JPAD) Trial Investigators. (2008). Low-dose aspirin for primary prevention of atherosclerotic events in patients with type 2 diabetes: A randomized controlled trial. *Journal of the American Medical Association, 300*(18), 2134–2141.

Okin, P. M., Wachtell, K., Devereux, R. B., Harris, K. E., Jern, S., Kjeldsen, S. E., . . . Dahlof, B. (2006). Regression of electrocardiographic left ventricular hypertrophy and decreased incidence of new-onset atrial fibrillation in patients with hypertension. *Journal of the American Medical Association, 296*(10), 1242–1248.

Otvos, J. D., Mora, S., Shalaurova, I., Greenland, P., Mackey, R. H., & Goff, D. C. (2011). Clinical implications of discordance between low-density lipoprotein cholesterol and particle number. *Journal of Clinical Lipidology, 5*(2), 105–113.

Packer, M., O'Connor, C. M., Ghali, J. K., Pressler, M. L., Carson, P. E., Belkin, R. N., . . . DeMets, D. L. (1996). Effects of amlodipine on morbidity and mortality in severe chronic heart failure. *The New England Journal of Medicine, 335,* 1107–1114.

Patel, A., MacMahon, S., Chalmers, J., Neal, B., Billot, L., Woodward, M., . . . ADVANCE Collaborative Group. (2008). Intensive blood glucose control and vascular outcomes in patients with type 2 diabetes. *The New England Journal of Medicine, 358*(24), 2560–2572.

Pereira, M. A., O'Reilly, E., Augustsson, K., Fraser, G. E., Heitmann, B. L., Hallman, G., . . . Ascherio, A. (2004). Dietary fiber and risk of coronary heart disease: A pooled analysis of cohort studies. *Archives of Internal Medicine, 164*(4), 370–376.

Pickering, T. G., Hall, J. E., Appel, L. J., Falkner, B. E., Graves, J., Hill, M. N., . . . Roccella, E. J. (2005). Recommendations for blood pressure measurement in humans and experimental animals Part 1: Blood pressure measurement in humans. *Hypertension, 45,* 142–161.

Pignone, M., Alberts, M. J., Colwell, J. A., Cushman, M., Inzucchi, S. E., Mukherjee, D., . . . the American Diabetes Association; American Heart Association; and American College of Cardiology Foundation. (2010). Aspirin for primary prevention of cardiovascular events in people with diabetes: A position statement of the American Diabetes Association, a scientific statement of the American Heart Association, and an expert consensus document of the American College of Cardiology Foundation. *Journal of the American College of Cardiology, 55*(25), 2878–2886.

Pitt, B., Zannad, F., Remme, W. J., Cody, R., Castaigne, A., Perez, A., . . . Wittes, J. (1999). The effect of spironolactone on morbidity and mortality in patients with severe heart failure. *The New England Journal of Medicine, 341,* 709–717.

Poole-Wilson, P. A., Swedberg, K., Cleland, J. G., Di Lenarda, A., Hanrath, P., Komaida, M., . . . Skene, A. (2003). Comparison of carvedilol and metoprolol on clinical outcomes in patients with chronic heart failure in the Carvedilol Or Metoprolol European Trial (COMET): Randomized controlled trial. *Lancet, 362* (9377), 7–13.

Puskas, J., Gerdisch, M., Nichols, D., Quinn, R., Anderson, C., Rhenman, B., . . . Graeve, A. (2014). Reduced anticoagulation after mechanical aortic valve replacement: Interim results from the prospective randomized On-X valve anticoagulation clinical trial randomized Food and Drug Administration investigational device exemption trial. *Journal of Thoracic and Cardiovascular Surgery, 147,* 1202–1211.

Raal, F. J., Honarpour, N., Blom, D. J., Hovingh, G. K., Xu, F., Scott, R., . . . the TESLA Investigators. (2014a). Inhibition of PCSK9 with evolocumab in homozygous familial hypercholesterolaemia (TESLA Part B): A randomised, double-blind, placebo-controlled trial. *The Lancet,* Early Online Publication, 2 October 2014. doi:10.1016/S0140-6736 (14)61374-X

Raal, F. J., Santos, R. D., Blom, D. J., Marais, A. D., Charng, M., Cromwell, W. C., . . . Crooke, S. T. (2011). Mipomersen, an apolipoprotein B synthesis inhibitor, for lowering of LDL cholesterol concentrations in patients with homozygous familial hypercholesterolaemia: A randomised, double-blind, placebo-controlled trial. *The Lancet, 375*(9719), 998–1006.

Raal, F. J., Stein, E. A., Dufour, R., Turner, T., Civeira, F., Burgess, L., . . . RUTHERFORD-2 Investigators. (2014b). PCSK9 inhibition with evolocumab (AMG 145) in heterozygous familial hypercholesterolaemia (RUTHERFORD-2): A randomised, double-blind, placebo-controlled trial. *The Lancet,* Early online publication, 1 October 2014. pii: S0140-6736(14)61399-4. doi:10.1016/S0140-6736(14)61399-4

Rauch, B., Schiele, R., Schneider, S., Diller, F., Victor, N., Gohlke, H., . . . OMEGA Study Group. (2010). OMEGA, a randomized, placebo-controlled trial to test the effect of highly purified omega-3 fatty acids on top of modern guideline-adjusted therapy after myocardial infarction. *Circulation, 122*(21), 2152–2159.

Ridker, P. M., Danielson, E., Fonseca, F. A. H., Genest, J., Gotto, A. M., Kastelein, J. J. P., . . . Glynn, R. J. (2008). Rosuvastatin to prevent vascular events in men and women with elevated C-reactive protein. *The New England Journal of Medicine, 359*, 2195–2207.

Risk and Prevention Study Collaborative Group. (2013). n–3 fatty acids in patients with multiple cardiovascular risk factors. *The New England Journal of Medicine, 368*(19), 1800–1808. The Lancet. 6736(14)61374-X.

Ritchy, M. D., Wall, H. W., Gillespie, C., George, M. S., & Jamal, A. (2014). Million hearts: Prevalence of leading cardiovascular risk factors—United States, 2005–2012. *Morbidity and Mortality Weekly Report, 63*(21), 462–467.

Rizos, C. V., Elisaf, M. S., & Liberopoulos, E. N. (2011). Effects of thyroid dysfunction on lipid profile. *The Open Cardiovascular Medicine Journal, 5*, 76–84.

Roger, V. L., Go, A. S., Lloyd-Jones, D. M., Benjamin, E. J., Berr, J. D., . . . Turner, M. B. (2012). Heart disease and stroke statistics—2012 update: A report from the American Heart Association. *Circulation, 125*, e2–e220.

Rossebo, A. B., Pedersen, T. R., Boman, K., Brudi, P., Chambers, J. B., Egstrup, K., . . . Willenheimer, R. (2008). Intensive lipid lowering with statin and ezetimibe in aortic stenosis. *The New England Journal of Medicine, 359*, 1343–1356.

Roth, E. M., Taskinen, M. R., Ginsberg, H. N., Kastelein, J. J., Colhoun, H. M., Robinson, J. G., . . . Baccara-Dinet, M. T. (2014). Monotherapy with the PCSK9 inhibitor alirocumab versus ezetimibe in patients with hypercholesterolemia: Results of a 24 week, double-blind, randomized Phase 3 trial. *The International Journal of Cardiology, 176*(1), 55–61.

Saikrishnan, N., Kumar, G., Sawaya, F. J., Lerakis, S., & Yoganathan, A. P. (2014). Accurate assessment of aortic stenosis: A review of diagnostic modalities and hemodynamics. *Circulation, 129*(2), 244–253.

Sattar, N., Preiss, D., Murray, H. M., Welsh, P., Buckley, B. M., de Craen, A. J., . . . Ford, I. (2010). Statins and risk of incident diabetes: A collaborative meta-analysis of randomized statin trials. *The Lancet, 375*(9716), 735–742.

Sayers, S. L., Riegel, B., Pawlowski, S., Coyne, J. C., & Samaha, F. F. (2008). Social support and self-care of patients with heart failure. *Annals of Behavioral Medicine, 35*, 70–79.

Sears, S. F., & Conti, J. B. (2002). Quality of life and psychological functioning of ICD patients. *Heart, 87*, 488–493.

Sesso, H. D., Lee, I. M., Gaziano, J. M., Rexrode, K. M., Glynn, R. J., & Buring, J. E. (2001). Maternal and paternal history of myocardial infarction and risk of cardiovascular disease in men and women. *Circulation, 104*(4), 393–398.

Shah, R. V., & Januzzi, J. L. (2014). Soluable ST2 and Galectin-3 in heart failure. *Clinics in Laboratory Medicine, 34*(1), 87–97.

Shah, S. A., Shapiro, R. J., Mehta, R., & Snyder, J. A. (2012). Impact of enhanced external counterpulsation on Canadian cardiovascular society angina class in patients with chronic stable angina: A meta-analysis, *Pharmacotherapy, 30*(7), 639–645.

Singh, J. P., Evans, J. C., Levy, D., Larson, M. G., Freed, L. A., Fuller, D. L., . . . Benjamin, E. J. (1999). Prevalence and clinical determinants of mitral, tricuspid, and aortic regurgitation. *The American Journal of Cardiology, 83*(6), 897–902.

Singh, S. N., Carson, P. E., & Fisher, S. G. (1997). Nonsustained ventricular tachycardia in severe heart failure. *Circulation, 96*(10), 3794–3795.

Skyler, J. S., Bergenstal, R., Bonow, R. O., Buse, J., Deedwania, P., Gale, E. A., . . . the American Diabetes Association, American College of Cardiology Foundation, and American Heart Association. (2009). Intensive Glycemic Control and the Prevention of Cardiovascular Events: Implications of the ACCORD, ADVANCE, and VA Diabetes Trials. A Position Statement of the American Diabetes Association and a Scientific Statement of the American College of Cardiology Foundation and the American Heart Association. *Circulation, 119*(2), 351–357.

Smolka, G., & Wojakowski, W. (2010). Paravalvular leak- important complication after implantation of prosthetic valve. *E-Journal of the European Society of Cardiology, 9*(8), obtained from http://escardio.org

Stassano, P., Di Tommaso, L., Monaco, M., Iorio, F., Pepino, P., Spampinato, N., & Vosa, C. (2009). A prospective randomized evaluation of mechanical versus biological valves in patients ages 55 to 70 years. *Journal of the American College of Cardiology, 54*(20), 1862–1868.

Stewart, G. C. (2012). Mechanical circulatory support for advanced heart failure: Patients and technology in evolution. *Circulation, 125*, 1304–1315.

Stoll, B. C., Ashcom, T. L., Johns, J. P., Johnson, J. E., & Rubal, B. J. (1995). Effects of atenolol on rest and exercise hemodynamics in patients with mitral stenosis. *The American Journal of Cardiology, 75*, 482–484.

Stone, N. J., Robinson, J. G., Lichtenstein, A. H., Merz, C. N., Blum, C. B., Eckel, R. H., . . . Wilson, P. W. (2013). 2013 ACC/AHA guideline on the treatment of blood cholesterol to reduce atherosclerotic cardiovascular risk in adults. *Circulation, 129*, s1–s45. doi:10.1161/01.cir.0000437738.63853.7a

Stromberg, A., Martensson, J., Fridlund, B., Levin, L. A., Karlsson, J. E., & Dahlstrom, U. (2003). Nurse-led heart failure clinics improve survival and self-care behavior in patients with heart failure. *European Heart Journal, 24*, 1014–1023.

Tamburino, C., Ussia, G. P., Maisano, F., Capodanno, D., La Canna, G., Scandura, S., . . . Alfieri, O. (2010). Percutaneous mitral valve repair with the MitraClip system: Acute results from a real world setting. *European Heart Journal, 1*, 1382–1389. doi:10.1093/eurheartj/ehq051

Tandon, N., Ali, M. K., & Narayan, V. (2012). Pharmacologic prevention of microvascular and macrovascular complications in diabetes mellitus: Implications of the results of recent clinical trials in type 2 diabetes. *The American Journal of Cardiovascular Drugs, 12*(1), 7–22.

Taylor, A. L., Ziesche, S., Yancy, C. W., Carson, P., D'Agostino, R., Ferdinand, K., . . . Cohn, J. N. (2004). Combination of isosorbide dinitrate and hydralazine in blacks with heart failure. *The New England Journal of Medicine, 351*, 2049–2057.

Threapleton, D. E., Greenwood, D. C., Evans, C. E., Cleghorn, C. L., Nykjaer, C., Woodhead, C., . . . Burley, V. J. (2013). Dietary fibre intake and risk of cardiovascular disease: Systematic review and meta-analysis. *The British Medical Journal, 347*, f6879.

TNT Steering Committee Members & Investigators. (2004). Treating new targets (TNT) study: Does lowering low-density lipoprotein cholesterol levels below currently recommended guidelines yield incremental clinical benefit? *The American Journal of Cardiology, 93*(2), 154–158.

U.S. Preventive Services Task Force. (2008). Screening for lipid disorders in adults: Selective update of 2001 U. S. Preventive Services Task Force review. Retrieved from http://www.uspreventiveservicestaskforce.org/uspst08/lipid/lipidrs.html

U.S. Preventive Services Task Force (USPSTF). (2009). Aspirin for the prevention of cardiovascular disease. Retrieved from http://www.uspreventiveservicestaskforce.org/uspstf/uspasasmi.htm

U.S. Preventive Services Task Force (USPSTF). (2014). Screening for lipid disorders in adults recommendation summary. U.S. Preventive Services Task Force. Retrieved from http://www.uspreventiveservicestaskforce.org/uspstf08/lipid/lipidrs.html

Van der Wal, M. H., Jaarsma, T., Moser, D. K., Veeger, N. J., van Gilst, W. H., & vanVeldhuisen, D. J. (2006). Compliance in heart failure patients: The importance of knowledge and beliefs. *European Heart Journal, 27*, 434–440.

van Veldhuisen, D. J., Cohen-Solal, A., Bohm, M., Anker, S. D., Babalis, D., Roughton, M., . . . Flather, M. D. (2009). Beta-blockade with nebivolol in elderly heart failure patients with impaired and preserved left ventricular ejection fraction: Data from SENIORS (Study of effects of nebivolol intervention on outcomes and rehospitalization in seniors with heart failure). *Journal of the American College of Cardiology, 53*, 2150–2158.

Varady, K. A., & Jones, P. J. (2005). Combination diet and exercise interventions for the treatment of dyslipidemia: An effective preliminary strategy to lower cholesterol levels? *Journal of Nutrition, 135*(8), 1829–1835.

Victor, R. (2012). Arterial hypertension. In L. Goldman & A. I. Schafer (Eds.), *Goldman's Cecil medicine* (24th ed., p. 378). Philadelphia, PA: Elsevier.

Vincentelli, A., Susen, S., Le Tourneau, T. L., Six, I., Fabre, O., . . . Jude, B. (2003). Acquired von Willebrand syndrome in aortic stenosis. *The New England Journal of Medicine, 349*(4), 343–349.

Wallentin, L., Becker, R. C., Budaj, A., Cannon, C. P., Emanuelsson, H., Held, C., . . . Harrington, R. A. (2009). Ticagrelor versus clopidogrel in patients with acute coronary syndromes. *The New England Journal of Medicine, 361*, 1045–1057.

Weber, L. P., Al-Dissi, A., Marit, J. S., German, T. N., & Terletski, S. D. (2011). Role of carbon monoxide in impaired endothelial function mediated by acute second-hand tobacco, incense, and candle smoke exposures. *Environmental Toxicology and Pharmacology, 31*(3), 453–459.

Whelton, S. P., Chin, A., Xin, X., & He, J. (2002). Effects of aerobic exercise on blood pressure: A meta-analysis of randomized, controlled trials. *Annals of Internal Medicine, 136*(7), 493–503.

Whitlow, P. L., Feldman, T., Pedersen, W. R., Lim, D. S., Kiperman, R., Smalling, R., . . . Kar, S. (2012). Acute and 12-month results with catheter-based mitral valve leaflet repair: The EVEREST II (endovascular valve edge-to edge repair) high risk study. *Journal of the American College of Cardiology, 59*(2), 130–139.

Wijns, W., Kolh, P., Danchin, N., Di Mario, C., Falk, V., Folliguet, T., . . . Tagart, D. (2010). Guidelines on myocardial revascularization. *European Heart Journal, 31*, 2501–2555.

Wiviott, S. D., Braunwald, E., McCabe, C. H., Montalescot, G., Ruzyllo, W., Gottilieb, S., . . . Antman, E. M. (2007). Prasugrel versus clopidogrel in patients with acute coronary syndromes. *The New England Journal of Medicine, 357*, 2001–2015.

Yancy, C. W., Jessup, M., Bozkurt, B., Masoudi, F. A., Butler, J., Casey, D. E., . . . Wilkoff, B. L. (2013). 2013 ACCF/AHA guideline for the management of heart failure. *Journal of the American College of Cardiology.* doi:10.1016/j.jacc.2013.05.019

Young, J. B., Abraham, W. T., Smith, A. L., Leon, A. R., Lieberman, R., Wilkoff, B., . . . Wheelan, K. (2003). Combined cardiac resynchronization and implantable cardioversion defibrillation in advanced chronic heart failure: The MIRACLE ICD Trial. *Journal of the American Medical Association, 289*, 2685–2694.

Yusuf, S., Pfeffer, M. A., Swedberg, K., Granger, C. B., Held, P., . . . Ostergren, J. (2003). Effects of candesartan in patients with chronic heart failure and preserved left ventricular ejection fraction: The CHARM-preserved trial. *The Lancet, 362*, 777–781.

Zannad, F., McMurray, J. J. V., Drum, H., van Veldhuisen, D. J., Swedberg, K., Shi, H., . . . EMPHASIS-HF Study Group. (2011). Eplerenone in patients with systolic heart failure and mild symptoms. *The New England Journal of Medicine, 364*, 11–21.

SECTION III

AFFIRM Investigators. (2002). A comparison of rate control and rhythm control in patients with atrial fibrillation. *The New England Journal of Medicine, 347*(23), 1825–1833.

American Heart Association. (2014). Atrial fibrillation. Retrieved from http://www.heart .org/HEARTORG/Conditions/Arrhythmia/AboutArrhythmia/Atrial-Fibrillation-AF-or AFib_UCM_302027_Article.jsp

Anderson, J. L., Halperin, J. L., Albert, N. M., Bozkurt, B., Brindis, R. G., Curtis, L. H., & Shen, W. K. (2013). Management of patients with atrial fibrillation (compilation of 2006

ACCF/AHA/ESC and 2011 ACCF/AHA/HRS guideline recommendations: A report of the American College of Cardiology Foundation/American Heart Association Task Force on Practice Guidelines. *Circulation, 127,* 1916–1926.

Baman, T. S., Lange, D. C., Ilg, K. J., Gupta, S. K., Liu, T., Alguire, C., . . . Bogun, F. (2010). Relationship between burden of premature ventricular complexes and left ventricular function. *Heart Rhythm, 7*(7), 865–869.

Bardy, G. H., Lee, K. L., Mark, D. B., Poole, J. E., Packer, D. L., . . . Sudden Cardiac Death in Heart Failure Trial (SCD-HeFT Investigators). (2005). Amiodarone or an implantable cardioverter-defibrillator for congestive heart failure. *The New England Journal of Medicine, 352,* 225–237.

Bernstein, A. D., Daubert, J., Fletcher, R. D., Hayes, D. L., Luderitz, B., Reynolds, D. W., . . . Sutton, R. (2002). NASPE position statement. The revised NASPE/BPEG generic code for antibradycardia, adaptive-rate and multisite pacing. *Journal of Pacing and Clinical Electrophysiology, 25*(2), 260–264.

Buxton, A. E., Lee, K. L., Fisher, J. D., Josephson, M. E., Prystowsky, E. N., & Hafley, G. (1999). A randomized study of the prevention of sudden death in patients with coronary artery disease. Multicenter unsustained tachycardia trial investigators. *The New England Journal of Medicine, 341,* 1882–1890.

CABANA Investigators. (2015). Catheter ablation versus anti-arrhythmic drug therapy for atrial fibrillation trial (NCT00911508). *ClinicalTrials.gov Website.* Retrieved from http://www.clinicaltrials.gov/.

Connolly, S. J., Camm, A. J., Halperin, J. L., Joyner, C., Allings, M., Amerena, J., . . . PALLAS investigators. (2011). Dronedarone in high-risk permanent atrial fibrillation. *The New England Journal of Medicine, 365,* 2268–2276.

Crossley, G. H., Poole, J. E., Rozner, M. A., Asirvatham, S. J., Cheng, A., Chung, M. K., & Thompson, A. (2011). The Heart Rhythm Society (HRS)/American Society of Anesthesiologists (ASA) expert consensus statement on the perioperative management of patients with implantable defibrillators, pacemakers and arrhythmia monitors. *Heart Rhythm, 8*(7), 1114–1154.

Ellis, E. R., & Josephson, M. E. (2013). Heart failure and tachycardia-induced cardiomyopathy. *Current Heart Failure Reports, 10*(4), 296–306.

Epstein, A. E., DiMarco, J. P., Ellenbogen, K. A., Estes, N. A. M., Freedman, R. A., . . . Sweeney, M. O. (2012). ACCF/AHA/HRS focused update incorporated into the ACCF/AHA/HRS 2008 guidelines for device-based therapy of cardiac rhythm abnormalities: A report of the American College of Cardiology Foundation/American Heart Association Task Force on Practice Guidelines and the Heart Rhythm Society. *Circulation, 127,* e283–e352.

Exner, D. V., Pinski, S. L., Wyse, D. G., Renfroe, E. G., Follmann, D., Gold, M., . . . Hallstrom, A. P. (2001). Electrical storm presages nonsudden death: The antiarrhythmic versus implantable defibrillators (AIVD) trial. *Circulation, 103*(16), 2066–2071.

Ezekowitz, M. D., Aikens, T. H., Nagarakanti, R., & Shapiro, T. (2011). Atrial fibrillation: Outpatient presentation and management. *Circulation, 124,* 95–99.

Fricchoine, G. L., Olson, L. S., & Vlay, S. C. (1989). Psychiatric syndromes in patients with automatic internal cardioverter defibrillator: Anxiety, psychological dependence, abuse, and withdrawal. *American Heart Journal, 117,* 1411–1414.

Gage, B. F., Waterman, A. D., Shannon, W., Boechler, M., Rich, M. W., & Radford, M. J. (2001). Validation of clinical classification schemes for predicting stroke: Results from the national registry of atrial fibrillation. *Journal of the American Medical Association, 285*(22), 2864–2870.

Ghanbari, H., Saint Phard, W., Al-Ameri, H., Latchamsetty, R., Jongnarngsin, K., Crawford, T., . . . Pelosi, F. (2012). Meta-analysis of safety and efficacy of uninterrupted warfarin compared to heparin-based bridging therapy during implantation of cardiac rhythm devices. *The American Journal of Cardiology, 110*(10), 1482–1488.

Hamner, M., Hunt, N., Gee, J., Garrell, R., & Monroe, R. (1999). PSTD and automatic implantable cardioverter defibrillators. *Psychosomatics, 40*, 82–85.

January, C. T., Wann, L. S., Alpert, J. S., Calkins, H., Cigarroa, J. E., Cleveland, J. C., . . . Yancy, C. W. (2014). 2014 AHA/ACC/HRS guideline for the management of patients with atrial fibrillation: A report of the American College of Cardiology/American Heart Association Task Force on Practice Guidelines and the Heart Rhythm Society. *Circulation, 130*, e199–e267.

Khasnis, A., Jongnarangsin, K., Abela, G., Veerareddy, S., Reddy, V., & Thakur, R. (2005). Tachycardia-induced cardiomyopathy: A review of literature. *Pacing and Clinical Electrophysiology, 28*(7), 710–721.

Kusumoto, F. M., Calkins, H., Boehmer, J., Buxton, A. E., Chung, M. K., Gold, M. R., . . . Welikovitch, L. (2014). HRS/ACC/AHA expert consensus statement on the use of implantable cardioverter-defibrillator therapy in patients who are not included or not well represented in clinical trials. *Circulation, 130*, 94–125.

Lampert, R., Hayes, D. L., Annas, G. J., Farley, M. A., Goldstein, N. E., Hamilton, R. M., . . . Zellner, R. (2010). Heart Rhythm Society (HRS) expert consensus statement on management of cardiovascular implantable electronic devices in patients nearing end of life or requesting withdrawal of therapy. *Heart Rhythm, 7*(7), 1008–1026.

Mirowski, M. (1985). The automatic implantable cardioverter-defibrillator: An overview. *Journal of the American College of Cardiology, 6*(2), 461–466.

Moss, A. J., Hall, W. J., Cannom, D. S., Daubert, J. P., Higgins, S. L., Klein, H., . . . Heo, M. (1996). Improved survival with an implanted defibrillator in patients with coronary disease at high risk for ventricular arrhythmia: Multicenter automatic defibrillator implantation trial investigators. *The New England Journal of Medicine, 335*, 1933–1940.

Moss, A. J., Zareba, W., Hall, W. J., Klein, H., Wilbur, D. J., Cannom, D. S., . . . Multicenter Automatic Defibrillator Implantation Trial II Investigators. (2002). Prophylactic implantation of a defibrillator in patients with myocardial infarction and reduced ejection fraction. *The New England Journal of Medicine, 346*, 877–883.

National Heart, Lung, and Blood Institute (NHLBI). (2014). Explore atrial fibrillation. Retrieved from http://www.nhlbi.nih.gov/health/health-topics/topics/af

O'Neill, M. D., Jais, P., Jonsson, A., Takahashi, Y., Sacher, F., Hocini, M., . . . Haissaguerre, M. (2006). An approach to catheter ablation of cavotricuspid isthmus dependent atrial flutter. *Indian Pacing and Electrophysiology Journal, 6*(2), 100–110.

Priori, S. G., Wilde, A. A., Horie, M., Cho, Y., Behr, E. R., Berul, C., . . . Tracy, C. (2013). HRS/EHRA/APHRS expert consensus statement on the diagnosis and management of patients with inherited primary arrhythmia syndromes. *Heart Rhythm, 10*(12), 1932–1963. Retrieved from www.QTdrugs.org

Raj, V., Rowe, A. A., Fleisch, S. B., Paranjape, S. Y., Arain, A. M., & Nicolson, S. E. (2014). Psychogenic pseudosyncope: Diagnosis and management. *Autonomic Neuroscience, 184*, 66–72.

Saklani, P., Krahn, A., & Klein, G. (2013). Syncope. *Circulation, 127*(12), 1330–1339.

Strickberger, S. A., Benson, D. W., Biaggioni, I., Callans, D. J., Cohen, M. I., Ellenbogen, K. A., . . . Sila, C. A. (2006). AHA/ACCF scientific statement on the evaluation of syncope: From the American Heart Association Councils on clinical cardiology, cardiovascular nursing, cardiovascular disease in the young, and stroke, and the quality of care and outcomes research interdisciplinary working group; and the American College of Cardiology Foundation in collaboration with the Heart Rhythm Society. *Circulation, 113*, 316–327.

Tracy, C. M., Epstein, A. E., Darbar, D., DiMarco, J. P., Dunbar, S. B., Estes, M., . . . Varosy, P. D. (2013). ACCF/AHA/HRS focused update incorporated into the ACCF/AHA/HRS 2008 Guidelines for device-based therapy of cardiac rhythm abnormalities: A report of the American College of Cardiology Foundation/American Heart Association Task Force on Practice Guidelines and the Heart Rhythm Society. *Journal of the American College of Cardiology, 61*(3), e6–e75. doi:10.1016/j.jacc.2012.11.007

Van Gelder, I. C., Groenveld, H. F., Crijns, H. J. G. M., Tuininga, Y. S., Tijssen, J. G. P., Alings, A. M., . . . Van Den Berg, M. P. (2010). Lenient versus strict rate control in patients with atrial fibrillation. *The New England Journal of Medicine, 362,* 1363–1373.

Wadke, R. (2013). Atrial fibrillation. *Disease-a-Month, 59*(3), 67–73.

Wazni, O., Epstein, L. M., Carrillo, R. G., Love, C., Adler, S. W., Riggio, D. W., . . . Wilkoff, B. L. (2010). Lead extraction in the contemporary setting: The LExICon Study: An observational retrospective study of consecutive laser lead extractions. *Journal of the American College of Cardiology, 55*(6), 579–586.

Yancy, C. W., Jessup, M., Bozkurt, B., Butler, J., Casey, D. E., Drazner, M. H., . . . Wilkoff, B. L. (2013). ACCF/AHA guideline for the management of heart failure: A report of the American College of Cardiology Foundation/American Heart Association Task Force on Practice Guidelines. *Journal of the American College of Cardiology, 62*(16), e147–e239. doi:10.1016/j.jacc.2013.05.019

SECTION IV

Aboyans, V., Criqui, M. H., Abraham, P., Allison, M. A., Creager, M. A., Diehm, C., . . . Treat-Jacobson, D. (2012). American Heart Association Council on Peripheral Vascular Disease; Council on Epidemiology and Prevention; Council on Clinical Cardiology; Council on Cardiovascular Nursing; Council on Cardiovascular Radiology and Intervention, and Council on Cardiovascular Surgery and Anesthesia. Measurement and interpretation of the ankle-brachial index: A scientific statement from the American Heart Association. *Circulation, 126,* 2890–2909.

Alhara, H., Soga, Y., Mii, S., Okazaki, J., Yamaoka, T., Kamoi, D., . . . Ishikawa, T., RECA-NALISE Registry Investigators. (2014). Comparison of long-term outcome after endovascular therapy versus bypass surgery in claudication patients with Trans-Atlantic Inter-society Consensus-II C and D femoropopliteal disease. *Circulation Journal, 78*(2), 457–464.

Allard, L., Cloutier, G., Durand, L. G., Roederer, G. O., & Langlois, Y. E. (1994). Limitations of ultrasonic duplex scanning for diagnosing lower limb arterial stenosis in the presence of adjacent segment disease. *Journal of Vascular Surgery, 19*(4), 650–657.

Andras, A., Stansby, G., & Hansrani, M. (2013). Homocysteine lowering interventions for peripheral arterial disease and bypass grafts. *Cochrane Database of Systematic Reviews, 7.* Article no. CD003285. doi:10.1002/14651858.CD003285.pub2

Antithrombotic Trialists' Collaboration. (2002). Collaborative meta-analysis of randomized trials of antiplatelet therapy for prevention of death, myocardial infarction, and stroke in high risk patients. *The British Medical Journal, 324,* 71–86.

Antoniou, G. A., Chalmers, N., Georgiadis, G. S., Lazarides, M. K., Antoniou, S. A., Serracino-Inglott, F., . . . Murray, D. (2013). A meta-analysis of endovascular versus surgical reconstruction of femoropopliteal arterial disease. *Journal of Vascular Surgery, 57*(1), 242–253.

Ballard, D. J., Filardo, G., Fowkes, G., & Powell, J. T. (2008). Surgery for small asymptomatic abdominal aortic aneurysms. *Cochrane Database Syst Rev, 4,* CD001835.

Banerjee, A. (1993). Atypical manifestations of abdominal aortic aneurysms. *The Fellowship of Postgraduate Medicine, 69,* 6–11.

Becquemin, J. P., Pillet, J. C., Lescalie, F., Sapoval, M., Goueffic, Y., Lermusiaux, P., . . . ACE trialists. (2011). A randomized controlled trial of endovascular aneurysm repair *versus* open surgery for abdominal aortic aneurysms in low- to moderate-risk patients. *Journal of Vascular Surgery, 53,* 1167–1173.e1.

Beebe, H. G., Dawson, D. L., Cutler, B. S., Herd, J. A., Strandness, D. E., Borley, E. B., & Forbes, W. P. (1999). A new pharmacological treatment for intermittent claudication:

Results of a randomized, multicenter trial. *Archives of Internal Medicine, 159*(17), 2041–2450.

Berger, J. S., Hochman, J., Lobach, I., Adelman, M. A., Riles, T. S., & Rockman, C. B. (2013). Modifiable risk factor burden and the prevalence of peripheral artery disease in different vascular territories. *Journal of Vascular Surgery, 58*(3), 673–681.

Blankensteijn, J. D., deJong, S. E., Prinssen, M., vanderHam, A. C., Buth, J., van Sterkenburg, S. M., . . . Dutch Randomized Endovascular Aneurysm Management (DREAM) Trial Group. (2005). Two-year outcomes after conventional or endovascular repair of abdominal aortic aneurysms. *The New England Journal of Medicine, 352*, 2398–2405.

Bown, M. J., Sweeting, M. J., Brown, L. C., Powell, J. T., & Thompson, S. G. (RESCAN Collaborators). (2013). Surveillance intervals for small abdominal aortic aneurysms: A meta-analysis. *Journal of the American Medical Association, 309*(8), 806–813.

Brewster, D. C., Cronenwett, J. L., Hallett, J. W., Johnston, K. W., Krupski, W. C., & Matsumura, J. S. (2003). Guidelines for the treatment of abdominal aortic aneurysms: Report of a subcommittee of the Joint Council of the American Association for Vascular Surgery and Society for Vascular Surgery. *Journal of Vascular Surgery, 37*, 1106–1117.

Centers for Disease Control and Prevention. (2013). *The state of aging and health in America* (6th ed.). Atlanta, GA: Centers for Disease Control and Prevention, U.S. Department of Health and Human Services. Retrieved from www.cdc.gov/aging

Centers for Disease Control and Prevention. (2014). *Crude and age-adjusted percentage of civilian, non-institutionalized population with diagnosed diabetes, United States, 1980–2011*. Atlanta, GA: U.S. Department of Health and Human Services, CDC, National Diabetes Surveillance System. Retrieved from www.cdc.gov/diabetes/statistics/prevalence

Chaikof, E. L., Brewster, D. C., Dalman, R. L., Makaroun, M. S., Illig, K. A., . . . Society for Vascular Surgery. (2009). The care of patients with an abdominal aortic aneurysm: The Society for Vascular Surgery practice guidelines. *Journal of Vascular Surgery, 50*(Suppl. 4), S2–S49.

Cosford, P. A., Leng, G. C., & Thomas, J. (2007). Screening for abdominal aortic aneurysm (Review). *Cochrane Database Systematic Review*, (2). Article no. CD002945. doi:10.1002/14651858.CD002945.pub2

Criqui, M. H., Denenberg, J. O., Langer, R. D., & Fronek, A. (1997). The epidemiology of peripheral arterial disease: Importance of identifying the population at risk. *Vascular Medicine, 2*(3), 221–226.

Criqui, M. H., Fronek, A., Barrett-Connor, E., Klauber, M. R., Gabriel, S., & Goodman, D. (1985). The prevalence of peripheral arterial disease in a defined population. *Circulation, 71*(3), 510–551.

Criqui, M. H., Langer, R. D., Fronek, A., Feigelson, H. S., Klauber, M. R., McCann, T. J., & Browner, D. (1992). Mortality over a period of 10 years in patients with peripheral arterial disease. *The New England Journal of Medicine, 326*(6), 381–386.

De Bruin, J. L., Baas, A. F., Buth, J., Prinssen, M., Verhoeven, E. L., Cuypers, P. W., . . . DREAM Study Group. (2010). Long-term 41 outcome of open or endovascular repair of abdominal aortic aneurysm. *The New England Journal of Medicine, 362*, 1881–1889.

Dean, R. H., Yao, J. S., Thompson, R. G., & Bergan, J. J. (1975). Predictive value of ultrasonically derived arterial pressure in determination of amputation level. *American Surgeon, 41*(11), 731–737.

Department of Health and Human Services, Centers for Medicare & Medicaid Services (DHHS/CMS). (2014). MLN matters: Medicare coverage of ultrasound screening for abdominal aortic aneurysms (AAA) and screening fecal-occult blood tests (FOBT). MLN Matters Number: MM8881, CR 8881, Transmittal # R3096CP, R176NCD, and R196BP.

Diehm, C., Allenberg, R. J., Pittrow, D., Mahn, M., Tepohl, G., Haberi, R. L., . . . Diehm, C. (2009). Mortality and vascular morbidity in older adults with asymptomatic versus symptomatic peripheral arterial disease. *Circulation, 120*(21), 2053–2061.

Dormandy, J. A., Heeck, L., & Vig, S. (1999). The fate of patients with critical leg ischemia. *Seminars in Vascular Surgery, 12*(12), 142–147.

Dormandy, J. A., & Rutherford, R. B. (2000). Management of peripheral arterial disease (PAD). TASC Working Group. TransAtlantic Inter-Society Consensus (TASC). *Journal of Vascular Surgery, 31*(1 Pt 2), S1–S296.

Dorweiler, B., Neufang, A., Kreitner, K. F., Schmiedt, W., & Oelert, H. (2002). Magnetic resonance angiography unmasks reliable target vessels for pedal bypass grafting in patients with diabetes mellitus. *Journal of Vascular Surgery, 35*(4), 766–772.

Egorova, N., Giacovelli, J. K., Gelijns, A., Greco, G., Moskowitz, A., McKinsey, J., & Kent, K. C. (2009). Defining high-risk patients for endovascular aneurysm repair. *Journal of Vascular Surgery, 50*, 1271–1279.

Eldrup, N., Budtz-Lilly, J., Laustsen, J., Bibby, B. M., & Paaske, W. P. (2012). Long-term incidence of myocardial infarct, stroke, and mortality in patients operated on for abdominal aortic aneurysms. *Journal of Vascular Surgery, 55*, 311–317.

Erb, W. (1911). Klinische Bietrage zur Pathologie des Intermittierenden Hinkens. *Munchener Medizinische Wochenschrift, 2*, 2487.

Faxon, D. P., Fuster, V., Libby, P., Beckman, J. A., Hiatt, W. R., Thompson, R. W., . . . American Heart Association. (2004). Atherosclerotic Vascular Disease Conference: Writing Group III: Pathophysiology. *Circulation, 109*(21), 2617–2625.

Ferket, B. S., Grootenboer, N., Colkesen, E. B., Visser, J. J., van Sambeek, M. R. H. M., Spronk, S., . . . Hunink, M. G. M. (2012). Systematic review of guidelines on abdominal aortic aneurysm screening. *Journal of Vascular Surgery, 55*, 1295–1305.

Filardo, G., Powell, J. T., Martinez, M. A. M., & Ballard, D. J. (2012). Surgery for small asymptomatic abdominal aortic aneurysms. *Cochrane Database of Systematic Reviews*, Issue 3. Art. No.: CD001835. doi:10.1002/14651858.CD001835.pub3

Fowkes, F. G. (1995). Fibrinogen and peripheral arterial disease. *European Heart Journal* (Suppl. A), 36–40.

Fowkes, F. G., Housley, E., Cawood, E. H., Macintyre, C. C., Ruckley, C. V., & Prescott, R. J. (1991). Edinburgh artery study: Prevalence of asymptomatic and symptomatic peripheral arterial disease in the general population. *International Journal of Epidemiology, 20*(2), 384–392.

Fowkes, F. G., Murray, G. D., Butcher, I., Heald, C. L., Lee, R. J., Chambless, L. E., . . . Ankle Brachial Index Collaboration. (2008). Ankle brachial index combined with Framingham risk score to predict cardiovascular events and mortality: A meta-analysis. *Journal of the American Medical Association, 300*(2), 197–208.

Fowkes, F. G., Rudan, D., Rudan, I., Aboyans, V., Denenberg, J. O., McDermott, M. M., . . . Criqui, M. H. (2013). Comparison of global estimates of prevalence and risk factors for peripheral arterial disease in 2000 and 2010: A systematic review and analysis. *The Lancet, 382*(9901), 1329–1340.

Freiberg, M. S., Arnold, A. M., Newman, A. B., Edwards, M. S., Kraemer, K. L., & Kuller, L. H. (2008). Abdominal aortic aneurysms, increasing infrarenal aortic diameter, and risk of total mortality and incident cardiovascular disease events 10-year follow-up data from the cardiovascular health study. *Circulation, 117*, 1010–1017.

Gardner, A. W., Montgomery, P. S., & Parker, D. E. (2008). Physical activity is a predictor of all-cause mortality in patients with intermittent claudication. *Journal of Vascular Surgery, 47*(1), 1176–1122.

Gardner, A. W., Parker, D. E., Montgomery, P. S., Scott, K. J., & Blevins, S. M. (2011). Efficacy of quantified home-based exercise and supervised exercise in patients with intermittent claudication: A randomized controlled trial. *Circulation, 123*(5), 491–498.

Giles, K. A., Schermerhorn, M. L., O'Malley, A. J., Cotterill, P., Jhaveri, A., Pomposelli, F. B., & Landon, B. E. (2009). Risk prediction for perioperative mortality of endovascular vs open repair of abdominal aortic aneurysms using the Medicare population. *Journal of Vascular Surgery, 50*, 256–262.

Glagov, S., Zarins, C., Bassiouny, H., & Giddens, D. (1995). New understanding of the patho-physiology of the atherosclerotic process. In J. Yao & W. Pearce (Eds.), *The ischemic extremity: Advances in treatment* (pp. 13–24). Norwalk, Connecticut: Appleton and Lange.

Golledge, J., Muller, R., Clancy, P., McCann, M., & Norman, P. E. (2011). Evaluation of the diagnostic and prognostic value of plasma D-dimer for abdominal aortic aneurysm. *European Heart Journal, 32*, 354–364.

Greenhalgh, R. M., Brown, L. C., Kwong, G. P., Powell, J. T., & Thompson, S. G.; & EVAR trial participants. (2004). Comparison of endovascular aneurysm repair with open repair in patients with abdominal aortic aneurysm (EVAR trial 1), 30-day operative mortality results: Randomised controlled trial. *The Lancet, 364*, 843–848.

Greenhalgh, R. M., Brown, L. C., Kwong, G. P., Powell, J. T., & Thompson, S. G.; & EVAR trial participants. (2005a). Endovascular aneurysm repair versus open repair in patients with abdominal aortic aneurysm (EVAR trial 1). *The Lancet, 365*, 2179–2186.

Greenhalgh, R. M., Brown, L. C., Kwong, G. P., Powell, J. T., & Thompson, S. G.; & EVAR trial participants. (2005b). Endovascular aneurysm repair and outcome in patients unfit for open repair of abdominal aortic aneurysm (EVAR trial 2): Randomised controlled trial. *The Lancet, 365*(9478), 2187–2192.

Greenhalgh, R. M., Brown, L. C., Kwong, G. P., Powell, J. T., Thompson, S. G., & Epstein, D.; & EVAR trial participants. (2010). Endovascular versus open repair of abdominal aortic aneurysm. *The New England Journal of Medicine, 362*, 1863–1871.

Grundy, S. M., Cleeman, J. I., Merz, C. N., Brewer, H. B., Clark, L. T., Hunninghake, D. B., . . . Coordinating Committee of the National Cholesterol Education Program. (2004). Impli-cations of recent clinical trials for the National Cholesterol Education Program Adult Treatment Panel III Guidelines. *Journal of the American College of Cardiology, 44*(3), 720–732.

Guessous, I., Periard, D., Lorenzetti, D., Cornuz, J., & Ghali, W. A. (2008). The efficacy of pharmacotherapy for decreasing the expansion rate of abdominal aortic aneurysms: A systematic review and meta-analysis. *PloS ONE, 3*, e1895, 1–10.

Guirguis-Blake, J. M., Beil, T. L., Senger, C. A., & Whitlock, E. P. (2014). Ultrasonography screening for abdominal aortic aneurysms: A systematic evidence review for the U.S. Preventive Services Task Force. *Annals of Internal Medicine*. doi:10.7326/M13-1844

Hawkins, I. F., Cho, K. J., & Caridi, J. G. (2009). Carbon dioxide in angiography to reduce the risk of contrast-induced nephropathy. *Radiology Clinics of North America, 47*(5), 813–825.

Heart Protection Study Collaboration Group. (2002). MRC/BHF heart protection study of cholesterol lowering with simvastatin in 20,536 high-risk individuals: A randomized placebo-controlled trial. *The Lancet, 360*(9326), 7–22.

Hellman, R. N. (2011). Gadolinium-induced nephrogenic systemic fibrosis. *Seminars in Nephrology, 31*(3), 310–316.

Hellmann, D. B., Grand, D. J., & Freischlag, J. A. (2007). Inflammatory abdominal aortic aneurysm. *Journal of the American Medical Association, 297*, 395–400.

Hill, R. D., & Smith, R. B., III. (1990). Examination of the extremities: Pulses, bruits, and phlebitis. In H. K. Walker, W. D. Hall, & J. W. Hurst (Eds.), *Clinical methods: The history, physical, and laboratory examinations* (Chapter 30, 3rd ed.). Boston: Butterworths.

Hills, A. J., Shalhoub, J., Shepherd, A. C., & Davies, A. H. (2009). Peripheral arterial disease. *The British Journal of Hospital Medicine, 70*(10), 560–565.

Hirsch, A., Criqui, M. H., Treat-Jacobson, D., Regensteiner, J. G., Creager, M. A., Olin, J. W., . . . Hiatt, W. R. (2001). Peripheral arterial disease detection, awareness, and treatment in primary care. *Journal of the American Medical Association, 286*(11), 1317–1324.

Hirsch, A. T., Haskal, Z. J., Hertzer, N. R., Bakal, C. W., Creager, M. A., Halperin, J. L., Riegel, B., . . . Vascular Disease Foundation. (2006). ACC/AHA 2005 guidelines for the manage-ment of patients with peripheral arterial disease (lower extremity, renal, mesenteric, and abdominal aortic): Executive summary a collaborative report from the American Asso-ciation for Vascular Surgery/Society for Vascular Surgery, Society for Cardiovascular

Angiography and Interventions, Society for Vascular Medicine and Biology, Society of Interventional Radiology, and the ACC/AHA Task Force on Practice Guidelines (Writing Committee to Develop Guidelines for the Management of Patients With Peripheral Arterial Disease) endorsed by the American Association of Cardiovascular and Pulmonary Rehabilitation; National Heart, Lung, and Blood Institute; Society for Vascular Nursing; TransAtlantic Inter-Society Consensus; and Vascular Disease Foundation. *Journal of the American College of Cardiology, 47,* 1239–1312.

Holt, P. J. E., Poloniecki, J. D., Gerrard, D., Loftus, I. M., & Thompson, M. M. (2007). Meta-analysis and systematic review of the relationship between volume and outcome in abdominal aortic aneurysm surgery. *The British Journal of Surgery, 94,* 395–403. doi:10.1002/bjs.5710

James, P. A., Oparil, S., Carter, B. L., Cushman, W. C., Dennison-Himmelfarb, C., Handler, J., . . . Ortiz, E. (2014). 2014 evidence-based guideline for the management of high blood pressure in adults: Report from the panel members appointed to the Eighth Joint National Committee (JNC-8). *Journal of the American Medical Association, 311*(5), 507–520.

Kaewlai, R., & Abujudeh, H. (2012). Nephrogenic systemic fibrosis. *The American Journal of Roentgenology, 199*(1), W17–W23.

Kannel, W. B., & McGee, D. L. (1985). DL. Update of some epidemiological features of intermittent claudication: The Framingham Study. *Journal of the American Geriatrics Society, 33*(1), 13–18.

Karthikesalingam, A., Al-Jundi, W., Jackson, D., Boyle, J. R., Beard, J. D., Holt, P. J. E., & Thompson, M. M. (2012). Systematic review and meta-analysis of duplex ultrasonography, contrast-enhanced ultrasonography or computed tomography for surveillance after endovascular aneurysm repair. *The British Journal of Surgery, 99,* 1514–1523.

Kent, K. C., Zwolak, R. M., Egorova, N. N., Riles, T. S., Manganaro, A., Moskowitz, A. J., . . . Greco, G. (2010). Analysis of risk factors for abdominal aortic aneurysm in a cohort of more than 3 million individuals. *Journal of Vascular Surgery, 52,* 539–548.

Kent, K. C., Zwolak, R. M., Jaff, M. R., Hollenbeck, S. T., Thompson, R. W., Schermerhorn, M. L., . . . Cronenwett, J. L. (2004). Screening for abdominal aortic aneurysm: A consensus statement. *Journal of Vascular Surgery, 39,* 267–269.

Khandanpour, N., Loke, Y. K., Meyer, F., Jennings, B., & Armon, M. P. (2009). Homocysteine and peripheral arterial disease: Systematic review and meta-analysis. *European Journal of Vascular and Endovascular Surgery, 38*(3), 316–322.

Koelemay, M. J., Lijmer, J. G., Stoker, J., Legemate, D. A., & Bossuyt, P. M. (2001). Magnetic resonance angiography for the evaluation of lower extremity arterial disease: A meta-analysis. *Journal of the American Medical Association, 285*(10), 1338–1345.

Kreitner, K. F., Kalden, P., Neufang, A., Duber, C., Krummenauer, F., Kustner, E., . . . Thelen, M. (2000). Diabetes and peripheral arterial occlusive disease: Prospective comparison of contrast-enhanced three-dimensional MR angiography with conventional digital subtraction angiography. *The American Journal of Roentgenology, 174*(1), 171–179.

Kronzon, I., & Saric, M. 2010. Cholesterol embolization syndrome. *Circulation, 122,* 631–641.

Kuivaniemi, H., Shibamura, H., Arthur, C., Berguer, R., Cole, C. W., Juvonen, T., . . . Tromp, G. (2003). Familial abdominal aortic aneurysms: Collection of 233 multiplex families. *Journal of Vascular Surgery, 37,* 340–345.

Lane, D. A., & Lip, G. Y. (2013). Treatment of hypertension in peripheral arterial disease. *Cochrane Database Systematic Review, 12.* Article no. CD003075. doi:10.1002/14651858. CD003075.pub3

Lederle, F. A., Freischlag, J. A., Kyriakides, T. C., Matsumura, J. S., Padberg, F. T., Kohler, T. R.; . . . OVER Veterans Affairs Cooperative Study Group. (2012). Long-term comparison of endovascular and open repair of abdominal aortic aneurysm. *The New England Journal of Medicine, 367,* 1988–1997.

Lederle, F. A., Freischlag, J. A., Kyriakides, T. C., Padberg, F. T., Matsumura, J. S., Kohler, T. R., . . . Open Versus Endovascular Repair (OVER) Veterans Affairs Cooperative Study Group. (2009). Outcomes following endovascular vs open repair of abdominal aortic aneurysm: A randomized trial. *Journal of the American Medical Association, 302,* 1535–1542.

Lederle, F. A., & Simel, D. L. (1999). Does this patient have abdominal aortic aneurysm? *Journal of the American Medical Association, 281,* 77–82.

Lederle, F. A., Wilson, S. E., Johnson, G. R., Reinke, D. B., Littooy, F. N., Acher, C. W.; . . . Aneurysm Detection and Management Veterans Affairs (ADAM VA) Cooperative Study Group. (2002). Immediate repair compared with surveillance of small abdominal aortic aneurysms. *The New England Journal of Medicine, 346,* 1437–1444.

LeFevre, M. L. (2014). Screening for abdominal aortic aneurysms: U.S. Preventive Services Task Force recommendation statement. *Annals of Internal Medicine, 161*(4), 281–290.

Leng, G. C., Lee, A. J., Fowkes, F. G., Whiteman, M., Dunbar, J., Housley, E., & Ruckley, C. V. (1996). Incidence, natural history and cardiovascular events in symptomatic and asymptomatic peripheral arterial disease in the general population. *International Journal of Epidemiology, 25,* 1172–1181.

Libby, P., Ridker, P. M., & Maseri, A. (2002). Inflammation and atherosclerosis. *Circulation, 105*(9), 1135–1143.

Liddington, M. I., & Heather, B. P. (1992). The relationship between aortic diameter and body habitus. *European Journal of Vascular Surgery, 6*(1), 89–92.

Lin, P. H., Bush, R. L., McCoy, S. A., Felkai, D., Pasnelli, T. K., Nelson, J. C., . . . Lumsden, A. B. (2003). A prospective study of a hand-held ultrasound device in abdominal aortic aneurysm evaluation. *The American Journal of Surgery, 186,* 455–459.

Lovegrove, R. E., Javid, M., Magee, T. R., & Galland, R. B. (2008). A meta-analysis of 21,178 patients undergoing open or endovascular repair of abdominal aortic aneurysm. *The British Journal of Surgery, 95,* 677–684.

Lu, L., Mackay, D. F., & Pell, J. P. (2014). Meta-analysis of the association between cigarette smoking and peripheral arterial disease. *Heart, 100*(5), 414–423.

Lynch, R. M. (2004). Accuracy of abdominal examination in the diagnosis of non-ruptured abdominal aortic aneurysm. *Accident and Emergency Nursing, 12,* 99–107.

Mani, K., Björck, M., Lundkvist, J., & Wanhainen, A. (2009). Improved long-term survival after abdominal aortic aneurysm repair. *Circulation, 120,* 201–211.

McKenna, M., Wolfson, S., & Kuller, L. (1991). The ratio of ankle and arm arterial pressure as an independent predictor of mortality. *Atherosclerosis, 87*(2–3), 119–128.

Menke, J., & Larsen, J. (2010). Meta-analysis: Accuracy of contrast-enhanced magnetic resonance angiography for assessing steno-occlusions in peripheral arterial disease. *Annals of Internal Medicine, 153*(5), 325–334.

Met, R., Bipat, S., Legemate, D. A., Reekers, J. A., & Koelemay, M. J. (2009). Diagnostic performance of computed tomography angiography in peripheral arterial disease: A 2014 systematic review and meta-analysis. *Journal of the American Medical Association, 301*(4), 415–424.

Moneta, G. L., Yeager, R. A., Lee, R. W., & Porter, J. M. (1993). Noninvasive localization of arterial occlusive disease: A comparison of segmental Doppler pressures and arterial duplex mapping. *Journal of Vascular Surgery, 17*(3), 578–582.

Mueller, T., Hinterreiter, F., Luft, C., Poelz, W., Haltmayer, M., & Dieplinger, B. (2014). Mortality rates and mortality predictors in patients with symptomatic peripheral artery disease stratified according to age and diabetes. *Journal of Vascular Surgery, 59*(5), 1291–1299.

Muluk, S. C., Muluk, V. S., Kelley, M. E., Whittle, J. C., Tierney, J. A., Webster, M. W., & Makaroun, M. S. (2001). Outcome events in patients with claudication: A 15-year study in 2777 patients. *Journal of Vascular Surgery, 33*(2), 251–257.

Munro, J. M., & Cotran, R. S. (1988). The pathogenesis of atherosclerosis: Atherogenesis and inflammation. *Lab Investigation, 58*(3), 249–261.

Ness, J., & Aronow, W. S. (1999). Prevalence of coexistence of coronary artery disease, ischemic stroke, and peripheral arterial disease in older persons, mean age 80 years, in an academic, hospital-based geriatrics practice. *Journal of the American Geriatrics Society, 47*(10), 1255–1256.

Newman, A. B., Arnold, A. M., Burke, G. L., O'Leary, D. H., & Manolio, T. A. (2001). Cardiovascular disease and mortality in older adults with small abdominal aortic aneurysms detected by ultrasonography: The cardiovascular health study. *Annals of Internal Medicine, 134,* 182–190. doi:10.7326/0003-4819-134-3-200102060-00008

Norgren, L., Hiatt, W. R., Dormandy, J. A., Nehler, M. R., Harris, K. A., Fowkes, F. G., . . . TASC II Working Group. (2007). Intersociety consensus for the management of peripheral arterial disease (TASC II). *Journal of Vascular Surgery, 45*(Suppl. S), S5–S67.

O'Hare, A. M., Glidden, D. V., Fox, C. S., & Hsu, C. Y. (2004). High prevalence of peripheral arterial disease in persons with renal insufficiency: Results from the National Health and Nutrition Examination Survey 1999–2000. *Circulation, 109*(3), 320–323.

Ortmann, C., Wüllenweber, J., Brinkmann, B., & Fracasso, T. (2010). Fatal mycotic aneurysm caused by *Pseudallescheria boydii* after near drowning. *International Journal of Legal Medicine, 124,* 243–247. doi:10.1007/s00414-009-0336-9

Ostchega, Y., Paulose-Ram, R., Dillon, C. F., Gu, Q., & Hughes, J. P. (2007). Prevalence of peripheral arterial disease and risk factors in persons aged 60 and older: Data from the National Health and Nutrition Examination Survey 1999–2004. *Journal of the American Geriatric Society, 55*(4), 583–589.

Poldermans, D., Bax, J. J., Kertai, M. D., Krenning, B., Westerhout, C. M., Schinkel, A. F., . . . Boersma, E. (2003). Statins are associated with a reduced incidence of perioperative mortality in patients undergoing major non-cardiac vascular surgery. *Circulation, 107*(14), 1848–1851.

Prinssen, M., Verhoeven, E. L., Buth, J., Cuypers, P. W. M., van Sambeek, M. R. H. M., Balm, R., . . . Dutch Randomized Endovascular Aneurysm Management (DREAM) Trial Group. (2004). A randomized trial comparing conventional and endovascular repair of abdominal aortic aneurysms. *The New England Journal of Medicine, 351,* 1607–1618.

Raij, L. (1991). Hypertension, endothelium, and cardiovascular risk factors. *The American Journal of Medicine, 90*(2A), 3S–18S.

Regensteiner, J. G., Ware, J. E., Jr., McCarthy, W. J., Zhang, P., Forbes, W. P., Heckman, J., & Hiatt, W. R. (2002). Effect of cilostazol on treadmill walking, community-based walking ability, and health-related quality of life in patients with intermittent claudication due to peripheral arterial disease: Meta-analysis of six randomized controlled trials. *Journal of the American Geriatric Society, 50*(12), 1939–1946.

Reis, P. E. O. (2005). Blue Toe syndrome. *Jornal Vascular Brasileiro, 4,* 391–393.

Ridker, P. M., Cushman, M., Stampfer, M. J., Tracy, R. P., & Hennekens, C. H. (2004). Plasma concentration of C-reactive protein and risk of developing peripheral vascular disease. *Circulation, 97*(5), 425–428.

Rooke, T. W., Hirsch, A. T., Misra, S., Sidawy, A. N., Beckman, J. A., Findeiss, L. K., . . . Zierler, R. E. (2011). 2011 ACCF/AHA focused update of the guidelines for the management of patients with peripheral artery disease (updating the 2005 guideline): A report of the American College of Cardiology Foundation/American Heart Association Task Force on Practice Guidelines. *Circulation, 124,* 2020–2045.

Rubano, E., Mehta, N., Caputo, W., Paladino, L., & Sinert, R. (2013). Systematic review: Emergency department bedside ultrasonography for diagnosing suspected abdominal aortic aneurysm. *Academic Emergency Medicine, 20,* 128–138.

Rughani, G., Robertson, L., & Clarke, M. (2012). Medical treatment for small abdominal aortic aneurysms. *Cochrane Database of Systematic Reviews,* Issue 9. Art. No.: CD009536. doi:10.1002/14651858.CD009536.pub2

Rutherford, R. B., Lowenstein, D. H., & Klein, M. F. (1979). Combining segmental systolic pressures and plethysmography to diagnose arterial occlusive disease of the legs. *The American Journal of Surgery, 138*(2), 211–218.

Sacks, D., Robinson, M. L., Marinelli, D. L., & Perlmutter, G. S. (1992). Peripheral arterial Doppler ultrasonography: Diagnostic criteria. *Journal of Ultrasound in Medicine, 11*(3), 95–103.

Sadat, U., Boyle, J. R., Walsh, S. R., Tang, T., Varty, K., & Hayes, P. D. (2008). Endovascular vs open repair of acute abdominal aortic aneurysms—A systematic review and meta-analysis. *Journal of Vascular Surgery, 48*, 227–236.

Sakalihasan, N., Limet, R., & Defawe, O. D. (2005). Abdominal aortic aneurysm. *The Lancet, 365*(9470), 1577–1589.

Salhiyyah, K., Senanayake, E., Abdel-Hadi, M., Booth, A., & Michaels, J. A. (2012). Pentoxifylline for intermittent claudication. *Cochrane Database of Systematic Reviews, 1.* Article no. CD005262. doi:10.1002/14651858.CD005262.pub2

Santilli, S. M., Littooy, F. N., Cambria, R. A., Rapp, J. H., Tretinyak, A. S., d'Audiffret, A. C., . . . Krupski, W. C. (2002). Expansion rates and outcomes for the 3.0-cm to the 3.9-cm infrarenal abdominal aortic aneurysm. *Journal of Vascular Surgery, 35*, 666–671.

Schermerhorn, M. L., O'Malley, A. J., Jhaveri, A., Cotterill, P., Pomposelli, F., & Landon, B. E. (2008). Endovascular vs. open repair of abdominal aortic aneurysms in the Medicare population. *The New England Journal of Medicine, 358*, 464–474.

Schousboe, J. T., Wilson, K. E., & Kiel, D. P. (2006). Detection of abdominal aortic calcification with lateral spine imaging using DEX. *Journal of Clinical Densitometry, 9*, 302–308.

Selvin, E., & Erlinger, T. P. (2004). Prevalence and risk factors for peripheral arterial disease in the United States: Results from the National Health and Nutrition Examination Survey, 1999–2000. *Circulation, 110*(6), 738–743.

Shaw, D. R., & Kessel, D. O. (2006). The current status of the use of carbon dioxide in diagnostic and interventional angiographic procedures. *Cardiovascular and Interventional Radiology, 29*(3), 323–331.

Silverstein, M. D., Pitts, S. R., Chaikof, E. L., & Ballard, D. J. (2005). Abdominal aortic aneurysm (AAA): Cost-effectiveness of screening, surveillance of intermediate-sized AAA, and management of symptomatic AAA. *Proceedings (Bayl Univ Med Cent), 18*(4), 345–367.

Spronk, S., White, J. V., Ryjewski, C., Rosenblum, J., Bosch, J. L., & Hunink, M. G. (2009). Invasive treatment of claudication is indicated for patients unable to adequately ambulate during cardiac rehabilitation. *Journal of Vascular Surgery, 49*(5), 1217–1225.

Sprouse, R. L., Meier, G. H., LeSar, C. J., DeMasi, R. J., Sood, J., Parent, F. L., . . . Gayle, R. G. (2003). Comparison of abdominal aortic aneurysm diameter measurements obtained with ultrasound and computed tomography: Is there a difference? *Journal of Vascular Surgery, 38*, 466–472.

Stather, P. W., Sidloff, D., Dattani, N., Choke, E., Bown, M. J., & Sayers, R. D. (2013). Systematic review and meta-analysis of the early and late outcomes of open and endovascular repair of abdominal aortic aneurysm. *The British Journal of Surgery, 100*, 863–872.

Stavropoulos, S. W., & Charagundla, S. R. (2007). Imaging techniques for detection and management of endoleaks after endovascular aortic aneurysm repair. *Radiology, 243*(3), 641–655. doi:10.1148/radiol.2433051649

Stewart, K., Hiatt, W. R., Regensteiner, J. G., & Hirsh, A. T. (2002). Exercise training for claudication. *The New England Journal of Medicine, 347*(24), 1941–1951.

Stone, N. J., Robinson, J., Lichtenstein, A. H., Bairey Merz, C. N., Blum, C. B., Eckel, R. H., Wilson, P. W. F., . . . Tomaselli, G. F. (2013). 2013 ACC/AHA guideline on the treatment of blood cholesterol to reduce atherosclerotic cardiovascular risk in adults: A report of the American College of Cardiology/American Heart Association Task Force on Practice Guidelines. *Circulation, 129*(25 Supplement 2), S1–S45.

Strandness, D. E., Dalman, R. L., Panian, S., Randell, M. S., Comp, P. C., Zhang, P., & Forbes, W. P. (2002). Effect of cilostazol in patients with intermittent claudication: A randomized, double-blind, placebo-controlled study. *Vascular and Endovascular Surgery, 36*(2), 83–91.

Sweeting, M. J., Thompson, S. G., Brown, L. C., & Powell, J. T. (2012). Meta-analysis of individual patient data to examine factors affecting growth and rupture of small abdominal aortic aneurysms. *The British Journal of Surgery, 99*, 655–665.

Thomas, S. M., Beard, J. D., Ireland, M., & Ayers, S. (2005). Results from the prospective registry of endovascular treatment of abdominal aortic aneurysms (RETA): Mid term results to five years. *European Journal of Vascular Endovascular Surgery, 29*(6), 563–570.

UK Small Aneurysm Trial Participants. (1998). Mortality results for randomised controlled trial of early elective surgery or ultrasonographic surveillance for small abdominal aortic aneurysms. *The Lancet, 352*, 1649–1655.

U.S. Preventive Services Task Force. (2005). Screening for abdominal aortic aneurysm: Recommendation statement. *Annals of Internal Medicine, 14*, 198–202.

U.S. Preventive Services Task Force. (2014). Retrieved from www.uspreventiveservices taskforce.org/Page/Document/UpdateSummaryFinal/abdominal-aortic-aneurysm-screening

Vincent, D. G., Salles-Cunha, S. X., Bernhard, V. M., & Towne, J. B. (1983). Noninvasive assessment of toe systolic pressures with special reference to diabetes mellitus. *Journal of Cardiovascular Surgery (Torino), 24*(1), 22–28.

Wattanakit, K., Folsom, A. R., Selvin, E., Coresh, J., Hirsch, A. T., & Weatherly, B. D. (2007). Kidney function and risk of peripheral arterial disease; results from the Atherosclerosis Risk in Communities (ARIC) study. *Journal of the American Society of Nephrology, 18*(2), 629–636.

Wessler, S., & Silberg, N. R. (1953). Studies in peripheral arterial occlusive disease: II Clinical findings in patients with advanced arterial obstruction and gangrene. *Circulation, 7*(6), 810–818.

White, J. V. (2010). Lower extremity arterial disease: General considerations. In J. L. Cronenwett & K. W. Johnston (Eds.), *Rutherford's vascular surgery* (pp. 1576–1592). Philadelphia: WB Saunders.

Whitehall, T. A. (1997). Role of revascularization in the treatment of intermittent claudication. *Vascular Medicine, 2*(3), 252–256.

Whitmore, A. D., & Belkin, M. (2000). Infrainguinal bypass. In R. B. Rutherford (Ed.), *Vascular surgery* (vol. 5; pp. 998–1018). Philadelphia: WB Saunders.

Willigendael, E. M., Teijink, J. A., Bartelink, M. L., Kuiken, B. W., Boiten, J., Moll, F. L., . . . Prins, M. H. (2004). Influence of smoking on incidence and prevalence of peripheral arterial disease. *Journal of Vascular Surgery, 40*(6),1158–1165.

Wilmink, A. B. M., Vardulaki, K. A., Hubbard, C. S., Day, N. E., Ashton, H. A., Scott, A. P., & Quick, C. R. G. (2002). Are antihypertensive drugs associated with abdominal aortic aneurysms? *Journal of Vascular Surgery, 36*, 751–757.

Wilson, A. M., Sadrzadeh-Rafie, A. H., Myers, J., Assimes, T., Nead, K. T., Higgins, M., . . . Cooke, J. P. (2011). Low lifetime recreational activity is a risk factor for peripheral arterial disease. *Journal of Vascular Surgery, 54*(20), 427–432.

Wilt, T. J., Lederle, F. A., MacDonald, R., Jonk, Y. C., Rector, T. S., & Kane, R. L. (2006). Comparison of endovascular and open surgical repairs for abdominal aortic aneurysm. Rockville (MD): Agency for Healthcare Research and Quality (US). (Evidence Reports/Technology Assessments, No. 144.) Retrieved from http://www.ncbi.nlm.nih.gov/books/NBK38176/

Wolf, Y. G., Johnson, B. L., Hill, B. B., Rubin, G. D., Fogarty, T. J., & Zarins, C. K. (2000). Duplex ultrasound scanning versus computed tomographic angiography for postoperative evaluation of endovascular abdominal aortic aneurysm repair. *Journal of Vascular Surgery, 32*, 1142–1148.

Xu, C., Zarins, C. K., & Glagov, S. (2001). Aneurysmal and occlusive atherosclerosis of the human abdominal aorta. *Journal of Vascular Surgery, 33*, 91–96.

Yao, S. T., Hobbs, J. T., & Irvine, W. T. (1969). Ankle systolic pressure measurements in arterial disease affecting the lower extremities. *The British Journal of Surgery, 56*(9), 676–679.

SECTION V

Abidov, A., Rozanski, A., Hachamovitch, R., Hayes, S. W., Aboul-Enein, F., Cohen, I., . . . Berman, D. S. (2005). Prognostic significance of dyspnea in patients referred for cardiac stress testing. *The New England Journal of Medicine, 353*(18), 1889–1898.

Abiomed. (2014). *Recovering hearts. Saving lives.* Retrieved from http://www.abiomed.com

Abraham, N. S., Hlatky, M. A., Antman, E. M., Bhatt, D. L., Bjorkman, D. J., Clark, C. B., . . . Tomaselli, G. F. (2010). ACCF/ACG/AHA 2010 expert consensus document on the concomitant use of proton pump inhibitors and thienopyridines: A focused update of the ACCF/ACG/AHA 2008 expert consensus document on reducing the gastrointestinal risks of antiplatelet therapy and NSAID use. *Journal of the American College of Cardiology, 56*(24), 2051–2066.

ACE Inhibitor Myocardial Infarction Collaborative Group. (1998). Indications for ACE inhibitors in the early treatment of acute myocardial infarction: Systematic overview of individual data from 100,000 patients in randomized trials. *Circulation, 97,* 2202–2212.

Adamopoulos, C., Ahmed, A., Fay, R., Angioi, M., Filippatos, G., Vincent, J., . . . Zannad, F. (2009). Timing of eplerenone initiation and outcomes in patients with heart failure after acute myocardial infarction complicated by left ventricular systolic dysfunction: Insights from the EPHESUS trial. *European Journal of Heart Failure, 11,* 1099–1105.

Adams, K. F., Fonarow, G. C., Emerman, C. L., LeJemtel, T. H., Costanzo, M. R., Abraham, W. T., . . . Horton, D. P. (2005). Characteristics and outcomes of patients hospitalized for heart failure in the United States: Rationale, design, and preliminary observations from the first 100,000 cases in the Acute Decompensated Heart Failure National Registry (ADHERE). *American Heart Journal, 149*(2), 209–216.

Agewall, S., Cattaneo, M., Collet, J. P., Andreotti, F., Lip, G. Y. H., Verheugt, F. W. A., . . . Storey, R. F. (2013). Expert position paper on the use of proton pump inhibitors in patients with cardiovascular disease and antithrombotic therapy. *European Heart Journal, 34*(23), 1708–1713.

Aggarwal, M., & Khan, U. (2006). Hypertensive crisis: Hypertensive emergencies and urgencies. *Cardiology Clinics, 24*(1), 135–146.

Ahmed, A., Bourge, R. C., Fonarow, G. C., Patel, K., Morgan, C. J., & Fleg, J. L. (2014). Digoxin use and lower 30-day all-cause readmission for medicare beneficiaries hospitalized for heart failure. *The American Journal of Medicine, 127*(1), 61–70.

Akhter, N., Milford-Beland, S., Roe, M. T., Plana, R. N., Kao, J., & Shroff, A. (2009). Gender differences among patients with acute coronary syndromes undergoing percutaneous coronary intervention in the American College of Cardiology-National Cardiovascular Data Registry (ACC-NCDR). *American Heart Journal, 157,* 141–148.

Aliti, G. B., Rabelo, E. R., Clausell, N., Rohde, L. E., Biolo, A., & Beck-da-Silva, L. (2013). Aggressive fluid and sodium restriction in acute decompensated heart failure: A randomized controlled trial. *JAMA Internal Medicine, 173*(12), 1058–1064.

American Heart Association. (2014). Get With The Guidelines—HF clinical tools library. Retrieved from http://www.heart.org/HEARTORG/HealthcareResearch/GetWithThe Guidelines/GetWithTheGuidelines-HF/Get-With-The-Guidelines-HF-Clinical-Tools-Library_UCM_305817_Article.jsp

Ammirati, F., Colivicchi, F., Di Battista, G., Garelli, F. F., Pandozi, C., & Santini, M. (1998). Variable cerebral dysfunction during tilt induced vasovagal syncope. *Pacing Clinical Electrophysiology, 21*(11), 2420–2425.

Amsterdam, E. A., Wenger, N. K., Brindis, R. G., Casey, D. E., Jr., Ganiats, T. G., Holmes, D. R., Jr., . . . Zieman, S. J. (2014). 2014 ACC/AHA guideline for the management of patients with non–ST-elevation acute coronary syndromes: A report of the American College of Cardiology/American Heart Association Task Force on Practice Guidelines. *Journal of the American College of Cardiology, 64*(24), e139–e228. doi:10.1016/j.jacc.2014.09.017

Ananth, C., Keyes, K., & Wapner, R. (2013). Pre-eclampsia rates in the United States, 1980–2010: Age-period-cohort analysis. *The British Medical Journal, 347*, f6564. Retrieved from http://www.bmj.com/content/347/bmj.f6564.full.pdf+html

Anderson, J. L., Adams, C. D., Antman, E. M., Bridges, C. R., Califf, R. M., Casey, D. E., Jr., . . . Wright, R. S. (2013). 2012 ACCF/AHA focused update incorporated into the guideline for the management of patients with unstable angina/non-ST-elevation myocardial infarction: A report of the American College of Cardiology Foundation/American Heart Association Task Force on Practice Guidelines. *Journal of the American College of Cardiology, 61*, e179–e347. doi:10.1016/j.jacc.2013.01.014

Antiarrhythmics Versus Implantable Defibrillator (AVID) Investigators. (1997). A comparison of antiarrhythmic-drug therapy with implantable defibrillators in patients resuscitated from near-fatal ventricular arrhythmias. *The New England Journal of Medicine, 337*, 1576–1584.

Antman, E. M. (2012). Chapter 54—ST-elevation myocardial infarction: Pathology, pathophysiology, and clinical features. In R. O. Bonow, D. L. Mann, D. P. Zipes, P. Libby, & E. Braunwald (Eds.), *Braunwald's heart disease: A textbook of cardiovascular medicine* (9th ed., pp. 1087–1109). Philadelphia, PA: Saunders-Elsevier.

Antman, E. M., Cohen, M., Bernink, P. J., McCabe, C. H., Horacek, T., Papuchis, G., . . . Braunwald, E. (2000). The TIMI risk score for unstable angina/non–ST elevation MI: A method for prognostication and therapeutic decision making. *Journal of the American Medical Association, 284*, 835–842.

Antman, E. M., & Morrow, D. A. (2012). Chapter 55—ST-elevation myocardial infarction: Management. In R. O. Bonow, D. L. Mann, D. P. Zipes, P. Libby, & E. Braunwald (Eds.), *Braunwald's heart disease: A textbook of cardiovascular medicine* (9th ed., pp. 1111–1177). Philadelphia, PA: Saunders-Elsevier.

Arbab-Zadeh, A., Nakano, M., Virmani, R., & Fuster, V. (2012). Acute coronary events. *Circulation, 125*, 1147–1156.

Arnar, D. (2013). Syncope in patients with structural heart disease. *Journal of Internal Medicine, 274*(4), 336–344.

Aronson, D., & Burger, A. J. (2004). Relation between pulse pressure and survival in patients with decompensated heart failure. *The American Journal of Cardiology, 93*, 785–787.

Assaad, M. C., Calle-Muller, C., Dahu, M., Nowak, R. M., Hudson, M. P., Mueller, C., . . . McCord, J. (2013). The relationship between chest pain duration and the incidence of acute myocardial infarction among patients with acute chest pain. *Critical Pathways in Cardiology, 12*(3), 150–153.

Austin, J. J. (2005). Chapter 30—Aortic dissection. In J. B. Hall, G. A. Schmidt, & L. H. Wood (Eds.), *Principles of critical care* (3rd ed.). Retrieved from http://accessmedicine.mhmedical.com/content.aspx?bookid=361&Sectionid=39866397

Backus, B. E., Six, A. J., Kelder, J. C., Bosschaert, M. A., Mast, E. G., Mosterd, A., . . . Doevendans, P. A. (2013). A prospective validation of the HEART score for chest pain patients at the emergency department. *International Journal of Cardiology, 168*(3), 2153–2158.

Backus, B. E., Six, A. J., Kelder, J. H., Gibler, W. B., Moll, F. L., & Doevendans, P. A. (2011). Risk scores for patients with chest pain: Evaluation in the emergency department. *Current Cardiology Reviews, 7*(1), 2–8.

Baddour, L. M., Wilson, W. R., Bayer, A. S., Fowler, V. G., Jr., Bolger, A. F., Levison, M. E., . . . Taubert, K. A. (2005). Infective endocarditis: Diagnosis, antimicrobial therapy, and management of complications: A statement for health care professionals from the Committee on Rheumatic Fever, Endocarditis, and Kawasaki Disease, Council on Cardiovascular Disease in the Young, and the Councils on Clinical Cardiology, Stroke, and Cardiovascular Surgery and Anesthesia, American Heart Association: Endorsed by the Infectious Diseases Society of America. *Circulation, 111*, e394–e434.

Bardy, G. H., Lee, K. L., Mark, D. B., Poole, J. E., Packer, D. L., Boineau, R., . . . Ip, J. H. (2005). Amiodarone or an implantable cardioverter-defibrillator for congestive heart failure. *The New England Journal of Medicine, 352,* 225–237.

Bart, B. A., Goldsmith, S. R., Lee, K. L., Givertz, M. M., O'Connor, C. M., Bull, D. A., . . . Heart Failure Clinical Research Network. (2012). Ultrafiltration in decompensated heart failure with cardiorenal syndrome. *The New England Journal of Medicine, 367,* 2296–2304.

Bawamia, B., Mehran, R., Qiu, W., & Kunadian, V. (2013). Risk scores in acute coronary syndrome and percutaneous coronary intervention: A review. *American Heart Journal, 165*(4), 441–450.

Bayes-Genis, A., deAntonio, M., Vila, J., Penafiel, J., Galan, A., Barallat, J., . . . Lupon, J. (2014). Head-to-head comparison of 2 myocardial fibrosis biomarkers for long-term heart failure risk stratification: ST2 versus galectin-3. *Journal of the American College of Cardiology, 63*(2), 158–166.

Berlin, D. (2014). Hemodynamic consequences of auto-PEEP. *Journal of Intensive Care Medicine, 29*(2), 81–86.

Betriu, A., Heras, M., Cohen, M., & Fuster, V. (1992). Unstable angina: Outcome according to clinical presentation. *Journal of the American College of Cardiology, 19*(7), 1659–1663.

Bhimji, S. (2013). Postinfarction ventricular septal rupture. *Medscape.* Retrieved from http://emedicine.medscape.com/article/428240-overview#a1

Bickley, L. S., & Szilagyi, P. G. (2013). *Bates' guide to physical examination and history taking* (11th ed.). Philadelphia, PA: Wolters Kluwer Health.

Birnbaum, Y., Chamoun, A. J., Anzuini, A., Lick, S. D., Ahmad, M., & Uretsky, B. F. (2003). Ventricular free wall rupture following myocardial infarction. *Coronary Artery Disease, 14,* 463–470.

Boersma, E., Pieper, K. S., Steyerberg, E. W., Wilcox, R. G., Chang, W., Lee, K. L., . . . PURSUIT Investigators. (2000). Predictors of outcome in patients with acute coronary syndromes without persistent ST-segment elevation. Results from an international trial of 9461 patients. *Circulation, 101,* 2557–2567.

Booher, A., Isselbacher, E., Nienaber, C., Trimarchi, S., Evangelista, A., Montgomery D., . . . Eagle, K. (2013). The IRAD classification system for characterizing survival after aortic dissection. *The American Journal of Medicine, 126*(8), 730, e19–730.e24.

Bradley, E. H., Nallamothu, B. K., Stern, A. F., Cherlin, E. J., Wang, Y., Byrd, J. R., . . . Krumholz, H. (2009). The door-to-balloon alliance for quality: Who joins national collaborative efforts and why? *Joint Commission Journal on Quality and Patient Safety, 35*(2), 93–99.

Braunwald, E., Antman, E. M., Beasley, J. W., Califf, R. M., Cheitlin, M. D., Hochman, J. S., . . . Theroux, P. (2000). ACC/AHA guidelines for the management of patients with unstable angina and non-ST-segment elevation myocardial infarction: A report of the American College of Cardiology/American Heart Association Task Force on Practice Guidelines (Committee on the Management of Patients with Unstable Angina). *Journal of the American College of Cardiology, 36*(3), 970–1062.

Brenyo, A., Barsheshet, A., Rao, M., Huang, D. T., Zareba, W., McNitt, S., . . . Goldenberg, I. (2013). Brain natriuretic peptide and cardiac resynchronization therapy in patients with mildly symptomatic heart failure. *Circulation: Heart Failure, 6,* 998–1004.

Brieger, D., Eagle, K. A., Goodman, S. G., Steg, P. G., Budaj, A., White, K., & Montelesot, G. (2004). Acute coronary syndromes without chest pain, an underdiagnosed and undertreated high-risk group: Insights from the global registry of acute coronary events. *Chest, 126*(2), 461–469.

Brignole, M., Menozzi, C., Bartoletti, A., Giada, F., Lagi, A., Ungar, A., . . . Scivales, A. (2006). A new management of syncope: Prospective systematic guideline-based evaluation of patients referred urgently to the general hospitals. *European Heart Journal, 27,* 76–82.

Brilakis, E., Scott Wright, R., Kopecky, S., Reeder, G. S., Williams, B. A., & Miller, W. L. (2001). Bundle branch block as a predictor of long-term survival after acute myocardial infarction. *The American Journal of Cardiology, 88*(3), 205–209.

Burke, A. P., Farb, A., Malcom, G. T., Liang, Y. H., Smialek, J., & Virmani, R. (1997). Coronary risk factors and plaque morphology in men with coronary disease who died suddenly. *The New England Journal of Medicine, 336,* 1276–1282.

Butterworth, J. F., Mackey, D. C., & Wasnick, J. D. (2013). Chapter 20—cardiovascular physiology & anesthesia. In J. F. Butterworth, D. C. Mackey, & J. D. Wasnick (Eds.), *Morgan & Mikhail's clinical anesthesiology* (5th ed.). New York, NY: McGraw-Hill. Retrieved from http://accessmedicine.mhmedical.com/content.aspx?bookid=564&Sectionid=42800552

Buxton, A. E., Calkins, H., Callans, D. J., DiMarco, J. P., Fisher, J. D., Greene, H. L., . . . Zimetbaum, P. J. (2006). ACC/AHA/HRS 2006 key data elements and definitions for electrophysiological studies and procedures. *Circulation, 114*(23), 2534–2570.

Calkins, H., & Zipes, D. P. (2015). Chapter 40—Hypotension and syncope. In D. L. Mann, D. P. Zipes, P. Libby, R. O. Bonow, & E. Braunwald (Eds.), *Braunwald's heart disease: A textbook of cardiovascular medicine* (10th ed., pp. 861–871). Philadelphia, PA: Elsevier-Saunders.

Cannon, C. P., Braunwald, E., McCabe, C. H., Rader, D. J., Rouleau, J. L., Belder, R., . . . Skene, A. M. (2004). Intensive versus moderate lipid lowering with statins after acute coronary syndromes. *The New England Journal of Medicine, 350*(15), 1495–1504.

Canto, J. G., Goldberg, R. J., Hand, M. M., Bonow, R. O., Sopko, G., Pepine, C. J., & Long, T. (2007). Symptom presentation of women with acute coronary syndromes. *Archives of Internal Medicine, 167*(22), 2405–2413.

Canto, J. G., Rogers, W. J., Goldberg, R. J., Peterson, E. D., Wenger, N. K., Vaccarino, V., . . . NRMI Investigators. (2012). Association of age and sex with myocardial infarction symptom presentation and in-hospital mortality. *Journal of the American Medical Association, 307*(8), 813–822.

Chan, T. C., Vilke, G. M., Pollack, M., & Brady, W. J. (2001). Electrocardiographic manifestations: Pulmonary embolism. *Journal of Emergency Medicine, 21*(3), 263–270.

Chobanian, A., Bakris, G., Blac, H., Cushman, W., Green, L., Izzo, J. L., . . . National High Blood Pressure Education Program Coordinating Committee. (2003). Seventh report of the Joint National Committee on Prevention, Detection, Evaluation, and Treatment of High Blood Pressure. *Hypertension, 42,* 1206–1252.

Cleland, J. G. F., Chattopadhyay, S., Khand, A., Houghton, T., & Kaye, G. C. (2002). Prevalence and Incidence of arrhythmias and sudden death in heart failure. *Heart Failure Reviews, 7,* 229–242.

Clopidogrel in Unstable Angina to Prevent Recurrent Events Trial Investigators. (2001). Effects of clopidogrel in addition to aspirin in patients with acute coronary syndromes without ST-segment elevation. *The New England Journal of Medicine, 345,* 494–502.

Colivicchi, F., Ammirati, F., Melina, D., Guido, V., Imperoli, G., & Santini, M. (2003). Development and prospective validation of a risk stratification system for patients with syncope in the emergency department: The OESIL risk score. *European Heart Journal, 24,* 811–819.

Consensus Committee of the American Autonomic Society & American Academy of Neurology. (1996). Consensus statement on the definition of orthostatic hypotension, pure autonomic failure, and multiple system atrophy. *Neurology, 146,* 1470.

Conti, C. R. (2011). Myocardial ischemia is not always due to epicardial atheromatous disease. *Clinical Cardiology, 34*(1), 8–9.

Costanzo, M. R., Guglin, M. E., Saltzberg, M. T., Jessup, M. L., Bart, B. A., Teerlink, J. R., . . . UNLOAD Trial Investigators. (2007). Ultrafiltration versus intravenous diuretics for patients hospitalized for acute decompensated heart failure. *Journal of the American College of Cardiology, 49*(6), 675–683.

Coxib and Traditional NSAID Trialists' Collaboration. (2013). Vascular and upper gastrointestinal effects of non-steroidal anti-inflammatory drugs: Meta-analyses of individual participant data from randomized trials. *The Lancet, 382,* 769–779.

Crawford, M. H. (2014). Chapter 22—Infective endocarditis. In M. H. Crawford (Ed.), *Current diagnosis & treatment: Cardiology* (4th ed.). Retrieved from http://accessmedicine .mhmedical.com.proxygw.wrlc.org/content.aspx?

Cullen, L., Mueller, C., Parsonage, W. A., Wildi, K., Greenslade, J. H., Twerenbold, R., . . . Than, M. (2013). Validation of high-sensitivity troponin I in a 2-hour diagnostic strategy to assess 30-day outcomes in emergency department patients with possible acute coronary syndrome. *Journal of the American College of Cardiology, 62*(14), 1242–1249.

Darby, A. E., & DiMarco, J. P. (2014). Chapter 15—Sudden cardiac death. In M. H. Crawford (Ed.), *Current diagnosis & treatment: Cardiology* (4th ed.). Retrieved from http:// accessmedicine.mhmedical.com.proxygw.wrlc.org/content.aspx?bookid=715&section id=48214547

De Backer, D., Biston, P., Devriendt, J., Madl, C., Chochrad, D., Adlecoa, C., . . . Vincent, J. (2010). Comparison of dopamine and norepinephrine in the treatment of shock. *The New England Journal of Medicine, 362*(9), 779–789.

de Jonge, P., van den Brink, R. H. S., Spijkerman, T. A., & Ormel, J. (2006). Only incident depressive episodes after myocardial infarction are associated with new cardiovascular events. *Journal of the American Medical Association, 48*(11), 2204–2208.

de Lemos, J. A., O'Rourke, R. A., & Harrington, R. (2011). Chapter 59—Unstable angina and non-ST-segment elevation myocardial infarction. In V. Fuster, R. A. Walsh, & R. A. Harrington (Eds.), *Hurst's the heart* (13th ed.). [McGraw-Hill Access Medicine version]. Retrieved from http://accessmedicine.mhmedical.com/book.aspx?bookid=376

de Moya, M. A. (2013). Shock. In R. S. Porter & J. L. Kaplan (Eds.), *The Merck manual for health care professionals.* Retrieved from http://www.merckmanuals.com/professional/critical_ care_medicine/shock_and_fluid_resuscitation/shock.html#v928145

de Zwaan, C., Barr, F. W., Janssen, J. H. A., Cheriex, E. C., Dassen, W. R. M., Brugada, P., . . . Wellens, H. J. J. (1989). Angiographic and clinical characteristics of patients with unstable angina showing an ECG pattern indicating critical narrowing of the proximal LAD coronary artery. *American Heart Journal, 117*(3), 657–665.

Depre, C., Vatner, S. F., & Gross, G. J. (2011). Chapter 54—Coronary blood flow and myocardial ischemia. In V. Fuster, R. A. Walsh, & R. A. Harrington (Eds.), *Hurst's the heart* (13th ed.). [McGraw-Hill Access Medicine version]. Retrieved from http://accessmedicine .mhmedical.com/book.aspx?bookid=376

Deshmukh, A., Furmar, G., Kurmar, N., Nachal, R., Gobal, F., Sakhuja, A., & Mehta, J. (2011). Effect of Joint National Committee VII report on hospitalizations for hypertensive emergencies in the United States. *The American Journal of Cardiology, 108*(9), 1277–1282.

Diercks, D., Promes, S., Schuur, J., Shah, K., Valente, J., & Cantrill, S. (2015). Clinical policy: Critical issues in the evaluation and management of adult patients with suspected acute nontraumatic thoracic aortic dissection. *Annals of Emergency Medicine, 65*, 32–42.

Doust, J. A., Pietrzak, E., Dobson, A., & Glasziou, P. (2005). How well does B-type natriuretic peptide predict death and cardiac events in patients with heart failure: Systematic review. *The British Medical Journal, 330*, 625. Retrieved from http://www.bmj.com/ content/330/7492/625.full.pdf+html. doi:http://dx.doi.org/10.1136/bmj.330.7492.625

Drazner, M. H., Rame, J. E., Stevenson, L. W., & Dries, D. L. (2001). Prognostic importance of elevated jugular venous pressure and a third heart sound in patients with heart failure. *The New England Journal of Medicine, 345*(8), 574–581.

Drory, Y. (2002). Sexual activity and cardiovascular risk. *European Heart Journal* [Suppl. H], 4, H13–H18.

Dumitru, I. (2014). Heart failure. *Medscape.* Retrieved from http://emedicine.medscape.com/ article/163062-overview

Eachempati, S. R. (2013). Oliguria. In R. S. Porter & J. L. Kaplan (Eds.), *The Merck manual for health care professionals.* Retrieved from http://www.merckmanuals.com/professional/ critical_care_medicine/approach_to_the_critically_ill_patient/oliguria.html

Echt, D. S., Liebson, P. R., Mitchell, L. B., Peters, R. W., Obias-Manno, D., Barker, A. H., . . . CAST Investigators. (1991). Mortality and morbidity in patients receiving encainide, flecainide, or placebo: The cardiac arrhythmia suppression trial. *The New England Journal of Medicine, 324,* 781–788.

Eckel, R. H., Jakicic, J. M., Ard, J. D., de Jesus, J. M., Houston Miller, N., Hubbard, V. S., . . . Yanovski, S. Z. (2014). 2013 AHA/ACC guideline on lifestyle management to reduce cardiovascular risk: A report of the American College of Cardiology/American Heart Association Task Force on Practice Guidelines. *Circulation, 129* (Suppl. 2), S76–S99.

Falk, E., Nakano, M., Betzon, J. F., Finn, A. V., & Virmani, R. (2013). Update on acute coronary syndromes: The pathologists' view. *European Heart Journal, 34,* 719–728.

Fang, J. C., & O'Gara, P. T. (2012). Chapter 12—The history and physical examination: An evidence-based approach. In R. O. Bonow, D. L. Mann, D. P. Zipes, P. Libby, & E. Braunwald (Eds.), *Braunwald's heart disease: A textbook of cardiovascular medicine* (9th ed., pp. 108–118). Philadelphia, PA: Saunders-Elsevier.

Farkouh, M. E., Domanski, M., Sleeper, L. A., Siami, F. S., Dangas, G., Mack, M., . . . Fuster, V. (2012). Strategies for multivessel revascularization in patients with diabetes. *The New England Journal of Medicine, 367,* 2375–2384.

Fava, S., Azzopardi, J., & Agius-Muscat, H. (1997). Outcome of unstable angina in patients with diabetes mellitus. *Diabetic Medicine, 14*(3), 209–213.

Fedorowski, A., & Melander, O. (2013). Syndromes of orthostatic intolerance: A hidden danger. *Journal of Internal Medicine, 273*(4), 322–335.

Fedullo, P. F. (2011). Chapter 72—Pulmonary embolism. In V. Fuster, R. A. Walsh, & R. A. Harrington (Eds.), *Hurst's the heart* (13th ed.). Retrieved from http://accessmedicine .mhmedical.com.proxygw.wrlc.org/content.aspx?bookid=376&Sectionid=40279805

Felker, G. M., Lee, K. L., Bull, D. A., Redfield, M. M., Stevenson, L. W., Goldsmith, S. R., . . . O'Connor, C. M. (2011). Diuretic strategies in patients with acute decompensated heart failure. *The New England Journal of Medicine, 364,* 797–805.

Ferri, F. (2014). Acute coronary syndromes. In F. Ferri (Ed.), *Ferri's clinical advisor 2014* (1st ed.). Philadelphia, PA: Elsevier-Mosby.

Finfer, S., Chittock, D. R., Su, S.Y-S., Blair, D., Foster, D., Dhingra, V., . . . Ronco, J. J. (2009). Intensive versus conventional glucose control in critically ill patients. *The New England Journal of Medicine, 360,* 1283–1297.

Finn, A. V., Nakano, M., Narula, J., Kolodgie, F. D., & Virmani, R. (2010). Concept of vulnerable/unstable plaque. *Arteriosclerosis, Thrombosis, and Vascular Biology, 30,* 1282–1292.

Fonarow, G. C., Abraham, W. T., Albert, N. M., Stough, W., Gheorghiade, M., Greenberg, B. H., . . . OPTIMIZE-HF Investigators and Hospitals. (2007). Factors identified as precipitating hospital admissions for heart failure and clinical outcomes: Findings from OPTIMIZE-HF. *Archives of Internal Medicine, 168,* 847–854.

Fonarow, G. C., Adams, K. F., Jr., Abraham, W. T., Yancy, C. W., Boscardin, W. J., ADHERE Scientific Advisory Committee, Study Group, and Investigators. (2005). Risk stratification for in-hospital mortality in acutely decompensated heart failure: Classification and regression tree analysis. *JAMA, 293,* 572–580.

Fonarow, G. C., & ADHERE Scientific Advisory Committee. (2005). Overview of acutely decompensated congestive heart failure: A report from the ADHERE Registry. *Heart Failure Reviews, 9*(3), 179–185.

Fonarow, G. C., Stough, W. G., Abraham, W. T., Albert, N. M., Gheorghiade, M., Greenberg, B. H., . . . Young, J. B. (2007). Characteristics, treatments, and outcomes of patients with preserved systolic function hospitalized for heart failure: A report from the OPTIMIZE-HF Registry. *Journal of the American College of Cardiology, 50*(8), 768–777.

Fox, K. A., Eagle, K. A., Gore, J. M., Steg, P. G., Anderson, F. A., & GRACE and GRACE2 Investigators. (2010). The global registry of acute coronary events, 1999 to 2009—GRACE. *Heart, 96,* 1095–1101.

Freda, B. J., Tang, W. H., Van Lente, F., Peacock, W. F., & Francis, G. S. (2002). Cardiac troponins in renal insufficiency: Review and clinical implications. *Journal of the American College of Cardiology, 40,* 2065–2071.

FRISC-II (FRagmin and Fast Revascularisation during InStability in Coronary artery disease) investigators. (1999). Invasive compared with non-invasive treatment in unstable coronary-artery disease: FRISC II prospective randomised multicentre study. *The Lancet, 354,* 708–715.

Furberg, C. D., Psaty, B. M., & Meyer, J. V. (1995). Nifedipine: Dose-related increase in mortality in patients with coronary heart disease. *Circulation, 92,* 1326–1331.

Fuster, V., Moreno, P. R., Fayad, Z. A., Corti, R., & Badimon, J. J. (2005). Atherothrombosis and high-risk plaque part I: Evolving concepts. *Journal of the American College of Cardiology, 46*(6), 937–954.

Galvani, M., Ottani, F., Ferrini, D., Ladenson, J. H., Destro, A., Baccos, D., . . . Jaffe, A. S. (1997). Prognostic influence of elevated values of cardiac troponin I in patients with unstable angina. *Circulation, 95,* 2053–2059.

Galvani, M., Ottani, F., Oltrona, L., Ardissino, D., Gensini, G. F., Maggioni, A. P., . . . Vecchio, C. (2004). N-terminal pro-brain natriuretic peptide on admission has prognostic value across the whole spectrum of acute coronary syndromes. *Circulation, 110,* 128–134.

Gheorghiade, M., Abraham, W. T., Albert, N. M., Gattis Stough, W., Greenberg, B. H., O'Connor, C. M., . . . Fonarow, G. C. (2007). Relationship between admission serum sodium concentration and clinical outcomes in patients hospitalized for heart failure: An analysis from the OPTIMIZE-HF registry. *European Heart Journal, 28,* 980–988.

Gheorghiade, M., Abraham, W. T., Albert, N. M., Greenberg, B. H., O'Connor, C. M., She, L., . . . OPTIMIZE-HF Investigators. (2006). Systolic blood pressure at admission, clinical characteristics, and outcomes in patients hospitalized with acute heart failure. *Journal of the American Medical Association, 296*(10), 2217–2226.

Gheorghiade, M., Filippatos, G. S., & Felker, G. M. (2012). Chapter 27—Diagnosis and management of acute heart failure syndromes. In R. O. Bonow, D. L. Mann, D. P. Zipes, P. Libby, & E. Braunwald (Eds.), *Braunwald's heart disease: A textbook of cardiovascular medicine* (9th ed., pp. 517–542). Philadelphia, PA: Saunders-Elsevier.

Gheorghiade, M., Konstam, M. A., Burnett, J. A., Grinfeld, L., Maggioni, A. P., Swedberg, K., . . . Orlandi, C. (2007). Short-term clinical effects of tolvaptan, an oral vasopressin antagonist, in patients hospitalized for heart failure: The EVEREST clinical status trials. *Journal of the American Medical Association, 297*(12), 1332–1343.

Gheorghiade, M., & Pang, P. S. (2009). Acute heart failure syndromes. *Journal of the American College of Cardiology, 53*(7), 557–573.

Gimenez, M., Relter, M., Twerenbold, R., Reichlin, T., Wildi, K., Haaf, P., . . . Mueller, C. (2014). Sex-specific chest pain characteristics in the early diagnosis of acute myocardial infarction. *JAMA Internal Medicine, 174*(2), 241–249.

Go, A. S., Mozaffarian, D., Roger, V. L., Benjamin, E. J., Berry, J. D., Blaha, M. J., . . . on behalf of the American Heart Association Statistics Committee and Stroke Statistics Subcommittee. (2014). Heart disease and stroke statistics—2014 update: A report from the American Heart Association. *Circulation, 129,* e28–e292. doi:10.1161/01.cir.0000441139.02102.80

Goldhaber, S. Z. (2015). Chapter 73—Pulmonary embolism. In D. L. Mann, D. P. Zipes, P. Libby, R. O. Bonow, & E. Braunwald (Eds.), *Braunwald's heart disease: A textbook of cardiovascular medicine* (10th ed., pp. 1664–1681). Philadelphia, PA: Saunders-Elsevier.

Golledge, J., & Engle, K. (2008). Acute aortic dissection. *The Lancet, 372,* 55–66.

Grady, D., Chaput, L., & Kristof, M. (2003). Results of systematic review of research on diagnosis and treatment of coronary heart disease in women. Evidence Report/Technology Assessment No. 80. AHRQ Publication No. 03-0035. Rockville, MD: Agency for Healthcare Research and Quality.

Grasso, A. W., & Brener, S. J. (2013). Cleveland Clinic Center for Continuing Education: Complications of acute myocardial infarction. Retrieved from http://www.cleveland clinicmeded.com/medicalpubs/diseasemanagement/cardiology/complications-of-acute-myocardial-infarction/

Grub, B. P. (2005). Neurogenic syncope. *The New England Journal of Medicine, 352*, 1004–1010.

Guttentag, A. (2005). Brain images [PowerPoint slides]. Retrieved from http://learningra diology.com/lectures/facultylectures/Basic%20Brain%20Imaging/player.html

Habib, G., Hoen, B., Tornos, P., Thuny, F., Prendergast, B., Vilacosta, I., . . . Zamorano, J. L. (2009). Guidelines on the prevention, diagnosis, and treatment of infective endocarditis (new version 2009). *European Heart Journal, 30*, 2369–2413.

Hagan, P., Nienaber, C., Isselbacher, E., Bruckman, D., Karavite, D., Russman, P., . . . Eagle, K. (2000). The International Registry of Acute Aortic Dissection (IRAD) new insights into an old disease. *Journal of the American Medical Association, 283*(7), 897–903.

Hall, J. E. (2011a). Chapter 13—Cardiac arrhythmias and their electrocardiographic inter-pretation. In J. E. Hall (Ed.), *Guyton and Hall textbook of medical physiology* (12th ed., pp. 143–153). Philadelphia, PA: Saunders Elsevier.

Hall, J. E. (2011b). Chapter 21—Muscle blood flow and cardiac output during exercise; the coronary circulation and ischemic heart disease. In J. E. Hall (Ed.), *Guyton and Hall textbook of medical physiology* (12th ed., pp. 243–253). Philadelphia, PA: Saunders Elsevier.

Hamm, C. W., Bassand, J. P., Agewall, S., Bax, J., Boersma, E., Bueno, H., . . . Widimsky, P. (2011). ESC guidelines for the management of acute coronary syndromes in patients without persistent ST-segment elevation: The task force for the management of acute coronary syndromes (ACS) in patients presenting without persistent ST-segment elevation of the European Society of Cardiology (ESC). *European Heart Journal, 32*, 2999–3054.

Hass, E. E., Yang, E. H., Gersh, B. J., & O'Rourke, R. A. (2011). Chapter 60—ST-segment ele-vation myocardial infarction. In V. Fuster, R. A. Walsh, & R. A. Harrington (Eds.), *Hurst's the heart* (13th ed.). New York, NY: McGraw-Hill.

Heran, B. S., Chen, J. M. H., Ebrahim, S., Moxham, T., Oldridge, N., Rees, K., . . . Taylor, R. S. (2011). Exercise-based cardiac rehabilitation for coronary heart disease. *Cochrane Data-base of Systematic Reviews*, (7), CD001800 doi:10.1002/14651858.CD001800pub2

Heywood, J. T., Fonarow, G. C., Costanzo, M. R., Mathur, V. S., Wigneswaran, J. R., & Wynne, J. (2007). High prevalence of renal dysfunction and its impact on outcome in 118,465 patients hospitalized with acute decompensated heart failure: A report from the ADHERE database. *Journal of Cardiac Failure, 13*(6), 422–430.

Hillis, L. D., Smith, P. K., Anderson, J. L., Bittl, J., Bridges, C. R., Byrne, J. G., . . . Winniford, M. D. (2011). 2011 ACCF/AHA guideline for coronary artery bypass graft surgery: Executive summary. *Journal of the American College of Cardiology, 58*(24), 2584–2614.

Hiratzka, L., Bakris, G., Beckman, J., Bersin, R., Carr, V., Casey, D., . . . Williams, D. (2010). 2010 ACCF/AHA/AATS/ACR/ASA/SCA/SCAI/SIR/STS/SVM guidelines for the diagnosis and management of patients with thoracic aortic disease: Executive summary. *Journal of the American College of Cardiology, 55*(14), 1509–1544.

Ho, K. T., Miller, T. D., Hodge, D. O., Bailey, K. R., & Gibbons, R. J. (2002). Use of a simple clinical score to predict prognosis of patients with normal or mildly abnormal resting electrocardiographic findings undergoing evaluation for coronary artery disease. *Mayo Clinic Proceedings, 77*, 515–521.

Hochman, J. S., & Ingbar, D. H. (2012). Chapter 272—Cardiogenic shock and pulmonary edema. In D. L. Longo, A. S. Fauci, D. L. Kasper, S. L. Hauser, J. Jameson, & J. Loscalzo (Eds.), *Harrison's principles of internal medicine* (18th ed.). Retrieved from http://accessmed icine.mhmedical.com.proxygw.wrlc.org/content.aspx?bookid=331&Sectionid=40727058

Hochman, J. S., Sleeper, L. A., White, H. D., Dzavik, V., Wong, S. C., Menon, V., . . . LeJemtel, T. H. for the SHOCK Investigators. (2001). One-year survival following revasculariza-tion for cardiogenic shock. *Journal of the American Medical Association, 285*, 190–192.

Hoit, B. D. (2011). Chapter 85—Pericardial disease. In V. Fuster, R. A. Walsh, & R. A. Harrington (Eds.), *Hurst's the heart* (13th ed.). Retrieved from http://accessmedicine .mhmedical.com.proxygw.wrlc.org/content.aspx?bookid=376&Sectionid=40279821

Hoit, B. D., & Walsh, R. A. (2011). Chapter 5—Normal physiology of the cardiovascular system. In V. Fuster, R. A. Walsh, & R. A. Harrington (Eds.), *Hurst's the heart* (13th ed.). [McGraw-Hill Access Medicine version]. Retrieved from http://accessmedicine.mh medical.com/book.aspx?bookid=376

Hollander, J. E., & Diercks, D. B. (2011). Chapter 53—Acute coronary syndromes: Acute myocardial infarction and unstable angina. In J. E. Tintinalli, S. Stapczynski, O. J. Ma, D. M. Cline, R. K. Cydulka, & G. D. Meckler (Eds.), *Tintinalli's emergency medicine: A comprehensive study guide* (7th ed.). New York, NY: McGraw-Hill. Retrieved from http:// accessmedicine.mhmedical.com/content.aspx?bookid=348&Sectionid=40381518

Hoo, G. W. (2013). Barotrauma and mechanical ventilation. *Medscape: Drugs & diseases*. Retrieved from http://emedicine.medscape.com/article/296625-overview#aw2aab6b3

Horwitz, J., Horwitz, N., & Noggle, C. A. (2012). Dysautonomia. In C. A. Noggle, R. S. Dean, & A. M. Horton, Jr. (Eds.), *The encyclopedia of neuropsychological disorders*. New York, NY: Springer.

Hreybe, H., & Saba, S. (2009). Location of acute myocardial infarction and associated arrhythmias and outcome. *Clinical Cardiology, 32*(5), 274–277.

Huff, J., Decker, W., Quinn, J., Perron, A., Napoli, A., Peeters, S., & Jagoda, A. (2007). Clinical policy: Critical issues in the evaluation and management of adult patients presenting to the emergency department with syncope. *Annals of Emergency Medicine, 49*(4), 431–444.

Imazio, M. (2014). Chapter 28—Pericardial diseases. In M. H. Crawford (Ed.), *Current diagnosis & treatment: Cardiology* (4th ed.). Retrieved from http://accessmedicine.mhmedical .com.proxygw.wrlc.org/content.aspx?bookid=715&Sectionid=48214562

Imazio, M., & Adler, Y. (2013). Treatment with aspirin, NSAID, corticosteroids and colchicine in acute and recurrent pericarditis. *Heart Failure Reviews, 18*, 355–360.

Jain, S., Ting, H. T., Bell, M., Bjerke, C. M., Lennon, R. J., Gersh, B., . . . Presad, A. (2011). Utility of left bundle branch block as a diagnostic criterion for acute myocardial infarction. *The American Journal of Cardiology, 107*, 1111–1116.

James, P. A., Oparil, S., Carter, B. L., Cushman, W. C., Dennison-Himmelfarb, C., Handler, J., . . . Ortiz, E. (2014). 2014 Evidence-based guideline for the management of high blood pressure in adults: Report from the panel members appointed to the Eighth Joint National Committee (JNC 8). *Journal of the American Medical Association, 311*(5), 507–520.

Januzzi, J. L., Mebazaa, A., & DiSomma, A. (2015). ST2 and prognosis in acutely decompensated heart failure: The international ST2 consensus panel. *The American Journal of Cardiology*. doi:10.1016/j.amjcard.2015.01.037

Jauch, E. C., Saver, J. L., Adams, H. P., Jr., Bruno, A., Connors, J. J., Demaerschalk, B. M., . . . Yonas, H. (2013). Guidelines for the early management of patients with acute ischemic stroke: A guideline for health care professionals from the American Heart Association/ American Stroke Association. *Stroke, 44*(3), 870–947.

Jneid, H., Anderson, J. L., Wright, R. S., Adams, C. D., Bridges, C. R., Casey, D. E., Jr., . . . Zidar, J. P. (2012). 2012 ACCF/AHA focused update of the guideline for the management of patients with unstable angina/non–ST-elevation myocardial infarction (updating the 2007 guideline and replacing the 2011 focused update): A report of the American College of Cardiology Foundation/American Heart Association Task Force on Practice Guidelines. *Journal of the American College of Cardiology, 60*, 645–681.

Johnson, W., Nguyen, M., & Patel, R. (2012). Hypertension crisis in the emergency department. *Cardiology Clinics, 30*, 533–543.

Jois, P. (2012). Hypertensive emergencies. *Critical Decisions in Emergency Medicine, 26*(8), 11–18.

Jolliffe, J. A., Rees, K., Taylor, R. S., Thompson, D., Oldridge, N., & Ebrahim, S. (2001). Exercise-based rehabilitation for coronary heart disease. *Cochrane Database of Systematic Reviews, 1*, CD001800.

Jones, J., & Stearley, S. (2011). Chapter 24—Chest trauma. In C. Stone & R. L. Humphries (Eds.), *Current diagnosis & treatment emergency medicine* (7th ed.). Retrieved from http://accessmedicine.mhmedical.com.proxygw.wrlc.org/content.aspx?bookid=385& Sectionid=40357239

Juul-Moller, S. (2013). Syncope—A complex syndrome of several causes. *Journal of Internal Medicine, 273*(4), 320–321.

Kapoor, W. (1990). Evaluation and outcome of patients with syncope. *Medicine* (Baltimore), *69,* 160–175.

Kapoor, W. (2000). Syncope. *The New England Journal of Medicine, 343*(25), 1856–1862.

Keys, T. F. (2014). Infective endocarditis. *Cleveland Clinic Center for Continuing Education.* Retrieved from http://www.clevelandclinicmeded.com/medicalpubs/diseasemanage ment/infectious-disease/infective-endocarditis/#s0015

Khan, N. A., Daskalopoulou, S. S., Karp, I., Eisenberg, M. J., Pelletier, R., Tsadok, M. A., . . . Pilote, L. (2013). Sex differences in acute coronary syndrome symptom presentation in young patients. *JAMA Internal Medicine, 173*(20), 1863–1871.

Killip, T., 3rd, & Kimball, J. T. (1967). Treatment of myocardial infarction in a coronary care unit. A two-year experience with 250 patients. *The American Journal of Cardiology, 20,* 457.

Kirklin, J. K., Naftel, D. C., Kormos, R. L., Stevenson, L. W., Pagani, F. D., Miller, M. A., . . . Young, J. B. (2011). Third INTERMACS annual report: The evolution of destination therapy in the United States. *Journal of Heart and Lung Transplantation, 30,* 115–126.

Kirklin, J. K., Naftel, D. C., Pagani, F. D., Kormos, R. L., Stevenson, L. W., Blume, E. D., . . . Young, J. B. (2014). Sixth INTERMACS annual report: A 10,000-patient database. *Journal of Heart and Lung Transplantation, 33*(6), 555–564.

Klompas, M. (2002). Does this patient have an acute thoracic aortic dissection? *Journal of the American Medical Association, 287,* 2262–2272.

Kociol, R. D., Horton, J. R., Fonarow, G. C., Reyes, E. M., Shaw, L. K., O'Connor, C. M., . . . Hernandez, A. F. (2011). Admission, discharge, or change in B-type natriuretic peptide and long-term outcomes: Data from Organized Program to Initiate Lifesaving Treat- ment in Hospitalized Patients with Heart Failure (OPTIMIZE-HF) linked to Medicare claims. *Circulation: Heart Failure, 4*(5), 628–636.

Konstam, M. A., Gheorghiade, M., Burnett, J. C., Grinfeld, L., Maggioni, A. P., Swedberg, K., . . . Efficacy of Vasopressin Antagonism in Heart Failure Outcome Study with Tol- vaptan (EVEREST) Investigators. (2007). Effects of oral tolvaptan in patients hospital- ized for worsening heart failure: The EVEREST outcome trial. *Journal of the American Medical Association, 297*(12), 1319–1331.

Korenstein, D., Wisnivesky, J. P., Wyer, P., Adler, R., Ponieman, D., & McGinn, T. (2007). The utility of B-type natriuretic peptide in the diagnosis of heart failure in the emer- gency department: A systematic review. *BMC Emergency Medicine, 7,* 6. doi:10.1186/ 1471-227X-7-6

Krahn, A., Klein, G., Yee, R., Hoch, J., & Skanes, A. (2003). Cost implication of testing strat- egy in patients with syncope: Randomized assessment of syncope trial. *Journal Ameri- can College of Cardiology, 42,* 495–501.

Lee, K. H., Jeong, M. H., Kim, H. M., Ahn, Y., Kim, J. H., Chae, S. C., . . . Park, S. J. (2011). Benefit of early statin therapy in patients with acute myocardial infarction who have extremely low low-density lipoprotein cholesterol. *Journal of the American College of Cardiology, 58*(16), 1664–1671.

Lemonick, D. (2010). Evaluation of syncope in the emergency department. *The American Journal of Clinical Medicine, 7*(1), 11–19.

Lentini, S., & Perrotta, S. (2011). Aortic dissection with concomitant acute myocardial infarction: From diagnosis to management. *Journal of Emergency, Trauma, and Shock, 4*(2), 273–278.

Lesperance, F., Frasure-Smith, N., Koszycki, D., Laliberte, M. A., van Zyl, L. T., Baker, B., . . . Guertin, M. C. (2007). Effects of citalopram and interpersonal psychotherapy on

depression in patients with coronary artery disease: The Canadian Cardiac Randomized Evaluation of Antidepressant and Psychotherapy Efficacy (CREATE) Trial. *Journal
of the American Medical Association, 297*, 367–379.

Levine, G. N., Steinkey, E. E., Bakaeen, F. G., Bozkurt, B., Cheitlin, M. D., Conti, J. B., . . .
Stewart, W. J. (2012). AHA scientific statement: Sexual activity and cardiovascular disease. *Circulation, 125*, 1058–1072.

LeWinter, M. M., & Hopkins, W. E. (2015). Pericardial diseases. In D. L. Mann, D. P. Zipes,
P. Libby, R. O. Bonow, & E. Braunwald (Eds.), *Braunwald's heart disease: A textbook of
cardiovascular medicine* (10th ed., pp. 1636–1657). Philadelphia, PA: Saunders-Elsevier.

Li, J. S., Sexton, D. J., Mick, N., Nettles, R., Fowler, V. G., Jr., Ryan, T., . . . Corey, G. R. (2000).
Proposed modifications to the Duke criteria for the diagnosis of infective endocarditis.
Clinical Infectious Diseases, 30, 633–638.

Libby, P. (2013). Mechanisms of disease: Mechanisms of acute coronary syndromes and their
implications for therapy. *The New England Journal of Medicine, 368*(21), 2004–2013.

Lilly/Daiichi Sankyo. (2013, November). Effient® (prasugrel) tablets prescribing information.
Retrieved from http://www.effienthcp.com/effient-prescribing-information.aspx

Little, W. C., & Oh, J. K. (2012). Pericardial diseases. In L. Goldman & A. I. Schafer (Eds.),
Goldman's Cecil medicine (24th ed., p. 480). Philadelphia, PA: Elsevier Saunders.

Litwin, S. E., & Benjamin, I. J. (2010). Evaluation of the patient with cardiovascular disease.
In T. E. Andreoli, I. J. Benjamin, R. C. Griggs, & E. J. Wing (Eds.). *Andreoli's and Carpenter's Cecil essentials of medicine* (8th ed., pp. 32–45). Philadelphia, PA: Saunders-Elsevier.

Lloyd-Jones, D. M., Camargo, C. A. J., Lapuerta, P., Giugliano, R. P., & O'Donnell, C. J.
(1998). Electrocardiographic and clinical predictors of acute myocardial infarction in
patients with unstable angina pectoris. *The American Journal of Cardiology, 81*, 1182–1186.

Madias, C., Maron, B. J., Weinstock, J., Estes, N. A. M., III, & Link, M. S. (2007). Commotio
Cordis—Sudden death with chest wall impact. *Journal of Cardiovascular Electrophysiology, 18*, 115–122.

Maisel, A. S., Clopton, P., Krishnaswamy, P., Nowak, R. M., McCord, J., Hollander, J. E., . . .
McCullough, P. A. (2004). Impact of age, race, and sex on the ability of B-type natriuretic
peptide to aid in the emergency diagnosis of heart failure: Results from the Breathing
Not Properly (BNP) multinational study. *American Heart Journal, 147*(6), 1078–1084.

Malmberg, K., Ryden, L., Wedel, H., Birkeland, K., Bootsma, A., Dickstein, K., . . .
Waldenstrom, A. (2005). Intense metabolic control by means of insulin in patients with
diabetes mellitus and acute myocardial infarction (DIGAMI 2): Effects on mortality and
morbidity. *European Heart Journal, 26*, 650–661.

Mancini, M. C. (2012). Tricuspid regurgitation clinical presentation. *Medscape: Drugs and
diseases*. Retrieved from http://emedicine.medscape.com/article/158484-overview

Mancini, M. C. (2014). Aortic dissection. *Medscape: Drugs and diseases*. Retrieved from
http://emedicine.medscape.com/article/2062452-overview

Mann, J., & Davies, M. J. (1999). Mechanisms of progression in native coronary artery disease:
Role of healed plaque disruption. *Heart, 82*, 265–268.

Marcus, G. M., Cohen, J., Varosy, P. D., Vessey, J., Rose, E., Massey, B. M., . . . Waters, D.
(2007). The utility of gestures in patients with chest discomfort. *The American Journal of
Medicine, 120*(1), 83–89.

Marik, P., & Varon, J. (2007). Hypertensive crisis challenges and management. *Chest, 131*(6),
1949–1962.

Martin, B. J., Arena, R., Haykowsky, M., Hauer, T., Austford, L. D., Knudtson, M., . . . Stone,
J. A. (2013). Cardiovascular fitness and mortality after contemporary cardiac rehabilitation. *Mayo Clinic Proceedings, 88*(5), 455–463.

Martin, L. (2013). Cyanosis. Medscape. Retrieved from http://emedicine.medscape.com/
article/303533-overview#aw2aab6b2

Martin, T., Hanusa, B., & Kapoor, W. (1997). Risk stratification of patients with syncope.
Annals of Emergency Medicine, 29, 459–466.

Martinez-Rumayor, A. A., Vazquez, J., Rehman, S. U., & Januzzi, J. L., Jr. (2010). Relative value of amino-terminal pro-B-type natriuretic peptide testing and radiographic standards for the diagnostic evaluation of heart failure in acutely dyspneic subjects. *Biomarkers, 15*(2), 175–182.

Mattu, A. (May 7, 2009). Syncope. (In) Head emergencies. *Audio-Digest Emergency Medicine, 26*(9). Retrieved from http://www.audiodigest.org/pages/htmlos/3449.4.4231252564761264740/EM2609

McCord, J., Jneid, H., Hollander, J. E., deLemos, J. A., Cercek, B., Hsue, P., . . . Newby, L. K. (2008). Management of cocaine-associated chest pain and myocardial infarction: A scientific statement from the American Heart Association Acute Cardiac Care Committee of the Council on Clinical Cardiology. *Circulation, 117*, 1897–1907.

McCullough, P. A., Thompson, R. J., & Tobin, K. J. (1998). Validation of a decision support tool for the evaluation of cardiac arrest victims. *Clinical Cardiology, 21*(3), 195–200.

McGee, S. (2012). *Evidence-based physical diagnosis*. Philadelphia, PA: Saunders-Elsevier.

McMurray, J. V., Adamopoulos, S., Anker, S. D., Auricchio, A., Bohm, M., Dickstein, K., . . . Zeiher, A. (2012). ESC guidelines for the diagnosis and treatment of acute and chronic heart failure. *European Heart Journal, 33*, 1787–1847.

McNulty, E. (2014). Chapter 9—Cardiogenic shock. In M. H. Crawford (Ed.), *Current diagnosis & treatment: Cardiology* (4th ed.). New York, NY: McGraw-Hill.

McSweeney, J. C., O'Sullivan, P., Cody, M., & Crane, P. B. (2004). Development of the McSweeney acute and prodromal myocardial infarction symptom survey. *Journal of Cardiovascular Nursing, 19*(1), 58–67.

Medicines Company. (2013). Angiomax prescribing information. Retrieved from http://www.angiomax.com/downloads/Angiomax_US_PI_June_2013.pdf

Medscape Reference. (2014). Enoxaparin. Retrieved from http://reference.medscape.com/drug/lovenox-enoxaparin-342174#0

Mehta, R., Suzuki, T., Hagan, P., Bossone, E., Gilon, D., Llovet, A., . . . Eagle, K. (2002). Predicting death in patients with acute type A aortic dissection. *Circulation, 105*, 200–206.

Mehta, R. H., Starr, A. Z., Lopes, R. D., Hochman, J. S., Widimsky, P., Pieper, K. S., . . . APEX AMI Investigators. (2009). Incidence of and outcomes associated with ventricular tachycardia or fibrillation in patients undergoing primary percutaneous coronary intervention. *Journal of the American Medical Association, 301*(17), 1779–1789.

Meine, T. J., Roe, M. T., Chen, A. Y., Patel, M. R., Washam, J. B., Ohman, E. M., . . . Peterson, E. D. (2005). Association of intravenous morphine use and outcomes in acute coronary syndromes: Results from the CRUSADE quality improvement initiative. *American Heart Journal, 149*, 1043–1049.

Menon, V., Webb, J. G., Hillis, L. D., Sleeper, L. A., Abboud, R., Dzavik, V., . . . Hochman, J. S. (2000). Outcome and profile of ventricular septal rupture with cardiogenic shock after myocardial infarction: A report from the SHOCK trial registry. *Journal of the American College of Cardiology, 36*(3s1), 1110–1116.

Merchant, R. M., Yang, L., Becker, L. B., Berg, R. A., Nadkarni, V., Nichol, G., . . . American Heart Association Get With The Guidelines-Resuscitation Investigators. (2011). Incidence of treated cardiac arrest in hospitalized patients in the United States. *Critical Care Medicine, 39*, 2401–2406.

Michaels, A. D. (2010). Coronary heart disease. In T. E. Andreoli, I. J. Benjamin, R. C. Griggs, & E. J. Wing (Eds.), *Andreoli's and Carpenter's Cecil essentials of medicine* (8th ed., pp. 106–117). Philadelphia, PA: Saunders-Elsevier.

Moradkhan, R., & Sinoway, L. I. (2010). Revisiting the role of oxygen therapy in cardiac patients. *Journal of the American College of Cardiology, 56*, 1013–1016.

Morise, A. P., Haddad, W. J., & Beckner, D. (1997). Development and validation of a clinical score to estimate the probability of coronary artery disease in men and women presenting with suspected coronary disease. *The American Journal of Medicine, 102*, 350–356.

Morrow, D. A., Cannon, C. P., Jessie, R. L., Newby, C. P., Ravkilde, J., Storrow, A. B., . . . Christenson, R. H. (2007). National Academy of Clinical Biochemistry laboratory medicine practice guidelines: Clinical characteristics and utilization of biochemical markers in acute coronary syndromes. *Clinical Chemistry, 53*(4), 552–574.

Morrow, D. A., Rifai, N., Antman, E. M., Weiner, D. L., McCabe, C. H., Cannon, C. P., & Braunwald, E. (1998). C-reactive protein is a potent predictor of mortality independently of and in combination with troponin T in acute coronary syndromes: A TIMI 11A substudy. Thrombolysis in myocardial infarction. *Journal of the American College of Cardiology, 31*(7), 1460–1465.

Moses, S. (2012). Medication causes of orthostatic hypotension. *Family Practice Notebook.* Retrieved from http://www.fpnotebook.com/cv/pharm/MdctnCsOfOrthstcHyptnsn .htm

Moss, A. J., Hall, W. J., Cannom, D. S., Daubert, J. P., Higgins, S. L., Klein, H., . . . Heo, M. (1996). Improved survival with an implanted defibrillator in patients with coronary disease at high risk for ventricular arrhythmia: Multicenter automatic defibrillator implantation trial investigators. *The New England Journal of Medicine, 335,* 1933–1940.

Moss, A. J., Zareba, W., Hall, W. J., Klein, H., Wilbur, D. J., Cannom, D. S., . . . Andrews, M. L. (2002). Prophylactic implantation of a defibrillator in patients with myocardial infarction and reduced ejection fraction. *The New England Journal of Medicine, 346,* 877–883.

Moya, A., Sutton, R., Ammirati, F., Blanc, J., Brignole, M., Dahm, J., . . . Wieling, W. (2009). Guidelines for the diagnosis and management of syncope (version 2009). *European Heart Journal, 30*(21), 2631–2671.

Muller, J. E., Mittleman, M. A., Maclure, M., Sherwood, J. B., & Tofler, G. H. (1996). Triggering myocardial infarction by sexual activity: Low absolute risk and prevention by regular physical exertion. *Journal of the American Medical Association, 275,* 1405–1409.

Multicenter Postinfarction Research Group. (1983). Risk stratification and survival after myocardial infarction. *The New England Journal of Medicine, 309*(6), 331–336.

Murdoch, D. R., Corey, G. R., Hoen, B., Miró, J. M., Fowler, V. G., Jr., Bayer, A. S., . . . Cabell, C. H. (2009). Clinical presentation, etiology, and outcome of infective endocarditis in the 21st century: The International Collaboration on Endocarditis–Prospective Cohort Study. *Archives of Internal Medicine, 169*(5), 463–473.

Myerburg, R. J., & Castellanos, A. (2015). Chapter 39—Cardiac arrest and sudden cardiac death. In D. L. Mann, D. P. Zipes, R. O. Bonow, & E. Braunwald (Eds.), *Braunwald's heart disease: A textbook of cardiovascular medicine* (10th ed., pp. 821–860). Philadelphia, PA: Saunders-Elsevier.

Nakano, J., Okabayashi, H., Hanyu, M., Soga, Y., Nomoto, T., . . . Kawatou, M. (2008). Risk factors for wound infection after off-pump coronary artery bypass grafting: Should bilateral internal thoracic arteries be harvested in patients with diabetes? *Journal of Thoracic and Cardiovascular Surgery, 135*(3), 540–545.

Narula, J., Nakano, M., Virmani, R., Kolodgie, F. D., Petersen, R., Newcomb, R., . . . Finn, A. V. (2013). Histopathologic characteristics of atherosclerotic coronary disease and implications of the findings for the invasive and noninvasive detection of vulnerable plaques. *Journal of the American College of Cardiology, 61*(10), 1041–1051.

Neumar, R. W., Otto, C. W., Link, M. S., Kronick, S. L., Shuster, M., Callaway, C. W., . . . Morrison, L. J. (2010). Part 8: Adult advanced cardiovascular life support, 2010 American Heart Association guidelines for cardiopulmonary resuscitation and emergency cardiovascular care. *Circulation, 122,* S729–S767.

Nichol, G., Thomas, E., Callaway, C. W., Hedges, J., Powell, J. L., Aufderheide, T. P., . . . Stiell, I. (2008). Regional variation in out-of-hospital cardiac arrest incidence and outcome. *Journal of the American Medical Association, 300,* 1423–1431.

Nieminen, M. S., Bohm, M., Cowie, M. R., Drexler, H., Filippatos, G. S., & Jondeau, G. (2005). Executive summary of the guidelines on the diagnosis and treatment of acute heart failure: The task force on acute heart failure of the European society of cardiology. *European Heart Journal, 26,* 384–416.

Nienaber, C. A., & Eagle, K. A. (2003). Aortic dissection: New frontiers in diagnosis and management: Part I: From etiology to diagnostic strategies. *Circulation, 108*(5), –628–635.

Nyman, H. A., Dowling, T. C., Hudson, J. Q., St. Peter, W. L., Joy, M. S., & Nolin, T. D. (2011). Comparative evaluation of the Cockcroft-Gault equation and the Modification of Diet in Renal Disease (MDRD) study equation for drug dosing. *Pharmacotherapy, 31*(11), 1130–1144.

O'Connor, C. M., Starling, R. C., Hernandez, A. F., Armstrong, P. W., Dickstein, K., Hasselblad, V., . . . Califf, R. M. (2011). Effect of nesiritide in patients with acute decompensated heart failure. *The New England Journal of Medicine, 365*(1), 32–43.

O'Gara, P. T., Kushner, F. G., Ascheim, D. D., Casey, D. E., Jr., Chung, M. K., de Lemos, J. A., . . . Zhao, D. X. (2013). ACC/AHA guideline for the management of ST-elevation myocardial infarction: A report of the American College of Cardiology Foundation/American Heart Association Task Force on Practice Guidelines. *Journal of the American College of Cardiology, 61,* e78–140. doi:10.1016/j.jacc2012.11.019

Oh, K. T. (2014). Opthalmologic manifestations of hypertension. *Medscape: Drugs & diseases.* Retrieved from http://emedicine.medscape.com/article/1201779-overview

Olshansky, B., & Sullivan, R. (2013). Sudden death risk in syncope: The role of the implantable cardioverter defibrillator. *Progress in Cardiovascular Diseases, 55,* 443–453.

Overgaard, C. B., & Dzavik, V. (2008). Inotropes and vasopressors: Review of physiology and clinical use in cardiovascular disease. *Circulation, 118*(10), 1047–1056.

Paterick, T. E., Paterick, T. J., Nishimura, R. A., & Steckelberg, J. M. (2007). Complexity and subtlety of infective endocarditis. *Mayo Clinic Proceedings, 82*(5), 615–621.

Peacock, W. F., IV, De Marco, T., Fonarow, G. C., Dierecks, D., Wynne, J., Apple, F. S., & Wu, A. H. B. for the ADHERE Investigators. (2008). Cardiac troponin and outcome in acute heart failure. *The New England Journal of Medicine, 358*(20), 2117–2126.

Peberdy, M. A., Callaway, C. W., Neumar, R. W., Geocadin, R. G., Zimmerman, J. L., Donnino, M., . . . Kronick, S. L. (2010). Part 9: Post–cardiac arrest care: 2010 American Heart Association guidelines for cardiopulmonary resuscitation and emergency cardiovascular care. *Circulation, 122*(Suppl. 3), S768–S786.

Pepine, C. J., Faich, G., & Makuch, R. (1998). Verapamil use in patients with cardiovascular disease: An overview of randomized trials. *Clinical Cardiology, 21,* 633–641.

Peterson, P. N., Rumsfeld, J. S., Liang, L., Albert, N. M., Hernandez, A. F., Peterson, E. D., Fonarow, G. C., . . . American Heart Association Get With the Guidelines—Heart Failure Program. (2010). A validated risk score for inhospital mortality in patients with heart failure from the American Heart Association Get With The Guidelines Program. *Circulation: Cardiovascular Quality Outcomes, 3,* 25–32.

Picard, M. H., Davidoff, R., Sleeper, L. A., Mendes, L. A., Thompson, C. R., Davidoff, R., . . . Hochman, J. S. (2003). Echocardiographic predictors of survival and response to early revascularization in cardiogenic shock. *Circulation, 107,* 279–284.

Picariello, C., Lazzeri, C., Valente, S., Chiostri, M., & Gensini, G. F. (2011). Procalcitonin in acute cardiac patients. *Internal and Emergency Medicine, 6*(3), 245–252.

Pinsky, L. E., & Wipf, J. E. (2014). Physical exam: Neck veins technique for examining hepatojugular reflux (HJR). University of Washington Department of Medicine. Retrieved from http://depts.washington.edu/physdx/neck/physical_hepa.html

Quinn, J., McDermott, D., Kramer, N., Yeh, C., Kohn, M. A., Stiell, I., & Wells, G. (2008). Death after emergency department visits for syncope: How common and can it be predicted. *Annals of Emergency Medicine, 51*(5), 585–590.

Quinn, J., McDermott, D., Stiell, I., Kohn, M., & Wells, G. (2006). Prospective validation of the San Francisco syncope rule to predict patients with serious outcomes. *Annals of Emergency Medicine, 47,* 448–454.

Quinn, J. V., Stiell, I. G., McDermott, D. A., Sellers, K. L., Kohn, M. A., & Wells, G. A. (2004). Derivation of the San Francisco Syncope Rule to predict patients with short-term serious outcomes. *Annals of Emergency Medicine, 43*(2), 224–232.

Rehman, S. U., Martinez-Rumayor, A., Mueller, T., & Januzzi, J. L. (2008). Independent and incremental prognostic value of multimarker testing in acute dyspnea: Results from the ProBNP investigation of dyspnea in the emergency department (PRIDE) study. *Clinica Chimica Acta, 392*(1–2), 41–45.

Ren, X. (2014). Cardiogenic shock. *Medscape Reference.* Retrieved from http://emedicine.medscape.com/article/152191-overview

Reynolds, H. R., & Hochman, J. S. (2008). Cardiogenic shock: Current concepts and improving outcomes. *Circulation, 117,* 686–697.

Rigotti, N. A., Clair, C., Munafo, M. R., & Stead, L. F. (2012). Interventions for smoking cessation in hospitalised patients. *Cochrane Database of Systematic Reviews, 5.* Art. No.: CD001837. doi:10.1002/14651858.CD001837.pub3. Retrieved from http://onlinelibrary.wiley.com

Robalino, B. D., Whitlow, P. L., Underwood, D. A., & Salcedo, E. E. (1989). Electrocardiographic manifestations of right ventricular infarction. *American Heart Journal, 118,* 138–144.

Rodger, M., Makropoulos, D., Turek, M., Quevillon, J., Raymond, F., Rasuli, P., & Wells, P. S. (2000). Diagnostic value of the electrocardiogram in suspected pulmonary embolism. *The American Journal of Cardiology, 86,* 807–809.

Roger, V. L., Go, A. S., Lloyd-Jones, D. M., Benjamin, E. J., Berry, J. D., Borden, W. B., . . . Turner, M. B. (2012). Heart disease and stroke statistics—2012 update: A report from the American Heart Association. *Circulation, 125,* e2–e220.

Sabatine, M. S., & Cannon, C. P. (2012). Chapter 53—Approach to the patient with chest pain. In R. O. Bonow, D. L. Mann, D. P. Zipes, P. Libby, & E. Braunwald (Eds.), *Braunwald's heart disease: A textbook of cardiovascular medicine* (9th ed., pp. 1076–1085). Philadelphia, PA: Saunders-Elsevier.

Saklani, P., Krahn, A., & Klein, G. (2013). Syncope. *Circulation, 127,* 1330–1339.

Salvador, D. R., Rey, N. R., Ramos, G. C., & Punzalan, F. E. (2005). Continuous infusion versus bolus injection of loop diuretics in congestive heart failure. *Cochrane Database Systematic Review, 3,* CD003178.

Sarasin, F., Hanusa, B., Perneger, T., Louis-Simonet, M., Rajeswaran, A., & Kapoor, W. N. (2003). A risk score to predict arrhythmias in patients with unexplained syncope. *Academic Emergency Medicine, 10*(12), 1312–1317.

Schoen, F. J., & Mitchell, R. N. (2015). The heart. In V. Kumar, A. K. Abba, & J. Aster (Eds.), *Robbins and Cotran pathologic basis of disease* (9th ed; pp. 540–550). Philadelphia, PA: Elsevier-Saunders.

Schreiber, D. (2013). Cardiac markers. *Medscape.* Retrieved from http://emedicine.medscape.com/article/811905-overview#aw2aab6b2

Shah, P. K., Falk, E., Badimon, J. J., Fernandez-Ortiz, A., Mailhac, A., Villareal-Levy, G., . . . Fuster, V. (1995). Human monocyte-derived macrophages induce collagen breakdown in fibrous caps of atherosclerotic plaques: Potential role of matrix-degrading metalloproteinases and implications for plaque rupture. *Circulation, 92*(6), 1565–1569.

Shah, R. V., Chen-Tournoux, A. A., Picard, M. H., van Kimmenade, R. R. J., & Januzzi, J. L. (2010). Galectin-3, cardiac structure and function, and long-term mortality in patients with acutely decompensated heart failure. *European Journal of Heart Failure, 12*(8), 826–832.

Sheldon, R., Hersi, A., Richie, F., Koshman, M., & Rose, S. (2010). Syncope and structural heart disease: Historical criteria for vasovagal syncope and ventricular dysrhythmia. *Journal Cardiovascular Electrophysiology, 21*(12), 1358–1364.

Sheldon, R., Morillo, C., Krahn, A., O'Neill, B., Thiruganasambandamoorthy, V., Parkash, P., . . . Leather, R. (2011). Standarized approaches to the investigation of syncope: Canadian Cardiovascular Society position paper. *Canadian Journal of Cardiology, 27*(2), 246–253.

Sheldon, R., Sheldon, A., Connolly, S., Morillo, C., Klingenheben, T., Krahn, A., . . . Investigators in the Syncope Symptom Study and the Prevention of Syncope Trial. (2006). Age of first faint in patients with vasovagal syncope. *Journal of Cardiovascular Electrophysiology, 17*(1), 49–54.

Slovis, C., & Reddi, A. (2008). Increased blood pressure without evidence of acute end organ damage. *Annals of Emergency Medicine, 52*(3), 57–59.

Smith, S. C., Jr., Benjamin, E. J., Bonow, R. O., Braun, L. T., Creager, M. A., Franklin, B. A., . . . Taubert, K. A. (2011). AHA/ACCF secondary prevention and risk reduction therapy for patients with coronary and other atherosclerotic vascular disease: 2011 update: A guideline from the American Heart Association and American College of Cardiology Foundation. *Journal of the American College of Cardiology, 58*, 2432–2446.

Soteriades, E. S., Evans, J. C., Larson, M. G., Chen, M. H., Chen, L., Benjamin, E., & Levy, D. (2002). Incidence and prognosis of syncope. *The New England Journal of Medicine, 347*(12), 878–885.

Sovari, A. A. (2012). Cardiogenic pulmonary edema clinical presentation. *Medscape*. Retrieved from http://emedicine.medscape.com/article/157452-overview#aw2aab6b2b2aa

Spangler, S. (2013). Acute pericarditis. *Medscape*. Retrieved from http://emedicine.medscape.com/article/156951-overview

Steg, P. G., Jolly, S. S., Mehta, S. R., Afzal, R., Xavier, D., Rupprecht, H., . . . FUTURA/OASIS-8 Trial Group. (2010). Low-dose vs standard-dose unfractionated heparin for percutaneous coronary intervention in acute coronary syndromes treated with fondaparinux: The FUTURA/OASIS-8 randomized trial. *Journal of the American Medical Association, 304*, 1339–1349.

Stein, P. D., Matta, F., Keyes, D. C., & Willyerd, G. L. (2012). Impact of vena cava filters on in-hospital case fatality rate from pulmonary embolism. *The American Journal of Medicine, 125*, 478–484.

Stone, G. W., Bertrand, M. E., Moses, J. W., Ohman, E. M., Lincoff, A. M., Ware, J. H., . . . ACUITY Investigators. (2007). Routine upstream initiation vs deferred selective use of glycoprotein IIb/IIIa inhibitors in acute coronary syndromes: The ACUITY Timing trial. *Journal of the American Medical Association, 297*, 591–602.

Stone, N. J., Robinson, J., Lichtenstein, A. H., Merz, N. B., Lloyd-Jones, D. M., Blum, C. B., . . . Wilson, P. W. F. (2013). 2013 ACC/AHA guideline on the treatment of blood cholesterol to reduce atherosclerotic cardiovascular risk in adults: A report of the American College of Cardiology/American Heart Association Task Force on Practice Guidelines. *Journal of the American College of Cardiology*. doi:10.1016/j.jacc.2013.11.002. Retrieved from http://content.onlinejacc.org/article.aspx?articleid=1879710

Sun, B. C., Emond, J. A., & Camargo, C. A. (2004). Characteristics and admission patterns of patients presenting with syncope to U.S. emergency departments, 1992–2000. *Academic Emergency Medicine, 11*(10), 1029–1034.

TACTICS (Treat Angina with Aggrastat and Determine Cost of Therapy with an Invasive or Conservative Strategy)—Thrombolysis in Myocardial Infarction - 18 Investigators. (2001). Comparison of early invasive and conservative strategies in patients with unstable coronary syndromes treated with the glycoprotein IIb/IIIa inhibitor tirofiban. *The New England Journal of Medicine, 344*(25), 1879–1887.

Taylor, R. S., Brown, A., Ebrahim, S., Jolliffe, J., Noorani, H., Rees, K., . . . Oldridge, N. (2004). Exercise-based rehabilitation for patients with coronary heart disease: Systematic review and meta-analysis of randomized controlled trials. *The American Journal of Medicine, 116*(10), 682–692.

Than, M., Aldous, S., Lord, S. J., Goodacre, S., Frampton, C. M. A., Troughton, R., . . . Richards, A. M. (2014). A 2-Hour diagnostic protocol for possible cardiac chest pain in the emergency department: A randomized clinical trial. *JAMA Internal Medicine, 174*(1), 51–58.

Than, M., Cullen, L., Aldous, S., Parsonage, W. A., Reid, C. M., Greenslade, J., . . . Richards, A. M. (2012). 2-Hour accelerated diagnostic protocol to assess patients with chest pain symptoms using contemporary troponins as the only biomarker: The ADAPT trial. *Journal of the American College of Cardiolology, 59*(23), 2091–2098.

Thiruganasambandamoorthy, V., Wells, G., Hess, E., Turko, E., Perry, J., & Stiell, U. (2014). Derivation of a risk scale and quantification of risk factors for serious adverse events in adult emergency department syncope patients. *Canadian Journal of Emergency Medicine, 16*(2), 120–130.

Thompson, P. D. (2005). Exercise prescription and proscription for patients with coronary artery disease. *Circulation, 112*, 2354–2363.

Thygesen, K., Alpert, J. S., Jaffe, A. S., Simoons, M. L., Chaitman, B. R., White, H. D., & the Writing Group on behalf of the Joint ESC/ACCF/AHA/WHF Task Force for the Universal Definition of Myocardial Infarction. (2012). Third universal definition of myocardial infarction. *Journal of the American College of Cardiology, 60*(16), 1581–1598.

Thygesen, K., Alpert, J. S., & White, H. D. (2007). Universal definition of myocardial infarction. *European Heart Journal, 28*, 2525–2538.

TIMI Study Group. (2011). TIMI risk score. Retrieved from http://www.timi.org/

Tomich, E. B. (2012). Takotsubo cardiomyopathy. *Medscape.* Retrieved from http://emedicine.medscape.com/article/1513631-overview

Tracy, C. M., Epstein, A. E., Darbar, D., DiMarco, J. P., Dunbar, S. B., Estes, M., III, . . . Varosy, P. D. (2013). 2012 ACCF/AHA/HRS focused update incorporated into the ACCF/AHA/HRS 2008 guidelines for device-based therapy of cardiac rhythm abnormalities. *Journal of the American College of Cardiology, 61*(3), e6–e75.

Tsai, T., Nienaber, C., & Eagle, K. (2005). Acute aortic syndromes. *Circulation, 112*, 3802–3813.

Tsai, T., Trimarchi, S., & Nienaber, C. (2009). Acute aortic dissection: Perspectives from the International Registry of Acute Aortic Dissection (IRAD). *European Journal Vascular and Endovascular Surgery, 37*, 149–159.

Turnipseed, S. D., Trythall, W. S., Diercks, D. B., Laurin, E. G., Kirk, J. J., Smith, D. S., . . . Amsterdam, E. A. (2009). Frequency of acute coronary syndrome in patients with normal electrocardiogram performed during presence or absence of chest pain. *Academic Emergency Medicine, 16*, 495–499.

University of Massachusetts Medical School. (2014). Center for outcomes research: Risk assessment models—original GRACE risk score. Retrieved from http://www.outcomes-umassmed.org/risk_models_grace_orig.aspx

Valle, R., Aspromonte, N., Giovinazzo, P., Carbonieri, E., Chiatto, M., diTano, G., . . . Milani, L. (2008). B-type natriuretic peptide-guided treatment for predicting outcome in patients hospitalized in sub-intensive care unit with acute heart failure. *Journal of Cardiac Failure, 14*(3), 219–224.

Varas-Lorenzo, C., Riera-Guardia, N., Calingaert, B., Castellsague, J., Salvo, F., Nicotra, F., . . . Perez-Gutthann, S. (2013). Myocardial infarction and individual nonsteroidal anti-inflammatory drugs meta-analysis of observational studies. *Pharmacoepidemiology and Drug Safety, 22*, 559–570.

Verma, S., Farkouh, M. E., Yanagawa, B., Fitchett, D., Ahsan, M. R., Ruel, M., . . . Friedrich, J. O. (2013). Comparison of coronary artery bypass surgery and percutaneous coronary intervention in patients with diabetes: A meta-analysis of randomized controlled trials. *The Lancet Diabetes & Endocrinology, 1*(4), 317–328. doi:10.1016/S2213–8587(13)70089–5

Virmani, R., Burke, A. P., Farb, A., & Kolodgie, F. D. (2006). *Pathology of vulnerable plaque. Journal of the American College of Cardiology, 47*(8), Suppl. C13–C18.

Wallace, S. M., Walton, B. I., Kharbanda, R. K., Hardy, R., Wilson, A. P., & Swanton, R. H. (2002). Mortality from infective endocarditis: Clinical predictors of outcome. *Heart, 88*, 53–60.

Wallmuller, C., Meron, G., Kurckciyan, I., Schober, A., Stratil, P., & Sterz, F. (2012). Causes of in-hospital cardiac arrest and influence on outcome. *Resuscitation, 83*(10), 1206–1211.

Webb, J. G., Lowe, A. M., Sanborn, T. A., White, H. D., Sleeper, L. A., Carere, R. G., . . . Hochman, J. S. (2003). Percutaneous coronary intervention for cardiogenic shock in the SHOCK trial. *Journal of the American College of Cardiology, 42*, 1380–1386.

Wieling, W., Krediet, C., Solari, D., de Lange, F., van Dijk, N., Thijs, R., . . . Jardine, D. (2013). At the heart of arterial baroreflex a physiologic basis for a new classification of carotid sinus hypersensitivity. *Journal of Internal Medicine, 273,* 345–358.

Wieling, W., Thijs, R. D., van Dijk, N., Wilde, A., Benditt, D., & van Dijk, J. (2009). Symptoms and signs of syncope: A review of the link between physiology and clinical clues. *Brain, 132*(10), 2630–2642.

Wijdicks, E. F., Hijdra, A., Young, G. B., Bassetti, C. L., & Wiebe, S. (2006). Practice parameter: Prediction of outcome in comatose survivors after cardiopulmonary resuscitation (an evidence-based review): Report of the Quality Standards Subcommittee of the American Academy of Neurology. *Neurology, 67,* 203–210.

Williams, M. E. (2009). The basic geriatric respiratory examination. *Medscape.* Retrieved from http://www.medscape.com/viewarticle/712242_2

Wilson, K., Gibson, N., Willan, A., & Cook, D. (2000). Effect of smoking cessation on mortality after myocardial infarction: Meta-analysis of cohort studies. *Archives of Internal Medicine, 160*(7), 939–944.

Wiviott, S. D., Braunwald, E., McCabe, C. H., Montelescot, G., Ruzyllo, W., Gottlieb, S., . . . Antman, E. M. for the TRITON-TIMI 38 Investigators. (2007). Prasugrel versus clopidogrel in patients with acute coronary syndromes. *The New England Journal of Medicine, 357*(20), 2001–2015.

Wolf, S., Lo, B., Shih, R., Smith, M., & Fesmire, F. (2013). Clinical policy: Critical issues in the evaluation and management of adult patients in the emergency department with asymptomatic elevated blood pressure. *Annals of Emergency Medicine, 62*(1), 59–64.

Wong, S. C., Sleeper, L. A., Monrad, E. S., Menegus, M. A., Palazzo, A., Dzavik, V., . . . Hochman, J. S. (2001). Absence of gender differences in clinical outcomes in patients with cardiogenic shock complicating acute myocardial infarction. A report from the SHOCK Trial Registry. *Journal of the American College of Cardiology, 38*(5), 1395–1401.

Woo, K. C., & Schneider, J. I. (2009). High-risk chief complaints: Chest pain—the big three. *Emergency Clinics of North America, 27,* 685–712.

Yancy, C. W., Jessup, M., Bozkurt, B., Butler, J., Casey, D. E., Drazner, M. H., . . . Wilkoff, B. L. (2013). 2013 ACCF/AHA guideline for the management of heart failure. *Journal of the American College of Cardiology, 62*(16), e147–e239.

Yeo, T., & Burrell, S. (2010). Hypertensive crisis in an era of escalating health care changes. *Journal for Nurse Practitioners, 6*(5), 338–346.

Yoshino, H., Yotsukura, M., Yano, K., Taniuchi, M., Kachi, E., Shimizu, H., . . . Ishikawa, K. (2000). Cardiac rupture and admission electrocardiography in acute anterior myocardial infarction: Implication of ST elevation in aVL. *Journal of Electrocardiology, 33,* 49–54.

Young, W. F., Jr. (2011). Chapter 11—Shock. In C. Stone & R. L. Humphries (Eds.), *Current diagnosis & treatment emergency medicine* (7th ed.). Retrieved from http://accessmedicine .mhmedical.com.proxygw.wrlc.org/content.aspx?bookid=385&Sectionid=40357225

Zampaglione, B., Pascale, C., Marchisio, M., & Cavalle-Perin, P. (1996). Hypertensive urgencies and emergencies: Prevalence and clinical presentation. *Hypertension, 27*(1), 144–147.

Zandbergen, E. G., Hijdra, A., Koelman, J. H., Hart, A. A., Vos, P. E., Verbeek, M. M., & de Haan, R. J. (2006). Prediction of poor outcome within the first 3 days of postanoxic coma. *Neurology, 66,* 62–68.

SECTION VI

Accurso, V., Winnicki, M., Shamsuzzaman, A. S., Wenzel, A., Johnson, A. K., & Somers, V. K. (2001). Predisposition to vasovagal syncope in subjects with blood/injury phobia. *Circulation, 104*(8), 903–907.

Ackerman, M. J., Priori, S. G., Willems, S., Berul, C., Brugada, R., Calkins, H., . . . Zipes, D. P. (2011). HRS/EHRA expert consensus statement on the state of genetic testing for the channelopathies and cardiomyopathies. *Europace, 13*, 1077–1109.

Agatston, A. S., Janowitz, W. R., Hildner, F. J., Zusmer, N. R., Viamonte, M., Jr., & Detrano, R. (1990). Quantification of coronary artery calcium using ultrafast computed tomography. *Journal of the American College of Cardiology, 15*(4), 827–832.

Allman, K. C. (2013). Noninvasive assessment myocardial viability: Current status and future directions. *Journal of Nuclear Cardiology, 20*(4), 618–637.

Amanullah, A. M., Berman, D. S., Kang, X., Cohen, I., Germano, G., & Friedman, J. D. (2000). Enhanced prognostic stratification of patients with left ventricular hypertrophy with the use of single-photon emission computed tomography. *American Heart Journal, 140*(3), 456–462.

American Diabetes Association. (2013). Tight diabetes control. Retrieved from http://www .diabetes.org/living-with-diabetes/treatment-and-care/blood-glucose-control/tight-diabetes-control.html

American Diabetes Association. (2014a). A1C and eAG. Retrieved from http://www.diabetes .org/living-with-diabetes/treatment-and-care/blood-glucose-control/a1c/

American Diabetes Association (ADA). (2014b). Standards of medical care in diabetes—2014. *Diabetes Care, 37*(Supplement 1), S14–S80.

American Heart Association. (2014). Homocysteine, folic acid and cardiovascular disease. Retrieved from http://www.heart.org/HEARTORG/GettingHealthy/NutritionCenter/ Homocysteine-Folic-Acid-and-Cardiovascular-Disease_UCM_305997_Article.jsp

Anderson, J. L., Adams, C. D., Antman, E. M., Bridges, C. R., Califf, R. M., Casey, D. E., . . . Wright, R. S. (2013). 2012 ACCF/AHA focused update incorporated into the ACCF/ AHA 2007 guidelines for the management of patients with unstable angina/non-ST-elevation myocardial infarction: A report of the American College of Cardiology Foundation/American Heart Association Task Force on Practice Guidelines. *Circulation, 127*, e000–e000.

Anderson, K. M., Murphy, D. L., & Balaji, M. (2014). Essentials of noninvasive cardiac stress testing. *Journal of the American Academy of Nurse Practitioners, 26*(2), 59–69.

Arena, R., & Sietsema, K. E. (2011). Cardiopulmonary exercise testing in the clinical evaluation of patients with heart and lung disease. *Circulation, 123*(6), 668–680.

Arepally, G., & Ortel, T. (2006). Heparin-induced thrombocytopenia. *The New England Journal of Medicine, 355*, 809–817.

Balady, G. J., Arena, R., Sietsema, K., Myers, J., Coke, L., Fletcher, G. F., . . . Interdisciplinary Council on Quality of Care and Outcomes Research. (2010). Clinician's guide to cardiopulmonary exercise testing in adults: A scientific statement from the American Heart Association. *Circulation, 122*(2), 191–225.

Banerjee, A., Newman, D. R., Van den Bruel, A., & Heneghan, C. (2012). Diagnostic accuracy of exercise stress testing for coronary artery disease: A systematic review and meta-analysis of prospective studies. *International Journal of Clinical Practice, 66*(5), 477–492.

Beanlands, R. S., & Youssef, G. (2010). Diagnosis and prognosis of coronary artery disease: PET is superior to SPECT: Pro. *Journal of Nuclear Cardiology, 17*(4), 683–695.

Bommer, W. J., Shah, P. M., Allen, H., Meltzer, R., & Kisslo, J. (1984). The safety of contrast echocardiography: Report of the Committee on Contrast Echocardiography for the American Society of Echocardiography. *Journal of American College of Cardiology, 3*(1), 6–13.

Breidthardt, T., Balmelli, C., Twerenbold, R., Mosimann, T., Espinola, J., Haaf, P., . . . Mueller, C. (2013). Heart failure therapy-induced early ST2 changes may offer long-term therapy guidance. *Journal of Cardiac Failure, 19*(12), 821–828.

Brignole, M., Menozzi, C., Gianfranchi, L., Oddone, D., Lolli, G., & Bertulla, A. (1991). Neurally mediated syncope detected by carotid sinus massage and head-up tilt test in sick sinus syndrome. *The American Journal of Cardiology, 68*(10), 1032–1036.

Brignole, M., Vardas, P., Hoffman, E., Huikuri, H., Moya, A., Ricci, R., . . . Botto, G. L. (2009). Indications for the use of diagnostic implantable and external ECG loop recorders. *Europace*, 11(5), 671–687.

Brown, K. A. (1995). Prognostic value of cardiac imaging in patients with known or suspected coronary artery disease: Comparison of myocardial perfusion imaging, stress echocardiography, and position emission tomography. *The American Journal of Cardiology*, 75(11), 35D–41D.

Brown, K. A. (1996). Prognostic value of myocardial perfusion imaging: State of the art and new developments. *Journal of Nuclear Cardiology*, 3(6 Pt 1), 516–537.

Bruce, R. A. (1974). Methods of exercise testing. Step test, bicycle, treadmill, isometrics. *The American Journal of Cardiology*, 33(6), 715–720.

Bruce, R. A., Blackmon, J. R., Jones, J. W., & Strait, G. (1963). Exercising testing in adult normal subjects and cardiac patients. *Pediatrics*, 32, SUPPL 742–756.

Bui, K. L., Horner, J. D., Herts, B. R., & Einstein, D. M. (2007). Intravenous iodinated contrast agents: Risks and problematic situations. *Cleveland Clinical Journal of Medicine*, 74(5), 361–364, 367.

Burwash, I. G., & Chan, K. (2012). Chapter 1—Transesophageal echocargiography. In C. M. Otto (Ed.), *Practice of clinical echocardiography* (4th ed.). Philadelphia, PA: Elsevier Saunders.

Cahalin, L. P., Chase, P., Arena, R., Myers, J., Bensimhon, D., Peberdy, M. A., . . . Guazzi, M. (2013). A meta-analysis of the prognostic significance of cardiopulmonary exercise testing in patients with heart failure. *Heart Fail Rev*, 18(1), 79–94.

Callister, T. Q., Cooil, B., Raya, S. P., Lippolis, N. J., Russo, D. J., & Raggi, P. (1998). Coronary artery disease: Improved reproducibility of calcium scoring with an electron-beam CT volumetric method. *Radiology*, 208(3), 807–814.

Canclini, S., Terzi, A., Rossini, P., Vignati, A., La Canna, G., Magri, G. C., Pizzocaro, C., & Giubbini, R. (2001). Gated blood pool tomography for the evaluation of global and regional left ventricular function in comparison to planar techniques and echocardiography. *Italian Heart Journal*, 2(1), 42–48.

Carson, J. L., Grossman, B. J., Kleinman, S., Tinmouth, A. T., Marques, M. B., Fung, M. K., . . . Djulbegovic, B. (2012). Red blood cell transfusion: A clinical practice guideline from the AABB. *Annals of Internal Medicine*, 157, 49–58.

Centers for Disease Control and Prevention (CDC). (2014). Recommendations to prevent and control iron deficiency in the United States. Retrieved from http://www.cdc.gov/mmwr/preview/mmwrhtml/00051880.htm#00003038.htm

Cerqueira, M. D. (2010). Diagnosis and prognosis of coronary artery disease: PET is superior to SPECT: Con. *Journal of Nuclear Cardiology*, 17(4), 678–682.

Cerqueira, M. D., Weissman, N. J., Dilsizian, V., Jacobs, A. K., Kaul, S., Laskey, W. K., . . . American Heart Association Writing Group on Myocardial Segmentation and Registration for Cardiac Imaging. (2002). Standardized myocardial segmentation and nomenclature for tomographic imaging of the heart. A statement for health care professionals from the Cardiac Imaging Committee of the Council on Clinical Cardiology of the American Heart Association. *Circulation*, 105(4), 539–542.

Cheitlin, M. D., Alpert, J. S., Armstrong, W. F., Aurigemma, G. P., Beller, G. A., Bierman, F. Z., . . . Gillam, L. D. (1997). ACC/AHA guidelines for the clinical application of echocardiography. A report of the American College of Cardiology/American Heart Association Task Force on Practice Guidelines (Committee on Clinical Application of Echocardiography). Developed in collaboration with the American Society of Echocardiography. *Circulation*, 95(6), 1686–1744.

Chong, B. H., Burgess, J., & Ismail, F. (1993). The clinical usefulness of the platelet aggregation test for the diagnosis of heparin-induced thrombocytopenia. *Journal of Thrombosis and Haemostasis*, 69(4), 344–350.

Cleveland HeartLab, Inc. (2013). VAP (The VAP® Test). Retrieved from http://www.cleveland heartlab.com/tests/vap-the-vap-test

Cohn, J. N., Johnson, G. R., Shabetai, R., Loeb, H., Tristani, F., Rector, T., . . . Fletcher, R. (1993). Ejection fraction, peak exercise oxygen consumption, cardiothoracic ratio, ventricular arrhythmias, and plasma norepinephrine as determinants of prognosis in heart failure. The V-HeFT VA cooperative studies group. *Circulation, 87*(6 Suppl), VI5–V16.

Cowper, S. E. (2008). Nephrogenic systemic fibrosis: An overview. *Journal of American College of Radiology, 5*(1), 23–28.

Crawford, M. H., Bernstein, S. J., Deedwania, P. C., DiMarco, J. P., Ferrick, K. J., Garson, A., Jr., . . . Smith, S. C., Jr. (1999a). ACC/AHA guidelines for ambulatory electrocardiography. A report of the American College of Cardiology/American Heart Association Task Force on Practice Guidelines (Committee to Revise the Guidelines for Ambulatory Electrocardiography). Developed in collaboration with the North American Society for Pacing and Electrophysiology. *Journal of American College of Cardiology, 34*(3), 912–948.

Crawford, M. H., Bernstein, S. J., Deedwania, P. C., DiMarco, J. P., Ferrick, K. J., Garson, A., Jr., . . . Smith, S. C., Jr. (1999b). ACC/AHA guidelines for ambulatory electrocardiography: Executive summary and recommendations. A report of the American College of Cardiology/American Heart Association Task Force on Practice Guidelines (committee to revise the guidelines for ambulatory electrocardiography). *Circulation, 100*(8), 886–893.

Daniel, W. G., Erbel, R., Kasper, W., Visser, C. A., Engberding, R., Sutherland, G. R., . . . Dennig, K. (1991). Safety of transesophageal echocardiography: A multicenter survey of 10,419 examinations. *Circulation, 83*(3), 817–821.

Daniels, L. B., Clopton, P., Bhalla, V., Krishnaswamp, P., Nowak, R. M., & McCord, J. (2006). How obesity affects the cut-points for B-type natriuretic peptide in the diagnosis of acute heart failure: Results from the breathing not properly multinational study. *American Heart Journal, 151*(5), 999–1005.

de Jong, M. C., Genders, T. S., van Geuns, R. J., Moelker, A., & Hunink, M. G. (2012). Diagnostic performance of stress myocardial perfusion imaging for coronary artery disease: A systematic review and meta analysis *European Radiology, 22*(9), 1881–1895.

Debatin, J. F., Nadel, S. N., Paolini, J. F., Sostman, H. D., Coleman, R. E., Evans, A. J., . . . Bashore, T. M. (1992). Cardiac ejection fraction: Phantom study comparing cine MR imaging, radionuclide blood pool imaging, and ventriculography. *Journal of Magnetic Resonance Imaging, 2*(2), 135–142.

Delwiche, F. A. (2003). Mapping the literature of clinical laboratory science. *Journal of the Medical Library Association, 91*, 303–310.

Desai, R. R., & Jha, S. (2013). Diagnostic performance of cardiac stress perfusion MRI in the detection of coronary artery disease using fractional flow reserve as the reference standard: A meta-analysis. *The American Journal of Roentgenology, 201*(2), W245–W252.

Dill, T. (2008). Contraindications to magnetic resonance imaging: Non-invasive imaging. *Heart, 94*(7), 943–948.

DiMarco, J. P., & Philbrick, J. T. (1990). Use of ambulatory electrocardiographic (Holter) monitoring. *Annals of Internal Medicine, 113*(1), 53–68.

Dolan, M. S., Gala, S. S., Dodla, S., Abdelmoneim, S. S., Xie, F., Cloutier, D., . . . Labovitz, A. Z. (2009). Safety and efficacy of commercially available ultrasound contrast agents for rest and stress echocardiography a multicenter experience. *Journal of American College of Cardiology, 53*(1), 32–38.

Douglas, P. S., Garcia, M. J., Haines, D. E., Lai, W. W., Manning, W. J., Patel, A. R., . . . Weiner, R. B. (2011). ACCF/ASE/AHA/ASNC/HFSA/HRS/SCAI/SCCM/SCCT/SCMR 2011 Appropriate use criteria for echocardiography. A report of the American College of Cardiology Foundation Appropriate Use Criteria Task Force, American Society of Echocardiography, American Heart Association, American Society of Nuclear Cardiology, Heart Failure Society of America, Heart Rhythm Society, Society for Cardiovascular Angiography and Interventions, Society of Critical Care Medicine, Society of Cardiovascular Computed Tomography, Society for Cardiovascular Magnetic Resonance American College of Chest Physicians. *Journal of American Society Echocardiography, 24*(3), 229–267.

Doust, J. A., Pietrzak, E., Dobson, A., & Glasziou, P. P. (2005). How well does B-type natriuretic peptide predict death and cardiac events in patients with heart failure: Systematic review. *The British Medical Journal, 330,* 625–633.

EGAPP Work Group. (2010). Recommendations from the EGAPP Working Group: Genomic profiling to assess cardiovascular risk to improve cardiovascular health. *Genetics in Medicine, 12,* 839–843.

Einstein, A. J., Henzlova, M. J., & Rajagopalan, S. (2007). Estimating risk of cancer associated with radiation exposure from 64-slice computed tomography coronary angiography. *The Journal of the American Medical Association. 298*(3), 317–323.

Elmholdt, T. R., Buus, N. H., Ramsing, M., & Olesen, A. B. (2011). Antifibrotic effect after low-dose imatinib mesylate treatment in patients with nephrogenic systemic fibrosis: An open-label non-randomized, uncontrolled clinical trial. *Journal of the European Academy of Dermatology and Venereology, 27*(6), 779–784.

Farwell, D. J., Freemantle, N., & Sulke, A. N. (2004). Use of implantable loop recorders in the diagnosis and management of syncope. *European Heart Journal, 25*(14), 1257–1263.

Fisch, C. (1989). Evolution of the clinical electrocardiogram. *Journal of American College of Cardiology, 14*(5), 1127–1138.

Fleischmann, K. E., Hunink, M. G., Kuntz, K. M., & Douglas, P. S. (1998). Exercise echocardiography or exercise SPECT imaging? A meta-analysis of diagnostic test performance. *JAMA, 280*(10), 913–920.

Fletcher, G. F., Mills, W. C., & Taylor, W. C. (2006). Update on exercise stress testing. *American Family Physician, 74*(10), 1749–1754.

Freeman, R., Wieling, W., Axelrod, F. B., Benditt, D. G., Benarroch, E., Biaggioni, I., . . . van Dijk, J. G. (2011). Consensus statement on the definition of orthostatic hypotension, neurally mediated syncope and the postural tachycardia syndrome. *Autonomic Neuroscience, 161*(1–2), 46–48.

Friedberg, C. K., & Zager, A. (1961). "Nonspecific" ST and T-wave changes. *Circulation, 23,* 655–661.

Friedewald, W. T., Levy, R. I., & Fredrickson, D. S. (1972). Estimation of the concentration of low-density lipoprotein cholesterol in plasma, without use of the preparative ultracentrifuge. *Clinical Chemistry, 18*(6), 499–502.

Furukawa, T., Maggi, R., Solano, A., Croci, F., & Brignole, M. (2011). Effect of clinical triggers on positive responses to tilt-table testing potentiated with nitroglycerin or clomipramine. *The American Journal of Cardiology, 107*(11), 1693–1697.

Gaggin, H. K., Motiwala, S., Bhardwaj, A., Parks, K. A., & Januzzi, J. L. (2013). Soluble concentrations of the interleukin receptor family member ST2 and β-blocker therapy in chronic heart failure. *Circulation, 6,* 1206–1213.

Geleijnse, M. L., Krenning, B. J., van Dalen, B. M., Nemes, A., Soliman, O. I., Bosch, J. G., . . . Boersma, E. (2009). Factors affecting sensitivity and specificity of diagnostic testing: Dobutamine stress echocardiography. *Journal of American Society Echocardiography, 22*(11), 1199–1208.

Gerhard-Herman, M., Gardin, J. M., Jaff, M., Mohler, E., Roman, M., & Naqvi, T. Z. (2006). Guidelines for noninvasive vascular laboratory testing: A report from the American Society of Echocardiography and the Society of Vascular Medicine and Biology. *Journal of American Society Echocardiography, 19*(8), 955–972.

Gibbons, R. J., Balady, G. J., Beasley, J. W., Bricker, J. T., Duvernoy, W. F., Froelicher, V. F., . . . Ryan, T. J. (1997). ACC/AHA guidelines for exercise testing. A report of the American College of Cardiology/American Heart Association Task Force on Practice Guidelines (committee on exercise testing). *Journal of American College of Cardiology, 30*(1), 260–311.

Gibbons, R. J., Balady, G. J., Bricker, J. T., Chaitman, B. R., Fletcher, G. F., Froelicher, V. F., . . . Smith, S. C., Jr. (2002). ACC/AHA 2002 guideline update for exercise testing: Summary article: A report of the American College of Cardiology/American Heart Association

Task Force on Practice Guidelines (Committee to Update the 1997 Exercise Testing Guidelines). *Circulation, 106*(14), 1883–1892.

Goff, D. C., Jr., Lloyd-Jones, D. M., Bennett, G., Coady, S., D'Agostino, R. B., Sr., Gibbons, R., . . . Wilson, P. W. (2014). 2013 ACC/AHA guideline on the assessment of cardiovascular risk: A report of the American College of Cardiology/American Heart Association Task Force on Practice Guidelines. *Journal of American College of Cardiology, 63*(25 Pt B), 2935–2959.

Goff, D. C., Lloyd-Jones, D. M., Bennett, G., Coady, S., D'Agostino, R. B., Gibbons, R., . . . Wilson, P. W. F. (2013). 2013 ACC/AHA guideline on the assessment of cardiovascular risk: A report of the American College of Cardiology/American Heart Association Task Force on Practice Guidelines. *Circulation, 129*, S49–S73.

Grant, E. G., Benson, C. B., Moneta, G. L., Alexandrov, A. V., Baker, J. D., Bluth, E. I., . . . Zierler, R. E. (2003). Carotid artery stenosis: Gray-scale and Doppler US diagnosis—Society of Radiologists in Ultrasound Consensus Conference. *Radiology, 229*(2), 340–346.

Greenland, P., Alpert, J. S., Beller, G. A., Benjamin, E. J., Budoff, M. J., Fayad, Z. A., . . . Jacobs, A. K. (2010). 2010 ACCF/AHA guideline for assessment of cardiovascular risk in asymptomatic adults: A report of the American College of Cardiology Foundation/American Heart Association Task Force on Practice Guidelines. *Circulation, 122*(25), e584–e636.

Greenland, P., LaBree, L., Azen, S. P., Doherty, T. M., & Detrano, R. C. (2004). Coronary artery calcium score combined with Framingham score for risk prediction in asymptomatic individuals. *JAMA, 291*(2), 210–215.

Grubb, B. P. (2008). Postural tachycardia syndrome. *Circulation, 117*(21), 2814–2817.

Hachamovitch, R., Rozanski, A., Shaw, L. J., Stone, G. W., Thomson, L. E., Friedman, J. D., . . . Berman, D. S. (2011). Impact of ischaemia and scar on the therapeutic benefit derived from myocardial revascularization vs. medical therapy among patients undergoing stress-rest myocardial perfusion scintigraphy. *European Heart Journal, 32*(8), 1012–1024.

Hahn, R. T., Abraham, T., Adams, M. S., Bruce, C. J., Glas, K. E., Lang, R. M., . . . Picard, M. H. (2013). Guidelines for performing a comprehensive transesophageal echocardiographic examination: Recommendations from the American Society of Echocardiography and the Society of Cardiovascular Anesthesiologists. *Journal of American Society Echocardiography, 26*(9), 921–964.

Hancock, E. W., Deal, B. J., Mirvis, D. M., Okin, P., Kligfield, P., Gettes, L. S., . . . Heart Rhythm Society. (2009). AHA/ACCF/HRS recommendations for the standardization and interpretation of the electrocardiogram: Part V: Electrocardiogram changes associated with cardiac chamber hypertrophy: A scientific statement from the American Heart Association Electrocardiography and Arrhythmias Committee, Council on Clinical Cardiology; the American College of Cardiology Foundation; and the Heart Rhythm Society: Endorsed by the International Society for Computerized Electrocardiology. *Circulation, 119*(10), e251–e261.

Hays, J. T., Mahmarian, J. J., Cochran, A. J., & Verani, M. S. (1993). Dobutamine thallium-201 tomography for evaluating patients with suspected coronary artery disease unable to undergo exercise or vasodilator pharmacologic stress testing. *Journal of American College of Cardiology, 21*(7), 1583–1590.

Heller, G. V., & Brown, K. A. (1994). Prognosis of acute and chronic coronary artery disease by myocardial perfusion imaging. *Cardiology Clinics, 12*(2), 271–287.

Hendel, R. C., Berman, D. S., Di Carli, M. F., Heidenreich, P. A., Henkin, R. E., Pellikka, P. A., . . . Society for Cardiovascular Magnetic Resonance; Society of Nuclear Medicine. (2009). ACCF/ASNC/ACR/AHA/ASE/SCCT/SCMR/SNM 2009 appropriate use criteria for cardiac radionuclide imaging: A report of the American College of Cardiology Foundation Appropriate Use Criteria Task Force, the American Society of Nuclear Cardiology, the American College of Radiology, the American Heart Association, the American Society of Echocardiography, the Society of Cardiovascular Computed

Tomography, the Society for Cardiovascular Magnetic Resonance, and the Society of Nuclear Medicine. *Journal of American College of Cardiology, 53*(23), 2201–2229.

Hendel, R. C., Patel, M. R., Kramer, C. M., Poon, M., Carr, J. C., Gerstad, N. A., . . . Society of Interventional Radiology. (2006). ACCF/ACR/SCCT/SCMR/ASNC/NASCI/SCAI/SIR 2006 appropriateness criteria for cardiac computed tomography and cardiac magnetic resonance imaging: A report of the American College of Cardiology Foundation Quality Strategic Directions Committee Appropriateness Criteria Working Group, American College of Radiology, Society of Cardiovascular Computed Tomography, Society for Cardiovascular Magnetic Resonance, American Society of Nuclear Cardiology, North American Society for Cardiac Imaging, Society for Cardiovascular Angiography and Interventions, and Society of Interventional Radiology. *Journal of American College of Cardiology, 48*(7), 1475–1497.

Henzlova, M. J., Cerqueira, M. D., Mahmarian, J. J., & Yao, S. S. (2006). Stress protocols and tracers. *Journal of Nuclear Cardiology, 13*(6), e80–e90.

Hill, J., & Timmis, A. (2002). Exercise tolerance testing. *BMJ, 324*(7345), 1084–1087.

Hoffmann, U., Ferencik, M., Cury, R. C., & Pena, A. J. (2006). Coronary CT angiography. *Journal of Nuclear Medicine, 47*(5), 797–806.

Hong, C., Bae, K. T., & Pilgram, T. K. (2003). Coronary artery calcium: Accuracy and reproducibility of measurements with multi-detector row CT—assessment of effects of different thresholds and quantification methods. *Radiology, 227*(3), 795–801.

Hylton, N. M. (2000). Suspension of breast-feeding following gadopentetate dimeglumine administration. *Radiology, 216*(2), 325–326.

Inaba, Y., Chen, J. A., & Bergmann, S. R. (2012). Carotid plaque, compared with carotid intima-media thickness, more accurately predicts coronary artery disease events: A meta-analysis. *Atherosclerosis, 220*(1), 128–133.

Iskander, S., & Iskandrian, A. E. (1998). Risk assessment using single-photon emission computed tomographic technetium-99m sestamibi imaging. *Journal of American College of Cardiology, 32*(1), 57–62.

Jaarsma, C., Leiner, T., Bekkers, S. C., Crijns, H. J., Wildberger, J. E., Nagel, E., . . . Schalla, S. (2012). Diagnostic performance of noninvasive myocardial perfusion imaging using single-photon emission computed tomography, cardiac magnetic resonance, and positron emission tomography imaging for the detection of obstructive coronary artery disease: A meta-analysis. *Journal of American College of Cardiology, 59*(19), 1719–1728.

Januzzi, J. L., Mebazaa, A., & DiSomma, A. (2015). ST2 and prognosis in acutely decompensated heart failure: The international ST2 consensus panel. *The American Journal of Cardiology.* doi:10.1016/j.amjcard.2015.01.037.

Januzzi, J. L., Peacock, W. F., Maisel, A. A., Chae, C. U., Jesse, R. L., & Baggish, A. L. (2007). Measurement of the interleukin family member ST2 in patients with acute dyspnea: Results from the PRIDE (Pro-brain natriuretic peptide investigation of dyspnea in the emergency department) study. *Journal of the American College of Cardiology, 50*(7), 607–613.

Januzzi, J. L., & Troughton, R. (2013). Are serial BNP measurements useful in heart failure management? *Circulation, 127,* 500–508.

Jneid, H., Anderson, J. L., Wright, R. S., Adams, C. D., Bridges, C. R., Casey, D. E., . . . Zidar, J. P. (2010). 2012 ACCF/AHA focused update of the guideline for the management of patients with unstable angina/non-ST-elevation myocardial infarction (updating the 2007 guideline and replacing the 2011 focused update): A report of the American College of Cardiology Foundation/American Heart Association Task Force on Practice Guidelines. *Circulation, 126,* 875–910.

Jones, G. R. D., & Lim, E. (2003). The National Kidney Foundation guideline on estimation of the glomerular filtration rate. *Clinical Biochemical Review, 24,* 95–98.

Jung, W., Zvereva, V., Hajredini, B., & Jackle, S. (2011). Initial experience with magnetic resonance imaging-safe pacemakers: A review. *Journal of Interventional Cardiac Electrophysiology, 32*(3), 213–219.

Kadish, A. H., Buxton, A. E., Kennedy, H. L., Knight, B. P., Mason, J. W., Schuger, C. D., . . . International Society for Holter and Noninvasive Electrocardiology. (2001). ACC/AHA clinical competence statement on electrocardiography and ambulatory electrocardiography: A report of the ACC/AHA/ACP-ASIM task force on clinical competence (ACC/AHA Committee to develop a clinical competence statement on electrocardiography and ambulatory electrocardiography) endorsed by the International Society for Holter and noninvasive electrocardiology. *Circulation, 104*(25), 3169–3178.

Kafi, R., Fisher, G. J., Quan, T., Shao, Y., Wang, R., Voorhees, J. J., & Kang, S. (2004). UV-A1 phototherapy improves nephrogenic fibrosing dermopathy. *Archives of Dermatology, 140*(11), 1322–1324.

Karagiannis, S. E., Bax, J. J., Elhendy, A., Feringa, H. H., Cokkinos, D. V., van Domburg, R., . . . Poldermans, D. (2006). Enhanced sensitivity of dobutamine stress echocardiography by observing wall motion abnormalities during the recovery phase after acute beta-blocker administration. *The American Journal of Cardiology, 97*(4), 462–465.

Kearon, C., Akl, E. A., Comerota, A. J., Prandoni, P., Bounameux, H., Goldhaber, S. Z., . . . American College of Chest Physicians. (2012). Antithrombotic therapy and prevention of thrombosis, 9th ed: American College of chest physicians evidence-based clinical practice guidelines. *Chest, 141*(2), 419S–494S.

Kempfert, J., Van Linden, A., Lehmkuhl, L., Rastan, A. J., Holzhey, D., Blumenstein, J., Mohr, F. W., & Walther, T. (2012). Aortic annulus sizing: Echocardiographic versus computed tomography derived measurements in comparison with direct surgical sizing. *European Journal of Cardiothoracic Surgery, 42*(4), 627–633.

Kenny, R. A., Ingram, A., Bayliss, J., & Sutton, R. (1986). Head-up tilt: A useful test for investigating unexplained syncope. *The Lancet, 1*(8494), 1352–1355.

Kim, R. J., de Roos, A., Fleck, E., Higgins, C. B., Pohost, G. M., Prince, M., . . . Society for Cardiovascular Magnetic Resonance (SCMR) Clinical Practice Committee. (2007). Guidelines for training in Cardiovascular Magnetic Resonance (CMR). *Journal of Cardiovascular Magnetic Resonance, 9*(1), 3–4.

Kintossou, R., D'Incan, M., Chauveau, D., Bens, G., Franck, F., Dauplat, M. M., . . . Souteyrand, P. (2007). [Nephrogenic fibrosing dermopathy treated with extracorporeal photopheresis: Role of gadolinium?]. *Annales de Dermatologie et de Venereologie, 134*(8–9), 667–671.

Kirk, R. (2014). Transplant kids information. Retrieved from www.transplantkids.org.uk.

Kligfield, P., Gettes, L. S., Bailey, J. J., Childers, R., Deal, B. J., Hancock, E. W., . . . Wellens, H. (2007). Recommendations for the standardization and interpretation of the electrocardiogram: Part I: The electrocardiogram and its technology: A scientific statement from the American Heart Association Electrocardiography and Arrhythmias Committee, Council on Clinical Cardiology; the American College of Cardiology Foundation; and the Heart Rhythm Society: Endorsed by the International Society for Computerized Electrocardiology. *Circulation, 115*(10), 1306–1324.

Kodali, S., Baher, A., & Shah, D. (2013). Safety of MRIs in patients with pacemakers and defibrillators. *Methodist Debakey Cardiovascular Journal, 9*(3), 137–141.

Koike, A., Itoh, H., Kato, M., Sawada, H., Aizawa, T., Fu, L. T., & Watanabe, H. (2002). Prognostic power of ventilatory responses during submaximal exercise in patients with chronic heart disease. *Chest, 121*(5), 1581–1588.

Krahn, A. D., Klein, G. J., Norris, C., & Yee, R. (1995). The etiology of syncope in patients with negative tilt table and electrophysiological testing. *Circulation, 92*(7), 1819–1824.

Lainchbury, J. G., Troughton, R. W., Strangman, K. M., Frampton, C. M., Pilbrow, A., Yandle, T. G., . . . Richards, A. M. (2010). N-terminal pro-B-type natriuretic peptide-guided treatment for chronic heart failure. Results from the BATTLESCARRED (NT-proBNP-assisted treatment to lessen serial cardiac readmissions and death) trial. *Journal of the American College of Cardiology, 55*(1), 53–60.

Langlois, Y., Roederer, G. O., Chan, A., Phillips, D. J., Beach, K. W., Martin, D., . . . Strandness, D. E., Jr. (1983). Evaluating carotid artery disease. The concordance between pulsed Doppler/spectrum analysis and angiography. *Ultrasound in Medicine and Biology, 9*(1), 51–63.

Langlois, Y., Roederer, G. O., Chan, A., & Strandness, D. E., Jr. (1983). The use of common carotid waveform analysis in the diagnosis of carotid occlusive disease. *Angiology, 34*(10), 679–687.

Langsted, A., Freiberg, J. J., & Nordestgaard, B. G. (2008). Fasting and nonfasting lipid levels: Influence of normal food intake on lipids, lipoproteins, apolipoproteins, and cardiovascular risk prediction. *Circulation, 118*, 2047–2056.

Levey, A. A., Bosch, J. P., Lewis, J. B., Greene, T., Rogers, N., & Roth, D. for the modification of diet in renal disease study group. (1999). A more accurate method to estimate glomerular filtration rate from serum creatinine: A new prediction equation. *Annals of Internal Medicine, 130*(6), 461–470.

Likoff, M. J., Chandler, S. L., & Kay, H. R. (1987). Clinical determinants of mortality in chronic congestive heart failure secondary to idiopathic dilated or to ischemic cardiomyopathy. *The American Journal of Cardiology, 59*(6), 634–638.

Mahajan, V. S., & Jarolim, P. (2011). How to interpret elevated cardiac troponin levels. *Circulation, 124*, 2350–2354.

Main, M. L., Ryan, A. C., Davis, T. E., Albano, M. P., Kusnetzky, L. L., & Hibberd, M. (2008). Acute mortality in hospitalized patients undergoing echocardiography with and without an ultrasound contrast agent (multicenter registry results in 4,300,966 consecutive patients). *The American Journal of Cardiology, 102*(12), 1742–1746.

Malinow, R., Bostom, A., & Krauss, R. (1999). Homocysteine, diet, and cardiovascular diseases: A statement for health care professionals from the Nutrition Committee, American Heart Association. *Circulation, 99*, 178–182.

Mancini, D. M., Eisen, H., Kussmaul, W., Mull, R., Edmunds, L. H., Jr., & Wilson, J. R. (1991). Value of peak exercise oxygen consumption for optimal timing of cardiac transplantation in ambulatory patients with heart failure. *Circulation, 83*(3), 778–786.

Manzano-Fernandez, S., Mueller, T., Pascual-Figal, D., Truong, Q. A., & Januzzi, J. L. (2011). Usefulness of soluble concentrations of interleukin family member ST2 as predictor of mortality in patients with acutely decompensated heart failure relative to left ventricular ejection fraction. *The American Journal of Cardiology, 107*(2), 259–267.

Martin, S. S., Blaha, M. J., Elshazly, M. B., Brinton, E. A., Toth, P. P., McEvoy, J. W., . . . Jones, S. R. (2013). Friedewald estimated versus directly measured low-density lipoprotein cholesterol and treatment implications. *Journal of the American College of Cardiology, 62*(8), 732–739.

Marwick, T. H. (2007). Stress echocardiography with nonexercise techniques: Principles, protocols, interpretation, and clinical applications. In C. M. Otto (Ed.), *The clinical practice of clinical echocardiography*. Philadelphia, PA: Saunders Elsevier.

Mason, J. W., Hancock, E. W., Gettes, L. S., Bailey, J. J., Childers, R., Deal, B. J., . . . Wellens, H. (2007). Recommendations for the standardization and interpretation of the electrocardiogram: Part II: Electrocardiography diagnostic statement list: A scientific statement from the American Heart Association Electrocardiography and Arrhythmias Committee, Council on Clinical Cardiology; the American College of Cardiology Foundation; and the Heart Rhythm Society: Endorsed by the International Society for Computerized Electrocardiology. *Circulation, 115*(10), 1325–1332.

Mathias, W., Jr., Tsutsui, J. M., Andrade, J. L., Kowatsch, I., Lemos, P. A., Leal, S. M., . . . Ramires, J. F. (2003). Value of rapid beta-blocker injection at peak dobutamine-atropine stress echocardiography for detection of coronary artery disease. *Journal of American College of Cardiology, 41*(9), 1583–1589.

Media, A. C. (2013). Administration of contrast media to breast-feeding mothers. In A. C. o. Radiology (Ed.), *ACR manual on contrast media* (Version 9 ed., pp. 97–98).

Merhige, M. E., Breen, W. J., Shelton, V., Houston, T., D'Arcy, B. J., & Perna, A. F. (2007). Impact of myocardial perfusion imaging with PET and (82)Rb on downstream invasive procedure utilization, costs, and outcomes in coronary disease management. *Journal of Nuclear Medicine, 48*(7), 1069–1076.

Mertes, H., Sawada, S. G., Ryan, T., Segar, D. S., Kovacs, R., Foltz, J., & Feigenbaum, H. (1993). Symptoms, adverse effects, and complications associated with dobutamine stress echocardiography: Experience in 1118 patients. *Circulation, 88*(1), 15–19.

Metz, L. D., Beattie, M., Hom, R., Redberg, R. F., Grady, D., & Fleischmann, K. E. (2007). The prognostic value of normal exercise myocardial perfusion imaging and exercise echocardiography: A meta-analysis. *Journal of American College of Cardiology, 49*(2), 227–237.

Mittal, S., Movsowitz, C., & Steinberg, J. S. (2011). Ambulatory external electrocardiographic monitoring: Focus on atrial fibrillation. *Journal of American College of Cardiology, 58*(17), 1741–1749.

Mohler, E. R., III, Gornik, H. L., Gerhard-Herman, M., Misra, S., Olin, J. W., Zierler, R. E., . . . Society for Vascular Surgery. (2012). ACCF/ACR/AIUM/ASE/ASN/ICAVL/SCAI/SCCT/SIR/SVM/SVS/SVU [corrected] 2012 appropriate use criteria for peripheral vascular ultrasound and physiological testing part I: Arterial ultrasound and physiological testing: A report of the American College of Cardiology Foundation appropriate use criteria task force, American College of Radiology, American Institute of Ultrasound in Medicine, American Society of Echocardiography, American Society of Nephrology, Intersocietal Commission for the Accreditation of Vascular Laboratories, Society for Cardiovascular Angiography and Interventions, Society of Cardiovascular Computed Tomography, Society for Interventional Radiology, Society for Vascular Medicine, Society for Vascular Surgery [corrected], and Society for Vascular Ultrasound [corrected]. *Journal of American College of Cardiology, 60*(3), 242–276.

Mosca, L., Benjamin, E. J., Berra, K., Bezanson, J. L., Dolor, R. J., Lloyd-Jones, D. M., . . . Wenger, N. K. (2011). Effectiveness-based guidelines for the prevention of cardiovascular disease in women—2011 update. A guideline from the American Heart Association. *Circulation, 123*, 1243–1262.

Moya, A., Sutton, R., Ammirati, F., Blanc, J. J., Brignole, M., Dahm, J. B, . . Wieling, W. (2009). Guidelines for the diagnosis and management of syncope (version 2009). *European Heart Journal, 30*(21), 2631–2671.

Mulvagh, S. L., Rakowski, H., Vannan, M. A., Abdelmoneim, S. S., Becher, H., Bierig, S. M., . . . American Society of Echocardiography. (2008). American Society of Echocardiography consensus statement on the clinical applications of ultrasonic contrast agents in echocardiography. *Journal of American Society Echocardiography, 21*(11), 1179–1201; quiz 1281.

Murdoch, D. R., Corey, G. R., Hoen, B., Miró, J. M., Fowler, V. G., Jr., Bayer, A. S., . . . International Collaboration on Endocarditis-Prospective Cohort Study (ICE-PCS) Investigators. (2009). Clinical presentation, etiology, and outcome of infective endocarditis in the 21st century: The international collaboration on endocarditis–prospective cohort study. *Archives of Internal Medicine, 169*(5), 463–473.

Nandalur, K. R., Dwamena, B. A., Choudhri, A. F., Nandalur, M. R., & Carlos, R. C. (2007). Diagnostic performance of stress cardiac magnetic resonance imaging in the detection of coronary artery disease: A meta-analysis. *Journal of American College of Cardiology, 50*(14), 1343–1353.

Narayana, S. K., Woods, D. R., & Boos, C. J. (2011). Management of amiodarone-related thyroid problems. *Therapeutic Advances in Endocrinology and Metabolism, 2*(3), 115–126. doi:10.1177/2042018811398516

National Institutes of Health. (2014). Medline plus. Retrieved from http://www.nlm.nih.gov/medlineplus/ency/article/003599.htm

National Kidney Foundation (NKF). (2002). NKF K/DOQI clinical practice guidelines for chronic kidney disease: Evaluation, classification, and stratification. *The American Journal of Kidney Disease, 39*, S1–S266. Retrieved from http://www2.kidney.org/professionals/KDOQI/guidelines_ckd/toc.htm

National Kidney Foundation. (2014a). Frequently asked questions about GFR estimates. Retrieved from https://www.kidney.org/sites/default/files/docs/12-10-4004_abe_faqs_aboutgfrrev1b_singleb.pdf

National Kidney Foundation. (2014b). Glomerular filtration rate (GFR). Retrieved from https://www.kidney.org/atoz/content/gfr

Neuberg, G. W., Friedman, S. H., Weiss, M. B., & Herman, M. V. (1988). Cardiopulmonary exercise testing: The clinical value of gas exchange data. *Archives of Internal Medicine, 148*(10), 2221–2226.

Newby, L. K., Jesse, R. L., Babb, J. D., Christenson, R. H., DeFer, T. M., Diamond, G. A., . . . Weintraub, W. S. (2012). ACCF 2012 expert consensus document on practical clinical considerations in the interpretation of troponin elevations. *Journal of the American College of Cardiology, 60*(23), 2419–2455.

Nielsen, L. H., Ortner, N., Norgaard, B. L., Achenbach, S., Leipsic, J., & Abdulla, J. (2014). The diagnostic accuracy and outcomes after coronary computed tomography angiography vs. conventional functional testing in patients with stable angina pectoris: A systematic review and meta-analysis. *European Heart Journal Cardiovascular Imaging, 15*(9), 961–971.

Nishimura, R. A., Otto, C. M., Bonow, R. O., Carabello, B. A., Erwin, J. P., III, Guyton, R. A., . . . ACC/AHA Task Force Members. (2014). 2014 AHA/ACC guideline for the management of patients with valvular heart disease: A report of the American College of Cardiology/American Heart Association Task Force on Practice Guidelines. *Circulation, 129*(23), 2440–2492.

O'Brien, P. J., Thiemann, D. R., McNamara, R. L., Roberts, J. W., Raska, K., Oppenheimer, S. M., & Lima, J. A. (1998). Usefulness of transesophageal echocardiography in predicting mortality and morbidity in stroke patients without clinically known cardiac sources of embolus. *The American Journal of Cardiology, 81*(9), 1144–1151.

O'Leary, D. H., Polak, J. F., Kronmal, R. A., Manolio, T. A., Burke, G. L., & Wolfson, S. K., Jr. (1999). Carotid-artery intima and media thickness as a risk factor for myocardial infarction and stroke in older adults. Cardiovascular Health Study Collaborative Research Group. *The New England Journal of Medicine, 340*(1), 14–22.

Pagana, K., & Pagana, T. (2012). *Mosby's diagnostic and laboratory test reference* (10th ed.). St. Louis: Mosby Elsevier.

Park, C., Ihm, S., Yoo, K., Kim, D., Chung, W., Seung, K., & Kim, J. (2010). Relation between C-reactive protein, homocysteine levels, fibrinogen, and lipoprotein levels and leukocyte and platelet counts, and 10-year risk for cardiovascular disease among healthy adults in the USA. *The American Journal of Cardiology, 105*(9), 1284–1288.

Parker, M. W., Iskandar, A., Limone, B., Perugini, A., Kim, H., Jones, C., . . . Heller, G. V. (2012). Diagnostic accuracy of cardiac positron emission tomography versus single photon emission computed tomography for coronary artery disease: A bivariate meta-analysis. *Circulation Cardiovascular Imaging, 5*(6), 700–707.

Patel, M. R., Bailey, S. R., Bonow, R. O., Chambers, C. E., Chan, P. S., Dehmer, G. J., . . . Ward, R. P. (2012). ACCF/SCAI/AATS/AHA/ASE/ASNC/HFSA/HRS/SCCM/SCCT/SCMR/STS 2012 appropriate use criteria for diagnostic catheterization: A report of the American College of Cardiology Foundation Appropriate Use Criteria Task Force, Society for Cardiovascular Angiography and Interventions, American Association for Thoracic Surgery, American Heart Association, American Society of Echocardiography, American Society of Nuclear Cardiology, Heart Failure Society of America, Heart Rhythm Society, Society of Critical Care Medicine, Society of Cardiovascular Magnetic Resonance, and Society of Thoracic Surgeons. *Journal of Thoracic and Cardiovascular Surgery, 143*, 39–71.

Pellikka, P. A., Nagueh, S. F., Elhendy, A. A., Kuehl, C. A., & Sawada, S. G. (2007). American Society of Echocardiography recommendations for performance, interpretation, and application of stress echocardiography. *Journal of American Society Echocardiography, 20*(9), 1021–1041.

Picard, M. H., Adams, D., Bierig, S. M., Dent, J. M., Douglas, P. S., Gillam, L. D., . . . Zoghbi, W. A. (2011). American Society of Echocardiography recommendations for quality echocardiography laboratory operations. *Journal of American Society Echocardiography, 24*(1), 1–10.

Piepoli, M. F., Corra, U., Agostoni, P. G., Belardinelli, R., Cohen-Solal, A., Hambrecht, R., & Vanhees, L. (2006). Statement on cardiopulmonary exercise testing in chronic heart failure due to left ventricular dysfunction: Recommendations for performance and interpretation Part II: How to perform cardiopulmonary exercise testing in chronic heart failure. *European Journal of Cardiovascular Prevention and Rehabilitation, 13*(3), 300–311.

Pignoli, P., Tremoli, E., Poli, A., Oreste, P., & Paoletti, R. (1986). Intimal plus medial thickness of the arterial wall: A direct measurement with ultrasound imaging. *Circulation, 74*(6), 1399–1406.

Raj, S. R. (2006). The Postural Tachycardia Syndrome (POTS): Pathophysiology, diagnosis & management. *Indian Pacing Electrophysiology Journal, 6*(2), 84–99.

Rautaharju, P. M., Surawicz, B., Gettes, L. S., Bailey, J. J., Childers, R., Deal, B. J., . . . Heart Rhythm Society. (2009). AHA/ACCF/HRS recommendations for the standardization and interpretation of the electrocardiogram: Part IV: The ST segment, T and U waves, and the QT interval: A scientific statement from the American Heart Association Electrocardiography and Arrhythmias Committee, Council on Clinical Cardiology; the American College of Cardiology Foundation; and the Heart Rhythm Society: Endorsed by the International Society for Computerized Electrocardiology. *Circulation, 119*(10), e241–e250.

Reed, S. L. (2009). Laboratory tests using blood. In S. L. Woods, E. S. S. Froelicher, S. A. Motzer, & E. J. Bridges (Eds.), *Cardiac nursing* (pp. 245–264). New York, NY: Wolters Kluwer, Lippincott Williams & Wilkins.

Reeves, S. T. (2013). Basic and comprehensive perioperative transesophageal echocardiography consensus statement documents. *Journal of American Society Echocardiography, 26*(7), 25A.

Rehman, S. U., Martinez-Rumayor, A., Mueller, T., & Januzzi, J. L. (2008). Independent and incremental prognostic value of multimarker testing in acute dyspnea: Results from the ProBNP investigation of dyspnea in the emergency department (PRIDE) study. *Clinica Chimica Acta, 392*(1–2), 41–45.

Richards, K. L. (1985). Doppler echocardiographic diagnosis and quantification of valvular heart disease. *Current Problems in Cardiology, 10*(2), 1–49.

Ridker, P. M., Danielson, E., Fonseca, F. A. H., Genest, J., Gotto, A. M., Kastelein, J. J. P., . . . Glynn, R. J. for the JUPITER Study Group. (2008). Rosuvastatin to prevent vascular events in men and women with elevated C-reactive protein. *The New England Journal of Medicine, 359*(21), 2195–2207.

Romero, J. R., Frey, J. L., Schwamm, L. H., Demaerschalk, B. M., Chaliki, H. P., Parikh, G., . . . Babikian, V. L. (2009). Cerebral ischemic events associated with 'bubble study' for identification of right to left shunts. *Stroke, 40*(7), 2343–2348.

Romero, J., Xue, X., Gonzalez, W., & Garcia, M. J. (2012). CMR imaging assessing viability in patients with chronic ventricular dysfunction due to coronary artery disease: A meta-analysis of prospective trials. *JACC Cardiovascular Imaging, 5*(5), 494–508.

Samson, W. E., & Scher, A. M. (1960). Mechanism of ST-segment alteration during acute myocardial injury. *Circulation Research, 8,* 780–787.

Sato, N., Gheorghiade, M., Kajimoto, K., Munakata, R., Minami, Y., Mizuno, M., . . . Takano, T. (2013). Hyponatremia and in-hospital mortality in patients admitted for heart failure (from the ATTEND registry). *The American Journal of Cardiology, 111*(7), 1019–1025. Retrieved from http://www.ajconline.org/article/S0002-9149%2812%2902925 63-5/abstract

Schijvenaars, B. J., Kors, J. A., van Herpen, G., Kornreich, F., & van Bemmel, J. H. (1997). Effect of electrode positioning on ECG interpretation by computer. *Journal of Electrocardiology, 30*(3), 247–256.

Schlant, R. C., Adolph, R. J., DiMarco, J. P., Dreifus, L. S., Dunn, M. I., Fisch, C., . . . Murray, J. A. (1992). Guidelines for electrocardiography. A report of the American College of Cardiology/American Heart Association Task Force on assessment of diagnostic and therapeutic cardiovascular procedures (committee on electrocardiography). *Circulation, 85*(3), 1221–1228.

Schmook, T., Budde, K., Ulrich, C., Neumayer, H. H., Fritsche, L., & Stockfleth, E. (2005). Successful treatment of nephrogenic fibrosing dermopathy in a kidney transplant recipient with photodynamic therapy. *Nephrology Dialysis Transplantation, 20*(1), 220–222.

Shaw, L. J., Raggi, P., Schisterman, E., Berman, D. S., & Callister, T. Q. (2003). Prognostic value of cardiac risk factors and coronary artery calcium screening for all-cause mortality. *Radiology, 228*(3), 826–833.

Shaw, L. J., Vasey, C., Sawada, S., Rimmerman, C., & Marwick, T. H. (2005). Impact of gender on risk stratification by exercise and dobutamine stress echocardiography: Long-term mortality in 4234 women and 6898 men. *European Heart Journal, 26*(5), 447–456.

Shellock, F. G., & Crues, J. V., III. (2014). MRI issues for implants and devices. *MRI Bioeffects, Safety, and Patient Management*. Playa Del Rey, CA: Biomedical Research Publishing Group.

Shiba, N., & Shimokawa, H. (2011). Chronic kidney disease and heart failure——Bidirectional close link and common therapeutic goal. *Journal of Cardiology, 57*(1), 8–17.

Shinbane, J. S., Colletti, P. M., & Shellock, F. G. (2011). Magnetic resonance imaging in patients with cardiac pacemakers: Era of "MR Conditional" designs. *Journal of Cardiovascular Magnetic Resononance, 13*, 63.

Smart, S. C., Knickelbine, T., Stoiber, T. R., Carlos, M., Wynsen, J. C., & Sagar, K. B. (1997). Safety and accuracy of dobutamine-atropine stress echocardiography for the detection of residual stenosis of the infarct-related artery and multivessel disease during the first week after acute myocardial infarction. *Circulation, 95*(6), 1394–1401.

Solano, A., Menozzi, C., Maggi, R., Donateo, P., Bottoni, N., Lolli, G., . . . Brignole, M. (2004). Incidence, diagnostic yield and safety of the implantable loop-recorder to detect the mechanism of syncope in patients with and without structural heart disease. *European Heart Journal, 25*(13), 1116–1119.

STARS-US. (2014). Syncope trust & reflex anoxic seizures. Retrieved from http://www.stars-us.org. Accessed October 14, 2014.

Stein, J. H., Korcarz, C. E., Hurst, R. T., Lonn, E., Kendall, C. B., Mohler, E. R., . . . American Society of Echocardiography Carotid Intima-Media Thickness Task Force. (2008). Use of carotid ultrasound to identify subclinical vascular disease and evaluate cardiovascular disease risk: A consensus statement from the American Society of Echocardiography Carotid Intima-Media Thickness Task Force. Endorsed by the Society for Vascular Medicine. *Journal of American Society Echocardiography, 21*(2), 93–111; quiz 189–190.

Stein, P. D., Yaekoub, A. Y., Matta, F., & Sostman, H. D. (2008). 64-slice CT for diagnosis of coronary artery disease: A systematic review. *The American Journal of Medicine, 121*(8), 715–725.

Stone, N., Robinson, J., Lichenstein, A., Merz, C., Blum, C., Eckel, R., . . . Levy, D. (2013). 2013 ACC/AHA guideline on the treatment of blood cholesterol to reduce atherosclerotic cardiovascular risk in adults. Retrieved from http://circ.ahajournals.org/content/early/2013/11/11/01.cir.0000437738.63853.7a

Strickberger, S. A., Benson, D. W., Biaggioni, I., Callans, D. J., Cohen, M. I., Ellenbogen, K. A., . . . American Autonomic Society. (2006). AHA/ACCF Scientific Statement on the evaluation of syncope: From the American Heart Association Councils on Clinical Cardiology, Cardiovascular Nursing, Cardiovascular Disease in the Young, and Stroke, and the Quality of Care and Outcomes Research Interdisciplinary Working Group; and the American College of Cardiology Foundation: In collaboration with the Heart Rhythm Society: Endorsed by the American Autonomic Society. *Circulation, 113*(2), 316–327.

Stuart, R. J., Jr., & Ellestad, M. H. (1980). National survey of exercise stress testing facilities. *Chest, 77*(1), 94–97.

Sun, R. R., Lu, L., Liu, M., Cao, Y., Li, X. C., & Liu, H. (2014). Biomarkers and heart disease. *European Review for Medical and Pharmacological Sciences, 18,* 2927–2935.

Surawicz, B., Childers, R., Deal, B. J., Gettes, L. S., Bailey, J. J., Gorgels, A., . . . Heart Rhythm Society. (2009). AHA/ACCF/HRS recommendations for the standardization and interpretation of the electrocardiogram: Part III: Intraventricular conduction disturbances: A scientific statement from the American Heart Association Electrocardiography and Arrhythmias Committee, Council on Clinical Cardiology; the American College of Cardiology Foundation; and the Heart Rhythm Society: Endorsed by the International Society for Computerized Electrocardiology. *Circulation, 119*(10), e235–e240.

Szlachcic, J., Massie, B. M., Kramer, B. L., Topic, N., & Tubau, J. (1985). Correlates and prognostic implication of exercise capacity in chronic congestive heart failure. *The American Journal of Cardiology, 55*(8), 1037–1042.

Tadamura, E., Yamamuro, M., Kubo, S., Kanao, S., Saga, T., Harada, M., …Togashi, K. (2005). Effectiveness of delayed enhanced MRI for identification of cardiac sarcoidosis: Comparison with radionuclide imaging. *American Journal of Roentgenology, 185*(1), 110–115.

Taylor, A. J., Cerqueira, M., Hodgson, J. M., Mark, D., Min, J., O'Gara, P., . . . Society for Cardiovascular Angiography and Interventions; Society for Cardiovascular Magnetic Resonance. (2010). ACCF/SCCT/ACR/AHA/ASE/ASNC/NASCI/SCAI/SCMR 2010 Appropriate Use Criteria for Cardiac Computed Tomography. A report of the American College of Cardiology Foundation Appropriate Use Criteria Task Force, the Society of Cardiovascular Computed Tomography, the American College of Radiology, the American Heart Association, the American Society of Echocardiography, the American Society of Nuclear Cardiology, the North American Society for Cardiovascular Imaging, the Society for Cardiovascular Angiography and Interventions, and the Society for Cardiovascular Magnetic Resonance. *Journal of Cardiovascular Computed Tomography, 4*(6), 407, e401–e433.

Thygesen, K., Alpert, J. S., Jaffe, A. S., Simoons, M. L., Chaitman, B. R., White, H. D., & Writing Group on behalf of the Joint ESC/ACCF/AHA/WHF Task Force for the Universal Definition of Myocardial Infarction. (2012). Third universal definition of myocardial infarction. *Journal of the American College of Cardiology, 60*(16),1581–1598.

Touboul, P. J., Hennerici, M. G., Meairs, S., Adams, H., Amarenco, P., Desvarieux, M., . . . Advisory Board of the 3rd Watching the Risk Symposium 2004, 13th European Stroke Conference. (2004). Mannheim intima-media thickness consensus. *Cerebrovascular Diseases, 18*(4), 346–349.

United States Preventive Services Task Force (USPSTF). September 2014. Retrieved from http://www.uspreventiveservicestaskforce.org/Page/Topic/recommendation-summary/lipid-disorders-in-adults-cholesterol-dyslipidemia-screening?ds=1&s=

van der Vleuten, P. A., de Jonge, G. J., Lubbers, D. D., Tio, R. A., Willems, T. P., Oudkerk, M., & Zijlstra, F. (2009). Evaluation of global left ventricular function assessment by dual-source computed tomography compared with MRI. *European Radiology, 19*(2), 271–277.

Wagner, G. S., Macfarlane, P., Wellens, H., Josephson, M., Gorgels, A., Mirvis, D. M., . . . Heart Rhythm Society. (2009). AHA/ACCF/HRS recommendations for the standardization and interpretation of the electrocardiogram: Part VI: Acute ischemia/infarction: A scientific statement from the American Heart Association Electrocardiography and Arrhythmias Committee, Council on Clinical Cardiology; the American College of Cardiology Foundation; and the Heart Rhythm Society: Endorsed by the International Society for Computerized Electrocardiology. *Circulation, 119*(10), e262–e270.

Wikstrand, J., & Wendelhag, I. (1994). Methodological considerations of ultrasound investigation of intima-media thickness and lumen diameter. *Journal of Internal Medicine, 236*(5), 555–559.

Yancy, C. W., Jessup, M., Bozkurt, B., Butler, J., Casey, D. E., Drazner, M. H., . . . Wilkoff, B. L. (2013). 2013 ACCF/AHA guidelines for the management of heart failure: A report of the American College of Cardiology Foundation/American Heart Association Task Force on Practice Guidelines. *Circulation, 128*(16), e240.

Yoshinaga, K., Chow, B. J., Williams, K., Chen, L., deKemp, R. A., Garrard, L., . . . Beanlands, R. S. (2006). What is the prognostic value of myocardial perfusion imaging using rubidium-82 positron emission tomography? *Journal of American College of Cardiology, 48*(5), 1029–1039.

Young, W. F., & Kaplan, N. M. (2014). Clinical presentation and diagnosis of pheochromocytoma. *UpToDate.* Retrieved from http://www.uptodate.com/contents/clinical-presentation-and-diagnosis-ofpheochromocytoma?source=search_result&search=pheochromocytoma &selectedTitle=1%7E150.

Zimetbaum, P. J., & Josephson, M. E. (1999). The evolving role of ambulatory arrhythmia monitoring in general clinical practice. *Annals of Internal Medicine, 130*(10), 848–856.

SECTION VII

ACTIVE Investigators. (2006). Clopidogrel plus aspirin versus oral anticoagulation for atrial fibrillation in the atrial fibrillation clopidogrel trial with irbesartan for prevention of vascular events (ACTIVE W): A randomized controlled trial. *The Lancet, 367,* 1903–1912.

ACTIVE Investigators. (2009). Effect of clopidogrel added to aspirin in patients with atrial fibrillation. *The New England Journal of Medicine, 360,* 2066–2078.

Ageno, W., Gallus, A. S., Wittkowsky, A., Crowther, M., Hylek, E. M., & Palareti, G. (2012). Antithrombotic therapy and prevention of thrombosis, 9th ed: American College of Chest Physicians evidence-based clinical practice guidelines. Oral anticoagulant therapy. *Chest, 141,* e44S–e88S.

Alderman, E. L., Bourassa, M. G., Cohen, L. S., Davis, K. B., Kaiser, G. G., Killip, T., . . . CASS Investigators. (1990). Ten-year follow-up of survival and myocardial infarction in the randomized coronary artery surgery study. *Circulation, 82*(5), 1629–1646.

ALLHAT. (2002). The antihypertensive and lipid-lowering treatment to prevent heart attack trial. Major outcomes in high-risk hypertensive patients randomized to angiotensin-converting enzyme inhibitor or calcium channel blocker vs diuretic: The antihypertensive and lipid. *Journal of the American Medical Association, 288,* 2981–2997.

Alving, B. (2003). How I treat heparin-induced thrombocytopenia. *Blood, 101,* 31–37.

Amabile, C., & Spencer, A. (2004). Keeping your patient with heart failure safe. *Archives of Internal Medicine, 164,* 709–714.

American Heart Association (AHA). (2013). The American Heart Association recommendations for physical activity in adults. Retrieved from http://www.heart.org/HEARTORG/GettingHealthy/PhysicalActivity/StartWalking/Physical-activity-improves-quality-of-life_UCM_307977_Article.jsp

American Heart Association (AHA). (2014a). Easy tips to get active. Retrieved from http://www.heart.org/HEARTORG/GettingHealthy/PhysicalActivity/StartWalking/Get-Moving-Easy-Tips-to-Get-Active_UCM_307978_Article.jsp

American Heart Association (AHA). (2014b). Physical activity and calories. Retrieved from http://www.heart.org/HEARTORG/GettingHealthy/PhysicalActivity/Fitness Basics/Moderate-to-Vigorous—What-is-your-level-of-intensity_UCM_463775_Article.jsp

American Heart Association (AHA). (2014c). The price of inactivity. Retrieved from http://www.heart.org/HEARTORG/GettingHealthy/PhysicalActivity/StartWalking/The-Price-of-Inactivity_UCM_307974_Article.jsp

American Massage Therapy Association (AMTA). (2006). Massage therapy can relieve stress: A position paper from the American Massage Therapy Association. Retrieved from http://www.amtamassage.org/statement2.html

Ammerman, A. S., Keyserling, T. C., Atwood, J. R., Hosking, J. D., Zayed, H., & Krasny, C. (2003). A randomized controlled trial of a public health nurse directed treatment program for rural patients with high blood cholesterol. *Preventive Medicine, 36*(3), 340–351.

AMPLIFY Investigators. (2013). Oral apixaban for the treatment of acute venous thromboembolism. *The New England Journal of Medicine, 369*(9), 799–808.

AMPLIFY-EXT Investigators. (2013). Apixaban for extended treatment of venous thromboembolism. *The New England Journal of Medicine, 368*(8), 699–708.

Amsterdam, E. A., Wenger, N. K., Brindis, R. G., Casey, D. E., Ganiats, T. G., Holmes, D. R., . . . Zieman, S. J. (2014). 2014 AHA/ACC guideline for the management of patients with non-ST-elevation acute coronary syndromes. *Journal of the American College of Cardiology, 64*, e139–e228.

Amsterdam, E. A., Wenger, N. K., Brindis, R. G., Casey, D. E., Jr., Ganiats, T. G., Holmes, D. H., . . . ACC/AHA Task Force Members. (2014). 2014 AHA/ACC guideline for the management of patients with non-ST-elevation acute coronary syndromes: A report of the ACC/AHA Task Force on practice guidelines. *Circulation, 130*, e344–e426.

Andersen, H., Nielsen, T., Rasmussen, K., Thuesen, L., Kelbaek, H., Thayssen, P., . . . Mortensen, L. S. (2003). A comparison of coronary angioplasty with fibrinolytic therapy in acute myocardial infarction. *The New England Journal of Medicine, 349*(8), 733–742.

Anderson, J. L., Adams, C. D., Antman, E. M., Bridges, C. R., Califf, R. M., Casey, D. E. . . . Wright, R. S. (2011). 2011 ACCF/AHA focused update incorporated into the ACC/AHA 2007 guidelines for the management of patients with unstable angina/non-ST-elevation myocardial infarction: A report of the American College of Cardiology Foundation/American Heart Association Task Force on Practice Guidelines. *Circulation, 123*, e426–e579.

Anderson, J. L., Adams, C. D., Antman, E. M., Bridges, C. R., Califf, R. M., Casey, D. E., . . . Wright, R. S. (2013a). 2012 ACCF/AHA focused update incorporated into the ACCF/AHA 2007 guidelines for the management of patients with unstable angina/non-ST-elevation myocardial infarction: A report of the American College of Cardiology Foundation/American Heart Association Task Force on Practice Guidelines. *Circulation, 127*: e636–e828.

Anderson, J. L., Halperin, J. L., Albert, N. M., Bozkurt, B., Brindis, R. G., Curtis, L. H., . . . Shen, W. K. (2013b). Management of patients with atrial fibrillation (compilation of 2006 ACCF/AHA/ESC and 2011 ACCF/AHA/HRS recommendations: A report of the American College of Cardiology/American Heart Association Task Force on Practice Guidelines. *Circulation, 127*, 1916–1926.

Antman, E. M., Cohen, M., Bernink, P. J., McCabe, C. H., Horacek, T., Papuchis, G., . . . Braunwald, E. (2000). The TIMI risk score for unstable angina/non-ST elevation MI: A method for prognostication and therapeutic decision making. *Journal of the American Medical Association, 284*(7), 835–842.

Arepally, G., & Ortel, T. (2006). Heparin-induced thrombocytopenia. *The New England Journal of Medicine, 355*, 809–817.

Armstrong, P. C., & Peter, K. (2012). GPIIb/IIIa inhibitors: From bench to bedside and back to bench again. *Thrombosis and Haemostasis, 107*, 808–814.

ARTEMIS Investigators. (2006). Efficacy and safety of fondaparinux for the prevention of venous thromboembolism in older acute medical patients: Randomised placebo controlled trial. *The British Medical Journal, 332*, 325–329.

Ashley, J. M., St. Jeor, S. T., Schrage, J. P., Perumean-Chaney, S. E., Gilbertson, M. C., McCall, N. L., & Bovee, V. (2001). Weight control in the physician's office. *Archives of Internal Medicine, 161*, 1599–1604.

ASTEROID Investigators. (2006). Effect of very high-intensity statin therapy on regression of coronary atherosclerosis: The ASTEROID trial. *Journal of the American Medical Association, 295*, 1556–1565.

Awtry, E. H., & Loscalzo, J. (2000). Aspirin. *Circulation, 101*, 1206–1218.

Bacon, C. G., Mittleman, M. A., Kawachi, I., Giovannucci, E., Glasser, D. B., & Rimm, E. B. (2006). A prospective study of risk factors for erectile dysfunction. *Journal of Urology, 176*(1), 217–221.

Bairey Merz, C. N., Dwyer, J., Nordstrom, C. K., Walton, K. G., Salerno, J. W., & Schneider, R. H. (2002). Psychological stress and cardiovascular disease: Pathophysiologic links. *Behavioral Medicine, 27*(4), 141–146.

Bala, M. M., Strzeszynski, L., Topor-Madry, R., & Cahill, K. (2013). Mass media interventions for smoking cessation in adults [update]. *Cochrane Database of Systematic Reviews, 6*, CD004704.

Balady, G. J., Ades, P. A., Comoss, P., Limacher, M., Pina, I. L., Southard, D., . . . Bazzarre, T. (2000). Core components of cardiac rehabilitation/secondary prevention programs: A statement for health care professionals from the American Heart Association and the American Association of Cardiovascular and Pulmonary Rehabilitation Writing Group. *Circulation, 102*, 1069–1073.

Bao, Y., Han, J., Hu, F. B., Giovannucci, E. L., Stampfer, M. J., Willett, W. C., & Fuchs, C. S. (2013). Association of Nut Consumption with Total and Cause-Specific Mortality. *The New England Journal of Medicine, 369*, 2001–2011.

Barefoot, J. C., & Schroll, M. (1996). Symptoms of depression, acute myocardial infarction, and total mortality in a community sample. *Circulation, 93*, 1976–1980.

Bashore, T. M., Balter, S., Barac, A., Byrne, J. G., Cavendish, J. J., Chambers, C. E., . . . Tommaso, C. L. (2012). 2012 American College of Cardiology Foundation/Society for Cardiovascular Angiography and Interventions Expert Consensus Document on Cardiac Catheterization Laboratory Standards Update. *Journal of the American College of Cardiology, 59*(24), 2221–2305.

Bates, S., Greer, I., Middeldorp, S., Veenstra, D., Prabulos, A., & Vandvik, P. (2012). VTE, thrombophilia, antithrombotic therapy, and pregnancy: Antithrombotic therapy and prevention of thrombosis, 9th ed: American College of Chest Physicians evidence-based clinical practice guidelines. *Chest, 141*, e691S–736S.

Bavry, A. A., Kumbhani, D. J., Rassi, A. N., Bhatt, D. L., & Askari, A. T. (2006). Benefit of early invasive therapy in acute coronary syndromes: A meta-analysis of contemporary randomized clinical trials. *Journal of the American College of Cardiology, 48*(7), 1319–1325.

Beckmann, S. L., Os, I., Kjeldsen, S. E., Eide, I. K., Westheim, A., & Hjermann, I. (1995). Effect of dietary counselling on blood pressure and arterial plasma catecholamines in primary hypertension. *The American Journal of Hypertension, 8*(7), 704–711.

Bell, E. J., Lutsey, P. L., Windham, B. G., & Folsom, A. R. (2013). Physical activity and cardiovascular disease in African Americans in atherosclerosis risk in communities. *Medicine and Science in Sports and Exercise, 45*(5), 901–907.

Bell, K. J., Hayen, A., Irwig, L., Takahaski, O., Ohde, S., & Glasziou, P. (2013). When to remeasure cardiovascular risk in untreated people at low and intermediate risk: Observational study. *The British Medical Journal, 346*, 1895.

Belsey, J., Savelieva, I., Mugelli, A., & Camm, A. J. (2015). Relative efficacy of antianginal drugs used as add-on therapy in patients with stable angina: A systematic review and meta-analysis. *European Journal of Preventative Cardiology, 22*(7), 837–848.

Bhatt, D. L., Fox, K. A., Hacke, W., Berger, P. B., Black, H. R., Boden, W. E., . . . Topol, E. J. (2006). Clopidogrel and aspirin versus aspirin alone for the prevention of atherothrombotic events (CHARISMA). *The New England Journal of Medicine, 354*, 1706–1717.

Bibbins-Domingo, K. (2014). The Institute of Medicine Report Sodium Intake in Populations: Assessment of evidence summary of primary findings and implications for clinicians. *JAMA Internal Medicine, 174*, 136–137.

Bjorkman, D. J. (1998). The effect of aspirin and nonsteroidal anti-inflammatory drugs on prostaglandins. *The American Journal of Medicine, 105*, 8S–12S.

Boden, W. E., O'Rourke, R. A., Teo, K. K., Hartigan, P. M., Maron, D. J., Kostuk, W. J., . . . COURAGE Trial Research Group. (2007). Optimal medical therapy with or without PCI for stable coronary disease. *The New England Journal of Medicine 356*, 1503–1516.

Boehringer Ingelheim Pharmaceuticals, Inc. (2012). *Aggrenox: Highlights of prescribing information*. Ridgefield, CT: Boehringer Ingelheim Pharmaceuticals, Inc.

Bohm, M., Baumhakel, M., Teo, K., Sleight, P., Probstfield, J., Gao, P., & Yusuf, S. (2010). Erectile dysfunction predicts events in high-risk patients receiving telmisartan, ramipril or both. *Circulation, 121*, 1439–1446.

Bonow, R. O., Mann, D. L., Zipes, D. P., & Libby, P. (2012). Toxins and the heart. In P. Libby, R. O. Bonow, D. L. Mann, & D. P. Zipes, *Braunwald's heart disease* (pp. 1805–1814). Philadelphia, PA: Saunders Elsevier.

Bragadottir, G., Redfors, B., Nygren, A., Sellgren, J., & Ricksten, S. (2009). Low-dose vasopressin increases glomerular filtration rate, but impairs renal oxygenation in post-cardiac surgery patients. *Acta Anasthesiologica Scandinavica, 53*, 1052–1059.

Brater, D. (2000). Pharmacology of diuretics. *The American Journal of Medical Science, 319*, 38–50.

Bristol-Myers Squibb Company. (2014a). *Coumadin: Highlights of prescribing information*. Princeton, NJ: Bristol-Myers Squibb Company.

Bristol-Myers Squibb Company. (2014b). *Eliquis: Highlights of prescribing information*. Princeton, NJ: Briston-Myers Squibb Company.

Brotman, D. J., Gloden, S. H., & Wittstein, I. S. (2007). The cardiovascular toll of stress. *The Lancet, 370*, 1089–1100.

Brown, C. G., Werman, H. A., Davis, E. A., Katz, S., & Hamlin, R. L. (1987). The effect of high-dose phenylephrine versus epinephrine on regional cerebral blood flow during CPR. *Annals of Emergency Medicine, 16*, 743–748.

Buller, D. B., Morrill, C., Douglas Taren, M., Aickin, L., Sennott-Miller, M. K., Buller, L. L., Alatorre, C., & Wentzel, T. M. (1999). Randomized trial testing the effect of peer education at increasing fruit and vegetable intake. *Journal of the National Cancer Institute, 91*(17), 1491–1500.

Büller, H. R., Davidson, B. L., Decousus, H., Gallus, A., Gent, M., Piovella, F., . . . Lensing, A. W. (2003). Subcutaneous fondaparinux versus intravenous unfractionated heparin in the initial treatment of pulmonary embolism. *The New England Journal of Medicine, 349*, 1695–1702.

Büller, H. R., Davidson, B. L., Decousus, H., Gallus, A., Gent, M., Piovella . . . Lensing, A. W. (2004). Fondaparinux or enoxaparin for the initial treatment of symptomatic deep venous thrombosis. *The New England Journal of Medicine, 140*, 867–873.

Cahill, K., Stead, L. F., & Lancaster, T. (2012). Nicotine receptor partial agonists for smoking cessation. *Cochrane Database of Systematic Reviews* 4:CD006103.

Callaham, M., Madsen, C. D., Barton, C. W., Saunders, C., & Pointer, J. (1992). A randomized clinical trial of high-dose epinephrine and norepinephrine vs standard-dose epinephrine in prehospital cardiac arrest. *Journal of the American Medical Association, 268*, 2667–2672.

Callaway, C. W., Hostler, D. H., Doshi, A. A., Pinchalk, M., Roth, R. N., Lubin, J., . . . Kelly, L. J. (2006). Usefulness of vasopressin administered with epinephrine during out-of-hospital cardiac arrest. *The American Journal of Cardiology, 98*, 1316–1321.

Campbell, T., & Williams, K. (1998). Therapeutic drug monitoring: Antiarrhythmic drugs. *The British Journal of Clinical Pharmacology, 46*, 307–319.

Cannon, C. P., Braunwald, E., McCabe, C. H., Rader, D. J., Rouleau, J. L., Belder, R., . . . Skene, A. M. (2004). Intensive versus moderate lipid lowering with statins after acute coronary syndromes. *The New England Journal of Medicine, 350*, 1495–1504.

Cannon, W. (1914). Emergency function of the adrenal medulla in pain and the major emotions. *The American Journal of Physiology, 33*, 356.

CAPRIE Steering Committee. (1996). A randomised, blinded, trial of clopidogrel versus aspirin in patients at risk of ischaemic events (CAPRIE). *The Lancet, 348*, 1329–1339.

Caspersen, C. J., Powell, K. E., & Christenson, G. M. (1985). Physical activity, exercise, and physical fitness: Definitions and distinctions for health related research. *Public Health Report, 100*, 126–131.

Cheng, J. Y., Ng, E. M., Ko, J. S., & Chen, R. Y. (2007). Physical activity and erectile dysfunction: Meta-analysis of population-based studies. *International Journal of Impotence Research, 19*, 245–252.

Chenoweth, D., & Leutzinger, J. (2006). The economic cost of physical inactivity and excess weight gain in American adults. *Journal of Physical Activity and Health, 3*, 148–163.

Chobanian, A. V., Bakris, G. L., Black, H. R., Cushman, W. C., Green, L. A., Izzo, J. L., . . . Rocella, E. J. (2003). The seventh report of the Joint National Committee on prevention, detection, evaluation, and treatment of high blood pressure. *Journal of the American Medical Association, 289*(19), 2560–1571.

CIBIS-II. (1999). The Cardiac Insufficiency Bisoprolol Study II (CIBIS-II): A randomised trial. *The Lancet, 353*, 9–13.

Cleland, J., Coletta, A., & Witte, K. (2006). Practical applications of intravenous diuretic therapy in decompensated heart failure. *The American Journal of Medicine, 119*, S26–S36.

CLOT Investigators. (2003). Low-molecular-weight heparin versus a coumarin for the prevention of recurrent venous thromboembolism in patients with cancer. *The New England Journal of Medicine, 349*, 146–153.

Cohen, B. (2014, January 14). *Angioplasty.org*. Retrieved from Angioplasty.org: http://www.ptca.org

Connolly, S. J., Camm, A. J., Halperin, J. L., Joyner, C., Alings, M., Amerena, J., . . . Hohnloser, S. H. (2011). Dronedarone in high-risk permanent atrial fibrillation. *The New England Journal of Medicine, 365*, 2268–2276.

Connolly, S. J., Eikelboom, J., Joyner, C., Diener, H. C., Hart, R., Golitsyn, S., . . . Yusuf, S. (2011). Apixaban in patients with atrial fibrillation (AVERROES). *The New England Journal of Medicine, 364*, 806–817.

Connolly, S. J., Ezekowitz, M. D., Yusuf, S., Eikelboom, J., Oldgren, J., Parekh, A., . . . Wallentin, L. (2009). Dabigatran versus warfarin in patients with atrial fibrillation. *The New England Journal of Medicine, 361*, 1139–1151.

CONSENSUS Trial Study Group. (1987). Effects of enalapril on mortality in severe congestive heart failure. Results of the Cooperative North Scandinavian Enalapril Survival Study (CONSENSUS). *The New England Journal of Medicine, 316*, 1429–1435.

Conti, A. A., & Macchi, C. (2013). Protective effects of regular physical activity on human vascular system. *Clinical Therapeutics, 164*(4), 293–294. doi:10.7417/CT.2013.1575

CURE Trial Investigators. (2001). Effects of clopidogrel in addition to aspirin in patients with acute coronary syndromes without ST-segment elevation. *The New England Journal of Medicine, 345*, 494–502.

CURRENT-OASIS 7 Investigators. (2010). Dose comparison of clopiodgrel and aspirin in acute coronary syndromes. *The New England Journal of Medicine, 363*, 930–942.

Dahabreh, I. J., & Paulus, J. K. (2011). Association of episodic physical and sexual activity with triggering of acute cardiac events: Systematic review and meta-analysis. *Journal of the American Medical Association, 305*, 1225–1233.

Dahlöf, B., Devereux, R., Kjeldsen, S., Julius, S., Beevers, G., de Faire, U., . . . Wedel, H. (2002). Cardiovascular morbidity and mortality in the Losartan Intervention For Endpoint reduction in hypertension study (LIFE): A randomised trial against atenolol. *The Lancet, 359*, 995–1003.

Daiichi Sankyo Co., LTD. (2015). *Savaysa: Highlights of prescribing information*. Parsippany, NJ: Daiichi Sankyo, Inc.

De Bruyne, B., Pijls, N. H., Kalesan, B., Barbato, E., Tonino, P. A., Piroth, Z., . . . Fearon, W. F. for the FAME2 Trial Investigators. (2012). Fractional flow reserve-guided PCI versus medical therapy in stable coronary disease. *The New England Journal of Medicine, 367*, 991–1001.

De Jaegere, P., Mudra, H., Figulla, H., Almagor, Y., Doucet, S., Penn, I., . . . van Es, G. A. (1998). Intravascular ultrasound-guided optimized stent deployment: Immediate and 6 months clinical and angiographic results from the Multicenter Ultrasound Stenting in Coronaries Study (MUSIC Study). *European Heart Journal, 19*, 1214–1223.

De Backer, D., Biston, P., Devriendt, J., Madl, C., Chochrad, D. A., Brasseur, A., . . . Vincent, J. L. (2010). Comparison of dopamine and norepinephrine in the treatment of shock. *The New England Journal of Medicine, 362*, 779–789.

Delaney, J. P., Leong, K. S., Watkins, A., & Brodie, D. (2002). The short-term effects of myofascial trigger point massage therapy on cardiac autonomic tone in healthy subjects. *Journal of Advanced Nursing, 37*, 364–371.

Dellinger, R. P., Levy, M. M., Rhodes, A., Annane, D., Gerlach, H., Opal, S. M., . . . Moreno, R. (2013). Surviving sepsis campaign: International guidelines for management of severe sepsis and septic shock. *Critical Care Medicine, 41*(2), 580–637.

Deo, R., Katz, R., Shlipak, M. G., Sotoodehnia, N., Psaty, B. M., Sarnak, M. J., & Kestenbaum, B. (2011). Vitamin D, parathyroid hormone, and sudden cardiac death: Results from the Cardiovascular Health Study. *Hypertension, 58*(6), 1021–1028.

Dhanunjaya, L., et al. (2013). Effect of yoga on arrhythmia burden, anxiety, depression, and quality of life in paroxysmal atrial fibrillation: The YOGA My Heart study. *Journal of the American College of Cardiology, 61*(11), 1177–1182.

Diener, H. C., Bogousslavsky, J., Brass, L. M., Cimminiello, C., Csiba, L., Kaste, M., . . . Rupprecht, H. J. (2004). Aspirin and clopidogrel compared with clopidogrel alone after recent ischaemic stroke or transient ischaemic attack in high-risk patients (MATCH): Randomized, double-blind, placebo-controlled trial. *The Lancet, 364*, 331–337.

Diener, H. C., Cunha, L., Forbes, C., Sivenius, J., Smets, P., & Lowenthal, A. (1996). European stroke prevention study 2. Dipyridamole and acetylsalicyclic acid in the secondary prevention of stroke. *Journal of the Neurological Sciences, 143*, 1–13.

Digitalis Investigation Group. (1997). The effect of digoxin on mortality and morbidity in patients with heart failure. *The New England Journal of Medicine, 336*, 525–533.

DiNicolantonio, J. J., Niazi, A. K., Sadaf, R., O'Keefe, J. H., Lucan, S. C., & Lavie, C. J. (2013). Dietary sodium: Take it with a grain of salt. *The American Journal of Medicine, 126*(11), 951–955.

Dong, C., Rundek, T., Wright, C. B., Anwar, Z., Elkind, M. S. V., & Sacco, R. S. (2012). Ideal cardiovascular health predicts lower risks of myocardial infarction, stroke, and vascular death across Whites, Blacks, and Hispanics: The Northern Manhattan Study. *Circulation, 125*, 2975–2984.

Duru, O. K., Sarkisian, C. A., Leng, M., & Mangione, C. M. (2010). Sisters in motion: A randomized controlled trial of a faith-based physical activity intervention. *Journal of the American Geriatric Society, 58*(10), 1863.

Dusek, J. A., & Benson, H. (2009). Mind-body medicine: A model of the comparative clinical impact of the acute stress and relaxation responses. *Minnesota Medicine, 92*(5), 47–50.

EAFT Study Group. (1993). Secondary prevention in non-rheumatic atrial fibrillation after transient ischaemic attack or minor stroke. *The Lancet, 342*, 1255–1262.

Echt, D. S., Liebson, P. R., Mitchell, L. B., Peters, R. W., Obias-Manno, D., Barker, A. H., . . . Richardson, D. W. (1991). Mortality and morbidity in patients receiving encainide, flecainide, or placebo: The cardiac arrhythmia suppression trial (CAST). *The New England Journal of Medicine, 324*, 781–788.

Eckel, R. H., Jakicic, J. M., Ard, J. D., Hubbard, V. S., de Jesus, J. M., Lee, I.-M., & Yanovski, S. Z. (2013). 2013 AHA/ACC guideline on lifestyle management to reduce cardiovascular risk: A report of the American College of Cardiology/American Heart Association Task Force on Practice Guidelines. Retrieved from http://circ.ahajournals.org/content/early/2013/11/11/01.cir.0000437740.48606.d1

EINSTEIN Investigators. (2010). Oral rivaroxaban for symptomatic venous thromboembolism. *The New England Journal of Medicine, 363*(26), 2499–2510.

EINSTEIN-PE Investigators. (2012). Oral rivaroxaban for the treatment of symptomatic pulmonary embolism. *The New England Journal of Medicine, 366*(14), 1287–1297.

Eli Lilly and Company. (2013). *ReoPro: Package insert.* Indianapolis, IN: Eli Lilly and Company.

Encyclopedia. Retrieved from http://en.wikipedia.org/w/index.php?title=Renin%E2%80%93angiotensin_system&oldid=640798030

ENHANCE Investigators. (2008). Simvastatin with or without ezetimibe in familial hypercholesterolemia. *The New England Journal of Medicine, 358*, 1431–1443.

Ernst, M., & Moser, M. (2009). Use of diuretics in patients with hypertension. *The New England Journal of Medicine, 361*, 2153–2164.

Estruch, R., Ros, E., Salas-Salvado, J., Covas, M.-I., Corella, D., Aros, F., & Martinez-Gonzalez, M. A. (2013). Primary prevention of cardiovascular disease with a Mediterranean diet. *The New England Journal of Medicine, 368*(14), 1279–1290.

Fagard, R. H., & Cornelissen, V. A. (2007). Effect of exercise on blood pressure control. *European Journal of Prevention and Rehabilitation, 14*, 12–17.

Feldman, T., Foster, E., Glower, D. D., Kar, S., Rinaldi, M. J., Fail, P. S., Smalling, R. W., . . . EVEREST II Investigators. (2011). Percutaneous repair or surgery for mitral regurgitation. *The New England Journal of Medicine, 364*, 1395–1406.

Felker, G. M., Lee, K. L., Bull, D. A., Redfield, M. M., Stevenson, L. W., Goldsmith, S. R., . . . O'Connor, C. M. (2011). Diuretic strategies in patients with acute decompensated heart failure. *The New England Journal of Medicine, 364*, 797–805.

Fenster, J. M. (2003). *Mavericks, miracles, and medicine: The pioneers who risked their lives to bring medicine into the modern age.* New York, NY: Carroll & Graf.

Field, T. (1996). Massage therapy reduces anxiety and enhances EEG pattern of alertness and math computation. *International Journal of Neuroscience, 86*, 197–205.

Field, T., Hernandez-Reif, M., Diego, M., Schanberg, S., & Kuhn, C. (2005). Cortisol decreases and serotonin and dopamine increases following massage therapy. *International Journal of Neuroscience, 115*, 1397–1413.

Fihn, S. D., Gardin, J. M., Abrams, J., Berra, K., Blankenship, J. C., Dallas, A. P., . . . Anderson, J. L. (2012). 2012 ACCF/AHA/ACP/AATS/PCNA/SCAI/STS guideline for the diagnosis and management of patients with stable ischemic heart disease: A report of the American College of Cardiology Foundation/American Heart Association Task Force on Practice Guidelines, and the American College of Physicians, American Association for Thoracic Surgery, Preventive Cardiovascular Nurses Association, Society for Cardiovascular Angiography and Interventions, and Society of Thoracic Surgeons. *Circulation, 126*, e354–e471.

Fischman, D. L., Leon, M. B., Baim, D. S., Schatz, R. A., Savage, M. P., Penn, I., . . . Goldberg, S. for the Stent Restenosis Study Investigators. (1994). A randomized comparison of coronary-stent placement and balloon angioplasty in the treatment of coronary artery disease. Stent restenosis study investigators. *The New England Journal of Medicine, 331*, 496–501.

Fletcher, G. F., Ades, P. A., Kligfield, P., Arena, R., Balady, G. J., & Bittner, V. A. (2013). Exercise standards for testing and training: A statement from the American Heart Association. *Circulation, 128*(8), 873–934.

Fletcher, G. F., Balady, G. J., Amsterdam, E. A., Chaitman, B., Eckel, R., Fleg, J., & Bazzarre, T. (2001). AHA scientific statement: Exercise standards for testing and training. A statement for health care professionals from the American Heart Association. *Circulation, 104*, 1694–1740.

Fletcher, G. F., Balady, G., Blair, S. N., Blumenthal, J., Caspersen, C., Chaitman, B., . . . Pollock, M. L. (1996). Statement on exercise: Benefits and recommendations for physical activity programs for all Americans. A statement for health professionals by the Committee on Exercise and Cardiac Rehabilitation of the Council on Clinical Cardiology, American Heart Association. *Circulation, 4*(4), 857–862.

Franklin, B. A., Gibbons, R. J., Grundy, S. M., Hiratzka, L. F., Jones, D. W., Smith, S. C., Jr., . . . World Heart Federation and the Preventive Cardiovascular Nurses Association. (2011). AHA/ACCF secondary prevention and risk reduction therapy for patients with coronary and other atherosclerotic vascular disease: 2011 update: A statement from the American Heart Association and the American College of Cardiology. *Circulation, 124,* 2458–2473.

Gailani, D., & Renne, T. (2007). Intrinsic pathway of coagulation and arterial thrombosis. *Atheriosclerosis, Thrombosis, and Vascular Biology, 27,* 2507–2513.

Gaziano, J. M., & Gaziano, T. (2012). Global burden of cardiovascular disease. In P. Libby, R. O. Bonow, D. L. Mann, & D. P. Zipes, *Braunwald's heart disease.* Philadelphia, PA: Saunders Elsevier, 1–22.

George, C. J., Baim, D. S., Brinker, J. A., Fischman, D. L., Goldberg, S., Holubkov, R., . . . Detre, K. M. (1998). One-year follow-up of the Stent Restenosis (STRESS I) Study. *The American Journal of Cardiology, 81*(7), 860–865.

Gersh, B. J., Maron, B. J., Bonow, R. A., Dearani, J. A., Fifer, M. A., Link, M. S., . . . American College of Cardiology Foundation/American Heart Association Task Force on Practice Guidelines. (2011). 2011 ACCF/AHA guidelines for the diagnosis and treatment of hypertrophic cardiomyopathy. *Journal of the American College of Cardiology, 58,* e212–e260.

Gibbons, R. J., Balady, G. J., Beasley, J. W., Bricker, J. T., Duvernoy, W. F., Froelicher, V. F., . . . Yanowitz, F. G. (1997). ACC/AHA guideline for exercise testing: A report of the American College of Cardiology/American Heart Association Task Force on Practice Guidelines (Committee on Exercise Testing). *Journal of the American College of Cardiology, 30*(1), 260–315.

GlaxoSmithKline. (2013). *Arixtra: Highlights of prescribing information.* Research Triangle Park, NC: GlaxoSmithKline.

Go, A. S., Mozaffarian, D., Roger, V. L., Benjamin, E. J., Berry, J. D., Blaha, M. J., . . . Turner, M. B. (2013). Heart disease and stroke statistics—2014 Update: A report from the American Heart Association. *Circulation, 129,* e28–e292.

Goff, D. C., Lloyd-Jones, D. M., Bennet, G., Coady, S., D'Agostino, R. B., Gibbons, R., . . . Wilson, P. W. F. (2014). 2013 ACC/AHA guideline on the assessment of cardiovascular risk: A report of the American College of Cardiology/American Heart Association Task Force on Practice Guidelines. *Circulation, 129,* S49–S73.

Goff, D. C., Lloyd-Jones, D. M., Bennett, G., Coady, S., D'Agostino, R. B., Gibbons, R., . . . Wilson, P. W. F. (2014). 2013 ACC/AHA guideline on the assessment of cardiovascular risk: A report of the American College of Cardiology/American Heart Association Task Force on Practice Guidelines. *Journal of the American College of Cardiology, 63*(5), 2935–2959. doi:10.1016/j.jacc.2013.11.005

Granger, C. B., Alexander, J. H., McMurray, J. J. V., Lopes, R., Hylek, E. M., Hanna, M., . . . Wallentin, L. (2011). Apixaban versus warfarin in patients with atrial fibrillation. *The New England Journal of Medicine, 365,* 980–992.

Granger, C. B., McMurray, J. J., Yusuf, S., Held, P., Michelson, E. L., Olofsson, B., . . . Swedberg, K. (2003). Effects of candesartan in patients with chronic heart failure and reduced left ventricular systolic function intolerant to angiotensin converting enzyme inhibitors: The CHARM-Alternative trial. *The Lancet, 362,* 772–776.

Greeson, J. M. (2009). Mindfulness research update: 2008. *Complementary Health Practice Review, 14*(1) 10–18.

Greinacher, A., & Warkentin, T. E. (2008). The direct thrombin inhibitor hirudin. *Thrombosis and Haemostasis, 99,* 819–829.

Grossman, P., Niemann, L., Schmidt, S., & Walach, H. (2004). Mindfulness-based stress reduction and health benefits: A meta-analysis. *Journal of Psychosomatic Research, 57,* 35–43.

Gruppo Italiano per lo Studio della Sopravvivenza nell'Infarto Miocardico. (1994). GISSI-3: Effects of lisinopril and transdermal glyceryl trinitrate singly and together on 6 week mortality and ventricular function after acute myocardial infarction. *The Lancet, 343,* 1115–1122.

Gueugniaud, P. Y., David, J. S., Chanzy, E., Hubert, H., Dubien, P. Y., Mauriaucourt, P., . . . Marret, E. (2008). Vasopressin and epinephrine vs. epinephrine along in cardiopulmonary resuscitation. *The New England Journal of Medicine, 359,* 21–30.

Gulliksson, M., Burell, G., Vessby, B., Lundin, L., Toss, H., & Svärdsudd, K. (2011). Randomized controlled trial of cognitive behavioral therapy vs standard treatment to prevent recurrent cardiovascular events in patients with coronary heart disease: Secondary Prevention in Uppsala Primary Health Care project (SUPRIM). *Archives of Internal Medicine, 171*(2), 134–140.

Guo, X., Zhou, B., Nishimura, T., Teramukai, S., & Fukushima, M. (2008). Clinical effect of qigong practice on essential hypertension: A meta-analysis of randomized controlled trials. *Journal of Alternative and Complementary Medicine, 14*(1), 27–37. doi:10.1089/acm.2007.7213

Guyton, J., & Bays, H. (2007). Safety considerations with niacin therapy. *The American Journal of Cardiology, 99,* 22C–31C.

Hafiz, A. M., Jan, M. F., Mori, N., Shaikh, F., Wallach, J., Bajwa, T., & Allaqaband, S. (2012). Prevention of contrast-induced acute kidney injury in patients with stable chronic renal disease undergoing percutaneous coronary and peripheral interventions: Randomized comparison of two prevention strategies. *Catheterization and Cardiovascular Interventions, 79,* 929–937.

Hagins, M., Rundle, Consedine, N. S., & Khalsa, S. B. (2014). A randomized controlled trial comparing the effects of yoga with the active control on ambulatory BP in individuals with pre-hypertension and stage 1 hypertension. *Journal of Clinical Hypertension, 16*(1), 54–62.

Hagins, M., States, R., Selfe, T., & Innes, K. (2013). Effectiveness of yoga for hypertension: Systematic review and meta-analysis. *Evidence Based Complementary and Alternative Medicine,* 1–13. Article no. 649836. doi:10.1155/2013/649836

Hambrecht, R., Adams, V., Erbs, S., Linke, A., Krankel, N., Shu, Y., & Schuler, G. (2003). Regular physical activity improves endothelial function in patients with coronary artery disease by increasing phosphorylation of endothelial nitric oxide synthase. *Circulation, 107*(25), 3152–3158.

Hamilton, M. T., Healy, G. N., Dunstan, D. W., Zderic, T. W., & Owen, N. (2008). Too little exercise and too much sitting: Inactivity physiology and the need for new recommendations on sedentary behavior. *Current Cardiovascular Report, 2*(4), 292–298.

Hammill, B. G., Curtis, L. H., & Whelihan, D. J. (2010). Relationship between cardiac rehabilitation and long-term risks of death and MI among elderly Medicare beneficiaries. *Circulation, 121,* 63–67.

Hanuksela, M. L., & Ellahham, S. (2001). Benefits and risks of sauna. *The American Journal of Medicine, 110*(2), 118–126.

Harper, C., & Jacobson, T. (2001). The fats of life: The role of omega-3 fatty acids in the prevention of coronary heart disease. *Archives of Internal Medicine, 161,* 2185–2192.

Harsha, D. W., & Bray, G. A. (2008). Controversies in hypertension: Weight loss and blood pressure control. *Hypertension, 51,* 1420–1425.

Hartley, L., Flowers, N., Holmes, J., Clarke, A., Stranges, S., Hooper, L., & Rees, K. (2013). Green and black tea for the primary prevention of cardiovascular disease. *Cochrane Database of Systematic Reviews, 6,* CD009934.

Heidenreich, P. A., McDonald, K. M., Hastie, T., Fadel, B. H. V., Lee, B. K., & Hlatky, M. A. (1999). Meta-analysis of trials comparing β-blockers, calcium antagonists, and nitrates for stable angina. *Journal of the American Medical Association, 281,* 1927–1936.

Hill, A. M., Fleming, J. A., & Kris-Etherton, P. M. (2009). The role of diet and nutrition supplements in preventing and treating cardiovascular disease. *Current Opinion in Cardiology, 24*(5), 433–441.

Hirsh, J., Anand, S. S., Halperin, J. L., & Fuster, V. (2001). Mechanism of action and pharmacology of unfractionated heparin. *Arteriosclerosis, Thrombosis, and Vascular Biology, 21,* 1094–1096.

Hirsh, J., Fuster, V., Ansell, J., & Halperin, J. L. (2003). American Heart Association/American College of Cardiology Foundation guide to warfarin therapy. *Circulation, 107,* 1692–1711.

Hochman, D. M., Feinstein, R. E., & Stauter, E. C. (2013). An office-based approach to emotional and behavioral risk factor reduction for cardiovascular disease. *Cardiology in Review, 21*(5), 213–221. doi:10.1097/CRD.0b013e3182918f57

Hochman, J. S., Sleeper, L. A., Webb, J. G., Sanborn, T. A., White, H. D., Talley, J. D., . . . SHOCK Investigators. (1999). Early revascularization in acute myocardial infarction complicated by cardiogenic shock. *The New England Journal of Medicine, 351,* 625–634.

Hohnloser, S., Crijns, H., Van Euckels, M., Gaudin, C., Page, R., Torp-Pedersen, C., & Connolly, S. J. (2009). Effects of dronedarone on cardiovascular events in atrial fibrillation. *The New England Journal of Medicine, 360,* 668–678.

Hooper, L., Thompson, R. L., Harrison, R. A., Summerbell, C. D., Ness, A. R., Moore, H. J., . . . Smith, G. D. (2006). Risks and benefits of omega 3 fats for mortality, cardiovascular disease, and cancer: Systematic review. *The British Medical Journal, 332*(7544), 752–760.

Hsia, J., Heiss, G., Ren, H., Allison, M., Dolan, N. C., Greenland, P., & Trevisan, M. (2007). Calcium/vitamin D supplementation and cardiovascular events. *Circulation, 115,* 846–854.

Hsu, S., Ton, V. K., Dominique Ashen, M., Martin, S. S., Gluckman, T. J., Kohli, P., & Blaha, M. J. (2013). A clinician's guide to the ABCs of cardiovascular disease prevention: The Johns Hopkins Ciccarone Center for the prevention of heart disease and American College of Cardiology Cardiosource Approach to the million hearts initiative. *Clinical Cardiology, 36*(7), 383–393.

Hsue, P. Y., Salinas, C. L., Bolger, A. F., Benowitz, N. L., & Waters, D. D. (2002). Acute aortic dissection related to crack cocaine. *Circulation, 105*(13), 1592–1595.

IMPROVE Investigators. (2007). Venous thromboembolism prophylaxis in acutely ill hospitalized medical patients: Findings from the International Medical Prevention Registry on Venous Thromboembolism. *Chest, 132,* 936–945.

Innes, K. E., & Vincent, H. K. (2007). The influence of yoga-based programs on risk profiles in adults with type 2 diabetes mellitus: A systematic review. *Evidence Based Complementary and Alternative Medicine, 4,* 469–486.

ISIS-4 Collaborative Group. (1995). ISIS-4: A randomized factorial trail assessing early oral captopril, oral mononitrate, and intravenous magnesium sulphate in 58050 patients with suspected acute myocardial infarction. *The Lancet, 345,* 669–685.

Jacobs, I. G., Finn, J. C., Jelinek, G. A., Oxer, H. F., & Thompson, P. L. (2011). Effect of adrenaline on survival in out-of-hospital cardiac arrest: A randomised double-blind placebo-controlled trial. *Resuscitation, 82,* 1138–1143.

Jamerson, K., Weber, M., Bakris, G., Dahlöf, B., Pitt, B., Shi, V., Hester, A., Gupte, J., Gatlin, M., & Velazquez, E. J. (2008). Benazepril plus amlodipine or hydrochlorothiazide for hypertension in high-risk patients. *The New England Journal of Medicine, 359,* 2417–2428.

James, P. A., Oparil, S., Carter, B., Cushman, W., Dennison-Himmelfarb, C., Handler, J., . . . Ortiz, E. (2013). 2014 evidence-based guideline for the management of high blood pressure in adults: Report from the panel members appointed to the Eighth Joint National Committee (JNC 8). *Journal of American Medical Association, 311,* 507–521.

January, C. T., Wann, L. S., Alpert, J. S., Calkins, H., Cigarroa, J. E., Cleveland, J. C., . . . Yancy, C. W. (2014). 2014 AHA/ACC/HRS guideline for the management of patients with atrial fibrillation. *Journal of the American College of Cardiology, 64,* e1–e76.

Jaunch, E. C., Saver, J. L., Adams, H. P., Bruno, A., Connors, J. J., Demaerschalk, B. M., . . . Yonas, H. (2013). Guidelines for the early management of patients with acute ischemic stroke: A guideline for health care professionals from the American Heart Association/American Stroke Association. *Stroke, 44,* 870–947.

Jensen, M. D., Ryan, D. H., Apovian, C. M., Ard, J. D., Comuzzie, A. G., Donato, K. A., . . . Yanovski, S. Z. (2013). 2013 AHA/ACC/TOS guideline for the management of overweight and obesity in adults: A report of the American College of Cardiology/American Heart Association Task Force on Practice Guidelines. Retrieved from http://circ.ahajournals.org/content/early/2013/11/11/01.cir.0000437739.71477

Jentzer, J., DeWald, T., & Hernandez, A. (2010). Combination of loop diuretics with thiazide-type diuretics in heart failure. *Journal of the American College of Cardiology, 56*, 1527–1534.

Jneid, H., Anderson, J. L., Wright, R. S., Adams, C. D., Bridges, C. R., Casey, D. E., . . . Zidar, J. P. (2012). 2012 ACCF/AHA focused update of the guideline for the management of patients with unstable angina/non–ST-elevation myocardial infarction (updating the 2007 guideline and replacing the 2011 focused update): A report of the American College of Cardiology Foundation/American Heart Association Task Force on Practice Guidelines. *Circulation, 126*, 875–910.

Joe, D. (2007). Wikimedia Commons. Retrieved from http://commons.wikimedia.org/wiki/File:Coagulation_full.svg

Johnson, E. S., Lanes, S. F., Wentworth, C. E., Satterfield, M. H., Abebe, B. L., & Dicker, L. W. (1999). A meta-regression analysis of the dose-response effect of aspirin on stroke. *Archives of Internal Medicine, 159*, 1248–1253.

Julius, S., Kjeldsen, S., Weber, M., Brunner, H., Ekman, S., Hansson, L., . . . Zanchetti, A. (2004). Outcomes in hypertensive patients at high cardiovascular risk treated with regimens based on valsartan or amlodipine: The VALUE randomised trial. *The Lancet, 363*, 2022–2031.

Kannel, W. (1995). Range of serum cholesterol values in the population developing coronary artery disease. *The American Journal of Cardiology, 76*, 69C–77C.

Kannel, W. B., Dawber, T. R., Kagan, A., Revotskie, N., & Stokes, J. (1961). Factors of risk in the development of coronary heart disease—Six year follow up experience. *Annals of Internal Medicine, 55*(1), 33–50.

Kaplan, N. M. (2012). Systemic hypertension: Therapy. In P. Libby, R. O. Bonow, D. L. Mann, & D. P. Zipes, *Braunwald's heart disease* (pp. 1049–1068). Philadelphia, PA: Saunders Elsevier.

Katch, V. L., McArdle, W. D., & Katch, F. I. (2011). Energy expenditure during rest and physical activity. In E. Lupash, R. Keifer, C. D. Murphy, & S. Bertling (Eds.), *Essentials of exercise physiology* (4th ed., pp. 237–262). Baltimore, MD: Lippincott Williams & Wilkins.

Katzmarzyk, P. T., & Lee, I. M. (2012). Sedentary behavior and life expectancy in the USA: A cause deleted life table analysis. *BMI Open, 2*, e000828.

Kearon, C., Akl, E. A., Comerota, A. J., Prandoni, P., Bounameux, H., Goldhaber, S. Z., . . . Kahn, S. R. (2012). Antithrombotic therapy for VTE disease: Antithrombotic therapy and prevention of thrombosis, 9th ed: American College of Chest Physicians evidence-based clinical practice guidelines. *Chest, 141*(2), 419S–494S.

Keeley, E. C., Boura, J. A., & Grines, C. L. (2003). Primary angioplasty versus intravenous thrombolytic therapy for acute myocardial infarction: A quantitative review of 23 randomized trials. *The Lancet, 361*, 13–20.

Kernan, W. N., Ovbiagele, B., Black, H. R., Bravata, D. M., Chimowitz, M. I., Ezekowitz, M. D., . . . Wilson, J. A. (2014). Guidelines for the prevention of stroke in patients with stroke and transient ischemic attack. *Stroke, 45*, 2160–2236.

Kihara, T., Biro, S., Imamura, M., Yoshifuku, S., Takasaki, K., Ikeda, Y., & Tei, C. (2002). Repeated sauna treatment improves vascular endothelial and cardiac function in patients with chronic heart failure. *Journal of the American College of Cardiology, 39*, 754–759.

King, D. E., Mainous, A. G., & Geesey, M. E. (2008). Adopting moderate alcohol consumption in middle age: Subsequent cardiovascular events. *The American Journal of Medicine, 121*(3), 201–206.

King, S. B. (1996). Angioplasty from bench to bedside to bench. *Circulation, 93*, 1621–1629.

Kirtane, A. J., Leon, M. B., Ball, M. W., Bajwa, H. S., Sketch, M. H., Coleman, P. S., . . . ENDEAVOR IV Investigators. (2013). The 'final' 5-year follow-up from the ENDEAVOR

IV trial comparing a zotarolimus-eluting stent with a paclitaxel-eluting stent. *JACC Cardiovascular Interventions, 6*(4), 325–333.

Kloner, R. A., Leor, J., Poole, W. K., & Perritt, R. (1997). Population based analysis of the effect of the Northridge earthquake on cardiac death in LA County CA. *Journal of the American College of Cardiology, 30*, 1174–1180.

Kober, L. K., Torp-Pedersen, C., McMurray, J. J., Gotzchhe, O., Levy, S., Crijns, H., Amlie, J., & Carlsen, J. (2008). Increased mortality after dronedarone therapy for severe heart failure. *The New England Journal of Medicine, 358*, 2678–2687.

Konstantinides, S., Heusel, G., Heinrick, F., & Kasper, W. (2002). Heparin plus alteplase compared with heparin alone in patients with submassive pulmonary embolism. *The New England Journal of Medicine, 347*, 1143–1150.

Krauss, R. M. (2012). Nutrition and cardiovascular disease. In P. Libby, R. O. Bonow, D. L. Mann, & D. P. Zipes, *Braunwald's heart disease*. Philadelphia, PA: Saunders Elsevier: 1107–1118.

Kris-Etherton, P. M., Harris, W. S., & Appel, L. J. (2002). Fish consumption, fish oil, omega-3 fatty acids, and cardiovascular disease. *Arteriosclerosis, Thrombosis & Vascular Biology, 23*(2), 20–30.

Kumar, R. S., Douglas, P. S., Peterson, E. D., Anstrom, K. J., Dai, D., . . . Shaw, R. E. (2013). Effect of race and ethnicity on outcomes with drug-eluting and bare metal stents: Results in 423 965 patients in the linked National Cardiovascular Data Registry and Centers for Medicare & Medicaid Services payer databases. *Circulation, 127*(13), 1395–1403.

Kutcher, M. A., Klein, L. W., Ou, F., Wharton, T. P., Dehmer, G. J., Singh, M., . . . National Cardiovascular Data Registry (NCDR). 2009. Percutaneous coronary interventions in facilities without cardiac surgery on site: A report from the National Cardiovascular Data Registry (NCDR). *Journal of the American College of Cardiology, 54*(1), 16–24.

Le Heuzey, J., de Ferrari, G., Radzik, D. S., Zhu, J., & Davy, J. (2010). A short-term, random-ized, double-blind, parallel group study to evaluate the efficacy and safety of drone-darone versus amiodarone in patients with persistent atrial fibrillation: The DIONYSOS study. *Journal of Cardiovascular Electrophysiology, 21*, 597–605.

Leape, L. L., Park, R. E., Bashore, T. M., Harrison, J., Davidson, C. J., & Brook, R. H. (2000). Effect of variability in the interpretation of coronary angiograms on the appropriateness of use of coronary revascularization procedures. *American Heart Journal, 139*(1), 106–113.

Lee, D. C. (2010). Mortality trends in the general population: The importance of cardiorespi-ratory fitness. *Journal of Psychopharmacology, 24*(11), 27–35.

Lee, I. M., Shiroma, E. J., Lobelo, F., Puska, P., Blair, S. N., & Katzmarzyk, P. T. (2012). Effect of physical inactivity on major non-communicable diseases worldwide: An analysis of burden of disease and life expectancy. *The Lancet, 380*, 219–229.

Leijon, M. E., Faskunger, J., Bendtsen, P., Festin, K., & Nilsen, P. (2011). Who is not adhering to physical activity referrals and why? *Scandinavian Journal of Primary Health Care, 29*, 234–240.

Leitzmann, M. F., Park, Y., Blair, A., Ballard-Barbash, R., Mouw, T., Hollenbeck, A. R., & Schatzkin, A. (2007). Physical activity recommendations and decreased mortality risk. *Archives of Internal Medicine, 167*(22), 2453–2460.

Leizorovicz, A., Cohen, A., Turpie, A., Olsson, C.-G., Vaikus, P., & Goldhaber, S. (2004). Ran-domized, placebo-controlled trial of dalteparin for the prevention of venous thrombo-embolism in acutely ill medical patients. *Circulation, 110*, 874–879.

Lenk, K., Uhlemann, M., Schuler, G., & Adams, V. (2011). Role of endothelial progenitor cells in the beneficial effects of physical exercise on atherosclerosis and coronary artery dis-ease. *Journal of Applied Physiology, 111*, 321–328.

Leon, M. B., Baim, D. S., Popma, J. J., Gordon, P. C., Cutlip, D. E., Ho, K. K., . . . Stent Anti-coagulation Restenosis Study Investigators. (1998). A clinical trial comparing three antithrombotic-drug regimens after coronary artery stenting. Stent Anticoagulation Restenosis Study Investigators. *The New England Journal of Medicine, 339*, 1665–1671.

Levine, G. N., Bates, E. R., Blankenship, J. C., Bailey, S. R., Bittl, J. A., Cercek, B., . . . Ting, H. H. (2011). 2011 ACCF/AHA/SCAI guideline for percutaneous coronary intervention: A report of the American College of Cardiology Foundation/American Heart Association Task Force on Practice Guidelines and the Society for Cardiovascular Angiography and Interventions. *Journal of the American College of Cardiology, 58*(24), e44–e122.

Levine, G. N., Steinke, E. E., Bakaeen, F. G., Bozkurt, B., Cheitlin, M. D., Conti, J. B., . . . Stewart, W. J. (2012). Sexual activity and cardiovascular disease: A scientific statement from the American Heart Association. *Circulation, 125*(8), 1058.

Li, J. X., Hong, Y., & Chan, K. M. (2001). Tai Chi: Physiologic characteristics and beneficial effects on health. *The British Journal of Sports Medicine, 35*(3), 148–156.

Libby, P., Bonow, R. O., Mann, D. L., & Zipes, D. P. (2012). *Braunwald's heart disease*. Philadelphia, PA: Saunders Elsevier.

Lim, S. S., Vos, T., Flaxman, A. D., Danaei, G., Shibuya, K., Adair-Rohani, H., & Ezzati, M. (2012). A comparative risk assessment of burden of disease and injury attributable to 67 risk factors and risk factor clusters in 21 regions, 1990–2010: A systematic analysis for the Global Burden of Disease Study 2010. *The Lancet, 380* (9859), 2224–2260.

Lin, G., Xiang, Q., Fu, X., Wang, S., Wang, S., Chen, S., & Wang, T. (2012). Heart rate variability biofeedback decreases blood pressure in prehypertensive subjects by improving autonomic function and baroreflex. *Journal of Alternative and Complementary Medicine, 18*(2), 143.

Linkins, L., Dans, A., Moores, L., Bona, R., Davidson, B., Schulman, S., & Crowther, M. (2012). Treatment and prevention of heparin-induced thrombocytopenia: Antithrombotic therapy and prevention of thrombosis, 9th ed: American College of Chest Physicians evidence-based clinical practice guidelines. *Chest, 141*, e495S–530S.

Lloyd-Jones, D. M., Hong, Y., Labarthe, D., Mozaffarian, D., Appel, L. J., & Van Horn, L. (2010). Defining and setting national goals for cardiovascular health promotion and disease reduction: The American Heart Association's strategic impact goal through 2020 and beyond. *Circulation, 121*(4), 586–613. doi:10.1161/circulationAHA.109.192703

Lopez-Garcia, E., van Dam, R. M., Li, T. Y., Rodriguez-Artalejo, F., & Hu, F. B. (2008). The relationship of coffee consumption with mortality. *Annals of Internal Medicine, 148*(12), 904–914.

Macaya, C., Serruys, P. W., Ruygrok, P., Suryapranata, H., Mast, G., Klugmann, S., . . . Morel, M. (1996). Continued benefit of coronary stenting versus balloon angioplasty: One year clinical follow-up of Benestent trial. *Journal of the American College of Cardiology, 27*(2), 255–261.

Mackman, N., Tilley, R. E., & Key, N. S. (2007). Extrinsic pathway of blood coagulation in hemostasis and thrombosis. *Atheriosclerosis, Thrombosis, and Vascular Biology, 27,* 1687–1693.

Makkar, R. R., Fontana, G. P., Jilaihawi, H., Kapadia, S., Pichard, A. D., Douglas, P. S., . . . PARTNER Trial Investigators. (2012). Transcatheter aortic-valve replacement for inoperable severe aortic stenosis. *The New England Journal of Medicine, 366*(18), 1696–1704.

Marik, P., & Varon, J. (2007). Hypertensive crisis: Challenges and management. *Chest, 131,* 1949–1962.

Marti-Carvajal, A. J., Sola, I., Lathyris, D., Karakitsiou, D. E., & Simancas-Racines, D. (2013). Homocysteine-lowering interventions for preventing cardiovascular events. *Cochrane Database of Systematic Reviews, 1,* CD006612.

McMurray, J., Ostergren, J., Swedberg, K., Granger, C., El, M., Olofsson, B., Yusuf, S., & Pfeffer, M. A. (2003). Effects of candesartan in patients with chronic heart failure and reduced left-ventricular systolic function taking angiotensin-converting-enzyme inhibitors: The CHARM-Added trial. *The Lancet, 362,* 767–771.

McNamara, R. L., Wang, Y., Herrin, J., Curtis, J. P., Bradley, E. H., Magid, D. J., . . . Krumholz, H. M. (2006). Effect of door-to-balloon time on mortality in patients with ST-segment elevation myocardial infarction. *Journal of the American College of Cardiology, 47*(11), 2180–2186.

MDPIT Research Group. (1988). The effect of diltiazem on mortality and reinfarction after myocardial infarction (MDPIT). *The New England Journal of Medicine, 219*, 385–392.

Mehran, R., Aymong, E. D., Nikolsky, E., Lasic, Z., Iakovou, I., Fahy, M., . . . Dangas, G. (2004). A simple risk score for prediction of contrast-induced nephropathy after percutaneous coronary intervention: Development and initial validation. *Journal of the American College of Cardiology, 44*, 1393–1399.

Menotti, A., Lanti, M., Nedeljkovic, S., Nissinen, A., Kafatos, A., & Kromhout, D. (2006). The relationship of age, blood pressure, serum cholesterol and smoking habits with the risk of typical and atypical coronary disease death in the European cohorts of the Seven Countries Study. *International Journal of Cardiology, 106*, 157–163.

Merck & Co., Inc. (2014a). *Zontivity: Highlights of prescribing information.* Whitehouse Station, NJ: Merck & Co.

Merck & Co., Inc. (2014b). *Integrilin: Highlights of prescribing information.* Whitehouse Station, NJ: Merck & Co.

MERIT-HF. (1999). Effect of metoprolol CR/XL in chronic heart failure: Metoprolol CR/XL randomised intervention trial in congestive heart failure (MERIT-HF). *The Lancet, 353*, 2001–2007.

Meschia, J. F., Bushnell, C., Boden-Albala, B., Braun, L. T., Bravata, D. M., Chaturvedi, S., . . . Wilson, J. A. (2014). Guidelines for the primary prevention of stroke. *Stroke, 45*, 3754–3832.

MIAMI Trial Research Group. (1985). Metoprolol in acute myocardial infarction (MIAMI). A randomized placebo controlled international trial. *European Heart Journal, 6*, 199–226.

Montalescot, G., Bolognese, L., Dudek, D., Goldstein, P., Hamm, C., Tanguay, J. F., . . . Widimsky, P. (2013). Pretreatment with prasugrel in non-ST-segment elevation acute coronary syndromes. *The New England Journal of Medicine, 369*, 999–1010.

Morice, M., Serruys, P. W., Sousa, J. E., Fajadet, J., Hayashi, E. B., Perin, M., . . . RAVEL Study Group. (2002). A randomized comparison of a sirolimus-eluting stent with a standard stent for coronary revascularization. *The New England Journal of Medicine, 346*, 1773–1780.

Morise, A. P., Haddad, W. J., & Beckner, D. (1997). Development and validation of a clinical score to estimate the probability of coronary artery disease in men and women presenting with suspected coronary artery disease. *The American Journal of Medicine, 102*(4), 350–356.

Morris, J. N., Heady, J. A., Raffle, P. A. B., Roberts, C. G., & Parks, J. W. (1953). Coronary heart disease and physical activity of work. *The Lancet, 265*, 1111–1120.

Morrow, D. A., Braunwald, E., Bonaca, M. P., Ameriso, S. F., Dalby, A. J., Fish, M. P., . . . Murphy, S. A. (2012). Vorapaxar in the secondary prevention of atherothrombotic events (TRA 2P-TIMI 50). *The New England Journal of Medicine, 366*, 1404–1413.

Moscucci, M. (2013). *Grossman & Baim's cardiac catheterization, angiography and intervention.* Baltimore: Williams & Wilkins.

Mostofsky, E., Rice, M. S., Levitan, E. B., & Mittleman, M. A. (2012). Habitual coffee consumption and risk of heart failure: A dose-response meta-analysis. *Circulation: Heart Failure, 5*(4), 401–405.

Mukamal, K. J., Tolstrup, J. S., Friberg, J., Jensen, G., & Gronbaek, M. (2005). Alcohol consumption and risk of atrial fibrillation in men and women: The Copenhagen City Heart Study. *Circulation, 112*(12), 1736–1742.

Murdoch, D. R., Corey, G. R., Hoen, B., Miro, J. M., Fowler, V. G., Bayer, A. S., . . . Cabell, C. H. (2009). Clinical presentation, etiology, and outcome of infective endocarditis in the 21st century: The international collaboration on endocarditis–prospective cohort study. *Archives of Internal Medicine, 169*(5), 463–473.

Myung, S. K., Wu, J., Cho, B., Oh, S. W., Park, S. M., Koo, B. K., & Park, B. J. (2013). Efficacy of vitamin and antioxidant supplements in prevention of cardiovascular disease: Systematic review and meta-analysis of randomised controlled trials. *The British Medical Journal, 346*, f10. doi:10.1136/bmj.f10

Naidu, S. S., Rao, S. V., Blankenship, J., Cavendish, J. J., Farhah, T., Moussa, I., . . . Yakubov, S. J. (2012). Clinical expert consensus statement on best practices in the cardiac catheterization laboratory. *Catheterization and Cardiovascular Interventions, 80*(3), 456–464.

Neter, J. E., Stam, B. E., Kok, F. J., Grobbee, D. E., & Geleijnse, J. M. (2003). Influence of weight reduction on blood pressure: A meta-analysis of randomized controlled trials. *Hypertension, 42*, 878–884.

Neumar, R. W., Otto, C. W., Link, M. S., Kronick, S. L., Shuster, M., Callaway, C., . . . Morrison, L. J. (2010). Adult advanced cardiovascular life support: 2010 American Heart Association guidelines for cardiopulmonary resuscitation and emergency cardiovascular care. *Circulation, 122*, S729–S767.

Nicholls, S., Ballantyne, C. M., Barter, P. J., Chapman, J., Erbel, R. M., Libby, P., . . . Nissen, S. E. (2011). Effect of two intensive statin regimens. *The New England Journal of Medicine, 365*, 2078–2087.

Nishimura, R. N., Otto, C. M., Bonow, R. A., Carabello, B. A., Erwin, J. P., III, Guyton, R. A., . . . ACC/AHA Task Force Members. (2014). 2014 ACC/AHA guideline for the management of patients with valvular heart disease: A report from the ACC/AHA Task Force on Practice Guidelines. *Circulation, 129*(23), e651.

Nishioka, T., Amanullah, A. M., Luo, H., Berglund, H., Kim, C., Nagai, T., . . . Siegel, R. J. (1999). Clinical validation of intravascular ultrasound imaging for assessment of coronary stenosis severity: Comparison with stress myocardial perfusion imaging. *Journal of the American College of Cardiology, 33*(7), 1870–1878.

O'Gara, P. T., Kushner, F. G., Ascheim, D. D., Casey, D. E., Chung, M. K., de Lemos, J. A., . . . Zhao, D. X. (2013a). 2013 ACCF/AHA guideline for the management of ST-elevation myocardial infarction: executive report: A report of the American College of Cardiology Foundation/American Heart Association Task Force on Practice Guidelines. *Circulation, 127*, 529–555.

O'Gara, P. T., Kushner, F. G., Ascheim, D. D., Casey, D. E., Chung, M. K., de Lemos, J. A., . . . Zhao, D. X. (2013b). 2013 ACCF/AHA guideline for the management of ST-elevation myocardial infarction: A report of the American College of Cardiology Foundation/American Heart Association Task Force on Practice Guidelines. *Circulation, 127*, e362–e425.

O'Gara, P. T., Kushner, F. G., Ascheim, D. D., Casey, D. E., Chung, M. K., deLemos, J. A., . . . Zhao, D. X. (2013c). 2013 ACCF/AHA guideline for the management of ST-elevation myocardial infarction: A report of the American College of Cardiology Foundation/American Heart Association Task Force on Practice Guidelines. *Journal of the American College of Cardiology, 61*, e78–e140.

OASIS-5 Investigators. (2006). Comparison of fondaparinux and enoxaparin in acute coronary syndromes. *The New England Journal of Medicine, 354*, 1464–1476.

Oh, B., Mitchell, J., Herron, J., Chung, J., Khan, M., & Keefe, D. (2007). Aliskiren, an oral renin inhibitor, provides dose-dependent efficacy and sustained 24-hour blood pressure control in patients with hypertension. *Journal of American College of Cardiology, 49*, 1157–1163.

Okuyemi, K. S., Nollen, N. L., & Ahluwalia, J. S. (2006). Interventions to facilitate smoking cessation. *American Family Physician, 74*(2), 262–271.

Packer, M., Bristow, R., Cohn, J., Colucci, W., Fowler, M., Gilbert, E., & Shusterman, N. H. (1996). The effect of carvedilol or morbidity and mortality in patients with chronic heart failure. US Carvedilol Heart Failure Study Group. *The New England Journal of Medicine, 334*, 1349–1355.

Packer, M., Fowler, M., Eb, R., Coats, A., Katus, H., Krum, H., Mohacsi, P., . . . DeMets, D. L. (2002). Effect of carvedilol on the morbidity of patients with severe chronic heart failure: Results of the carvedilol prospective randomized cumulative survival (COPERNICUS) study. *Circulation, 106*, 2194–2199.

Palmore, E. B. (1982). Predictors of longevity difference: 25 years follow-up. *Gerontologist, 22*(6), 513–518.

Parswani, M. J., Sharma, M. P., & Iyengar, S. S. (2013). Mindfulness-based stress reduction program in coronary heart disease: A randomized controlled trial. *International Journal of Yoga, 6*(2), 111–117.

Patel, M. R., Bailey, S. R., Bonow, R. O., Chambers, C. E., Chan, P. S., Dehmer, G. J., . . . Ward, R. P. (2012). ACCF/SCAI/AATS/AHA/ASE/ASNC/HFSA/HRS/SCCM/SCCT/SCMR/STS 2012 appropriate use criteria for diagnostic catheterization: A report of the American College of Cardiology Foundation Appropriate Use Criteria Task Force. *Journal of the American College of Cardiology, 59*, 1–33.

Patel, M. R., Mahaffey, K. W., Garg, J., Pan, G., Singer, D. E., Hacke, W., . . . Califf, R. M. (2011). Rivaroxaban versus warfarin in nonvalvular atrial fibrillation. *The New England Journal of Medicine, 365*, 883–891.

Patel, T., Shah, S., & Pancholy, S. (2013). Balloon-assisted tracking of a guide catheter through difficult radial anatomy: A technical report. *Catheterization and Cardiovascular Interventions, 81*(5), E215–E218.

Pearson, T. A., Palaniappan, L. P., Artinian, N. T., Carnethon, M. R., Criqui, M. H., . . . Sasson, C. (2013). American Heart Association Guide for improving cardiovascular health at the community level, 2013 update. *Circulation 127*(16), 1730–1753.

Pescatello, L. S. (2004). American College of Sports Medicine Position Stand. *Exercise and Hypertension, 36*(3), 533–553.

Peterson, E. D., Dai, D., DeLong, E. R., Brennan, J. M., Singh, M., Rao, S., . . . NCDR Registry Participants. (2010). Contemporary mortality risk prediction for percutaneous coronary intervention: Results from 588,398 procedures in the National Cardiovascular Data Registry. *Journal of the American College of Cardiology, 55*(18), 1923–1932.

Peto, R., Emberson, J., Landray, M., Baigent, C., Collins, R., Clare, R., & Califf, R. (2008). Analyses of cancer data from three ezetimibe trials. *The New England Journal of Medicine, 359*, 1357–1366.

Pfeffer, M., Swedberg, K. G. C., Held, P., McMurry, J., Michelson, E., Olofsson, B., . . . Pocock, S. (2003). Effects of candesartan on mortality and morbidity in patients with chronic heart failure: The CHARM-Overall programme. *The Lancet, 362*, 759–766.

Pfisterer, M., Brunner-La Rocca, H. P., Buser, P. T., Rickenbacher, P., Hunziker, P., Mueller, C., . . . Kaiser, C. (2006). Late clinical events after clopidogrel discontinuation may limit the benefit of drug-eluting stents: An observational study of drug-eluting versus bare-metal stents. *Journal of the American College of Cardiology, 48*(12), 2584–2591.

Pijls, N. H., De Bruyne, B., Peels, K., van der Voort, P. H., Bonnier, H. J., Bartunek, J., & Koolen, J. J. (1996). Measurement of fractional flow reserve to assess the functional severity of coronary stenoses. *The New England Journal of Medicine, 334*, 1703–1708.

Pijls, N. H., van Schaardenburgh, P., Manoharan, G., Boersma, E., Bech, J., van't Veer, M., . . . de Bruyne, B. (2007). Percutaneous coronary intervention of functionally nonsignificant stenoses: 5-year follow-up of the DEFER study. *Journal of the American College of Cardiology, 49*(21), 2105–2111.

Pitt, B., Remme, W., Zannad, F., Martinez, F., Roniker, B., Bittman, R., . . . Gatlin, M. (2003). Eplerenone, a selective aldosterone blocker, in patients with left ventricular dysfunction after myocardial infarction. *The New England Journal of Medicine, 348*, 1309–1321.

Pitt, B., Zannad, F., Remme, W., Cody, R., Castaigne, A., Perez, A., Palensky, J., & Wittes, J. (1999). The effect of spironolactone on morbidity and mortality in patients with severe heart failure. Randomized aldactone evaluation study investigators. *The New England Journal of Medicine, 341*, 709–717.

Pories, W. J. (2008). Bariatric surgery: Risks and rewards. *Journal of Clinical Endocrinology and Metabolism, 93*(11), S89–S96.

Prochaska, J. O., & Norcross, J. C. (2001). Stages of change. *Psychotherapy: Theory, Research, Practice, Training, 38*(4), 443–448. doi:10.1037/0033-3204.38.4.443

PROGRESS. (2001). Randomised trial of a perindopril-based blood-pressure-lowering. *The Lancet, 66*, 1033–1041.

Qaseem, A., Fihn, S., Dallas, P., Williams, S., Owens, D. K., & Shekelle, P. (2012). Management of stable ischemic heart disease: Summary of a clinical practice guideline from the American College of Physicians/American College of Cardiology Foundation/American Heart Association/American Association for Thoracic Surgery/Preventive Cardiovascular Nurses Association/Society of Thoracic Surgeons. *Annals of Internal Medicine, 157,* 735–743.

Rad, A. (2006). Renin-angiotensin-aldosterone system. From Wikimedia Commons, the free media repository. Retrieved from commons.wikimedia.org

Ramos, A. P., & Varon, J. (2014). Current and newer agents for hypertensive emergencies. *Current Hypertension Report, 16,* 450.

RE-COVER Study Group. (2009). Dabigatran versus warfarin in the treatment of acute venous thromboembolism. *The New England Journal of Medicine, 361,* 2342–2352.

Rees, K., Dyakova, M., Ward, K., Thorogood, M., & Brunner, E. (2013). Dietary advice for reducing cardiovascular risk. *Cochrane Database of Systematic Reviews, 6,* CD009874.

Rees, K., Hartley, L., Day, C., Flowers, N., Clarke, A., & Stranges, S. (2013). Selenium supplementation for the primary prevention of cardiovascular disease. *Cochrane Database of Systematic Reviews,* CD009671. doi:10.1002/14651858.CD009671.pub2

Rees, K., Hartley, L., Flowers, N., Clarke, A., Hooper, L., Thorogood, M., & Stranges, S. (2013). "Mediterranean" dietary pattern for the primary prevention of cardiovascular disease. *Cochrane Database of Systemic Reviews, 8,* CD009825. doi:10.1002/14651858.CD009825.pub2

Rhoney, D., & Peacock, W. (2009a). Intravenous therapy for hypertensive emergencies, part 1. *The American Journal of Health-System Pharmacists, 66,* 1343–1352.

Rhoney, D., & Peacock, W. (2009b). Intravenous therapy for hypertensive emergencies, part 2. *The American Journal of Health-System Pharmacists, 66,* 1448–1457.

Ridker, P. M., & Libby, P. (2008). Risk factors for atherothrombotic disease. In P. Libby, R. O. Bonow, D. L. Mann, & D. P. Zipes (Eds.), *Braunwald's heart disease* (pp. 1003–1026). Philadelphia, PA: Saunders Elsevier.

Ries, A. L., Bauldoff, G. S., Carlin, B. W., Casaburi, R., Emery, C. F., Mahler, D. A., & Herrerias, C. (2007). Pulmonary rehabilitation guidelines panel. Pulmonary rehabilitation: Joint ACCP/AACVPR evidence-based guidelines. *Chest, 131*(Supp 5), 4S–42S.

Riley, R. F., Don, C. W., Powell, W., Maynard, C., & Dean, L. S. (2011). Trends in coronary revascularization in the United States from 2001 to 2009: Recent declines in percuatneous coronary intervention volumes. *Circulation: Cardiovascular Quality and Outcomes, 4,* 193–197.

Roca-Rodriguez, M. M., Garcia-Almeida, J. M., Ruiz-Nava, J., Alcaide-Torres, J., Saracho-Dominquez, H., Rioja-Vazquez, R., . . . (2014). Impact of outpatient cardiac rehabilitation program on clinical and analytical variables in cardiovascular disease. *Journal of Cardiopulmonary Rehabilitation and Prevention, 34*(1), 43–48. doi:10.1097/HCR.00000000 00000026

Rodriguez, M. A., Kumar, S. K., & DeCaro, M. (2010). Hypertensive crisis. *Cardiology in Review, 18*(2), 102–107.

Roe, M. T., Armstrong, P. W., Fox, K. A., White, H. D., Prabhakaran, D., Goodman, S. G., . . . Ohman, E. M. (2012). Prasugrel versus clopidogrel for acute coronary syndromes without revascularization. *The New England Journal of Medicine, 367,* 1297–1309.

Ros, E., & Hu, F. B. (2013). Consumption of plant seeds and cardiovascular health: Epidemiological and clinical trial evidence. *Circulation, 128*(5), 553–565.

Rosendorff, C., Black, H., Cannon, C., Gersh, B., Gore, J., Izzo, J., . . . Oparil, S. (2007). Treatment of hypertension in the prevention and management of ischemic heart disease. *Circulation, 115,* 2761–2788.

Rossebo, A. B., Pedersen, T. R., Boman, K., Brudi, P., Chambers, J. B., Egstrup, K., . . . Willenheimer, R. (2008). Intensive lipid lowering with simvastatin and ezetimibe in aortic stenosis. *The New England Journal of Medicine, 359,* 1343–1356.

Russell, J. A., Walley, K. R., Singer, J., Gordon, A. C., Hébert, P. C., Cooper, D. J., . . . Ayers, D. (2008). Vasopressin versus norepinephrine infusion in patients with septic shock. *The New England Journal of Medicine, 358,* 877–887.

Ryan, D. H., & Bray, G. A. (2013). Pharmacologic treatments for weight loss: What is old is new again. *Current Hypertension Reports, 15*(3), 182–189.

Sacco, R, L., Diener, H. C., Yusuf, S., Cotton, D., Ounpuu, S., Lawton, W. A., . . . Yoon, B. W. (2008). Aspirin and extended-release dipyridamole versus clopidogrel for recurrent stroke. *The New England Journal of Medicine, 359,* 1238–1251.

Samama, M., Darmon, J., Desjardins, L., Eldor, A., Janbon, C., Leizorovicz, A., . . . Weisslinger, N. (1999). A comparison of enoxaparin with placebo for the prevention of venous thromboembolism in acutely ill medical patients. *The New England Journal of Medicine, 341,* 793–800.

Samieri, C., Feart, C., Proust-Lima, C., Peuchant, E., Tzourio, C., Stapf, C., & Barberger-Gateau, P. (2011). Olive oil consumption, plasma oleic acid, and stroke incidence: The Three-City Study. *Neurology, 77*(5), 418–425.

Schwartz, G. G., Olsson, A. G., Ezekowitz, M. D., Ganz, P., Oliver, M. F., Waters, D., . . . Stern, T. (2001). Effects of atorvastatin on early recurrent ischemic events in acute coronary syndromes. *Journal of the American Medical Association, 285,* 1711–1718.

Selye, H. (1956). *The stress of life.* New York, NY: McGraw-Hill.

Serruys, P. W., Morice, M., Kappetein, A. P., Colombo, A., Holmes, D. R., Mack, M. J., . . . SYNTAX Investigators. (2009). Percutaneous coronary intervention versus coronary-artery bypass grafting for severe coronary artery disease. *The New England Journal of Medicine, 360,* 961–972.

Sjostrom, C. D., Peltonen, M., Wedel, H., & Sjostrom, L. (2000). Differentiated long-term effects of intentional weight loss on diabetes and hypertension. *Hypertension, 36*(1), 20–25.

Smith, S. C., Benjamin, E. J., Bonow, R. O., Braun, L. T., Creager, M. A., Franklin, B. A., . . . Taubert, K. A. (2011). AHA/ACCF secondary prevention and risk reduction therapy for patients with coronary and other atherosclerotic vascular disease: 2011 Update: A statement from the American Heart Association and the American College of Cardiology. *Circulation, 124,* 2458–2473.

Stead, L. F., Buitrago, D, Preciado, N., Sanchez, G., Hartmann-Boyce, J., & Lancaster, T. (2013). Physician advice for smoking cessation. *Cochrune Database of Systematic Reviews, 5,* CD000165. doi:10.1002/14651858.CD000165.pub4

Steinke, E. E., Jaarsma, T., Barnason, S. A., Byrne, M., Doherty, S., Dougherty, C. M., & Moser, D. K. (2013). Sexual counseling for individuals with cardiovascular disease and their partners: A consensus document from the American Heart Association and the ESC council on cardiovascular nursing and allied professions. *Circulation, 128*(18), 2075–2096.

Steptoe, A., & Kivimaki, M. (2012). Stress and cardiovascular disease. *Nature Reviews Cardiology, 9,* 360–370.

Stone, N., Robinson, J., Lichtenstein, A. H., Bairey, M. C. N., Blum, C. B., Eckel, R. H., . . . Wilson, P. W. (2013). 2013 ACC/AHA guideline of the treatment of blood cholesterol to reduce atherosclerotic cardiovascular risk in adults: A report of the American College of Cardiology/American Heart Association Task Force of Practice Guidelines. *Circulation, 129,* S1–S45.

Strath, S. J., Kaminsky, L. A., Ainsworth, B. E., Ekelund, U., Freedson, P. S., Gary, R. A., & Swartz, A. M. (2013). Guide to the assessment of physical activity: Clinical and research applications: A scientific statement from the American Heart Association. *Circulation, 128*(20), 2259–2279. doi:10.1161/01.cir.0000435708.67487.da

Suaya, J. A., Shepard, D. S., Normand, S. T., Prottas, P. A., & Stason, W. B. (2007). Use of cardiac rehab by Medicare beneficiaries after MI or CABG surgery. *Circulation, 116,* 1653–1662.

Tanaka, H., Dinenno, F. A., Monahan, K. D., Clevenger, C. M., DeSouza, C. A., & Seals, D. R. (2000). Aging, habitual exercise, and dynamic arterial compliance. *Circulation, 102,* 1270–1275.

Taylor, A., Ziesche, S., Yancy, C., Carson, P., D'Agostino, R., Ferdinand, K., . . . Cohn, J. N. (2004). Combination of isosorbide dinitrate and hydralazine in Blacks with heart failure. *The New England Journal of Medicine, 351,* 2049–2057.

Taylor, R. S., Ashton, K. E., Moxham, T., Hooper, L., & Ebrahim, S. (2011). Reduced dietary salt for the prevention of cardiovascular disease. *The American Journal of Hypertension, 24*(8), 843–853.

Thompson, I. M., Tangen, C. M., Goodman, P. J., Probstfield, J. L., Moinpour, C. M., & Coltman, C. A. (2005). Erectile dysfunction and subsequent cardiovascular disease. *Journal of the American Medical Association, 294*(23), 2996–3002.

Thornley, S., Tayler, R., & Sikaris, K. (2012). Sugar restriction: The evidence for a drug-free intervention to reduce cardiovascular disease risk. *Internal Medicine Journal, 42,* 46–58. doi:10.1111/j.1445-5994.2012.02902

Toise, S., Sears, S. F., Schoenfeld, M. H., Blitzer, M. L., Marieb, M. A., Drury, J. H., & Donohue, T. J. (2014). Psychosocial and cardiac outcome of yoga for ICD patients: A randomized clinical control trial. *Pacing and Clinical Electrophysiology, 37,* 48–62.

Tonino, P. A., De Bruyne, B., Pijls, N. H., Siebert, U., Ikeno, F., van't Veer, M., . . . FAME Study Investigators. (2009). Fractional flow reserve versus angiography for guiding percutaneous coronary intervention. *The New England Journal of Medicine, 360,* 213–224.

Tricoci, P., Huang, Z., Held, C., Moliterno, D. J., Armstrong, P. W., Van de Werf, F., . . . Mahaffey, K. W. (2012). Thrombin-receptor antagonist vorapaxar in acute coronary syndromes (TRACER). *The New England Journal of Medicine, 366,* 20–33.

Turpie, A., Chin, B., & Lip, G. (2002). Venous thromboembolism: Pathophysiology, clinical features, and prevention. *The British Medical Journal, 325,* 887–890.

University of Utah Health Care, Thrombosis Service. (2007). *My warfarin therapy—a patient's guide.* Salt Lake City, Utah. Retrieved from http://healthcare.utah.edu/thrombosis/images/tablet_chart.jpg

Valgimigli, M., Campo, G., Penzo, C., Tebaldi, M., Biscaglia, S., & Ferrari, R. (2014). Transradial coronary catheterization and intervention across the whole spectrum of Allen test results. *Journal of the American College of Cardiology, 63*(18), 1833–1841.

Van Sluijs, E. M., van Poppel, M. N. M., & van Mechelen, W. (2004). Stage-based lifestyle interventions in primary care: Are they effective? *American Journal of Preventive Medicine, 26*(4), 330–343.

Vescovi, P. P., Casti, A., Michelini, M., Maninetti, L., Pedrazzoni, M., & Passeri, M. (1992). Plasma ACTH, beta-endorphin, prolactin, growth hormone and luteinizing hormone levels after thermal stress, heat and cold. *Stress Medicine, 8,* 187–191.

Vincent-Baudry, S., Defoort, C., Gerber, M., Bernard, M. C., Verger, P., Helal, O., Portugal, H., & Lairon, D. (2005). The Medi-RIVAGE study: Reduction of cardiovascular disease risk factors after a 3-mo intervention with a Mediterranean-type diet or a low-fat diet. *The American Journal of Clinical Nutrition, 82,* 964–971.

Wallace, R. K., Benson, H., & Wilson, A. F. (1971). A wakeful hypometabolic physiologic state. *The American Journal of Physiology, 221,* 795–799.

Wallentin, L., Becker, R. C., Budaj, A., Cannon, C. P., Emanuelsson, H., Held, C., . . . Harrington, R. A. (2009). Ticagrelor versus clopidogrel in patients with acute coronary syndromes. *The New England Journal of Medicine, 361,* 1045–1057.

Wang, C. W., Chan, C. H., Ho, R. T., Chan, J. S., Ng, S. M., & Chan, C. L. (2014). Managing stress and anxiety through qigong exercise in healthy adults: A systematic review and meta-analysis of randomized controlled trials. *BMC Complementary and Alternative Medicine, 14,* 8.

Wang, Y., Wang, Y., Zhao, X., Liu, L., Wang, D., Wang, C., . . . Johnston, S. C. (2013). Clopidogrel with aspirin in acute minor stroke or transient ischemic attack. *The New England Journal of Medicine, 369,* 11–19.

Warburton, D. E., McKenzie, D. C., Haykowsky, M. J., Taylor, A., Shoemaker, P., Ignaszewski, A. P., & Chan, S. Y. (2005). Effectiveness of high-intensity interval training for the rehabilitation of patients with coronary artery disease. *The American Journal of Cardiology, 95,* 1090.

Wark, D. M. (2008). What we can do with hypnosis: A brief note. *The American Journal of Clinical Hypnosis, 51,* 1.

Warkentin, T., Greinacher, A., Koster, A., & Lincoff, A. (2008). Treatment and prevention of heparin-induced thrombocytopenia: American College of Chest Physicians Evidenced-Based Clinical Practice Guidelines (8th ed.). *Chest, 133*, 340S–380S.

Warner, M. M. (2012). Cardiac rehab past present and future: An overview. *Cardiovascular Diagnosis and Therapy, 2,* 1.

Weber, M., Schriffin, E., White, W., Mann, S., Lindholm, L., Kenerson, J., . . . Harrap, S. B. (2013). Clinical practice guidelines for the management of hypertension in the community: A statement by the American Society of Hypertension and the International Society of Hypertension. *Journal of Clinical Hypertension, 16,* 1–13.

Wenzel, V., Krismer, A. C., Arntz, R., Sitter, H., Stadlbauer, K. H., Lindner, K. H., & European Resuscitation Council Vasopressor During Cardiopulmonary Resuscitation Study. (2004). A comparison of vasopressin and epinephrine for out-of-hospital cardiopulmonary resuscitation. *The New England Journal of Medicine, 350,* 105–113.

Willenheimer, R. (2008). Intensive lipid lowering with simavastatin and ezetimibe in aortic stenosis. *The New England Journal of Medicine, 359,* 1343–1356.

Williams, D. M., Fraser, A., & Lawlor, D. A. (2011). Associations of vitamin D, parathyroid hormone and calcium with cardiovascular risk factors in US adolescents. *Heart (British Cardiac Society), 97,* 315–320.

Wing, R., Bolin, P., Brancati, F. L., Bray, G. A., Clark, J. M., Coday, M., . . . Yanovski, S. Z. (2013). Cardiovascular effects of intensive lifestyle intervention in type 2 diabetes. *The New England Journal of Medicine, 369,* 145–154. doi:10.1056/NEJMoa1212914

Wiviott, S. D., Braunwald, E., McCabe, C. H., Montalescot, G., Ruzyllo, W., Gottlieb, S., . . . Antman, F. M. (2007). Prasugrel versus clopidogrel in patients with acute coronary syndromes. *The New England Journal of Medicine, 357,* 2001–2015.

World Health Organization. (2013). WHO report on the global tobacco epidemic, 2011: Warning about the dangers of tobacco. Retrieved from http://www.who.int/tobacco/global_report/2013/en/

World Health Organization. (2014). Draft guideline: Sugars intake for adults and children. Retrieved from http://www.who.int/nutrition/sugars_public_consultation/en

Yancy, C. W. (2012). Heart disease in varied populations. In Libby, P., Bonow, R. O., Mann, D. L., & Zipes, D. P. *Braunwald's heart disease.* Philadelphia, PA: Saunders Elsevier: 1003–1026.

Yancy, C. W., Jessup, M., Bozkurt, B., Butler, J., Casey, D. E., Drazner, M. H., . . . Wilkoff, B. L. (2013). 2013 ACCF/AHA guideline for the management of heart failure: A report of the American College of Cardiology Foundation/American Heart Association Task Force on Practice Guidelines. *Circulation, 128,* e240–e327.

Yeh, G. Y., McCarthy, E. P., Wayne, P. M., Stevenson, L. W., Wood, M. J., Forman, D., & Phillips, R. S. (2011). Tai Chi exercise in patients with chronic heart failure: A randomized clinical trial. *Archives of Internal Medicine, 171,* 750–757.

Yusuf, S., Hawken, S., Ounpuu, S., Dans, T., Avezum, A., Lanas, F., & Lisheng, L. (2004). Effect of potentially modifiable risk factors associated with myocardial infarction in 52 countries (the INTERHEART study): Case-control study. *The Lancet, 364,* 937–952.

Yusuf, S., Sleight, P., Pogue, J., Bosch, J., Davies, R., & Dagenais, G. (2000). Effects of an angiotensin-converting-enzyme inhibitor, ramipril, on cardiovascular events in high-risk patients. The Heart Outcomes Prevention Evaluation Study Investigators. *The New England Journal of Medicine, 342,* 145–153.

Yusuf, S., Teo, K., Pogue, J., Dyal, L., Copland, I., Schumaker, H., . . . Anderson, C. (2008). Telmisartan, ramipril, or both in patients at high risk for vascular events. *The New England Journal of Medicine, 358,* 1547–1559.

Zannad, F., McMurray, J., Krum, H., Veldhuisen, D., Swedberg, K., Shi, H., . . . Pitt, B. (2011). Eplerenone in patients with systolic heart failure and mild symptoms. *The New England Journal of Medicine, 364,* 11–21.

Index

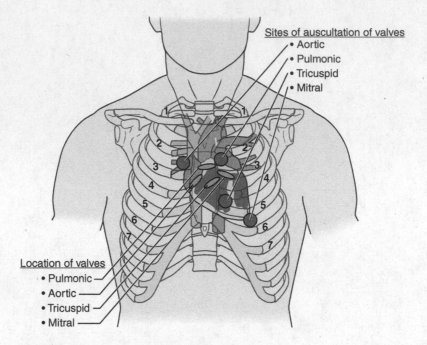

Sites of auscultation of valves
- Aortic
- Pulmonic
- Tricuspid
- Mitral

Location of valves
- Pulmonic
- Aortic
- Tricuspid
- Mitral

FIGURE 3.2 Cardiac auscultation locations.

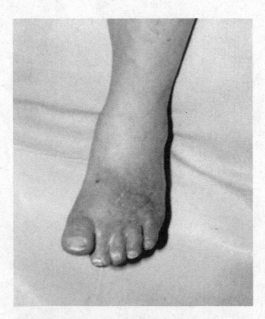

FIGURE 15.1 Dependent rubor of the lower extremity.

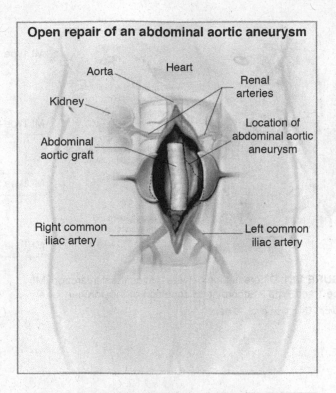

Open repair of an abdominal aortic aneurysm

Aorta

Heart

Renal arteries

Kidney

Location of abdominal aortic aneurysm

Abdominal aortic graft

Right common iliac artery

Left common iliac artery

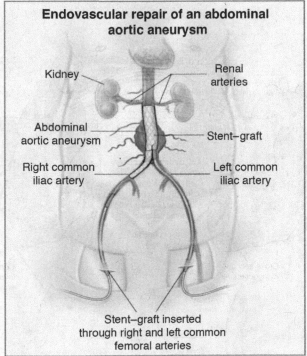

Endovascular repair of an abdominal aortic aneurysm

Kidney

Renal arteries

Abdominal aortic aneurysm

Stent–graft

Right common iliac artery

Left common iliac artery

Stent–graft inserted through right and left common femoral arteries

FIGURE 16.1 Open repair and endovascular repair of an infrarenal abdominal aortic aneurysm. See color insert.

Reprinted from Schermerhorn et al. (2008, p. 465), with permission from Massachusetts Medical Society.

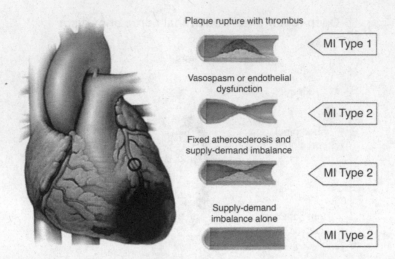

FIGURE 18.1 Differentiation between myocardial infarction (MI) Type 1 and Type 2 according to condition of the coronary artery.

Source: Thygesen et al. (2012).

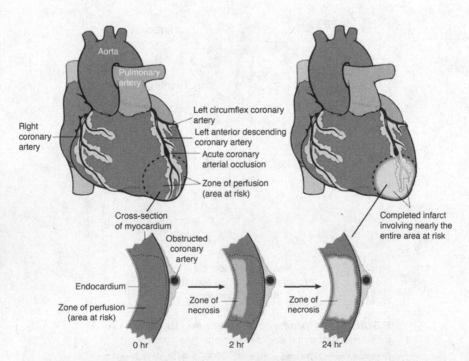

FIGURE 18.2 Progression of myocardial necrosis after coronary artery occlusion.

Reprinted from Schoen and Mitchell (2015, pp. 540–550), with permission from Elsevier.

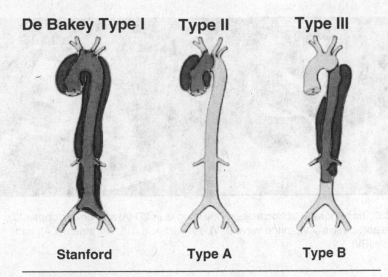

De Bakey

Type I   Originates in the ascending aorta, propagates at least to the aortic arch and often beyond it distally

Type II   Originates in and is confined to the ascending aorta.

Type III   Originates in the descending aorta and extends distally down the aorta or, rarely, retrograde into the aortic arch and ascending aorta.

Stanford

Type A   All dissections involving the ascending aorta, regardless of the site of origin.

Type B   All dissections not involving the ascending aorta.

FIGURE 21.1 The most common classification systems of thoracic aortic dissection: Stanford and De Bakey.

Reprinted from Nienaber and Eagle (2003, pp. 628–635), with permission from Wolters Kluwer Health.

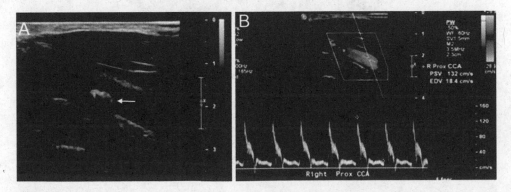

FIGURE 26.4 Carotid ultrasound images of the proximal right internal carotid artery. (A) Demonstrates plaque (arrow) with only mildly elevated velocities on Doppler imaging (B) Suggestive of mild stenosis (<50%).

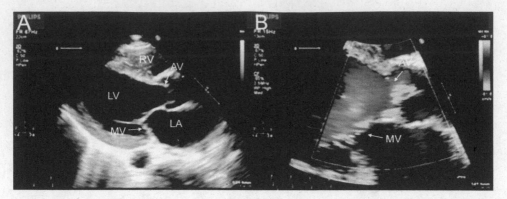

FIGURE 26.6 Transthoracic echocardiography images in 2D (A) and color doppler (B), showing the aortic valve (AV), mitral valve (MV), left ventricle (LV), left atrium (LA), and right ventricle (RV).

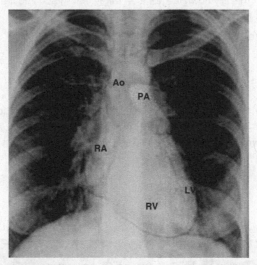

FIGURE 27.1 Chest x-ray showing approximate location of heart structures.

Ao, ascending aorta; LV, left ventricle; PA, pulmonary artery; RA, right atrium; RV, right ventricle.

Reprinted from Kirk (2014), with permission www.transplantkids.org.uk

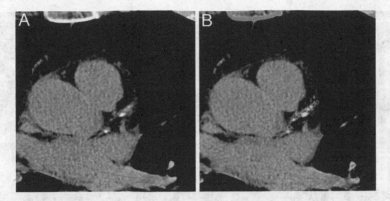

FIGURE 27.2 Non-contrast cardiac CT scan performed for calcium scoring (A). Postprocessing software identifies coronary artery calcification lesions for scoring (B).

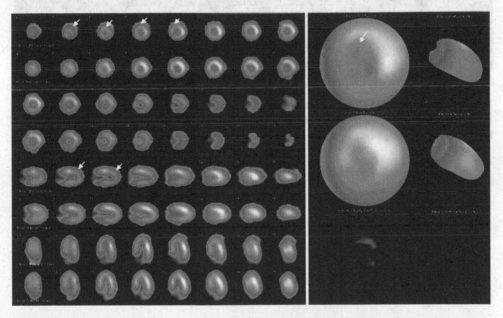

FIGURE 27.6 SPECT MPI study showing reversible perfusion defect involving the mid- and apical anterior walls (arrows) suggestive of ischemia in the LAD territory.

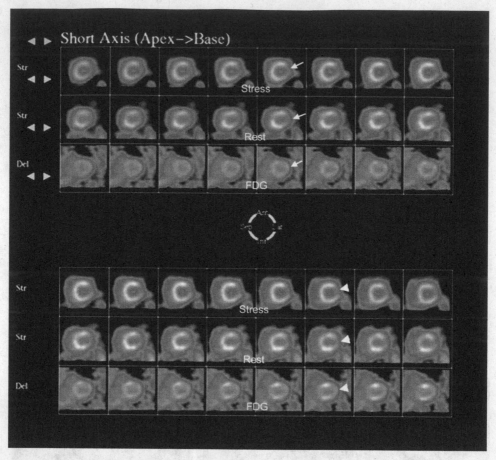

FIGURE 27.7 Rest and stress PET MPI with metabolic FDG imaging showing ischemia (arrowheads) and viability (arrow) in the lateral wall.

FDG, fluorodeoxyglucose; MPI, myocardial perfusion imaging; PET, positron emission tomography.

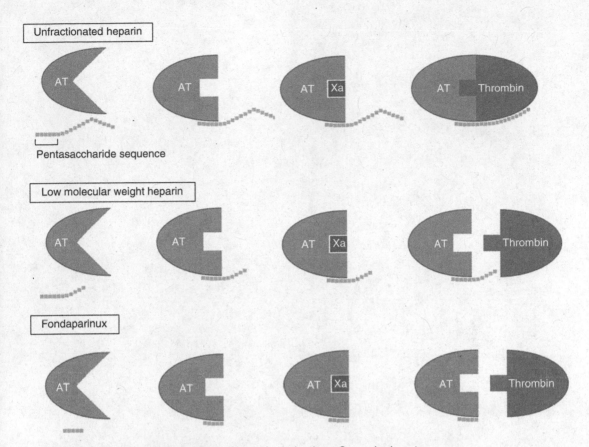

FIGURE 31.2 Mechanism of heparin and heparin derivatives. See color insert.

AT, antithrombin; Xa, factor Xa; UFH, unfractionated heparin, LMWH, low molecular weight heparin.

UFH: The pentasaccharide sequence binds to antithrombin, inducing a conformational change to increase its affinity for factor Xa or IIa. Inactivation of factor IIa requires UFH chains of sufficient length to bind to both antithrombin and thrombin.

LMWH: Similar to UFH, the pentasaccharide sequence activates antithrombin, which binds and inactivates factor Xa. Due to the shorter chain length, its activity against thrombin is limited.

Indirect factor Xa inhibitor/Fondaparinux: Only the pentasaccharide sequence is present; thus, only factor Xa can be inactivated through the antithrombin-dependent mechanism utilized by UFH and LMWH.

Printed in the United States
By Bookmasters